GERIATRIC PHYSICAL THERAPY

THIRD EDITION

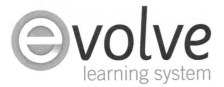

evolve
learning system

To access your Student Resources, visit:

http://evolve.elsevier.com/Guccione/geriatricP

REGISTE

Register today and gain access to:

Evolve Student Learning Resources for Guccione: Geriatric Physical Therapy, Third Edition offers the following features:

- **References** – All of references referred to in each chapter are posted and where applicable, linked to the PUBMED abstract.
- **Weblinks** – An exciting resource that lets you link to hundreds of websites carefully chosen to supplement the content of the textbook.

Evolve Instructor Resources for Guccione: Geriatric Physical Therapy, Third Edition offers the following features:

- **Image Collection** – Search, view, and download the large selection of images from the textbook.

NOTE: Instructors should check with their Elsevier sales representative for further information.

THIRD EDITION

GERIATRIC
PHYSICAL
THERAPY

ANDREW A. GUCCIONE, PT, PhD, DPT, FAPTA
Deputy Director
Health Services Research & Development Service
Department of Veterans Affairs
Washington, DC

RITA A. WONG, EdD, PT
Physical Therapy Department Chairperson
Professor of Physical Therapy
Marymount University
Arlington, Virginia

DALE AVERS, PT, DPT, PhD
Associate Professor
Director, Post Professional DPT Program
Department of Physical Therapy Education
College of Health Professions
SUNY Upstate Medical University
Syracuse, New York

ELSEVIER
MOSBY

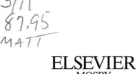

3251 Riverport Lane
St. Louis, Missouri 63043

GERIATRIC PHYSICAL THERAPY, THIRD EDITION   ISBN: 978-0-323-02948-3
Copyright © 2012, 2000, 1993 by Mosby, Inc., an affiliate of Elsevier Inc.

ISBN: 978-0-323-02948-3

Vice President and Publisher: Linda Duncan
Executive Editor: Kathy Falk
Senior Developmental Editor: Christie M. Hart
Publishing Services Manager: Catherine Jackson
Senior Project Manager: Mary Pohlman
Book Designer: Jessica Williams

Printed in the United States of America

Last digit is the print number: 9 8 7 6 5 4 3 2 1

Thrice again – for Nancy, Katie, and Nicole

Andrew A. Guccione

To my husband Al for his unwavering support and encouragement; and to my children and grandchildren who grow more precious every day

Rita A. Wong

To Patrick VanBeveren, my husband, partner and best friend

Dale Avers

Alia A. Alghwiri, PT, MS
PhD candidate
University of Pittsburgh
Physical Therapy Department
Pittsburgh, Pennsylvania

Dale Avers, PT, DPT, PhD
Associate Professor
Director, Post Professional DPT
 Program
Department of Physical Therapy
 Education
College of Health Professions
SUNY Upstate Medical University
Syracuse, New York

Katherine Beissner, PT, PhD
Professor
Department of Physical Therapy
Ithaca College
Ithaca, New York

Diane Borello-France, PT, PhD
Associate Professor
Department of Physical Therapy
Rangos School of Health Sciences
Duquesne University
Pittsburgh, Pennsylvania

Richard Briggs, MA, PT
Hospice Physical Therapist
Enloe Medical Center, Hospice and
 HomeCare
Chico, California

Marybeth Brown, PT, PhD, FAPTA
Professor
Physical Therapy Program,
 Biomedical Sciences
University of Missouri
Columbia, Missouri

Sabrina Camilo, PT, MSPT, GCS
Private Practitioner
São Paulo, Brazil

Cory Christiansen, PT, PhD
Assistant Professor
Physical Therapy Program
Department of Physical Medicine
 & Rehabilitation
School of Medicine
University of Colorado
Aurora, Colorado

**Charles D. Ciccone, PT, PhD,
 FAPTA**
Professor
Department of Physical Therapy
Ithaca College
Ithaca, New York

Rhea Cohn, PT, DPT
Health Care Consultant
Washington, DC metro area

**Joan E. Edelstein, PT, MA, FISPO,
 CPed**
Special Lecturer
Program in Physical Therapy
Columbia University
New York, New York

Cathy S. Elrod, PT, PhD
Associate Professor
Department of Physical Therapy
Marymount University
Arlington, Virginia

Christine E. Fordyce, PT, DPT
Rehab Director
Gentiva Health Services
Auburn, New York

**Claire Gold, MSPT, MBA, COS-C,
 CPHQ**
Home Health Agency Administrator
Gentiva® Home Health
San Diego, California

**Andrew A. Guccione, PT, PhD,
 DPT, FAPTA**
Deputy Director
Health Services Research
 & Development Service
Department of Veterans Affairs
Washington, DC

Greg W. Hartley, PT, DPT, GCS
Director of Rehabilitation &
 Assistant Hospital
 Administrator,
Geriatric Residency Program
 Director
St. Catherine's Rehabilitation
 Hospitals and Villa Maria
 Nursing Centers
Miami, Florida;
Adjunct Assistant Professor
University of Miami Miller School
 of Medicine
Department of Physical Therapy
Coral Gables, Florida

**Barbara J. Hoogenboom, PT,
 EdD, SCS, ATC**
Associate Professor
Program in Physical Therapy
Grand Valley State University
Grand Rapids, Michigan

Catherine E. Lang PT, PhD
Assistant Professor
Program in Physical Therapy
Program in Occupational
 Therapy
Department of Neurology
Washington University
Saint Louis, Missouri

Tanya LaPier, PT, PhD, CCS
Professor
Eastern Washington University
Cheney, Washington

Paul LaStayo, PT, PhD, CHT
Associate Professor
Department of Physical Therapy
University of Utah
Salt Lake City, Utah

Carleen Lindsey, PT, MScAH, GCS
Physical Therapist
Bones, Backs & Balance
Bristol, Connecticut

Toby M. Long, PT, PhD, FAPTA
Associate Professor
Department of Pediatrics
Director of Training
Center for Child and Human
    Development
Georgetown University
Washington, DC

Michelle M. Lusardi, PT, DPT, PhD
Professor Emerita
Department of Physical Therapy and
    Human Movement Science
College of Education and Health
    Professions
Sacred Heart University
Fairfield, Connecticut

Robin L. Marcus, PT, PhD, OCS
Assistant Professor
Department of Physical Therapy
University of Utah
Salt Lake City, Utah

Carol A. Miller, PT, PhD, GCS
Professor
Doctorate Program in Physical
    Therapy
North Georgia College & State
    University
Dahlonega, Georgia

Justin Moore, PT, DPT
Vice President, Government and
    Payment Advocacy
American Physical Therapy
    Association (APTA)
Alexandria, Virginia

Karen Mueller, PT, PhD
Professor
College of Health and Human
    Services
Department of Physical Therapy
Northern Arizona University
Flagstaff, Arizona

Jean Oulund Peteet, PT, MPH, PhD
Clinical Assistant Professor
Department of Physical Therapy and
    Athletic Training
Boston University College of Health
    and Rehabilitation Sciences–
    Sargent
Boston, Massachusetts

**John Rabbia, PT, DPT, MS, GCS,
CWS**
Visiting Nurse Association of
    Central New York

**Barbara Resnick, PhD, CRNP,
FAAN, FAANP**
Professor
Sonya Ziporkin Gershowitz Chair in
    Gerontology
University of Maryland School of
    Nursing
College Park, Maryland

Julie D. Ries, PT, PhD
Associate Professor
Program in Physical Therapy
Marymount University
Arlington, Virginia

Kathleen Toscano, MHS, PT, PCS
Pediatric Physical Therapist
Montgomery County Infant and
    Toddler Program
Olney, Maryland

**Patrick J. VanBeveren, PT, DPT,
MA, OCS, GCS, CSCS**
Director of Physical Therapy Services
St. Camillus Health and
    Rehabilitation Center
Syracuse, New York

**Michael Voight, PT, SCS, OCS,
ATC, CSCS**
Professor
School of Physical Therapy
Belmont University
Nashville, Tennessee

Martha Walker, PT, DPT
Clinical Instructor
Physical Therapy and Rehabilitation
    Science
University of Maryland
Baltimore, Maryland

**Chris L. Wells, PhD, PT, CCS,
ATC**
Assistant Professor–Part Time,
Department of Physical Therapy
    & Rehabilitation Science
University of Maryland School of
    Medicine
College Park, Maryland

Karin Westlen-Boyer, DPT, MPH
Intermountain Health & Fitness
    Institute at LDS Hospital
Salt Lake City, Utah

Mary Ann Wharton, PT, MS
Associate Professor and
    Curriculum Coordinator
Department of Physical Therapy
Saint Francis University
Loretto, Pennsylvania;
Adjunct Associate Professor
Physical Therapist Assistant
    Program
Community College of Allegheny
    County, Boyce Campus
Monroeville, Pennsylvania

**Susan L. Whitney, PT, DPT, PhD,
NCS, ATC, FAPTA**
Associate Professor
Program in Physical Therapy and
    Otolaryngology
University of Pittsburgh
Pittsburgh, Pennsylvania

Ann K. Williams, PT, PhD
Adjunct Professor
College of Health Professions and
    Biomedical Sciences
The University of Montana
Missoula, Montana

Rita A. Wong, EdD, PT
Physical Therapy Department
    Chairperson
Professor of Physical Therapy
Marymount University
Arlington, Virginia

Although the content of previous editions has been substantially revised, it is remarkable that the overall purpose of this textbook has not changed since the first edition 18 years ago. The editors' intent for undertaking the third edition of *Geriatric Physical Therapy* is to assist the development of reflective physical therapists who can use the available scientific evidence and objective tools to integrate health and functional status information with examination data, formulate an accurate diagnosis, and design effective treatment plans that can be implemented at all levels of care and across all settings to produce optimal outcomes. We further believe that this practitioner can serve both patients and society as an informed advocate for older adults. What has changed throughout the years is that the original publication was intended only as a textbook for entry-level students. In the intervening years we have expanded the vision of this text to include individuals studying for the examination to be certified as geriatric clinical specialist as well as practicing clinicians. The last group is perhaps the most surprising and the most gratifying. Geriatric physical therapy has come into its own in the last two decades. The emergence of the specialty, the growth of certified specialists, and the number of practicing clinicians in the area all attest to the fact that physical therapist practice oriented toward older adults is no longer a novelty, confined to a few physical therapists whose good hearts and intentions led them to concerns about America's aging population. On the contrary, geriatric physical therapy is bursting with innovation in practice and cutting edge research that will enable physical therapists to exercise the full range of their education, experience, and expertise across the full continuum of the health care system from primary prevention to end-of-life care.

The new edition of *Geriatric Physical Therapy* has been arranged in six parts. In Part I, we organize the foundational sciences of geriatric physical therapy, which range from basic physiology of aging to clinical epidemiology of disease and disability. Next, our contributors explore the personal and environmental contexts of examination and intervention, particularly as these factors provide nuance to examination findings or modulate the outcomes of intervention. Part III provides the scientific basis for evaluation and diagnosis of prototypical health conditions and patient problems that are emblematic of geriatric physical therapy as well as the design of plans of care for effective treatment and optimal outcomes. In the next section, the chapters cover some health conditions that are not common to the entire population of older adults but represent points of substantial health impact requiring specific expertise to be addressed effectively. The practice of physical therapists in our application of specific education, experience, and expertise in the health problems of older adults across spectrum of healthcare delivery is presented in Part V. Finally, the last section tackles the societal issues affecting physical therapist practice that can propel or obstruct the profession's ability to address the health of older adults and optimize the health of the nation: reimbursement and advocacy.

What started as an attempt to update a well-received resource was infused with a new vision and turned into a substantial revision to reflect the changes in geriatric physical therapy and the profession itself in the last 20 years. The goals which we first described in 1993 and repeated in the second edition remain: to define the scientific basis of physical therapy; to describe how physical therapist practice with older adults differs from physical therapist practice in general; and to promote the adoption of evidence-based principles of clinical care that advance geriatric physical therapist practice. It is clear now that the best scientific thoughts are being translated into clinical actions. We are pleased to think that we have contributed to this phenomenon.

Andrew A. Guccione, PT, PhD, DPT, FAPTA
Rita A. Wong, EdD, PT
Dale Avers, PT, DPT, PhD

ACKNOWLEDGMENTS

This is truly a textbook that reunites an old team with some long-term colleagues, but also introduces a substantial number of new contributors that allows us to appreciate the vitality of geriatric physical therapy and the profession itself. Their vibrant contributions, joined with cutting-edge expertise, have expanded the horizons of this text and enriched us as professionals committed to practice with older adults.

The editorial team exemplifies the essence of collaborative practice in geriatric physical therapy. As it happens, we had worked together before on what was, and still is, a professional career highlight for all of us: the development of the geriatric specialty examination. During that venture, our special contributor and friend, Marybeth Brown, was a full member of the team. For this venture, our "silent" partner in developing the examination, Dale Avers, switched places with Marybeth, taking the on-stage role while Marybeth contributed her singular expertise from the wings. It seemed fortuitous to find each other then; we know now we were blessed with an exciting intellectual partnership and professional friendship.

We are indebted to Christie Hart for encouraging us to undertake a third edition. While the response to the previous editions was very positive, we knew the scope of geriatric physical therapist practice had evolved substantially necessitating a global revision. The team at Mosby/Elsevier has supported us each step of the way.

Ultimately, we recognize that whatever we might know about geriatric physical therapy is the summation of countless interactions with scientists, clinicians, educators and students, but most of all our patients. It is in recognition of their primary role in teaching us as well as our families in supporting us that this work is dedicated.

Andrew A. Guccione, PT, PhD, DPT, FAPTA
Rita A. Wong, EdD, PT
Dale Avers, PT, DPT, PhD

x

CONTENTS

PART V
Special Populations and the Continuum of Care

PART VI
Societal Issues

PART I

Foundations

Geriatric Physical Therapy in the 21st Century:
Overarching Principles and Approaches to Practice

Rita A. Wong, EdD, PT

INTRODUCTION

This book promotes the reflective, critical, objective, and analytical practice of physical therapy applied to the older adult. All physical therapists, not just those working in settings traditionally identified as "geriatric," should possess strong foundational knowledge about geriatrics and be able to apply this knowledge to a variety of older adults. Indeed, older adults comprise at least 40% of patients across physical therapy clinical settings.[1] Although the fundamental principles of patient management are similar regardless of patient age, there are unique features and considerations in the management of older adults that can greatly improve outcomes.

This chapter starts with a brief discussion of the key principles and philosophies upon which the book is grounded: evidence-based practice; optimal aging; the slippery slope of aging; clinical decision making in geriatrics; the role of exercise and physical activity for optimal aging; objectivity in the use of outcome assessment tools; and the importance of patient values and motivation. The chapter continues with a discussion of the geriatric practitioner of the future and mechanisms required to prepare adequate numbers of practitioners for this expanding role; it then moves to the key principles of locating, analyzing, and applying best evidence in the care of older adults. The chapter ends with a discussion of ageism and the impact of ageism on health care services to older adults.

KEY PRINCIPLES UNDERLYING CONTEMPORARY GERIATRIC PHYSICAL THERAPY

Evidence-Based Practice

Evidence-based practice is an approach to clinical decision making about the care of an individual patient that integrates three separate but equally important sources of information in making a clinical decision about the care of a patient. Figure 1-1 illustrates these three information sources: (1) best available scientific evidence, (2) clinical experience and judgment of the practitioner, and (3) patient preferences and motivations.[2] The term *evidence-based practice* sometimes misleads people into thinking that the scientific evidence is the only factor to be considered when using this approach to inform a patient-care decision. Although the scientific literature is an essential and substantive component of credible clinical decision making, it is only one of the three essential components.[2,3] An alternative, and perhaps more accurate, label for this approach is evidence-informed practice.

The competent geriatric practitioner must have a good grasp of the current scientific literature and be able to interpret and apply this literature in the context of an individual patient situation. This practitioner must also have the clinical expertise to skillfully perform the appropriate tests and measures needed for diagnosis, interpret the findings in light of age-related and condition-specific characteristics of the patient, and then to skillfully

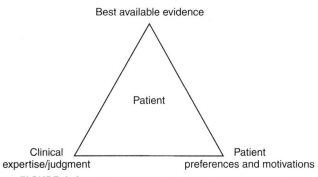

FIGURE 1-1 Key elements of evidence-informed practice.

apply the appropriate interventions to best manage the problem. This is all done with clear and full communication with the patient to assure the goals and preferences of the patient are a central component of the development of a plan of care.

Optimal Aging

Rowe and Kahn[4] first introduced the terms *successful* and *usual* aging in the mid-1980s as a mechanism to remind practitioners and researchers that the typical changes in physiological functioning observed in older adults (usual aging) are quite variable and generally represent a combination of unavoidable aging-related changes and modifiable (avoidable) lifestyle factors such as physical activity, nutrition, and stress management. Their perspective encourages practitioners to consider that for many older adults, a substantial proportion of apparent age-related changes in functional ability may be partially reversible with lifestyle modification programs.

Ten years later, Rowe and Kahn[5] provided further clarification of the key components that make up their model for successful aging. The specific elements they present as the signs of an individual who is aging successfully are (1) absence of disease and disability, (2) high cognitive and physical functioning, and (3) active engagement with life. Rowe and Kahn describe a usual aging syndrome as one in which suboptimal lifestyle leads to chronic health problems that affect function and thus the ability to readily engage in family or community activities. Improving healthy lifestyle is encouraged as a means of achieving successful aging.

Although helping older adults avoid disease and disease-related disability is a central consideration for all health care practitioners, the reality is that the majority of older adults do have at least one chronic health condition and many, particularly among the very old, live with functional limitations and disabilities associated with the sequela of one or more chronic health conditions. For this large group of individuals, Rowe and Kahn's model needs to stretch beyond the concept of avoidance of disease and disability.

Brummel-Smith[6] expanded the concepts of Rowe and Kahn in the depiction of *optimal* aging as a more inclusive term than *successful* aging. Brummel-Smith defines optimal aging as "the capacity to function across many domains—physical, functional, cognitive, emotional, social, and spiritual—to one's satisfaction and in spite of one's medical conditions."[6] This conceptualization recognizes the importance of optimizing functional capacity in older adults regardless of the presence or absence of a chronic health condition. Functional limitations associated with chronic health conditions often lead to a vicious downward cycle with increasing levels of disability leading to greater deconditioning that further decreases functional ability. These declines lead to secondary conditions associated with chronic conditions and, often, to additional new diseases. Physical therapists can be particularly instrumental in reducing the disabling effects of chronic disease processes by promoting restorative and accommodative changes that stop or reverse the vicious downward functional cycle, allowing the individual to achieve optimal aging in the presence of chronic health conditions.

Slippery Slope of Aging

Closely linked to the concept of optimal aging is the concept of a "slippery slope" of aging (Figure 1-2). The slope, originally proposed by Schwartz,[7] represents the general decline in overall physiological ability (that Schwartz expressed as "vigor") that is observed with increasing age. The curve is arbitrarily plotted by decade on the x-axis so the actual location of any individual along the y-axis—regardless of age—can be modified (in either a positive or negative direction) based on

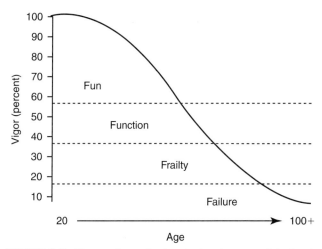

FIGURE 1-2 Slippery slope of aging depicts the general decline in overall physiological ability observed with increasing age and its impact on function. *(Adapted from Schwartz RS: Sarcopenia and physical performance in old age: introduction. Muscle Nerve Suppl5: S10-S12, 1997.)*

lifestyle factors and illness that influence physiological functioning.

Schwartz has embedded functional status thresholds at various points along this slope. Conceptually, these thresholds represent key impact points where small changes in physiological ability can have a large impact on function, participation, and disability. These four distinctive functional levels are descriptively labeled fun, function, frailty, and failure. Fun, the highest level, represents a physiological state that allows unrestricted participation in work, home, and leisure activities. The person who crosses the threshold into function continues to accomplish most work and home activities but may need to modify performance and will substantially self-restrict leisure activities (fun) because of declining physiological capacity. Moving from function into frailty occurs when managing basic activities of daily living (BADLs; walking, bathing, toileting, eating, etc.) consumes a substantial portion of physiological capacity, with substantial limitations in ability to participate in community activities and requiring outside assistance to accomplish many home or work activities. The final threshold into failure is reached when an individual requires assistance with BADLs as well as instrumental daily activities and may be completely bedridden.

The concept of functional thresholds and the downward movement from fun to frailty helps explain the apparent disconnect that is often observed between the extent of change of physiological functions (impairments) and changes in functional status. For example, for a person who is teetering between the thresholds of function and frailty, a relatively small physiological challenge (a bout of influenza or a short hospitalization) is likely to drop them squarely into the level of "frailty," with its associated functional limitations. Once a person moves to a lower functional level (down the curve of the y-axis) it requires substantial effort to build physiological capacity to move back up to a higher level (back up the y-axis). Lifestyle changes including increased exercise activities may enhance efforts for an upward movement along the slippery slope. Moreover, the further the person is able to move above a key threshold, the more physiological reserve is available for protection from an acute decline in a physiological system. A major role of physical therapy is to maximize the movement-related physiological ability (vigor) of older adult patients/clients to keep them at their optimal functional level and with highest physiological reserve.

Clinical Decision Making in Geriatric Physical Therapy

The primary purpose of physical therapy practice is the enhancement of human performance as it pertains to movement and health. Providing a framework for clinical decision making in geriatric physical therapy is particularly important because of the sheer volume of information that must be brought to bear on a clinical decision. Several conceptual frameworks are presented in Chapter 6 and integrated into a model to guide physical therapy clinical decision making in geriatrics. The model is grounded in the patient-client management model of the *Guide to Physical Therapist Practice*[8] and emphasizes the central role of functional movement task analysis in establishing a physical therapy diagnosis and guiding choice of interventions. The enablement–disablement concepts of the World Health Organization's International Classification of Functioning, Disability and Health (ICF) model of disability[9] are also incorporated into this model, using ICF language to communicate the process of disablement and placing a substantial emphasis on describing and explaining personal, medical, and environmental factors likely to enable functional ability or increase disability.

Crucial Role of Physical Activity and Exercise in Maximizing Optimal Aging

Lack of physical activity (sedentary lifestyle) is a major public health concern across age groups. Only 22% of older adults report engaging in regular leisure-time physical activity.[10] Sedentary lifestyle increases the rate of age-related functional decline and reduces capacity for exercise sustainability to regain physiological reserve following an injury or illness. It is critical that physical therapists overtly address sedentary behavior as part of the plan of care for their older adult patients.

Exercise may well be the most important tool a physical therapist has to positively affect function and increase physical activity toward optimal aging. Despite a well-defined body of evidence to guide decisions about optimal intensity, duration, and mode of exercise prescription, physical therapists often underutilize exercise, with a negative impact on the potential to achieve optimal outcomes in the least amount of time. Underutilization of appropriately constructed exercise prescriptions may be associated with such factors as age biases that lower expectations for high levels of function, lack of awareness of age-based functional norms that can be used to set goals and measure outcomes, and perceived as well as real restrictions imposed by third-party payers regarding number of visits or the types of interventions (e.g., prevention) that are covered and reimbursed under a person's insurance benefit. Physical therapists should take every opportunity to apply evidence-based recommendations for physical activity and exercise programs that encourage positive lifestyle changes and, thus, maximize optimal aging.

Objectivity in Use of Outcome Tools

Older adults become increasingly dissimilar with increasing age. A similarly aged person can be frail and reside in a nursing home or be a senior athlete participating in a triathlon. Dissimilarities cannot be attributed to age alone and can challenge the therapist to set appropriate goals and expectations. Functional markers are useful to avoid inappropriate stereotyping and undershooting of an older adult's functional potential. Functional tests, especially those with normative values, can provide a more objective and universally understood description of actual performance relative to similarly aged older adults, serving as a common language and as a baseline for measuring progress. For example, describing an 82-year-old gentleman in terms of gait speed (0.65 m/s), 6-minute walk test (175 m), Berg balance test (26/56), and Timed 5-repetition chair rise (0) provides a more accurate description than "an older man who requires mod assistance of two to transfer, walks 75 feet with a walker, and whose strength is WFL." Reliable, valid, and responsive tests, appropriate for a wide range of abilities, enhance practice and provide valuable information for our patients and referral sources.

THE PATIENT-CENTERED PHYSICAL THERAPIST ON THE GERIATRIC TEAM

Physical therapists working with older adults must be prepared to serve as autonomous primary care practitioners, and as consultants, educators (patient and community), clinical researchers (contributors and critical assessors), case managers, patient advocates, interdisciplinary team members, and practice managers.[11] Although none of these roles is unique to geriatric physical therapy, what is unique is the remarkable variability among older adult patients and the regularity with which the geriatric physical therapist encounters patients with particularly complex needs. Unlike the typical younger individual, older adults are likely to have several complicating comorbid conditions in addition to the condition that has brought them to physical therapy. Patients with similar medical diagnoses often demonstrate great variability in baseline functional status and may be simultaneously dealing with significant psychosocial stresses such as loss of a spouse, loss of an important aspect of independence, or a change in residence. Thus, cognitive issues such as depression, fear, reaction to change, and family issues can compound the physical aspects and provide an additive challenge to the physical therapist. The physical therapist must be creative, pay close attention to functional clues about underlying modifiable or accommodative impairments, and listen carefully to the patient to assure goal setting truly represents mutually agreed-upon goals.

In addition, the older patient is likely to be followed by multiple health care providers, thus making the physical therapist a member of a team (whether that team is informally or formally identified). As such, the physical therapist must share information and consult with other team members; recognize signs and symptoms that suggest a need to refer out to other practitioners; coordinate services; provide education to patient and caretaker/family; and advocate for the needs of patients and their families.

Physical therapists who find geriatrics particularly rewarding and exciting tend to be practitioners who dislike a clinical world of "routine" patients. These practitioners enjoy being creative and being challenged to guide patients through a complex maze to achieve their highest level of optimal aging; and enjoy making a more personal impact on the care of their patients. Navigating an effective solution in the midst of a complex set of patient issues is professionally affirming and rarely dull or routine.

Need for Physical Therapists in Geriatrics

The year 2011 marks a critical date for the American population age structure, representing the date when the first wave of the baby-boomer generation turned age 65 years. This group, born post–World War II, is much larger than its preceding generation, both in terms of number of children born during this era (1946 to 1965) and increased longevity of those in that cohort. Interestingly, although health services researchers have long forecasted the substantial impact of this demographic shift on the health care system and encouraged coordinated planning efforts, inadequate preparation has been made to assure sufficient numbers of well-prepared health care practitioners to meet the needs of this large group of older adults. The 2008 landmark report of the Institute of Medicine (IOM) *Retooling for an Aging America*[12] provides a compelling argument for wide-ranging shortages of both formal and informal health care providers for older adults across all levels of the health care workforce (professional, technical, unskilled direct care worker, and family caregiver). These shortages include shortages of physical therapists and physical therapist assistants. The report provides numerous recommendations for enhancing the number of health care practitioners and the depth of preparation of these practitioners. The goal of this textbook is to provide a strong foundation to support physical therapists who work with older adults.

A sizeable proportion of the caseload of most physical therapy practices is the older adult. A recent large-scale physical therapist practice analysis[1] reported that 40% to 43% of the caseload of physical therapists, aggregated across clinical practice settings, are patients age 66 years or older. Undoubtedly, with very few exceptions, the majority of the caseload of the average physical therapist will soon consist of older adults. Despite this, physical therapists still tend to think about geriatrics only as care provided in a nursing home or, perhaps, in home care. Although these are major and important practice settings for geriatric physical therapy, physical therapists must recognize and be ready to provide effective services for the high volume of older adult patients across all practice settings. Every physical therapist should be well grounded in the science of geriatrics and gerontology in order to be effective in making evidence-based clinical decisions related to older adults.

Clinical Expertise in Physical Therapy

Clinical expertise is one of the three anchors to EBP. Jensen and colleagues,[13] through a series of well-planned qualitative studies using grounded theory methodology, identified four core dimensions of expert physical therapist practice: knowledge, clinical reasoning, virtue, and movement. These four dimensions provide a theoretical model to examine professional development from novice to expert. As depicted in Figure 1-3, the novice practitioner (physical therapy student) typically examines each dimension as a discrete entity. As professional development progresses, the practitioner begins to see the interrelationships among the dimensions, with recognition of overlap becoming obvious as clinical competence develops. Expert practitioners describe these four dimensions as closely interwoven concepts and explain their relationships in terms of a well-articulated philosophy of practice. The core of the expert physical therapist's philosophy of practice is patient-centered care that values collaborative decision making with the patient.

This model for expert-practice professional development was examined for each of four physical therapy specialty areas (orthopedics, neurology, pediatrics, geriatrics) using board-certified clinical specialists recommended by peers as expert clinicians. All specialists were found to be highly motivated, with a strong commitment to lifelong learning. Experts sought out mentors and could clearly describe the role each mentor had in their development, whether for enhanced decision making, professional responsibilities, personal values, or technical skill development. Experts had a deep knowledge of their specialty practice and used self-reflection regularly to identify strengths and weaknesses in their knowledge or thought processes to guide their ongoing self-improvement. The expert did not "blame the patient" if a treatment did not go as anticipated. Rather, the expert reflected deeply about what he or she could have done differently that would have allowed the patient to succeed.

Expert Practice in Geriatric Physical Therapy. The geriatric clinical specialists interviewed by Jensen and colleagues each provided reflections about how he or she progressed from novice to expert. Figure 1-4 illustrates the conceptual model for the development of expertise expressed by geriatric physical therapy experts.

In describing their path from new graduate generalist to geriatric clinical specialist, none of the geriatric experts started their careers anticipating specialization in geriatrics. They each sought a generalist practice experience as a new graduate and found themselves gradually gravitating toward the older adult patient as opportunities came their way. They came to recognize the talent they had for working with older adults and were called to action by their perceptions that many at-risk older adults were receiving inadequate care. They became

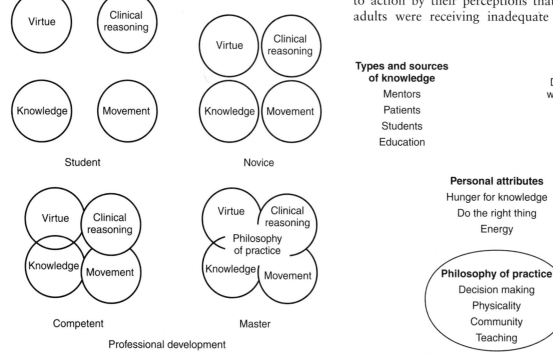

FIGURE 1-3 Developing clinical expertise: Moving from novice to expert practice. *(From Jensen GM, Gwyer J, Hack LM, Shepard KF. Expertise in physical therapy practice: applications for practice, teaching, and research. ed 2, Philadelphia, PA, 2007, Saunders Elsevier.)*

FIGURE 1-4 Conceptual model illustrating the factors contributing to the development of expertise in geriatric physical therapy. *(From Jensen GM, Gwyer J, Hack LM, Shepard KF. Expertise in physical therapy practice: applications for practice, teaching, and research. ed 2, Philadelphia, PA, 2007, Saunders Elsevier. p. 105.)*

firm believers in the principles of optimal aging and had a genuine high regard for the capabilities of older adults if given the opportunity to fully participate in rehabilitation.

Geriatric experts are high-energy people who firmly believe in their role and responsibility as a patient advocate, and they thrive on the challenge of the complex patient who needs creativity and individualization of approach, good interpersonal skills, and deep knowledge of the specialty content.

These specialists model clinical excellence by not settling for less than what the patient is capable of. Physical therapists are essential practitioners in geriatrics. The physical therapist must embrace this essential role—and recognize the positive challenge—of mastering the management of a complex and variable group of patients.

Skill acquisition in any specialty area consists of technical, perceptual, and decision-making components during which the learner starts with uncomplicated standard situations and progresses to complex and variable ones. Performing in a highly complex and variable environment requires the highest level of decision making—typically mastered after the lower levels. Part of the transition from novice to expert is the increasing ease with which a person can enter a new and complex situation, quickly (and increasingly implicitly) analyze the various components, and then make effective and efficient decisions. Because the typical older adult patient is more complex and variable than the typical younger patient, the level of expertise required is particularly high. Less experienced physical therapists should seek mentorship and residency opportunities and engage in active and frequent reflection with peers to develop these skills.

FINDING, ANALYZING, AND APPLYING BEST EVIDENCE

Incorporation of best evidence into clinical decision making is the second major anchor of evidence-based practice. We live in an information age. For almost any topic, an overwhelming amount of information can be accessed in seconds using computer technology. The challenge, as evidence-based practitioners, is to quickly identify and apply best evidence. The best evidence is credible, clinically important, and applicable to the specific patient situation.

When faced with an unfamiliar clinical situation, a clinician reflects on past knowledge and experience, and may identify missing evidence needed to guide their decision making. A four-step process is typically used to locate and apply best evidence: (1) asking a searchable clinical question, (2) searching the literature and locating evidence, (3) critically assessing the evidence, and (4) determining the applicability of the evidence to a specific patient situation. The following section describes each step in this process and provides insights into applying these principles in geriatric physical therapy.

Asking an Answerable Question

Converting a need for information into a searchable clinical question is the first step of an evidence-based approach. Taking a few moments to formulate a clear search question can considerably facilitate the search process. A poorly formulated question often leads to frustration as thousands of possible pieces of evidence may be identified, most of which are only tangentially related to the real question. Strauss et al.[2] identify four major components of a clinical question that should guide a search for evidence: the patient, the intervention (or diagnosis/prognosis), the comparison intervention (diagnosis, prognosis), and the outcome. Some common themes when considering an answerable question related to older adults are as follows:

1. The Patient. This component should narrow the search to an applicable subgroup of older adults. For example, a clinician may be working with two different patients, each with a diagnosis of spinal stenosis. One patient is 92 years old and frail; the other is a very fit and generally healthy senior athlete. The best evidence to guide the clinical approach to the frail older adult with spinal stenosis is likely to be different from the best evidence for the senior athlete. Consider a more complete description of the patient beyond spinal stenosis. For example, include modifiers as appropriate such as community-dwelling or nursing home resident (institutional); well-older adult, generally healthy, or frail older adult; independently functioning or dependent; young-old (age 60 to 75 years), old (age 75 to 85 years), old-old (older than age 85 years).

2. Intervention: This portion of the answerable question represents the patient management focus of a question (therapy, diagnosis or diagnostic tool, prognostic factors, etc.). The information delimiting the patient section will help to focus the evidence on the unique considerations of the older adult.

3. Comparison intervention: A question about the effectiveness of a given intervention or diagnostic procedure is often asking one of two questions: (a) "Does a new intervention have better outcomes than the commonly accepted usual care?" or (b) "Does a new intervention have a better outcome than no intervention at all?" Either question may be important given the likelihood that alternative interventions are typically available and recommended.

4. Outcomes: Carefully considering the specific outcomes of interest is a good way of focusing the search for the evidence that is most useful in guiding the specific episode of care. For example, does the primary question relate to the best approach to remediate a key impairment, improve functional mobility, increase the patient's ability to participate in activities, or improve overall quality of life? Typically, there are more studies addressing specific

impairments and functional activity than participation and quality of life.

Searching the Literature

Sources of Evidence. The scientific literature is divided into two broad categories: primary and secondary sources. The primary sources are the original reports of research studies. Secondary sources represent reviews and analyses of these primary studies. The ideal evidence source is a trusted resource that is readily available, easily accessed, and formatted to answer your specific questions quickly and accurately. Physical therapists must be competent in finding and assessing the quality, importance, and applicability of primary research articles as well as being able to choose appropriate secondary evidence from trusted sources. Geriatric physical therapy is a broad specialty area requiring an expansive range of knowledge and clinical expertise and, therefore, a wide variety of evidence sources.

As depicted in Box 1-1, each piece of evidence falls along a continuum from foundational concepts and theories to the aggregation of high-quality and clinically applicable empirical studies. On casual review of published studies, it is sometimes difficult to determine just where a specific type of evidence falls within the continuum of evidence and a closer review is often required.

The highest quality research to answer a clinical question (i.e., providing the strongest evidence that offers the most certainty about the implications of the findings) is typically derived from the recommendations emerging from a valid systematic review that aggregates numerous high-quality studies directly focusing on the clinical question. However, only a very small proportion of evidence associated with the physical therapy management of older adults is well enough developed to support systematic reviews yielding definitive and strong recommendations. More commonly, best evidence consists of the integration of the findings of one or several individual studies of varying quality by practitioners who incorporate this evidence into their clinical judgments. The evidence-based practitioner must be able to quickly locate, categorize, interpret, and synthesize the available evidence and also judge its relevance to the particular situation.

Figure 1-5 and Box 1-1 provide an organizational schematic depicting the scientific literature as a pyramid with foundational studies at the bottom of the pyramid and the systematic integration and synthesis of multiple high-quality studies at the top of the pyramid. The literature is replete with both foundational and initial (early) clinical studies (the first two levels of the pyramid). Foundational studies provide theories, frameworks, and observations that spur empirical investigations of topics with clinical applicability but, in and of themselves, have little direct and generalizable clinical applicability. Similarly, early empirical studies provide direction to future research and suggest potential impact but, by themselves, do not provide definitive answers to clinical questions.

Studies with a more definitive influence on clinical decisions are higher up on the pyramid. High-quality primary studies that examine typical patients under typical conditions and provide sufficiently long follow-up are the most valuable in our search for best primary evidence. These studies, termed effectiveness studies, are

---

BOX 1-1	Continuum of Evidence: Studies Representing Early Foundational Concepts Through Integration of Findings Across Multiple Studies

Foundational Concepts and Theories →	**Initial Testing of Foundational Concepts** →	**Definitive Testing of Clinical Applicability** →	**Aggregation of the Clinically Applicable Evidence**
Descriptive studies	Single-case design studies	Well-controlled studies with high internal validity and clearly identified external validity:	Systematic review and meta-analysis
Case reports	Testing on "normals" (no real clinical applicability)	• Diagnosis	Evidence-based clinical practice guideline
Idea papers (based on theories and observations)	Small cohort studies (assessing safety and potential for benefit with real patients)	• Prognosis	
"Bench research" (cellular or animal model research for initial testing of theories)	Clinical trials,* phase I and II	• Intervention	
Opinions of experts in the field (based on experience and review of literature)		• Outcomes	
		• Clinical trials,* phase III and IV	

*Clinical trials:
Phase I: examines a small group of people to evaluate treatment safety, determine safe dosage range, and identify side effects.
Phase II: examines somewhat larger group of people to evaluate treatment efficacy and safety.
Phase III: examines a large group of people to confirm treatment effectiveness, monitor side effects, compare it to commonly used treatments, and further examine safety.
Phase IV: postmarketing studies delineate additional information including the documented risks, benefits, and optimal use.

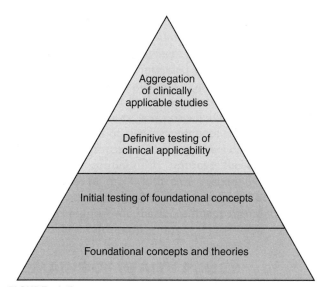

FIGURE 1-5 Pyramid depicting the organization of scientific evidence from low to high clinical applicability.

few and far between in geriatric physical therapy. The highest category of evidence (top of the pyramid) is a systematic review of the existing literature performed using unbiased and transparent methodology that directly addresses the clinician's specific question.

Searching the Literature for Best Evidence. Locating evidence is typically a two-step process: (1) finding the citation and (2) locating the full text of the reference.

Finding the Citations. The biomedical literature is cataloged and indexed according to their citations (title, authors, and identifying information about the source). An abstract of the article is often provided with the citation as well as information about how to access the full text of the article and whether access is free or requires membership or payment of a fee. PubMed (pubmed. com) is generally the best database to use to search for biomedical evidence. PubMed is a product of the United States National Library of Medicine (NLM) at the National Institutes of Health (NIH). This database provides citations and abstracts from an expansive list of biomedical journals, most in English, but also including major non-English biomedical journals. All journals indexed in PubMed must meet high-quality standards, thus providing a certain level of comfort about using PubMed-indexed journals as trusted sources.

The PubMed database can be searched online free of charge. PubMed provides a link to the full text or to a link to the publisher who controls access to the article if there is a publisher-controlled charge for access. PubMed utilizes a powerful search engine organized to easily narrow or expand a search as needed for efficiency. PubMed provides many free online tutorials that help the user maximize their efficiency and effectiveness using this database. The Medical Subject Heading terminology (MeSH) used by PubMed also automatically searches for words that are known synonyms (e.g., a search of *high*

blood pressure also retrieves articles on *hypertension*). In the "advance search" mode, you can limit your search to studies focused on older adults (65+) or, even more narrowly, to individuals aged 80 years and above. Or you can limit the search to studies in the highest level of the pyramid (randomized controlled trials, phase 3 or 4 clinical trials, systematic reviews). All these features make the search faster and more focused.

Cumulative Index of Nursing and Allied Health Literature (CINAHL) is a database that focuses specifically on nursing and allied health. You must either pay to subscribe to CINAHL or gain access through membership in a library or a professional organization that subscribes to it. The CINAHL database is available free of charge to members of the American Physical Therapy Association (APTA). The criteria for being indexed in CINAHL are less stringent than PubMed. Thus, although there is an overlap with many journals indexed in both databases, those indexed in CINAHL but not PubMed tend to be smaller journals containing studies more likely to be located lower on the pyramid with a greater need to be assessed for design flaws that make findings suspect. The search engine for CINAHL is also less powerful than PubMed.

Finding Full Text. Accessing through PubMed provides an automatic link to the full text if it is available free of charge. In this electronic era, most biomedical journals (at least the volumes published over the past decade or so) are accessed electronically either from the publisher or from companies that purchase the rights to include the journal's holdings in a bundled set of journals made available to libraries and other entities for an annual fee. Frequently, university and medical libraries provide a link to PubMed directly from their websites. Accessing PubMed through one of the linked library websites allows an immediate link to the full text of any articles that are available to library patrons. Members of the APTA may similarly access a broad array of journals through *Open Door* as a member benefit.

Staying Updated with Evidence. Practitioners (across all health care fields) are often unaware of new evidence applicable to their practice, or ignore new evidence because it is inconsistent with their accustomed approach. Although both consumers and payers expect practice based on valid evidence, the Institute of Medicine reports long lag times between publication of important new evidence and the incorporation of evidence into practice.[14]

All health care practitioners should have a strategy to regularly review current evidence in their specialty area. A simple review of the table of contents of core journals in the topic area can be useful. Core journals in geriatrics and geriatric physical therapy are listed in Box 1-2. In addition, choose one or two core journals in a professionally applicable subspecialty area (stroke, arthritis, osteoporosis, etc.). It is a simple process to request the monthly table of contents of these journals; scan the table of contents and carefully select a small number of particularly applicable articles to read full-text. The higher the article is on the pyramid of evidence, the more likely its findings can be readily applied to clinical practice.

A second approach is to go to a site such as AMEDEO (www.amedeo.com). This is a free service providing weekly e-mails aggregating article citations specific to any interest across a wide range of health care specialties. The citations are typically taken from ongoing searches of newly published issues of core journals in the specialty area (or a subset of these journals as requested). A third option is to set up a free PubMed account that allows an individual to identify and save a specific search strategy within PubMed, have the search automatically run periodically to identify any new citations, and have the new citations automatically forwarded via e-mail. The PubMed approach allows you to be the most specific about the characteristics of the studies of interest and searches across the widest variety of journals.

Sources that Translate Evidence into Practice Recommendations.
Systematic reviews that provide evidence of objective and unbiased synthesis of the full body of literature on a topic, providing unambiguous and well-grounded recommendations, are important sources for translating evidence into practice recommendations. Clinical practice guidelines, particularly those based on a systematic review of the literature and expert consensus in applying the evidence to clinical practice, can be efficient sources of evidence. The National Guideline Clearinghouse of the Agency for HealthCare Research and Quality (AHRQ) of the U.S. Department of Health and Human Services provides a central and searchable guideline database. When examining the Practice Guidelines, confirm the comprehensiveness and objective analysis of the literature on which the guideline is based. Strength of the evidence should be based on quality, consistency, and number of studies supporting the recommendation.

Critically Assessing the Evidence

"Best available evidence" has become a catch phrase to describe preferred information sources for evidence-informed practice. But what exactly does best evidence really mean? Best evidence is evidence that is credible (collected, analyzed, and reported using unbiased and valid processes), is clinically important (the study's findings demonstrate a large enough change to have a clinically meaningful impact), and the credible and important findings are directly applicable to your patient or situation.

Credibility. Searching for credible evidence starts out using the procedures described in the previous section to locate studies likely to provide the highest level of evidence. Credibility (quality) is assessed through a critical assessment of the internal and external validity of the potential studies. Regardless of its general category (i.e., therapy, prognosis, diagnosis, or systematic review), the study should provide convincing evidence that data were collected, analyzed, and reported in an unbiased fashion. A full review of the concepts of critical assessment of the biomedical literature is available in several well-organized textbooks.[2,15,16] A brief summary of selected points is provided below.

Diagnosis studies compare the performance of a new diagnostic test against the current gold standard or its equivalent,[17] typically testing the test. Diagnosis studies should confirm representativeness of the subjects in the study and present a solid argument that justifies the choice of gold standard.[18] Assessors for reference and target tests should be independent and blinded to the findings of the other to avoid any biasing influence, all subjects should undergo the gold standard, and, ideally, the study should be repeated with a new set of subjects to confirm the findings.

Prognosis studies follow subjects with a target disorder or risk factor over time and monitor the occurrence of the outcome of interest. Prognosis studies may follow either one or two groups of patients (cohort or case–control, respectively), preferably prospectively, to examine the impact of various factors on the target disorder. The findings of prognosis studies inform judgments about such things as who is most likely to benefit from rehabilitation or the length of time to achieve rehabilitation goals. Key indicators of credibility and validity of prognosis studies[19] include the representativeness of the subjects, length of follow-up, and prospective design. Were subjects assembled at a common point in the course of the disease, are subjects reasonably representative of the typical patient at this point in the disease, and are subjects followed for a sufficiently long time period, without large attrition, to capture everyone who experienced the predicted outcome? Were the outcomes criteria free of patient or practitioner biases and responsive enough to capture the outcome if it occurred?

Therapy studies assess the impact of specific interventions on subjects chosen because they possess the specific characteristics or condition of interest in the study. Key indicators of quality in a therapy study are the presence of a control or a comparison group to which subjects were randomly assigned, reasonable between-group similarity at baseline, and low attrition over the course of the study. The methods used in the study should minimize risk of researcher bias or confounding variables providing plausible alternative explanations for the observed outcomes.

There are several distinguishing features of quality in a systematic review. A systematic review should confirm that a comprehensive search of the appropriate literature has been performed using a transparent and reproducible process for identifying studies and confirming that included studies meet established inclusion criteria. At least two reviewers should independently assess quality and applicability of each study considered for the review. Meta-analysis across studies is performed if sufficient numbers of studies with sufficient homogeneity are identified. The recommendations and statement of the strength of the evidence are well grounded and clearly justified based on the quality, findings, and applicability of the included studies.

Determining the Importance of the Findings of the Study

Diagnosis Studies. Sensitivity, specificity, and likelihood ratios are the most commonly reported findings of studies aimed at establishing the accuracy of diagnostic tools. Several references provide excellent reviews of this topic.[2,17] When sensitivity is high, a negative test result is likely to rule out the condition, whereas, when specificity is high, a positive test result is likely to rule in the condition. Likelihood ratios (LRs) are best for increasing the therapist's confidence in the ability to associate a positive or negative test effect with having the target condition/disorder (posttest probability).[20] A high positive likelihood ratio (LR+) (arbitrarily identified as a score above 7 or 10) indicates that the condition is very likely to be present in the person with a positive test. Conversely, a very low likelihood ratio (LR−) (arbitrarily identified as a score below 0.2) indicates that it is very unlikely that the person with a negative test has the condition.

Prognosis Studies. Prognosis studies examine the ability of selected factors to predict an outcome of interest. Most commonly, although not exclusively, the statistical analysis of choice is a regression analysis. Logistic regression is utilized more commonly than linear regression because many of the key explanatory variables (e.g., "sex" or "presence or absence of surgical history") as well as the outcome of interest are categorical variables. The aim of prognostic studies using logistic regression is to determine the extent to which the presence or absence of selected variables predicts a patient's outcome or risk of belonging to a target group. For example, how accurately does a set of prognostic variables predict which subjects are likely to go home at the end of rehabilitation (as compared to those who go to a nursing home or other setting)? These predictions provide an estimate of the "odds" of belonging in the target outcome group. Typically, several predictor variables are examined and, in combination, provide a statistically more robust assessment of the odds of obtaining an outcome (i.e., belong to the target group) than one variable alone. By convention (and fairly arbitrarily

defined) an odds ratio greater than 3 is generally interpreted as a moderate increase in odds of being in the target group; an odds ratio greater than 10 as a very large increase. Odds ratios less than 1 (identified as negative odds ratios) indicate that the presence of the predictor variables is related to decreased odds of being in the target group. The full range of possible scores for negative odds ratios is 1 to 0. An odds ratio of 0.7 is generally described as representing a moderate decrease in odds of being in the target group, and an odds ratio of 0.2 as a very large decrease in odds of being in the target group. The confidence interval (CI), most commonly reported as the 95% CI, must also be considered. In order for an odds ratio to be considered statistically significant (and thus generalizable), the scores within the bracketed CI must NOT include 1, as a score of 1 represents equal odds of being in either group. A more detailed discussion of statistical analysis and prognosis studies is found elsewhere.[20]

In comparison to logistic regression, linear regression examines outcomes along a continuum. Rather than focusing on whether or not a set of variables can predict patient location within one of two identified groups, a linear regression analysis wants to determine a specific score across a linear continuum of scores based on scores on predictor variables. For example, patient age, heart rate, and number of chronic health conditions might be hypothesized to predict the gait speed of community-dwelling older adults. The outcome of linear regression would be an equation that can be used to predict the specific gait speed of comparable patients given their scores on each of the predictor variables. The proportion of variance explained by the model indicates the degree to which all the variables included in the model account for the outcome or dependent variable. A model that predicts the outcome score perfectly would be described as explaining all the variance; however, realistically, there is always unexplained variance. Linear regression provides useful information about trends in the population but is often not very useful in predicting the scores of one specific patient. Variability among and between subjects may be too great in small, convenience samples, which is typically the case in the rehabilitation literature. Generally, statistically significant predictions that account for as little as 40% of the variance may have some value in guiding judgments about the relative contributions of a set of predictor variables, and a study that constructed a predictive model accounting for 70% of the variance would be perceived as very compelling findings.

The more variability in the predictor variables—as is commonly the case in studies of older adults—the less robust the prediction, thus lowering the odds ratio or percentage of variance explained, which decreases confidence in the accuracy of the prediction. Studies may need particularly large sample sizes combined with a large number of well-chosen predictor variables to explain enough of the variance to be clinically useful. Underpowered studies are of particular concern for prognosis studies of adults aged 75 years and older.

Therapy Studies. Therapy studies typically use statistical analyses to evaluate the relative impact of one or more interventions within or across groups of subjects. The concepts of statistical significance and clinical importance both need to be examined in assessing the findings of a study. Differences between or among groups that are deemed statistically significant are considered real, that is, not occurring by chance, and provide a reasonable level of confidence that similar outcomes would be obtained for comparable groups receiving comparable interventions. Only findings deemed statistically significant should be further evaluated for clinical importance.

Although a finding must demonstrate statistically significant differences to be further evaluated for clinical importance, statistical significance alone does not assume clinical importance. An outcome deemed to represent a statistically significant improvement may, nonetheless, have such a small impact on the patient that the amount of change is clinically unimportant. The term *minimum clinically important difference* (MCID) represents the smallest amount of change deemed clinically important for the patient. An MCID has been established for many commonly used outcome tools, and the number of tools with established MCID scores is growing annually.

A common approach for establishing a tool's MCID is to link the patient's reported statement of outcome with the amount of change obtained in a tool. The Global Rating of Change (GRC) tool,[21] or a variation of it, is often used as an anchor for patient-reported outcomes. The GRC is a 15-point rank-ordered scale, with −7 representing "a very great deal worse"; 0 representing "no change"; and +7 representing "a very great deal better." Box 1-3 lists all descriptors commonly used as labels across this scale. For example, this tool has been used to link the amount of change on the 6-minute walk test (6MWT) and patient-reported outcomes of change; in community-dwelling older adults, a 20-m increase in distance walked during the 6MWT represents a small but clinically meaningful improvement.[22] This MCID was established from the average change in distance walked for patients who reported their improvements as 2 (a little better) or 3 (somewhat better) on the GRC scale during an exercise intervention. Thus, using the MCID of 20 m on the 6MWT as an example, the finding of a study must be both statistically significant AND demonstrate a change of at least 20 m on the (6MWT) to be deemed clinically important for the community-dwelling older adult.

For the many tools that do not have an established MCID, the person critically appraising a study would simply identify the amount of change represented in the study (pretest to posttest change; or amount of change in one group versus amount of change in the comparison group) and make a clinical judgment, based on experience and an understanding of the condition, about the likelihood that the amount of reported change would be clinically meaningful to the patient.

Systematic Reviews. The purpose of a systematic review is to aggregate the findings across studies to provide a recommendation about the "strength" (certainty) of the body of evidence on a given topic. The strength of the recommendation for each outcome being reviewed in the systematic review is based on the quality level of each included article as well as the effect size (magnitude of the change or the correlation of scores). Effect size may be calculated for each individual article and then descriptively discussed and synthesized by the authors, or quantitatively aggregated through a meta-analysis into one mathematically derived effect size across all studies. The specific meta-analysis used to calculate an effect size will vary based on the statistical analyses performed in the original studies. A commonly applied rule of thumb is that an effect size of at least 0.2 represents a small effect; 0.5, a medium effect; and more than 0.8, a large effect. A confidence interval is also calculated with the meta-analysis, which provides a range of effect sizes likely across the population.

Many grading schemes are available to categorize the strength of the recommendations that one can draw from a systematic review. Some are fairly elaborate

BOX 1-3	Common Descriptors Used for Each of 15 Possible Responses to Patient-Reported Outcomes Using a Global Rating of Change Tool, as Described by Jaeschke et al.[21]
+7 = a very great deal better	−1 = almost the same, hardly any worse at all
+6 = a great deal better	−2 = a little worse
+5 = a good deal better	−3 = somewhat worse
+4 = moderately better	−4 = moderately worse
+3 = somewhat better	−5 = a good deal worse
+2 = a little better	−6 = a great deal worse
+1 = almost the same, hardly any better at all	−7 = a very great deal worse
0 = no change	

ranking systems and others fairly simple. Box 1-4 provides this author's suggestion for a simple and useful categorization of evidence to qualify the recommendations. Using this system, a reviewer could conclude that the findings of the systematic review provided good, fair, or weak evidence to support or refute an outcome, or one could conclude that there is insufficient evidence to allow one to draw any conclusions.

Applicability to a Specific Patient. Although examining a study for the applicability of the findings of the study to particular patients is very straightforward, it is a step that is often forgotten. A thoughtful comparison of the similarity of the subjects of the study and the clinical environment in which the care is delivered to the target conditions of specific patients and clinical environment will allow you to answer this question. The inclusion and exclusion criteria for a study as well as the general characteristics of subjects who chose to participate in the study should be reviewed. Are these subjects reasonably similar to the patient spurring the clinician's search for evidence? Or are the differences too large to apply the findings with confidence? What equipment, specialized knowledge, or availability of resources was necessary to apply the findings of the study to your clinical world? Is this feasible? If the conclusion is that the approach is not feasible in a particular clinic, the physical therapist should continue to look for alternative approaches with similar outcomes. If, indeed, a determination is made that the outcomes achieved from this approach are far superior to the alternatives available at your clinic, then a mechanism should be adopted to either refer the patient out when this approach is required or for the clinic to obtain the capability or the equipment to provide the approach.

Generalizing findings across broad groups of older adults can be particularly difficult in geriatrics. As stated earlier, older adults as a group are extraordinarily variable. Researchers must balance inclusiveness with homogeneity. The more homogeneous the subjects in a study, the fewer are the confounding factors to mask real change. However, the greater the number of exclusion criteria, the narrower the generalizability. Often, the exclusion criteria include those patients the clinician is most interested in applying the findings to. It is fairly common for studies to exclude subjects older than age 70 or 75 years, those with commonly occurring comorbid conditions, or individuals who have any cognitive impairment. Was everyone who had heart disease, diabetes, or high blood pressure excluded from a study involving exercise? In a group of older adults, this requirement would likely exclude at least half of the patients treated in physical therapy practices. Consider the impact of the exclusion criteria on the ability to apply the findings to your typical patient world.

The terms efficacy and effectiveness are frequently used to describe the aim of a study, particularly an intervention study. These terms give you a clue to the expectations of the researchers about the generalizability of the findings. The terms, commonly used in conjunction with the four levels of clinical trials as described by NIH, suggest that the aim of an efficacy study is to determine if a given intervention *can* work. Meaning, given an ideal situation and ideal patient, is the intervention successful? An effectiveness study is one that aims to determine if the intervention *will* work in the typical clinical world with typical patients including all their variability. Effectiveness studies are particularly applicable to everyday clinical practice and, therefore, are worthy of particularly close review and consideration.

A challenge, and reality check, is the likely differences between the current cohort of older adults (on which current research is based) and the next generation of older adults. Much of the current evidence is based on studies that emerged from landmark investigations completed 20 to 40 years ago. The older adult of prior years is not the same older adult we anticipate in the next 20 years. Baby boomers are approaching old age with a different perspective and set of experiences with physical activity and exercise than prior generations of older adults. Medical science has decreased the impact of many chronic health conditions and increased the likelihood of other conditions associated with a longer life span.

BOX 1-4	One Framework for Assigning Strength to Recommendations Emerging from a Systematic Review
Good evidence	Reasonably consistent findings from several high-quality definitive studies of clinical applicability. Unlikely that further research will change the recommendation in any important way.
Fair evidence	Reasonably consistent findings from several moderate-quality studies (initial studies evaluating foundational concepts) or one definitive study of clinical applicability. Although there is support for the recommendation, there is a reasonable possibility that further research will modify the recommendation in some important way.
Weak evidence	Reasonably consistent findings from primarily foundational studies with findings not yet rigorously tested on relevant patient groups. It is quite likely that further research will modify the recommendation in some important way.
Inconclusive evidence	There is insufficient or markedly conflicting evidence that does not allow a recommendation to be made for or against the intervention.

PATIENT-CLIENT PREFERENCES AND MOTIVATIONS

Patient-client preference and motivation is the third information stream making up evidence-based (evidence-informed) practice. The scientific evidence and the expertise of the practitioner are combined with the preferences and motivations of the patient to reach a shared and informed decision about goals and interventions. Patient autonomy is grounded in the principle that patients have the right to make their own decisions about their health care. There is a tendency for health care providers to behave paternalistically toward older adult patients, assuming these patients are less capable than younger adults to make decisions about their health and rehabilitation. The reality of clinical practice is that physical therapists encounter a wide variety of decision-making capabilities in their older adult patients. Physical therapists have a responsibility to ensure their patients (and family/caretakers, as appropriate) have all pertinent information needed to make therapy-related health care decisions, and that this information is shared in a manner that is understandable to the patient and free of clinician bias. The patient should understand the potential risks, benefits, and harms; amount of effort and compliance associated with the various options; and the likely prognosis.

Patients should have the opportunity to express their preferences and be satisfied that the practitioner has heard them accurately and without bias. The goals and preferences of the older adult patient may be very different from what the physical therapist assumes (or believe they would want for themselves under similar circumstances). Part of the "art" of physical therapy is creatively addressing the patient's goals using appropriate evidence, clinical skills, and available resources.

THE INFLUENCE OF AGEISM

The perception of someone as being old or geriatric is a social construct that can differ greatly among cultures and social groups. A recent Pew Foundation survey[23] found that, on average, a representative sample of the U.S. population perceives age 68 years as the age at which a person crosses the threshold to be classified as old. However, the age of the survey respondent influenced perceptions: Respondents under the age of 30 years identified old age as starting at 60 years; those between 30 and 64 years indicated 70 years as the beginning of old age; and those older than age 64 years indicated that old age starts at 74 years. The age of 65 years, which is the typical age when individuals in the United States become eligible for Medicare, is probably the most common age identified by medical researchers and social policy advocates when categorizing individuals as old.

In reality, perceiving a specific individual as old is often more associated with the person's physical appearance and health status than his or her chronological age. An 80-year-old who is independent, fit, and healthy may not be described as old by those around her, whereas a 60-year-old who is unfit, has multiple chronic health problems, and needs help with daily activities that are physically challenging is likely to be perceived and described as old.

Age bias, a negative perception of older adults based on their age alone, is endemic in Western culture, including health care settings.[24] Kite and Johnson,[25] in a meta-analysis of 43 studies on age bias, concluded that attitudes toward older people are more negative than toward younger people. The subtle negative attitudes toward older adults that are often identified among health care practitioners become more obvious and influential when old age is combined with a perception of the patient as having low motivation, poor compliance, or poor prognosis.

Rybarczyk et al[25a] considered age plus other patient characteristics in a study of bias in nearly 1000 rehabilitation professionals, including physical therapists. One core clinical scenario was developed representing a patient receiving rehabilitation postamputation. However, multiple variations of this core scenario were presented. The identically involved patient was either young or old and further divided into male or female. The young or old patient was (1) ideally motivated and cooperative with rehabilitation, (2) depressed, or (3) noncompliant. The study found little age bias when the ideally motivated old patient was compared to the ideally motivated young patient. However, when two noncompliant or depressed patients were compared, those responding to the scenario describing an old patient demonstrated more negative attitudes than those responding to the scenario describing a young patient.

In the hectic and often stressful acute care setting, nurses admit that older patients are often marginalized with their needs given lower priority, and less time spent making a human connection with the patient.[26] Age bias has been identified as a reason for undertreating older adults with cancer based on unsupported assumptions that treatments are unsafe for the older adult, or at times, despite evidence supporting the use of the intervention for older adults.[24,27,28]

Typically, physical therapists are drawn to the profession by a strong desire to help people in a very tangible and interactive way, often expressing low interest in patients they perceive as having low potential for improvement.[29,30] Stereotypes about older adults inaccurately suggest that, as a group, older adults have low potential for improvement, are unmotivated, noncompliant and set in their ways, confused, and permanently dependent on others.

Many interactions with physical therapists occur at very vulnerable points in an older adult's life. For example, it is common to first evaluate an older adult in the midst of an acute hospitalization from a sudden and significant illness; in a skilled nursing facility for rehabilitation after hip fracture or knee replacement; or in the outpatient department during a disabling bout of back pain. When formulating a prognosis and making recommendations for the aggressiveness of interventions, it is easy to fall back on stereotypes suggesting old patients have low potential for improvement and low motivation for rehabilitation. It is true that some older adults enter physical therapy very low on the slippery slope of aging (frailty and failure stages). Rehabilitation may be particularly challenging given prior functional level, requiring the individual to make conscious decisions about where they want to place their efforts in the presence of substantially limited energy reserves; in which case goals not achievable through physical rehabilitation may guide their decisions. However, for most older patients, appropriately aggressive physical therapy can substantially affect functional ability and quality of life. Physical therapists who let ageist stereotypes influence their judgment are likely to make assumptions that underestimate prior functional ability of individuals and future potential for improvement. Do not let stereotypes cloud judgment about the capacity of older adults and the benefit to be achieved by appropriately aggressive rehabilitation.

Hausdorff et al.,[31] in a study examining the influence of ageist messages on older adults, found significant differences in gait parameters (gait speed and swing time) in community-dwelling older adults exposed to negative versus positive reinforcement of age stereotypes during a 30-minute interaction. In the clinical environment, most patients will look to the professional for guidance in the likely outcome of various therapies. Thorough consideration of the patient's goals, and objective (unbiased) assessment and communication of the likely efforts required to meet those goals will help reduce stereotyping.

SUMMARY

The key principles underlying contemporary geriatric physical therapy practice described in this chapter are woven throughout the remainder of this book. The need is great and opportunities abound for talented physical therapists committed to optimal aging and ready to apply best evidence, fully develop their clinical expertise, and work collaboratively with their patients and other health care providers. It is a challenging time full of opportunity to be a geriatrically focused physical therapist. However, whether as a geriatrically focused physical therapist or simply a physical therapist who frequently/occasionally treats older patients, the number and complexity of the older adult patients among the caseload of all physical therapists will increase in the decades to come, emphasizing the clinical relevance of the material in this book.

REFERENCES

To enhance this text and add value for the reader, all references are included on the companion Evolve site that accompanies this text book. The reader can view the reference source and access it online whenever possible. There are a total of 31 cited references and other general references for this chapter.

Implications of an Aging Population for Rehabilitation:
Demography, Mortality, and Morbidity of Older Adults

Andrew A. Guccione, PT, PhD, DPT, FAPTA

What are the implications of an increase in the number of older persons in American society, particularly as it affects rehabilitation specialists such as physical therapists? Some have portrayed the "graying" of America during the past 60 years as a social problem of vast numbers of resource-guzzling older adults who threaten to strip the health care system of its scarce resources. Others have portrayed this same group as a rich resource to their families and their communities: a group still very much engaged in life as healthy, active older adults. Is it possible that these two contrasting representations of America's older persons refer to the same set of individuals?

The purpose of this chapter is to review the sociodemographic characteristics of older adults in American society, then relate these factors to mortality and morbidity in this population. In doing so, we shall find that conflicting portrayals of older persons as active and healthy, or as sick and frail, are neither incorrect nor contradictory, but more appropriately applied to only some segments of a heterogeneous population.

Although physical therapists implement interventions in a plan of care designed for individual patients or clients, each of us has physical, psychological, and social characteristics by which we can be categorized into groups. Knowing that individuals with certain characteristics—for example, being a particular age or sex—are more likely to experience a particular health problem can assist physical therapists in anticipating some clinical presentations, placing an individual's progress in perspective, and even sometimes altering outcomes through preventive measures. It is also useful to know the prevalence of a particular condition (i.e., the number of cases of that condition in a population) and its incidence (the number of new cases of a

condition in a population within a specified time period). Taken beyond examination of a single person, physical therapists can use this information to plan and develop services that will meet the needs of an aging society whose members span a continuum across health, infirmity, and death.

There is one critical caveat to any of the inferences about aging or older persons that may be drawn from the data below. Much of what we in the United States know in gerontology and geriatrics has been derived from two specific cohorts. The first cohort was born near the end of the 19th century, many of them impoverished child immigrants or born into families recently arrived in America. Thus the initial emergence of gerontological research in the 1970s is based largely on these individuals whose early health and vitality into adulthood were determined long before the medical advances and economic prosperity that marked the "American Century." Their children comprise the second cohort, whose experiences define our current-day understanding of aging. Geriatric and gerontological research in this group is also contextually situated in the defining events of the first half of the 20th century: two world wars and the Great Depression. Thus, whenever we choose to explicate aging and the status of older adults, be it their physical health or social well-being, we must also appreciate that what we understand is based on what either has been or is currently the case, not necessarily what will be the norm in the future. As the adults of the post–World War II "baby boom" begin to retire in 2011, we can expect that gerontological theories and geriatric practice—geriatric physical therapy included—will change markedly by mid–21st century to accommodate new findings that emerge from scientific study of this third and markedly distinct cohort.

SUCCESSFUL VS. OPTIMAL AGING

"Successful aging" was a multidimensional concept first articulated in the late 1980s and further elaborated in the 1990s to distinguish between individuals with the characteristics of usual aging and those adults who had managed successful aging. The concept of successful aging encompassed three elements: avoiding disease and disability, maintaining high physical and cognitive function, and sustaining engagement in social and productive activities.[1,2] The research that supported the concept suggested that biological orientations to aging in gerontological research were biased toward "usual" or "average" aging but ignored the equally important long-term effects of diet, exercise, and lifestyle that characterized the successful aging of many who had escaped the usual decline and disability of average aging. Physical therapists can assist the promotion of successful aging by encouraging modification of some extrinsic factors, particularly in teenagers and young adults, which lead to less disease and disability in the later years. For those with disease and disability, the physical therapist should work within the concept of "optimal aging," which allows an individual to achieve life satisfaction in multiple domains—physical, psychological, and social—despite the presence of disabling medical conditions. Physical therapists can promote optimal aging by reducing the disabling effects of disease and stopping a vicious cycle of "disease–disability–new incident disease" to maintain quality of life.

DEMOGRAPHY

Defining "Older" Adult

The first gerontological question is how a particular segment of a population comes to be categorized as "older"? The chronological criterion that is presently used for identifying the older adult in America is strictly arbitrary and usually has been set at age 65 years. However, the onset of some of the "geriatric" health problems of older individuals may occur as soon as they enter their early 50s, and, as detailed elsewhere, "older" athletes may be only in their 40s. As the mean age of the population increases and more individuals live into their ninth and tenth decades, we can expect that our notion of who is "older" will change.

Population Estimates and Age Structure

The number of Americans age 65 years and older continues to grow at an unprecedented rate. In 2007 the best available estimate of persons age 65 years or older was 37.3 million,[3] reflecting the major changes in the population structure of the United States in the past century. Individuals who had reached their 65th birthday accounted for only 4% of the total population in

1900. In 1940 they were 6.9% of the population, and by 1950 they were equal to 8.2%. Although they represented just fewer than 10% of the population in 1970, they currently account for almost 13% of the U.S. population.[4] Individuals born between the years 1946 and 1964 are frequently referred to as the "Baby Boomers" and will be responsible for a sharp rise in the number of older people between 2010 and 2030, when the older population is predicted to account for nearly 20% of the total U.S. population.[4] Individuals older than age 85 years currently represent just under 10% of people older than age 65 years (5.3 million people in 2006), but their representation within the general populace is likely to quadruple by 2050 (Figure 2-1).[4] The number of individuals older than 100 also continues to increase, even though the actual proportion of the total population (1 of every 10,000) is relatively small.[5]

Two concurrent factors that have affected the increase in the proportion of aged in our society are a declining birthrate and a declining death rate. With fewer births overall and more survivors at older ages, the age structure of the population changes from a triangular shape, with a larger number of younger individuals at the base, to a more rectangular distribution of the population by age, with a trend over time for a larger proportion of older individuals at the top, especially among the oldest old.[6] In 1990 and 2000, the shape of the age pyramid shows remnants of the traditional triangular structure as well as the beginning "rectangularization" (Figure 2-2).

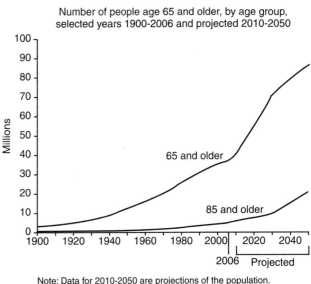

Number of people age 65 and older, by age group, selected years 1900-2006 and projected 2010-2050

Note: Data for 2010-2050 are projections of the population.
Reference population: These data refer to the resident population.
Source: U.S. Census Bureau, Decennial Census, Population Estimates and Projections.

FIGURE 2-1 Growth of the population age 65 years and older, past and projected, with projected growth of adults age 85 years and older to midcentury. *(From Federal Interagency Forum on Aging-Related Statistics: Older Americans 2008: key indicators of well-being. Washington, DC: U.S. Government Printing Office, March 2008.)*

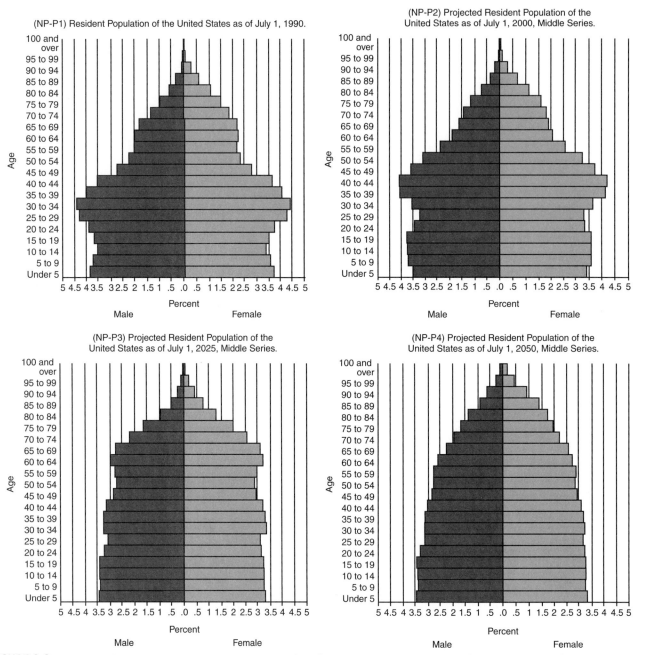

FIGURE 2-2 Change in the population age structure by age and sex from 1990 to 2050 showing shifts in proportions of younger individuals to older individuals. *(Source: National Estimates Program, Population Division, U.S. Census Bureau, Washington, DC, 20233. From U.S. Census Bureau: U.S. population projects: population pyramids [website]: http://www.census.gov/population/www/projections/natchart.html; Accessed February 27, 2010.)*

By 2050, the age structure "pyramid" is relatively rectangular except among the older age groups.

Life Expectancy

In 2007, the median age of the total population of the United States was 36.4 years, whereas the median age of individuals 65 years and older was 74.8 years.[3] In the first half of the 20th century, mortality declined primarily as a result of advances in health at birth and younger ages, especially infant mortality. However, by 2000 the

changes in life expectancy were primarily the result of reduced mortality at older ages, not the least of which was the dramatic increase in the number of adults who lived to age 85 years.[6] In 1900, a person who lived until age 65 years might expect another 12 years of life. Additional life expectancy for individuals age 65 years in 2000 had grown to 18 years. However, female life expectancy continues to outpace male life expectancy, despite gains made for both sexes, although the gap has begun to decrease. Racial differences in life expectancy have also been demonstrated, as white women generally live the longest, whereas black women and white men live about the same and black men have the lowest survivorship.[6] There has been a long-standing controversy in the literature regarding whether there is a racial crossover at the oldest ages, where black survivorship may improve. Some have argued that the phenomenon is actually a statistical artifact of misreporting and data inconsistencies, or not accounting for confounding variables; other researchers have drawn conclusions about "survival of the fittest," arguing that individuals who surmount racial, socioeconomic, and health disadvantages early in life represent the most "fit" to survive into old age.

Race and Ethnicity

Racial and nonwhite ethnic minorities are currently underrepresented among the nation's older adults relative to the distribution of these subgroups in the general population. In 2006, approximately 81% of the population age 65 years and older was non-Hispanic white, whereas blacks accounted for 9%, Asians 3%, and Hispanics of any race 6%.[4] Hispanic representation in the older population has the fastest overall growth rate of any subgroup, likely to surpass the black subpopulation of older adults by 2028, and anticipated to be 15 million in 2050, or nearly eight times as large as it was in 2005.[4] More recent immigrations in the 1990s of peoples from Southeast Asia will likely add to the relatively small number (about 1 million) of older Asians in the United States to a projected 7 million by 2050.[4] Clearly, the geriatric physical therapist must recognize that the older adult of the future, especially those who will be considered the "oldest old," will be more racially and culturally diverse than those patients currently served, and culturally competent care will literally require a global appreciation of diversity.

Sex Distribution and Marital Status

Simply put, there is a marked sex differential in mortality, and a number of social and life factors beyond biologic predisposition may lead to shorter lives for men overall.[6,7] Married people have a lower mortality at all ages than their unmarried peers, and married men appear to derive a greater survival advantage than married women.[6] However, because women typically live longer than men, the problems of America's older adults are largely the problems of women, of whom fewer will have a living spouse at the age of 65 years and older in contrast to their male counterparts (Figure 2-3).[8] Older men are more likely to be married than older women and married men are generally older than their wives, who have a greater life expectancy by virtue of their sex across all racial and ethnic groups.[6] Women age 65 years and older are three times more likely to be widowed as comparably aged men, with the proportion growing with each decade of aging.[3] There have been many theories proposed to explain the salutary effects of marriage

on longevity, generally focusing on social support and shared resources. However, like most social institutions, marriage or partnered relationships defy easy characterizations, suggesting that one must look at the specific attributes of a particular relationship before drawing conclusions.

In addition to the caregiving burdens and socioeconomic implications of being partnered, loss of a significant other brings its own set of psychosocial challenges to the individual in contemporary society. Any individual whose identity is linked to being a couple or part of a long-term relationship may experience a severe disruption of social roles when left alone. This disruption complicates the search for self-validation through the recognition, esteem, and affection of another that may have been present in a marital or partnered relationship.

Living Arrangements

In 2000, 28% of the population age 65 years and older lived alone,[9] noting that older non-Hispanic white women and black women were more likely to live alone than other racial or ethnic groups.[4] Older black, Asian, and Hispanic women are more likely than non-Hispanic white women to live with nonspousal relatives.[4] When older adults need assistance in basic and instrumental activities of daily living (ADLs), spouses and children often provide the majority of help. Decline in functional abilities strongly predicts the likelihood that an older adult living alone will seek other arrangements.

Nursing home utilization has changed since the mid-1980s, especially with respect to racial and ethnic diversity.[10] Many more of these individuals now have short-term admissions and return to their premorbid living arrangements compared with 20 years ago.[10] In 2004, older adults in nursing homes were predominately female; age 75 years and older (82%); white, non-Hispanic, and not married.[11]

Family Roles and Relationships. Despite many social advances for younger generations of women, the degree to which female older adults are still bound by society to traditional roles such as homemaking and caretaking should not be underestimated. Furthermore, an older woman is more likely to live alone when compared to a male counterpart and must continue to function independently, whatever her level of physical function. Women are therefore more likely than men to report disability with respect to social roles. The relative unavailability of assistance with home chores in comparison with other social support services may be a subtle discrimination against older women, although the level of unmet need in this area is not well documented. These home services can often be the essential element in allowing an older adult to remain living independently at home when functional abilities are compromised. Physical therapists will need to continue working with other health professionals to advocate for access to a wide

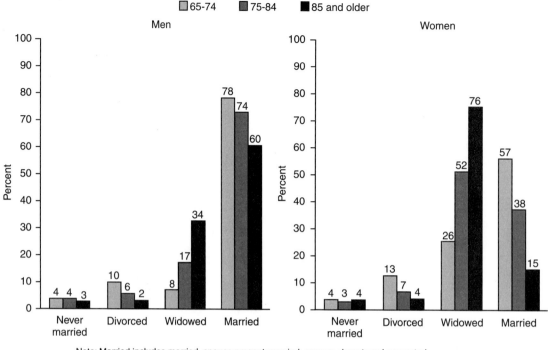

Marital status of the population age 65 and older, by age group and sex, 2007

Note: Married includes married, spouse present; married, spouse absent; and separated.
Reference population: These data refer to the civilian noninstitutionalized population.
Source: U.S. Census Bureau, Current Population Survey, Annual Social and Economic Supplement.

FIGURE 2-3 Marital status by age and sex of adults age 65 years and older. *(From Federal Interagency Forum on Aging-Related Statistics: Older Americans 2008: key indicators of well-being. Washington, DC: U.S. Government Printing Office, March 2008.)*

range of services that support the highest level of independent living for the aged.

Although findings from a number of studies during the past 20 years have been treated as "common wisdom" about families and aging, the simple fact is that the magnitude of variation in "family" as a social construct is very great and cannot easily be generalized into evidence-based statements about the nature of families, the influence of ethnicity, or gender-specific roles in caring for older family members. Fertility rates and immigration patterns also influence the proportion of family members able to support aging parents.[6] Older adults who do live with family can often find themselves in multigenerational families, growing old with their children. Spouses are the most likely individuals to care for their partners in old age and sickness. When a spouse is unable or unavailable to provide assistance, it is not easily determined who will do what for an aging parent in need. The actual provision of direct care to older parents has traditionally been described as "women's work," which is as much a function of traditional social mores as a lack of evidence to the contrary. Research has not elucidated the role of men in caring for older parents as investigators have often assumed that the responsibility of caregiving falls to daughters and daughters-in-law, often to the

exclusion of men as subjects in many studies. Recommendations that increase the tasks of caregiving among selected family members (e.g., assisting with a home exercise program) may be perceived as either a burden or as an opportunity[12,13]; thus evaluation of caregiving impact of rehabilitation interventions may be required. Many stereotypes exist about different racial and ethnic groups, but the data do not support a facile conclusion that one group is more "predisposed" to offer assistance. Physical therapists must evaluate each family situation for its unique characteristics.

The societal roles of grandparenting also continue to evolve. Increased longevity increases the amount of one's life that might be spent being a grandparent. It is not unusual for an aging individual to witness a grandchild's movement through the life course from birth up to the grandchild's adulthood. Healthy older adults still provide substantial financial and emotional support to their children. Many grandparents find themselves taking on additional babysitting and child-rearing responsibilities. Therefore, an examination and evaluation of an older person's functional abilities in this social context might need to consider whether a grandparent has the dexterity to change a diaper, the strength to lift a toddler, and the stamina to walk young children home from the school bus.

Economic Status

The tendency to regard older adults as a homogeneous group biases any understanding of their economic status. The heterogeneity of this population group is perhaps best illustrated by considering who is financially well-off and who is economically disadvantaged among older adults. Overall, the entrance of the youngest stratum of older adults, who benefit from private and workers' pension programs, has improved the economic well-being of older adults as a whole, as the proportion of older adults living in poverty has shrunk from 35% in 1959 to 9% in 2006 (Figure 2-4).[4] In comparison with poverty among children younger than age 18 years, people age 65 years and older have experienced a relatively steady decline in poverty.[4] These group figures, however, do obscure the realities of poverty among older people; poverty increases with age; women are more often in poverty than men; and older Hispanics and older blacks experience greater economic deprivation than non-Hispanic whites.[4] Furthermore, although older adults may be less likely to enter into poverty than individuals younger than age 18 years, people age 65 years and older who do enter poverty are less likely to transition out than their younger counterparts.[6] Housing expenditures account for about 33% of expenses, whereas health care and food each account for about 13%.[4] Although expenditures for housing, food, and transportation remain relatively constant for noninstitutionalized older adults, health care expenses continue to rise after age 65 years (Figure 2-5).

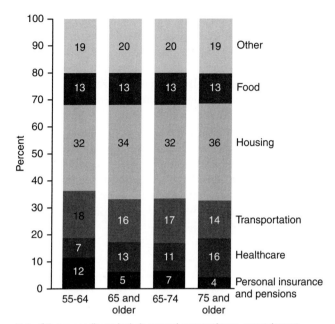

Note: Other expenditures include apparel, personal care, entertainment, reading, education, alcohol, tobacco, cash contribtions, and miscellaneous expenditures.
Reference population: These data refer to the resident noninstiutionalized population.
Source: Bureau of Labor Statistics, Consumer Expenditure Survey.

FIGURE 2-5 Total household expenditures by category and age group. *(From Federal Interagency Forum on Aging-Related Statistics: Older Americans 2008: key indicators of well-being. Washington, DC: U.S. Government Printing Office, March 2008.)*

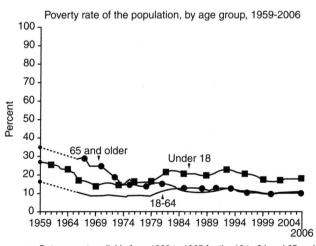

········ Data are not available from 1960 to 1965 for the 18 to 64 and 65 and older age groups.
Reference population: These data refer to the civilian noninstitutionalized population.
Source: U.S. Census Bureau, Current Population Survey, Annual Social and Economic Supplement, 1960-2007.

FIGURE 2-4 Poverty rates by age group. *(From Federal Interagency Forum on Aging-Related Statistics: Older Americans 2008: key indicators of well-being. Washington, DC: U.S. Government Printing Office, March 2008.)*

MORTALITY

Causes of Death

The five most common causes of death for all individuals age 65 years or older are heart diseases, malignant neoplasms, cerebrovascular disease, chronic lower respiratory diseases, and pneumonia and influenza.[4,6] Despite its position as the leading cause of death, age-adjusted death rates in the United States from heart disease and stroke mortality have declined remarkably in the past 30 years, most likely because of improvements in the detection and treatment of hypertension as well as improvements in emergency and critical care.[4] However, age-adjusted death rates for both diabetes and respiratory diseases increased markedly in the same period. Given the role of exercise in the primary and secondary prevention as well as rehabilitation of all of these conditions, physical therapists are able to make a major contribution to the well-being of the geriatric population.

Active Life Expectancy

Adults who survive to age 65 years can expect to live almost 19 years longer, which is about 7 years longer than what would have been expected in 1900.[4] Although gains in overall life expectancy are important indicators of a nation's well-being, active life expectancy, that is, the years spent without a major infirmity or disabling condition, may provide more meaningful information for health professionals. More accessible health care, improved understanding of genetic predisposition, and preventive behaviors such as increased physical activity and balanced nutrition have all contributed to more years spent in better health. Although medical advances have improved the survivorship of individuals with multiple impairments in old age, the data support the notion that each successive generation of older adults enjoys a slightly greater active life expectancy prior to entering permanent functional decline.[4,6]

MORBIDITY

Prevalent Chronic Conditions

The proportion of older adults at any age without any chronic conditions is small. About 80% have at least one chronic condition and 50% have two or more.[6] Among these, arthritis is the most prevalent self-reported condition causing an activity limitation. Hypertension, heart disease, stroke, diabetes, hearing and vision impairments, and fractures also take their toll on activity.[4,6] Chronic conditions are not randomly dispersed throughout the population (Figure 2-6). Arthritis is more common among women. Hypertension is more prevalent among women and blacks than men and whites. Heart disease is more prevalent among men than women, whereas non-Hispanic blacks tend to experience stroke more often than other subgroups. Diabetes affects men and women about equally, but prevalence among older Hispanics and non-Hispanic blacks is greater than older non-Hispanic whites. Osteoporosis is four times more likely among women and substantially increases the risk of fracture.[4,6]

Prevalent Activity Limitations

Estimates from a number of national surveys indicate that a substantial proportion of older adults are hampered in their ability to perform a major life activity or are limited in mobility, and despite some studies that suggested this trend was improving, it may actually be worsening.[14] Furthermore, these surveys indicate that these limitations in function increase with age, and they are generally worse for women (who may contract more disabling conditions such as arthritis), nonwhites, and obese individuals.[6,14] As has been noted in the overall health status of the general population, it is commonly agreed that the risks of physical disability are higher for nonwhites and individuals with lower socioeconomic status.[6]

As we shift from exploring population characteristics associated with biological phenomena such as mortality

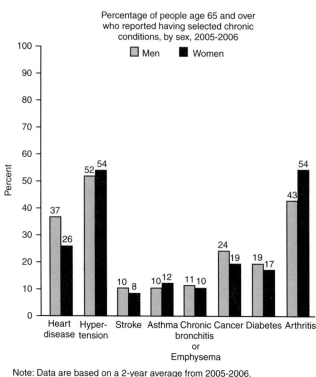

Percentage of people age 65 and over who reported having selected chronic conditions, by sex, 2005-2006

Note: Data are based on a 2-year average from 2005-2006.
Reference population: These data refer to the civilian noninstitutionalized population.
Source: Centers for Disease Control and Prevention, National Center for Health Statistics, National Health Interview Survey.

FIGURE 2-6 Chronic conditions among adults age 65 years and older by sex. *(From Federal Interagency Forum on Aging-Related Statistics: Older Americans 2008: key indicators of well-being. Washington, DC: U.S. Government Printing Office, March 2008.)*

to consider the functional status of various groups, which is a biopsychosocial phenomenon, a word of caution is always in order when interpreting subgroup statistics. First, the definitions for complex concepts such as race/ethnicity or socioeconomic status may shift over time from survey to survey, or have been imperfectly applied during data collection so that some subgroups are over- or underrepresented in statistical analyses. The concepts themselves may be proxy measures of other factors that affect health status and function, such as educational advantage, lifetime employment opportunity, or living environment, but are very difficult to measure directly and rarely studied.[15] Statistically, these findings may be highly correlated, which, for example, leaves demographers uncertain as to whether race/ethnicity or poverty or educational attainment better explains poor health status from a statistical point of view (i.e., greater explanatory power of a particular variable in a more robust statistical model). Furthermore, even highly correlated relationships among variables may not be linear or parallel and may disproportionately affect individuals at different points on the intersecting continua of education, income, or health status. Alternatively, the models that are used to explain functional deficits or activity limitations may not be robust and multidimensional so that the statistical analyses incorporate data gathered from multiple domains such as socioeconomic status and physiological impairment.[16] Therefore, at the level of the individual person, which is the level at which we measure activity limitation, functional deficit, or disability, inferences from these models about the interplay between broad sociodemographic factors and health status or quality of life are more tentative and, more than occasionally, not particularly useful to clinical decision making as they represent factors outside the clinician's control.

Disease and Disability

The six most common chronic health conditions that result in activity limitations are arthritis and other musculoskeletal conditions, heart and other circulatory problems, vision or hearing impairments, fractures and joint injuries, diabetes, and mental illness (Figure 2-7).[6]

Increasing age is associated with increasing prevalence of activity limitations, with the exception of mental illness. Importantly for physical therapists, exercise and physical activity are not only critical interventions once health conditions develop[17-19] but they provide broad health promotion opportunities. Physical therapists can assume a key role in public health by instruction in exercise and physical activity to achieve primary prevention and risk reduction for development of several health conditions (heart and circulatory disorders, fractures associated with falls, and diabetes).[20-22]

Comorbidity and Disability

It is not unusual for physical therapists to find that the patients with the most disability are also likely to have a number of medical or health conditions that complicate not only understanding of the genesis of functional deficit but treatment as well. For example, the individual

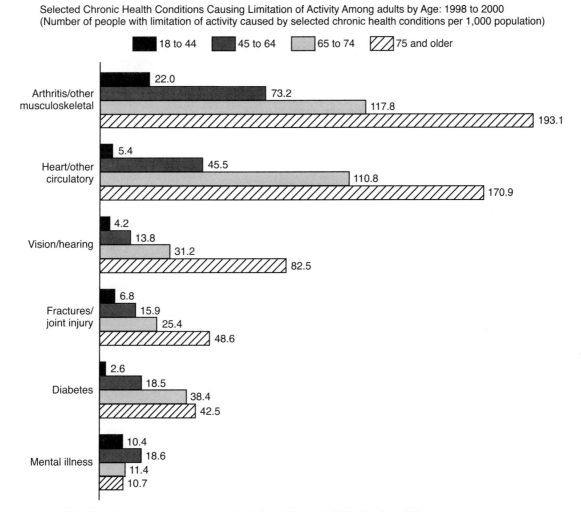

Selected Chronic Health Conditions Causing Limitation of Activity Among adults by Age: 1998 to 2000
(Number of people with limitation of activity caused by selected chronic health conditions per 1,000 population)

Note: The reference population for these data is the civillian noninstitutionalized population.
Source: National Center for Health Statistics, 2002a, Figure 17. For full citation, see references at end of chapter.

FIGURE 2-7 Chronic health conditions causing activity limitations by age group. *(From He W, Sengupta M, Velkoff VA, Debarros, KA: U.S. Census Bureau population reports, P23–209, 65+ in the United States: 2005. Washington, DC: U.S. Government Printing Office, 2005.)*

with a stroke, who also has degenerative changes in the foot and low tolerance for stressful activity secondary to angina with exertion, can present a particular challenge to the geriatric physical therapist's knowledge and skill.

Although there is an emerging body of knowledge on the effects of disease on function, less is known about the effects of coexistent disease on function. Older adults vary a great deal in the degree to which their chronic comorbidity affects their functional capacities. However, one comorbidity that has a documented negative effect on function is obesity.[23-26] Physical therapists working with other health professionals can have a major impact on functional decline by applying their evidence base in exercise and physical activity to this threat to public health.

FUNCTION

Physical Function and Disability

Physical, psychological, and social function are all dimensions of function that are included in the measurement of a person's overall health status. Physical therapists address issues of physical function. In general, independent physical function declines with age, and this decline is influenced by a host of biological, psychological, and social factors. Function is not a static phenomenon and individual transitions in functional status are more the norm than the exception. Function is also a sociological phenomenon. Functional assessment does not only measure the individual's abilities to perform tasks that are personally meaningful to the individual, but it also measures performance essential to meeting social expectations of what is "normal" functioning for an adult. It is therefore necessary that the overall approach to functional assessment of an older adult include items that take into account what is "normal" in that person's social and cultural sphere. Physical functional activities can be subdivided into five areas: mobility, which includes transfers and ambulation; basic self-care and personal hygiene (ADLs); more complex activities essential to an adult's living in the community, known as instrumental ADLs (IADLs); work; and recreation.

Mobility. A primary concern of physical therapists in performing a physical functional assessment of any adult individual is to identify any functional limitations in mobility that can range from the ability to move independently in bed, transfer from bed to chair, ambulation on level surfaces within the home, stair climbing, negotiating uneven terrain, and walking for longer distances in the community. Mobility is a component of ADLs, work, and recreational activities.

Activities of Daily Living

Basic Activities of Daily Living. Basic ADLs include all of the fundamental tasks and activities necessary for survival, hygiene, and self-care within the home. A typical ADL battery, which may be administered by a physical therapist alone or cooperatively with other health professionals, covers eating, bathing, grooming, dressing, bed mobility, and transfers. Incontinence and the ability to use a bathroom are especially important elements in the assessment of physical function in some older individuals. The ability of an adult in three aspects of independent toileting function may require exploration of specific task accomplishment: to get to the bathroom in an appropriate time period, to move safely on and off the receptacle, and to perform self-hygiene tasks.

Instrumental Activities of Daily Living. An examination and evaluation of IADLs addresses multiple areas that are essential to living independently as an adult: cooking, shopping, washing, housekeeping, and ability to use public transportation or drive a car. For some individuals, it may also be appropriate to investigate the ability to perform home chores such as shoveling snow or yardwork.

Relationship between ADLs and IADLs. Most older adults living in the community are generally independent in both ADLs and IADLs (Figure 2-8). The relationship between ADL and IADL is generally hierarchical; that is, limitations in ADL usually predict limitations in IADL. Thus, a home-care physical therapist working with a patient recently returning home from an acute care hospital after a hip fracture would first explore the individual's ability to do the tasks and activities encompassed by basic ADL, such as transfers, ambulation, and toileting. If deficits were found, independence in these activities would serve as the first goals of intervention. If the patient was independent in basic ADL upon initial examination, or became independent through the physical therapist's intervention, the therapist would then examine the older person's limitations in performing IADL, which supports a person's ability to live independently in the community. As part of the plan of care, as the patient progresses to greater levels of independence, the physical therapist will play an important role in identifying the patient's needs for formal caregivers, such as homemakers and home health aides, and in teaching families how to manage a person's limitations well enough so that the individual may continue to reside in the community.

Work. One measure of adult competence is employment. Previously, it has been assumed that older adults did not need to or want to work, based on data trends that appear to have ended in the 1980s.[4] Changes in federal regulations have raised the minimum age at which individuals may receive full Social Security benefits and mandatory retirement at a specific age for most occupations is not typically permitted. Therefore, older adults who want to, or need to, remain in the workforce may do so if they are physically able to perform the tasks of their employment. A substantial proportion of civilian noninstitutionalized individuals older than age 65 years are still counted in the workforce.[4] Specifically, 34.4% of the men and 24.2% of the women age 65 to 69 years

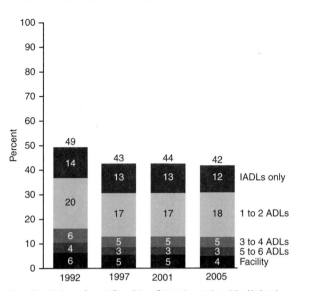

Note: The Medicare Current Beneficiary Survey has replaced the National Long Term Care Survey as the data source for this indicator. Consequently, the measurement of functional limitations (previously called disability) has changed from previous editions of *Older Americans*. ADL limitations refer to difficulty performing (or inability to perform for a health reason) one or more of the following tasks: bathing, dressing, eating, getting in/out of chairs, walking, or using the toilet. IADL limitations refer to difficulty performing (or inability to perform for a health reason) one or more of the following tasks: using the telephone, light housework, heavy housework, meal preparation, shopping, or managing money. Rates are age adjusted using the 2000 standard population. Data for 1992 and 2001 do not sum to the totals because of rounding. Reference: These data refer to Medicare enrollees. Source: Centers for Medicare and Medicaid Services, Medicare Current Beneficiary Survey.

FIGURE 2-8 Percentage of Medicare enrollees with limitations in activities of daily living (ADLs) or instrumental ADLs (IADLs) or residing in a facility. *(From Federal Interagency Forum on Aging-Related Statistics: Older Americans 2008: key indicators of well-being. Washington, DC: U.S. Government Printing Office, March 2008.)*

were labor force participants in 2006. There is a striking reduction among women age 70 years or older (7.1%) in comparison to their male peers (24.2%). Overall, the rates of labor force participation for older Americans have grown for both men and women, with a much steeper increase for women most likely due to generational changes in roles and societal expectations for women working outside the home, particularly during the past four decades.[4]

Physical limitations impacting one's ability to work can be examined by comparing an individual's work participation against the general conditions of work itself: Is the individual working the anticipated number of hours each week? Have the requirements of the job been modified in any respect to allow the individual to work? Does the quantity or quality of work completed meet the anticipated standard of performance? Another approach to assessing work performance, first described by Nagi,[27] is to examine an individual's ability to perform 10 particular physical tasks associated with work disability: (1) walking up 10 steps without resting; (2) walking a quarter of a mile; (3) sitting for 2 hours; (4) standing for 2 hours; (5) stooping, crouching, or kneeling; (6) reaching up overhead; (7) reaching out to shake hands; (8) grasping with fingers; (9) lifting or carrying 10 pounds; and (10) lifting

or carrying 25 pounds. Using these data on "advanced" mobility, one can infer what an individual's capacity to work would be. Interestingly, recent studies of the ability to perform these kinds of physical functional tasks indicated increasing disability with every decade and a significant difference between men and women that persisted in every age group (Figure 2-9).[4]

Recreation. Recreational activities are no less important than work to maintain a sense of well-being. Clearly, more older men and women today are maintaining interests in recreational sports that they developed earlier in life. Others are discovering the pleasures of recreational sports as older adults. Functional assessment of recreational activities, however, is not limited to sports. Many adults enjoy dancing and gardening, which require a relatively high degree of balance, flexibility, and strength. Even sedentary activities, such as stamp collecting or playing chess, require a certain degree of physical ability in the hand and upper extremity and therefore may be functional measures of the outcomes of intervention for some patients.

Heath and Health Care

Utilization of Services. Functional deficits are important markers for increased utilization of services, especially with the use of formal services such as home health care. Older patients in home health care tend to be women, white, widowed, between the ages of 75 and 84 years, and living in a private residence. Almost half of these receive care from family members.[4]

In contrast, nursing home residents are likely to be women, especially those older than age 85 years.[6] Nursing home utilization is generally on the decline, probably attributable to emerging alternative care options such as assisted living. Currently, it appears that any racial disparities in nursing home usage that may have previously existed are disappearing especially among nursing home residents aged 85 years and older.[6] The vast majority of nursing home residents need assistance with three or more basic ADLs, particularly bathing and dressing.[6] A distinct racial disparity in functional status has been documented among black nursing home residents, who are more likely to be functionally limited in basic ADLs than their nonblack peers.[28]

The majority portion of health care expenditures is paid by public programs such as Medicare or Medicaid.[6] Yet nearly 20% is paid out of pocket and a smaller proportion out of private insurance. Older adults in poverty or near poverty have the worst health status (Figure 2-10) and also incur the greatest health care costs.[6,29]

Current Trends and Future Possibilities. Changes in the demographic characteristics of the U.S. population represent a critical challenge to geriatric physical therapists. Older adults are expected to live longer than ever before, but the quality of their lives in these added years

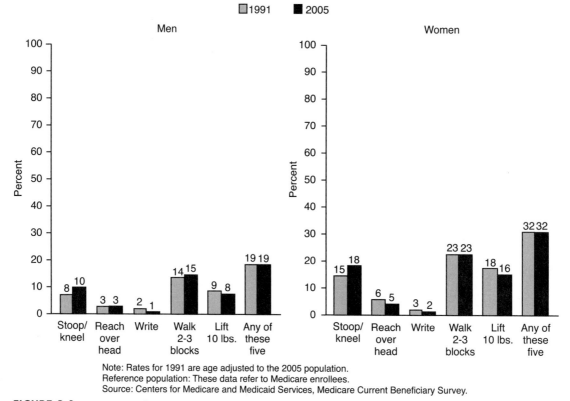

Percentage of Medicare enrollees age 65 and older who are unable
to perform certain physical functions, by sex, 1991 and 2005

Note: Rates for 1991 are age adjusted to the 2005 population.
Reference population: These data refer to Medicare enrollees.
Source: Centers for Medicare and Medicaid Services, Medicare Current Beneficiary Survey.

FIGURE 2-9 Percentage of Medicare enrollees who cannot perform selected physical tasks by sex. *(From Federal Interagency Forum on Aging-Related Statistics: Older Americans 2008: key indicators of well-being. Washington, DC: U.S. Government Printing Office, March 2008.)*

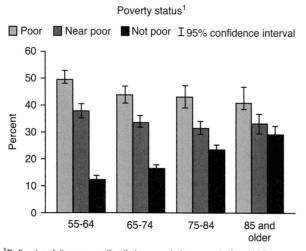

[1]Defined as follows; *poor* (family incomes below poverty threshold);
near poor (family incomes 100% to less than 200% of poverty threshold);
and *not poor* (family incomes 200% of poverty threshold or greater).
Note: Data are based on household interviews of a sample of the civilian noninstitutionalized population.
Data source: CDC/NCHS, National Health Interview Survey, 2004-2007.

FIGURE 2-10 Percentage of adults age 55 years and older in fair or poor health by age group and poverty status. *(From Schoenborn CA, Heyman KM: Health characteristics of adults aged 55 years and over: United States, 2004–2007. National health statistic reports, no. 16. Hyattsville, MD: National Center for Health Statistics, 2009.)*

is still a matter of conjecture. Aging with multiple diseases further aggravates a propensity toward physical decline with advanced age. Function deficits are the expected outcomes of disease; in turn, functional limitations predict increased utilization of services, further morbidity, and death. Future research must establish the ability of physical therapy to delay the onset of disease and disability and to prolong optimal function well into old age.

REFERENCES

To enhance this text and add value for the reader, all references are included on the companion Evolve site that accompanies this text book. The reader can view the reference source and access it online whenever possible. There are a total of 29 cited references and other general references for this chapter.

The Physiology of Age-Related and Lifestyle-Related Decline

Marybeth Brown, PT, PhD, FAPTA

INTRODUCTION

Aging is a fundamental process that affects all of our systems and tissues. The rate and magnitude of change in each system may differ person to person, but total body decline is an inevitable part of life for everyone. Ironically, we spend about 75% of our entire life span undergoing the process of decline.

Although there are hundreds of theories on why we age there is no one unifying theory that satisfactorily accounts for all the changes the body undergoes. Indeed, the study of aging is still in its infancy. Although enormous strides have been made in our understanding of the aging process, there is still much to discover about the science of age-related decline. A recent advancement is the recognition that whole-body inflammation is an important contributor to aging-related decline: a significant shift from concepts such as wear and tear and the biological clock based on genetic programming. Also it has only recently been realized that approximately half of the decline with age has a genetic basis.[1-5] The remainder of age-related change is the consequence of lifestyle, primarily physical inactivity that can account for the other half of the decline with age. Coupling sedentary lifestyle with inadequate nutrient intake, excess body weight (which puts stresses on tissues, increases inflammation, predisposes toward disease), and variables such as smoking and excessive alcohol intake, the biological decline is more precipitous and greater in magnitude.[6-8]

Even though age-related decline may result in the loss of lung capacity, renal clearance, or aerobic endurance, we have enough tissue reserve in each of our systems to get through 80 to 90 years without infirmity. Indeed, those who surgically donate a kidney or lung, which obviously results in the loss of half of the tissue function, still have a normal life span. As examples of normal aging there are 90-year-olds who can run marathons, do finger-tip push-ups, and dance vigorously.

Because so much of the decline with aging is lifestyle related, physical therapists have ample opportunity to intervene along the way, with successful results likely at any age. Indeed, there is a growing body of evidence indicating that exercise is a powerful modifier of inactivity-related decline, even for sarcopenia, the age-related wasting of muscle.[9-13] Loss of skeletal muscle mass and force is inevitable with aging and can be further exacerbated by a host of variables, such as nutrition and disease. However, sedentary lifestyle is likely to take the greatest toll.[2,3,7,14-16] By and large, men and women who include physical activity in their daily routine should have sufficient muscle mass and force to achieve all of the fundamental activities of daily living for 90 to 100 years. Sarcopenia is distinct from another muscle wasting condition, cachexia. Cachexia is rapid and relentless muscle wasting that frequently occurs before death. Cachexia occurs with terminal disease such as cancer. Physical therapy is highly successful for the modification of sarcopenia; however, physical therapist intervention cannot remediate cachexia, as will be discussed below.

Aging is manifested by cellular and subcellular changes within all tissues. The intent of this chapter is to describe what occurs in selected systems for the purpose of understanding the functional consequences of aging as they present to the physical therapist clinically. For example, the natural decline in bone mineral content may predispose patients to osteoporosis. It is not uncommon for those with osteoporosis to manifest postural changes that affect balance, diminish lung capacity, and shorten step and stride length. Once cellular changes are described, other inactivity- and lifestyle-related events that further contribute to systemic decline will be addressed. Thus, physical therapists must consider all the sequelae of health disorders.

There is not a single tissue or system that does not undergo age-related changes. However, only those systems that physical therapists treat directly or affect the ability to render optimal care will be discussed in this chapter. Gastrointestinal or genitourinary systems, for example, will not be discussed in detail, except with respect to the issue of drug clearance through the kidney. Skeletal muscle is also excluded, as it will be covered in a separate chapter. Finally, some attention will be given to age-related issues that are amenable to change with exercise: sleep, sexual function, depression, gastroesophageal reflux disease (GERD), gastric motility, and constipation.

AGING: A DECLINE IN HOMEOSTASIS

Homeostasis is a critical concept that summarizes all of aging from a functional standpoint. Homeostasis refers to the physiological processes that maintain a stable internal environment of the body. The extent to which the body can adapt to physiological stressors and maintain homeostasis will influence susceptibility to illness and injury. As we age the capacity to tolerate stressors decreases but remains partially modifiable with lifestyle adaptations. The physical stress theory (PST) proposed by Mueller and Maluf[17] captures the essence of homeostasis. Figure 3-1 illustrates the relationship between various levels of physical stress and the adaptive responses of tissue. Figure 3-2 provides a conceptual picture of the relationship of successful and unsuccessful aging to a tolerance for challenges to homeostasis and the effect of varying levels of challenge on homeostasis.

The successfully aging older adult maintains a high capacity to tolerate physiological stress, whereas the person who is aging unsuccessfully generally has a low tolerance to physiological stressors that challenge homeostasis. The ability to improve tolerance for physiological stress and, thus, provide a wider homeostasis window is possible using principles incorporated in the

PST. Tolerance range increases in response to exercise, and decreases with the addition of chronic disease and greater inactivity. The older individual with very low tolerance to physiological stressors is highly susceptible to illness and has low capacity to combat the effects of the illness: a bout of influenza may kill.

When a person is in homeostasis, exercise results in robust positive change with systemic adaptation. Strength and balance can increase as can aerobic and muscle endurance. When the inactive older adult with stable chronic diseases engages in exercise, positive change also occurs, albeit more slowly and of smaller magnitude. Under both sets of circumstances, a widening of the window of homeostasis occurs, providing greater tolerance to physiological stress, thus reducing the possibility of moving out of homeostasis into cachexia and death. The wider the window of homeostasis, the greater the chance of survival and of maintaining independence in physical function. Furthermore, the wider the window, the greater the physical reserve as well as the capacity of the body to draw on a "well" of immune function, strength, and endurance among other resources in order to meet the demands of another day.

The natural corollary of homeostasis is survival. Those who maintain homeostasis will continue to thrive, whereas men and women unable to maintain homeostasis against even small stressors may become cachexic, or succumb to a devastating illness such as pneumonia. One of the biggest challenges of current practice is to promote wellness and enhance survival through the maintenance of a large physiological reserve that maintains homeostasis even in the presence of large stressors.

It is necessary to define several terms that characterize many older adults. *Cachexia* typically refers to an inexorable decline in muscle (and body) wasting that cannot be arrested nutritionally.[18-20] Cachexia is associated with end-stage cancer, AIDS, tuberculosis, and certain infectious diseases and is a response to one or more pathologies that overwhelm the body. Although some young adults with more "reserve" may recover from a cachectic state, most people do not, and rarely do older adults recover from cachexia. The cachexia of old age typically precedes death and is the final stage of chronic obstructive pulmonary disease (COPD), chronic heart failure (CHF), and other terminal pathologies. Although the cause of cachexia is not well defined, it is believed to be the consequence of a massive increase in inflammatory cytokines, which will be discussed later in this chapter.[18-21]

The other term that must be defined is *sarcopenia*, which is the muscle wasting of old age.[19] Sarcopenia is present if muscle mass as determined by dual-energy x-ray absorptiometry is two or more standard deviations below values obtained for young adults.[22-26] Approximately 22% of all men and women older than age 70 years have sarcopenia; for those older than age 80 years the number of sarcopenic individuals approaches 50%, with a higher percentage for men than women.[27]

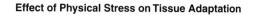

Effect of Physical Stress on Tissue Adaptation

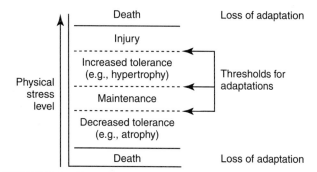

FIGURE 3-1 Effect of varying levels of physical stress (inadequately low to excessively high) on tissue's ability to adapt and to maintain homeostasis. *(Reprinted with permission, from Mueller MJ, Maluf KS: Tissue adaptation to physical stress: a proposed "Physical Stress Theory" to guide physical therapist practice, education, and research. Phys Ther 82(4):383-403, 2002.)*

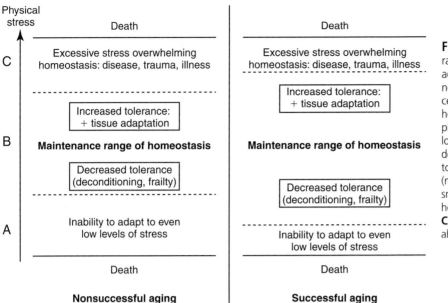

FIGURE 3-2 A depiction of the differences in range of homeostasis tolerance and ability to adapt to stress in individuals who have aged nonsuccessfully and those who have aged successfully. The dotted lines represent the limits of homeostasis centered around the range of physical stress that maintains tissue at physiological equilibrium and effect of increased or decreased stress on tolerance to challenges to homeostasis. **A,** Inadequate ability to adapt (maintain tissue homeostasis) against even small stresses. **B,** Level of stress that maintains homeostasis tolerance at the same level. **C,** Level of stress that overwhelms the tissue's ability to maintain homeostasis

The major distinction between the muscle wasting of sarcopenia versus cachexia is that sarcopenia is amenable to change. Indeed, sarcopenic muscle is completely capable of responding to strength-training exercise, with significant increases in muscle mass and strength.[10,12,28] In contrast, cachexic muscle will not respond to exercise, and physical therapy treatment to improve strength at this phase of old age is generally unwarranted.

In the United States and around the world, the fastest growing segment of the population are those adults who are age 85 years and older. Although longevity continues to increase, quality of life frequently does not. Indeed, approximately half of all individuals in the 85+ years age group are physically dependent on others for basic essentials such as shopping, cooking, housekeeping, medication management, walking, and bathing. Some of the decline in functional ability is secondary to sarcopenia; for others, accumulated declines in strength, balance, and endurance—often the consequence of inactivity—have resulted in frailty. Sarcopenia is frequently the hallmark of frailty and the number of men and women with frailty is growing exponentially.[19] The increasing incidence of sarcopenia and frailty provides limitless opportunities for positive impact through physical therapy. Further discussion of sarcopenia is included in the chapter on impaired muscle performance.

Physical decline occurs in all systems. The age-related changes in the systems most applicable to physical therapy are presented in the following sections. The potential for enhanced tissue and organ function through physical therapy is also discussed.

Skeletal Tissue

Skeletal tissue is remarkably susceptible to change in response to day-to-day nutrient intake, inactivity, weight bearing, hormones, and medications.[29-34] These day-to-day changes occur in addition to the ongoing decline in bone mineral that begins in the 3rd decade and continues on through life (Figure 3-3). It is well known that women have a faster rate of bone mass loss during the menopause, where the typical yearly decrease of 0.5% to 1% doubles to about 2% per year

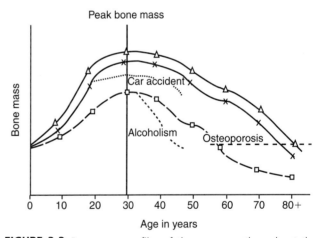

FIGURE 3-3 Bone mass profiles of three women throughout the course of a lifetime. The *top line* (△) represents usual lifestyle, including adequate nutrition including calcium, occasional or no weight-bearing exercise, some outdoor time (vitamin D exposure), minimal inactivity-related diseases, including obesity, modest alcohol intake, no drugs that diminish bone. The *middle line* (X) reflects optimal bone mass in a woman who embraced a healthy lifestyle over the course of her lifetime. Healthy lifestyle includes adequate nutrition including protein and calcium intake, a regular weight-bearing exercise program, routine exposure to sunshine, minimal disease burden, modest alcohol consumption, no drugs that diminish bone. The *bottom line* (□) reflects one of several possibilities: inadequate calcium during the teenage years and/or amenorrhea as a teen or early adult stage of life, or anorexia as a teenager with inadequate calcium and protein intake. Anorexia often results in low estrogen values as well. Major points: Calcium intake during adolescence is critical; loss of normal serum estrogen results in accelerated bone loss with age or failure to maximize bone stock in youth; poor lifestyle choices (e.g., alcoholism, sedentary lifestyle, poor nutrition) diminishes bone at all ages; and serious physical compromise (e.g., car accident with prolonged bed rest) has lifelong consequences.

for the 5-year peri- and menopausal era. Given the smaller bone size of women compared to men, women are much more susceptible to developing osteopenia with menopause. The current estimated risk for osteoporosis in the postmenopausal woman is a staggering 50% (International Osteoporosis Foundation).

Bone is composed of three cell types: the osteoclast, which breaks down bone; the osteoblast, which produces and increases bone mineral; and the osteocyte, which maintains bone. These three cell types form the basic metabolic unit (BMU) of bone as suggested by Frost.[35] Under normal circumstances, there is a balance between osteoblastic and osteoclastic activity such that the loss/gain ratio each day is one-to-one. With aging, there is a shift, believed to have a hormonal basis, that causes either a higher bone breakdown rate or reduced bone accretion rate, which is what causes age-related bone decline.[29,31] Thus, with advancing age, the BMU favors bone catabolism rather than bone anabolism which, of course, is what occurs during growth.

Factors other than aging may affect the health and well-being of men and women throughout the life span and account for more decline in bone mass than aging alone. Some of these factors are nonmodifiable, but many factors affecting bone mass are modifiable with lifestyle. Factors that are modifiable with lifestyle and those that are not modifiable are summarized in Box 3-1.

It is important to realize that estrogen is critical for the maintenance of bone mass in both men and women. Recently, it has become evident that testosterone and estrogen are independent mediators of bone health in men.[26] Thus, any condition affecting sex hormones (e.g., prostate cancer, breast cancer) automatically affects skeletal health in both sexes.

The fact that tomorrow's osteoporotic women are being created among the youth of today gravely concerns the Centers for Disease Control and Prevention (CDC).[36] Young women are not drinking milk, are highly sedentary, are not using their muscles, are not going outside routinely for sun exposure, and are eating nutritionally poor foods without adequate calcium, protein, and vitamin D. Each day spent without the building blocks of bone robs the skeletal system of more mineral. During the teenage years, bone mass increases tremendously and it is during the ages of 12 to 18 that the ultimate skeletal profile is determined. Thus, if a teenager drinks no milk, eats pizza and burgers most days of the week, and gets no exercise outside, chances increase that these adolescents will emerge from their teens with a skeletal profile of a 60-year-old. At the other end of the age spectrum is the older women in a nursing home who spends 23.5 hours per day lying in bed or sitting inside.[33,34] These women, who already are at unusually high risk for fracture, are becoming more osteoporotic and frail, and more predisposed to falling and bone breakage with each passing day.[37,38]

BOX 3-1   Nonmodifiable and Modifiable Risk Factors for Bone Loss

Nonmodifiable Risk Factors for Bone Loss
Genetics: women with small frames
Caucasian race
Hispanic women
Age: female older than age 50 years
Family history of osteoporosis
Premature at birth
Low estrogen: menopause
Childhood malabsorption disease
Seizure disorder—using Dilantin
Age-associated loss of muscle mass

Modifiable Risk Factors
Calcium intake: 1200 mg/day or more is required
Excessive alcohol intake: maximum allowable is not defined
Smoking cigarettes
Low body mass index (<18.5)
Low estrogen: amenorrhea, anorexia
Low estrogen: ovariohysterectomy
Inactivity, immobilization
Substituting soda for milk, especially among children
Insufficient protein at all ages
Inadequate vitamin D
Hyperthyroidism
Prednisone and cortisone use, hyperparathyroidism

Exercise is critical to the health and well-being of skeletal tissue. The natural pull of contracting muscles is what maintains bone mineral density; inactivity robs bone of a critical stimulus for osteoblastic activity. A classic example is the remarkable amount of bone loss that occurs when someone is immobilized in a cast or goes into space. The loss of bone in space has been estimated at 0.5% to 1.0% *per day* because muscle contractions are not producing any demand on bone.[39]

Several studies have indicated that exercise or hormone replacement therapy (dehydroepiandrosterone [DHEA], testosterone, estrogen, or estrogen/progesterone combined), either alone or in combination, can add bone mineral density to the osteopenic framework of older men and women. Dalsky,[40] for example, used loading exercise as the stimulus in 60- to 70-year-old women during a 1-year study and observed a 3% to 6% increase in bone mineral content.[38,41] Kohrt and colleagues found that older women who were already on hormone replacement therapy (HRT) gained additional bone mineral density (BMD) in the spine and hip with loading exercise. Activities consisted of weight training and wearing a weighted vest while ascending stairs.[42] Furthermore, Villareal demonstrated that frail older women (older than age 75 years) on HRT also had significant increases of approximately 3.5% in lumbar spine BMD with 9 months of resistance and aerobic exercise training.[43,44]

Thus, the evidence suggests that bone in women of all ages is able to respond to HRT and to exercise with additive effects. In one of the few studies that included men, DHEA was given for 2 years to subjects of both sexes aged 65 to 75 years. Women on DHEA increased spine BMD 1.7% the first year and by 3.6% after 2 years of supplementation. No increases in bone were observed for men.[45] Given the current trend of increasing osteoporosis in men, successful therapies are needed. Natural alternatives such as genistein and other food additives are being investigated in both sexes. It is also still unclear whether exercise coupled with selective estrogen receptor modulators (SERMs) such as tamoxifen or raloxifene affect bone in a synergistic and additive fashion.

Body Composition

Throughout the decades there is a gradual shift in body composition such that lean mass decreases and fat mass proportionately increases (Figure 3-4). To provide a typical example, it is not uncommon for a man in his 20s to have a lean body mass/fat mass ratio of 85/15. Even if this same man maintains body weight for the next 50 years he is likely to have a lean/fat ratio of 70/30. For women, it is not uncommon to observe a fat mass of 50% at age 80 years even though the individual appears to be no more than "pleasingly plump." Of considerable significance is the fact that most of the fat increase occurs inside the peritoneum,[7,46-51] which is now believed to be a significant contributor to the increased inflammation that occurs with age. The increase in intra-abdominal fat is also believed to predispose older individuals, particularly women, to elevated lipids and prediabetes.[51,52] Fat is an extraordinarily active metabolic tissue, and its contribution to age-related decline and disease is just beginning to be understood.

The more intra-abdominal fat the greater the risk for heart disease, metabolic syndrome, diabetes, and cancer. Women are particularly vulnerable to these diseases after menopause as the protective effects of estrogen are gone and women have more fat than men at all ages.[50] Exercise plays an important role in controlling intra-abdominal fat.[49,52,53] Every mile walked is about 100 calories burned. When the heart rate goes up in response to exercise and muscles are engaged, metabolic rate increases and fat is burned as fuel. Men and women of all ages who are consistently active do not add intra-abdominal fat to the same extent as those who are sedentary.[52] Consequently, active men and women have less whole-body inflammation and less disease.[43]

Collagenous Tissues

Collagen is probably the most ubiquitous tissue type in the body, comprising the skin, tendons, ligaments, fascia, and a host of lesser entities. Essentially, collagenous tissues hold us together while still permitting freedom of

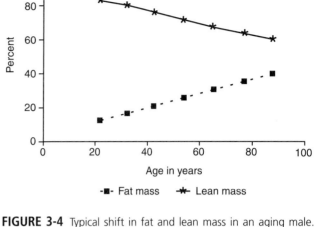

FIGURE 3-4 Typical shift in fat and lean mass in an aging male. Lean mass, which is mostly muscle, declines continuously after the 3rd decade. Fat mass increases concomitantly. In this individual, body weight has not changed over the 60 years that are represented.

movement in all directions. Over the decades, subtle change occurs in all collagenous tissues, but only three of these changes will be discussed here: loss of water from matrix, increase in crosslinks, and loss of elastic fibers.[54-57]

Collagenous tissues are composed of collagen, which provides substantial tensile strength, and a surrounding semiliquid matrix that binds water and permits collagen fibers to easily glide past one another. Matrix composition changes over the years such that water content decreases considerably. The most obvious consequence of the water loss is body shrinking or height loss primarily because of water loss from the intervertebral discs. Articular cartilage also loses water and becomes more susceptible to breakdown (osteoarthritis). Clinically, the loss of water manifests itself in two ways: reduced range of motion and loss of "bounce," that is, the ability to absorb shock. From an exercise standpoint, working toward end range becomes more and more important with advancing age to prevent range losses from limiting function. Exercises too should be shifted away from activities that are jarring such as jumping from high surfaces. Although plyometric exercises are recommended as an excellent stimulus to increase bone mass, care should be taken to choose exercises that act as a stimulus to bone without being too stressful on an older body less able to absorb the impact.

Because the number of collagen crosslinks also increases with age, two observable clinical changes become manifest: a decreased range of motion and an increase in stiffness. Even though end range is diminished with advancing years, range should still be sufficient to accomplish all activities of daily living, including reaching into high cupboards and down to the floor. Range loss should *not* preclude accomplishing any basic activities—it merely reduces the potential for extremes. Stiffness, on the other hand, has several clinical implications. From a biomechanical perspective, stiffness implies a lack of "give" that translates, for example, to a greater likelihood of tendon avulsion rather than rupture.[58,59] Stiffness also means that the passive tension within tissues is increased. Phrased another way, the proportion of total tension (i.e., total muscle tension as the sum of active and passive tension) that can be attributed to passive stiffness is increased with age. Couple the increase in passive "drag" with the decline in muscle force that occurs with aging, the consequence is greater muscular effort required for less output. Increased tissue stiffness is one factor contributing to less muscle endurance with age.

Box 3-2 summarizes the three major age-related changes in collagenous tissues: decreased water content from the matrix, increase in number of collagen crosslinks, and loss of elastic properties. Loss of elasticity is abundantly evident in aging skin which no longer has its turgor and tends to hang. Tendons, ligaments, and muscles also lose their elasticity, further contributing to change in function. As inconceivable as it is to regard a 35-year-old baseball or basketball player as "too old" for the sport, age-related change in connective tissue is one of the major contributors to "losing one's edge" in athletics. In addition to tendons and muscles, internal organs are no longer held in place as well as they were, and age-related changes in connective tissues contribute to the tendency for uterine prolapse, bladder issues, constipation, and hernia with advancing years.

Cardiovascular Tissues

Fundamental changes in vascular tissues that occur with aging, summarized in Box 3-3, have a profound effect on function. Probably the most notable and clinically

BOX 3-2	Major Age-Related Changes in Collagenous Tissues and Associated Clinical Consequences
Age-Related Change	**Clinical Consequence**
Loss of water from the matrix	Shrinkage of articular cartilage, vertebral discs
	Decreased ability to absorb shock
	Reduced range of motion
Increase in number of collagen crosslinks	"Stiffer" tissues, greater passive tension within tissues
	More effort required to move
	Loss of end range of motion
Loss of elastic fibers	Sagging skin and organs; Less "give" to tendons, ligaments, fascia.

BOX 3-3	Major Age-Related Changes in Cardiovascular Tissues and Associated Clinical Consequences
Anatomic/Physiological Change with Age	**Clinical Consequences**
Decline in maximum heart rate	Smaller aerobic workload possible
Decline in $\dot{V}o_2$max	Smaller aerobic workload possible
Stiffer, less compliant vascular tissues	Higher blood pressures
	Slower ventricle filling time with reduced cardiac output
Loss of cells from the SA node	Slower heart rate
	Lower HRmax
Reduced contractility of the vascular walls	Slower HR
	Lower $\dot{V}o_2$max
	Smaller aerobic workload possible
Thickened basement membrane in capillary	Reduced arteriovenous O_2 uptake

important change is the decline in maximum heart rate.[60-62] The typical formula of 220 minus age provides a relative guideline for an expected change in maximum heart rate. Thus, an 80-year old individual is likely to have a maximum heart rate (HRmax) of 140 bpm which obviously limits the extent of cardiovascular challenge that can be endured for any duration. One of the primary reasons for the slowing of aerobic performance with age is the reduction in maximum heart rate. Even though 90-year-olds are still capable of completing the New York City marathon, their times are typically 7 to 8 hours, which is analogous in speed to a 3-mph walk.

Does participation in lifelong exercise prevent the decline in maximum heart rate? Although it was believed that long-term aerobic participation would stave off decline for approximately a decade, more recent study does not support this contention.[60,61] At this juncture, scientists do not fully understand what causes the decline in maximum heart rate, although factors contributing to the process have been identified. For example, increased stiffness of the heart with slower filling of the left ventricle, is one factor,[63] and age-related decrease in the number of cells in the sinoatrial (SA) node is another factor. Regardless of the cause of lower maximum HR, it is a fundamental feature of older age, which translates to lower possible aerobic workload.

Coupled with the decline in maximum HR is a concomitant and related decline in $\dot{V}o_2$max. Both decline in a collinear fashion at a rate of approximately 10% per decade.[64-67] Thus, a healthy, reasonably active 80-year-old woman who had an HRmax of 200 bpm as a 20-year-old and a $\dot{V}o_2$max of ~45 mL O_2/kg/min now has a maximum HR of 140 and a $\dot{V}o_2max$ of ~20 to 25 mL O_2/kg/min. The presence of vascular and cardiovascular disease, however, can decrease the maximum by another 50% to values as low as 10% or 15%.

There is also a correlation between muscle mass and $\dot{V}o_2max$, which is the primary reason men have higher max values than women.[67,68] The higher the lean mass at any age, the higher the maximal aerobic capacity. Those who are sarcopenic have very low aerobic capacity.[69-71] Hypothetically, adding muscle mass to the sarcopenic individual will enhance adaptation to aerobic exercise[69,72]—another compelling reason for frail older adults with sarcopenia to participate in resistance training.

Physical therapists regularly treat older adults who have a long history of inactivity and periodic bouts of disease- or illness-related bed rest. These patients are likely to have gained weight over the years and live in a society that poses little to no physical challenges. Thus, it is quite common for patients older than age 60 years to have $\dot{V}o_2max$ values in the 13 to 18 mL O_2/kg/min range, which translates to inability to climb a flight of stairs without resting and inability to walk a quarter of a mile.[73,114] Nearly all physical therapists have faced the challenge of the deconditioned older adult who is hospitalized, further imposing inactivity-related decline on a system that has nearly run out of cardiovascular capacity, and who reaches an unacceptably high HR just getting from bed to the bathroom. This scenario, reflecting enormous loss in cardiovascular reserve, is one major contributor to loss in homeostasis as well as loss of independence.

Because of the fundamental changes in connective tissues, increased crosslinking of collagen, altered matrix composition, and loss of elastin, the entire vascular system, including the heart and peripheral vessels, is stiffer and less compliant.[65,74] Most noticeable is the increase in blood pressure that occurs with age, the consequence of stiffer connective tissues within the vascular walls.[62,65] Contractility of the left ventricle is compromised as well, which results in a reduction of cardiac output, one of the major components of $\dot{V}o_2max$.[70,75] In the author's clinical experience, most (approximately 65%) of the clients older than age 70 years are medicated for hypertension. Rarely has the patient's medication dosage been examined beyond a fundamental baseline blood pressure ascertained while the patient was sitting in the physician's office. It is not uncommon to see patients overwhelm their hypertension medications during exercise. Consequently, from the standpoint of exercise safety, the physical therapist must watch for blood pressure increases that are unacceptably high. It is imperative that older adults perform warm-ups prior to aerobic exercise to accommodate for the slower arteriovenous oxygen exchange, stiffer vascular tissues, reduction in sympathetic nervous system output, and lower aerobic capacity associated with older age.

Perhaps as a consequence of connective tissue changes, or other factors, the basement membrane in the capillary wall thickens with age.[63,65,74] Thus, the exchange of oxygen and nutrients from the vasculature to working tissues occurs more slowly. Because tissue perfusion occurs more slowly, the "burn" in working muscles takes longer to subside during the initial phases of exercise, necessitating a warm-up longer than the usual requisite 3 minutes prior to more rigorous work. Thickening of the basement wall occurs in sedentary people but *not* in master athletes, which suggests that this aspect of "age-related" decline is actually a lifestyle modification.[76] Indeed, an aerobic exercise training study of older (age 60 to 70 years), previously sedentary men and women revealed that basement membrane thickening was no longer present after 3 months of training at 70% or more of $\dot{V}o_2max$.[5] Whether membrane thickening occurs at older ages in men and women with a lifetime history of exercise is not known. Diseases of the peripheral vasculature such as diabetes and peripheral vascular disease (PVD) further increase basement membrane thickness, which can result in sufficient lack of oxygen perfusion to skin tissues for breakdown and nonhealing of ulcers. Lack of perfusion to skeletal muscle results in additional loss of fibers, and lack of perfusion to nerves leads to neuropathy.[66]

There is controversy in the literature as to whether the goal in the management of age-related increases in blood pressure is to achieve a blood pressure in the 120/80 range.[77] Because of the increase in connective tissue stiffness within the vascular tree, there is currently a question if blood pressures of 140/80 should be considered as more "normal." This should not be interpreted to suggest that increased blood pressure is not problematic. There is a substantial body of literature indicating that blood pressures that are too high can lead to stroke, and treating this condition increases life span.[70] From a physical therapy perspective, the more important question is whether a patient is safe in our care. In a patient who is overmedicated, hypotension can result in dizziness and heightened risk for falling. Changes in medication are likely indicated. If patients have exercise pressures that are exceptionally high, medication modification is probably needed here as well. More clarity on what constitutes "normal" blood pressure for an 80-year-old versus that of a 60-year-old and a centenarian is needed. What are acceptable and safe blood pressures for sleeping, waking, exercising, and postprandial conditions for patients with heart disease is not known. Also unknown is whether age affects the effectiveness of treatments for hypertension.

Peripheral to the discussion of age-related decline in the cardiovascular system is an issue of enormous importance to physical therapy: anesthesia. Men and women of all ages are affected by inhalation anesthesia, but the effects are most noticeable in older adults who have already lost a significant amount of cardiovascular reserve. Although the mechanism is unknown, inhalation anesthesia obliterates mitochondria and, thus, the ability to deliver ATP during exercise is severely compromised.[78] Thus, in our patients, after surgery with inhalation anesthesia, muscular and cardiovascular endurance is severely compromised.[78] Physical therapists often see patients the day after total joint replacement surgery, often the day after fractured hip and, inevitably, these men and women become exhausted with minimal effort. It is no surprise that spontaneous improvement begins to manifest 2 months after the initial surgery or insult, long after physical therapy has come to an end. The initial phase of physical therapy following hip fracture is effective for teaching patients the essentials: transfers, walker use, home exercise, proper gait pattern, and mobility strategies. Evidence strongly suggests that therapy aimed at strengthening and endurance adaptations given to patients in the days immediately following surgery for hip fracture is ineffectual.[79] The enormous devastation to the energy delivery system, coupled with bed rest, the trauma of surgery, and inactivity indicate that perhaps physical therapy intervention would be more effective 2 to 3 months after hospital discharge. As a profession, physical therapists need to reevaluate intervention effectiveness under these treatment conditions.

One aspect of aging needs to be emphasized. Even though maximum heart rates and aerobic capacity are reduced, there is no reason that exercise in healthy older adults should be restricted to a low-intensity level for fear of a heart attack or stroke. The aging heart is fully capable of reaching HR zones of 70% to 80% of maximum.[61,62,65,66,69,72] The Cooper Institute and other cardiac programs around the country have recorded tens of thousands of hours of strenuous exercise for older adults of all ages and for patients with blatant cardiovascular disease.[80,81] To enhance cardiovascular endurance, exercise programs must challenge older adults. Walking a patient in the hallway 100 feet does not constitute an acceptable aerobic challenge for most people, unless heart rate is within a training zone of 60% to 80% of the HRmax estimated. For training to occur, elevated HRs have to be sustained for 20 minutes or more, which many older adults cannot achieve. Nonetheless, it is not unreasonable to accumulate 20 minutes of aerobic challenge throughout the course of a daily treatment. Five minutes of exercise bike followed by a rest followed by 5 minutes of alternating normal/brisk gait is an example of accumulating aerobic exercise.[72] The heart, like any other muscle, must be challenged to grow stronger. Treating older adults like fragile objects is inadequate treatment.

Nervous System

There are fundamental changes within the central and peripheral nervous systems that have significant import for function. Slowing of the nervous system is an inherent aspect of aging. Nerve conduction studies of young and older adults confirm anatomic observations. Many years ago, Norris and colleagues stimulated the ulnar nerve 5 cm below the axilla, at the elbow, and at the wrist; and recorded the latency response at the hypothenar eminence. Response times were on average about 10 ms slower in men in the oldest age group (80 to 90 years) compared to 20- to 30-year-olds. Gradual change was apparent with each successive decade.[82]

Slowing of movement speed is one of the major clinical manifestations of a slowing nervous system. Examples abound but two will be given here. Alexander and colleagues identified the fact that even men and women in the young-old category (65 to 74 years) are already at heightened risk for falling as response time to an induced fall was too slow for recovery.[83] In this instance, subjects were leaning forward into a harness that was preventing them from falling forward. Next, however, the harness was released and subjects were allowed to stumble and fall (an overhead suspension system prevented anyone from actually striking the ground). Their study found that most of the young-old healthy adults studied could not get their legs back underneath the body quickly enough and step appropriately to prevent a fall. Other studies from the same lab have indicated that response times to external perturbations to balance are slowed, which may explain the noticeable increase in number of falls per year in those older than age 60 years.[84] In the author's lab, reaction times have been assessed in hundreds of young and old healthy individuals. The task involved simulated driving, where the person being tested must respond as quickly as possible to a red light by moving the foot from the gas pedal to the brake pedal. The clock begins the instant the light changes from green to red and stops as soon as the brake pedal is depressed. Times for young adults ranged between 150 and 250 ms, which is well within the 500 ms cut-off time imposed by many Motor Vehicle departments for the same task. Reaction times for the approximately 150 healthy older adults (ranging 70 to 85 years old) tested ranged from 350 to 1200 ms.

Exercise has a modest effect on speed of reaction but the increase in speed is not likely to attain sufficient magnitude to make an impact on function.[85,86] Toe tap times, for example, increased after exercise from 27 to 30 in 10 seconds, which is still a long way from the 47 taps in 10 seconds expected of younger adults. Several investigators have demonstrated a slight exercise-induced increase in peg board times in that the number of pegs that could be moved in 30 seconds increased. Most of the slowing occurs centrally, but sloughing of myelin has been demonstrated anatomically in peripheral nerves, which will certainly slow conduction velocity. It should be borne in mind that most studies on changes in movement speed were performed on healthy individuals, not those with disease that would also affect movement speed further. Studies done to date have also not considered the potential blunting effects of many drugs.

Although the aging of muscle is covered thoroughly in another chapter, it should be mentioned here that another facet of age-related decline is a fallout or loss of neurons.[87,88] Roughly half of the decline in muscle mass is the consequence of neuronal, specifically, axonal loss.[87] Indeed, muscle is not the only tissue that experiences loss of innervation; innervation declines in all tissues, with far-reaching outcomes that affect the sympathetic, parasympathetic, sensory, and motor systems.

Before age-related decline begins, the yin–yang of the parasympathetic and sympathetic nervous systems is delicately balanced and poised to participate in flight or fight. With age, the balance of the parasympathetic and sympathetic nervous system output is altered (although poorly defined) and likely related to the slowing of gastric motility, possible issues with bladder control, hypertension and hypotension, and deficits in control of blood flow to and from the periphery.[89] The failure of the sympathetic nervous system to adequately respond to heat and cold is responsible for the deaths of many seniors each summer and winter as they failed to perceive the need to cool down or warm up.

One of the most complex and poorly understood phenomena with aging is altered somatic sensory input.[89,90] It is common for vague symptoms of pain in one area of the body to represent a totally unrelated event. It is a tremendous challenge for physical therapists to discern if and when something is wrong with an older patient based on vague somatic complaints. Abdominal pain could reflect a host of possible issues ranging from simple indigestion to pancreatitis, cancer, intestinal obstruction, peritonitis, impending heart attack, or inguinal hernia. Back pain could reflect a simple muscle or joint irritation but could also reflect an abdominal aorta aneurysm, appendicitis, bladder infection, and cancer. Carefully noting these complaints is important, particularly if complaints are coupled with sudden change in function, sensorium, the emergence of fever, or an increase or sharpening of symptoms.

Peripheral sensation gradually diminishes in older adults, even those individuals without vascular diseases or neuropathy secondary to diabetes. To illustrate, Semmes-Weinstein testing on 125 older adults without diabetes revealed the absence of normal sensation (6.13-g monofilament) in all persons tested (M. Brown, unpublished data). Protective sensation was still present in these individuals (5.07-g monofilament), but fine discrimination was lacking. The blunting of peripheral sensation undoubtedly contributes to the inability to perceive excessive heat or cold. Box 3-4 summarizes physiological changes of the nervous system and impact on function.

The Immune System

There are literally hundreds of theories on why we age, ranging from accumulated wear and tear to programmed apoptosis to the accumulation in errors during translation

| BOX 3-4 | Major Age-related Changes in the Nervous System and Associated Clinical Consequences |

Anatomic/Physiological changes	Clinical Consequences
Sloughing/loss of myelin	Slowed nerve conduction
Axonal loss	Fewer muscle fibers
	Loss of fine sensation
Autonomic nervous system dysfunction	Slower systemic function (e.g., C-V, GI) with altered sensory input
Loss of sensory neurons	Reduced ability to discern hot/cold, pain
Slowed response time (speed of reaction)	Increased risk of falls

of messages from the DNA. Although many of the current theories are likely to have some veracity, few of the current theories have import for physical therapy. Recently, however, one aspect of age-related decline has emerged as a major contributor to the loss of muscle and organ reserve that has considerable import for physical therapy. It is now evident that with advancing age, there is an increase in systemic inflammation because of changes in the immune system. Major increases in known proinflammatory cytokines such as interleukin 1 and 10 (IL-1, IL-10), C-reactive protein (CRP), and tumor necrosis factor-α (TNF-α) occur with advancing age, which is significantly associated with muscle wasting and loss of physical function.[6,7,14,46,72,91,92] The increase in systemic inflammation is also an underlying factor in the development of age-related diseases such as Alzheimer's disease, atherosclerosis, cancer, and diabetes.[91,93] Thus, it is hypothesized that controlling inflammatory status may allow for more successful aging.[8,94,95]

Four approaches to the management of total-body inflammation have been considered: anti-inflammatory drugs, use of antioxidants, caloric restriction, and exercise.[6,94-96] Of the three, exercise is far superior to the minimal impact noted from anti-inflammatory drugs and antioxidants.[21,27,48,53] One exercise bout results in a significant reduction in markers of inflammation such as IL-1 and TNF-α.[48,50,92,93] Cumulative exercise sessions further reduce inflammation, which should enable chronic exercisers to resist fatal infections and aggressive pathogens.[97] Men and women who are habitually physically active have less systemic inflammation than those who are sedentary, which may be the major reason for the enhanced well-being of exercisers, who also have a wider window of homeostasis. These current findings suggest that physical therapy can play an important role in the management of systemic inflammation, enhancing systemic "reserve," reducing risk for disease, and delaying functional decline through the use of exercise. An example of the power of exercise is that many fewer men and women who consistently exercise have Alzheimer's disease than those who are sedentary.[91,93]

One of the probable contributors to the rise in inflammation is the shift in fat mass from the periphery to the abdomen coupled with the general increase in total intra-abdominal fat with advancing years.[27,51] Abdominal fat is metabolically active and is an inflammatory organ. Not only do inflammatory cytokines result in muscle wasting, they diminish the function of other organ systems as well, which reduces reserve and shrinks the window of homeostasis. The increase in inflammatory cytokines is also associated with metabolic syndrome.[98]

The Hormonal Axis

One of the realities of aging is a loss of hormones, a loss in responsiveness of hormone target tissues, or both.[27,31,99] It is not uncommon for older adults to develop "senile" diabetes because insulin sensitivity, particularly in skeletal muscle, is reduced.[99] Women after menopause have little estrogen, and men lose testosterone throughout the course of a lifetime, such that the majority of men in the 8th decade are hypogonadal.[99,100] Recently, the loss of sex hormones has been determined to be a contributor to the reduction in muscle mass and, in particular, muscle strength.[100,101] Indeed, older hypogonadal men given testosterone replacement gain a significant amount of lean mass although data suggest that the increase in mass is not accompanied by much strength change unless resistance exercise and testosterone are given together.[99]

Loss of estrogen has only recently received interest. A meta-analysis concluded that estrogen is an anabolic steroid that is associated with an increase in strength and lean mass in postmenopausal women.[102] Taafe and co-workers conducted a double-blind study of 80 women (50 to 57 years) who were randomly assigned to one of four groups: control, hormone replacement therapy (HRT), exercise, or HRT plus exercise. Subjects were in the research study for 1 year and exercised two to three times a week. Prior to and following the year enrollment, lean mass of quadriceps and hamstrings, strength, vertical jump height, and running speed were assessed. Those in the HRT and exercise plus HRT groups (not the exercise only group) had significant increases in running speed, muscle mass in both compartments and vertical jump height compared to controls. No strength measures were reported. A recent study of postmenopausal twins, one of whom was on HRT whereas the other was not, has further substantiated estrogen effectiveness.[101] The women taking HRT were between 5 and 15 years postmenopause. Vertical jump height, fast gait, and grip strength were higher in the twin taking hormones. Curiously, knee extension strength was not greater. Other studies of older postmenopausal women suggest the same important outcome: more muscle mass and strength with HRT.[103]

One of the most interesting findings in muscle deprived of estrogen was reported in several studies of rats. When ovaries were removed, simulating menopause,

specific muscle force (force/unit of muscle mass) almost immediately declined by about 15%.[104] When estrogen was returned to the system, specific force normalized back to baseline values.[105] It is not uncommon to hear complaints of weakness from women who have undergone ovariohysterectomy. Perhaps these findings from rats provide an explanation for these complaints. Findings also suggest that strength training for postmenopausal women at any age is particularly important.

From a rehabilitation perspective, several important findings have been reported on estrogen-deficient muscle from rodents. When muscle atrophy is induced in rats (simulated bed rest), recovery of muscle mass and strength fails to occur or occurs more slowly in estrogen-deficit rats.[106-108] These findings may provide an explanation for why women do not progress as well as men with spinal injury, severe trauma, or head injury, all conditions that cause estrogen values to plummet to undetectable ranges. Rodent studies also indicate that estrogen-deficient muscle is more susceptible to injury, which may be another factor influencing recovery of muscle mass and strength in women who are estrogen-deficient.[109-112]

Replacement of one hormone may not be sufficient to overcome a specific deficit as hormones tend to work in concert with one another. For example, testosterone has been shown to increase insulin-like growth factor-I (IGF-I), which stimulates protein synthesis in muscle.[100] However, if IGF-I levels are already low, then perhaps the utility of testosterone is limited. One scientist has recommended hormone replacement, particularly for men as they lose muscle mass at a more rapid rate than women. His conclusion was that perhaps in future studies multiple hormones should be administered simultaneously as low values in one hormone are likely to reflect deficiencies in other hormones.[113] Hormone supplementation is in its infancy and should bring considerable change. An enhanced understanding of how hormones can influence health and well-being is to be expected in the years ahead.

EXERCISE FOR REVERSING DECLINE AND PREVENTING DISEASE

It is becoming evident that a lifestyle that includes routine exercise can be extremely influential in preventing physical decline and disease. Those who exercise routinely (at *any* age) have less cardiovascular disease, osteoarthritis, diabetes, vascular disease, metabolic syndrome, pain, and Alzheimer's disease, to name a few. Studies of Masters athletes and habitual exercisers indicate that physical activity promotes optimal well-being and enhanced self-efficacy.[114,115] Physical therapists have more potential to promote healthy aging than any health care professional, and it should be the profession's mission to do so.

Is there a threshold for physical activity that is protective? The answer to this question is unclear but evidence suggests a dose–response aspect of benefit. For example, it is possible to gain strength with a stimulus that is 50% of 1-repetition maximum (1 RM).[116] However, more strength will be gained if the demand is higher. The same holds true for cardiovascular conditioning; additional reserve will be gained with higher intensity training but any stimulus over and above what is encountered on a day-to-day basis will result in positive change. Several interesting findings have emerged from the research of Paffenbarger and Blair that may influence decision making on this issue.[117-119] In their studies, subjects were divided into three categories of "fitness" based upon number of minutes spent in physical activity per week. In addition, subjects were divided into three categories based upon body mass index. As expected, those with the highest body mass had the highest rate of disease (e.g., cardiovascular) and mortality and those who were the most physically active had the least. What was not expected was that the incidences of disease and mortality were not that different for those in the moderate and vigorously active categories. Moreover, those with high BMIs were protected from disease and premature mortality if they were moderately or vigorously active.[117] In all likelihood, there is a threshold of activity that is protective but it differs from individual to individual based upon natural endowment of muscle mass and cardiovascular capability, genetic predisposition to disease based upon family history, self-efficacy, soft-tissue integrity, and a host of other factors. Thus, discussing an identifiable level of physical activity for the older individual is premature, but the evidence in favor of a physically active lifestyle is overwhelming.

SUMMARY

Aging is an inevitable process and decline occurs in all tissues and systems. Nonetheless, with a thoughtful lifestyle approach, it is possible to prevent or attenuate the severity of some diseases, and delay (possibly avoid) the condition of frailty.

Indeed, physical activity is the most potent tool of physical therapists to optimize function throughout the entire life span. Inactivity should be considered as much a contributor to impairments and loss of function as pathology or disease. Physical therapists can utilize the principles espoused in the physical stress theory to help guide the modulation of exercise for older adults to the appropriate level to achieve positive gains in tissue functioning and homeostasis; while avoiding, both the tissue damages of excessively high stress and the physiological decline of inadequately low stress.

It is appropriate for physical therapists to consider the impact of age-related changes on the rehabilitation and wellness plan for their older adult patients. However, physical therapists must take care not to underutilize active rehabilitation; rather, they need to adjust the rehabilitation to meet the unique needs of the older patient. Physical therapists should use their understanding of age- and disease-related changes in tissue functioning to focus a rehabilitation and wellness plan. This plan should be based on a careful examination of the specific impairments, tasks, and activities affecting function; an integration of all evaluation data (including patient goals and preferences) to inform prognosis; then careful targeting of the structures and tasks that can provide greatest functional gain; and finally determination of the intensity of the intervention to optimize positive adaptation to stress.

REFERENCES

To enhance this text and add value for the reader, all references are included on the companion Evolve site that accompanies this text book. The reader can view the reference source and access it online whenever possible. There are a total of 119 cited references and other general references for this chapter.

Geriatric Pharmacology

Charles D. Ciccone, PT, PhD, FAPTA

INTRODUCTION

Physical therapists working with any patient population must be aware of the drug regimen used in each patient. Therapists must have a basic understanding of the beneficial and adverse effects of each medication and must be cognizant of how specific drugs can interact with various rehabilitation procedures. This idea seems especially true for geriatric patients receiving physical therapy. Older adults are generally more sensitive to the adverse effects of drug therapy, and many adverse drug reactions (ADRs) impede the patient's progress and ability to participate in rehabilitation procedures. An adequate understanding of the patient's drug regimen, however, can help physical therapists recognize and deal with these adverse effects as well as capitalize on the beneficial effects of drug therapy in their geriatric patients.

The purpose of this chapter is to discuss some of the pertinent aspects of geriatric pharmacology with specific emphasis on how drug therapy can affect older individuals receiving physical therapy. This chapter begins by describing the pharmacologic profile of the geriatric patient, with emphasis on why ADRs tend to occur more commonly in older adults. Specific ADRs that commonly occur in the older adult are then discussed. Finally, the beneficial and adverse effects of specific medications are examined, along with how these medications can have an impact on the rehabilitation of older adults.

PHARMACOLOGIC PROFILE OF THE GERIATRIC PATIENT

Older adults are more likely than younger adults to experience an ADR, and these adverse reactions are typically more severe in older adults.[1] The increased incidence of adverse drug effects in older adults is influenced by two principal factors: the pattern of drug use that occurs in a geriatric population and the altered response to drug therapy in older adults.[2,3] A number of other contributing factors, such as multiple disease states, lack of proper drug testing, and problems with drug education and compliance also increase the likelihood of adverse effects in older adults. The influence of each of these factors on drug response in older adults is discussed briefly here.

Pattern of Drug Use in Older Adults: Problems of Polypharmacy

Older adults consume a disproportionately large amount of drugs relative to younger people.[1] Adults older than age 65 years, for example, compose about 13% of the U.S. population, but they receive 34% of all prescription drugs.[3] Given that more and more of the population is reaching advanced age, it seems certain that older adults will continue to receive a disproportionate share of drugs over the next several decades.[3]

A logical explanation for this disproportionate drug use is that older adults take more drugs because they suffer more illnesses.[1] Indeed, more than 80% of individuals older than age 65 years suffer from one or more chronic conditions, and drug therapy is often the primary method used to treat these conditions.[3] In a large sample of community-dwelling people age 57 to 85 years, 81% reported using at least one prescription medication, and 29% used at least five prescription medications simultaneously.[4] Drug use in certain older subpopulations is even higher, with nursing home residents and frail older patients often receiving five or more prescription medications each day.[3] Use of nonprescription (over-the-counter) products is also an important factor in geriatric pharmacology, especially among the community-dwelling older adults who have greater access to these products.[4,5]

Older adults therefore rely heavily on various prescription and nonprescription products, and medications are often essential in helping resolve or alleviate some of the illnesses and other medical complications that occur commonly in older adults. A distinction must be made, however, between the reasonable and appropriate use of drugs and the phenomenon of polypharmacy. Although sources may vary somewhat in exactly how they define this term, *polypharmacy* typically refers to the excessive or inappropriate use of medications.[6] Owing to the extensive use of medications in this population, older adults are often at high risk for polypharmacy.[7,8]

Polypharmacy can be distinguished from a more reasonable drug regimen by the criteria listed in Table 4-1. Of these criteria, the use of drugs to treat ADRs is especially important. The administration of drugs to treat drug-related reactions often creates a vicious cycle in

TABLE 4-1	Characteristics of Polypharmacy in Older Adults	
Characteristic	**Example**
Use of medications for no apparent reason	Digoxin use in patients who do not exhibit heart failure
Use of duplicate medications	Simultaneous use of two or three laxatives
Concurrent use of interacting medications	Simultaneous use of a laxative and an antidiarrheal agent
Use of contraindicated medications	Use of aspirin in bleeding ulcers
Use of inappropriate dosage	Failure to use a lower dose of a benzodiazepine sedative-hypnotic
Use of drug therapy to treat adverse drug reactions	Use of antacids to treat aspirin-induced gastric irritation
Patient improves when medications are discontinued	Withdrawal of a sedative-hypnotic results in clearer sensorium

(Adapted from Simonson W: Medications and the Elderly: A Guide for Promoting Proper Use. Rockville, MD: Aspen Publications, 1984.)

which additional drugs are used to treat ADRs, thus creating more adverse effects, thereby initiating the use of more drugs, and so on (Figure 4-1).[3,9] This cycle, known also as a "medication cascade effect," can rapidly accelerate until the patient is receiving a dozen or more medications.

In addition to the risk of creating the vicious cycle seen in Figure 4-1, there are several obvious drawbacks to polypharmacy in older adults. Because each drug will inevitably produce some adverse effects when used alone, the number of adverse effects will begin to accumulate when several agents are used concurrently.[9] More importantly, the interaction of one drug with another (drug–drug interaction) increases the risk of an untoward reaction because of the ability of one agent to modify the effects and metabolism of another drug. If many drugs are administered simultaneously, the risk of ADRs increases exponentially.[9,10] Other negative aspects of polypharmacy are the risk of decreased patient adherence to the drug regimen[11] and the increased financial burden of using large numbers of unnecessary drugs.[12]

Polypharmacy can occur in older adults for a number of reasons. In particular, physicians may rely on drug therapy to accomplish goals that could be achieved through nonpharmacologic methods; that is, it is often relatively easy to prescribe a medication to resolve a problem in the older adult even though other methods that do not require drugs could be used. For instance, the patient who naps throughout the day will probably not be sleepy at bedtime. It is much easier to administer a sedative-hypnotic agent at bedtime rather than institute activities that keep the patient awake during the day and allow nocturnal sleep to occur naturally.

In some cases, the patient may also play a contributing role toward polypharmacy. Patients may obtain prescriptions from various practitioners, thus accumulating a formidable list of prescription medications. Older individuals may receive medications from friends and family members who want to "share" the benefits of their prescription drugs. Some older adults may also use over-the-counter and self-help remedies to such an extent that these agents interact with one another and with their prescription medications.

Polypharmacy can be prevented if the patient's drug regimen is reviewed periodically and any unnecessary or harmful drugs are discontinued.[13,14] Also, new medications should only be administered if a thorough patient evaluation indicates that the drug is truly needed in that patient.[15] When several physicians are dealing with the same patient, these practitioners should make sure that they communicate with one another regarding the patient's drug regimen.[16] Physical therapists can play a role in preventing polypharmacy by recognizing any changes in the patient's response to drug therapy and helping to correctly identify these changes as drug reactions rather than disease "symptoms." In this way, therapists may help prevent the formation of the vicious cycle illustrated in Figure 4-1.

Altered Response to Drugs

There is little doubt that the response to many drugs is affected by age and that the therapeutic and toxic effects of any medication will be different in an older adult than in a younger individual. Alterations in drug response in older adults can be attributed to differences in the way the body handles the drug (pharmacokinetic changes) as well as differences in the way the drug affects the body

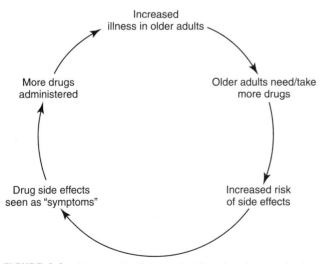

FIGURE 4-1 Vicious cycle of drug administration that can lead to polypharmacy in the older adult.

(pharmacodynamic changes).[17] The effects of aging on drug pharmacokinetics and pharmacodynamics are discussed briefly here.

Pharmacokinetic Changes. Pharmacokinetics is the study of how the body handles a drug, including how the drug is absorbed, distributed, metabolized, and excreted. Several changes in physiological function occur as a result of aging that alter pharmacokinetic variables in older adults. The principal pharmacokinetic changes associated with aging are summarized in Figure 4-2 and are discussed briefly here. The effects of aging on pharmacokinetics has been the subject of extensive research, and the reader is referred to several excellent reviews for more information on this topic.[17-19]

Drug Absorption. Several well-documented changes occur in gastrointestinal (GI) function in the older adult that could potentially affect the way drugs are absorbed from the GI tract. Such changes include decreased gastric acid production, decreased gastric emptying, decreased GI blood flow, diminished area of the absorptive surface, and decreased intestinal motility.[18,20] The effect of these changes on drug absorption, however, is often inconsistent; that is, aging does not appear to significantly alter the absorption of most orally administered drugs. This may be due in part to the fact that the aforementioned changes may offset one another. For instance, factors that tend to decrease absorption (e.g., decreased GI blood flow, decreased absorptive surface area) could be counterbalanced by factors that allow the drug to remain in the gut for longer periods (decreased GI motility), thus allowing more time for absorption. Hence, altered drug absorption does not appear to be a major factor in determining pharmacokinetic changes in older adults.

Drug Distribution. After a drug is absorbed into the body, it undergoes distribution to various tissues and body fluid compartments (e.g., vascular system, intracellular fluid, and so forth). Drug distribution may be altered in older adults because of several physiological changes such as decreased total body water, decreased lean body mass, increased percentage body fat, and decreased plasma protein concentrations.[17,18,21] Depending on the specific drug, these changes can affect how the drug is distributed in the body, thus potentially changing the response to the drug. For instance, drugs that bind to plasma proteins (e.g., aspirin, warfarin) may produce a greater response because there will be less drug bound to plasma proteins and more of the drug will be free to reach the target tissue. Drugs that are soluble in water (e.g., alcohol, morphine) will be relatively more concentrated in the body because there is less body water in which to dissolve the drug. Increased percentages of body fat can act as a reservoir for lipid-soluble drugs, and problems related to drug storage may occur with these agents. Hence, these potential problems in drug distribution must be anticipated, and dosages must be adjusted accordingly in older individuals.

Drug Metabolism. The principal role of drug metabolism (biotransformation) is to inactivate drugs and create water-soluble by-products (metabolites) that can be excreted by the kidneys. Although some degree of drug metabolism can occur in tissues throughout the body, the liver is the primary site for metabolism of most medications. Several distinct changes in liver function occur with aging that affect hepatic drug metabolism. The total drug-metabolizing capacity of the liver decreases with age because of a reduction in liver mass, a decline in hepatic blood flow, and decreased activity of drug-metabolizing enzymes.[20,22] As a result, drugs that undergo inactivation in the liver will remain active for longer periods because of the general decrease in the hepatic metabolizing capacity seen in older adults.

Drug Excretion. The kidneys are the primary routes for drug excretion from the body. Drugs reach the kidney in either their active form or as a drug metabolite after biotransformation in the liver. In either case, it is the kidney's responsibility to filter the drug from the circulation and excrete it from the body via the urine. With aging, declines in renal blood flow, renal mass, and function of renal tubules result in a reduced ability of the kidneys to excrete drugs and their metabolites.[23,24] These changes in renal function tend to be one of the most important factors affecting drug pharmacokinetics in older adults, and reduced renal function should be taken into account whenever drugs are prescribed to these individuals.[17,21]

The cumulative effect of the pharmacokinetic changes associated with aging is that drugs and drug metabolites often remain active for longer periods, thus prolonging

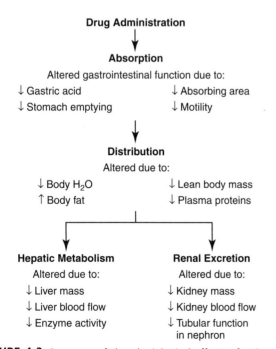

Drug Administration

↓

Absorption

Altered gastrointestinal function due to:

↓ Gastric acid   ↓ Absorbing area
↓ Stomach emptying   ↓ Motility

↓

Distribution

Altered due to:

↓ Body H$_2$O   ↓ Lean body mass
↑ Body fat   ↓ Plasma proteins

Hepatic Metabolism   **Renal Excretion**

Altered due to: Altered due to:

↓ Liver mass   ↓ Kidney mass
↓ Liver blood flow   ↓ Kidney blood flow
↓ Enzyme activity   ↓ Tubular function
                                  in nephron

FIGURE 4-2 Summary of the physiological effects of aging that may alter pharmacokinetics in older adults.

drug effects and increasing the risk for toxic side effects. This is evidenced by the fact that drug half-life (the time required to eliminate 50% of the drug remaining in the body) is often substantially longer in an older individual versus a younger adult.[25] For example, the half-life of certain medications such as the benzodiazepines (e.g., diazepam [Valium], chlordiazepoxide [Librium]) can be increased as much as fourfold in older adults.[26] Obviously, this represents a dramatic change in the way the older adult's body deals with certain pharmacologic agents. Altered pharmacokinetics in older adults must be anticipated by evaluating changes in body composition (e.g., decreased body water, increased percentages of body fat) and monitoring changes in organ function (e.g., decreased hepatic and renal function) so that drug dosages can be adjusted and ADRs minimized in older individuals.[17,18]

Finally, it should be noted that the age-related pharmacokinetic changes described here vary considerably from person to person within the geriatric population.[19] These changes are, however, considered part of the "normal" aging process. Any disease or illness that affects drug distribution, metabolism, or excretion will cause an additional change in pharmacokinetic variables, thus further increasing the risk of ADRs in older adults.[20,23]

Pharmacodynamic Changes. Pharmacodynamics is the study of how drugs affect the body, including systemic drug effects as well as cellular and biochemical mechanisms of drug action. Changes in the control of different physiological systems can influence the systemic response to various drugs in older adults.[27,28] For instance, deficits in the homeostatic control of circulation (e.g., decreased baroreceptor sensitivity, decreased vascular compliance) may change the response of older adults to cardiovascular medications. Other age-related changes, such as impaired postural control, decreased visceral muscle function, altered thermoregulatory responses, and declines in cognitive ability, can alter the pharmacotherapeutic response as well as the potential side effects that may occur when various agents are administered to the older adult.[28] The degree to which systemic drug response is altered will vary depending on the magnitude of these physiological changes in each individual.

In addition to these systemic changes, the way a drug affects tissues on a cellular level may be different in the older adult. Most drugs exert their effects by first binding to a receptor that is located on or within specific target cells that are influenced by each type of drug. This receptor is usually coupled in some way to the biochemical "machinery" of the target cell, so that when the drug binds to the receptor, a biochemical event occurs that changes cell function in a predictable way (Figure 4-3). For instance, binding of epinephrine (adrenaline) to β1-receptors on myocardial cells causes an increase in the activity of certain intracellular enzymes, which in turn causes an increase in heart rate and contractile force.

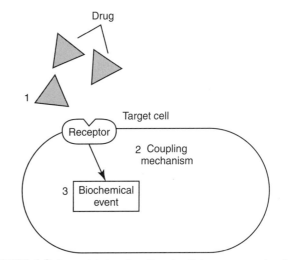

FIGURE 4-3 Potential sites for altered cellular responses in older adults. Changes may occur (1) in drug-receptor affinity, (2) in the coupling of the receptor to an intracellular biochemical event, and (3) in the cell's ability to generate a specific biochemical response.

Similar mechanisms can be described for other drugs and their respective cellular receptors. The altered response to certain drugs seen in older adults may be caused by one or more of the cellular changes depicted in Figure 4-3. For instance, alterations in the drug–receptor attraction (affinity) could help explain an increase or decrease in the sensitivity of the older adult to various medications.[17,27] Likewise, changes in the way the receptor is linked or coupled to the cell's internal biochemistry have been noted in certain tissues as a function of aging.[29,30] Finally, the actual biochemical response within the cell may be blunted because of changes in subcellular structure and function that occur with aging.[27] Age-related declines in mitochondrial function, for example, could influence how the cell responds to various medications.[31,32]

Changes in cellular activity, however, vary according to the tissue and the drugs that affect that tissue. Although some tissues might be more sensitive to certain drugs (e.g., increased sensitivity of CNS tissues to psychotropics and opioids), other tissues may be less responsive (e.g., decreased sensitivity of the cardiovascular system to β-adrenergic agents).[17] Age-related changes in cellular response must therefore be considered according to each tissue and the specific drugs that affect that tissue.

Consequently, pharmacodynamics may be altered in older adults as a result of systemic physiological changes acting in combination with changes in drug responsiveness that occur on a cellular or even subcellular level. These pharmacodynamic changes along with the pharmacokinetic changes discussed earlier help explain why the response of a geriatric individual to drug therapy often differs from the analogous response in a younger individual.

Other Factors That Increase the Risk of Adverse Drug Reactions in Older Adults

In addition to the pattern of drug use and the altered response to drugs seen in older adults, several other factors may contribute to the increased incidence of ADRs seen in these individuals. Several of these additional factors are presented here.

Presence of Multiple Disease States. The fact that older people often suffer from several chronic conditions greatly increases the risk of ADRs.[1] The presence of more than one disease (comorbidity) often necessitates the use of several drugs, thus increasing the risk of drug–drug interactions. Even more important is the fact that various diseases and illnesses usually alter the pharmacokinetic and pharmacodynamic variables discussed earlier. For instance, the age-related changes in hepatic metabolism and renal excretion of drugs are affected to an even greater extent if liver or kidney disease is present. Many older patients suffer from diseases that further decrease function in both of these organs as well as cause diminished function in other physiological systems. The involvement of several organ systems, combined with the presence of several different drugs, makes the chance of an ADR almost inevitable in older adult patients with multiple disease states.

Lack of Proper Drug Testing and Regulation. The Food and Drug Administration (FDA) is responsible for monitoring the safety and efficacy of all drugs marketed in the United States. The FDA requires all drugs to undergo extensive preclinical (animal) and clinical (human) trials before they receive approval. With regard to older adults, some question has been raised about the evaluation of drugs in geriatric individuals prior to FDA approval. It has been recognized that an adequate number of patients older than age 65 years should be included at various stages of the clinical testing, especially for drugs that are targeted for problems that occur primarily in older adults (e.g., dementia, Parkinson's disease, and so forth).[33] It is unclear, however, whether efforts to increase drug testing in geriatric subjects have been successful in providing improved information about drug safety in older adults.[34,35] Clinical trials, for example, may lack adequate numbers of older subjects, especially subjects who are older than age 75 years.[36] Additional efforts on the part of the FDA and the drug manufacturing companies may be necessary to help reduce the risk of adverse effects through better drug testing.

There also has been concern that many drugs are overprescribed and misused in older adults. This concern seems especially true for certain classes of psychotropic agents (e.g., antipsychotics, sedative-hypnotic agents).[37] Fortunately, efforts have been made to institute government regulations and guidelines that limit the use of these medications.[38] It is hoped that enforcement of existing regulations and development of guidelines for other types of drugs will reduce the incidence of inappropriate drug use in older adults.

Problems with Patient Education and Nonadherence to Drug Therapy. Even the most appropriate and well-planned drug regimen will be useless if the drugs are not taken as directed. Patients may experience an increase in adverse side effects, especially if drugs are taken in excessive doses or for the wrong reason.[39] Conversely, older patients may stop taking their medications, resulting in a lack of therapeutic effects and a possible increase in disease symptoms. The fact that older patients often neglect to take their medications is one of the most common types of drug nonadherence.[39,40]

Many factors can disrupt the older individual's adherence (compliance) to drug therapy. A decline in cognitive function, for example, may impair the older person's ability to understand instructions given by the physician, nurse practitioner, or pharmacist. This can hamper the ability of the geriatric patient to take drugs according to the proper dosing schedule, especially if several medications are being administered, with a different dosing schedule for each medication.[9,41] Other factors such as poor eyesight may limit the older person's ability to distinguish one pill from another, and arthritic changes may make it difficult to open certain "childproof" containers.

Some patients may fail to adhere to drug therapy because they feel that their medications are simply not effective; that is, they fail to see any obvious benefit from the drugs.[41,42] The older adult may also stop taking a medication because of an annoying but unavoidable side effect.[40] For instance, older patients with hypertension may refuse to take a diuretic because this particular medication increases urinary output and may necessitate several trips to the bathroom in the middle of the night. To encourage patient self-adherence, it must be realized that these annoying side effects are not trivial and can represent a major source of concern to the patient. Hence, health care professionals should not dismiss these complaints but should make an extra effort to help the patient understand the importance of adhering to the drug regimen whenever such unavoidable side effects are present.

Use of Inappropriate Medications. Because of the physiological changes described earlier, certain medications pose an especially high risk for ADRs in older adults. To identify these medications, an expert panel developed criteria and compiled a specific list of medications that should probably be avoided in people older than age 65 years.[43] These criteria and the related list are known commonly as the Beers criteria (or Beers list) because they were created originally by geriatrician Mark Beers. The Beers criteria/list has been updated periodically to indicate medications that should be avoided and thus help improve geriatric prescribing.[44,45] Hopefully, physicians and pharmacists can refer to this list to avoid use of these drugs in older adults, thereby reducing the risk of serious adverse effects in this population.

Additional Factors. Other factors, including poor diet, excessive use of over-the-counter products, cigarette smoking, and consumption of various other substances (e.g., caffeine, alcohol), may help contribute to the increased risk of adverse drug effects in older adults.[3,46-48] These factors must be taken into consideration when a prescription drug program is implemented for older individuals. For instance, it must be realized that the older adult with a protein-deficient diet may have extremely low plasma protein levels, thus further altering drug pharmacokinetics and increasing the risk of an adverse drug effect. It is therefore important to consider all aspects of the lifestyle and environment of the older adult that may affect drug therapy in these individuals.

COMMON ADVERSE DRUG REACTIONS IN OLDER ADULTS

An ADR is any unwanted and potentially harmful effect caused by a drug when the drug is given at the recommended dosage.[9] Listed here are some of the more common ADRs that may occur in older adults. Of course, this is not a complete list of all the potential ADRs, but these are some of the responses that physical therapists should be aware of when dealing with geriatric patients in a rehabilitation setting.

Gastrointestinal Symptoms

Gastrointestinal problems such as nausea, vomiting, diarrhea, and constipation are among the most commonly occurring adverse drug reactions in older adults.[49,50] These reactions can occur with virtually any medication, and GI symptoms are especially prevalent with certain medications such as the opioid (narcotic) and nonopioid (nonsteroidal anti-inflammatory drugs [NSAIDs]) analgesics. Although these symptoms are sometimes mild and transient in younger patients, older individuals often require adjustments in the type and dosage of specific medications that cause gastrointestinal problems.

Sedation

Older adults seem especially susceptible to drowsiness and sleepiness as a side effect of many medications. In particular, drugs that produce sedation as a primary effect (e.g., sedative-hypnotics) as well as drugs with sedative side effects (e.g., opioid analgesics, antipsychotics) will often produce excessive drowsiness in older adults.

Confusion

Various degrees of confusion ranging from mild disorientation to delirium may occur with a number of medications, such as antidepressants, narcotic analgesics, and drugs with anticholinergic activity.[51,52] Confusion can also indicate that certain drugs, such as lithium and digoxin, are accumulating and reaching toxic levels in the body. Older individuals who are already somewhat confused

may be more susceptible to drugs that tend to further increase confusion.

Depression

Symptoms of depression (e.g., intense sadness and apathy, as described elsewhere in this text) may be induced in older adults by certain medications. Drugs such as barbiturates, antipsychotics, alcohol, and several antihypertensive agents (e.g., clonidine, reserpine, propranolol) have been implicated in producing depression as an ADR in older adults.[53,54]

Orthostatic Hypotension

Orthostatic (postural) hypotension is typically described as a 20-mmHg or greater decline in systolic blood pressure or a 10-mmHg or greater decline in diastolic blood pressure that occurs when an individual assumes a more upright posture (e.g., moving from lying to sitting or from sitting to standing).[55] Owing to the fact that many older adults are relatively sedentary and have diminished cardiovascular function, these individuals tend to be more susceptible to episodes of orthostatic hypotension, even without the influence of drug therapy.[55,56] A number of medications, however, augment the incidence and severity of this blood pressure decline.[57,58] In particular, drugs that tend to lower blood pressure (e.g., antihypertensives, antianginal medications) are a common cause of orthostatic hypotension in older adults. Orthostatic hypotension often leads to dizziness and syncope, because blood pressure is too low to provide adequate cerebral perfusion and oxygen delivery to the brain. Hence, orthostatic hypotension may precipitate falls and subsequent injury (e.g., hip fractures, other trauma) in older individuals.[58] Because older patients are especially susceptible to episodes of orthostatic hypotension during certain rehabilitation procedures (e.g., gait training, functional activities), physical therapists should be especially alert for this ADR.

Fatigue and Weakness

Strength loss and muscular weakness may occur for a number of reasons in response to drug therapy. Some agents, such as the skeletal muscle relaxants, may directly decrease muscle contraction strength, whereas other drugs, such as the diuretics, may affect muscle strength by altering fluid and electrolyte balance. Older individuals who are already debilitated will be more susceptible to strength loss as an ADR.

Dizziness and Falls

Drug-induced dizziness can be especially detrimental in older adults because of the increased risk of loss of balance and falling. Problems with dizziness result from drugs that produce sedation or from agents that directly affect vestibular function. Examples of such agents include sedatives, antipsychotics, opioid analgesics, and antihistamine drugs.[59-61] Dizziness may also occur secondary to drugs that cause orthostatic hypotension (see previous discussion). Drug-induced dizziness and increased risk of falling may be especially prevalent in older adults who already exhibit balance problems, and physical therapists should be especially alert for these ADRs in these individuals.

Anticholinergic Effects

Acetylcholine is an important neurotransmitter that controls function in the central nervous system and also affects peripheral organs such as the heart, lungs, and GI tract. A number of drugs exhibit anticholinergic side effects, meaning that these agents tend to diminish the response of various tissues to acetylcholine. In particular, antihistamines, antidepressants, and certain antipsychotics tend to exhibit anticholinergic side effects. Acetylcholine affects several diverse physiological systems throughout the body, and drugs with anticholinergic effects are therefore associated with a wide range of ADRs. Drugs with anticholinergic effects may produce central nervous system effects, such as confusion, nervousness, drowsiness, and dizziness. Peripheral anticholinergic effects include dry mouth, constipation, urinary retention, tachycardia, and blurred vision. Older adults seem to be more sensitive to anticholinergic effects, possibly because of the fact that acetylcholine influence has already started to diminish as a result of the aging process. In any event, physical therapists should be aware that a rather diverse array of potentially serious ADRs may arise from drugs with anticholinergic properties.

Extrapyramidal Symptoms

Drugs that produce side effects that mimic extrapyramidal tract lesions are said to exhibit extrapyramidal symptoms. Such symptoms include tardive dyskinesia, pseudoparkinsonism, akathisia, and other dystonias. Antipsychotic medications are commonly associated with an increased risk of extrapyramidal symptoms. The problem of extrapyramidal symptoms as an antipsychotic ADR is presented in more detail later in this chapter.

DRUG CLASSES COMMONLY USED IN OLDER ADULTS: IMPACT ON PHYSICAL THERAPY

This section provides a brief overview of drug therapy in older adults. Included are some of the more common groups of drugs that are prescribed to older adults. For each group, the principal clinical indication or indications are listed, along with a brief description of the

mechanism of action of each type of drug. The primary adverse effects and any specific concerns for physical therapy in older patients receiving these drugs are also discussed. Examples of typical drugs found in each of the major groups are indicated in several tables in this section. For additional information about specific agents listed here, the reader can refer to one of the sources listed at the end of this chapter.[62-64]

Psychotropic Medications

Psychotropic drugs include a variety of agents that affect mood, behavior, and other aspects of mental function. As a group, older adults exhibit a high incidence of psychiatric disorders.[65,66] Psychotropic drugs are therefore commonly used in older individuals and are also associated with a high incidence of adverse effects that can have an impact on rehabilitation.[66] The major groups of psychotropic drugs are listed in Table 4-2, and pertinent aspects of each group are discussed here.

Sedative-Hypnotic and Antianxiety Agents. Sedative-hypnotic drugs are used to relax the patient and promote a relatively normal state of sleep. Antianxiety drugs are intended to decrease anxiety without producing excessive sedation. Insomnia and disordered sleep may occur in older individuals concomitant to normal aging or in response to medical problems and lifestyle changes that occur with advanced age.[67,68] Likewise, medical illness, depression, and other aspects of aging may result in increased feelings of fear and apprehension in older adults.[69,70] Hence, use of sedative-hypnotic and antianxiety drugs is commonly encountered in older adults.

Historically, a group of agents known as the benzodiazepines have been the primary drugs used to promote sleep and decrease anxiety in older adults (see Table 4-2).[71,72] Benzodiazepines exert their beneficial effects by increasing the central inhibitory effect of the neurotransmitter γ-aminobutyric acid (GABA).[73] This increase in GABA-mediated inhibition seems to account for the decreased anxiety and increased sleepiness associated with these drugs.

Despite their extensive use, benzodiazepines are associated with several problems, especially when administered to older adults. When treating insomnia, for example, residual or "hangover" effects may occur, producing drowsiness and sluggishness the morning after a sedative-hypnotic is used. These effects seem especially prevalent if a relatively long-acting benzodiazepine, such as chlordiazepoxide, diazepam, or flurazepam, is administered to an older patient.[74] Physical therapists should be especially aware of the possibility of residual effects of sedative-hypnotic drugs when scheduling older patients for rehabilitation first thing in the morning. Other potential adverse effects include "anterograde amnesia," in which patients have lapses in short-term memory for the period immediately preceding drug administration, and "rebound insomnia," in which sleeplessness increases when the drug is discontinued.[74]

TABLE 4-2 | Psychotropic Drug Groups

Group	Common Examples	
	Generic Name	**Trade Name**
Sedative-Hypnotic Agents		
Benzodiazepines	Estazolam	ProSom
	Flurazepam	Dalmane
	Temazepam	Restoril
	Triazolam	Halcion
Others	Eszopiclone	Lunesta
	Ramelteon	Rozerem
	Zaleplon	Sonata
	Zolpidem	Ambien
Antianxiety Agents		
Benzodiazepines	Chlordiazepoxide	Librium
	Diazepam	Valium
	Lorazepam	Ativan
Azapirones	Buspirone	BuSpar
Antidepressants		
Tricyclics	Amitriptyline	Elavil, Endep
	Imipramine	Norfranil, Tofranil
MAO* inhibitors	Isocarboxazid	Marplan
	Phenelzine	Nardil
Second-generation agents	Bupropion	Wellbutrin
	Escitalopram	Lexapro
	Fluoxetine	Prozac
	Maprotiline	Ludiomil
	Paroxetine	Paxil
	Sertraline	Zoloft
	Venlafaxine	Effexor
Antipsychotics		
Conventional agents	Chlorpromazine	Thorazine
	Haloperidol	Haldol
	Prochlorperazine	Compazine
	Thioridazine	Mellaril
Second generation (atypical antipsychotics)	Clozapine	Clozaril
	Olanzapine	Zyprexa
	Quetiapine	Seroquel
	Risperidone	Risperdal

*MAO, monoamine oxidase.

Use of benzodiazepines to treat sleep disorders can also result in problems associated with addiction if these drugs are used indiscriminately for prolonged periods (4 weeks or longer).[75,76] These problems include the need to progressively increase dosage to achieve beneficial effects (tolerance) and the onset of withdrawal symptoms when the drug is discontinued (physical dependence). Clearly, benzodiazepines can help the older patient cope with occasional sleep disturbances, but these drugs should be used at the lowest possible dose and for only short periods while trying to find nonpharmacologic methods (e.g., counseling and decreased caffeine use) to deal with the patient's insomnia.[72,76,77]

Benzodiazepines are also associated with specific adverse responses when used to treat anxiety in older adults. As previously described, these agents can cause tolerance and physical dependence when used for prolonged periods. Likewise, sedation and cognitive impairment are possible side effects when benzodiazepines are used to treat anxiety in older adults.[68] Physical therapists should therefore realize that the use of benzodiazepines in older patients is a two-edged sword. Decreased anxiety may enable the patient to be more relaxed and cooperative during rehabilitation, but any benefits will be negated if the patient experiences significant psychomotor slowing and is unable to remain alert during the therapy session.

In order to treat insomnia and anxiety more effectively in older adults, several newer strategies have been explored. Regarding sleep disorders, nonbenzodiazepine agents such as eszopiclone, zolpidem, and zaleplon are now available (see Table 4-2).[72,78,79] Although these newer drugs also affect the GABA receptor, they appear to bind somewhat more selectively to this receptor than the benzodiazepines. Moreover, these newer drugs tend to produce fewer residual effects, such as the hangover effect, and may be less likely to cause tolerance and dependence.[78,80] In addition, ramelteon (Rozerem) is a drug that stimulates CNS melatonin receptors, and this drug may also be effective in promoting sleep in older adults with less risk of residual effects and addiction.[81,82] Hence, several new options are now available to treat sleep disorders in older adults, and many patients are being prescribed these newer drugs instead of the more traditional benzodiazepines.

Regarding treatment of anxiety, agents known as the azapirones (e.g., buspirone) have been developed.[70] These agents appear to decrease anxiety by directly stimulating serotonin receptors in certain parts of the brain (dorsal raphe nucleus) rather than by increasing GABA-mediated inhibition like the benzodiazepines.[83] More importantly, azapirones such as buspirone do not cause sedation, do not impair cognition and psychomotor function, and appear to have a much lower potential for the patient developing tolerance and physical dependence than traditional agents such as the benzodiazepines.[83]

Likewise, certain antidepressants are currently regarded as effective treatments for anxiety disorders in older adults. In particular, antidepressants such as escitalopram and paroxetine selectively affect serotonin activity (see later), and these drugs may also be effective in treating anxiety.[84,85] Certain patients have symptoms of depression combined with anxiety, and these drugs certainly seem like a good option for these patients. It appears, however, that these antidepressants may also be effective in treating anxiety even in the absence of depression.[70]

Treatment of anxiety has therefore evolved to where agents such as the azapirones and certain antidepressants may be used in favor of benzodiazepines. These newer options seem to be better tolerated in older adults and continue to be used increasingly in the treatment of various forms of anxiety in older adults.[70]

Antidepressants. Depression is the most common form of mental illness in the general population as well as the most commonly observed mental disorder in older adults.[69,86] Feelings of intense sadness, hopelessness, and other symptoms may occur in older adults after a specific event (e.g., loss of a spouse, acute illness) or in response to the gradual decline in health and functional status often associated with aging. Drug therapy may be instituted to help resolve these symptoms, along with other nonpharmacologic methods, such as counseling and behavioral therapy.

There are several distinct groups of antidepressant medications: tricyclics, monoamine oxidase (MAO) inhibitors, and the newer "second-generation" drugs (see Table 4-2). All antidepressant drugs share a common goal—to increase synaptic transmission in central neural pathways that use amine neurotransmitters such as norepinephrine, dopamine, or 5-hydroxytryptamine (serotonin). The rationale is that symptoms of depression are due to an imbalance in the activity of certain central amine neurotransmitter pathways, especially pathways where serotonin receptors regulate dopamine activity in the brain.[87] Drugs that overstimulate these receptors bring about a compensatory decrease (downregulation) in the number of functioning receptors, thereby restoring the balance of amine neurotransmitters in the brain.[88] As receptor sensitivity stabilizes, the clinical symptoms of depression appear to be resolved.

A primary focus in treating depression in older adults has been identifying which agents produce the best effects with the least side effects.[89,90] In the past, tricyclic antidepressants were often the drugs of choice, though these drugs tend to produce anticholinergic and other side effects (see the following discussion). Certain second-generation drugs, however, appear to be as effective as the tricyclics but may be better tolerated in older adults. In particular, agents such as fluoxetine (Prozac), sertraline (Zoloft), and paroxetine (Paxil) have been advocated as drugs of choice in older adults because they generally have fewer severe side effects than other antidepressants.[89,91] These agents are known collectively as selective serotonin reuptake inhibitors (SSRIs) because they tend to preferentially affect CNS synapses that use serotonin as a neurotransmitter rather than affect synapses using other amine transmitters, such as norepinephrine or dopamine. Considerable debate still exists, however, and optimal use of SSRIs and other antidepressants in older adults remains under investigation.[89,92]

Antidepressants produce various side effects, depending on the particular type of drug. As indicated earlier, tricyclic antidepressants produce anticholinergic effects and may cause dry mouth, constipation, urinary retention, and central nervous system (CNS) symptoms such

as confusion, cognitive impairment, and delirium. Tricyclics also cause sedation and orthostatic hypotension, and these drugs can produce serious cardiotoxic effects after overdose.[93] Monoamine oxidase inhibitors also produce orthostatic hypotension and tend to cause insomnia. Side effects associated with the second-generation drugs vary depending on the specific agent. As previously noted, certain effects that are particularly troublesome in older adults (i.e., sedation, anticholinergic effects, orthostatic hypotension) tend to occur less frequently with the SSRIs. SSRIs, however, have a greater tendency to cause other bothersome effects, such as GI irritation and upper GI bleeding.[89,94]

Physical therapists should be aware that antidepressants may help improve the patient's mood and increase the patient's interest in physical therapy. Certain side effects, however, such as sedation and confusion, may impair the patient's cognitive ability and make it difficult for some older patients to participate actively in rehabilitation procedures. Hence, selection of drugs that minimize these effects may be especially helpful. Therapists should also be aware that some patients may respond fairly rapidly to the antidepressant effects of these drugs; that is, some patients receiving SSRIs experience beneficial effects within 1 week after beginning drug treatment.[95] Other patients, however, may take 6 or more weeks from the onset of drug therapy until an improvement occurs in the depressive symptoms. This substantial time lag is critical because the patient may actually become more depressed before mood begins to improve. Therapists should therefore look for signs that depression is worsening, especially during the first few weeks of antidepressant drug therapy. A suspected increase in depressive symptoms should be brought to the attention of the appropriate member of the health care team (e.g., physician or psychologist).

Treatment of Bipolar Disorder. Bipolar disorder, known also as manic depression, is a form of mental illness characterized by mood swings from an excited, hyperactive state (mania) to periods of apathy and dysphoria (depression). Although the cause of bipolar disorder is unknown, this condition responds fairly well to the drug lithium. It is not exactly clear how lithium prevents episodes of manic depression, but this drug may prevent the excitable, or manic, phase of this disorder, thus stabilizing disposition and preventing the mood swings characteristic of this disease.[96,97]

It is important to be aware of older patients taking lithium to treat manic depression because this drug can rapidly accumulate to toxic levels in these individuals.[98] Lithium is an element and cannot be degraded in the body to an inactive form. The body must therefore rely solely on renal excretion to eliminate this drug. Because renal function is reduced in older adults, the elimination of this drug is often impaired. Accumulation of lithium beyond a certain level results in lithium toxicity.[98] Symptoms of mild lithium toxicity include a metallic taste in the mouth, fine hand tremor, nausea, and muscular weakness and fatigue. These symptoms increase as toxicity reaches moderate levels, and other CNS signs such as blurred vision and incoordination may appear. Severe lithium toxicity may cause irreversible cerebellar damage, and prolonged lithium neurotoxicity can lead to coma and even death.[98,99]

Hence, physical therapists working with older patients who are taking lithium must continually be alert for any signs of lithium toxicity. This idea is especially important if there is any change in the patient's health or activity level that might cause an additional compromise in lithium excretion.

In addition to lithium, several other medications can be used to help treat bipolar disorder. In particular, antipsychotic medications such as quetiapine and olanzapine can help stabilize mood, especially during the acute manic phase of this disorder.[97] Likewise, aripiprazole (Abilify) is a relatively new antipsychotic that has shown promise in treating acute manic episodes and in the long term or maintenance of bipolar disorder.[100] The neurochemistry of these newer antipsychotics is addressed in the next section.

Antipsychotics

Antipsychotic medications are often used to help normalize behavior in older adults. *Psychosis* is the term used to describe the more severe forms of mental illness that are characterized by marked thought disturbances and altered perceptions of reality.[101] Aggressive, disordered behavior may also accompany symptoms of psychosis. In older adults, psychotic-like behavior may occur because of actual psychotic syndromes (e.g., schizophrenia, severe paranoid disorders) or may be associated with various forms of dementia.[101,102] In any event, antipsychotic drugs may be helpful in improving behavior and compliance in older patients.

Further, antipsychotic drugs are often characterized as either conventional or second-generation (atypical) agents (see Table 4-2). Conventional agents have been on the market for some time, and they tend to produce different side effects than the newer, second-generation antipsychotic drugs (see later). Regardless of their classification, these drugs all share a common mechanism in that they impair synaptic transmission in central dopamine pathways.[103] It is theorized that psychosis may be due to increased central dopamine influence in cortical and limbic system pathways. Antipsychotic drugs are believed to reduce this dopaminergic influence, thus helping to decrease psychotic-like behavior. Some second-generation antipsychotics also appear to strongly block serotonin receptors, with a more moderate effect on dopamine receptors.[103,104] This simultaneous effect on serotonin and dopamine may explain why these newer agents exert antipsychotic effects with less risk of certain side effects (see later).

Antipsychotic drugs are associated with several annoying but fairly minor side effects, such as sedation and anticholinergic effects (e.g., dry mouth, constipation). Orthostatic hypotension may also occur, especially within the first few days after drug treatment is initiated. A more serious concern with antipsychotic drugs is the possibility of extrapyramidal side effects.[105,106] As discussed earlier in this chapter, motor symptoms that mimic lesions in the extrapyramidal tracts are a common ADR associated with these medications, especially in older adults.[105] For instance, patients may exhibit involuntary movements of the face, jaw, and extremities (tardive dyskinesia), symptoms that resemble Parkinson's disease (pseudoparkinsonism), extreme restlessness (akathisia), or other problems with involuntary muscle movements (dystonias).[107] Early recognition of these extrapyramidal signs is important because they may persist long after the antipsychotic drug is discontinued, or these signs may even remain permanently. This fact seems especially true for drug-induced tardive dyskinesia, which may be irreversible if antipsychotic drug therapy is not altered when these symptoms first appear.[106]

Fortunately, newer agents such as clozapine and risperidone are less likely to produce extrapyramidal symptoms than older or more conventional agents (see Table 4-2). As indicated earlier, these newer drugs are often classified as second-generation or "atypical" antipsychotics because of their reduced risk of certain side effects.[104] Although tardive dyskinesia and other motor side effects can still occur with newer agents, especially at higher doses, the incidence of these problems is lower than more conventional drugs.[107] Second-generation antipsychotics, however, may produce other serious problems such as cardiovascular toxicity, weight gain, and metabolic disturbances that resemble diabetes mellitus.[107,108]

The use of antipsychotic drugs may have beneficial effects on rehabilitation outcomes because patients may become more cooperative and less agitated during physical therapy. Therapists should be especially alert for the onset of any extrapyramidal symptoms because of the potential that these symptoms may result in long-term or permanent motor side effects. Therapists should realize, however, that antipsychotics may sometimes be used inappropriately in older adults.[38,109] These medications are approved to help control certain psychotic-related symptoms, including behavioral problems such as aggression and severe agitation. These drugs, however, should not be used indiscriminately as "tranquilizers" to control all unwanted behaviors in older adults. As indicated earlier, government regulations have been instituted to help decrease the inappropriate and unnecessary use of these medications in older adults.[102]

Treatment of Dementia. *Dementia* is a term used to describe a fairly global decline in intellectual function, with marked impairments in cognition, speech, personality, and other skills.[110] Some forms of dementia may be due to specific factors such as an infection, metabolic disorder, or an adverse reaction to drugs that have psychoactive side effects.[111] These so-called reversible dementias are often resolved if the precipitating factor is identified and corrected. Irreversible dementia is typically associated with progressive degenerative changes in cortical structure and function, such as those occurring in Alzheimer's disease. Drug treatment of irreversible dementia follows two primary strategies: improving cognitive function and treating behavioral symptoms. These strategies are discussed briefly here.

In the past, attempts to improve cognitive function using various medications resulted in only limited success in persons with irreversible dementia. Recent drug development, however, has focused on the use of agents that increase acetylcholine function in the brain.[112] It is known that acetylcholine influence in the brain begins to diminish because of the neuronal degeneration inherent to Alzheimer's disease. Therefore, drugs that increase cholinergic activity may help improve intellectual and cognitive function in persons with Alzheimer-type dementia. As a result, agents such as tacrine (Cognex) and donepezil (Aricept), galantamine (Reminyl), and rivastigmine (Exelon) have been developed to specifically improve cognition and behavioral function in persons with Alzheimer's disease.[113,114] These drugs inhibit the acetylcholinesterase enzyme, thus decreasing acetylcholine breakdown and prolonging the activity of this neurotransmitter in the brain.

Regrettably, cholinergic stimulants provide only moderate benefits in patients who are in the relatively early stages of this disease[113,115]; that is, these drugs may help patients retain more cognitive and intellectual function during the mild to moderate stages of Alzheimer's disease, but these benefits are eventually lost as the disease progresses. Likewise, side effects such as GI distress and liver toxicity may limit the use of these drugs in some patients.[110,114] Still, these agents may help sustain cognitive function during the early course of Alzheimer's disease, thus enabling patients to continue to participate in various activities, including physical therapy.

A newer pharmacotherapeutic option for treating Alzheimer's disease is memantine (Namenda). This drug blocks the N-methyl-D-aspartate (NMDA) receptor in the brain.[116] This receptor normally responds to glutamate, an amino acid neurotransmitter that is important in memory and learning.[117] Evidently, glutamate overstimulation of the NMDA receptor can contribute to the neurodegenerative changes associated with Alzheimer's disease. By reducing this glutamate activity, memantine may help improve memory and cognition and reduce symptoms of agitation and aggression.[117] Moreover, this drug may offer some protection for CNS neurons and thus help decrease the progression of Alzheimer's disease.[116] Hence, memantine offers an additional therapeutic option, and use of this drug alone or in combination with cholinesterase inhibitors may help improve symptoms in people with Alzheimer's

disease.[118] Likewise, other pharmacologic strategies that enhance cognition or delay the degenerative changes in Alzheimer's disease are currently being explored, and these strategies may help provide more long-lasting effects in the future.[112]

Finally, other drugs already discussed in this chapter may be used to help normalize and control behavior in patients with Alzheimer's disease and other forms of dementia. In particular, antipsychotic drugs may help improve certain aspects of behavior, such as decreased hallucinations and diminished feelings of hostility and suspiciousness.[102,119] Response to these drugs, however, is highly variable, and side effects are quite common when these drugs are given to older people.[101,119]

As noted earlier, efforts are also being made to decrease the indiscriminate use of antipsychotics in persons with Alzheimer's disease. For example, nonpharmacologic interventions such as therapeutic activities, environmental modification, and caregiver support/education should be considered before resorting to drug therapy.[110,112] If drug therapy is required, choice of a specific medication should be based on the specific symptoms exhibited by each patient.[120] For example, the severely anxious patient may respond better to an antianxiety drug, the depressed patient may respond to an antidepressant, and so on.[121] The idea that antipsychotics are not a panacea for all dementia-like symptoms is certainly worth considering, and the use of alternative interventions may decrease the incidence of polypharmacy and antipsychotic-related side effects.

Neurologic Agents

In addition to the drugs that affect mood and behavior, there are specific agents that are important in controlling certain neurologic conditions in older adults. Drug treatment of two of these conditions, Parkinson's disease and seizure disorders, is discussed here.

Drugs Used for Parkinson's Disease. Parkinson's disease is one of the more prevalent disorders in older adults, with more than 1% of the population older than age 60 years being afflicted.[122] This disease is caused by the degeneration of dopamine-secreting neurons located in the basal ganglia.[123,124] Loss of dopaminergic influence initiates an imbalance in other neurotransmitters, including an increase in acetylcholine influence. This disruption in transmitter activity ultimately results in the typical parkinsonian motor symptoms of rigidity, bradykinesia, resting tremor, and postural instability.[125]

Drug treatment of Parkinson's disease usually focuses on restoring the balance of neurotransmitters in the basal ganglia.[126] The most common way of achieving this is to administer 3,4-dihydroxyphenylalanine (dopa), which is the immediate precursor to dopamine. Dopamine itself will not cross the blood–brain barrier, meaning that dopamine will not move from the bloodstream into the brain, where it is ultimately needed. However, levodopa (the L-isomer of dopa) will pass easily from the bloodstream into the brain, where it can then be transformed into dopamine and help restore the influence of this neurotransmitter in the basal ganglia.

Levodopa is often administered orally with a drug known as carbidopa. Carbidopa inhibits the enzyme that transforms levodopa to dopamine in the peripheral circulation, thus allowing levodopa to cross into the brain before it is finally converted to dopamine. If levodopa is converted to dopamine before reaching the brain, the dopamine will be useless in Parkinson's disease because it becomes trapped in the peripheral circulation. The simultaneous use of carbidopa and levodopa allows smaller doses of levodopa to be administered, because less of the levodopa will be wasted as a result of the premature conversion to dopamine in the periphery.

Levodopa therapy often produces dramatic beneficial effects, especially during the mild to moderate stages of Parkinson's disease. Nonetheless, levodopa is associated with several troublesome side effects.[125] In particular, levodopa may cause GI distress (e.g., nausea, vomiting) and cardiovascular problems (e.g., arrhythmias, orthostatic hypotension), especially for the first few days after drug therapy is initiated. Neuropsychiatric problems (e.g., confusion, depression, anxiety, hallucinations) and problems with involuntary movements (e.g., dyskinesia) have also been noted in patients on levodopa therapy.[127,128] Perhaps the most frustrating problem, however, is the tendency for the effectiveness of levodopa to diminish after 4 or 5 years of continuous use.[129,130] The reason for this diminished response is not fully understood but may be related to the fact that levodopa replacement simply cannot adequately restore neurotransmitter dysfunction in the final stages of this disease; that is, levodopa therapy may help supplement endogenous dopamine production in early to moderate Parkinson's disease, but this effect is eventually lost when the substantia nigra neurons degenerate beyond a certain point. Other fluctuations in the response to levodopa have been noted with long-term use.[131] These fluctuations include a spontaneous decrease in levodopa effectiveness in the middle of a dose interval (on–off phenomenon) or loss of drug effects toward the end of a dose cycle (end-of-dose akinesia). The reasons for these fluctuations are poorly understood but may be related to problems in the absorption and metabolism of levodopa in the later stages of Parkinson's disease.

Fortunately, several other agents are currently available to help alleviate the motor symptoms associated with Parkinson's disease (Table 4-3).[122,132] Drugs such as bromocriptine (Parlodel), pergolide (Permax), and other dopamine agonists mimic the effects of dopamine and can be used to replace the deficient neurotransmitter. Anticholinergic drugs (e.g., biperiden, ethopropazine) act to decrease acetylcholine influence in the brain and can attenuate the increased effects of acetylcholine that occur when dopamine influence is diminished. Amantadine

TABLE 4-3	Neurologic Drug Groups	
	Generic Name	**Trade Name**
Drugs Used in Parkinson's Disease		
Dopamine precursors	Levodopa	Sinemet*
Dopamine agonists	Bromocriptine	Parlodel
	Pergolide	Permax
	Pramipexole	Mirapex
	Ropinirole	Requip
Anticholinergic drugs	Benztropine	Cogentin
	Biperiden	Akineton
	Ethopropazine	Parsidol
	Procyclidine	Kemadrin
COMT† inhibitors	Entacapone	Comtan
	Tolcapone	Tasmar
Others	Amantadine	Symmetrel
	Selegiline	Deprenyl, Eldepryl
Drugs Used in Seizure Disorders		
Barbiturates	Mephobarbital	Mebaral
	Phenobarbital	Solfoton
Benzodiazepines	Clonazepam	Klonopin
	Clorazepate	Tranxene
Carboxylic acids	Divalproex	Depakote
Hydantoins	Ethotoin	Peganone
	Mephenytoin	Mesantoin
	Phenytoin	Dilantin
Succinimides	Ethosuximide	Zarontin
	Methsuximide	Celontin
Iminostilbenes	Carbamazepine	Tegretol
	Oxcarbazepine	Trileptal
Newer (second-generation) agents	Felbamate	Felbatol
	Gabapentin	Neurontin
	Lamotrigine	Lamictal
	Levetiracetam	Keppra
	Pregabalin	Lyrica
	Topiramate	Topamax

*Indicates trade name for levodopa combined with carbidopa, a peripheral decarboxylase inhibitor.
†*COMT*, catechol-*O*-methyltransferase.

(Symmetrel) is actually an antiviral drug that also exerts antiparkinson effects, presumably by blocking the NMDA receptor and decreasing the excitatory effects of CNS amino acids. Selegiline (Eldepryl) inhibits the monoamine oxidase (MAO) enzyme that degrades dopamine, thus prolonging the effects of any dopamine that exists in the basal ganglia. Finally, drugs such as entacapone (Comtan) and tolcapone (Tasmar) inhibitor the catechol-*o*-methyltransferase enzyme, thereby preventing premature destruction of levodopa in the bloodstream and allowing more levodopa to reach the brain.

Consequently, levodopa therapy is still the cornerstone of treatment in persons with Parkinson's disease, but several other agents are now available that can be used in combination with or instead of levodopa to create an optimal drug regimen for each patient.[133] Nonetheless, current pharmacotherapy of Parkinson's disease has some considerable shortcomings, and treatment of patients is often limited by inadequate effects or toxic side effects, especially during the advanced stages of this disease. Additional drug treatments are being considered that may actually help delay the neurodegenerative changes inherent to Parkinson's disease.[134,135] If proven effective, these treatments would offer substantial benefits because they would help slow the progression of this disease rather than merely treat the parkinsonian symptoms.

Physical therapists working with patients with Parkinson's disease should attempt to coordinate rehabilitation sessions with the peak effects of drug therapy whenever possible. For instance, scheduling physical therapy when levodopa and other antiparkinson drugs reach peak effects (usually 1 hour after oral administration) will often maximize the patient's ability to actively participate in exercise programs and functional training. Therapists should also be cognizant of the potential side effects of levodopa, including the tendency for responses to fluctuate or diminish with prolonged use. Physical therapists may also play an important role in documenting any decline or alteration in drug effectiveness while working closely with patients with Parkinson's disease.

Drugs Used to Control Seizures. Seizure disorders such as epilepsy are characterized by the sudden, uncontrolled firing of a group of cerebral neurons.[136] This uncontrolled neuronal excitation is manifested in various ways, depending on the location and extent of the neuronal involvement, and seizures are classified according to the motor and sensory symptoms that occur during a seizure. In the general population, the exact cause of the seizure disorder is often unknown. In older adults, however, seizure activity may be attributed to a fairly well-defined cause such as a previous CNS injury (e.g., stroke, trauma), tumor, or degenerative brain disease.[137] If the cause cannot be treated by surgical or other means, pharmacologic management remains the primary method of preventing recurrent seizures.

The primary goal of antiseizure drugs is to normalize the excitation threshold in the group of hyperexcitable neurons that initiate the seizure.[138,139] Ideally, this can be accomplished without suppressing the general excitation level within the brain. Several groups of chemically distinct antiseizure drugs are currently in use, and each group uses a different biochemical mechanism to selectively decrease excitability in the seizure-prone neurons (see Table 4-3). The selection of a particular antiseizure drug depends primarily on the type of seizure present in each patient.[138]

Sedation is the most common side effect that physical therapists should be aware of when working with older patients who are taking seizure medications.[140] Other annoying side effects include GI distress, headache, dizziness, incoordination, and dermatologic reactions

(e.g., rashes). More serious problems, such as liver toxicity and blood dyscrasias (aplastic anemia), may occur in some patients. In addition to monitoring these side effects, physical therapists can play an important role in helping assess the effectiveness of the antiseizure medications by observing and documenting any seizures that may occur during the rehabilitation session.

Treatment of Pain and Inflammation

Pharmacologic treatment of pain and inflammation is used in older adults to help resolve symptoms of chronic conditions (e.g., rheumatoid arthritis and osteoarthritis) as well as acute problems resulting from trauma and surgery.[141] Drugs used for analgesic and anti-inflammatory purposes include the opioid analgesics, nonopioid analgesics, and glucocorticoids (Table 4-4). These medications are discussed briefly here.

Opioid Analgesics. Opioid analgesics compose the group of drugs used to treat relatively severe, constant pain. These agents, also known as *narcotics*, are commonly used to reduce pain in older patients after surgery or trauma, or in more chronic situations such as cancer.[142] Opioids vary in terms of their relative analgesic strength, with drugs such as morphine and meperidine (Demerol) having strong analgesic properties, and drugs such as codeine having a more moderate ability to decrease pain. These drugs exert their beneficial effects by binding to opioid receptors in the brain and spinal cord, thereby altering synaptic transmission in pain-mediating pathways.[143,144] Opioid analgesics are often characterized by their ability to alter pain perception rather than completely eliminating painful sensations. This effect allows the patient to focus on other things rather than being continually preoccupied by the painful stimuli.

Physical therapists should be aware that the analgesic effects of opioid drugs tend to be accompanied by many side effects that can influence the patient's participation in rehabilitation.[145] Adverse side effects such as sedation, mood changes (e.g., euphoria or dysphoria), and GI problems (e.g., nausea, vomiting, constipation) are quite common. Orthostatic hypotension and respiratory depression are also common side effects, especially for the first few days after opioid analgesic therapy is started. Confusion may be a problem, particularly in older adults. Finally, aspects of drug addiction, including tolerance and physical dependence, are always a concern when opioid analgesics are used for prolonged periods.

Nonopioid Analgesics. Treatment of mild to moderate pain is often accomplished by the use of two types of nonopioid agents: NSAIDs and acetaminophen. NSAIDs compose a group of drugs that are therapeutically similar to aspirin (see Table 4-4). These aspirin-like drugs produce four therapeutic effects: analgesia, decreased inflammation, decreased fever (antipyresis), and decreased platelet aggregation (anticoagulant effects). Acetaminophen appears to have analgesic and antipyretic properties

TABLE 4-4 | Analgesic and Anti-inflammatory Drugs Groups

Category	Common Examples Generic Name	Trade Name
Opioid Analgesics		
	Codeine	Many trade names
	Meperidine	Demerol
	Morphine	Many trade names
	Oxycodone	OxyContin, Roxicodone
	Propoxyphene	Darvon, others
Nonopioid Analgesics		
NSAIDs*	Aspirin	Many trade names
	Ibuprofen	Advil, Motrin, others
	Ketoprofen	Orudis, others
	Naproxen	Naprosyn, Anaprox
	Piroxicam	Feldene
	Sulindac	Clinoril
COX-2 inhibitor	Celecoxib	Celebrex
Acetaminophen	—	Tylenol, Panadol
Corticosteroids	Betamethasone	Celestone, others
	Cortisone	Cortone
	Hydrocortisone	Cortef, Hydrocortone, others
	Prednisone	Deltasone, others
Disease-Modifying Drugs†		
Gold compounds	Auranofin	Ridaura
	Aurothioglucose	Solganal
	Gold sodium thiomalate	Myochrysine
Antimalarials	Chloroquine	Aralen
	Hydroxychloroquine	Plaquenil
Tumor necrosis factor inhibitors	Adalimumab	Humira
	Etanercept	Enbrel
Interleukin-1 inhibitor	Anakinra	Kineret
Others	Azathioprine	Imuran
	Cyclophosphamide	Cytoxan
	Methotrexate	Rheumatrex, others
	Penicillamine	Cuprimine, Depen

*NSAIDs, nonsteroidal anti-inflammatory drugs.
†Drugs used to slow the progression of rheumatoid arthritis.

similar to the NSAIDs, but acetaminophen lacks any significant anti-inflammatory or anticoagulation effects. NSAIDs and acetaminophen exert most, if not all, of their beneficial effects by inhibiting the synthesis of a group of compounds known as the *prostaglandins*. Prostaglandins are produced locally by many cells and are involved in mediating certain aspects of pain and inflammation.[146,147] Aspirin and other NSAIDs inhibit the cyclooxygenase (COX) enzyme that synthesizes prostaglandins in the central nervous system as well as peripheral tissues, thus diminishing the painful and inflammatory effects of these compounds throughout the body.[147] Acetaminophen also inhibits prostaglandin biosynthesis, but this inhibition may only occur in the central nervous system, thus accounting for the differences in acetaminophen and NSAID effects.[148]

Because certain prostaglandins produce beneficial or cytoprotective effects in the body, efforts were made to produce a type of NSAID that impaired the production of only the harmful prostaglandins. These efforts lead to the development of COX-2 inhibitors such as celecoxib (Celebrex). These drugs are so-named because they tend to inhibit the COX-2 form of the enzyme that synthesizes prostaglandins that cause pain and inflammation while sparing the production of the beneficial prostaglandins produced by the COX-1 enzyme.[147] Indeed, COX-2 inhibitors can reduce pain and inflammation in some patients with less chance of adverse effects such as gastric irritation.[149] These benefits, however, are not universal and some patients experience serious gastric toxicity from COX-2 drugs.[150] Moreover, COX-2 inhibitors are associated with potentially serious cardiovascular problems in some people, including myocardial infarction and stroke.[151,152] These adverse effects were the reason that certain COX-2 drugs such as rofecoxib (Vioxx) and valdecoxib (Bextra) were removed from the market. Hence, COX-2 selective drugs may be an attractive alternative to traditional NSAIDs in some patients, but the actual use of these drugs may be limited by serious side effects. Patients should be screened carefully before using these drugs, and COX-2 drugs should be avoided in patients with cardiovascular disease.[153]

NSAID use in older patients tends to be fairly safe when these drugs are used in moderate doses for short periods.[154] The most common side effect is gastrointestinal irritation, and problems ranging from minor stomach upset to serious gastric ulceration can occur in older adults.[155] Renal and hepatic toxicity may also occur, especially if higher doses are used for prolonged periods or in patients with preexisting kidney or liver disease.[156,157] As mentioned above, cardiovascular problems are a major concern for the COX-2 drugs, but traditional NSAIDs can also cause cardiovascular toxicity especially in people with hypertension and heart failure.[157] NSAIDs can impair bone healing, and should be avoided after fractures and certain surgeries such as spinal fusions.[154] Other problems that may occur in older patients include allergic reactions (e.g., skin rashes) and possible CNS toxicity (e.g., confusion, hearing problems). In particular, tinnitus (a ringing or buzzing sound in the ears) may develop with prolonged aspirin use, and this side effect may be especially annoying and distressing to older adults.

Acetaminophen does not produce any appreciable gastric irritation and may be taken preferentially by older patients for that reason.[153,157] It should be noted, however, that acetaminophen lacks anti-inflammatory effects and may be inferior to NSAIDs if pain and inflammation are present. Acetaminophen may also be more hepatotoxic than the NSAIDs in cases of overdose or in persons who are dehydrated, consume excessive amounts of alcohol, and so forth.

Glucocorticoids. Glucocorticoids are steroids produced by the adrenal cortex that have a number of physiological effects, including a potent ability to decrease inflammation.[158] Synthetic derivatives of endogenously produced glucocorticoids can be administered pharmacologically to capitalize on the powerful anti-inflammatory effects of these compounds. These agents are used to treat rheumatoid arthritis and a variety of other disorders that have an inflammatory component. Glucocorticoids exert their anti-inflammatory effects through several complex mechanisms, including the ability to suppress leukocyte function and to inhibit the production of proinflammatory substances, such as cytokines, prostaglandins, and leukotrienes, at the site of inflammation.[159,160]

The powerful anti-inflammatory effects of glucocorticoids must be balanced against the risk of several serious adverse effects. In particular, physical therapists should be aware that these drugs produce a general catabolic effect on supporting tissues throughout the body.[161,162] Breakdown of bones, ligaments, tendons, skin, and muscle can occur after prolonged systemic administration of glucocorticoids. This breakdown can be especially devastating in older adult patients who already have some degree of osteoporosis or muscle wasting.[163] Glucocorticoids also produce other serious adverse effects, including hypertension, peptic ulcer, aggravation of diabetes mellitus, glaucoma, increased risk of infection, and suppression of normal corticosteroid production by the adrenal cortex. Adrenocortical suppression can have devastating or even fatal results if the exogenous (drug) form of the glucocorticoid is suddenly withdrawn because the body is temporarily incapable of synthesizing adequate amounts of these important compounds. Finally, it should be realized that glucocorticoids often treat a disease manifestation (inflammation) without resolving the underlying cause of the disease. For instance, older patients with rheumatoid arthritis may appear quite healthy as a result of this "masking" effect of glucocorticoids, whereas other sequelae of this disease (e.g., bone erosion, joint destruction) continue to worsen.

Other Drugs Used in Inflammatory Disease: Disease-Modifying Agents. Because NSAIDs and other anti-inflammatory drugs do not usually slow the disease process in rheumatoid arthritis, efforts have been made to develop drugs that try to curb the progression of this disease.[164,165] These so-called disease-modifying antirheumatic drugs (DMARDs) include an assortment of agents with different chemical and pharmacodynamic properties (see Table 4-4).[166] In general, these agents have immunosuppressive effects that blunt

the autoimmune response that is believed to underlie rheumatic joint disease. Some drugs in this category, such as methotrexate, produce a fairly nonselective effect on the immune system, and attempt to slow the proliferation of lymphocytes and reduce the production of various chemicals that promote autoimmune destruction of joint tissues.[167] More recently, several strategies have been developed to limit a specific component in the immune response. Etanercept (Enbrel), for example, selectively inhibits the effects of tumor necrosis factor-α, and anakinra (Humira) inhibits the effects of interleukin-1.[168,169] These agents and similar biologic response modifiers (see Table 4-4) may help slow the progression of rheumatoid arthritis when used alone or in combination with other DMARDs.[170]

Disease-modifying antirheumatic drugs have therefore been successful in arresting or even reversing some of the arthritic changes in certain patients with this disease.[171] Hence, DMARDs should be used fairly early in the course of rheumatoid arthritis so that these drugs can help prevent some of the severe joint destruction associated with this disease.[165,166] Regrettably, use of these DMARDs is limited in some patients because of toxic effects such as GI distress and renal impairment.[170] Research continues to determine which DMARDs or combinations of these agents will provide optimal benefits in people with rheumatoid arthritis.[172]

Cardiovascular Drugs

Cardiovascular disease is one of the leading causes of morbidity and mortality in older individuals. Various drugs are therefore used to prevent and treat cardiovascular problems in older adults, and many of these medications can directly affect rehabilitation of older adults. Cardiovascular drugs are often categorized according to the types of diseases they are used to treat. The pharmacotherapeutic management of some common cardiovascular problems seen in older adults is presented below, and drugs used to treat these problems are also summarized in Table 4-5.

Drugs Used in Geriatric Hypertension. An increase in blood pressure is commonly observed in older adults, and this increase is believed to be due to changes in cardiovascular function (e.g., decreased compliance of vascular tissues, decreased baroreceptor sensitivity) and diminished renal function (e.g., decreased ability to excrete water and sodium) that normally occur with aging.[173] A mild increase in blood pressure may not necessarily be harmful in the older adult and may in fact have a protective effect in maintaining adequate blood flow to the brain and other organs.[174] It is clear, however, that an excessive increase in blood pressure is associated with various cardiovascular problems such as stroke, coronary artery disease, and heart failure, and that efforts should be made to keep blood pressure within an acceptable range.[173,175] Current guidelines suggest that systolic

TABLE 4-5	Cardiovascular Drug Groups		
		Common Examples	
Drug Group	**Primary Indications**	**Generic Name**	**Trade Name**
α-Blockers	Hypertension	Phenoxybenzamine Prazosin	Dibenzyline Minipress
Angiotensin-converting enzyme inhibitors	Hypertension, CHF	Captopril Enalapril Quinapril	Capoten Vasotec Accupril
Angiotensin II receptor blockers	Hypertension, CHF	Irbesartan Losartan Valsartan	Avapro Cozaar Diovan
Anticoagulants	Overactive clotting	Heparin Warfarin	Liquaemin, Lovenox, others Coumadin
β-Blockers	Hypertension Angina Arrhythmias	Atenolol Metoprolol Nadolol Propranolol	Tenormin Lopressor Corgard Inderal
Calcium channel blockers	Hypertension Angina Arrhythmias	Diltiazem Nifedipine Verapamil	Cardizem Adalat, Procardia Calan, Isoptin
Centrally acting sympatholytics	Hypertension	Clonidine Methyldopa	Catapres Aldomet
Digitalis glycosides	CHF	Digoxin	Lanoxin
Diuretics	Hypertension, CHF	Chlorothiazide Furosemide Spironolactone	Diuril Lasix Aldactone
Drugs that prolong repolarization	Arrhythmias	Amiodarone Bretylium	Cordarone Bretylol
Organic nitrates	Angina	Nitroglycerin	Nitrostat, others
Presynaptic adrenergic depleters	Hypertension	Guanethidine Reserpine	Ismelin Serpalan
Sodium channel blockers	Arrhythmias	Quinidine Lidocaine	Cardioquin, others Xylocaine, others
Statins	Hyperlipidemia	Atorvastatin Fluvastatin Rosuvastatin Simvastatin	Lipitor Lescol Crestor Zocor
Vasodilators	Hypertension	Hydralazine Minoxidil	Apresoline Loniten

CHF, congestive heart failure.

and diastolic values in older adults should be less than 140 and 90 mmHg, respectively, or less than 130/80 in older adults with comorbidities such as chronic renal insufficiency or diabetes mellitus.[176]

Fortunately, a large and diverse array of antihypertensive agents is available for treating older adults with hypertension (see Table 4-5). Diuretic agents act on the kidneys to increase the excretion of water and sodium, thereby diminishing blood pressure by reducing the volume of fluid in the vascular system. Sympatholytic agents (e.g., β-blockers, α-blockers) work in various ways to interrupt sympathetic stimulation of the heart and peripheral vasculature. Vasodilators reduce peripheral vascular resistance by directly relaxing

vascular smooth muscle. Angiotensin-converting enzyme (ACE) inhibitors block the formation of angiotensin II, a potent vasoconstrictor that also produces adverse structural changes in vascular tissues. Likewise, angiotensin receptor blockers prevent angiotensin II from reaching vascular tissues, thereby reducing the harmful effects of angiotensin II on the heart and vasculature. Finally, calcium channel blockers inhibit the entry of calcium into cardiac muscle cells and vascular smooth muscle cells, thus reducing contractility in these tissues.

Which antihypertensive agent or agents will be used in a given older patient depends on several factors, such as the magnitude of the hypertension and any other medical problems existing in that patient. Often, two or more drugs are combined to provide optimal effects.[177,178] Concurrent use of a diuretic and β-blocker, for example, may provide better effects than could be achieved using either drug alone.[179] Other common antihypertensive strategies include a calcium channel blocker combined with an ACE inhibitor, or an ACE inhibitor combined with a diuretic.[180] In some situations, two antihypertensive drugs can be combined in the same pill to make it easier and more convenient to administer, and thus improve, patient adherence.[177] Other antihypertensive drugs can be added or substituted based on the individual needs of each patient.[181,182] Regardless of which agents are used initially, a successful antihypertensive drug regimen should be designed specifically for each patient and should incorporate the "low-and-slow" philosophy of starting with low doses of each drug and slowly increasing dosages as needed.

The various drugs that could be used to manage hypertension are all associated with specific side effects. A common concern, however, is that blood pressure will be reduced pharmacologically to the point where symptoms of hypotension become a problem. Therapists should always be aware that dizziness and syncope may occur as a result of low blood pressure when the patient is stationary and especially when the patient stands (orthostatic hypotension). Also, any physical therapy intervention that causes an additional decrease in blood pressure should be used very cautiously in geriatric patients who are taking antihypertensive drugs. Treatments such as systemic heat (e.g., large whirlpool, Hubbard tank) and exercise using large muscle groups may cause peripheral vasodilation that exaggerates the effects of the antihypertensive drugs to produce a profound and potentially serious decrease in blood pressure.

Drugs Used in Congestive Heart Failure. Congestive heart failure is a common disorder in older adults and is characterized by a progressive decline in cardiac pumping ability.[183,184] As the pumping ability of the heart diminishes, fluid often collects in the lungs and extremities (hence the term *congestive heart failure*). Treatment of this disorder typically consists of using drugs that improve myocardial pumping ability (e.g., digitalis glycosides, β-blockers) combined with drugs that reduce fluid volume and vascular resistance (e.g., diuretics, ACE inhibitors, angiotensin receptor blockers, vasodilators).[185-187] Digitalis glycosides such as digoxin cause an increase in myocardial pumping ability by a complex biochemical mechanism that increases the calcium concentration in myocardial cells. β-Blockers reduce excessive sympathetic stimulation of the heart, thus stabilizing heart rate and allowing more normal ventricular function in certain types of heart failure. Diuretics such as the aldosterone receptor blockers (e.g., spironolactone) are used to increase renal excretion of water and sodium, thus decreasing some of the excess fluid in the lungs and body tissues. ACE inhibitors, angiotensin receptor

blockers, and vasodilators, such as the organic nitrates, reduce peripheral vascular tone, thus decreasing the pressure the heart must pump against.

Each drug category used to treat heart failure is associated with specific adverse effects. Diuretics, for example, can cause fluid and electrolyte imbalances if too much water, sodium, or potassium is excreted by the kidneys. β-Blockers and nitrates can cause hypotension, thus leading to dizziness and syncope. These adverse effects, however, are typically dose-related and the agents are relatively safe at doses used to treat heart failure in older adults. Likewise, ACE inhibitors and angiotensin receptor blockers are often tolerated fairly well in older adults, although hypotension and orthostatic hypotension may occur when these drugs are first administered to older individuals. On the other hand, digoxin and similar drugs are often associated with some common and potentially serious adverse effects. These agents can accumulate rapidly in the bloodstream of an older patient, resulting in digitalis toxicity.[188] Digitalis toxicity is characterized by gastrointestinal symptoms (e.g., nausea, vomiting, diarrhea), CNS disturbances (e.g., confusion, blurred vision, sedation), and cardiac arrhythmias. Arrhythmias can be quite severe and may result in cardiac fatalities if digitalis toxicity is not quickly rectified. Physical therapists should be alert for signs of digitalis toxicity because early recognition is essential in preventing the more serious and potentially fatal side effects of these drugs.

Treatment of Cardiac Arrhythmias. Disturbances in cardiac rhythm—that is, a heart rate that is too slow, too fast, or irregular—may occur in older adults for various reasons.[189,190] Although some cardiac arrhythmias are asymptomatic and do not require any intervention, certain rhythm disturbances such as atrial fibrillation and complex ventricular arrhythmias should be treated to decrease the risk of stroke and sudden cardiac death in older adults.[190,191] A variety of different drugs can be used to stabilize heart rate and normalize cardiac rhythm, and these agents are typically grouped into four categories.[192] Sodium channel blockers (lidocaine, quinidine) control myocardial excitability by stabilizing the opening and closing of membrane sodium channels. β-Blockers (metoprolol, propranolol) normalize heart rate by blocking the effects of cardioacceleratory substances such as norepinephrine and epinephrine. Drugs that prolong cardiac repolarization (bretylium) stabilize heart rate by prolonging the refractory period of cardiac action potentials. Calcium channel blockers (diltiazem, verapamil) decrease myocardial excitability and conduction of action potentials by limiting the entry of calcium into cardiac muscle cells. Although different antiarrhythmic drugs have various side effects, the most common adverse reaction is an increased risk of cardiac arrhythmias[193]; that is, drugs used to treat one type of arrhythmia may inadvertently cause a different type of rhythm disturbance. Physical therapists should be alert for changes in cardiac rhythm by monitoring heart rate in older patients who are taking antiarrhythmic drugs.

Treatment of Angina Pectoris. Older adults often develop chest pain (angina pectoris) as a symptom of coronary artery disease. Organic nitrates such as nitroglycerin are the primary drugs used to prevent episodes of angina pectoris.[194] Angina typically occurs when myocardial oxygen demand exceeds myocardial oxygen supply. Nitroglycerin decreases myocardial oxygen demand by vasodilating the peripheral vasculature.[195] Peripheral vasodilation causes a decrease in the amount of blood returning to the heart (cardiac preload) as well as the amount of pressure in the vascular system that the heart must pump against (cardiac afterload). Consequently, cardiac workload and oxygen demand are temporarily reduced, thus allowing the anginal attack to subside.[196]

Nitrates can be administered at the onset of an anginal attack by placing the drug under the tongue (sublingually). These drugs can also be administered transdermally using drug-impregnated patches that allow slow, steady absorption of nitrate into the bloodstream. The use of nitrate patches has gained favor because the continuous administration of small amounts of drug may help prevent the onset or reduce the severity of anginal attacks.[194]

Several other drug strategies can also be used to reduce cardiac workload and prevent the onset of angina pectoris. These strategies include β-blockers, calcium channel blockers, and drugs that moderate the renin–angiotensin system (ACE inhibitors, angiotensin-receptor blockers).[194,196] Likewise, use of low-dose aspirin therapy or other platelet inhibitors can help prevent angina attacks from progressing to myocardial infarction.[194] It must be realized, however, that drug therapy often treats the symptoms of coronary artery disease (i.e., angina pectoris) but does not necessarily resolve the underlying issues that created an imbalance in the supply and utilization of oxygen in the heart (e.g., coronary artery atherosclerosis). Hence, drug therapy should always be combined with exercise and lifestyle changes that help restore a more normal balance between myocardial oxygen supply and demand.[194]

The primary adverse effects that may affect physical therapy are related to the peripheral vasodilating effects of the nitrates. Blood pressure may decrease in patients taking nitroglycerin, and dizziness due to hypotension is a common problem. Likewise, orthostatic hypotension may occur if the patient stands suddenly. Headache may also occur due to vasodilation of meningeal vessels. These side effects are most common immediately after the patient takes a rapid-acting sublingual dose. Hence, therapists should be especially concerned about hypotensive effects from the first minutes to 1 hour after a patient self-administers a sublingual dose of nitrates. Finally, patients who take nitrates sublingually must be sure to bring their medications with them to physical therapy so that the patient can self-administer the nitrate

if anginal symptoms occur during the rehabilitation session.

Treatment of Hyperlipidemia. Older adults may have high cholesterol levels and other plasma lipid disorders that can lead to atherosclerotic lesions and cardiovascular disease.[197] Hence, drug therapy should be combined with dietary changes to help improve plasma lipid profiles and reduce the risk of myocardial infarction and stroke.[198] Statins are the primary drug group used to manage lipid disorders[198,199] (see Table 4-5). These drugs, known also as hydroxymethylglutarate coenzyme A (HMG/ Co-A) reductase inhibitors, block a key enzyme responsible for cholesterol biosynthesis in the liver.[200] Reduced cholesterol production can help lower total cholesterol and produce other beneficial effects on plasma lipids such as reduced low-density lipoproteins and increased high-density lipoproteins. These agents may also produce a number of other favorable effects such as improving function of the vascular endothelium and stabilizing atherosclerotic plaques within the vascular wall.[200,201]

Statins are generally well tolerated, but some patients may develop serious muscle pain and inflammation (myopathy) when taking these drugs.[202,203] Although the exact reason for these myopathic changes is not clear, these drugs may impair skeletal muscle mitochondrial function and energy production in susceptible individuals.[204] Clinicians should therefore be alert for any muscle pain and weakness in patients taking statin drugs. Patients with these symptoms should be referred back to the physician immediately to consider whether these myopathic changes are drug induced and if drug therapy needs to be changed or discontinued.

Drugs Used in Coagulation Disorders. Excessive hemostasis, or a tendency for the blood to clot too rapidly, is a common and serious problem in older adults.[205] Formation of blood clots may result in thrombophlebitis and thromboembolism. These problems are especially important in the older patient after surgery and prolonged bed rest.[206] The use of two anticoagulants, heparin and warfarin, is a mainstay in preventing excessive hemostasis.[207,208] These agents work by different mechanisms to prolong and normalize the clotting time of the blood.[208,209] Although warfarin is taken orally, heparins must be administered by parenteral (nonoral) routes. The traditional or "unfractionated" form of heparin is usually administered via intravenous injection, whereas the newer or "low-molecular-weight" heparins such as enoxaparin (Lovenox) and dalteparin (Fragmin) can be administered by subcutaneous injection. Low-molecular-weight heparins are also safer than the traditional forms, thus offering a more convenient route of administration as well as decreased risk of adverse effects such as hemorrhage. Regardless of the type of heparin used, anticoagulant treatment often starts with heparin to achieve a rapid decrease in blood clotting, followed by long-term management of excessive coagulation through oral warfarin administration. Newer anticoagulant therapies include drugs like fondaparinux, an agent that directly inhibits clotting factor X, thus normalizing clotting time.[210] Clinical studies are helping to determine how these newer agents can be incorporated into anticoagulant regimens for older adults.

The most common problem with anticoagulant drug therapy is an increased tendency for hemorrhage.[209,211] Use of heparin and warfarin can result in too much of a delay in blood clotting, so that excessive bleeding occurs. Physical therapists should be cautious when dealing with open wounds or procedures that potentially induce tissue trauma (e.g., chest percussion, vigorous massage) because of the increased risk for hemorrhage.

Respiratory and Gastrointestinal Drugs

Drugs Used in Respiratory Disorders. Older adults may take drugs to treat fairly simple respiratory conditions associated with the common cold and seasonal allergies. Such drugs include cough medications (antitussives), decongestants, antihistamines, and drugs that help loosen and raise respiratory secretions (mucolytics and expectorants). Drugs may also be taken for more chronic, serious problems such as chronic obstructive pulmonary disease (COPD) and bronchial asthma.[212,213] Drug therapy for asthma and COPD includes bronchodilators such as β-adrenergic agonists (albuterol, epinephrine), xanthine derivatives (aminophylline, theophylline), and anticholinergic drugs (ipratropium, tiotropium). Corticosteroids may also be given to treat inflammation in the respiratory tracts that is often present in these chronic respiratory problems.

These respiratory drugs are associated with various side effects that may affect physical therapy of the older adult. In particular, older adults may be more susceptible to sedative side effects of drugs such as antihistamines and cough suppressants. For some of the prescription medications, side effects are often reduced if the medication can be applied directly to the respiratory tissues by inhalation.[214] For instance, even corticosteroids can be used fairly safely in older adults if these drugs are inhaled rather than administered orally and distributed into the systemic circulation. Inhaled forms of respiratory medications, however, can cause systemic side effects, especially when applied in higher doses or when used excessively.[215] Likewise, when these medications are administered systemically, lower doses of the prescription bronchodilators may be necessary in older adults. This fact is especially true in older patients with reduced liver or kidney function, because metabolism and elimination of the active form of the drug will be impaired. Finally, some older patients may use excessive amounts of certain over-the-counter products. Physical therapists should question the extent to which their geriatric patients routinely take large doses of cough suppressants, antihistamines, and other over-the-counter respiratory drugs.

Drugs Used in Gastrointestinal Disorders. Gastrointestinal drugs such as antacids and laxatives are among the most commonly used medications in older adults.[216,217] Antacids typically consist of a base that neutralizes hydrochloric acid, thus helping to alleviate stomach discomfort caused by excess gastric acid secretion. Other drugs that decrease gastric acid secretion include the H_2 blockers (e.g., cimetidine, ranitidine), which work by blocking certain histamine receptors (H_2 receptors) that are located in the gastric mucosa, and proton pump inhibitors (esomeprazole, omeprazole) that decrease formation of hydrochloric acid in the stomach by inhibiting transport of H^+ ions across the gastric lining. Laxatives stimulate bowel evacuation and defecation by a number of different methods depending on the drug used. Drugs used to treat diarrhea are also commonly taken by older patients. These drugs consist of agents such as opioids (diphenoxylate, loperamide) that help decrease GI motility and products such as the adsorbents (e.g., kaolin, pectin) that help sequester toxins and irritants in the GI tract that may cause diarrhea.

The major concern for GI drug use in older adults is the potential for inappropriate and excessive use of these agents.[218] Most of these drugs are readily available as over-the-counter products. Older individuals may self-administer these agents to the extent that normal GI activity is compromised. For instance, the older person who relies on daily laxative use (or possibly even several laxatives each day) may experience a decline in the normal regulation of bowel evacuation. Drugs may also be used as a substitute for proper eating habits. Antacids, for example, may be taken routinely to disguise the irritant effects of certain foods that are not tolerated well by the older adult. Physical therapists can often advise their geriatric patients that most GI drugs are meant to be used for only brief episodes of GI discomfort. Therapists can discourage the long-term use of such agents and advise their patients that proper nutrition and eating habits are a much safer and healthier alternative than prolonged use of GI drugs.

Hormonal Agents

General Strategy: Use of Hormones as Replacement Therapy. The endocrine glands synthesize and release hormones that travel through the blood to regulate the physiological function of various tissues and organs. If hormonal production is interrupted, natural or synthetic versions of these hormones can be administered pharmacologically to restore and maintain normal endocrine function. This replacement therapy is commonly used in older adults when endocrine function is diminished because of age-related factors (e.g., loss of ovarian hormones after menopause) or if endocrine function is lost after disease or surgery.[219] Some of the more common hormonal agents used in older adults are listed in Table 4-6 and are discussed here.

TABLE 4-6	Endocrine Drugs Groups		
		Common Examples	
Category	**Indication**	**Generic Name**	**Trade Name**
Androgens	Androgen deficiency	Methyltestosterone	Android, others
		Testosterone	AndroGel, others
Estrogens	Osteoporosis	Conjugated estrogens	Premarin, others
	Severe postmenopausal symptoms	Estradiol	Estrace, others
	Some cancers		
Insulin	Diabetes mellitus	—	Humulin, Novolin, others
Oral antidiabetics	Diabetes mellitus	Acarbose	Precose
		Chlorpropamide	Diabinese
		Glipizide	Glucotrol
		Metformin	Glucophage
		Repaglinide	Prandin
		Tolbutamide	Orinase
Antithyroid agents	Hyperthyroidism	Methimazole	Tapazole
		Propylthiouracil	Propyl-Thyracil
Thyroid hormones	Hypothyroidism	Levothyroxine (T$_4$)	Synthroid, others
		Liothyronine (T$_3$)	Cytomel

Estrogen Replacement. The primary female hormones—estrogen and progesterone—are normally produced by the ovaries from puberty until approximately the fifth or sixth decade when menopause occurs. Loss of these hormones is associated with a number of problems, including vasomotor symptoms (hot flashes), atrophic vaginitis, and atrophic dystrophy of the vulva. Replacement of the ovarian hormones, especially estrogen, can help resolve all these symptoms.[220] In addition, estrogen replacement can substantially reduce the risk of osteoporosis in postmenopausal women.[221,222] The effects of estrogen replacement on other physiological systems, however, is less clear. Some studies, for example, suggest that estrogen replacement can improve plasma lipid profile and might therefore reduce the risk of coronary heart disease when relatively low doses of estrogen are administered fairly soon after the onset of menopause.[223] Other studies, however, discovered an increased risk of stroke and venous thromboembolism, especially when higher doses were administered to older women (mid-60s).[224] Likewise, preliminary evidence suggested that estrogen may improve cognition and reduce the incidence of Alzheimer's disease in older women, but more recent studies have failed to confirm this effect.[225,226]

Estrogen replacement is therefore associated with certain beneficial effects, but there is concern that estrogen therapy may increase the risk of some forms of cancer, including breast and endometrial cancer, and that estrogen replacement may increase the risk of stroke and venous thromboembolic disease.[222,227] However, the exact relationship between estrogen replacement and the risk of cancer and cardiovascular disease remains uncertain.[228,229] The risks of these problems vary substantially from person to person, and other variables such as estrogen dose, combining estrogen with progesterone, the patient's age, and so forth, may greatly influence the adverse effects of estrogen replacement.[227,230]

At the present time, there is consensus that estrogen replacement therapy is not indicated for every woman after menopause, but that the risk–benefit ratio should be considered individually for each woman.[231,232] A woman, for example, with severe postmenopausal symptoms who is also at high risk for developing osteoporosis may be a good candidate for short-term estrogen replacement, provided, of course, that she does not have other risk factors that predispose to cancer or cardiovascular disease.[232] Likewise, newer estrogen-like compounds such as raloxifene and tamoxifen are an option for certain women. These agents, known also as selective estrogen-receptor modulators (SERMs), stimulate estrogen receptors on bone and certain cardiovascular tissues, while blocking estrogen receptors on breast and uterine tissues.[233] This selectivity may provide beneficial effects on bone and postmenopausal symptoms while decreasing the risk of breast cancer.[234] Efforts continue to develop effective and safer hormonal strategies for women who require estrogen replacement.

Androgen Replacement. In a situation analogous to postmenopausal women, certain older men may have reduced production of male hormones (androgens) such as testosterone. Testosterone production slowly declines with aging, but in certain men it may decline faster than normal.[235,236] Inadequate testosterone production is associated with several problems, including decreased lean body mass, increased body fat, decreased bone density, lack of energy, and decreased libido.[237] It therefore makes sense to identify men who might benefit from androgen replacement and provide small doses of testosterone-like drugs.[235]

Research suggests that androgen replacement can indeed improve body composition, bone density, mood, libido, and quality of life in older men who lack adequate endogenous testosterone production.[238,239] The primary concern, of course, is that androgen replacement may stimulate prostate growth and perhaps lead to prostate cancer. This risk, however, seems to be acceptable if specific, low-dose androgens are used to treat testosterone deficiencies in older men.[237,240] Future research will help confirm the best ways to screen potential candidates for androgen replacement and exactly which replacement strategies provide the best risk–benefit ratio in older men.

Diabetes Mellitus. Insulin is normally synthesized by pancreatic β cells, and this hormone regulates the metabolism of glucose and other energy substrates. Diabetes mellitus is a complex metabolic disorder caused by inadequate insulin production, decreased peripheral effects of insulin, or a combination of inadequate insulin production and decreased insulin effects. Diabetes mellitus consists of two principal types: type 1 and type 2 (known formerly as insulin-dependent and non-insulin-dependent diabetes mellitus, respectively). Type 1 diabetes mellitus is commonly associated with younger individuals, whereas type 2 diabetes mellitus occurs quite commonly in older adults.[241] Likewise, type 2 diabetes often occurs in older adults as part of a "metabolic syndrome" that consists of impaired glucose metabolism, obesity, hyperlipidemia, and hypertension.[242] If diabetes mellitus is not managed appropriately, acute effects (e.g., impaired glucose metabolism, ketoacidosis) and chronic effects (e.g., neuropathy, renal disease, blindness, poor wound healing) may occur.

Ideally, type 2 diabetes mellitus in older adults is managed successfully through diet, exercise, and maintenance of proper body weight.[242] When drug therapy is required, it is usually in the form of oral drugs (see Table 4-6).[243,244] These agents are taken orally to lower blood glucose levels, hence the term *oral hypoglycemic* or *oral antidiabetic*. Depending on the exact agent, these drugs help improve glucose metabolism by enhancing the release of insulin from the pancreas, increasing the sensitivity of peripheral tissues to insulin, stabilizing hepatic glucose output, or delaying absorption of glucose from the GI tract. In some people with type 2 diabetes, insulin can also be added to the drug regimen to provide optimal glucose control, especially in patients who are unable to achieve target glucose values with the oral drugs.[245]

The principal problem associated with drug therapy in older diabetic patients is that the blood glucose level may be reduced too much, resulting in symptoms of hypoglycemia.[246] Physical therapists should be alert for signs of a low blood glucose level, such as headache, dizziness, confusion, fatigue, nausea, and sweating.

Thyroid Disorders. The thyroid gland normally produces two hormones: thyroxine and triiodothyronine. These hormones affect a wide variety of tissues and are primarily responsible for regulating basal metabolic rate and other aspects of systemic metabolism. Thyroid dysfunction is quite common in older adults and can be manifested as either increased or decreased production of thyroid hormones.[247,248] Excess thyroid hormone production (hyperthyroidism, thyrotoxicosis) produces symptoms such as nervousness, weight loss, muscle wasting, and tachycardia. Inadequate production of the thyroid hormones (hypothyroidism) is characterized by weight gain, lethargy, sleepiness, bradycardia, and other features consistent with a slow body metabolism.

Hyperthyroidism can be managed with drugs that inhibit thyroid hormone biosynthesis, such as propylthiouracil, methimazole, or high doses of iodide.[249] The primary problems associated with these drugs are transient allergic reactions (e.g., skin rashes) and blood dyscrasias, such as aplastic anemia and agranulocytosis. A more permanent treatment of hyperthyroidism can be accomplished by administering radioactive iodine.[250] The radioactive iodine is taken up by the thyroid gland, where it selectively destroys the overactive thyroid tissues.

Hypothyroidism is usually managed quite successfully by replacement therapy using natural and synthetic versions of one or both of the thyroid hormones.[251,252] The most significant problem associated with thyroid hormone replacement in older patients is that older adults require smaller doses of these hormones than younger individuals.[252] Replacement doses that are too high evoke symptoms of hyperthyroidism, such as nervousness, weight loss, and tachycardia. Physical therapists should be alert for these symptoms when working with older patients who are receiving thyroid hormone replacement therapy.

Treatment of Infections

Various microorganisms such as bacteria, viruses, fungi, and protozoa can invade and proliferate in older individuals. Often the immune system is able to combat these microorganisms successfully, thus preventing infection. Occasionally, however, drugs must be used to supplement the body's normal immune response in combating infection caused by pathogenic microorganisms. Older adults are often susceptible to such infections, especially if their immune system has already been compromised by previous illness, a general state of debilitation, or prolonged use of immunosuppressant drugs such as the glucocorticoids. Two of the more common types of infections, bacterial and viral, are presented along with a brief description of the related drug therapy.

Antibacterial Drugs. Although some bacteria exist in the body in a helpful or symbiotic state, infiltration of pathogenic bacteria may result in infection. If the immune system is unable to contain or destroy these bacteria, antibacterial drugs must be administered. Some of the principal groups of antibacterial drugs are shown in Table 4-7. These agents are often grouped according to how they inhibit or kill bacterial cells. For instance, certain drugs (e.g., penicillins, cephalosporins) act by inhibiting bacterial cell-wall synthesis. Other drugs (e.g., aminoglycosides, tetracyclines) specifically inhibit the synthesis of bacterial proteins. Drugs such as the fluoroquinolones (e.g., ciprofloxacin) and sulfonamides (e.g., sulfadiazine) work by selectively inhibiting the synthesis and function of bacterial DNA and RNA. The selection of a specific agent from one of these groups is based primarily on the type of bacterial infection present in each patient.

The side effects that tend to occur with these agents vary from drug to drug, and it is not possible in this limited space to discuss all the potential antibacterial ADRs. With regard to their use in older patients, many of the precautions discussed earlier tend to apply. For instance, ADRs tend to occur more frequently because of the decreased renal clearance of antibacterial drugs in older adults.[253,254] Hence, physical therapists should be alert for any suspicious reactions in older patients who are taking antibacterial drugs, especially if renal function is already somewhat compromised. Resistance to antibacterial drugs is also a major concern in all age groups, including older adults.[255] Overuse and improper use of these agents have enabled certain bacterial strains to develop antidrug mechanisms, thus rendering these drugs ineffective against these bacteria. Physical therapists should be aware of the need to prevent the spread of bacterial infections through the use of frequent handwashing and other universal precautions.

Antiviral Drugs. Viruses are small microorganisms that can invade human (host) cells and use the biochemical machinery of the host cell to produce more viruses. As a result, the virus often disrupts or destroys the function of the host cell, causing specific symptoms that are indicative of viral infection. Viral infections can cause disease syndromes ranging from the common cold to serious conditions such as acquired immunodeficiency syndrome (AIDS). Because the viral invader usually functions and coexists within the host cell, it is often difficult to administer a drug that will kill the virus without simultaneously destroying the host cell. The number of antiviral agents is therefore limited (see Table 4-7), and these drugs often attenuate viral replication rather than actually destroy a virus that already exists in the body.

Because of the relatively limited number of effective antiviral agents, pharmacologic management of viral disease often focuses on preventing viral infection through the use of vaccines. Vaccines are usually a modified, inactive form of the virus that stimulates the patient's immune system to produce specific antiviral antibodies. When exposed to an active form of the virus, these antibodies help destroy the viral invader before an infection is established.

TABLE 4-7	Infection Drug Groups	
	Common Examples	
	Generic Name	Trade Name
Antibacterial Drugs		
Major Groups		
Aminoglycosides	Gentamicin	Garamycin; others
	Streptomycin	—
Cephalosporins	Cefaclor	Ceclor
	Cephalexin	Keflex; others
Erythromycins	Erythromycin	Many trade names
Fluoroquinolones	Ciprofloxacin	Cipro
	Norfloxacin	Noroxin
Penicillins	Penicillin G	Bicillin, many others
	Penicillin V	V-Cillin K, many others
	Amoxicillin	Amoxil, many others
	Ampicillin	Polycillin, many others
Sulfonamides	Sulfadiazine	Silvadene
	Sulfisoxazole	Gantrisin
Tetracyclines	Doxycycline	Vibramycin, others
	Tetracycline	Achromycin V, others
Antiviral Drugs		
Principal Indication		
Herpesviruses	Acyclovir	Zovirax
	Vidarabine	Vira-A
Cytomegalovirus	Foscarnet	Foscavir
	Ganciclovir	Cytovene
Influenza A	Amantadine	Symadine, Symmetrel
Human immunodeficiency virus (HIV)	Delavirdine	Rescriptor
	Didanosine	Videx
	Efavirenz	Sustiva
	Nelfinavir	Viracept
	Ritonavir	Norvir
	Saquinavir	Invirase
	Zalcitabine	Hivid
	Zidovudine (AZT)	Retrovir

Physical therapists should realize that the antiviral agents shown in Table 4-7 are often poorly tolerated and produce a number of adverse side effects, especially in older or debilitated patients.[256] Hence, prevention of viral infection through the use of vaccines is especially important in older adults. For instance, influenza vaccines are often advocated for older individuals before seasonal outbreaks of the "flu."[257,258] Of course, some vaccines are not always completely effective in preventing viral infections, and an appropriate vaccine has yet to be developed for certain viral diseases such as AIDS. Still, vaccines represent the most effective method of preventing viral infections in older individuals.

Cancer Chemotherapy

Cancer is the term used to describe diseases that are characterized by a rapid, uncontrolled cell proliferation and conversion of these cells to a more primitive and less functional state. Cancer is often treated aggressively through the use of a combination of several different techniques, such as surgery, radiation, and one or more cancer chemotherapeutic agents.

Older adults represent the majority of patients who will ultimately require some form of anticancer medication.[259] In general, the cancer chemotherapy regimens in older adults are similar to those used in younger individuals, with the exception that dosages are adjusted according to changes in liver and kidney function or other changes that affect drug pharmacokinetics.[260,261] The results of cancer chemotherapy in the older patient also parallel those seen in the younger individual, with the possible exception that some hematologic malignancies (certain leukemias) do not appear to respond as well to drug therapy in older adults.[262] The principal chemotherapeutic strategies and types of anticancer agents are presented here.

Basic Strategy of Cancer Chemotherapy. Traditional anticancer drugs work by inhibiting the synthesis and function of DNA and RNA. This action impairs the proliferation of cancer cells because they must rely on the rapid replication of genetic material in order to synthesize new cancer cells. Of course, DNA and RNA function is also impaired to some extent in healthy noncancerous cells, and this accounts for the many severe side effects and high level of toxicity associated with cancer chemotherapeutic agents.[263] Cancer cells, however, should suffer to a relatively greater degree because these cells typically have a greater need to replicate their genetic material in order to sustain a high rate of cell reproduction. Recently, however, several "targeted" drug strategies have been developed to better focus the effects of certain anticancer drugs on the malignant cells while sparing normal human tissues. Some of the general drug strategies used in cancer chemotherapy are outlined below.

Types of Anticancer Drugs. Anticancer medications are classified according to their biochemical characteristics and mechanism of action (Table 4-8).[264] For example, alkylating agents form strong bonds between nucleic acids in the DNA double helix so that the DNA strands within the helix are unable to unwind and allow replication of the cell's genetic code. Antimetabolites impair the normal biosynthesis of nucleic acids and other important cellular metabolic components necessary for cell function. Antimitotic agents directly inhibit the mitotic apparatus that is responsible for controlling the actual division of one cell into two identical cells (mitosis). Certain antibiotics are effective as anticancer agents because they become inserted (intercalated) directly into the DNA double helix and either inhibit DNA function or cause the helix to break at the point

TABLE 4-8	Cancer Drug Groups	
Major Groups	**Common Examples**	
	Generic Name	**Trade Name**
Alkylating agents	Busulfan	Myleran
	Carmustine	BCNU, BiCNU
	Cyclophosphamide	Cytoxan, Neosar
	Mechlorethamine	Mustargen
Antimetabolites	Cytarabine	Cytosar-U, others
	Floxuridine	FUDR
	Fluorouracil	Adrucil
	Methotrexate	—
Plant alkaloids	Paclitaxel	Taxol
	Vinblastine	Velban, Velsar
	Vincristine	Oncovin, Vincasar
Antineoplastic antibiotics	Daunorubicin	Cerubidine, others
	Doxorubicin	Adriamycin, others
	Idarubicin	Idamycin
Hormones		
Estrogens	Conjugated estrogens	Premarin, others
	Estradiol	Estrace, others
Antiestrogens	Tamoxifen	Nolvadex
Androgens	Testosterone	Many trade names
Antiandrogens	Flutamide	Eulexin
Biologic response modifiers	Interferon α-2a	Roferon-A
	Interferon α-2b	Intron A
	Interleukin-2	Proleukin
Monoclonal antibodies	Bevacizumab	Avastin
	Rituximab	Rituxan
Tyrosine kinase inhibitors	Imatinib	Gleevec
	Gefitinib	Iressa

where the drug is inserted. Hormones and drugs that block hormonal effects (antiestrogens, antiandrogens) are often used to attenuate the growth of hormone-sensitive tumors such as breast cancer and prostate cancer. Certain agents such as interferons, interleukin-2, and monoclonal antibodies are classified as biologic response modifiers because these drugs enhance the immune system's ability to destroy cancerous cells, or they selectively inhibit mechanisms within the cancer cells that cause proliferation of the cancer. Finally, several other "targeted" strategies such as angiogenesis inhibitors and tyrosine kinase inhibitors attempt to inhibit a specific biochemical trait of the cancer cell or tumor, thus focusing the drug's effect on the cancer cell with less harm to normal cells.

Anticancer drugs therefore inhibit replication and function of the cancer cell through one of the mechanisms just described. Likewise, several different drugs are often used simultaneously to achieve a synergistic effect between the antiproliferative actions of each drug.
Adverse Effects and Concerns for Rehabilitation. As mentioned, patients receiving cancer chemotherapy

typically experience a number of severe adverse drug effects. Side effects such as GI distress (e.g., anorexia, vomiting), skin reactions (e.g., hair loss, rashes), and toxicity of various organs are extremely common. Older patients receiving cancer chemotherapy are especially prone to certain adverse effects such as cardiotoxicity, neurotoxicity, and blood disorders (e.g., anemia, thrombocytopenia).[265,266] Unfortunately, these adverse effects must be tolerated because of the serious nature of cancer and the fact that death will ensue if these drugs are not used. In terms of rehabilitation of older patients, physical therapists must recognize that these adverse effects will inevitably interfere with rehabilitation procedures. There will be some days that the patient is simply unable to participate in any aspect of physical therapy. Still, the therapist can provide valuable and timely support for older adults receiving cancer chemotherapy and reassure the patient that these drug-related effects are often unavoidable because of the cytotoxic nature of the drugs.

General Strategies for Coordinating Physical Therapy with Drug Treatment in Older Adults

Based on the preceding discussion, it is clear that various medications can produce beneficial and adverse effects that may affect physical therapy of older adults in many different ways. There are, however, some basic strategies that therapists can use to help maximize the beneficial aspects of drug therapy and minimize the detrimental drug effects when working with geriatric individuals. These general strategies are summarized here.

Distinguishing Drug Effects from Symptoms

When evaluating a geriatric patient, therapists must try to account for the subjective and objective findings that may be due to ADRs rather than true disease sequelae and the effects of aging. For instance, the patient who appears confused and disoriented during the initial physical therapy evaluation may actually be experiencing an adverse reaction to a psychotropic drug, cardiovascular medication, or some other agent. The correct distinction of true symptoms from ADRs allows better treatment planning and clinical decision making.

As discussed earlier, therapists can also take steps to prevent inappropriate drug use and polypharmacy by helping distinguish ADRs from true disease symptoms. Distinguishing drug-related signs from true patient symptoms may require careful observation and consultation with family members or other healthcare professionals to see whether these signs tend to increase after each dosage. Periodic reevaluation should also take into account any changes in drug therapy, especially if new medications are added to the patient's regimen. Finally, the medical staff should be alerted to any change in the patient's response that may indicate an ADR.

Scheduling Physical Therapy Sessions Around Dosage Schedule

Physical therapy should be coordinated with peak drug effects if the patient's active participation will be enhanced by drug treatment. For instance, drugs that improve motor performance (e.g., antiparkinson agents), improve mood and behavior (e.g., antidepressants, antipsychotics), and decrease pain (e.g., analgesics) may increase the older patient's ability to take part in various rehabilitation procedures. Conversely, physical therapy should be scheduled when drug effects are at a minimum for older patients receiving drugs that produce excessive sedation, dizziness, or other adverse effects that may impair the patient's cognitive or motor abilities. Unfortunately, there is often a tradeoff between desirable effects and adverse effects with the same drug, such as the opioid analgesic that also produces sedation. In these cases, it may take some trial and error in each patient to find a treatment time that capitalizes on the drug's benefits with minimum interference from the adverse effects.

Promoting Synergistic Effects of Physical Therapy Procedures with Drug Therapy

One must not lose sight of the fact that many of the rehabilitation procedures used with geriatric clients may augment drug therapy. For instance, the patient with Parkinson's disease may experience an optimal improvement in motor function through a combination of physical therapy and antiparkinson drugs. In some cases, drug therapy may be reduced through the contribution of physical therapy procedures (e.g., reduction of pain medications through the simultaneous use of TENS, physical agents, and so forth). This synergistic relationship between drug therapy and physical therapy can help achieve better results than if either intervention is used alone.

Avoiding Potentially Harmful Interactions Between Physical Therapy Procedures and Drug Effects

Some physical therapy interventions used in older adults could potentially have a negative interaction with some medications. For instance, the use of rehabilitation procedures that cause extensive peripheral vasodilation (e.g., large whirlpool, some exercises) may produce severe hypotension in the patient receiving certain antihypertensive medications. These negative interactions must be anticipated and avoided when working with geriatric patients.

Improving Education and Compliance with Drug Therapy in Older Adults

Proper adherence to drug therapy is one area where physical therapists can have a direct impact. Therapists can reinforce the need for adhering to the prescribed regimen, and therapists can help monitor whether drugs have been taken as directed. Therapists can also help educate their geriatric patients and their families as to why specific drugs are indicated and what side effects should be expected and tolerated as opposed to side effects that may indicate drug toxicity.

CASE 4-1   PARKINSON'S DISEASE

Brief History

A 71-year-old male patient was diagnosed with Parkinson's disease 15 years ago. Drug therapy was initiated in the form of the dopamine agonist bromocriptine (Parlodel). Levodopa therapy was added to the drug regimen approximately 5 years ago when symptoms became incapacitating. Levodopa dosage was progressively increased over the next few years as the patient's condition gradually worsened. Recently, symptoms of bradykinesia and rigidity increased to the point that the patient's spouse was no longer able to care for him, and he was admitted to a nursing home. At the time of admission, the patient was receiving 500 mg of levodopa given in combination with 50 mg of carbidopa three times per day. Dosages were administered at mealtimes to decrease stomach irritation caused by these drugs. Upon admission, the patient began receiving daily physical therapy to help maintain mobility and joint range of motion.

Problem/Influence of Medication

The therapist began seeing the patient each morning in the physical therapy clinic at the nursing home. Although symptoms of rigidity and bradykinesia were fairly marked, the therapist found that the patient was able to actively participate to some extent in range-of-motion exercises and some ambulation activities. During the second session, however, the patient suddenly became extremely rigid and exhibited a complete loss of all voluntary movement. The therapist found this surprising because the patient had started the physical therapy session with a reasonable amount of voluntary motor activity. The patient had also completed the entire session on the preceding day without any such akinetic episodes. Upon further consideration, the therapist realized that the patient was seen later in the morning on the second day and that the akinetic episode occurred about 1 hour before the patient's next dose of levodopa.

Decision/Solution

The therapist realized that the patient was exhibiting end-of-dose akinesia. Patients who have been on levodopa therapy for several years often exhibit this phenomenon, in which the effectiveness of levodopa appears to wear off before the next dose. To prevent a recurrence of this problem, the therapist made a point of scheduling this patient about 1 hour after his initial (breakfast) dose of antiparkinson medications. This at least allowed the patient to participate as much as possible in his daily exercise regimen. The therapist also notified the patient's physician of the end-of-dose akinesia. This problem was ultimately resolved by increasing the levodopa dosage so that a sufficient amount of drug was available to maintain motor function throughout each dosing cycle.

CASE 4-2   LITHIUM TOXICITY

Brief History

A 76-year-old woman living at home fell and fractured her right hip. She was admitted to the hospital, where she underwent total hip arthroplasty. The patient had been in relatively good health before her fall but had been receiving treatment for bipolar syndrome (manic depression) for several years. At the time of admission, she was maintained on a dosage of 300 mg of lithium taken three times daily. The patient began receiving physical therapy in the hospital on the day after her hip surgery and was ambulating independently with a walker within 1 week after admission to the hospital. She was discharged to her home, but physical therapy was recommended at home to ensure continued progress and full recovery.

Problem/Influence of Medication

The physical therapist visiting this patient at home initially found her to be alert and enthusiastic about resuming her rehabilitation. By the second visit, however, the therapist noticed some confusion and slurred speech in this patient. Upon closer inspection, the therapist also observed symptoms such as hand tremors and muscle weakness. When ambulating, the patient exhibited some incoordination and became fatigued very easily.

Decision/Solution

The therapist became concerned of the potential for lithium toxicity in this patient. Apparently, the hip surgery and subsequent change in activity level in this patient had altered renal excretion of lithium to the extent that this drug was slowly accumulating in the patient's body. The therapist immediately notified the patient's physician. Laboratory tests revealed a serum concentration of 2.1 mEq/L, indicating moderate levels of lithium toxicity. The patient's dosage of lithium was decreased until serum levels returned to values that were within the therapeutic range. The patient continued to receive physical therapy at home and completed her recovery from hip surgery without any further incidents.

SUMMARY

Drug intervention in older adults can be regarded as a two-edged sword: The beneficial and therapeutic effects of any given medication must be balanced against the risk that the older adult will experience an adverse reaction to that drug. There is no doubt that many illnesses and afflictions that typically occur in a geriatric population can be alleviated through appropriate pharmacologic measures. However, the risk of ADRs is increased in older adults as a result of factors such as disproportionate drug use and an altered response to many medications. The potential for beneficial drug effects therefore coexists with an increased chance for serious adverse effects in the older adult.

Physical therapists must be aware of the drug regimen used in their older patients and how the beneficial and adverse effects of each medication can affect rehabilitation of these individuals. Physical therapists can also play an important role in recognizing ADRs in older adults. Finally, therapists can help encourage proper adherence to drug therapy and discourage the excessive and inappropriate use of unnecessary medications in their older patients. New drugs are regularly becoming available as well as new information about existing drugs. Box 4-1 provides a list of websites that are useful references for updated information about specific medications.

BOX 4-1 | Websites for Medication Updates

Drugs.com: www.drugs.com
Features:
Search box
News
Drugs A-Z
Drugs by condition
Pill identifier
Interactions checker

Epocrates*: http://online.epocrates.com/home
Features:
Search box
Alphabetical drug list
Drugs by class/subclass
Check drug interactions
Pill identifier

FDA website: www.fda.gov
Click on DRUGS
Features:
Spotlight (on current issues)
Recalls and alerts
Approvals and clearances

News and announcements
Drug safety
Search drugs box
Others

PubMed: www.ncbi.nlm.nih.gov/PubMed
National Library of Medicine's computerized bibliographic database; 3000+ peer-reviewed journals; covered since 1966.
Features:
Search articles by topic, author, or journals
Combine search terms (AND, OR, etc.), and use "limits" feature to refine search.

WebMD: www.webmd.com
Click on DRUGS & SUPPLEMENTS
Features:
Find a drug
Pill identifier
Drug news
Mobile drug information (downloads to certain handheld devices)
Vitamins and supplements
Others

*Note: this site offers other features including an option to download drug information to handheld devices. Some options require a subscription and fee to access.

REFERENCES

To enhance this text and add value for the reader, all references are included on the companion Evolve site that accompanies this text book. The reader can view the reference source and access it online whenever possible. There are a total of 266 cited references and other general references for this chapter.

CHAPTER 5

Exercise and Physical Activity for Older Adults

Patrick J. VanBeveren, PT, DPT, MA, OCS, GCS, CSCS,
Dale Avers, PT, DPT, PhD

Exercise is the single most efficacious intervention for older adults used by physical therapists. Exercise is known to simultaneously impact and mediate chronic disease, many impairments, functional deficits, quality of life, and cognition and prevent the negative sequelae associated with sedentary lifestyles. Combined with regular physical activity, appropriately prescribed exercise is the mainstay of the geriatric physical therapists' toolbox of interventions. This chapter discusses the role of physical activity and exercise, effects of a sedentary lifestyle, elements of an effective exercise prescription, and the different types of exercise applications for older adults.

ROLE OF PHYSICAL ACTIVITY

Physical activity is defined as any bodily movement that involves skeletal muscle contraction and that substantially increases energy expenditure.[1] Physical activity is typically leisurely activity, requires little to no supervision, is of lower intensity (3 to 6 metabolic equivalents [METs]) than exercise, and may be thought of as usual activity. In addition to leisure activities, often quoted guidelines for physical activity for older adults include the recommendation for 10,000 steps on a daily basis.[2] Exercise differs from physical activity in its intensity, and uses planned and repetitive body movements that are performed to achieve a goal such as increased strength, increased flexibility, or aerobic conditioning. Physical activity subsumes exercise, is not a skilled intervention, and should be encouraged with any exercise prescription.

The Centers for Disease Control and Prevention (CDC) has established specific physical activity recommendations for older adults to achieve important health benefits.[3] Older adults are encouraged to attain at least 150 minutes of *moderate-intensity* physical activity per week, recognizing that more activity has more robust health benefits. The CDC also recommends muscle strengthening exercise on 2 or more days per week that address all the major muscle groups

of the body.[3] Box 5-1 summarizes the CDC's physical activity recommendations for older adults.

The central role of physical activity and exercise is illustrated in the World Health Organization's International Classification of Function (Figure 5-1). The WHO model not only makes activity central but it also considers the role of environmental and personal factors that may pose barriers to physical activity and exercise. The WHO model is a useful reminder for physical therapists to incorporate physical activity into their plan of care while addressing impairments, activity limitations, and barriers to participation, including attitudes and self-efficacy.[4-6]

BOX 5-1 | CDC Physical Activity Guidelines for Older Adults

All older adults should engage in at least one of the following options on a regular basis to achieve the recommended amount of physical activity:

Option 1
- 2 hours 30 minutes (150 minutes) of *moderate-intensity* aerobic activity (i.e., brisk walking) every week
- Muscle strengthening exercise on 2 or more days a week that works all major muscle groups (legs, hips, back, abdomen, chest, shoulders, and arms)

Option 2
- 1 hour 15 minutes (75 minutes) of *vigorous-intensity* aerobic activity (i.e., jogging or running) every week
- Muscle strengthening exercise on 2 or more days a week that works all major muscle groups (legs, hips, back, abdomen, chest, shoulders, and arms)

Option 3
- An equivalent mix of moderate- and vigorous-intensity aerobic activity
- Muscle strengthening exercise on 2 or more days a week that works all major muscle groups (legs, hips, back, abdomen, chest, shoulders, and arms)

(http://www.cdc.gov/physicalactivity/everyone/guidelines/olderadults.html)

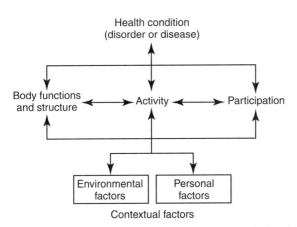

Health condition
(disorder or disease)

Body functions
and structure ⟷ Activity ⟷ Participation

Environmental
factors

Personal
factors

Contextual factors

FIGURE 5-1 World Health Organization's International Classification of Function.

Physical inactivity is a significant risk factor for developing many chronic conditions that impact functional mobility in older adults, and for increasing the risk of additional disability in someone who already has a chronic condition (Box 5-2). Physical activity is so vital to health and function that Lees and Booth have coined

BOX 5-2   Common Chronic Conditions and the Impact of Physical Inactivity

Physical Inactivity Is a Significant Risk Factor for the Development of Many Chronic Health Conditions
Heart disease
Cancer: breast, colon, prostate, and
    pancreatic
Congestive heart disease
Depression
Hypertension
Cognitive disease
Type 2 diabetes
Obesity
Osteoporosis
Peripheral vascular disease
Physical frailty
Sleep apnea
Osteoarthritis
Stroke
Balance problems and falls
Physical Inactivity Increases the Risk of Disability in Individuals with Various Chronic Health Conditions Including
Chronic back pain
Balance problems and falls
Stroke
Arthritis
Frailty
Debilitating illness
Long-term chemotherapy
Total joint arthroplasties
Lower extremity fracture
Parkinson's disease

the term *sedentary death syndrome* to dramatize the deleterious effects of inactivity.[7] Many of these conditions are prevalent in older adults and therefore often seen by physical therapists. The successful therapist is aware of the central role of physical activity in any treatment plan. For many of the conditions listed, inactivity has a direct physiological effect on pathology/disease (e.g., the deconditioning of the cardiovascular system). However, for some of the conditions listed, the pathology is made worse because of impairments that develop affect function. Accelerated loss of strength that impairs balance and mobility is often the end result of inactivity. The loss of function is from the weakness and not directly from the disease/pathology. The loss of mobility rather than the medical condition becomes the functional consequence that causes the individual's disability. In all of the conditions listed, inactivity increases the mobility disability associated with the condition. For physical therapists, the ultimate goal of activity/exercise may not be to affect the pathology but rather to improve mobility and function and thereby decrease the patient's mobility disability.

Mobility disability encompasses a common set of impairments and functional deficits that combine to interfere with one's normal ability to walk and move about in the community. Gill et al defined mobility disability as an inability to walk one quarter of a mile and to climb a flight of stairs.[8] Mobility disability is most often brought about through a temporary sedentary lifestyle such as may occur as a consequence of a hospitalization or prolonged recovery.[8]

Physical activity protects against mobility disability. Simonsick et al found that the likelihood of a new mobility disability increased by 65% in men and 37% in women for each 30-second increase over 5 minutes needed to complete a 400-m walk test.[9] Yet, only 23% of older adults achieve the CDC's physical activity recommendations and only 12% participate in strengthening exercises.[10] Clearly, as the population of older adults increases, the role of physical activity becomes even more critical for prevention and intervention.

THE SLIPPERY SLOPE OF AGING

Even with physical activity, there are physical effects of growing older. The age-related loss of strength is one of the most critical factors contributing to mobility disability and therefore greatly interests physical therapists working with older adults. In the average adult, strength decreases at a rate of 10% per decade starting at age 30 years, accelerating to 15% per decade after age 60 years or so.[11] If older adults are not physically active or did not build a reserve of strength in their younger years through physical activity and exercise, the result of this strength loss can be significant mobility disability.[8,12,13] Some authors believe that the concurrent but accelerated loss of power that occurs with age at a rate of 20% to 30% per decade is even more critical to the onset of mobility disability.[14-18]

Interestingly, the other physiological systems decline at approximately the same rate. These include the cardiac and respiratory systems, the hepatic and renal systems, and the cognitive and sensory systems (vision and hearing).[19,20] Figure 5-2 depicts this systemic loss graphically, implying that with age comes a risk of a downward trajectory through categories that Schwartz has defined as fun, function, frailty, and failure.[21] *Fun* is the physical ability to do whatever one wants, whenever one desires, for as long as desired. The *function* category represents those who have to make choices about their activities based on some decreased physical capacity. The functional category represents those who are at risk for mobility disability or have some degree of mobility disability. An example would be taking a motorized cart through the airport instead of walking, for fear of fatigue or inability to make one's plane on time. The *frail* category includes those who require help with instrumental and basic activities of daily living (IADLs and BADLs). Fried et al[135] has characterized frailty as a clinical syndrome whose characteristics are well known to physical therapists working with older adults, especially in nursing homes (Box 5-3). Finally, the *failure* category includes those who are completely dependent and often bedbound.

Bassey et al have determined that 24% of baseline strength is required to walk, underscoring the functional impact of the dramatic loss of strength that many individuals in nursing homes have sustained.[24] Leg strength has been shown to be the single most important predictor of subsequent institutionalization, and it is more important than physiological markers or disease.[25] Because no other organ system affects mobility as directly as skeletal muscle does, the muscular system can be characterized as the entryway to frailty.[20] The relationship between

| BOX 5-3 | Criteria for Frailty as a Clinical Syndrome as Proposed by Fried et al[135] |

Frailty Criteria:
- Unintentional weight loss of 10 lb or more in the past year
- Self-reported exhaustion (person states they are exhausted 3 or more days per week)
- Muscle weakness (grip strength in lowest 20%: <23 lb for women; <32 lb for men)
- Walking speed in the lowest 20% (<0.8 m/sec)[22]
- Low level of activity (kcal/week–lowest 20%: 270 kcal/wk for women; 383 kcal/wk for men equivalent to sitting quietly and/or lying down for the vast majority of the day)

A person is considered *frail* if he or she meets 3 of these 5 frailty criteria.

A person is considered *prefrail* if he or she meets one or two of these frailty criteria.

strength and well-being, including functional mobility, places enormous responsibility on physical therapists to create and deliver an effective strengthening exercise program.

Aging is not an automatic descent into frailty, as reflected by the high level of function of many older athletes. It is desirable and possible for older adults to stay functioning in the "fun" category well into very old age. Indeed, many aging adults are able to maintain a very high, active lifestyle that includes tennis, skiing, hiking, biking, and running well into late life. A continuous, high level of physical activity is the key to maintaining a quality of life that allows individuals "to die young at a very old age."

Taking into account the slippery slope of functional decline in aging, the role of physical activity and muscular strength is clear. To appropriately set goals that will have long-range health benefits and reduce or prevent mobility disability, physical therapists should be aware of the normative values of mobility, including usual and fast gait speed, distance walked in 6 minutes, chair rise time, stair climbing, and floor rise (Table 5-1).

Applying the appropriate principles of an exercise prescription should seek not only to return an individual to his or her previous level of function but also to increase physical reserves to return the individual to a higher level of function. Physical therapists need to recognize that a patient's "prior level of function" is not always that good and is the reason that the patient is in the care of a physical therapist. In addition, building reserve through exercise may help decrease the relapse so often seen after discharge from physical therapy.

In light of the overwhelming and compelling role of physical activity in protecting from disability and the strong evidence for the effects of exercise, physical therapists have a professional responsibility to apply exercise in the most efficacious manner possible. Understanding the principles of the exercise prescription is a necessary first step.

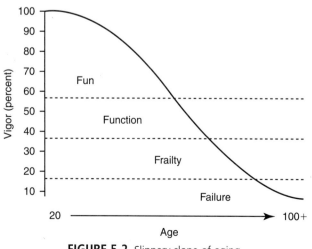

FIGURE 5-2 Slippery slope of aging.

TABLE 5-1	Estimated Values for Functional Markers			
	Fun	**Function**	**Frail**	**Failure**
Gait speed	>1.5 m/sec	0.8–1.5 m/sec	0.3–0.8 m/sec	<0.3 m/sec
Six-minute walk test	>500 m	350–500 m	200–350 m	<200 m
Chair rise 30 sec without hands	>15 repetitions	8–15 repetitions	<8 repetitions	Unable
Stair climbing 10 stairs	<10 sec without rails	10–30 sec with or without rails	30–50 sec with rails	Unable
Floor transfer	<10 sec without assist	10–30 sec with or without assist	>30 sec with assist	Unable

The categories indicate what may be necessary to move an older adult to the next higher category, a worthwhile goal if physical therapists are to have a significant impact on mobility disability.
m, meters; *m*/sec, meters per second; *sec*, seconds.

HISTORY OF STRENGTHENING EXERCISE

Some of the earliest recorded literature regarding strengthening exercise occurred after World War II when there was an urgent need to rehabilitate injured veterans returning from the war. An early seminal author was Thomas DeLorme, who wrote about his method to increase strength.[26] He suggested three progressive sets of each exercise based on a 10 repetition maximum (RM; i.e., a weight that can be lifted only 10 times with good form). DeLorme suggested a weight of 50% of a 10 RM for the first set, 75% of a 10 RM for the second set, and 100% of a 10 RM for the third set. He believed that the first two sets only served as warm-ups, and the third set was the actual stimulus to cause the strength increase.

In spite of DeLorme's efforts, little was written about exercise and fitness until the early 1970s when a strong link was made between aerobic conditioning and cardiovascular health. At that time, the United States was experiencing an unprecedented rise in cases of cardiovascular disease. The 1970s was a time of urban migration to the suburbs, increasing the use of automobiles and decreasing walking. The fitness recommendations from the American College of Sports Medicine (ACSM) in 1978 focused on cardiac fitness and body composition. Starting in the mid-1980s, there was a boom in the fitness industry and a concurrent renewed interest in strengthening as a component of fitness. The late 1980s and early 1990s saw increased research about strengthening exercises that has persisted through today. However, the ACSM did not add strengthening to its recommendations for adult fitness until the early 1990s.

At about the same time that the ACSM included strengthening in their fitness recommendations, Fiatarone et al authored a landmark study on the effects of a strengthening exercise program in older adults age 90 years or older living in a nursing home.[27] Although the number of subjects was small, the reported strength gains were on the order of 200% with a concurrent improvement in function. Her results were achieved using a strengthening stimulus of 80% of a 1 RM. A few years later, Evans offered strength-training guidelines for older

adults that also suggested high-intensity exercise.[28] These two researchers began the line of research that informs our current knowledge of strengthening and exercise for older adults. Fiatarone Singh reviewed the multiple benefits of strength training in older adults for nearly all chronic diseases common to aging.[29] Based on the compelling effects of strengthening exercise and the insidious loss of strength with age, we believe strengthening exercise would be the *first* type of exercise prescribed. Strengthening exercises improve joint integrity, which reduces pain from osteoarthritis. There is also evidence that strengthening exercises improve endurance more than aerobic exercises do in patients with chronic obstructive pulmonary disease.[30]

PHYSICAL STRESS THEORY

The physical stress theory (PST) has been the foundation of exercise prescription for many years. The PST is the predictable response of tissues, organs, and systems to mechanical and physiological stressors.[31] The PST explains the effect of overload or insufficient load on tissues, organs or systems, as well as the lack of change in tissues, organs, and systems if a "usual" stress is applied consistently. If more than usual stress (overload) is put on a tissue, the tissue responds by increasing its ability to absorb and dissipate that stress. If too much stress is placed on a tissue, the tissue is susceptible to injury (or even death, as in the case of integumentary tissue). Conversely, if too little stress is consistently placed on a tissue, the tissue loses its ability to absorb and dissipate stresses; that is, the tissue atrophies (Box 5-4).

Every tissue, organ, or system predictably responds to stress or a lack of stress in a like manner. For example, the PST predicts how skin will respond to stressors placed on it. If usual stress is placed on the skin and all other factors remain constant, the skin will not change; if less than usual stress is placed on the skin, the skin softens and loses its ability to absorb mechanical stress. This softening or atrophying of the skin is then susceptible to blistering even under the condition of usual stress

BOX 5-4	**Physical Stress Theory**	
Too much stress	(>100% of maximum)	→ Injury or tissue death
Appropriate overload	(60% to 100% of maximum)	→ Strengthening
Usual stress	(40% to 60% of maximum)	→ No change in tissue
Too little stress	(< 40% of maximum)	→ Atrophy
No stress	(0% of maximum)	→ Loss of ability to adapt (death)

such as when doing gardening or shoveling. If greater than usual stress is gradually applied to the skin over a period of time, the skin will toughen and eventually form a callus that further protects itself from high-level forces. The same principles apply to the cardiorespiratory and musculoskeletal systems. The effects of too little stress on the cardiorespiratory system are well known to physical therapists, appearing in the form of deconditioning that eventually increases the risk of some diseases. The effects of too little stress on the skeletal system manifest itself in osteoporosis. Therefore, physical therapists use the principles of the PST when they prescribe aerobic exercise to improve cardiovascular capacity or weight-bearing and resistive exercises to improve bone strength in the presence of osteoporosis. Physical activity and exercise that appropriately stress tissues can be modified to achieve the desired result, for example, strength, flexibility, or muscular endurance.

The ability of tissue to absorb and dissipate forces is dependent on many variables, including the time over which the stressor is applied; the direction, magnitude, and combination of stressors applied; the physiological condition of the tissue, organ, or system; the frequency of the application of a stressor and length of time between the applications; and even the psychological state of the person and the "environment" in which the stressor is applied. In the clinic, physical therapists can modify these variables within an exercise program to achieve a desired outcome. For example, the PST can be used to positively impact the cardiopulmonary, musculoskeletal, and vestibular systems in a frail older woman who has been sedentary for several years and now has increased fall risk and an inability to tolerate walking 1000 feet (community distance) at a reasonable pace. The physical therapist may choose initially to promote safety and reduce the risk of falling by having her use a walker for support and to decrease her unsteadiness, thus reducing the demand of the task to a level that matches the patient's current capabilities. Resistance exercise of an appropriate intensity, based on a 10 RM can then be prescribed to stress the tissue beyond what is typically experienced and at a level that will promote

change in muscle tissue. Physical activity in the form of walking may be encouraged through the use of a pedometer to monitor required levels of physical activity to promote conditioning of the cardiopulmonary system. The standard of a percentage of $\dot{V}o_2$ max can be used to determine the appropriate level of response, monitored through vital signs and/or pulse oximetry. Walking activity several times a day over increasingly longer distances can be monitored and supported by caregivers including family members, paid, and/or voluntary support personnel. Balance activities that address a hypoactive vestibular and somatosensory system can be incorporated in a gradually challenging manner to increase response time and accurate reactions. Self-efficacy and motor learning feedback principles can be incorporated to appropriately stress the psychological system. As each system responds, challenges (stressors) are added to that system for continuous adaptation. However, if too little challenge occurs, such as in too little resistance, too short a walking distance, or too slow a pace, little to no change will occur.

The concept of progression is also inherent in the PST. Once the tissue, organ, system, and person adapt to being able to absorb and dissipate a certain level of stressor, this level becomes the usual or maintenance level, and increased levels of stress are needed to achieve further gains. For example, a patient may achieve the ability to ambulate without an assistive device. Continued ambulation without greater challenge for the patient will be insufficient to provide a stimulus for further improvement. However, stimulating the patient's ability by having him or her carry a weight or walk on uneven surfaces may further overload the patient, making continued improvement possible.

ELEMENTS OF AN EXERCISE PRESCRIPTION

An exercise prescription should incorporate all necessary parameters to promote the desired change to a system. Appropriately designed exercise is a powerful intervention. Moreover, when attention is paid to appropriately manipulating the type of exercise, intensity, duration, frequency, type of contraction, speed of contraction, and concepts of motor learning, the outcome of exercise can be more accurately predicted. This section discusses the critical parameters of an exercise prescription that can be manipulated to achieve the most benefit from an exercise program.

Overload

In 1970, Moffroid and Whipple proposed that overload was the critical parameter needed to extend the limits of muscular performance and that appropriate intensity of exercise was needed to achieve high levels of function.[32] In 2000, the ACSM noted a necessary dose–response relationship such that muscle tissue must be exposed to a stimulus of at least 60% of the muscle's maximum force-generating capacity, to improve that muscle's force. The dose–response relationship states that the greater the stimulus, the greater the improvement.[33] To achieve improvement from any type of exercise, the exercise prescription must meet this minimal requirement of 60% of maximum tissue capability. It is easy to see how the application of the PST occurs for all exercise. In the case of aerobic exercise, a minimum stimulus of 60% of maximum capacity is necessary to achieve improved conditioning,[1] and in the case of a resistance exercise, an overload of at least 60% or a 15 RM is necessary to create significant strength gains that will also translate to functional gains.[34-36] Although it may be advisable to start with lower intensities in frail or severely deconditioned older adults to allow for gradual accommodation, a stimulus below 60% of maximum will not produce significant change.[37] Therefore, slow walking or lifting light weights such as 2 lb ankle weights to stimulate the quadriceps will not appreciably improve aerobic capacity or strength in most individuals. The ACSM and others have suggested that an intensity of 80% of a 1 RM is a preferred workload to obtain optimal results,[1,10] although a gradual increase beginning at 50% (usual stimulus) would provide a threshold for a progressive increase in workload stimulus for an individual who has been sedentary.

Assessment of Overload Stimulus. Determining the appropriate overload stimulus to achieve an adaptive response requires knowledge of thresholds for adaptation for the aerobic and muscular systems. For example,

the aerobic stimulus that is required to achieve a conditioning response is determined by a percentage of a $\dot{V}o_2$ max and can be calculated using a variety of methods. Measuring aerobic overload will be discussed in the section on aerobic exercise. For strengthening, the appropriate stimulus is classically determined by the 1 RM—defined as the resistance that can be moved one time and one time only before muscular fatigue to the degree of failure or loss of form has occurred.[1] One repetition maximum is the inability to generate enough force to move the resistance through full range again. Further discussion about measuring strength occurs later in this chapter.

Other useful ways of assessing overload are the Borg Scale of Perceived Exertion (RPE),[38] modified scale of perceived exertion, and the talk test[39,40] (Table 5-2). These scales are used interchangeably to determine overload in both the cardiovascular and muscular systems for all aged individuals, as explained later in this chapter.

Specificity

Specificity is achieved by prescribing exercises that match the type of muscle contraction, the speed of contraction, and consideration of the functional movement inherent in the desired outcome. Most authors agree that functional improvement occurs when the exercise stimulus closely matches the desired result.[32,41] Therefore, if you are attempting to strengthen the quadriceps to improve a client/patient's ability to get out of a chair, it would be more effective to work on overloading a squatting

TABLE 5-2	Rate of Perceived Exertion			
Modified Scale	**Ordinal Scale[38]**	**Percentage Effort Scale**	**Perceived Workload Scale**	**Talk Test[39]**
	6	20% effort	Very, very light	Rest
	7	30% effort		
	8	40% effort		
1	9	50% effort	Very light	Gentle walking or "strolling"
2	10	55% effort		
3	11	60% effort	Fairly light	Steady pace, not breathless
	12	65% effort		
4	13	70% effort	Somewhat hard	Brisk walking, able to carry on a conversation
	14	75% effort		
5	15	80% effort	Hard	Very brisk walking, must take a breath between groups of 4–5 words
	16	85% effort		
7	17	90% effort	Very hard	Unable to talk and keep pace
8	18	95% effort		
9	19	100% effort	Very, very hard	
10	20	Exhaustion		

movement or adapting the chair height than to strengthen the lower limb with open-chain, full-arc extension. The importance of specificity in strength training was documented by Sale in investigating squat performance.[42] Subjects who trained by performing a squat exercise improved twice as much as those performing either the leg press or open-chain knee extension, when squatting was *used as the outcome measure*. And those doing the leg press improved more so than those doing knee extension when squatting was used as the outcome measure (Figure 5-3), presumably because the leg press more closely mimics the squat compared to open-chain knee extension. Thus, there would be little basis for the use of straight leg raises to achieve a functional movement such as walking or stair climbing. Similarly, there is little basis for performing knee extension in a sitting position, unless one is training the older individual to kick from a sitting position. Current knowledge of the specific actions of the muscles involved in a movement is critical to apply the specificity concept. For example, years ago, it was thought that the vastus medialis contracted independently of the other quadriceps muscles, justifying a need to strengthen it separately. Many therapists advocated and were taught to use the adductors and an adduction movement to facilitate the vastus medialis's contraction. An exercise of wall sits with a ball between the legs was created based on this former understanding. However, more recently it has been discovered that the entire quadriceps contract as a whole and the vastus medialis does not contract separately. Furthermore, it is now hypothesized that the gluteus medius and maximus are critical in controlling the varus/valgus moment of the knee.[43]

The specificity concept has led to the contemporary practice of functional strengthening. Functional strengthening is the concept of strengthening a movement rather than a muscle.[41] An analysis of any movement shows that functional activities are multiplanar and asymmetrical, incorporate rotation, and are speed and balance dependent. Therefore, exercise aimed at improving function should meet the same criteria. Athletes have known for some time that the most efficient use of training-time and effort is to practice the event in which they are competing. We have been slow to incorporate that practice into rehabilitation. Table 5-3 and Figures 5-4 through 5-8 provide some suggestions of exercises that are critical to specific functional movements. Many of these exercises are illustrated later in this chapter.

In addition to specificity, the concepts of overload and a training stimulus of at least 60% to promote functional strength gains are critical in designing the exercise program. Simply walking a patient may not improve the patient's performance in walking above a critical threshold if there is no overload or challenge present. To overload the patient's gait, challenge their speed of walking, ambulate on unlevel surfaces, incorporating head turns while walking, and/or carry a large object that blocks direct vision of the patient's feet or have the patient move through an obstacle course.

Functional Training

Physical therapists have long recognized that any functional activity is a complex neuromuscular event that incorporates multiple systems. These systems include but are not limited to the muscular and articular systems, proprioceptive and cutaneous sensory systems, and vestibular and visual systems. Functional training refers to overloading the movement or activity of interest to challenge this whole neuromuscular system rather than simply challenging a muscle. Instead of breaking down a movement into individual muscle actions, functional training challenges the patient to use multiple joints through multiple axes of motion incorporating body weight and balance. For example, to improve the skill of transferring, the patient can be challenged throughout the transfer movement while he or she holds on to an object or weight[44] (Figure 5-8). Historically, functional training has been applied by physical therapists to injured workers in work hardening programs. Similarly, the approach could be used for an older adult who is having difficulty with outdoors ambulation by having the patient walk as quickly as possible through an obstacle course that incorporates uneven surfaces, different heights and kinds of surfaces and obstacles. Rose's concept of mall walking whereby a person moves through other people walking past the person is an example of functional training incorporating the visual, proprioceptive, vestibular, and muscular systems by manipulating environmental challenges. Progression of a functional exercise program is obtained by moving from

1. simple movements to more complex movements,
2. normal speed to either quicker or slower movements,
3. stable surfaces to unstable or compliant surfaces,
4. eyes open to eyes closed, and

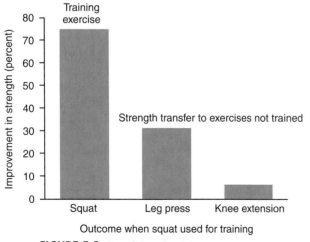

FIGURE 5-3 Specificity of training on outcome.

TABLE 5-3	Functional Movements, Key Muscle Groups, and Sample Exercises	
Functional Movement	**Key Muscles**	**Exercises**
Bed mobility	Abdominals, erector spinae, gluteus maximus	Bridge progression (Figure 5–4, A–D) Sit backs Plank (modified and full) Prone hip extension (single and double) Side plank (regular and modified) (Figure 5–5)
Transfers and squats	Gluteus maximus, medius, and obturator externus, piriformis, quadriceps	Sit to stand Squats with knees abducted and hips externally rotated Leg press, wall slides
Ambulation and stair climbing	Abdominals, erector spinae, gluteus maximus and medius, obturator externus, piriformis, quadriceps, and anterior tibialis and gastroc-soleus	Bridge progression (Figure 5–4, A–D) Sit backs Plank (modified and full) (Figure 5–5) Prone hip extension (single and double) Step ups (varied heights) Eccentric step downs (Figure 5–6) Forward and backward stepping with and without resistance Heel raises (single and double) Toe tapping with and without resistance and speed Concentric followed by eccentric dorsiflexion (Figure 5–7)
Floor transfers	Abdominals, erector spinae, gluteus maximus and medius, obturator externus, piriformis, quadriceps, and gastroc-soleus	Kneeling with trunk rotations, extension, upper extremity movements, quadriped trunk rotations and hip extensions
Fast gait and jumping	Gastroc-soleus, gluteus maximus and medius, quadriceps	Skipping, fast foot placement on target, hopping, fast walking and jogging for short distances

5. an emphasis on form to an emphasis on intensity and the working over from base of support to working outside the base of support.

Functional training can be used for balance and strengthening by having the patient progress from parallel stance to a staggered stance to tandem stance and finally to unilateral stance. At the same time, the patient can be challenged to perform activities further and further away from his or her base of support through multiple planes of movement, then with eyes closed, moving his or her head, and progressing to a compliant surface. Squats and lunges can also be incorporated into functional training using the same base of support and principles of progression. Finally, functional training can be incorporated into gait training by having the patient move in various directions (front, back, sideways, or diagonally), using walking, marching, jogging, skipping, jumping, or bounding movements while also using obstacles, head turns, changes in visual input, and on various compliant or uneven surfaces.

Speed and Power. Power is defined as the time rate of force development. The more powerful a muscle contraction, the more rapidly the muscle can produce a given level of force. Loss of speed and power is associated with frailty, falls, and slow gait speed; slow gait speed is predictive of loss of ADL ability and future institutionalization.[45-49] Many authors have suggested that power rather than force is a better predictor of

function.[17,45,46,50,51] Some authors have suggested that the slowness of movements and gait that so commonly occurs with age may occur because of a predilection for the loss of type II or fast-twitch muscle fibers. Other authors feel that generalized slowing might be in response to disuse. Because higher training speed produces improvement in power in older adults who train, more credibility has been given to the second theory.[52-54]

Speed is a necessary component of certain functional movements such as crossing a street with a timed traffic signal, getting to the bathroom in time, and walking with pedestrian traffic. Training for speed is an application of specificity and a necessary component of functional activities. Speed of movement can be used to challenge patients. Having patients perform an activity such as changing the speed of tandem walking can challenge balance. Another way to "overload" the speed of a functional movement is to time the patient as they perform the task. For example, rising from the floor is an essential task for older adults so a fear of not being able to rise from the floor is strongly related to a fear of falling.[55] Timing the patient's transfer from floor to standing can motivate the individual and provide an additional challenge after the individual can achieve the basic floor transfer independently. Having the patient perform the transfer on a compliant surface and then adding a timed component could achieve further overload.

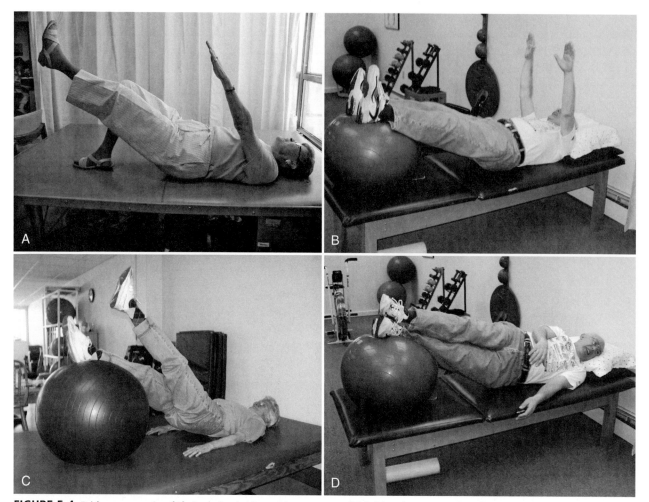

FIGURE 5-4 Bridge progression **(A)** single-leg bridge without arms to **(B)** bridge dynamic surface (ball) without arms (moderate difficulty). **(C)** Bridge progression single leg using dynamic surface (ball) with arms (most difficult). **(D)** Bridge progression side-lying bridge using dynamic surface.

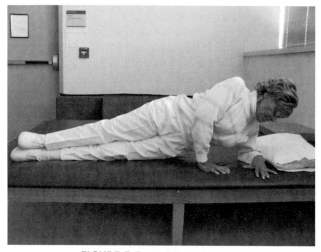

FIGURE 5-5 Modified side plank.

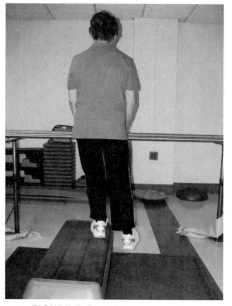

FIGURE 5-6 Eccentric step down.

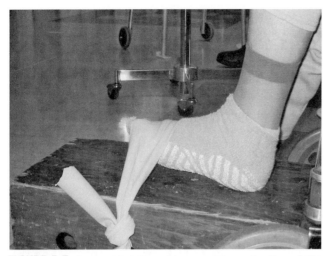

FIGURE 5-7 Concentric followed by eccentric contraction of tibialis anterior.

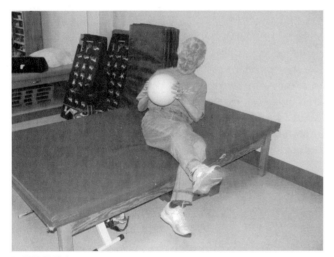

FIGURE 5-8 Overload principle applied to supine to sit transfer.

Types of Contractions

Incorporating the way the muscle is used in training programs meets the requirement of specificity. Functional activities can be analyzed to determine whether the type of muscle contraction needed to complete the activity is concentric, eccentric, or isometric. For example, trunk muscles are often used as stabilizers during movement and therefore should be trained isometrically. Because the gait cycle has been estimated as being composed of about 60% eccentric contractions, specific muscle groups should be trained eccentrically to improve the gait cycle.[56] For example, the dorsiflexors contract eccentrically at heel strike to foot flat and the gluteus medius contracts eccentrically during midstance. Training methods should take this into account. If the right gluteus medius is weak, having a patient stand on the right leg while performing a rapid contraction of the left gluteus medius against an elastic band causes the right gluteus medius to contract both rapidly and eccentrically, similar to the way it is used in gait. When performing an eccentric contraction, slowing the speed of the movement overloads the activity, as in having a patient sit down as slow as possible.

Motor Learning

A minimum of 6 weeks is needed to achieve a true strengthening response in muscle tissue. However, many patients demonstrate improved performance almost immediately. This change is due to motor learning rather than the strengthening response. Motor learning occurs with repetition and sufficient stimulus. Repeating a movement over and over again results in improving the patient's ability to perform that movement and that movement alone. Recent research suggests that it takes thousands of repetitions to achieve a learning response that is considered long term.[57,58] Random practice, that is, performing different tasks in variable orders and environments may achieve transferable performance to other environments. Random practice may improve the older adult's ability to use that muscle or movement in any situation. This varied performance is referred to as skill acquisition, an ability of interest to physical therapists because patients need to use a muscle or movement in multiple ways to address all their functional demands. Therefore, training the knee extensors in various and movement-specific ways so that they can be used for the tasks of sit to stand, stand to sit, squatting, split squatting, and going up and down stairs is achieved through random and repetitive practice.

Frequency

Frequency refers to the number of exercise sessions per week that are necessary or advisable to obtain optimum results (Table 5-4). Frequency of exercise sessions varies with the type of exercise being done. For example, the ACSM recommends aerobic exercise be performed three to five times per week. If patients are working at an intensity of 70% to 85% of their maximum heart rate, ACSM recommends 3 days per week as being sufficient to obtain maximum outcomes.[33] Alternatively, skill and balance exercise/activities can be practiced daily. Some variation as to intensity level should be incorporated such as having the patient work at a hard intensity on a particular skill 2 to 3 days per week; work at a moderate level 2 to 3 days per week; and at a low workload 1 to 2 days per week. This variable intensity prevents overtraining and a deterioration in performance. Stretching can be done on a daily basis without deleterious effects. Strengthening, at a high intensity (80% of a 1 RM) to the same muscle group need only be done 2 to 3 days per week.[59] Varying the muscle groups that you are strengthening may be necessary if the patient is being seen on a daily basis.

TABLE 5-4	Recommended Frequency for Types of Exercise
Activity	**Frequency**
Aerobic (cardiovascular conditioning)	3–5 times per week. With higher intensity, frequency can be decreased
Skills (motor learning) and balance	Daily
Stretching	5–7 times per week
Strengthening	2–3 times per week for each muscle group

Sets

The initial research that explored the recommended number of sets of a particular exercise found three sets to be more effective for strength gains than one or two sets. However, the difference in strength gain between one and three sets was only 2.9%.[60] This small difference would appear to be important only for highly trained competitive athletes. Many authors since have recommended one set of each exercise as effective for the first 3 months of training, in untrained and novice weight lifters, and in older adults because most of the strength gain occurs in the first set and fewer sets may avoid boredom or injury.[61-66] It would seem to make sense, given the available information on sets, specificity, and intensity, that instead of having the patient perform multiple sets of the *same* exercise, the therapist would devise several functional exercises that would challenge the muscle in different ways. For example, if the patient required increased strength of their quadriceps, the first set might be sit to stands, followed by a second set of lunges, and a third set of leg presses.

Duration

Duration refers to the amount of time of each exercise bout or the length of time of an exercise session. Typically, skill and balance activities are practiced 20 to 30 minutes per session. Although no research exists quantifying the length of bouts or sessions, motor learning theory suggests several thousand repetitions or several hours of practice are needed on a daily basis to learn a new movement pattern. The apparent brevity of typical exercise sessions compared with what the literature suggests most likely has to do with the practical problems of resource use as well as the current levels of reimbursement.[67]

Aerobic exercise durations are 30 minutes, with short periods of 5 to 10 minutes of warm-up and cool-down. Optimum duration of a stretching exercise has been shown to be 30 seconds in younger people compared to four repetitions of 60 seconds in older adults. One set of a 10 RM has been shown to be an appropriate stimulus

for strengthening exercises. Some literature suggests a 15 RM for untrained individuals with gradual progression to 10 RM. As a patient approaches his maximum capacity, more than one set of an exercise may be needed to achieve a high-level strength goal.

Conclusions

There are numerous variables to consider when designing an exercise prescription. The first and foremost consideration should be whether or not the exercises will challenge or overload a patient's ability. Secondarily, specificity of type of exercise, speed of exercise, and type of muscle contraction are all further considerations. Use of functional training meets these criteria. In addition, consideration needs to be given to motor learning theory, whether the exercise program is aimed at adaptation or improvement, and the frequency and length of the exercise bout or exercise sessions.

Improving and enhancing the manner in which an individual absorbs and dissipates physical and physiological stressors leads to improved function. The creative challenge of exercise prescription is how the physical therapist manipulates the variables. All of the variables in an exercise prescription can be varied to achieve the desired outcome. Patients can be asked to lift a heavier load (intensity), increase the number of transfers performed (repetitions), work for a longer period of time (duration), perform multiple movement patterns at one time to complete a single task (specificity), work on a compliant surface (environmental challenge), or work more quickly or slowly (time rate of force development), all to effect an appropriate overload and improved function.

TYPES OF EXERCISES FOR OLDER ADULTS

Aerobic Exercise

Measurement. Target heart rate is the most clinically applicable measure to determine aerobic exercise intensity. A subjective measure of exercise intensity is the rate of perceived exertion. Clinical functional measures of aerobic capacity include the 6-minute walk test (6MWT) and the 400-m walk test. The ACSM has suggested the exercise stimulus of 60% to 80% to achieve cardiovascular adaptation and fitness.

The simple equation for determining target heart rate is to determine 60% to 80% of the predicted maximum heart rate (60% to 80% × [220 − age]). More recently, authors have suggested using a percentage of heart rate reserve because the traditional formula may underestimate the heart rate load. Heart rate reserve subtracts a person's resting heart rate from his or her predicted maximum. The formula used to obtain this target heart rate is referred to as the Karvonen method ([60% to 80% × (220 − age − resting heart rate)] + resting heart rate). The Karvonen method will yield a slightly higher target heart rate than the traditional method (Table 5-5).

Subjective Measures of Perceived Exertion. The Borg Rating of Perceived Exertion (RPE) scale was originally established with young adults by correlating verbal descriptors of perceived workload effort with corresponding heart rate (e.g., perceived exertion described as "fairly light" corresponded to heart rate of 110; perceived exertion of "very hard" corresponded to a heart hare of 170.) The RPE scale as a tool to monitor exercise intensity has been validated in older adults,[69] and is particularly useful in those who may have a blunted heart rate response, such as those taking β-blockers. A rate of 11 to 15 on the Borg RPE corresponds to a percentage of 60% to 80%.[70] Other subjective measures include the modified RPE scale, which uses a simpler 0 to 10 scale and the talk test (see Table 5-2). The talk test represents the ability to engage in a conversation during exercise that represents work at or near a steady state and closely reflects actual heart rate and $\dot{V}o_2$ levels.[39] When the exerciser reaches an intensity at which he or she can "just barely respond in conversation," the intensity is considered to be safe and appropriate for cardiovascular adaptation. The talk test is considered somewhat conservative but may be useful for older adults beginning an aerobic program.

Exercise Stress Test. The diagnostic exercise test is the gold standard for determining readiness to exercise. The ACSM has developed risk stratification criteria that should be reviewed before establishing an aerobic exercise program.[1] However, in apparently healthy individuals without known heart disease and with two or fewer cardiovascular risk factors, the ACSM recommends only a medical examination prior to engaging in *vigorous* exercise.

Six-Minute Walk Test. The 6-minute walk test (6MWT) is a measure of how far a person can walk in 6 minutes and is a valid and reliable indicator of aerobic fitness.[71-73] The 6MWT can serve as a useful objective baseline measure and has normative results and minimal clinically important differences established for a range of older individuals.[74-79] Vital signs are taken before and after the test and an RPE also recorded at the end of the test to determine exercise capacity. The individual may stop and rest during the test but may not sit down.[80] If the person has to sit or stop the test before the end of 6 minutes, the distance walked is the person's test result. In this case, the time walked should also be noted. Standardized encouragement is provided at 1-minute intervals, and the person should not be paced. Individuals may use assistive devices during the test.

400-m Walk Test. The 400-m walk test is similar to the 6MWT but defines a distance to walk versus a length of time. Some have suggested that knowing the length to walk makes it easier for the patient to pace themselves and therefore achieves a greater effort.[81] Similar to the 6MWT, vital signs are taken prior to the test and vital signs and a measure of perceived exertion are taken following the test, recording the time it took to complete the 400 m.[82]

Indications for Aerobic Exercise. Aerobic exercise is indicated for patients who lack the ability to sustain activity for a desired period of time because of decreased cardiovascular efficiency. Oftentimes, these patients have complaints of fatigue with a given level of exercise. Aerobic exercise increases the body's capacity to absorb, deliver, and utilize oxygen. However, there are some limitations to being able to use aerobic conditioning for older adults. Joint pain and/or muscle weakness may preclude a patient from being able to perform the multiple contractions needed to provide a cardiovascular stimulus. In those cases, strengthening exercises may be needed prior to attempting aerobic exercise. For example, when an individual who is not on β-blockers walks 200 m on the 6MWT, but the heart rate only increases 10 beats per minute (bpm), the assumption can be made that the individual was not able to exert enough effort to

TABLE 5-5	Calculating Target Heart Rate for a 70–Year-Old Individual with a Resting Heart Rate of 75 bpm		
Traditional (ACSM) Method	**Karvonen Method**	**Aquatic Reduction**	
220	220	220	
−70	−70	−70	Age
		−5	Pulse reduction of 5 bpm (difference between land and water heart rate)
= 150	= 150	= 145	Maximum heart rate
	−75	−75	Resting heart rate
	= 75	= 70	Heart rate reserve
× .80	× .80	× .80	% of maximum
	= 60	= 56	
	+75	+75	Resting heart rate
= 120	= 135	= 131	Target heart rate

increase heart rate and that a lack of muscle strength may exist.[30]

Contraindications and Safety. Absolute contraindications for aerobic exercise include resting heart rate greater than 100 bpm, systolic blood pressure higher than 200 mmHg, and/or diastolic blood pressure higher than 120 mmHg.[1] For patients with unstable cardiac conditions or risk signs for cardiac disease, monitoring of blood pressure and heart rates should be routinely performed. Individuals can be instructed in how to self-monitor their status and to take their own heart rate and blood pressure. Patients should be instructed to report untoward effects of lightheadedness, dizziness, profuse sweating, or nausea. Physical therapists should be knowledgeable about an individual's medications, particularly those that have a potential effect on an individual's ability to exercise or that affect the response to exercise. β-blockers decrease both the force of contraction of heart muscle and heart rate, keeping the heart rate artificially low during exercise. As mentioned previously, an RPE is an acceptable alternate to taking a pulse in the presence of β-blockers. Exercise also changes the need for insulin in patients with diabetes; therefore, close monitoring of the patient with insulin-dependent diabetes is required. Chapter 12 on impaired aerobic capacity provides a comprehensive list of absolute and relative contraindications to aerobic exercise.

Equipment and Opportunities. A host of equipment can be used indoors for aerobic conditioning of the older individual, including a treadmill, elliptical trainer, stair stepper, rower, stationary bike, and recumbent-type bikes. Outdoor activities include walking or hiking, cross-country skiing, skating, jogging, and cycling. Each activity has advantages and disadvantages. The individual's preference should be the basis for recommending a specific type of aerobic exercise. In addition, the physical requirements for each activity should be considered, matching the requirements with the person's abilities. The best activity is the one that the individual will do consistently. Once an aerobic exercise program is established, there is typically little need for physical therapist supervision other than to periodically adjust the intensity of the program as the patient progresses.

Conclusion. Aerobic exercise may be one aspect of a complete exercise program for an older adult. Considerations as to patient physical impairments, functional deficits, and patient goals need to be considered. Strengthening exercises may need to be done prior to participation in aerobic conditioning to achieve the most optimum result, especially if the person complains of pain or fatigue.

Aquatic Exercise

Aquatic exercise allows the application of the physical stress theory for individuals who cannot tolerate the stresses of land-based exercises. The buoyancy of the water allows a deconditioned individual or an individual with significant joint pathology to exercise by decreasing the forces needed to move and decreasing the forces on the joint.

Measurement. Measurements of aquatic exercise are similar to land-based exercise. Target heart rate can be determined using the same formulas as for land-based exercise. However, because heart rate is lower in the pool, an "aquatic heart rate reduction" should be included in the formula. The heart rate reduction model was determined by Fernado Martins Kruel and is sometimes referred to as the Kruel protocol.[83] An aquatic heart rate reduction is determined by subtracting a 1-minute in-pool heart rate from a 1-minute land-based heart rate. The difference is referred to as the aquatic reduction. Subjective perceived exertion scales can also be used to determine the intensity of an aquatic exercise program. Land-based functional assessments are used to determine the benefits of an aquatic exercise program.

Indications for Aquatic Exercise. The buoyancy of water decreases compressive forces within joints while offering hydrostatic support to the upright position. The buoyancy effect may allow some patients who have painful joints in weight bearing to exercise. Patients who have osteoarthritis, who are overweight, or who have recently undergone surgery may initially benefit from this form of exercise.[84] Also, those patients who have significant balance disorders or a fear of falling may have some initial benefits before progressing to land-based exercises.

Contraindications and Safety. There are obvious safety issues with having patients move into and out of the water as well as issues of preventing drowning.[85] Patients need to be monitored walking over wet slippery surfaces, going up and down ladders or steps when entering or leaving the pool and while in the water. Otherwise, the same contraindications and safety monitoring as aerobic exercise apply to aquatic exercise. Individuals with open wounds should not be allowed in the water until the wound is well healed. Occasionally, individuals may develop an allergic skin reaction to the chemicals in the water.

Equipment. There are many types of flotation devices that can be used in the water to either provide support or resistance while exercising. Devices to promote ambulation in the pool range from sling-type walking devices that are relatively simple to underwater treadmill systems (Figure 5-9). Access to the pool can consist of ramps, hydraulic lifts, stairs, or ladders. Equipment for emergency communication should be in the pool area as should an automated external defibrillator (AED).

Conclusion. The use of aquatic exercise allows a patient, who may otherwise be unable to exercise because of pain or instability, the ability to be more physically active and to gain initial levels of strength to permit land-based exercise. However, as soon as possible, patients should be progressed to land-based exercise. Improving

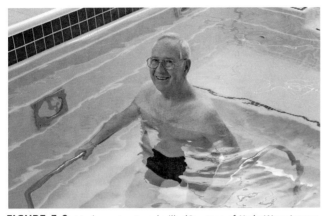

FIGURE 5-9 Underwater treadmill. *(Courtesy of HydroWorx International, Inc., Middleton, Penn.)*

function in water is only the first step to having the patient be able to complete functioning on land.

Strengthening Exercise

Older adults gain strength the same way that younger people gain strength. By applying an appropriate exercise prescription, numerous authors have documented quite significant strengthening effects even in very old adults, which may be related to how much strength they have lost.[28,29,37,52,86-89] Loss of strength can be associated with loss of function in older adults. The relationship between strength and function appears to be curvilinear (Figure 5-10); that is, strength is directly related to function only up to a certain threshold and then further increases in strength, though adding to reserve, will not appreciably improve function and the strength–function curve flattens out. The curvilinear relationship with respect to strength's effect on function may be due to function being a relatively low level of activity. The strength gain rate is different for trained and untrained older

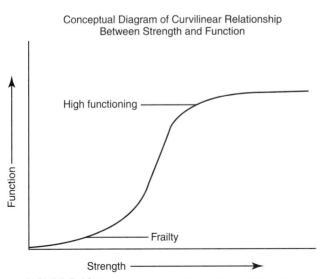

Conceptual Diagram of Curvilinear Relationship Between Strength and Function

FIGURE 5-10 Curvilinear strength–function relationship.

adults. Untrained older adults, those who are sedentary and are not participating in exercise, will have a steeper ascent before the curve flattens out compared to those who are trained. In trained individuals, strength gains are harder to detect because of the higher threshold of strength. Conceivably the point at which the strength gain curve flattens out is when a person achieves the level of strength needed to perform a task. For example, an individual needs a certain level of strength (about 45% of his or her body weight) to rise from a chair.[90] If a person is unable to rise from a chair unassisted because of weakness in the lower extremity, strengthening will help to improve that function. However, once an adequate level of strength is achieved and the person is able to rise from the chair unassisted, further strengthening will not necessarily have a direct linear effect on further improving chair rises. However, further strengthening will make the task more efficient, will allow a person to rise more quickly, and will create a strength reserve to help preserve the function of chair rise in the future.

Measurement. Strength testing using traditional manual muscle testing can be very subjective with substantial ceiling effects. Muscle dynamometry, isokinetic dynamometers, and a repetition maximum test are options that provide more objective scores. As will be discussed later, manual muscle testing grades of 4/5 and 5/5 have very low validity.[91-93]

Numerous types of muscle dynamometry exist, each with its own advantages and disadvantages. Hand-held muscle dynamometry, for example, is fairly quick and easy to use but the examiner must be able to exert enough force for a break test, similar to a manual muscle test. This may be difficult when testing large muscles or muscle groups in the lower extremity, creating a ceiling effect over the grade of 3/5. However, with proper technique and tester strength, a quantitative value can be achieved that will be more responsive to change than a manual muscle testing grade.[94] Hand-held muscle dynamometers, because of their quantitative nature, have norms that can be useful for therapists. Some of these values are listed in Table 5-6. Isokinetic dynamometers can be a reliable and valid way to test strength but they can be very expensive to purchase and because they have a mechanical axis, it is sometimes difficult to align the axis of movement at a particular joint. In addition, isokinetic dynamometers may not measure functional strength because of the lack of specificity for a given movement.[42]

Using a repetition maximum has been the gold standard to measure strength across a variety of individuals, including athletes. A repetition maximum can be for 1 RM or for multiple repetitions. A repetition maximum is documented by determining the maximum number of times a person can move a weight (including body weight) with good form. Let us say an individual can leg press 200 lb for six repetitions before losing form or being unable to complete another repetition.

TABLE 5-6	Key Hand-held Dynamometry Norms for Older Adults on Dominant Side in Newtons[136]			
Movement	Age	Gender	Mean Force (SD)	Mean Force/Body Weight (SD) (%)
Hip abduction	50–59	Men	308.9 (74.7)	36.2 (7.8)
		Women	214.8 (40.0)	34.7 (7.8)
	60–69	Men	258.9 (49.4)	32.8 (6.8)
		Women	172.3 (43.8)	28.2 (7.7)
	70–79	Men	250.8 (42.7)	33.6 (7.2)
		Women	152.7 (34.4)	26.7 (6.7)
Knee extension	50–59	Men*	470.9 (92.3)	55.7 (11.1)
		Women	334.7 (75.8)	53.7 (12.8)
	60–69	Men	386.9 (94.3)	48.9 (12.4)
		Women	273.6 (80.0)	44.6 (13.6)
	70–79	Men	360.3 (72.6)	47.7 (8.4)
		Women	210.1 (45.6)	36.6 (8.8)
Ankle dorsiflexion	50–59	Men	323.2 (90.8)	36.9 (13.5)
		Women	252.9 (53.3)	41.3 (12.1)
	60–69	Men	269.0 (76.9)	33.8 (10.4)
		Women	235.7 (74.9)	38.9 (15.2)
	70–79	Men	240.0 (47.3)	32.1 (7.2)
		Women	166.2 (48.7)	29.1 (9.9)

*Authors report that knee extensor force met or surpassed 650 N and was recorded as 650 N in three men in their 50s, creating a possibility that values for this decade may be depressed.

Two hundred pounds is then said to be this person's 6 RM. There are numerous tables that then can convert a multiple RM to a 1 RM or a 10 RM for the purpose of comparing the strength levels of different individuals or of the same individual over time and for determining the weight that will equate to a percentage maximum for training purposes. An example of a conversion is listed in Table 5-7.

The minimum training stimulus for strengthening exercise is 60% of a 1 RM.[1] To determine the amount of resistance needed to achieve a 60% training stimulus, you would need to know the weight a person can lift one time and one time only in a controlled manner and with good form, and then use 60% of that weight for exercise. Alternatively, you can estimate how much weight an older adult is likely to move, given his or her body weight– or age-based norms, and ask the individual to move that weight as many times as he or she can. We have had most success determining a repetition maximum on the leg press by starting with body weight. If the individual is able to move that load, determine how many times he or she can move it and determine

the RM. Sixty percent of a 1 RM is similar to or the same as a 15 RM. If the individual is able to move the resistance more than 15 times, you have dropped below an adequate stimulus for strength training. Although the ACSM recommends that the most accurate 1 RM is determined from no more than three trials in any session given a 30- to 60-second rest between trials, we find older adults have a better response with a multiple RM of 6 to 10. This may be because older adults may not be used to exerting maximum effort and need experience to learn to generate that type of force. We have also found that the RM changes quite rapidly in many untrained older adults, necessitating frequent assessment to maintain an adequate training stimulus. A very typical and effective strengthening exercise stimulus goal is 80% of a 1 RM. Eighty percent of a 1 RM is similar to or the same as a 8 RM. Table 5-8 includes the norms for leg press for individuals older than age 50 years.

Subjective perceived exertion scales can also be helpful in measuring effort during strength training exercise. Rates of perceived exertion of 11 to 15 on a

TABLE 5-7	Determining Intensity from a 1 RM[137]									
If the Desired % of 1 RM is	100%	95%	93%	90%	87%	85%	83%	80%	77%	75%
Then the desired number of repetitions are	1 RM	2 RM	3 RM	4 RM	5 RM	6 RM	7 RM	8 RM	9 RM	10 RM

TABLE 5-8	ACSM 1 RM for Leg Press[1] (p. 83)		
Percentile	Gender	50–59	60+
90	Men	1.80	1.73
	Women	1.37	1.32
80	Men	1.71	1.62
	Women	1.25	1.18
70	Men	1.64	1.56
	Women	1.17	1.13
60	Men	1.58	1.49
	Women	1.10	1.04
50	Men	1.52	1.43
	Women	1.05	0.99
40	Men	1.46	1.38
	Women	0.99	0.93
30	Men	1.39	1.30
	Women	0.95	0.88
20	Men	1.32	1.25
	Women	0.88	0.85
10	Men	1.22	1.16
	Women	0.78	0.72

1 RM bilateral leg press with leg press ratio = weight pushed/body weight.

6- to 20-point scale usually represents stimulus levels of 60% to 80% (see Table 5-2) and are validated against repetition maximum.[69,70] We have found large charts placed around the clinic area or carried on a clipboard helpful when asking older adults to determine their effort.

Manual muscle testing (MMT) has been used in the clinic to quantify strength, but its application is somewhat limited. Although MMT is a valid way to determine strength below or at a grade of 3/5, it is not valid above the grade of 3, especially when considering the strength required for functional, mobility-type movements. Bohannon found a large discrepancy in the actual forces recorded for muscles graded 4 and 5 (Good and Normal).[95] A grade of 4/5 or Good for a given muscle encompassed forces between 55.6 and 261.1 N and a grade of 5/5 or Normal had force ranges between 97.9 and 422.6 N. Bohannon has determined that the minimum amount of force necessary to rise from a chair unassisted and without the use of the individual's arms is 45% of a person's body weight, equating to a bilateral MMT of the quadriceps of 5/5 and 4+/5. Clearly, an MMT has a ceiling effect, especially for functional movements involving lower extremities.

Measuring a RM for a functional movement such as a chair rise requires some creativity. For example, if an older individual is not able to rise from a standard chair without using his or her arms, the therapist must create a situation where the person can be successful, such as raising the surface to allow the individual to complete the task independently. However many times the person can rise from the raised surface then becomes that person's repetition maximum and the appropriate training stimulus can be determined. So if the raised surface is 21 in. and the person can stand 10 times without using his or her arms, that is the 10 RM and represents the 80% training stimulus. If the person does more or less than 10 repetitions, the surface can be raised or lowered. With some creativity, this method can be used for any movement such as bridges, lunges, wall squats, and step ups and step downs.

A few MMT tests can be valuable to determine functional strength. For example, Lunsford and Perry determined holding a standing heel rise on one leg to be equal to an MMT grade of 3/5.[96] Because many older adults cannot generate this force, the heel rise test can be informative, especially because gastrocnemius and soleus strength are associated with gait speed. Similarly, these authors found that Normal or a grade of 5/5 was equal to 25 repetitions. Perry et al developed and quantified a supine hip extensor test that may be easier to perform in the clinic because so many older adults have difficulty lying prone.[97] Their method showed distinct difference between the forces elicited at each muscle grade (grade 5, 175.6 N; grade 4, 103.1 N; grade 3, 66.7 N; and grade 2, 19.1 N) but was not validated against the gold standard of hand-held dynamometry in the prone position.

Finally, a number of authors have suggested "functional" tests to grade muscle strength. Rikli and Jones, in their book *Senior Fitness Test*, documented norms for various strength tests including sit to stands and arm curls.[98] Timed movements such as floor transfers and stair climbing have also been suggested as a measure of lower extremity strength and power, similarly to usual and fast gait speed.

Indications. Strength has been implicated in most functional movements. Because of the insidious loss of strength with age, it can be assumed that strength training should be addressed where there are functional deficits. Strength training should also be used to add reserve to provide a protective effect in the event that the person has a period of enforced bed rest. Much recent research has determined that strength training is a first-line intervention for many of the symptoms and consequences of chronic diseases such as chronic obstructive pulmonary disease, osteoporosis, balance, and falls.[99-109] Strength training should never be overlooked and should be applied in as efficacious a manner as possible to achieve the best functional result. Our experience has been that strength training has been underutilized and undermanaged, depriving the older adult of the highest level of function possible.

Slowness of movement, a hallmark of frailty, should be addressed with a combination of strength and power training. Many movements intrinsic to balance require a response in milliseconds. Many authors have associated improved gait speed, stair climb time, chair rise time, and ADL function with improved power.[18,45,51,110-112] Overloaded repetitions done quickly are necessary to improve power and reaction time. Conventional wisdom would suggest that to increase the speed of movement you would need to decrease the amount of weight lifted. However, optimal results occur when the healthy older adult is both moving quickly and lifting a maximum amount of weight. De Vos et al used resistances of 30%, 50%, and 80% of a 1 RM; and although he found that power was increased at all these levels of resistance, the higher levels of resistance produced the most robust results.[113] Similarly, Earles et al used 50%, 60%, and 70% of body weight for resistance for the leg press during rapid contractions and saw power gains of 50%, 77%, and 141%, respectively.[114]

Contraindications/Safety. There are no absolute contraindications for strengthening exercises. Although care must be taken to have the person use proper form and avoid holding his or her breath, there have been very few reported problems with strength training. This is despite the fact that fairly high levels of systolic and diastolic pressures have been reported.[115] Even with high-intensity training of 80% of 1 RM, no long-term injuries have been reported. In fact, in many studies where control groups are used to measure the effects of strength training in older adults, the control group has more injuries and falls than the exercising group, presumably because of the continued, insidious strength loss that occurs with age and sedentary behavior.[87] Care should be used regarding proper form, especially when using high intensities and speed. We make it a practice to never leave an older adult exercising on his or her own when using high intensities of 70% to 90% of 1 RM. An older adult may need encouragement to maintain proper form, to breathe properly, and to attend to his or her level of joint or muscle discomfort.

Equipment and Exercises. Overload, which results in strength gains, can be achieved through a variety of means beginning with body weight and moving through the use of added resistance, such as elastic bands, cuff and hand weights, barbells, dumbbells, hand-held blades, etc. There is a remarkable amount of equipment that can be used creatively to provide an optimal training stimulus and to keep the program fun and interesting. Box 5-5 lists many types of equipment that have been used to achieve strengthening effects.

Each method of overload offers comparative advantages and disadvantages, such as safety, ease of use, and expense. However, the basic concepts of overload and specificity should always be honored and incorporated. Variety often helps clients maintain their enthusiasm for the strengthening exercise program. Mixing and matching the equipment and the type of exercise

---

BOX 5-5 | Equipment That Can Be Used for Strength Training

- Body weight in a variety of positions with or without climbing ropes, fixed straps, or chin up bars
- External weights such as a pulley system, weight machine, dumbbells and barbells, kettlebells, weight bars, weighted balls, and power bags
- Compliant surfaces (foam pads, air bladders, wobble boards)
- Elastic bands and tubing such as Theraband
- Inflated balls or stability balls
- Variable resistance (isokinetic) exercise machines (Cybex, BTE, etc.)
- Flexible rods (BodyBlade) (Figure 5–11)
- Immovable surfaces for isometric contractions
- Punching bags
- Weight sleds
- Steps
- Pilates table

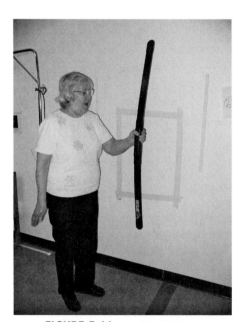

FIGURE 5-11 Hand-held blade.

---

that you prescribe can achieve variety in addition to achieving functional strengthening by training a given muscle to react in many different ways. Some authors have referred to this phenomenon of changing the exercise stimulus to prevent "staleness" as muscle confusion. Although it does appear that the muscle does respond better to changing stimulus for strengthening such as using concepts of martial arts, Pilates, Tai Chi, plyometrics, etc., there is still controversy about the concept and little supportive data in the literature. Providing a variety of strengthening options may have an additional advantage of keeping the program interesting, which may have positive effects on adherence.

Conclusion. Strengthening exercises at sufficient intensity to achieve a strength training effect is the hallmark of any skilled physical therapy intervention for older adults. The variety of strength-training exercises is endless and only requires creativity and knowledge of functional movements and specificity. It is our opinion that many older adults become uninterested in their exercise program because of insufficient challenge, lack of progress, or the appearance of irrelevancy of the exercise program to their personal goals. This is unfortunate because of the preponderance of evidence that describes the effectiveness of well-designed strengthening exercise programs to achieve improved function, decreased impact of chronic disease, and improved balance, coordination, speed of movement, and overall mobility. Physical therapists who treat older adults would do well to become exercise experts in applying the strengthening exercise evidence to programs for older adults in all practice settings and across all functional levels of their patients.

Stretching Exercises

Older adults adopt certain movement patterns and positioning as they age. Oftentimes, these movement patterns and acquired postures result in muscles and other soft tissue that is continuously held in a shortened or lengthened position. Stretching is indicated to promote adaptation of shortened muscles to a more lengthened position to achieve better posture and movement patterns. Muscles held in shortened positions appear to have a biased muscle spindle that may lead to active and passive resistance to increased length, resulting in muscle imbalance during movement and even painful movement patterns.[116] Research has shown that with increasing age and a loss of extensibility, effective stretching exercises require longer holding times. Although a 30-second hold is sufficient to achieve a long-term effect of muscle lengthening in a younger adult, 60 seconds is necessary for adults age 65 years and older.[117] Four repetitions of a 60-second hold performed regularly, 5 to 7 days a week, appear to be most effective. Some have suggested the use of ballistic or dynamic stretching to increase immediate muscle performance. There are data to suggest, however, that static stretching is preferred to dynamic stretching to improve muscle length. However, not all loss of joint range of motion is attributable to the muscle-tendon complex. Often other soft tissue, including the joint capsule or ligaments, fascia, and connective tissue may be involved. Slow static stretching is likewise recommended for stretching the collagen tissue that is the substance of these structures.

Measurement. Age-based normal ranges of motion have been recorded in a variety of publications. Functional ranges have also been recorded such as the modified sit and reach and the back scratch (Apley's) tests from the senior fitness test[98] (Table 5-9).

Indications. Joint range of motion limitations can lead to pain syndromes, painful postures, abnormal movement patterns, and loss of function. Consideration of the potential for future painful conditions and loss of function also may indicate a need for stretching intervention even when losses of motion have not yet led to pain or disability. For example, the pectoralis minor muscle, a muscle that commonly shortens because of typical, sedentary posture, has the potential to lead to shoulder impingement and pain by decreasing the subacromial space. Left untreated, the impingement may lead to rotator cuff tendinitis and eventually even frank tearing of the rotator cuff muscles. In either case, the ensuing pain or loss of movement results in decreased function of the shoulder, such as for overhead reaching or dressing activities. A prophylactic stretching program may eliminate or lessen these future problems. Typical muscles requiring stretching in older adults include the suboccipital muscles; the pectoralis minor and downward rotators and protractors of the shoulder girdle, the extensors of the lumbar spine, the hip flexors and external rotators, and the ankle plantar flexors (Table 5-10).

Contraindications. Some research suggests that stretching may cause at least a short-term decrease in muscle strength. Otherwise, the only absolute contraindication to stretching exercises is the presence of joint instability. Stretching exercises in this case would further contribute to the instability. During stretching exercises care should be taken to ensure that the stretching force is only exerted on the target muscle or joint and not neighboring joints or muscles. In addition, neural tissue is susceptible to stretching forces and may present as pins and needles or numbness. This may require altering the stretching position, using supports to localize the stretching force, or requiring an external stretching force. For example, while attempting to stretch the hamstrings by using trunk forward flexion, one may inadvertently be causing flexion forces to the lumbar spine. An alternate method may be to lie supine and use a rope on the foot to pull the lower extremity into a straight leg raise (Figure 5-12). Figures 5-12 to 5-15 illustrate some common stretches. There is no contraindication for the long-term effect of stretching muscles that are maintained habitually in a shortened position.

Conclusion. Muscle shortening often occurs from the lack of movement through its full range, a common effect of a sedentary lifestyle. Often, physical activity, especially when accompanied by strengthening exercises, will improve flexibility,[118] whereby specific stretching may not be necessary for those postural conditions that arise from prolonged positioning such as sitting. When specific stretching is indicated, a longer hold time is necessary to change the muscle tissue.

TABLE 5-9	Normative Data for Two Tests of Flexibility[98]							
Exercise	Gender	60–64	65–69	70–74	75–79	80–84	85–89	90–94
Chair sit and reach (inches +/-)	Men	−2.5 to +4.0	−3.0 to +3.0	−3.5 to +2.5	−4.0 to +2.0	−5.5 to +1.5	−5.5 to +0.5	−6.5 to −0.5
	Women	−0.5 to +5.0	−0.5 to +4.5	−1.0 to +4.0	−1.5 to +3.5	−2.0 to +3.0	−2.5 to +2.5	−4.5 to +1.0
Back scratch (Apley's)	Men	−6.5 to +0.0	−7.5 to −1.0	−8.0 to −1.0	−9.0 to −2.0	−9.5 to −2.0	−10.0 to −3.0	−10.5 to −4.0
	Women	−3.0 to +1.5	−3.5 to +1.5	−4.0 to +1.0	−5.0 to +0.5	−5.5 to +0.0	−7.0 to −1.0	−8.0 to −1.0

Normal range of scores for men and women. Normal is defined as the middle quartiles (middle 50% of rank ordered scores) of the population. Those scoring above this range (top 25%) would be considered above average for their age, and those scoring below this range (bottom 25%) are considered below average. The reader is referred to the Senior Fitness Test Manual[98] for instructions on how to perform and score these tests.[98]

TABLE 5-10	Typical Posturing in Older Adults and Related Shortened Muscles		
Posture	Shortened Muscles	Lengthened or Weak Muscles	Movement to Correct Posture
Forward head	Suboccipital	Prevertebrals	Chin tucks (Figure 5–13)
Forward downward sloping shoulders	Pectoralis minor	Serratus anterior	Shoulder retraction and upward rotation
Excessive lumbar lordosis — hip flexion tightness	Erector spinae and ilio-psoas, rectus femoris	Abdominals and hip extensors	Abdominal bracing and hip flexor stretch (Thomas Test) (Figure 5–14)
Hip external rotation	Piriformis, gluteus maximus, obturator externus	Gluteus minimus, tensor fascia lata, gracilis, pectineus	Internal rotation with hip and knee bent to 90 degrees, prone, supine, or in sitting
Plantarflexion tightness	Gastrocnemius and soleus	Dorsiflexors and tightness of ankle mortise	Heel cord stretch into dorsiflexion, or with foot off stair (Figure 5-15)

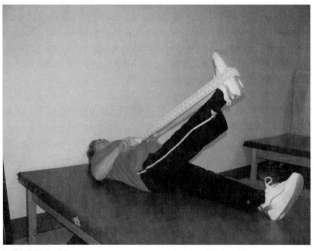

FIGURE 5-12 Stretching of hamstrings with lumbar spine stabilized.

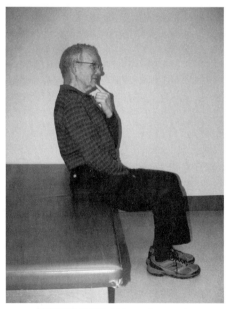

FIGURE 5-13 Chin tuck stretch.

Plyometrics

Plyometric exercise is an attempt to use the stretch reflex of the muscle spindle and the elastic energy that is stored in a stretched muscle to enhance an immediate reciprocal contraction in that muscle. Plyometrics usually consists of an eccentric (lengthening) contraction followed by a concentric (shortening) contraction of the same muscles. For example, a patient would rapidly squat and then follow that by a ballistic contraction to achieve a jumping motion. In this example, energy is stored in the gastrocnemius as the ankle dorsiflexes and in the quadriceps as the knee flexes. As

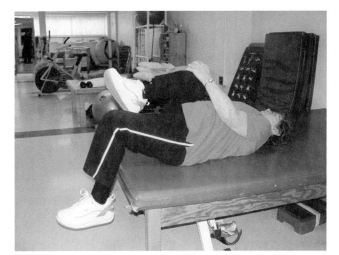

FIGURE 5-14 Left hip flexor stretch in a Thomas test position.

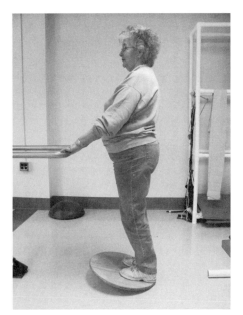

FIGURE 5-15 Heel cord stretch on Rocker Board.

the person begins to jump, a strong and rapid contraction of the gastrocnemius and quadriceps propels the patient into a jumping motion.

Measurement. Plyometric exercise is meant to result in an increase in the ballistic ability of the muscle, that is, the ability to increase the explosiveness of the muscle contraction. Testing for muscle power on an isokinetic dynamometer or similar device is a method of determining the effectiveness of this exercise approach. Alternately, any functional testing done by measuring the time taken to complete a task, that is, gait speed, floor transfer, or stair climbing, would also be a measure of improvement. Rose's Fullerton balance test, a higher-level balance assessment, includes a jumping task that indicates the muscle's capability to produce a rapid forceful contraction.[119] Obviously, the more powerful the contraction, the farther the patient jumps.

Indications. The loss of power with aging is even greater than the loss of muscle strength, occurring at 20% to 30% per decade after the age of 30 resulting in the classic view of older adults getting slower. The loss of power is seen in how relatively few older adults can run stairs or jump. An exercise approach that encourages increased speed of movement is desirable to help aging adults gain and maintain muscle power. Many authors have suggested that muscle power, or speed of muscle contraction, is a much better indicator of functional status than muscle strength.[46-48,112,120] In addition, plyometrics may aid in bone formation, according to Wolff's law, by increasing the compressive forces that the bone is required to absorb.[121,122] Jumping has been shown to have a positive effect on decreasing fall risk in long-term-care residents when combined with strengthening, stretching, and aerobic conditioning.[123] Other authors have suggested that using plyometrics for increasing upper extremity power, such as in a boxing-type movement aids in decreasing hip and head injuries associated with falling by allowing the person to get their arms out to absorb some of the force from the fall.[124,125]

Application. Beginning exercisers may not have the soft tissue and muscle integrity that is required by plyometric exercise. Therefore as older adults progress in their exercise program, speed of contraction should be used as a method of overload. Quick reciprocal movements performed functionally, as in plyometric exercise, is one way to achieve increased speed of muscle contraction. Initially, this may simply be having the patient jump in place. As the patient progresses, jumping off of and then back onto a low step further increases the challenge. Jumping from foot to foot may be progressed to jumping foot to foot in a forward or sideways progression. Figures 5-16 to 5-18 illustrate some plyometric exercises. In addition to creating a challenge to produce a quick contraction, plyometrics may also impose an overload to the cardiopulmonary system that may need to be monitored.

Conclusion. Although many therapists may not conceive of adding plyometrics to an exercise program for older adults, there are several advantages for this type of exercise. Older adults of all abilities need to be encouraged to move quickly, a form of explosive power. Although jumping may not always be realistic, asking a patient to walk as quickly but as safely as possible is an important safety training strategy. Incorporating rapid foot movements may aid in balance reactions. Also increasing the quickness or response in the upper extremities may minimize the risk of injury following a fall and may even prevent contact with the floor if the individual can block descent.

Tai Chi

Tai Chi originated as a form of marshal arts but now has multiple forms and styles that have been adapted from the original form. Whereas Tai Chi was traditionally

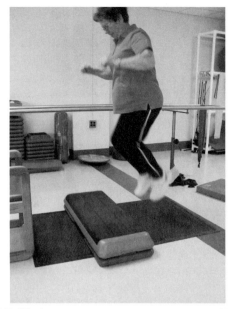

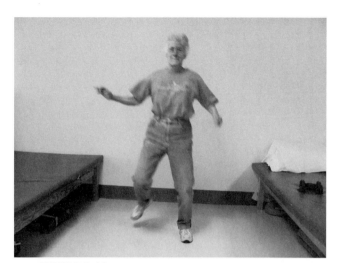

FIGURE 5-18 Plyometrics, jumping from foot to foot.

FIGURE 5-16 Plyometric exercise jumping onto and off of a step.

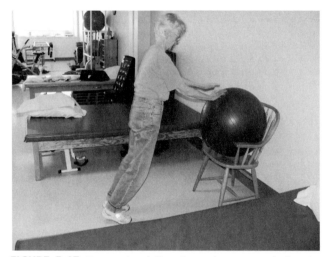

FIGURE 5-17 Plyometrics, falling forward onto gym ball to increase upper extremity power.

used in sports and competition, more recently Tai Chi has been advocated to have multiple medical benefits. The largest body of research about Tai Chi focuses on fall risk benefits.

Tai Chi involves learning multiple poses that are linked together with slow movements that emphasize control and balance. These routines or "forms" can range from the classic 109 postures to as few as 42. The focus required to complete the movements and postures and recalling the sequence of postures has been credited with both the mental calm and the cognitive benefits associated with Tai Chi. Improvement in balance and decreased fall risk are attributed to the slow repetitive

work and the emphasis on control and coordination especially at the ankle.

Measurement. No direct measurement of Tai Chi has been reported; however, research studying the effects of Tai Chi have used balance measurements such as the Berg balance score, the four-square step test, the senior fitness test, and one-legged stance time.

Indications. Practitioners of Tai Chi have suggested that Tai Chi mediates the effects of chronic conditions such as arthritis, cancer, cardiovascular disease, and diabetes and decreases stress, lessens depression, improves mental health and cognitive function while improving balance and fitness, thus decreasing falls and lessening fall risks. Researchers have studied the potential health benefit claims for Tai Chi. Unfortunately, the evidence supporting these claims is still lacking. Lee et al have performed systematic reviews on the effects of Tai Chi practice for rheumatoid arthritis, cancer, ankylosing spondylitis, osteoarthritis, osteoporosis, Parkinson's disease, and aerobic capacity.[126-132] These authors generally conclude that, based on small samples, poor methodology, lack of statistical significance, and publication in non–peer-reviewed articles, the evidence was insufficient to conclude that the practice of Tai Chi improved the management of disease process, decreased pain, or increased function. However, there is moderate evidence that Tai Chi does decrease the number of falls, lowers the risk of falling, and improves balance and physical functioning in older inactive adults.[133] Although it is unclear how Tai Chi improves balance and decreases fall risk, we believe the slow body movements superimposed on the ankle musculature that must react rapidly to maintain the position provides an overload stimulus for ankle power and proprioception. The decrease in fall risk also may be more robust in relatively younger nonfrail older adults.[134] Most patients enjoy the practice of Tai Chi and are compliant with its practice resulting in the benefit of the increased activity in general.

Resources/Exercises/Equipment. Typically, highly and knowledgeable practitioners in community venues teach Tai Chi in "schools." There appears to be some benefit of learning Tai Chi from experienced teachers who appreciate the skill, balance, coordination, mental application, and rigor that is necessary to obtain optimal benefit from this discipline. That is not to say that there is no benefit from learning Tai Chi from the many commercially available books and videos, some of which are specifically designed for physical therapists. Because of the evidence for improving fall risk, many therapists have learned Tai Chi and teach it to their patients as well as in classes.

Conclusion. Although there is good evidence for the use of Tai Chi in fall risk reduction, the evidence for other medical benefits is less consistent. Tai Chi's values lie in balance training and mental focus and can provide an interesting addition to a comprehensive exercise program.

SUMMARY

Exercise is *the* most powerful intervention for maintaining well-being, the remediation of impairment, and the promotion of function in all age groups. For older adults, exercise is a robust application for the prevention and treatment of chronic diseases and mobility disability and maintaining quality of life. As exercise, particularly strengthening, becomes more recognized for its beneficial effects on the aging process and thus demand for its skillful application is increased, physical therapists will be called upon to answer this need. Geriatric physical therapists are compelled to be exercise experts across all practice settings by applying our knowledge of the relationships between physical activity, pathology, impairment, functional abilities, and disability. Applying evidence-based principles can be challenging in geriatric settings, particularly when seeing the patient daily or twice daily. Table 5-11 provides an example of utilizing evidence-based exercise in an inpatient environment.

TABLE 5-11	Example of Using Evidence-based Recommendations in an Inpatient Environment			
	Monday	**Tuesday**	**Wednesday**	**Thursday**	**Friday**
Strengthening High intensity	Ankle and knee Quadriceps Dorsiflexors Gastrocnemius	Core strength Abdominals Gluteus maximus Gluteus medius Erector spinae	Ankle and knee Quadriceps Dorsiflexors Gastrocnemius	Core strength Abdominals Gluteus maximus Gluteus medius Erector spinae (Measure 10 RM/RPE)	Ankle and knee Quadriceps Dorsiflexors Gastrocnemius
Endurance Ambulation	Short bouts of fast gait speed (Measure: gait speed)	Ambulation distance (Measure: endurance 6 MWT or 400 MWT)	Work on gait speed	Ambulation distance	Short bouts of fast gait speed (Measure: gait speed)
Balancing Challenging	Static balance (reaching, head turns, eyes closed) Dynamic balance Stability ball	Dynamic gait (head turning, obstacle course, ramps, curbs, uneven and compliant surfaces)	Static balance Dynamic balance (squats, lunges, reaching with foot, ARROM with elastic while balancing on other foot) (Measure: balance, i.e., BBS)	Dynamic gait (head turning with forward, backward, and sideways stepping), obstacle course, uneven and compliant surfaces)	Static balance (reaching, head turns, eyes closed) Dynamic balance Stability ball
Task specific High intensity	Task specific (ADLs, transfers, bed mobility, wheelchair mobility) timed or weighted	Task specific (reaching, squatting, bending, lifting, rotation, etc.) timed or weighted	Task specific (ADLs, transfers, bed mobility, wheel chair mobility) timed or weighted	Task specific (reaching, squatting, bending, lifting, rotation, etc.) timed or weighted	Task specific (ADLs, transfers, bed mobility, wheelchair mobility) timed or weighted

This sample exercise program could be utilized with a patient requiring BID physical therapy treatments five days per week consistent with a functional profile of usual gait speed of .5 meters per second; Berg Balance Score of 40/56; a Timed Up and Go of 20 seconds; a 30 second sit-to-stand test of 5 repetitions; and a Four Square Step Test of 25 seconds.

REFERENCES

To enhance this text and add value for the reader, all references are included on the companion Evolve site that accompanies this text book. The reader can view the reference source and access it online whenever possible. There are a total of 137 cited references and other general references for this chapter.

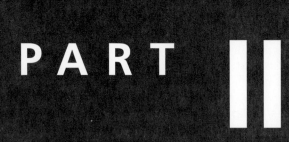

PART II

Contexts
for Examination
and Intervention

Health and Function:
Patient Management Principles

Andrew A. Guccione, PT, PhD, DPT, FAPTA, Cathy S. Elrod, PT, PhD

INTRODUCTION

Many different concepts are required to capture the broad dimensions of an older adult's eventual experience with disease and illness. Terms such as *health status, well-being,* and *quality of life* have all been used at various times to describe a facet of the human condition of individuals as they age. Physical therapists direct a substantial proportion of their clinical attention toward understanding the relationships among health, disease, and function, especially how the processes of normal aging and medical morbidity interact to alter a person's physical ability to do even the simplest activities of daily living (ADLs) and fulfill the role obligations associated with living independently as an adult.

One of the greatest challenges of geriatric physical therapy is to collect complete, but only pertinent, data and to categorize these clinical findings in a way that helps the therapist to understand what the patient's problems are; how they have come about; and what, if anything at all, could and should be done by a physical therapist to remedy the patient's situation. This chapter is intended to review existing patient management principles and to elucidate an integrated model for clinical decision making to meet this challenge effectively and efficiently. First, the chapter presents the concepts of health, disablement, and enablement and the primary purpose of physical therapist practice to enhance human performance as it pertains to movement and health. Subsequently, the process of making a clinical decision is discussed in the context of each of the components of patient management. Finally, a specific decision-making framework is presented for hypothesizing the causes of the patient's conditions (i.e., establishing a diagnosis) and designing a plan of care that integrates all pertinent information to achieve specific outcomes.

HEALTH, FUNCTION, AND DISABLEMENT

Health

The World Health Organization (WHO) defines *health* as a "state of complete physical, psychological, and social well-being, and not merely the absence of disease or infirmity."[1]

According to this definition, "health" is best understood as an end point in the major domains of human existence: physical, psychological, and social. In contrast to assuming "complete health" as the expected end point of an episode of care, physical therapists work across the spectrum, from wellness to the end of life to ensure outcomes associated with achieving the highest level of function possible wherever someone may be placed on that spectrum. The physical therapist's approach to optimizing "health" is typically grounded in objective tests and measures. In contrast, the patient's frame of reference is typically organized around the concept of *illness*, which refers to (1) the internal subjective experience of the individual who is aware that personal well-being has been jeopardized and (2) how the individual responds to the stressors on their well-being. The patient's concept of *illness* is a personal construct that represents an individual's response and interpretation of health status and its impact on particular roles.

When working with the older adult, it is also important to understand the concept of aging. Successful aging is considered to have three core elements: absence of disease and disability, high cognitive and physical functioning, and active engagement with life.[2] Although successful aging is ideal, it is unattainable for many older adults. Concurrently, optimal aging has been defined as "the capacity to function across many domains—physical, functional, cognitive, emotional, social, and spiritual—to one's satisfaction and in spite of one's medical conditions."[2] As optimal aging does not require the absence of disease, it fits well with the focus of most physical therapists who are working with the older adult.

Disablement and Enablement Applied to Function and Health

There have been several attempts to construct a model of health status that describes the relationship between health and function, or more precisely, describes the process of how individuals come to be disabled (disablement) and identifies factors, including therapeutic interventions, that can mitigate disablement (enablement process). The term *disablement* as defined in the *Guide to Physical Therapist Practice* refers to the "various impact(s) of chronic and acute conditions on the functioning of specific body systems, on basic human performance, and on people's functioning in necessary, usual, expected, and personally desired roles in society."[3]

The traditional medical model of disablement assumes a causal relationship between disease and illness. In this narrow perspective, disablement is primarily dependent on the characteristics of the individual (i.e., his or her pathology) that requires an intervention that can only be provided by a health care professional to alleviate it. The emerging social model of disability fundamentally broadens the focus away from an exclusive concentration on the disease-related physical impairments of the individual to also include the individual's physical and social environments that can impose both disabling limitations and enabling mitigation of limitations.[4]

Subsequent models of the twin processes of disablement and enablement have further explored the relationship of the environment to functional independence. In the 1960s, sociologist Saad Nagi characterized disablement as having four distinct components that evolve sequentially as an individual loses well-being: disease or pathology, impairments, functional limitations, and disability.[5,6] His work is associated with the biopsychosocial model, which recognizes the importance of psychological and social factors on the patient's experience of illness. In the late 1980s and early 1990s, Jette, Verbrugge, and Guccione began exploring the process of disablement as

a framework for physical therapists to assist them in clarifying the domains of practice.[7-11]

They proposed a multifactorial disablement framework that included the influence of environmental demand and individual capabilities on disability (Figure 6-1). Collectively, they have identified scientifically grounded factors associated with the development of disability that are organized into categories physical therapists should consider during examination. These categories include biological (e.g., genetic predisposition), demographic (e.g., age, education, income), medical and behavioral (e.g., medical care, comorbidities, health habits), psychological (e.g., motivation, coping), and the physical and social environments.

A further elaboration of Nagi's model was presented by Brandt and Pope in a 1997 report from the Institute of Medicine (IOM).[12] This revised model introduced the concept of enablement that explicated the balance between inevitable and reversible disablement depending on the confluence of disabling and enabling factors at the interface of a person with the environment. If ramps were introduced to allow access to the home or therapeutic exercises implemented that improved functional performance, then the individual with a neuromuscular condition precluding their ability to negotiate stairs has experienced a "disabling–enabling process." The IOM model has three dimensions: the person, the environment, and the interaction between the person and the environment. The "person" dimension shows a bidirectional connection between no disabling condition, pathology, impairment, and functional limitation. The physical, social, and psychological components of the environment are depicted in Figure 6-2 as a three-dimensional mat to

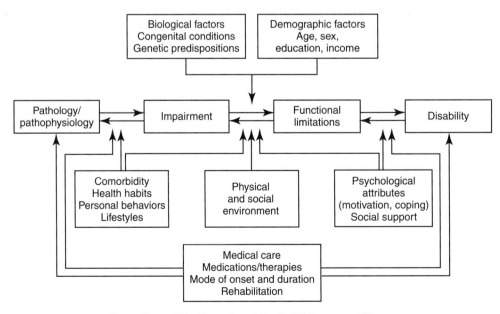

FIGURE 6-1 An expanded disablement model. *(Adapted with permission from Guccione AA. American physical therapy: Arthritis and the process of disablement. Phys Ther 1994;74:410.)*

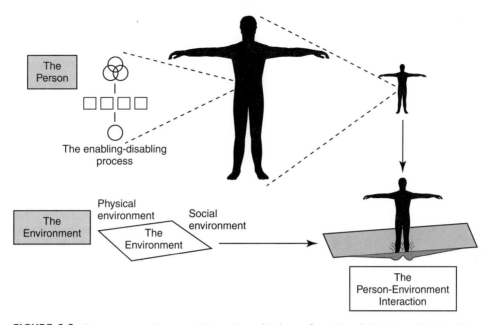

FIGURE 6-2 The person–environment interaction. *(Redrawn from Brandt EN, Pope AM: Enabling America: assessing the role of rehabilitation science and engineering. Washington, DC: National Academies Pres, 1997, p. 69.)*

indicate the magnitude of support provided by these systems and the importance of the person–environment interaction. This conceptualization allows us to understand how two older adults presenting with similar impairments associated with a right cerebrovascular accident can have different levels of disability according to the uniqueness of each individual and the environment in which they live. Physical therapists can use this information to promote optimal aging in the older adult.

International Classification of Functioning, Disability, and Health

The WHO also independently took on the task of developing a conceptual framework for describing and classifying the consequences of diseases. In 1980, they presented the *International Classification of Impairments, Disabilities, and Handicaps* (ICIDH).[13]

In response to concerns about the ICIDH, the WHO developed a substantially revised *International Classification of Functioning, Disability and Health* (ICF) in 2001 to "provide a unified and standard language and framework for the description of health and health-related states."[14] In 2007, the Institute of Medicine endorsed the adoption of this framework "as a means of promoting clear communication and building a coherent base of national and international research findings to inform public and private decision making."[15] The 2008 House of Delegates for the American Physical Therapy Association also embraced terminology of the ICF and initiated the process of incorporating ICF language into all relevant

Association publications, documents, and communications [HOD P06-08-11-04].

The ICF model, illustrated in Figure 6-3, employs a biopsychosocial approach that is compatible with many of the concepts from Nagi and the Institute of Medicine's work on enablement and disablement. Box 6-1 provides a comparison of the disablement terminology used by Nagi and ICF models. The ICF model is designed to encompass all aspects of health and include all situations that are associated with human functioning and its restrictions. Key operational definitions that allow interpretation and application of the ICF model are listed in Box 6-2. There are varying levels within the ICF's taxonomic classification schema of human functioning and disability. The first level consists of the broad categories of Body Functions, Body Structures, Activities and Participation, and Environmental Factors. Physical therapists will typically be

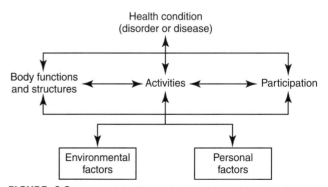

FIGURE 6-3 ICF model. *(From the World Health Organization: International classification of functioning, disability, and health: ICF. Geneva, Switzerland: World Health Organization, 2001, p. 18.)*

BOX 6-1	**Comparison of Disablement Concepts**
Nagi	**ICF**
Pathology	Health condition
Impairment	Body functions and structure
	Impairment
Functional limitation	Activity
	Activity limitation
Disability	Participation
	Participation restriction

ICF, International Classification of Functioning, Disability and Health.

BOX 6-2 | **ICF Definitions**

Health Condition: umbrella term for disease (acute or chronic), disorder, injury, or trauma; may also include other circumstances such as pregnancy, aging, stress, congenital anomaly, or genetic predisposition; coded using ICD-10

- *Body Functions:* the physiological functions of body systems, including psychological functions
- *Body Structures:* the structural or anatomic parts of the body such as organs, limbs, and their components classified according to body systems
- *Impairment:* a loss or abnormality in body structure or physiological function (including mental functions)
- *Activity:* the execution of a task or action by an individual; represents the individual perspective of functioning
- *Activity Limitation:* difficulties an individual may have in executing activities
- *Participation:* a person's involvement in a life situation; represents the societal perspective of functioning
- *Participation Restriction:* are problems an individual may experience in involvement in life situations
- *Functioning:* umbrella term for body functions, body structures, activities, and participation; denotes the positive aspects of the interaction between an individual (with a health condition) and that individual's contextual factors (environmental and personal factors)
- *Disability:* umbrella term for impairments, activity limitations, and participation restrictions; denotes the negative aspects of the interaction between an individual (with a health condition) and that individual's contextual factors (environment and personal factors)
- *Contextual Factors:* factors that together constitute the complete context of an individual's life, and in particular the background against which health states are classified in the ICF; there are two components of contextual factors: Environmental Factors and Personal Factors
- *Environmental Factors:* constitute a component of the ICF, and refer to all aspects of the external or extrinsic world that form the context of an individual's life and, as such, have an impact on that person's functioning; they include the physical world and its features, the human-made physical world, other people in different relationships and roles, attitudes and values, social systems and services, and policies, rules, and laws
- *Personal Factors:* contextual factors that relate to the individual such as age, gender, social status, life experience, and so on that are not currently classified in ICF but which users may incorporate in their application of the classification

(From: World Health Organization: International classification of functioning, disability, and health: ICF. Geneva: World Health Organization, 2001.)

most interested in the chapters contained within Activities and Participation. More specifically, the chapter on mobility delineates actions associated with (1) changing and maintaining body position; (2) carrying, moving, and handling objects; (3) walking and moving; and (4) moving around using transportation. The ICF taxonomy also denotes the severity of the problem with a set of standardized qualifiers that provide further description. Using the example in Box 6-3, a classification of d4104 indicates there is no problem (0 to 4%) in the ability of the individual in regard to "getting into and out of a standing position or changing body position from standing to any other position, such as lying down or sitting down."[14]

In contrast at the opposite end, a classification of d4104.3 indicates that there is a complete problem (96% to 100%) with the ability to perform this task. For further discussion of the application of this model to clinical practice, refer to the WHO's comprehensive publication on the ICF.[14] Thus, the ICF attempts to provide a common language to describe patients' behaviors and environmental situations that need to be taken into consideration when making clinical decisions, especially in regard to optimizing human performance in the older adult.

Disease/Health Condition. In Nagi's model, the term *disease* refers to an ongoing pathologic state that is delineated by a particular cluster of signs and symptoms and is recognized externally by either the individual or a practitioner as abnormal. Nagi's concept of disease is rooted in the principle of homeostasis: The human organism responds to an active pathologic state by mobilizing its resources to respond to a threat and to return to its normal state.[5]

Disease may be the result of infection, trauma, metabolic imbalance, degenerative processes, or other etiologic factors. Whatever the cause, Nagi's concept of disease emphasizes two features: (1) an active threat to the organism's normal state from a *single* active pathology and (2) an active response internally by the organism to that threat, which may be aided externally by therapeutic interventions. Nagi's concept of disease does not cover all scenarios that could necessitate the services of a physical therapist. There are numerous medical conditions that affect an individual's ability to function that are not related to any *single* active pathology. Congestive heart failure (CHF), for example, is a medical syndrome that is a recognized cluster of signs and symptoms. Although CHF evolves from active pathologic factors over time, it is the coexistence of these pathologic factors over the same time period that may explain CHF in the older individuals.[16] A physical therapist's caseload may also include individuals whose medical diagnoses indicate fixed lesions, which identify previous insults to a body

BOX 6-3 | Structure of ICF: An Example

Component	Activities and Participation (d)
Chapter	Mobility (4)
Category: Level 1	Changing and maintaining body position (d410-d429)
Category: Level 2	Changing basic body position (d410)
Category: Level 3	Standing (d4104)
Qualifier	Severe problem (d4104.3)

ICF, International Classification of Functioning, Disability and Health.

part or organ and sites of dysfunction but are not presently associated with any active processes. A patient who has had a stroke is a common example of an individual with a fixed neuroanatomic lesion that is no longer associated with any ongoing pathologic process but still experiences an alteration in his health.

The ICF expands beyond Nagi's concept of disease to include any *health condition* that takes the individual away from the "state of complete physical, psychological, and social well-being" and builds upon the evolving acceptance of wellness as an attainable goal.[1] The *International Classification of Disease, Tenth Revision* (ICD-10), also a product of the WHO, provides a classification schema that incorporates both diseases and related health problems into a comprehensive listing of "health conditions."

Impairment of Body Structure or Function. Impairments, defined as alterations in anatomic, physiological, or psychological structures or functions, typically evolve as the consequence of disease, pathologic processes, or lesions, altering the person's normal health state and contributing to the individual's illness. For example, physical impairments, such as pain and decreased range of motion (ROM) in the shoulder, may be the overt manifestations (or symptoms and signs) of either temporary or permanent disease or pathologic processes for some, but not necessarily all, older adult patients. The genesis of an impairment can often be unclear. Poor posture, for example, is neither a disease nor a pathologic state, yet the resultant muscle shortening and capsular tightness may present as major impairments in a clinical examination. Thus, not all older adults are patients because they have a disease. Some individuals are treated by physical therapists because their impairments are sufficient enough cause for intervention regardless of the presence (or absence) of disease or active pathology.

Given that much of physical therapy is directed toward remediating or minimizing impairments, additional elaboration of the concept of impairment is particularly useful in geriatric physical therapy. Schenkman and Butler have proposed that impairments can be classified in three ways: direct, indirect, and composite effect.[17,18] Direct impairments are the effect of a disease, syndrome, or lesion and are relatively confined to a single system. For example, they note that weakness can be classified as a neuromuscular impairment that is a direct effect of a peripheral motor neuropathy in the lower extremity. Indirect impairments are impairments in other systems that can "indirectly" affect the underlying problem. For example, ambulation training of a patient with a peripheral motor neuropathy may put excessive strain on joints and ligaments, resulting in new musculoskeletal impairments. The combination of weakness from the primary motor neuropathy and ligamentous strain from excessive forces on the joints may lead to a composite effect, the impairment of pain.

Using neurologic dysfunction as the vehicle, Schenkman and Butler described this three-category concept of impairment by categorizing clinical signs and symptoms into impairments that have a direct, indirect, or composite effect, thus bringing together into a cohesive relationship the diverse data of the medical history and the findings of the clinical examination. For example, consider a 79-year-old woman with severe peripheral vascular disease (PVD). Upon clinical examination, the physical therapist notes that this individual has lost sensation below the right knee. Sensory loss is an impairment that would be classified as a direct effect of PVD. As the individual is ambulating less and cannot sense full ankle ROM, loss of ROM may be an indirect effect of the patient's PVD on the musculoskeletal system. The combination of the direct impairment—sensory loss below the knee—and the indirect impairment—decreased ROM in the ankle—may help to explain another clinical finding, poor balance, which can be understood as a composite effect of other impairments. Piecing clinical data together in this fashion allows the therapist to uncover the interrelationships among a patient's PVD, loss of sensation, limited ROM, and balance deficits. Without a framework that sorts the patient's clinical data into relevant categories, the therapist might never comprehend how the patient's problems came to be and thus how to intervene. Treatment consisting of balance activities alone would be inappropriate, because the therapist must also address the loss in ROM as well as teach the patient to compensate for the sensory loss to remediate the impairments.

Activity Limitation. Although most of us anticipate that our body systems will deteriorate somewhat as we age, an inability to do for one's self from day to day perhaps most clearly identifies when adults are losing their health. Activity limitations result from impairments and consist of an individual's inability to perform his or her usual functions and tasks such as reaching for something on an overhead shelf or carrying a package. As measures of behaviors at the level of a person, and not anatomic or physiological conditions, limitations in the performance of activities should not be confused with diseases or impairments that encompass aberrations in specific tissues, organs, and systems that present clinically as the patient's signs and symptoms.

Activity limitations are typically grouped into distinct functional domains: physical, psychological, and social. *Physical function* covers an individual's sensorimotor performance in the execution of particular actions. Rolling, getting out of bed, transferring, walking, climbing, bending, lifting, and carrying are all examples of actions that are components of physical functional activities. These motoric acts underlie the fundamental daily organized patterns of behavioral tasks that are further classified as basic ADL such as feeding, dressing, bathing, grooming, and toileting. The more complex activities associated with independent community living, for example, using public transportation or grocery shopping, are categorized as instrumental activities of daily living, often abbreviated as IADLs. Successful performance of complex physical functional activities, such as personal hygiene and housekeeping, typically requires integration of cognitive and affective abilities as well as physical ones.[19]

Psychological function has two components: mental and affective. *Mental function* covers a range of cognitive activities such as telling time and performing money calculations that are essential to living independently as an adult. Attention, concentration, memory, and judgment are all elements of mental function. *Affective function* broadly refers to both the everyday "hassles" of daily existence that are part of every individual's experience as well as the more traumatic events such as death of a spouse. A person's emotional state and effectiveness in coping with the stresses attributable to disease or negative impacts of the aging process are indicators of the patient's affective function. Self-esteem, anxiety, depression, and coping are also represented in the construct of affective functioning.

Social function encompasses an individual's social activities such as church attendance or family gatherings as well as performance of social roles and obligations. Grandparenting and being employed outside the home are two examples of social role functioning relevant to an older individual and therefore are potential problems to be considered in the physical therapist's initial examination. Although physical therapists are chiefly concerned with physical functional activities, individuals typically conceive their personal identities in terms of specific social roles: worker, father, grandmother, wife, community volunteer. All of these roles demand a certain degree of physical ability. Many opportunities for social interaction for retired adults occur around volunteer and leisure activities, even if it means only the manual dexterity required to dial a telephone. The patient's goals and preferences, major contributors of the choice of therapeutic goals, are typically presented in terms of their desired social roles. Therefore, the positive effect of improved physical functional status with older persons has importance to the patient primarily in relationship to the concomitant positive effect these improvements have on social functioning.

Although most every patient under geriatric care is likely to carry at least two medical diagnoses, each of which will manifest itself in particular impairments of the cardiopulmonary, integumentary, musculoskeletal, or neuromuscular systems, impairment does not always entail activity limitations. One cannot assume that an individual will be unable to perform the actions and roles of usual daily living by virtue of having an impairment alone. For example, an adult with osteoarthritis (disease) may exhibit loss of range of motion (impairment) and experience great difficulty in transferring from a bed to a chair (action). Another individual with osteoarthritis and equal loss of ROM may transfer from bed to chair easily by choosing to use an appropriate assistive device, or participating in a supervised muscle strengthening program. Sometimes patients will overcome multiple, and even permanent, impairments by the sheer force of their motivation.

The degree to which limitations in physical functional activities may be linked to impairments has not been fully determined through research, and there is a critical need to update the epidemiology of impairment and action/function among older adults. The relatively few studies that have been reported in the literature support a generally linear but modest relationship between impairments and functional status. These need to be replicated or updated with more recent data on the health status of contemporary older adults.[20-24] Such data are essential to both (1) identifying relevant functional outcomes of an intervention and (2) establishing the dose–response relationship for an efficacious intervention that is known to remediate impairments to a particular degree or magnitude and is sufficient to produce a clinically important change in an individual's functional status.

Participation Restriction. In revising the ICIDH, WHO rejected the term *handicap* and introduced an alternative concept, *participation*, which is associated with their specific definition of *activity* and *activity limitation*.[14] In the ICF framework activity limitation bears some resemblance to functional limitation in the Nagi model, in which a person experiences a limitation in performing an action, task, or activity. In contrast, *participation* in the ICF is defined as "involvement in life situations" and is characterized by a person's performance of actions and tasks in that individual's actual environment. In this sense, participation restriction is most similar to Nagi's term *disability* that identified limitations in executing a specific social role in a particular sociocultural context (e.g., spouse, worker, grandparent, or caregiver). *Activity* and *participation* in the ICF do not admit Nagi's distinction between failure to perform a specific function and an inability to meet role expectations in which performing a particular function is essential to fulfilling the requirements of the role. In fact, the ICF uses the same list of actions and tasks to describe both *activity* and *participation*, an approach that has its critics and is likely to be refined on the basis of further research.[14,25]

The Concept of Disability. Nagi reserved the term *disability* for patterns of behavior that emerged over long periods of time during which an individual experienced functional limitations to such a degree that an inability to fulfill desired social roles resulted. Although a person may have a significant limitation in shoulder motion, this impaired state is *not* considered disabling if the individual is able to adapt performance (perhaps altering movement at other joints or using assistive devices) to achieve activities that allow them to continue performing social roles despite the limited shoulder movement. Compensation using an individual's other capabilities and abilities as well as task adaptation are "enabling" and thus offsets disablement through the process of enablement.

Although each of the terms that have been presented so far involves some consensus about what is "normal," the concept of a disability is socially constructed. Nagi's concept of disability or the ICF's *participation restriction* is characterized by discordance between the actual performance of an individual in a particular role and the expectations of the community for what is normal or typically expected behavior for an adult. The meaning of *disabled* is taken from the community in which the individual lives and the criteria for normal within that social group. The term *disabled* connotes a particular status in society. Labeling a person as disabled requires a judgment, usually by a professional, that an individual's behaviors are somehow inadequate based on the professional's understanding of the expectations that the activity should be accomplished in ways that are typical for a person's age and gender as well as cultural and social environment.

The ICF has redefined the term *disability* to reflect the summative negative aspects of the interaction between an individual who has a health condition and that individual's environment and personal factors. It encompasses impairment, activity limitations, and participation restrictions. Thus, disability is the broadest term in the ICF framework and harkens back to the IOM conceptualization that locates disability at the interface of a person's capabilities and abilities, personal factors, and the biopsychosocial environment. The evidence suggests that activity limitations and participation restrictions in a geriatric population change over time, and not all older adults exhibit functional decline. If we follow any cohort of older adults over time, there will be more activity limitations and subsequent restrictions in participation overall within the group, but some individuals will actually improve and others will maintain their functional level. Restricting the use of the term *disabled* to describe only long-term overall functional decline in geriatric populations encourages us to understand a particular older adult's activity limitations and participation restrictions in a dynamic context subject to change, particularly after therapeutic intervention. Participation restrictions depend on both the capacities of the individual

and the expectations that are imposed on the individual by those in the immediate social environment, most often the patient's family and caregivers. Physical therapists who apply a health status perspective to the assessment of patients draw on a broad appreciation of an older adult as a person living in a particular social context as well as having individual characteristics. Changing the expectations of a social context—for example, explaining to family members what level of assistance is appropriate to an older adult after stroke—may help to diminish disability as much as supplying the patient with assistive devices or increasing the physical ability to use them.

Granger was among the first to note that although the pathways from disease to disability are thought to be unidirectional, disability may itself initiate further impairments and activity limitations that foster disease.[26] Perhaps no clearer example of disability among older persons exists than the individual who has been incapacitated by cardiac disease because rehabilitation has not encouraged resumption of a level of activity that is normal for that person. Lack of activity may result in further impairment in both the cardiopulmonary and musculoskeletal systems, which may further put the individual at risk of recurrent cardiac episodes.

CLINICAL DECISION MAKING

The primary purpose of physical therapist practice with older adults is to enhance human performance as it pertains to movement and health. The concepts within the enablement/disablement process and the ICF can be used to inform diagnostic decisions that guide physical therapists to plan and direct treatment.[27-31] Functional status is the lens through which the physical therapist analyzes impairments to identify activities and participation deficits and subsequent interventions to enhance performance as it is mediated through movement. Analysis of human performance draws upon all domains of a physical therapist's knowledge to examine the complex interaction of systems that permits an individual to maintain a posture, transition to other postures, or sustain safe and efficient movement as an underlying dimension of an individual's ability to pursue and perform goal-directed and personally desired tasks and activities under natural conditions.

To provide physical therapy interventions that will achieve the goal of restoring, improving, or minimizing the loss of function, the physical therapist must know more than the patient's signs and symptoms, which are expressions of the individual's health conditions and impairments. The physical therapist must analyze the patient's movements and determine which activities have an undesirable effect on human performance. The tasks and actions that comprise these activities as well as the impairments that contribute to activity limitations must be discerned. The physical therapist then places these findings in the context of the individual's motivation to perform the action or task, and whether the physical and sociocultural environment facilitates goal achievement

A challenge for physical therapists is to accurately interpret the underlying reason for the patient/client's presentation and then effectively achieve optimal outcomes. To do this, the clinician must incorporate the judicious use of examination findings into the decision-making process to generate hypotheses for the cause of the patient's presenting complaint. Various factors influence clinical reasoning and choice of assessment methods. These factors include the therapist's knowledge, expertise, goals, values, beliefs, and use of evidence; the patient's age, diagnosis, medical history as well as his or her own goals, values, and beliefs; available resources; clinical practice environment; level of financial and social support; and the intended use of the collected information.[32,33] During the past two decades, several frameworks to guide patient management have

been articulated specifically to address physical therapist practice. In the following section, we will discuss three of these frameworks in detail.

The *Guide*'s Patient/Client Management Model

The *Guide to Physical Therapist Practice* describes a patient/client management model composed of five components: examination, evaluation, diagnosis, prognosis, and intervention (Figure 6-4).[3] The *Guide* was constructed initially in the mid-1990s with two underlying premises: (1) the process of disablement is a useful model for understanding and organizing physical therapist practice and (2) diagnosis by physical therapists is an essential element of practice requiring a classification scheme that directs intervention. Each component of the *Guide*'s model was intended to make a vital contribution to the

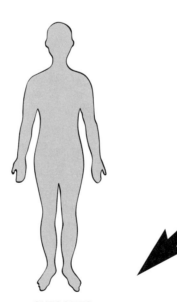

DIAGNOSIS
Both the process and the end result of evaluating examination data, which the physical therapist organizes into defined clusters, syndromes, or categories to help determine the prognosis (including the plan of care) and the most appropriate intervention strategies.

**PROGNOSIS
(Including Plan of Care)**
Determination of the level of optimal improvement that may be attained through intervention and the amount of time required to reach that level. The plan of care specifies the interventions to be used and their timing and frequency.

EVALUATION
A dynamic process in which the physical therapist makes clinical judgments based on data gathered during the examination. This process also may identify possible problems that require consultation with or referral to another provider.

INTERVENTION
Purposeful and skilled interaction of the physical therapist with the patient/client and, if appropriate, with other individuals involved in care of the patient/client, using various physical therapy procedures and techniques to produce changes in the condition that are consistent with the diagnosis and prognosis. The physical therapist conducts a reexamination to determine changes in patient/client status and to modify or redirect intervention. The decision to reexamine may be based on new clinical findings or on lack of patient/client progress. The process of reexamination also may identify the need for consultation with or referral to another provider.

EXAMINATION
The process of obtaining a history, performing a systems review, and selecting and administering tests and measures to gather data about the patient/client. The initial examination is a comprehensive screening and specific testing process that leads to a diagnostic classification. The examination process also may identify possible problems that require consultation with or referral to another provider.

OUTCOMES
Results of patient/client management, which include the impact of physical therapy interventions in the following domains: pathology/pathophysiology (disease, disorder, or condition); impairments, functional limitations, and disabilities; risk reduction/prevention; health, wellness, and fitness; societal resources; and patient/client satisfaction.

FIGURE 6-4 The elements of patient/client management. *(Redrawn from the American Physical Therapy Association: Guide to physical therapist practice. Alexandria, VA: American Physical Therapy Association, 2001, p. 32.)*

achievement of positive outcomes whereby activity limitations and disability are diminished or eliminated, patient satisfaction is attained, and secondary prevention is successful. This framework clearly delineates the major component of decision making that the physical therapist proceeds through in an organized fashion. However, it does not provide recommendations for decision-making approaches to guide the practitioner.

The first component of the patient/client management model, *examination*, has three parts: history, systems review, and specific tests and measures. Information about the patient's past and current health history can be obtained from the medical record, the patient, and/or caregivers. According to the *Guide*, the different types of data that can be generated from the patient history include general demographics, social history, employment/work, growth and development, general health status, social/health habits, family history, medical/surgical history, current condition(s)/chief complaint(s), functional status and activity level, medications, and other clinical tests.[3]

After organizing one's thoughts around whatever historical information about the patient is available, the therapist begins the "hands-on" component of the clinical encounter. The systems review is a brief examination of the anatomic and physiological status of the cardiopulmonary, integumentary, musculoskeletal, and neuromuscular systems, especially as each of these affects a person's ability to initiate and sustain purposeful movement directed toward performance of a task or activity pertinent to the patient's function. The data generated by the systems review is then used by the physical therapist to select specific tests and measures that, in turn, will be used to establish a diagnosis and prognosis and to develop the plan of care. The tests and measures that are done as part of an initial examination should only be those necessary to confirm or reject a hypothesis about the factors that contribute to making the patient's current level of function less than optimal.

The data that have been gathered from the examination portion is then organized and analyzed for the second component of patient management, *evaluation*. When evaluating the data, the therapist must use his or her clinical judgment to identify possible problems as those requiring either the skilled interventions provided by physical therapists or referral to other health care professionals. The relationship between impairment and function forms the tentative basis for a system of classification for diagnosis by physical therapists, which is the third component of patient management, *diagnosis*.[9]

The *Guide* established, through an extensive consensus process, preferred practice patterns that describe a cluster of impairments associated with health conditions that impede optimal function. After evaluation of the examination data, the physical therapist uses the classification scheme of the preferred practice patterns to complete the diagnostic process and applies a label (diagnosis) for the patient's clinical presentation. As constructed on the basis of impairments, the preferred practice patterns fulfill a major requirement of professional diagnosis, that is, the label (diagnosis) applied as the end result of the diagnostic process directs intervention within the scope of practice of the professional applying the label.[9] Specifically, each of the preferred practice patterns identifies the most characteristic impairments associated with a target condition that are likely to be the primary concerns of the physical therapist's plan of care.

Step four is to determine the *prognosis* or "the level of optimal improvement that may be attained through intervention and the amount of time required to reach that level."[3] Within this context, the plan of care is developed which identifies the specific interventions to be performed as well as the time frame in which they will occur.

Component five of the patient/client management model, *intervention*, as explicated by the *Guide*, has three parts: (1) coordination, communication, and documentation; (2) patient-related instruction; and (3) direct intervention. Effective and comprehensive care that addresses the patient's needs is promoted through the processes of coordination, communication, and documentation. The range of an older adult's needs can be very broad and often exceed a physical therapist's scope of practice. Health care can be conceived of as a continuum of services. At one end are medical and nursing care, which deal with the patient's disease and illness. At the other end of the continuum are social care and a system to facilitate reentry of a patient with a permanent disability into the community. Although some overlap will always exist, each of these professionals has a primary relationship with the patient that is predicated on the professional's domain of expertise. Superimposing the continuum of health care onto the patient's clinical needs may provide some clues as to which other practitioners should be consulted in a well-coordinated plan of care. The *Guide* also describes nine major groups of direct interventions, all of which are relevant to geriatric physical therapy: therapeutic exercise; functional training in self-care and home management; functional training in community and work integration or reintegration; manual therapy techniques; prescription, application, and as appropriate, fabrication of devices and equipment; airway clearance techniques; wound management; electrotherapeutic modalities; and physical agents and mechanical modalities. Specific applications of these direct interventions are discussed at length in other chapters of this text. Throughout the intervention step, the physical therapist engages in continuous reexamination of the patient to determine the effectiveness of the interventions and accuracy of the diagnostic process. A determination is made as to whether the patient has achieved the desired outcome or if further revision of the plan of care is needed.

Although the fundamental details of diagnosis and classification contained in the *Guide* are sufficient to its purpose as a general description of practice, the *Guide*'s patient/client management model is not explicit enough to guide actual clinical decisions. To explicate clinical decision making, it is worthwhile to consider several specific approaches to gathering and clustering data as a part of, and subsequent to, the initial clinical examination. These approaches will be described below.

Hypothesis-Oriented Algorithm for Clinicians

Rothstein and Echternach's work provides a framework for *how* one goes about making a clinical decision. Their Hypothesis-Oriented Algorithm for Clinicians (HOAC) was developed in 1986.[34]

At that time, the concept for clinical decision making had not been clearly articulated in physical therapy, but the approach used in the HOAC bears many similarities to the ideas articulated by Sackett[35] and Guyatt[36] among others that later became cornerstones of evidence-based practice and its emphasis on probabilistic strategies in diagnosis and intervention. Rothstein and Echternach stated that "it seems obvious that this process of examination of a patient, treatment planning, implementation of treatment, and treatment reevaluation needs an overall clinical decision-making scheme to allow the physical therapist to function in a changing environment."[37]

In 2003, they revised their original model into the Hypothesis-Oriented Algorithm for Clinicians II (HOAC II).[38] The HOAC II incorporated the disablement terminology used in the *Guide to Physical Therapist Practice* and the more recent emphasis on prevention in physical therapist practice. The fundamental component of both the original and revised model is the development of a hypothesis about the cause of the patient's problem. The term *hypothesis* is used "because it has a mechanism for therapists to test whether their ideas about causes of problems (i.e., their diagnoses) may be correct."[38] A systematic approach to patient management such as the one described by the HOAC allows the therapist to delineate a clear pathway for examining, evaluating, and monitoring the effects of all interventions and to reevaluate and, as necessary, to refine a treatment plan to ensure optimal outcomes.

Schenkman's Model of Integration and Task Analysis

Schenkman, Deutsch, and Gill-Body[39] proposed a systematic strategy for making clinical decisions that integrates enablement–disablement concepts, the HOAC II, and task analysis principles to interpret clinical findings within the patient/client management model proposed in the *Guide* (Figure 6-5). Although their strategies focused specifically on neurologic physical therapist practice, the framework is generally applicable to the broad range of diagnostic reasoning employed in geriatric physical ther-

apist practice. Instead of the process focusing around the health condition and resultant disability, this approach is patient-centered and emphasizes the patient's capabilities, not just limitations, to achieve the desired outcomes. Task analysis is the first step in understanding the relationship between activity limitation and impairment as task analysis further characterizes the nature and extent of the patient's limitation.

AN INTEGRATED STRATEGY FOR DECISION MAKING

The complexity of clinical decision making can be daunting because of the sheer volume of information and detailed considerations unique to the individual. However, physical therapists who make movement-related human performance the central focus of their decision-making process and approach each decision-making step systematically with a clear organizational strategy for gathering and utilizing information will find it easier to identify and apply pertinent information.

This final section describes a decision-making strategy that integrates key features of several decision-making models and frameworks discussed earlier. The model emphasizes the relationship between impairment and function as the central component of physical therapist practice that addresses human performance mediated through movement. Our model (Figure 6-6) remains generally organized around the five components of the *Guide to Physical Therapist Practice*'s Patient/Client Management Model incorporating Schenkman and colleagues' arguments that task analysis in the environmental context is one of the skills that define the physical therapist and is essential for effective decision making. Our strategy for evidence-based practice identifies the previously described enablement–disablement process as a fundamental organizing principle to formulate clinical hypotheses that guide the analysis, synthesis, and judgments made by physical therapists about the physical therapy management of their individual patients. The remainder of this chapter describes each patient management step in this integrated strategy.

Examination

The examination considers all the components identified in the *Guide to Physical Therapist Practice*, as described earlier. Older adults typically enter physical therapy with a referral that may contain a few useful facts about the patient's medical history or the medical reason for the referral. In these circumstances the first question to ask oneself is, Given the facts about the patient that are available before the examination, have any impairments or activity limitations been identified even before the patient is seen for the first time? The collection of two kinds of clinical data should be integrated into the format for the first clinical encounter. First, as summarized

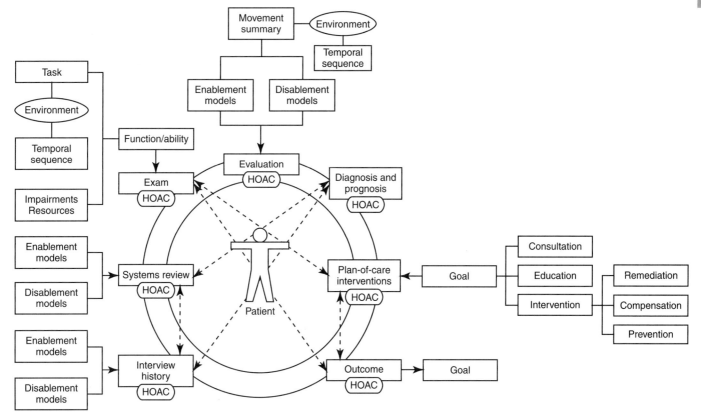

FIGURE 6-5 Schenkman's model of integration and task analysis. *HOAC,* Hypothesis-oriented algorithem for clinicians. *(Redrawn from Schenkman M, Duetsch JE, Gill-Body KM: An integrated framework for decision making in neurologic physical therapist practice. Phys Ther 2006;86:1683.)*

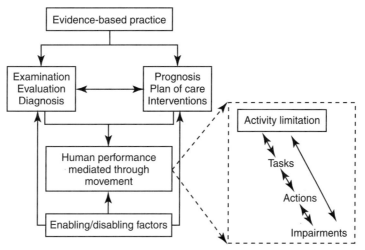

FIGURE 6-6 Integrated strategy for clinical decision making.

in Box 6-4, there are a number of factors identified in the literature and reviewed elsewhere in this text that may influence the trajectory of a patient from disease to disability. Physical therapists should always account for these potentially enabling–disabling influences as part of the patient examination. Additional information that would assist in setting goals and designing intervention and information from other disciplines can also be very helpful. Data on the individual's current medical condi-

tions and medications, for example, are extremely relevant.

If the overall goal is to optimize patient function, then one of the first steps is to ascertain the patient's current level of function. Whenever the patient's communication ability is intact, the initial interview begins by allowing patients to identify what they see as the primary activity limitations that have prompted the need for physical therapy. In their formulation of a

BOX 6-4   Components of Patient History

HISTORY

Previous
- Demographics
- Social history
- Work/school/play
- Living environment
- General health status
- Health habits
- Behavioral health
- Family history
- Medical/surgical history

Current
- Current conditions
- Chief complaint
- Current function
- Activity level
- Medications
- Clinical labs/tests
- Review of other systems

hypothetico-deductive strategy for making clinical judgments, Rothstein and Echternach emphasize the value of listening as patients identify their problems and allowing the individuals to express the desired goal of treatment in their own terms.[34] By talking with the patient, the therapist begins to develop not only a professional rapport but also an appreciation of the patient's understanding of the situation. The input of the patient in terms of preferences, motivations, and goals are central pieces of "evidence" in an evidence-based approach to decision making.[35] This is especially pertinent to care provided to older individuals who may find their ability to control their own personal destinies compromised by professional judgments made "in their best interests." When the patient is unable to communicate effectively, the therapist may turn to proxy information. The patient's family and friends may be able to give some insight as to what the patient would regard as the goals of intervention. The therapist may also hypothesize about a patient's functional deficits based on previous experience with similar patients.

Data from the history, as well as data on how the patient's problems have been treated in the past, allow the therapist to hypothesize that certain impairments or activity limitations might exist by virtue of the individual's medical condition(s) and sociodemographic and other personal characteristics. For example, suppose that the physical therapist learns from the patient's history that the patient has a medical diagnosis of Parkinson's disease, that she is 81 years old, and that she lives alone. The diagnosis of Parkinson's disease suggests the possibility of the following impairments: loss of motor control and abnormal tone, ROM deficits, faulty posture, and decreased endurance for functional activities. Using epidemiologic research about what activity limitations are likely for women living alone, specific questions about independence in IADLs, with specific tests and measures as indicated, would be appropriate to include in the examination. Social isolation, for example, may lead to depression,

which could further aggravate a person's functional difficulties.

Because there is a lot of variability (e.g., physical fitness, cognition, chronic conditions) in older adults, a screen of all systems is crucial to ensure the physical therapist does not miss a critical finding. Screening begins with a thorough patient history as the physical therapist relies heavily on the clinical presentation of the patient and any signs or symptoms that indicate the need for specific screening tests or questions.[40] Therapists must recognize, for example, when integumentary signs may be indicative of systemic connective tissue disorders or oncologic disease, when the patient would concomitantly benefit from the services of other health care professionals, and when additional signs and symptoms may also suggest other impairments that would benefit from physical therapy. The combination of the patient history and screening of systems leads to more focused tests and measures. As physical therapists strive to be efficient, they realize that performing all tests to rule in or out a potential diagnosis is time prohibitive. Expert clinicians rely on "pattern recognition" as well as early generation of hypotheses for interpreting collected data.[41] Concurrent with these observations and interim judgments, the physical therapist may reach a conclusion that the signs and symptoms are not consistent with any pattern of disease or illness that is in the scope of physical therapist practice and may refer the patient to another health care professional.

During the examination, the therapist should begin by performing a detailed analysis of functional activities (e.g., transferring from the bed to a chair) that also takes into consideration the environment in which the task is being performed. Task analysis is at the crux of establishing a diagnosis that can point to an intervention in the domain of physical therapist practice. The ICF organizes actions and tasks into an implicit hierarchy of functioning. Physical therapists are well prepared to identify dysfunction at the level of actions by examining the action- or movement-oriented component of tasks. Tests and measures of actions are particularly relevant, and using self-report assessment instruments such as the American Physical Therapy Association's (APTA's) OPTIMAL may facilitate identification of problem areas.[42] Difficulties in any part of this process could result in activity limitations that require the skills of a physical therapist to remediate.

The therapist initially makes a working hypothesis regarding the underlying cause of any deficits noted during the history and systems review and then selects specific tests and measures that would most likely confirm his or her suspicions about a tentative diagnosis. Specific tests and measures are used in the examination to clarify and characterize the nature and extent of activity limitations and further implicate impairments and other factors that impede performance. Is the inability to climb stairs in an older adult associated with knee and hip extensor weakness? What about balance deficits due to sensory loss in the feet and ankles? Thus, broadening the examination to focus on observing and critiquing the performance of actions and tasks is crucial to ensure a thorough evaluation of the patient's inability to perform specific goal-directed activities. The inability to perform movements needed to execute specific goal-directed activities is particularly relevant to physical therapist practice as they capture the complex integration of systems that permits an individual to maintain a posture, transition to other postures, or sustain safe and efficient movement.

Tests and measures will vary in the precision of measurement, yet useful data may be generated through various means. Data generated from either a gross test, such as "break" test for strength, or from a much more precise measure of a dynamometer could be used to reject the hypothesis that muscle performance is a contributing factor to the patient's functional deficit, depending on particular circumstances. Similarly, a functional assessment instrument may quantify a large number of ADLs or IADLs yet fail to detect a particular task and action deficit that is most crucial to the patient's limitation. The "correct" test or measure is the one that yields data that are sufficiently accurate and precise to allow the therapist to make a correct inference about the patient's condition. Therefore, the therapist must consider the quality of the data, the likelihood of error, and, most importantly, the risk to the patient associated with making a clinical judgment with less-than-acceptable certainty when evaluating the meaning of the data collected on examination.

Evaluation and Diagnosis

After the examination, the therapist evaluates the data by making clinical judgments about their meaning and their relevance to the patient's condition, and to confirm or reject hypotheses posed during the examination. The therapist then hypothesizes which findings contribute to the patient's functional deficits and will be the focus of patient-related instruction and direct intervention.

It is not unusual for older patients to have multiple impairments and activity limitations, many of which can be identified by a physical therapist and treated using physical therapy procedures. However, the overall purpose of evaluation is twofold: (1) to indicate which deficiencies in functioning prevent a person from achieving optimal well-being and (2) to identify the actions and tasks that are most associated with the patient's current level of function and must be remediated for the patient to reach an optimal functional level. An element of assessing data on the patient's ability to perform functional activities is to determine whether the manner in which actions and tasks are done represents an important quantitative or qualitative deviation from the way in which most people of similar age would perform them.

In the absence of norms for age-stratified functional performance, the therapist must bring previous experience with similar patients to bear on this judgment. Even if the therapist concludes that the patient's performance is other than "normal," this judgment does not imply that a person cannot meet socially imposed expectations of what it means to be independent or that an individual is permanently disabled. Furthermore, identifying the impairment alone may not fully explain the inability to perform an activity as the individual's motivation to perform the activity as well as the environment in which it is performed may affect goal achievement. Thus, the physical therapist must review activity limitations in light of other clinical findings that identify the patient's impairments and other psychological, social, and environmental factors that modify function in determining whether a patient will become disabled. Upon completion of the evaluation, physical therapists hypothesize as to the cause of the patient's need for physical therapy. The hypothesis, otherwise known as a diagnosis, allows the therapist to accurately and effectively direct the plan of care.

Approaches to Clinical Diagnosis. Physical therapists engage in the diagnostic process every time they assess a patient, cluster findings, interpret data, and label patient problems.[3] Several different approaches, previously described by Sackett et al., are used by practitioners to arrive at a clinical diagnosis.[35]

One strategy uses a *decision tree* to progress the initial examination along one of a large number of potential paths. A patient's response to each inquiry or clinical assessment procedure automatically determines the next inquiry. The major disadvantage of this approach is that all contingencies have to be worked out explicitly in advance. If a patient's response or clinical presentation has not been included on the tree, then the next step of the examination remains unknown. Matching all the possible responses that could be exhibited by an older adult to specific routines of clinical examination is a daunting challenge. Furthermore, as the profession of physical therapy seeks to establish its scientific credibility, each step of the decision tree must be validated empirically.

A second approach for clinical diagnosis is the *complete history and physical*, which has also been termed by Sackett as the *strategy of exhaustion*: "the painstaking invariant search for, but paying no immediate attention to, all medical facts about the patient followed by sifting through the data for the diagnosis."[35] Generally, this is the method of the novice and is abandoned with experience. Sackett et al. have commented that all medical students should be taught how to do both a complete history and physical and then, once they have mastered its components, never to do one. A similar admonition may be appropriate for physical therapy students and clinicians, especially those with an interest in caring for older adults. Students and clinicians must have mastery of all the components of a complete history and physical examination. Performing every clinical test and measure that a practitioner knows as an initial examination is, however, time-consuming, fiscally irresponsible, and likely to yield an uninterpretable catalog of abnormal findings. This does not mean that only cursory clinical examinations are indicated. On the contrary, optimal clinical examination may require in-depth tests and measures of certain aspects of a patient's clinical presentation in order to understand the factors contributing to the patient's functional deficits. The salient point is that examination will be limited to only those aspects.

A third approach to clinical diagnosis is called *pattern recognition*. Pattern recognition can be defined as the "instantaneous realization that the patient's presentation conforms to a previously learned picture."[35] Two examples of patterns recognized by many physical therapists are the upper extremity position of the adult with spastic hemiplegia and the bilateral swelling and ulnar deviation of the metacarpals of an individual with rheumatoid arthritis. These patterns represent something immediately identifiable to the experienced therapist that has been learned over time. Unfortunately, pattern recognition is a reflexive approach to categorizing a patient's problems that is not always a reflective process as well. The drawback of pattern recognition is that it can place too much reliance on the therapist's previous experience and lead to a narrow set of premature conclusions. If, for example, we are examining someone with shortened bilateral step length in a shuffling pattern, previous clinical experience might suggest that this is a neuromuscular impairment. On the other hand, previous exposure to patients with the bony changes associated with rheumatic diseases, who may exhibit the same nonspecific gait abnormalities, may lead to concerns about structural deformities of the metatarsals and pain (metatarsalgia). Neither conclusion would be correct without further corroborating evidence. Experienced clinicians must guard against a tendency to see patterns and assign a diagnostic interpretation to the patient's signs and symptoms prematurely. There is, however, great value to pattern recognition as part of a clinical diagnostic strategy, especially at the start of the diagnostic process. By suggesting that a patient's clinical presentation might conform to some previously encountered pattern, the therapist is able to limit the search for corroborating evidence to substantiate the clinical impression.

The fourth diagnostic method identified by Sackett is called the *hypothetico-deductive strategy*. Guyatt et al.[36] further refined this approach by having clinicians consider the evidence from clinical research and use a more probabilistic mode of diagnostic thinking. *Probabilistic diagnostic reasoning* consists of the formulation of a list of potential diagnoses or actions from the earliest clues about the patient, estimation of the probability associated with each, followed by performance of specific clinical tests and measures that will best result in the answer. This method corrects for the flaw in pattern recognition by not structuring the search for corroborating evidence too narrowly. Neither does it open the search too widely, requiring the therapist to consider every abnormal clinical finding that might be identified through a "complete" history and physical, especially one performed on a geriatric patient. Figure 6-7, from Guyatt et al.[36] compares pattern recognition and probabilistic diagnostic reasoning strategies. The probabilistic approach incorporates knowledge of human anatomy and pathophysiology, results of clinical research, and clinical experience.

Upon completing the examination of the individual during which data are collected to evaluate and form clinical judgment, therapists often group findings into meaningful clusters or clinical problems.[36] From these clusters, the process of differential diagnoses begins so the therapist can determine the most effective treatment to alleviate the health condition. At this time, the probable target disorders/causes are ranked according to which ones are most likely (probabilistic list) as the therapist is trying to determine the single best explanation/leading hypothesis for the patient's problem. The therapist then estimates the probability of each hypothesis (pretest probability) based on previous experience with similar conditions (which may be minimal or extensive), evidence from research, and clinical decision or prediction rules. As new information is generated, the ordering of target causes can change as one considers the strengths of the diagnostic tests and the uniqueness of the patient (posttest probability). The therapist also has in mind a treatment threshold level that once crossed leads to the decision to stop any further testing and begin treatment to address the identified hypothesized cause of the patient's problem.[36,43] Figure 6-8 provides a schematic illustration of the use of pretest and posttest

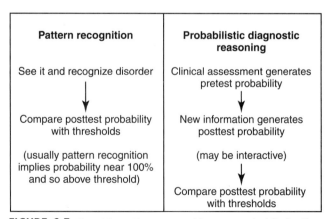

FIGURE 6-7 Guyatt's pattern recognition vs. probabilistic diagnostic reasoning. *(Redrawn from Guyatt GH, Mead MO, Rennie D, Cook DJ: User's guide to the medical literature: essentials of evidence-based clinical practice. New York, 2008, McGraw-Hill.)*

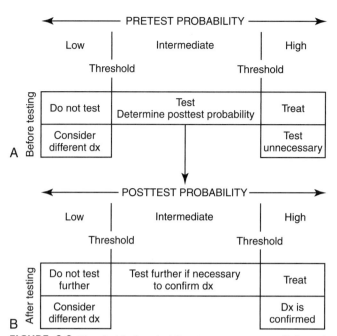

FIGURE 6-8 Thresholds for deciding to test or treat. *(Adapted from Straus SE, Richardson WSS, Glasziou P, et al: Evidence based medicine: how to practice and teach EBM, ed 3. Edinburgh, 2005, Churchill Livingstone.)*

probability thresholds to guide decisions to stop intervention and initiate treatment. When determining this threshold, the patient's values as well as the costs associated with being wrong versus the benefits of being right must be taken into consideration.

Evidence from the literature also assists the therapist with this process of diagnosis. The ideal diagnostic test would accurately discriminate between those with a condition and those without the target condition. In actual practice most tests are not 100% accurate so the therapist must appreciate the validity of a diagnostic test in order to make defensible inferences from examination data. Ultimately, the therapist should be concerned with the probability that the result is accurate enough for the certainty that the situation demands and the negative consequences for the patient of being less accurate than desirable. Chapter 1 provides an overview of key probabilistic considerations for diagnostic testing. Unfortunately, these psychometric properties have not been typically reported in the rehabilitation literature until recently, and therefore diagnostic accuracy in physical therapist practice is not as empirically grounded as it might be.

Structuring the Evaluation of Clinical Findings.
Following the evaluative process pertinent examination findings must be aggregated into categories using a relevant classification scheme that will communicate the cause of the individual's activity limitations and participation restrictions. Classification schemes must meet certain criteria that apply to all diagnoses provided by any professional: (1) the scheme must be consistent with the legal and regulatory boundaries of the profession's

focus and society's approbation of the profession's expertise to identify and treat specific kinds of problems; (2) the tests and measures that are used to validate the diagnosis are within the purview of the profession; and most importantly for clinical practice, (3) the particular diagnostic label must describe the problem in a way that implies or directs intervention.[9]

Because of the orientation of physical therapists toward examining movement deficits and the profession's singular expertise in movement dysfunction, there has been a substantial attempt to mold diagnosis by physical therapists toward categories of "movement diagnoses." However, these efforts have not been fully successful or broadly accepted, despite the utility of some formulations that have been constructed, especially since the concept was introduced in the 1980s. Overall, these formulations have fallen short of their goal to describe the totality of diagnosis by physical therapists because there are a sufficient number of instances in which the physical therapist must further deconstruct the movement dysfunction. The analysis of the dysfunction, which is identified first as an activity limitation at the level of the person, must cascade down to specific organ systems and perhaps even to implicating specific tissues, or at the opposite end of the spectrum of clinical hypotheses, attribute the dysfunction to limited behavioral repertoires or environmental challenges. In fact, what is first captured as a "movement dysfunction" in the diagnostic process is most often an observation about the ability to perform a particular action (e.g., rolling, bending, sitting, standing, walking, reaching, lifting) that is a requisite component of a task that must be completed as part of some larger activity. Structural inadequacies such as biomechanical faults or pathophysiological occurrences such as cardiac or ventilatory pump dysfunction mitigate efforts that constrain diagnosis by physical therapists to choosing among labels for "movement dysfunction" as the ultimate cause of an activity limitation. Conversely, using insights gleaned from the ICF and the IOM's emphasis on the interface between person and environment, other diagnostic hypotheses may be derived from data concerning a person's self-efficacy and motivation as well as environmental barriers to optimal functioning. Although all physical therapist interventions affect the movement system and a person's ability to sequence and execute actions, tasks, and activities to achieve goal-directed outcomes, contemporary physical therapist practice may require a more robust concept than "movement diagnoses" to define the domain of physical therapist practice, such as human performance, which stretches the reach of the profession from the most disease-afflicted states of health status to primary prevention.

Integrated Diagnostic Schema. Physical therapists should take an integrated approach to diagnosing deficits in human performance. Deconstructing movement in the context of human performance requires the examination of the complex interaction of sensoriperceptual, biomechanical, neuromotor, respiratory, and circulatory capabilities as well as the influence of personal motivation, cognition, behavior, and the environment on movement. Physical therapists must determine if the limitation in activity is at the level of task, action, and/or impairment. Ultimately, the physical therapist will pose a hypothesis or several hypotheses linking an inability to perform an action to a specific impairment or cluster of impairments. Consider, for example, the range of impairments that might explain the deficit in performing the required actions to accomplish the tasks that comprise the activity limitation that is reported as "I can't get to my mailbox to get my mail." Furthermore, suppose that we know that individual has low vision, lives in a second floor walk-up, is somewhat reluctant to go outside particularly in strong daylight, and has had osteoarthritis in one knee and is currently on medication for early stages of CHF. Each component of this activity (getting the mail) involves a series of tasks to be accomplished (e.g., opening a door, descending stairs, negotiating terrain, handling latches) that require specific actions (e.g., standing, walking, stepping, turning, pulling, grasping, carrying). It is highly likely that several impairments such as decreased muscle strength, reduced joint mobility, limited dynamic balance, or diminished endurance will need to be hypothesized and confirmed to account for this activity limitation.

Prognosis and Plan of Care. The next task of the physical therapist is to state a prognosis, which is a prediction about the optimal level of function that the patient will achieve and the time that will be required to reach that level. Having done that, the therapist and the patient can then mutually agree upon anticipated goals of treatment, which generally are related to expected outcomes of care. Therefore the functional outcomes of treatment should be stated in behavioral terms. On the basis of these anticipated goals and expected outcomes, the physical therapist then completes a plan of care that specifies the interventions to be implemented, including their frequency, intensity, and duration.

When the therapist's attention turns toward planning intervention, the key question is, Of the impairments that are hypothesized to be causal to the patient's activity limitations, which ones can also be remediated by physical therapist intervention? Furthermore, if the patient's impairments cannot be remediated initially or even with extensive treatment, the physical therapist then seeks to determine how the patient may compensate by using other abilities to accomplish the action or task and also how can the task be adapted so that the activity can be performed within the restrictions that the patient's condition imposes on the situation. The current evidence base for determining the optimal proportion, timing, and sequence of remediation, compensation, and adaptation of both initial and subsequent plans of care is shallow. Therefore, physical therapists must consider the balance among each of these three intervention

approaches dynamically, depending upon the persistence of deficits in structure or function, availability of compensatory resources without unintended negative consequences for other functioning, likelihood of full recovery with further remediation, and surmountability of environmental challenges. If it is decided that an individual's impairments and activity limitations are amenable to physical therapy intervention, the therapist should establish a schedule for evaluating the effectiveness of the intervention. If the patient achieves the anticipated goals for changes in impairments but does not also achieve the expected functional outcomes, this is an indication that the therapist has incorrectly hypothesized the relationship between the patient's impairments and functional status.[44] In this instance, the therapist may reexamine the patient to modify the plan of care.

Although a host of procedures and techniques might be used to remediate an impairment or minimize an activity limitation, only those that are most likely to promote the outcome in a cost-effective manner should be chosen for inclusion in the plan of care. The combination of direct interventions used with any particular patient will vary according to the impairments and activity limitations that are addressed by the plan of care for that individual. Three patients may have the same activity limitation, that is, inability to transfer independently from bed to chair, yet require entirely different programs of intervention. If the first individual lacked sufficient knee strength to come to a standing position, then the plan of care would incorporate strengthening exercises to remedy the impairment and improve the patient's function. If the second patient lacked sufficient range of motion (ROM) at the hip due to flexion contractures to allow full upright standing, then intervention would focus on increasing ROM at the hip to improve function. The third individual may possess all the musculoskeletal and neuromuscular prerequisites to allow function but still require appropriate instruction to do it safely and with minimal exertion. Each individual may achieve a similar level of functional independence, yet none of the three would have received the exact same treatment to achieve the same outcome.

Most of the direct interventions used by physical therapists are aimed at remediating impairments that underlie activity limitations; however, only two of the direct interventions (i.e., functional training in self-care and home management and functional training in community and work integration or reintegration) listed in the *Guide to Physical Therapist Practice* consider the activity limitation itself. Although physical therapists sometimes apply therapeutic exercise in the position of function—for example, standing balance exercises—or try to simulate the environment in which the functional activity is performed—for example, a staircase—the functional activity in and of itself should not be confused with the core elements of a physical therapist's plan of care, that is, therapeutic exercise and functional training.

It is particularly helpful for the therapist working with geriatric patients to appreciate that there are some impairments that will not change, no matter how much direct intervention is provided. This realization will diminish unnecessary treatment. In these instances, physical therapists may still achieve positive patient outcomes by teaching patients how to compensate for their permanent impairments by capitalizing on other capabilities or by modifying the environment to reduce the demands of the task. One of the beneficial consequences of a careful deconstruction of an activity limitation into tasks and actions is that this analysis indicates what kinds of outcomes are most suitable to demonstrating the success of the intervention. The most proximate outcomes of the remediation of impairments can be found in an improved ability to perform actions, somewhat irrespective of personal and environmental factors that are outside of the physical therapist's control. In comparison, activity limitations are typically measured with respect to broader outcome measures such as basic and instrumental ADLs. Relevant chapters of this book provide recommendations for valid and reliable functional measures to assess the outcomes of a physical therapy episode of care.

SUMMARY

The twin processes of disablement and enablement conceptualize health status into components that form a framework for geriatric examination, evaluation, diagnosis, and treatment planning. Physical therapists have particular expertise in the clinical analysis of human performance by deconstructing the relationship between impairments and activity limitations and in the application of direct interventions to address the older adult's problems by enhancing human performance mediated through movement, most immediately in the realm of remediating deficits in the ability to perform actions essential to successful task completion. Ultimately, the expected outcome of physical therapy for older patients is to sustain or improve their functional status and promote overall quality of life.

REFERENCES

To enhance this text and add value for the reader, all references are included on the companion Evolve site that accompanies this text book. The reader can view the reference source and access it online whenever possible. There are a total of 44 cited references and other general references for this chapter.

Environmental Design:
Accommodating Sensory Changes in the Older Adult

Mary Ann Wharton, PT, MS

INTRODUCTION

The ability to function in the everyday environment is essential to older individuals. Maintaining independence and quality of life, however, may be compromised by sensory changes that individuals experience over their life span. Changes in vision, hearing, taste, smell, and touch may deprive older persons of necessary sensory cues to perceive the environment and may influence both their behavior and the behavior of others toward them. This may be even truer when the older individual has dementia and sensory changes that affect the ability to interpret environmental cues. The ability of physical therapists to recognize the relationship between sensory changes and environmental interaction, to recommend adaptations to accommodate those changes, and to teach intervention strategies will promote continued independent functioning of older individuals and improve their overall quality of life.

Most individuals experience gradual sensory loss with age. Such changes are normal and irreversible and may not be uniform within the same individual. For example, visual loss may occur primarily in one eye, or an individual may have poor vision but excellent hearing. Moreover, loss of the different senses may be experienced at different ages. Changes in some senses, specifically hearing, may begin as early as age 40 years, whereas others, including vision, taste, and smell, may not decline until age 50 or 60 years.[1-3] The important point is that the sensory declines experienced with aging are highly individualized, with some people experiencing relatively minor declines and maintaining optimal functional ability and other individuals experiencing significant declines with resultant increased functional dependency. Typically, the declines occur gradually and may be unnoticed until older individuals are no longer capable of independent functioning within the environment.

Throughout life, individuals rely on sensory cues to perceive and interpret information from their surroundings and then respond appropriately. As one ages, both the reception and perception of the sensory stimulus diminish, with a resultant slowing of information processing. This factor leads to increased variability in reception, integration, and response to sensory stimuli. Consequently, older persons may misinterpret cues from the environment or may experience sensory deprivation. The consequences may be loss of independence or diminished quality of life by older individuals. Therefore, individuals may need higher thresholds of stimulation to continue to function in the environment. As individuals experience loss in functional ability, they may also become increasingly reliant on sensory cues from the environment. An interdependence develops between the senses and the environment: one relies on one's senses to perceive and derive pleasure from the environment, and one relies on the environment to promote and support functional ability as age-related sensory declines are experienced.

As physical therapists interact with the older adult, it is critical to recognize the importance of the balance between sensory perception and ability to function effectively in the environment. Therapists need to evaluate older individuals for sensory changes and to recommend appropriate interventions and modifications to enhance optimal functional performance in an environment without creating dependence (Table 7-1).

SENSORY CHANGES: RELATIONSHIP TO FUNCTIONAL ABILITY WITHIN THE ENVIRONMENT

Vision

Vision is important in identifying environmental cues and distinguishing environmental hazards. As people age, changes in vision and visual perception may lead to misinterpretation of visual cues and result in functional dependence.

TABLE 7-1	Examples of Accommodations to Enhance Functioning for Older Individuals Experiencing Sensory Loss
Sensory Change	**Examples of Accommodations**
Vision	
Visual field	Lower height for directional and informational signs
Acuity	Visual aids (glasses, contact lenses); magnifiers; large-print books and devices; large-print computer software
Illumination	UV-absorbing lenses; increased task illumination; gooseneck lamps; 200- to 300-watt light bulbs
Glare	Lamp shades, curtains, or blinds to soften light; cove lighting to conceal light source; nonglare wax on vinyl floors; carpeting; wallpaper or flat paints; avoid shiny materials such as glass or plastic furniture and metal fixtures
Dark adaptation	Night-lights with red bulbs; pocket flashlights, automatic light timers, light switches at point of entry to a room
Color	Bright, warm colors (reds, oranges, yellows); avoid pastel hues; avoid monotones
Contrast	Bright detail on dark backgrounds (white lettering/black background); warm colors to highlight handrails, steps; place mats or table coverings that contrast with plates, floor
Depth perception	Avoid patterned floor surfaces
Hearing	
	Hearing aids; pocket amplifiers; increasing bass and turning down treble on radios, televisions; smoke alarms, telephones, and doorbells with visual cues such as flashing lights; insulating acoustic materials to minimize background noise
Taste and smell	
Taste	Color to increase perceived flavor intensity; use of spices, herbs, and flavorings to enhance foods; feel for bulges in canned goods to detect spoilage; check date stored of frozen foods
Smell	Adapt smoke detectors with loud buzzers; safety-spring caps for gas jets on stoves; vent kitchens in institutions to allow residents to experience cooking aromas, and place flowers in living areas
Touch	
Tactile sensitivity	Introduce texture into the environment through wall hangings, carpet, textured upholstery; use soft blankets and textured clothing
Thermal sensitivity	Avoid temperature extremes from air conditioning, hot bathwater, heating pads

Physiologically, this decline in vision can result from age-related changes in the structures of the eye and in external ocular structures. Neuronal changes, perceptual changes, and pathologic conditions also contribute to vision and visual perceptual changes in the older person. The ability to function in the environment, in spite of changes in vision and visual perception, is dependent on the ability to adapt to visual impairment, including decreasing visual efficiency and low vision. Older individuals must adapt to problems such as decreased visual field, changes in visual acuity, increased needs for illumination balanced by needs to reduce glare, delayed dark–light adaptation, increased needs for contrast, decreased power of accommodation, and changes in color vision and depth perception.

Visual Field. A decrease in both peripheral and upper visual fields accelerates with aging. Decreased pupil size, resulting in admittance of less light to the peripheral retina, may be responsible for early changes. Later changes may result from decreased retinal metabolism. Mechanical causes are due to relaxation of the upper eyelid and loss of retrobulbar fat, which results in the eyes sinking more deeply into the orbits. As a result, upper gaze can be compromised with aging.[4,5]

Within the environment, this decrease in upper visual field may cause older individuals to miss cues above head level. Common examples of cues found above head level may include traffic and street signs, direction or information signs in public buildings (Figure 7-1), hanging light fixtures, and environmental hazards such as hanging tree limbs.

Lateral field, or peripheral vision, deficits—described as the inability to detect motion, form, or color on either side of the head while looking straight ahead—are particularly significant for older persons. For safety in the environment, older persons must be able to detect people or objects in the lateral field, and older drivers must possess adequate lateral awareness.[1,2]

Visual Acuity. Visual acuity, the capacity of the eye to discriminate fine details of objects in the visual field, generally declines with age, although this decline is not universal or inevitable. The 20/20 standard for "normal" vision occurs around age 18 years and typically remains unchanged until the sixth decade. Slight diminution of visual acuity has been documented to occur between the ages of 50 and 70 years and at a greater rate after age 70 years. Factors responsible for decreased visual acuity include increased thickness of the lens, which affects the amount of light allowed to reach the retina, and the loss of elasticity of the lens. These changes result in decreased ability to see clearly and particularly affect near objects. In addition, changes in the iris and pupil

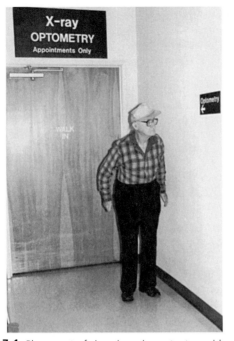

FIGURE 7-1 Placement of signs is an important consideration for older individuals. The wall sign is placed at eye level to accommodate changes in visual field. The door sign is a better size and has better contrast, but it is too high for an older individual to see clearly. *(From Melore GG: Visual function changes in the geriatric patient and environmental modifications. In Melore GG, editor: Treating vision problems in the older adult. St Louis, MO, 1997, Mosby. Used with permission.)*

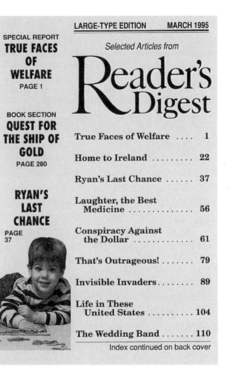

FIGURE 7-2 Large-print *Reader's Digest.* The 18-point type provides 2.0× relative size magnification compared with the 9-point type of a standard edition. *(From Williams DR: Functional adaptive devices. In Cole RG, Rosenthal BP, editors: Remediation and management of low vision. St Louis, MO, 1996, Mosby. Used with permission.)*

may decrease acuity. As one ages, the iris loses its ability to change width, and pupil size remains small in both dim and bright light. One specific consequence is decreased night vision. It is likely that optical factors alone are insufficient to account for acuity loss and that age-related changes in the retina and brain are also contributing factors. These include a loss of photoreceptors, bipolar cells, or ganglion cells within the retina and anatomical or functional changes in the geniculostriate pathway.[1-6]

Visual aids can be beneficial in improving visual acuity for older adults. Glasses and contact lenses can enhance vision when worn properly, especially in the early stages of vision loss. Hand-held magnifiers are adequate for use over short periods, for example, when reading a telephone book. Table stand magnifiers are beneficial when a person is reading books or newspapers because they cause less eye fatigue by maintaining a constant distance between the object being magnified and the magnifier. Illuminated magnifiers that hang from the neck are useful when a person is sewing or performing craft work. Other low-vision aids can be obtained at low-vision clinics.[3]

In addition to visual aids, certain modifications to environmental stimuli can enhance visual functioning for older persons. Use of large print is suggested for signs and labels, including medication schedules, telephone lists, and home programs. Large-print books (Figure 7-2) and

newspapers are also available, as are other large-print devices such as measuring tapes and rulers, measuring cups and spoons, cookbooks, wristwatches, phone dialers, and games. Local agencies for the blind are helpful in identifying such resources.[7-9]

Large-print typewriters are available that provide an effective means of personal communication for visually impaired older adults. This technology may be less intimidating than computers for some older individuals, and they may be more cost-effective. The National Braille Association has recommended three single space lines per vertical inch as the maximum acceptable pitch for large-print. To be considered "large print," lowercase letters should measure at least 1/8 inch to approximate 18-point type.[9]

Computer adaptations are available for older individuals who are visually impaired. Difficulties lie both in viewing what is on the computer screen as well as in navigating through documents and websites. Specially designed physical devices (i.e., hardware) may be used in addition to, or instead of, traditional components. These devices include full-page monitors that magnify images and text, special pointing devices, Braille-enhanced devices, and microphones for speech input among other items. Most hardware also requires installation of associated software. Compatibility with the computer system to be used should always be determined before purchase.

Modern operating systems provide computer users with access to system settings that control overall screen resolution, font selection, and color combinations. Relatively recent versions of Microsoft Windows or Apple Macintosh have a number of built-in accessibility features that have the advantage of requiring no additional cost. Built-in adaptations include accessibility options to control the display, keyboard, and the mouse and its cursor. They may even allow the addition of sounds that may help to confirm that a program has been launched or that an e-mail message has been received by the computer's application. Other examples of adaptations include the option to change the width of the cursor to make it easier to locate, the ability to select a background that allows easier viewing of items and icons on the desktop, the ability to adjust color schemes to increase contrast and make it easier to read the computer screen, and a simplified screen magnifier to enlarge text and graphics.[10]

In many cases, a software-only solution may provide sufficient adaptation. Microsoft Word provides easy on-screen enlargement of print via a zoom capability that allows significant enlargement exceeding 200%. Screen magnification software, which not only allows adjustment of font size to fit the viewer's need, enlarges the entire computer display and can be installed to run automatically when a computer is in use (Figure 7-3). It should be noted that some graphic-oriented programs may not be compatible with this software. Other types of adaptive software include screen-reading programs, such as JAWS, Window-Eyes, and ZoomText with NeoSpeech, which uses computer-synthesized speech to "read" the computer screen, and speech-recognition software, such as Dragon Naturally Speaking and MacSpeech Dictate, which can be used to verbally input text and commands. Barriers to the use of these programs include their cost and complexity and the relative speed with which enhancements are developed, requiring frequent upgrades.[9,11-13]

Illumination. Within the environment, declining visual acuity necessitates a stronger stimulus or light source. This was originally thought to be primarily related to senile miosis (an age-related decrease in pupillary size), changes in the refractory media, and a reduction in retinal cones and rods. More recent studies, conducted under varying light conditions, argue that the effects of aging are neural rather than optical in origin. These studies further suggest that it is the neural changes that have the greatest effects on vision under low illumination.

As a result of these optical and neural changes, it has been estimated that older individuals require as much as two to four times more light than their younger counterparts. Wall-mounted light fixtures and peripheral lighting from floor lamps are superior to a central ceiling source because they do not foster formation of shadows on critical corner and furniture areas. Background lighting should not be as bright as that in the area on which attention is directed. Lighting that focuses directly on the task, rather than overhead lighting, is recommended to meet the needs of older individuals for reading, task performance, and other close work. Using 200- or 300-watt light bulbs in reading lamps instead of the more typical 100-watt bulb is one of the simplest ways to provide adequate task illumination. Another way to modify the necessary amount of illumination independent of light bulb wattage is to simply move the light source closer to the task material, because the effective amount of illumination is inversely proportional to the distance of the light source to the surface. Gooseneck lamps (Figure 7-4) or small, high-intensity lamps with three-way switches are also helpful in achieving the proper ratio of background-to-task lighting.[1-6,14-16]

Glare. When illumination is increased, care must be exercised to avoid excessive and intensive illumination, which can create a hazard for older persons in the form of glare. Glare results from diffuse light scattering on the retina as it passes through mildly opaque refractive

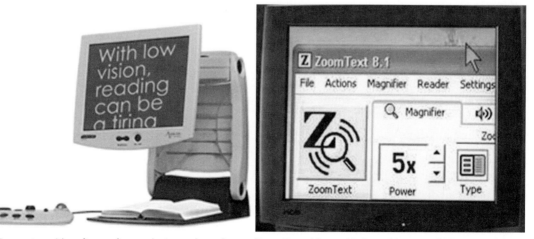

FIGURE 7-3 Computer with software for producing enlarged text. *(From Rosenbloom AJ: Rosenbloom and Morgan's vision and aging, St Louis, 2007, Butterworth-Heinemann.)*

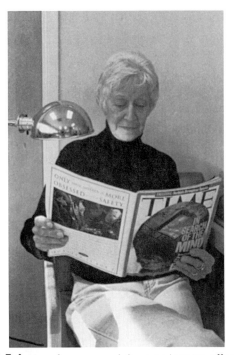

FIGURE 7-4 Use of a gooseneck lamp to increase effective task lighting without increasing light bulb wattage. *(From Melore GG: Visual function changes in the geriatric patient and environmental modifications. In Melore GG, editor: Treating vision problems in the older adult. St Louis, MO, 1997, Mosby. Used with permission.)*

media, inhibiting clear vision. A primary cause of glare sensitivity is the increasing opacity of the lens, which diffuses the incoming light. Degenerative changes that take place in the cornea also contribute to glare.[1-4,14]

Direct glare occurs when light reaches the eye directly from its source. An example of direct glare is uncontrolled natural light that enters a darkened room through a window. Another example of direct glare is excessive light from exposed light bulbs. Indirect glare can be the result of light reflecting off another surface. Examples include light reflecting off highly polished surfaces including waxed floors; plastic-covered furniture; polished silverware; or stainless steel assistive devices, including grab bars and walkers.[1-4,14]

Glare can be lessened by modifying light sources. Diffuse, soft lighting is preferable to single-light sources. Lamp shades should be used to soften the light. Glare from windows can be minimized by use of sheer curtains, venetian blinds, tinted-glass windows, or drapes. Wall-mounted valance or cove lighting that conceals the light source is also recommended. Fluorescent fixtures can be used to reduce glare, but they must be checked to ensure that they do not create another hazard for older individuals in the form of flickering. Also, "white" fluorescent lights are recommended because they make it possible to choose a "cool" light to eliminate the harshness and minimize accentuation of the blues, greens, and yellows created by older-style fluorescent lights.[9,16,17]

Another method of controlling glare is reducing the number of reflective surfaces. Positioning light sources to avoid reflection from shiny surfaces, such as waxed floors, is helpful. Use of carpeting, wallpaper, flat paints, and paneling is preferable to use of high-gloss paints. Glass, plastic, and glossy furniture should be avoided or covered with textured surfaces to minimize the effects of glare. Gleaming metal fixtures can be replaced with wood or plastic fixtures. Assistive devices, including grab bars and walkers, should not be constructed of shiny materials.

Care should be taken to control the sources of glare in public areas. For example, mall directories and bus signs should be covered with nonglare materials rather than highly reflective plastics. Grocery stores and drugstores should refrain from displaying products wrapped in plastic. Name tags, street signs, and publicity for older individuals should be prepared on dull surfaces to minimize glare.

Outdoor areas are also vulnerable to glare, especially with bright sunlight or with wet, shiny surfaces on rainy or snowy days. Sunscreens and adequate shade from trees are recommended to limit glare from direct sunlight. If it is not possible to provide adequate control for glare, older individuals should be encouraged to use sunglasses, visors, brimmed hats, or umbrellas. Glare that occurs at dusk as poorly illuminated objects are contrasted against a bright, postsunset sky can be particularly troublesome for older individuals. Night glare that occurs from oncoming headlights can also be hazardous. Use of well-lit routes and divided highways can minimize this hazard for older individuals.[2,3,5,18]

Dark Adaptation. Dark adaptation, or the ability of the eye to become more visually sensitive after remaining in darkness for a period of time, is delayed in older persons. One reason for this visual change is the smaller, miotic pupil, which limits the amount of light reaching the periphery of the retina. It is this area of the retina that contains the rods, which are sensitive to low light intensities. Another reason for delayed dark adaptation in older individuals is the metabolic changes in the retina. The oxygen supply to the rod-dense area of the retina diminishes as a result of vascular changes, which, in turn, affect the efficiency of the rods to respond to low levels of illumination. As a result of these changes, older persons have difficulty adapting to darkness and to abrupt and extreme changes in light.[2-5]

Use of a night-light is recommended to assist in overcoming the decreased ability for the eyes to adapt to the dark. Red light stimulates the cones but not the rods, allowing an older person to see well enough by red light to function in the dark. Therefore, a red bulb is suggested because it reduces the time required for adaptation to the dark and while permitting the older individual to see well enough to function. It is also recommended that older individuals carry a pocket flashlight to aid in transition to dimly lit environments. Improving lighting at the point of entry to an area, through pull cords or light switches near the entrance to a room, is also recommended. Automatic timers or keeping a light on at all times in dimly lit areas can prevent older individuals from having to enter a darkened room.[3,5,15]

Accommodation. Accommodation, the ability of the eye to focus images on the retina independent of object distances, is impaired with aging. Functionally, this results in the inability to focus clearly over a range of distances. The decrease in this ability, referred to as *presbyopia*, occurs gradually and affects near vision first.

Loss of accommodation is the result of several factors. Both the cornea and lens lose transparency with aging. In addition, the lens thickens, flattens, and yellows and becomes rigid. The ciliary muscle weakens and relaxes. As a result, the lens gradually loses its ability to change shape and focus at varying distances. Difficulty is encountered by older individuals when they attempt to read small print or detail, unless the material is held at a distance. Reading glasses are initially indicated. Later, bifocals are needed to compensate for the inability of the lens to change shape and focus on objects of varying distances.[1-4,14,17]

Color. The ability to perceive, differentiate, and distinguish colors declines with aging as a result of changes in retinal cones, the retinal bipolar and ganglion cells, the visual pathways that terminate in the occipital cortex, and the lens. As the lens thickens and yellows with age, it becomes less sensitive to colors that have shorter wavelengths. The ability to distinguish cool colors—blues, greens, and violets—is particularly impaired because they have the shorter wavelengths. Hue and saturation levels are particularly affected by aging, but brightness appears to be spared. Warm colors with longer wavelengths, including the reds, oranges, and yellows, are easier to differentiate and should therefore be used as focal points against sharply contrasting backgrounds. In addition to loss of color discrimination at the blue end of the color spectrum, a loss of sensitivity over the entire spectrum occurs. As a result, light pastel colors may be difficult to distinguish. Monotones also provide difficulty for older individuals, as may dark shades, which tend to blend into shadows. As a result, older persons may have trouble negotiating around dark furniture or in areas where dark floor surfaces and dark walls or doorways come together. Optimal lighting is needed to minimize this hazard.

Both warm and cool colors can be included in a color scheme when living environments are designed for aging individuals. Even though cool colors are more difficult to distinguish, they may be preferred for their soothing effects, particularly with agitated older persons. These cool colors are particularly suited for bedrooms because they promote calm and peacefulness. The use of bright, warm colors, which are better seen, should be encouraged for sensory stimulation. They are considered to be welcoming and uplifting and are suitable for entrances, day rooms, and dining rooms, particularly in residential care facilities. Contrasting bright yellows, reds, and oranges with cool blue, green, and violet colors may help minimize difficulties associated with loss of depth perception. The goal with the use of color is to use contrast to assist older individuals in distinguishing objects from their backgrounds. It is also important that the use of color be aesthetically pleasing.[3-5,14,17,19,20]

Contrast. The ability to discriminate between degrees of brightness appears to decrease in individuals age 60 years and older. In particular, contrast sensitivity to medium and high spatial frequencies declines progressively with age, and contrast sensitivity to low spatial frequencies remains unchanged. Typically, older individuals have difficulty seeing objects that have low contrast, especially with a bright background. Older persons require greater than two times as much light to see low-contrasting objects with the same degree of clarity as younger people. Earlier studies attributed this decreased ability to discriminate between degrees of brightness to be the result of an increase in light scatter secondary to age-related eye changes. More recent studies indicate that changes in the retina and the brain or neuronal loss within the visual pathways are responsible.[5,6]

Tone is one way to facilitate contrast in the environment. An example of contrasting tones is pairing a lighter shade against a dark shade. Another strategy is to use two colors, for example, choosing a pale pink against a brown. This principle should be applied in any area where the older individual needs a sensory cue to navigate safely such as doors, door handles, and handrails, and furniture coverings.[21]

Use of sharp contrast enhances the visual performance of older individuals. Bright detail on dark backgrounds is easier to distinguish than low contrast or dark detail on light background. Recommendations include white lettering on the telephone dial of a black telephone (Figure 7-5) or white lettering on a black background for reference dials on appliances. Use of warm colors—reds, oranges, and yellows—is recommended to highlight important visual targets such as handrails, steps, intersections, and traffic signs. Floors and rugs should contrast with woodwork and walls. To enhance eating, plates should contrast with tablecloths or tabletops. Colored rims on dishes and glasses can provide sufficient contrast to avoid spills. The table covering should also contrast with the floor to enhance the reference point of older individuals and help prevent falls.[3,8,15,17]

Depth Perception. Related to loss of color discrimination is change in depth perception, or the ability to estimate the relative distance and relief of objects. Lack of color contrast results in a flat visual effect, or decreased depth perception and inability to judge distances.[1,22] As a result of the inability to judge distances, older persons may have difficulty estimating the height of curbs and steps and may have difficulty with activities of daily

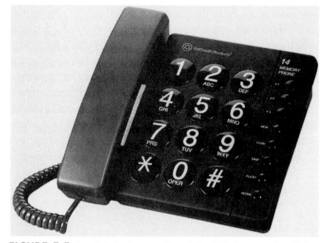

FIGURE 7-5 Black telephone with white lettering on the dial to enhance visual contrast. Large-button phone numbers also enhance visual acuity. *(From Williams DR: Functional adaptive devices. In Cole RG, Rosenthal BP, editors: Remediation and management of low vision. St Louis, MO, 1996, Mosby. Used with permission.)*

living that require distance judgment, including feeding tasks.

Related to depth perception is figure–ground, which is the object of focus from a diffuse background. It is difficult for older individuals to recognize a simple visual figure when it is embedded in a complex figure background. Specific implications for older persons are in selection of floor coverings. When a pattern is present on a floor surface, it may create a hazard as older individuals perceive it as one object or several objects. The avoidance of patterns is therefore recommended for floor surfaces, particularly in hallways or living areas.

Hearing

Hearing provides a primary link that allows individuals to identify with the environment and communicate effectively. Age-related hearing loss can lead to decreased awareness of environmental cues; poor communication skills; and ultimately, social isolation. With aging, there are both physiological and functional changes in the auditory system. Both the peripheral auditory system, which includes the structures of the ear itself, and the central nervous system, which integrates and gives meaning to sound, are affected. Age-related hearing loss can be attributed to three factors: conductive loss, sensorineural loss, and combined conductive and sensorineural loss. Changes that typically occur with aging and are detrimental to the older individual's ability to function independently in the environment include high-tone hearing loss, decreased speech discrimination, and difficulty in detecting and appropriately filtering background noise.

Conductive Hearing Loss. Conductive hearing loss results from dysfunction of the external ear, the middle ear, or both. Factors responsible for this type of hearing loss

include impacted cerumen, perforation of the tympanic membrane, serum or pus in the middle ear, and otosclerosis. Conductive hearing loss occurs when sound transmission to the inner ear is lost because the intensity of the signal is not sufficient. Even though the signal is weakened, sound received by the inner ear can still be analyzed because the inner ear itself is not affected. Therefore, increasing the intensity of the signal through louder speech or through mechanical amplification, such as a hearing aid, may help restore the ability to hear.

With a conductive loss, some impairment will occur in the ability to hear sounds of all frequencies. The specific pattern is dependent on the etiology of the hearing loss. An appropriate intervention when speaking to older individuals with a conductive hearing loss is to increase the speaker's volume to enable the person to hear the signal more clearly and to understand the speech. For individuals with profound hearing loss, an appropriate strategy may be to speak directly into the individual's ear. Devices such as timers, alarm clocks, smoke detectors, and doorbells can be modified or changed so that the signal is within the hearing range of older persons.[1,2,4,14]

Sensorineural Hearing Loss. Sensorineural hearing loss occurs when there is a dysfunction in conversion of sound waves to electrical signals by the inner ear or dysfunction in transmission of nerve impulses to the brain. Age-related sensorineural hearing loss is referred to as *presbycusis*. *Sensory* presbycusis is due to epithelial atrophy and degeneration of hair cells at the basal end of the organ of Corti and results in loss of high-frequency hearing. *Neural* presbycusis is due to degenerative changes in nerve fibers of the cochlea and neuron loss along the auditory pathway. It leads to loss in speech discrimination but not in pure-tone thresholds. As a result, the person continues to hear tone but cannot understand what is heard, particularly in loud settings. Amplifications may be of limited benefit, because these devices can amplify unintelligible sounds. *Strial* presbycusis results from atrophy and degeneration of the stria vascularis. It is most likely the result of arteriosclerotic vascular changes. It results in a relatively uniform reduction in pure-tone sensitivities for all frequencies and is accompanied by recruitment, which is a rapid increase in loudness as the sound intensity increases. *Cochlear conductive* presbycusis is caused by a disorder in the motion mechanics of the cochlear duct. The result is increasing hearing loss from low to high frequencies. The ability to understand speech is affected. High-pitched consonants such as *s, t, f,* and *g* are increasingly difficult to understand, especially in the presence of background noise, which masks the weak consonant sounds, or with rapid articulation.[1]

Older individuals with a sensorineural hearing loss may have significant difficulty maintaining independent function in the environment. In addition to difficulty in hearing and/or understanding speech, these individuals may have great difficulty hearing and interpreting key signals from the environment. Recommendations to assist these individuals incorporate strategies to address the hearing loss. Lower frequency and pitch of signals from television, stereo systems, or radio can be achieved by adjusting the treble and bass to compensate for loss of high frequency, that is, by tuning the bass up and the treble down. Use of microphones by speakers and entertainers will also cut out some of the high-frequency sound, making it easier for individuals to hear. Devices that have high-frequency sound, such as smoke alarms, telephones, and doorbells, should also have a visual cue, such as a flashing light.

For individuals with presbycusis, a traditional hearing aid may be of limited benefit, because this device may only amplify a distorted signal. Newer technology that allows frequency-selective amplification is indicated with sensorineural loss. Some assistive listening devices, such as pocket amplifiers with external earphones, microphones, and earphones, may also be beneficial[3,12] (Figure 7-6). As with profound conductive loss, speaking directly into the individual's ear may be of benefit for the person without a device.

Individuals with severe to profound bilateral sensorineural hearing loss may be candidates for cochlear implants (Figure 7-7) if they are unable to benefit from conventional amplification. With these implants, the level of speech perception is predicted by the duration of deafness, duration of implant use, and hearing ability before implantation. As the technology for implants improves, better outcomes, including improved ability to detect sound at lower intensities and improved lip-reading ability, are reported.[3] Adults who were deafened postlinguistically have significantly improved word recognition and many are able to converse on the telephone.

Environmental background noise that competes with the older person's ability to hear can be minimized by use of acoustic materials such as drapes, upholstered furniture, and carpets, which absorb noise. Insulating sheet rock should be installed in noisy areas such as kitchens or maintenance rooms. Tight window seals can minimize exterior noise.

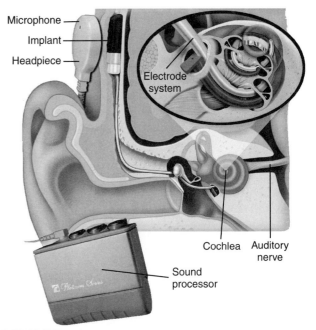

FIGURE 7-7 Cochlear implants may be used to improve amplification for individuals with severe sensorineural hearing loss who are unable to benefit from conventional amplification. *(From Lemmi FD, Lemmi CAE: Physical assessment findings CD-ROM. Philadelphia, PA, 2000, Saunders.)*

In institutions and public buildings, noise from telepages, radios, televisions, dishwashers, and air conditioners should be eliminated where possible. Background music should be eliminated, because it contributes to the older individual's inability to hear. Fluorescent lighting should be used with discretion, because the buzzing sound that is produced may also interfere with hearing.[1,3]

Taste and Smell

Taste and smell intertwine to provide additional links with the environment. These senses allow individuals to appreciate foods and pleasant odors in the environment, such as fresh-baked bread, the smell of newly cut grass,

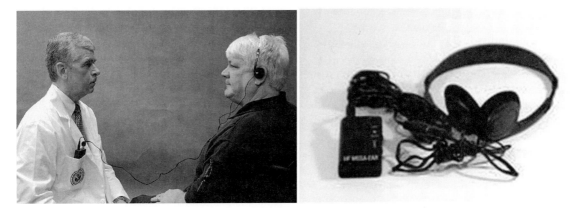

FIGURE 7-6 A hand-held pocket amplifier increases the ability to communicate with a hearing-impaired individual. *(From Rosenbloom AJ: Rosenbloom and Morgan's vision and aging, St Louis, 2007, Butterworth-Heinemann.)*

and roses. They also allow detection of unpleasant odors that can serve as warning to environmental hazards. Examples include unsafe drink and foods, fire, and noxious gases. Research on age-related changes in these senses is limited and often contradictory, but there is evidence that they are diminished. Research indicates that smell has more significant change and that taste changes are relatively minimal. This decline in taste and smell can affect the older individual's behavior, safety in the environment, and nutrition.

Taste. Although there is no agreement on the cause, it is known that the number of taste buds decreases with age. By age 60 years, most people have lost approximately half of their taste buds. This loss further accelerates after age 70 years. This loss of functioning taste buds, combined with neuron reduction in taste centers, changes in the levels of specific receptor proteins, ion channels, or signaling molecules may account for changes in taste with aging. Other age-related changes that affect taste may include changes in the elasticity of the mouth and lips, decreased saliva flow, alterations in the composition of nasal mucus, changes in oral secretions, increased incidence of gingivitis and periodontitis, use of dentures, and tongue fissures. Smoking and chronic diseases such as diabetes or cancer and the effects of therapeutic interventions including medications, radiation, and surgery may also contribute to the decline of taste sensitivity. Regardless of cause, age-related changes in taste acuity are thought to be small. Taste buds located in the front of the tongue that are responsible for sweet and salty tastes are the first to atrophy. Stronger stimuli are needed to appreciate these tastes, and older people may use excessive amounts of salt or may prefer sweets. These preferences can pose problems for older individuals suffering from hypertension or diabetes. Taste buds located on the posterior surface of the tongue that are responsible for bitter tastes and allow rejection of bitter toxins are lost later. In addition, older persons may experience an increased sensitivity to bitterness, with the resultant complaint that food tastes bitter or sour.

Recommendations to enhance the taste experience include suggestions to compensate with other senses. One study demonstrated that an increase in color caused a significant increase in the perceived flavor intensity of beverages for older individuals. This study speculated that older persons depend heavily on visual cues to determine characteristics of food products because they are less sensitive to changes in flavor.[23] Other suggestions include encouraging older individuals to stimulate smell with the aroma of cooking foods because smell is so closely intertwined with taste and to prepare meals using a variety of aromas, temperatures, and textures. Oral hygiene should be encouraged before eating to rid the mouth of unpleasant tastes. Supplemental flavors including spices, herbs, flavor extracts, and sugar and salt substitutes can be used to produce an equivalent intensity of taste and enhance the flavor of foods. Also,

adding tiny amounts of highly aromatic ingredients such as wine or butter immediately before serving rather than during the cooking process will increase the odor impact more than adding these ingredients during cooking. Use of food supplementation has been shown to improve food intake and satisfaction, thereby decreasing the nutritional risk that results when food selection becomes less varied with age. One study demonstrated that repeated consumption of flavor-enhanced cooked meals led to an increase in dietary intake of this meal and a subsequent increase in body weight, suggesting that adding flavor enhancers might improve appetite and dietary intake in older individuals.[1-3,14,24-26]

When dealing with canned foods, older persons should be taught to feel for any bulges in the can and to discard any suspicious cans. Stored foods should be dated and checked for spoilage. Defrosted foods should be used promptly, because thawing and refreezing affects flavor and texture. Individuals who cannot detect spoilage through the sense of smell should be encouraged to adhere to a strict schedule of removal so that the risk of eating spoiled food is minimized.[3,24,26]

Smell. Research on olfactory sensitivity and smell is contradictory, but sensation appears to decline as a result of age, as well as a result of other factors associated with age. These factors may include continuous exposure to odor, leading to decreased acuity, or exposure to environmental pollutants or smoking. Structural causes may include fiber loss in the olfactory bulb, with a loss of approximately three-fourths of the olfactory fibers by age 80 or 90 years. Alterations in nasal anatomy and physiology may also occur secondary to diseases of the respiratory system. In addition, sensory deficits may be an early indication of neurologic disorders such as Parkinson's or Alzheimer's disease.

A critical factor related to the actual sense of smell is the confidence that individuals have in their olfactory sense. One study has looked at the relationship between metacognitive awareness of olfactory ability and age, and demonstrated that the gradual loss of smell that occurs secondary to aging may result in an older individual being unaware of an olfactory loss. This lack of awareness may place that individual at risk of injury from undetected fire, fumes, or spoiled food, and from reduced nutritional intake.[27]

The sense of smell serves as an important early warning system to alert individuals to environmental dangers, including smoke or gas fumes. For older persons who experience a decline in the ability to smell and are living alone, it is critical that environmental adaptations be considered. One recommendation is to use smoke detectors with loud buzzers. Because declining sensitivity to odor may limit the individual's ability to detect mercaptans (foul-smelling additives) used to warn of natural gas leaks, safety-spring caps for gas jets of a stove are also recommended. If the sensory loss is profound, switching from gas to electrical appliances may be indicated.

Social interaction of older persons may be affected by a declining sense of smell. Individuals may not be able to detect body odor, so particular attention must be given to bathing patterns. Perfumes may be overutilized, making the scent overpowering and offensive to others.

For the institutionalized older person, unpleasant odors from cleaning equipment, sanitizing sprays, and substances designed to mask offensive odors abound. Pleasant odors associated with positive life experiences are often overlooked. Absence of "good" smells adversely affects the quality of life for these individuals. Opportunities should be created to stimulate positive life experiences with pleasant smells. Kitchens can be vented to allow the aroma of cooking food to permeate residential hallways and dining areas. Flowers with fragrant scents can be placed in living areas to enhance the older person's sensory experience.[1,3]

Touch

The sense of touch is a complicated human response that involves many separate processes—including touch, temperature, pain, as well as vibration sensitivity, kinesthesia, and stereognosis. Sensory input is subdivided into touch and tactile systems. Touch is used for awareness and protective responses. It can be determined culturally and is often lacking in the older person's environment, contributing to the individual's diminished sensorium. Tactile input is used to interact with the environment and allows individuals to perceive multiple characteristics of an object.[2-4] For example, a surface may feel smooth or rough, soft or hard, warm or cold.

Little conclusive research has been done on the sense of touch. However, evidence suggests that touch decreases with age and varies from individual to individual. Many of the losses in somatesthetic sensitivity are the result of diseases that occur with greater frequency in the older persons, rather than a result of aging per se. Increased thresholds for touch, especially textures, temperature, and kinesthesia, have implications for the older individual's ability to obtain needed sensory input from the environment.

Tactile Sensitivity. Degenerative changes in Meissner corpuscles may result in decreased sensitivity of the skin on the palm of the hand and sole of the foot but not of hairy skin. The resultant decrease in touch acuity can affect the ability of older individuals to localize stimuli. As a result, older individuals may have problems differentiating or manipulating small objects, including buttons and coins. The decrease in speed of reaction to tactile stimulation can cause harm to older persons, as they take longer to become aware of harmful or noxious stimuli, such as temperature extremes, chemical irritants, or simple pressure from a stone in a shoe.[1]

Introducing texture into the environment can be valuable in assisting independent function of older individuals, especially if there is impairment in other senses. Wall hangings, carpet, and textured upholstery on furniture can enhance tactile input and add warmth. Use of texture on handrails or doorknobs can give environmental cues and enhance safety. Tactile deprivation can be minimized by the use of soft blankets and sheets and textured clothing.

Thermal Sensitivity. Changes in vascular circulation and loss of subcutaneous tissue in older individuals may result in changes in thermal sensitivity and impaired ability to cope with extreme environmental temperatures. One consequence is that older persons may feel cold and uncomfortable, even on a day that seems warm to a younger person. Air conditioning may not be tolerated, especially in the institutional environment.

In addition, extremes in hot temperatures, for example, from hot bathwater or a heating pad, may not be readily detected by older individuals. As a consequence, individuals may suffer a burn from the inability to react quickly to the temperature extreme.

GENERAL PRINCIPLES OF DESIGN

Environmental design principles that accommodate age-related changes in sensation can enhance independent functioning of older individuals. The ideal environment will vary according to the needs of individuals but should be supportive of sensory changes while promoting satisfaction, safety, and security. Design that accommodates sensory changes that occur with age should enhance the ability of individuals to function at the maximum level of competence. Overuse and underuse of sensory cues should be avoided, because both create dependence and result in a mismatch between the individual and the environment.

The extent to which an environment demands a behavioral response is defined as *environmental press*. The ability of the individual to respond adaptively in areas of functional health, social roles, sensory-motor and perceptual functions, and cognition is referred to as *competence*. As the demanding physical environment fails to support aging individuals, safety, self-image, and interactions with others may be adversely affected, and stress may result. In this circumstance of high environmental demand, individuals with high competence levels will withstand greater levels of press, whereas individuals with the least capabilities will likely exhibit maladaptive behavior. Individuals in such situations must either change their competence through rehabilitation or alter their physical environment. Although rehabilitation to improve competence may be a sound solution, it is acknowledged that environmental adaptations are generally easier. Simple environmental changes, such as increased lighting, easily identifiable landmarks for cuing, or decreased background noise, may foster meaningful changes in behavior and interaction within the environment.[28]

Recommending too many changes in sensory stimuli within the environment may lead to sensory distortion, resultant overload, and decreased environmental press. This excessive decrease in environmental press may result in lack of challenge for some individuals, leading to marginal performance and dependent behavior. The optimal environment for older persons is one that provides a measure of challenge and, at the same time, provides the necessary supports for the individual.[28]

Numerous environmental checklists can be found in the literature that address physical barriers in the home and institution. However, special consideration must also be given to accommodating sensory changes. Each area of the physical environment in which older persons function must be addressed, with a focus on this interdependence of sensory loss, functional ability, and reliance on the environment for support. In addition to recommendations cited previously in this text, several areas deserve further emphasis. These include comments on personal/living space, long-term-care residencies, physical therapy clinics, stairs, escalators, and driving. Finally, special considerations must be addressed for adapting an environment for individuals with dementia.

Personal/Living Space

Because the home is the hub of most activity for older individuals, creating an environment to support sensory loss and enhance maximum functional independence is critical. Incorporating the previously outlined design principles that accommodate losses in vision, hearing, taste, smell, and touch will not only facilitate independence but may also minimize the occurrence of accidents leading to death or disability. Adhering to these design principles will facilitate aging in place when constructing new dwellings or retrofitting existing residences. Examples of accommodations that should be considered include use of enhanced lighting and provision of contrast in personal living space to deter falls that result from decreased vision and the use of smoke detectors with visual cues to decrease vulnerability to death from fires in older individuals with decreased ability to hear and smell.[15]

Residential Facilities

Residential facilities that were designed using traditional concepts derived from the medical model may fail to meet the needs of today's frail older population who suffer from multiple chronic conditions. To enhance the quality of life for these individuals, architects and administrators are challenged to incorporate design principles that create environments to support age-related changes and enhance functional performance of individuals with sensory losses.

Appropriate lighting can support greater independence and enhance the safety of older individuals with visual deficits. Although direct, incandescent lighting adds warmth, it may not provide adequate illumination and may also create light pools and shadows. Therefore, direct lighting is not recommended for use in corridors. It is, however, appropriate as supplemental task lighting. Desk lamps and table lamps by chairs should be provided for reading and close work. Indirect "white" fluorescent lighting is recommended for use in corridors, because this type of lighting provides adequate, even illumination and minimizes glare. Warm white bulbs are recommended because they give a softer tint. Care should be taken to minimize flickering, which can be a hazard. A regular schedule for checking ballasts on fluorescent lights and replacing worn-out bulbs can minimize this problem.[9]

Long-term-care facility design should be attentive to choices in materials for window coverings, ceilings, wall coverings, and floors. Window treatments should be chosen to minimize the effect of glare, because this is often a problem in residential facilities. Curtains or blinds can be used for this purpose. Draperies should be considered because they not only minimize glare but also serve to absorb extraneous background noise and assist in lowering energy costs.

Ceilings and wall coverings in residential facilities should be chosen to support sensory deficits of older residents. Ceilings should be covered with acoustic tile specially designed to absorb noise and extraneous sounds that interfere with speech discrimination. Use of these materials is particularly recommended in corridors, dining rooms, and other areas where background noise is prevalent. Wall coverings can be chosen to serve multiple purposes. Color can be used for resident orientation and cuing. Choosing paint or fabric of different colors for various areas within the facility can provide meaning, especially for residents with cognitive deficits. Use of contrast on door frames can serve as added landmarks and assist residents in locating their personal room. Color contrast between walls and floors can provide valuable sensory information to minimize falls in ambulatory individuals. Textured wall coverings that are soft to touch have the added benefit of providing tactile cues for older individuals deprived of touch and for visually impaired residents. Repetitive, random, and vivid patterns that create visual illusions and unstable figure–ground relationships should be avoided.

Floor coverings should be selected to enhance the mobility of older residents. Vinyl or linoleum is often chosen because it is easy to clean and provides little resistance for wheelchair mobility. One problem with vinyl surface is that it is a major source of glare. This can be controlled to an extent with use of nonglare wax. An alternative to vinyl is the use of carpet, which has traditionally been avoided because of stains and odor. Newer design, including solution-dyed fibers and liquid-barrier backing, has minimized these problems.

One older study recommends the use of carpeting to enhance walking for hospital inpatients. This study determined that gait speed and step length were significantly greater on carpeted than on vinyl surfaces. Although this study is dated, the recommendations are still valid.[29] Mobility of wheelchair-bound individual need not be hampered by use of carpeting, because low-looped pile that is very tightly woven can minimize friction.

Another study looked at the role of carpeted and vinyl floors in relation to injuries older individuals sustained as a result of a fall in a hospital. The study retrospectively reviewed a random sample of accident forms. Out of the group of patients who fell on carpet, only 17% sustained injuries. In the group of patients who fell on vinyl, 46% sustained injuries. Statistical analysis indicated less than 1% probability that the reduced rate of injury for those patients who fell on carpet was due to chance. Results of this study support the hypothesis that individuals who fall on carpet are less likely to be injured than those who fall on vinyl flooring.[30] However, results of this investigation should be viewed in light of a more recent study that investigated the effects of flooring on standing balance among older persons. The results of this study indicate that the more compliant—that is, the softer—the floor covering, the greater the effect on sway during moving visual environments. This may be a function of the sensitivity of older individuals to visual and proprioceptive inputs and of difficulty in handling sensory conflicts to the postural control system. The results of this study suggest that the type of floors could affect the potential for falling. High-softness (plush) flooring modules increase the potential for destabilizing balance and increase risk of a fall, even though these more compliant floors are more comfortable and may reduce the potential for hip fracture in the event of a fall. The fact that the moving environments were particularly destabilizing with highly compliant surfaces suggests that floor compliance will cause even greater instability during walking. However, additional studies are needed to verify this assumption.[31] This study supports the use of low-pile carpeting in geriatric facilities to improve balance of older individuals.

Furniture selected for residential facilities should be functional and, at the same time, supportive of sensory changes. Use of fabric upholstery can provide tactile cues and eliminate problems of glare created by vinyl upholstery. Choosing color that contrasts with flooring can serve as a valuable visual cue for residents with visual deficits. Repetitive and illusionary patterns should be avoided.

Particular consideration should be given to design of resident rooms in residential facilities. Beds and chairs should be comfortable and stable and support functional ability of residents.[4] Adequate illumination should be provided, with provisions included for task lighting. Glare should be controlled through use of appropriate window treatments, floor surfaces, and furniture choices. Color and contrast should be considered during the selection of wall coverings, and even furniture coverings. For example, bedspreads should be chosen to contrast with floor coverings so that a visually impaired resident will be able to safely transfer on and off the bed.

Special considerations for personal bathrooms and central bathing areas focus on features to enhance resident safety. One important consideration is to control glare, which is a particular problem with vinyl flooring, porcelain sinks, bathtubs, toilets, chrome towel bars, and grab bars. Suggestions to minimize glare include use of colored fixtures that can additionally provide contrast with floor and wall coverings. These are aesthetically pleasing and can serve as an important safety feature for older individuals with visual deficits and who may experience difficulty in judgment when the toilet, bathtub, or grab bar is of the same color as the floor.

Communal dining areas can pose several design challenges in residential facilities. In addition to the usual problems with lighting and control of glare, there is the added problem of noise control. Because dining areas are commonly located adjacent to the kitchen, background noise from dishwashers and food processors can contribute to difficulty with hearing-impaired residents and can cause further social isolation of these individuals. Use of good insulating materials or locating dining areas away from kitchens is recommended to minimize this problem. Further reduction in background noise can be attained through use of tablecloths and placement of paper pads between cups and saucers.

Physical Therapy Clinics

If older adults are to receive maximum benefit from physical therapy intervention, it is crucial that design principles incorporating recommendations to accommodate for sensory loss with aging be utilized when new facilities are built or existing space is renovated. Concepts previously discussed that accommodate sensory changes must be implemented. These include controlling light sources; minimizing glare; and choosing appropriate ceilings, wall coverings, and floor coverings. Specific recommendations for physical therapy clinics include choosing walkers and other assistive devices that are constructed of nonshiny materials in an effort to control glare. Some pieces of equipment, such as parallel bars, some whirlpools, and various other modalities, are, by design, constructed of shiny material. When using this equipment, light sources should be controlled to minimize the effect of glare.

When mat tables and treatment tables are being chosen, the overall design of the physical therapy space should be considered. These surfaces should be covered with material that provides contrast to floor coverings, so that older clients are afforded a specific visual cue that will enhance safety in transfers.

One significant problem in many physical therapy clinics is background noise. Suggestions to minimize this noise include confining whirlpool areas to separate rooms that are insulated with acoustic material. Another recommendation is to provide individual treatment booths rather than sectioning treatment areas with curtains. Not only will this afford privacy for older individuals, it will also serve as a means of limiting background noise. Background music from radios and use of intercom devices should be discouraged, because they serve as further distracters for the older persons with hearing loss.

Finally, use of texture is encouraged to enhance tactile sensation. When possible, linens should be used on mats and treatment tables rather than paper coverings. These should also contrast with floor coverings to enhance visual perception. Low-pile carpeting should be considered to enhance ambulation, absorb sound, and minimize glare.

Stairs

Stairs are one area within the environment not previously discussed that require special consideration, because they are common sites of accidents leading to injury, hospitalization, and even death. Safe negotiation of stairs requires integration of visual and kinesthetic tests of the conditions of the stairs. This is particularly critical for descent, which is generally more hazardous than ascent. Successful stair negotiation requires that individuals make a transition from free-form movement on level surfaces to the highly circumscribed foot placement that is required on stairs. Visual feedback is used initially in order to judge the position of the stair treads and maximize accuracy of foot placement. Looking at the steps then allows the user to scan the flight of steps for hazards, including broken treads, irregularities, or other obstacles. Once the visual test is accomplished, individuals rely on kinesthetic tests to obtain a feel of the treads and ensure accurate foot placement. In older individuals, visual distractions drawing the user's attention away from the stairs as well as visual deceptions built into the design of the stairs are identified as leading causes of stair accidents (Figure 7-8). Furthermore, the most critical piece of visual information for successful descent of steps was identified as a singular and unambiguous indication of the edge of each step. Optical illusions created by patterned carpeting overpower the ability of individuals to detect tread edges and create a significant hazard. Similar hazards are created by three-dimensional textures, including shag carpeting, because these textures cause treads to appear to merge into a continuous surface.[3,14]

Other environmental considerations on stairs include use of adequate lighting to enhance visual feedback. Light switches should be located at both the top and bottom of the flight of steps. Night-lights should also be

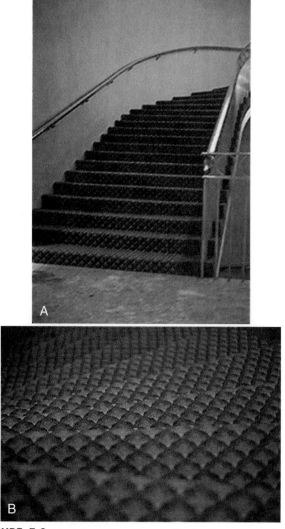

FIGURE 7-8 The visual deception built into the design of this staircase (**A**) and the visual distraction created by the carpeting with a visual figure embedded in a complex figure background (**B**) illustrate how staircase hazards can lead to an accident or fall in an older individual challenged by depth perception and figure–ground discrimination. *(Reprinted with permission of L. Allison.)*

located near the first and last steps to provide cuing during darkness. Glare reflecting from floor surfaces should be minimized by the use of nonglare surfaces, including appropriate types of carpeting. Light from windows located near stairs should be controlled with window coverings. Glare derived directly from light sources should be minimized by positioning and by avoiding exposed light bulbs. Kinesthetic feedback may be enhanced by use of carpeting; however, the addition of ribbed vinyl or rubber stair nosing of a contrasting color should be considered to aid in reducing the risk of falls by enhancing detection of the edge of the step. Stairs without carpeting can be marked by a strip of paint or tape in a contrasting color.[5]

Multifocal glasses (bifocals, trifocals, progressive lenses) may contribute to inability of older individuals to deal with challenges in the environment, especially on stairs. These multifocal glasses require the wearer to view the environment through the lower lenses, which have a typical focal length of 0.6 m. Normally, people view the environment at a distance approximating two steps ahead, at a critical focal distance of ~1.5 to 2 m, which is the focal distance needed for detecting and discriminating floor-level objects. As a result, vision may blur and contrast sensitivity and depth perception may be adversely affected for individuals wearing multifocal glasses, thereby increasing fall risk. One study verified that wearers of multifocal lens had significantly greater odds of falling than nonmultifocal lens wearers. In this study, the falls were more likely to occur outside the home and when the individuals were walking up- or downstairs.[22]

Escalators

Escalators have been identified as a hazardous environment for older persons because their use may result in accidents involving falls. It is thought that the repeated optical image that is a critical design feature of escalators may induce visual depth illusion, resulting in disorientation. This phenomenon, referred to as "wallpaper illusion," can occur when a person with normal binocular vision views a pattern that is periodic in the horizontal meridian of the visual field. This pattern can produce disorientation and result in loss of balance. More research is needed to determine whether the illusion adversely affects postural stability of older individuals more than that of younger people. However, it is theorized that the higher proportion of falls on escalators for older people may be a result of age-related declines in vision and a suspected relationship to postural stability. Older individuals should be alerted to the potential hazards of escalator use, and individuals with vision and visual perceptual deficits should be encouraged to avoid use of escalators. In addition, these individuals should be cautioned to avoid similar surfaces such as carpeting or linoleum that use repeated patterns.[32]

Driving

Because driving is a privilege that enhances independent functioning in the environment, it is important to consider the impact that age-related sensory changes might have on this skill. Vision is a critical sensory modality that undergoes changes with age. Older drivers must learn to give careful consideration to this system in relationship to specific skills needed for driving.

Although it seems logical that good vision is necessary for safe driving, there are no data to support the idea that poor vision results in unsafe driving. Studies linking vision and accident involvement have provided mixed results and are based more on theoretical considerations rather than empirical data. It is generally believed that there is a weak relationship between visual performance and accident involvement for multiple reasons. These reasons include facts such as most accidents have multiple causes (the most frequently cited human causes of accidents are attentional or higher-order perceptual failings), many large-scale studies rely on relatively unreliable vision data obtained from gross driver screenings, and drivers with reduced capacities may restrict driving to times when light conditions are favorable. Nevertheless, several studies link specific visual impairments and theoretically related driving tasks or accident-causing behaviors. These studies have found positive relationships between driver skills and visual acuity, depth perception, and contrast sensitivity.[3,33]

It is generally recognized that age-related decline in visual acuity is highly individualistic and that deterioration in static acuity under optimal illumination, reduced illumination, and glare is not significant before age 60 years. Studies have found small but consistent correlations between photopic static acuity, or day vision, and accident involvement, particularly for older drivers. Between 5% and 10% of 60- to 65-year-old drivers have corrected acuity worse than the 20/40 minimum acuity level required by most states and the District of Columbia. Although not as extensively studied, static acuity under reduced illumination may be more relevant to the visual requirements of older drivers. One study indicated that low-level static acuity was one of the best predictors of accident involvement among older drivers.[33] This is particularly relevant, because the onset is earlier and magnitude much larger than decline in photopic static acuity.[33] Older drivers should recognize the importance of adequate visual correction with glasses or contact lenses and may need to modify driving patterns in low-light conditions.

Dynamic visual acuity, or the ability to detect a moving object, is a more complex task than static visual acuity. Deterioration in this ability begins earlier and accelerates faster with increasing age. Studies have demonstrated a significant relationship between dynamic visual acuity and amount of driving and accident involvement. It is theorized that this correlation is due to the fact that this requires the combination of multiple visual sensory and motor skills, including fine oculomotor control. Another skill that is conceptually critical to safe driving is motion perception. The ability to detect movement relative to the driver is critical to detecting imminently dangerous situations. This ability is primarily limited by neural mechanisms, although the ability of the eye to effect smooth tracking also involves the oculomotor system. Studies have shown that visual training can be effective in enhancing motion discrimination in older persons and that some effects can be generalized to driving situations.[33] Older drivers should be encouraged to participate in visual training sessions that include complex, dynamic visual skills.

Declining visual field is another factor that must be given consideration. Older individuals must be aware of pedestrians or vehicles in the lateral field, and individuals who experience declines in peripheral vision must be taught to compensate by turning their heads or by using car mirrors. Similarly, drivers who have experienced loss in the upper visual field must be alerted to the need to look upward to avoid missing overhead road signs and traffic signals.

Depth perception is also known to decline with age and is additionally affected by increased susceptibility to glare, loss of visual acuity, dark adaptation, changing needs for illumination and contrast, and altered color perception. Older drivers need the ability to judge distances between their vehicle and other moving or stationary objects. This is critical for judging distances from oncoming cars, maintaining appropriate distances, safely passing other vehicles, merging onto a highway, or braking before reaching an intersection. Older drivers who experience difficulty with depth perception and are unable to compensate for this loss should be strongly cautioned to avoid driving.

Because older individuals have problems with dark adaptation, they may experience difficulty with changes in illumination coming from oncoming headlights or streetlights. As a result, night driving may pose a safety hazard, and older individuals may need to confine driving to daylight hours. In addition, older drivers may be limited in night driving by glare intolerance. They should be instructed to compensate for this by avoiding looking at oncoming headlights, traveling on divided highways, or traveling on well-lit roads. Vehicle design modifications introduced beginning with 1986 models have proved beneficial for older drivers who experience decreased night vision and difficulty with glare. These include changes in headlights, rear lights, and directional signals that can be seen on the side of the vehicle. They also include design concepts that result in reduction in windshield and dashboard glare and installation of rear-window defrosters and wipers.[4,33]

The impact of diminished color discrimination on driving is questionable. However, it has been suggested that it may take some older drivers twice as long as younger drivers to detect the flash of a brake light because red colors may appear dimmer as individuals age. The high-mounted rear brake light introduced in 1986 vehicle models may serve as an accommodation for older drivers.

In addition to visual loss, older drivers may experience difficulty because of age-related changes in hearing. Specifically, they may be unable to hear horns from other motorists warning of oncoming hazards, or they may be unable to localize the source of such signals. Vehicle malfunction warnings, such as brake sensors, may also go undetected with diminished hearing. Older drivers can compensate for this loss by adhering to a strict vehicle maintenance schedule.

The final deterrents to safe driving for older individuals that must be given consideration are hazards specific to the road environment itself, for example, poorly placed and poorly designed road signs. Signs should be of sufficient size and should provide adequate color contrast to be seen by older drivers. Traffic lights pose another difficulty. Hazards pertaining to traffic light changes at intersections occur when older drivers react slowly to light changes from green to red. It has been suggested that older drivers would benefit if engineering slowed the speed at which a traffic light changes to 10% less than the current recommended speed of change. Because night drivers rely on median and roadside delineator lines as visual cues, increasing the width of these markers from 4 to 8 in. has also been speculated to be of benefit to older night drivers. Older drivers with visual deficits may have difficulty on two-lane highways and older highways that have closely placed on-ramps and off-ramps. Newer highway design that includes four-lane highways with wide separation and better delineation of on-ramps and off-ramps should prove valuable for older drivers.[4,33] Finally, because older individuals are thought to have difficulty with visual depth illusion created by repeated optical patterns, repetitive patterns that occur in bridges, tunnels, and expressways may pose hazards. Some older drivers should avoid these environments to foster safe driving.

Special Considerations for Older Individuals with Dementia

The ability to perceive and interpret the environment is significantly altered by Alzheimer's disease and related dementias. The extent of the changes is highly individual and depends on multiple factors, including neuropathologic changes, sensory loss, time of day, medications, and the social and physical environment. One constant is that individuals with dementia are affected by the amount, type, and variety of stimuli found in the environment. Both under- and overstimulation can lead to confusion, illusions, frustration, and agitation. On the other hand, a well-planned environment suited for individuals with dementia can enhance functional independence and improve the quality of life for those individuals experiencing sensory loss and changes in judgment and memory.

Individuals with dementia are known to experience changes in visual ability. These may be associated with problems in depth perception, glare, and visual misinterpretation. Dementia-associated fall risk may be reduced when care is exercised to choose floor coverings or carpeting that avoids patterns or borders that increase visual–spatial difficulties. In addition, strong color contrast can enhance functional ability by highlighting environmental features between floors and walls, chairs and flooring, and even utensils and tabletops, thereby facilitating more meaningful interpretation of the environment.

Agitation associated with dementia may be related to inadequate lighting levels. Increasing light levels during activities may be effective in reducing these agitation levels. Visual misperceptions where individuals with dementia have difficulty differentiating reality from representation may also contribute to agitation. They may perceive photographs as family members watching them or perceive television shows as reality. Removing photos and turning television off are effective strategies for curbing this associated agitation. In addition, reflected glare may contribute to illusions and misperceptions. Taking care to minimize or control glare may reduce these misperceptions.

Another problem associated with dementia is auditory hallucinations. Excess noise is a known stressor. To minimize these hallucinations and the associated stress, it is important to reduce background noise. Suggestions include use of sound-absorbing fabrics such as drapes, carpeting, and wall hangings; using place mats on dining tables; choosing upholstered furniture; and eliminating or minimizing the use of overhead call systems in institutional environments.

Introducing music and pleasant sounds is considered therapeutic and is known to help individuals with dementia retrieve lost memories. Care must be exercised to ensure that content and volume is appropriate and that loud, discordant sounds are avoided.

Touch is important, and can have a therapeutic effect for individuals with dementia. Hand massages, the warm touch from a hug, and the presence of pets can have a positive effect on individuals with dementia. Related to the sensation of touch is thermoregulation. It is important to consider comfort levels, especially during activities of daily living. Use of heat lamps, sweat suits, layered clothing, and warming blankets can increase comfort level. One situation in which agitation may result from discomfort associated with the perception of being cold is during bathing. Suggestions to avoid this associated agitation are to reduce chill by use of terry-cloth robes and incorporating pleasant sensory stimulation to reduce the trauma of bathing. Specific suggestions are to control light levels in the bathing area with dimmer switches; to use rich apricot, yellow, or blue tones on bathroom walls; add a fragrance to bathwater; and play soothing, favorite music.

Because individuals with dementia experience sensory declines in taste and smell, it is important to enhance nutrition with flavor-enhanced food and to choose design influences that positively affect nutritional status. This may include ensuring adequate lighting, choosing table and tableware that allow color and contrast between the tabletop and dinnerware, using place mats and tablecloths with plain patterns to enhance contrast but avoid figure–ground confusion.[34-36]

TEACHING/CONSULTING STRATEGIES

Physical therapists working with the older adult are challenged to incorporate teaching strategies to accommodate sensory loss into treatment programs. Their unique knowledge of sensory changes that accompany aging, coupled with knowledge of appropriate interventions, will maximize the rehabilitation experience and afford older people an opportunity to utilize newly acquired skills in an environment that maintains reasonable control over functional ability and enhances quality of life.

Simply indicating which changes accompany normal aging may encourage older individuals to seek appropriate interventions and avoid the resignation that often accompanies a sense of helplessness at thoughts of "growing old." The physical therapist should encourage use of adaptive equipment and assistive technology to compensate for specific sensory loss. For example, individuals with visual loss should be supported in use of glasses and other low-vision aids, and persons with hearing loss should be encouraged to use hearing aids or other amplification devices that have been prescribed. Where indicated, physical therapists should support and encourage referral to appropriate specialists for evaluation of specific deficits and prescription of needed devices. They should also be knowledgeable of service agencies within the community that specialize in assistive technologies and support services for older individuals with sensory loss and assist individuals in contacting and using these agencies. In addition, therapists should instruct older persons in environmental modifications that are unique to their individual needs.

Physical therapists can use their knowledge and skills related to movement dysfunction and ergonomics to further enhance the functional independence of older individuals who require accommodations for sensory changes. For example, physical therapists can be particularly helpful in providing posture recommendations to enhance comfort for older individuals who use accommodations for low vision. This is important because the maintenance of focal distance, line of sight, head tilt, back position, and body posture determine the comfort and efficiency of many recommended low-vision systems. Suggestions may include modification of head position and line of sight to successfully use the device. Similar suggestions may be made for computer users who are visually impaired. In addition, therapists may serve a valuable role in recommending adaptations to prescribed devices that address concurrent problems often experienced by older, visually impaired patients. These may include the use of adjustable reading stands to hold large-print reading material or special ring stands, clamps, or headbands to position magnifying devices for individuals with arthritis, stroke, or Parkinson's disease, who may otherwise have difficulty using the prescribed device. Finally, physical therapists can be essential in assisting with mobility training for individuals who require the use of mobility assistive devices such as canes or dog guides.[9,37]

Specific teaching strategies that incorporate instruction in techniques to strengthen the sensory stimulus should be part of the physical therapy intervention for older individuals with sensory impairment. Examples might include adjustments to volume and tone of radios and televisions for hearing-impaired individuals or use of large-print books for the visually impaired. Another technique is to teach older individuals to compensate with other senses. For example, individuals with a diminished sense of smell can be taught to inspect food visually for signs of spoilage, or individuals with visual impairments can be encouraged to use auditory substitutions, including talking books and other talking products. The final strategy is to teach older individuals to modify behavior. One example is to pause when entering a darkened room from a bright, outdoor environment.[9]

Because of their knowledge of age-related sensory changes and environmental modifications, physical therapists should assume active roles as consultants. Providing information to architects and designers will foster safe access of facilities by older individuals. This is particularly important in public buildings, including churches, hospitals, outpatient clinics, and senior centers. In addition, independence of individuals in retirement complexes, senior housing, and long-term-care facilities can be enhanced when design principles are incorporated. Therapists should assist in plans for construction of new facilities and renovation of existing facilities. Encouraging architects and builders to incorporate universal design and aging in place concepts and design considerations to allow adaptability of structures to accommodate sensory changes related to age and disability may allow older individuals to remain in their own homes, and may be more economically feasible than renovating structures that do not incorporate such principles. Also, therapists should take an active role in purchase of supplies for existing facilities. Quality of life for older residents can be maximized by selecting such items as furniture, wall and floor coverings, and window treatments that enhance, rather than impede, functional performance. Finally, physical therapists can encourage development of appropriate products to meet the needs of older individuals with sensory loss by serving as consultants to companies that design and manufacture these devices.[12,38]

SUMMARY

It is important for physical therapists who work with the older adult to recognize sensory changes that occur with aging and to understand the effects that these changes have on the ability of older individuals to function in the environment. Knowledge of adaptations within the environment to accommodate and support losses that occur in vision, hearing, taste, smell, and touch can maximize the rehabilitation experience, promote optimal functional independence, and enhance quality of life.

Physical therapists should be able to apply this information concerning sensory losses and environmental adaptations to general principles of design in order to create meaningful environments for older persons. Consideration should be given to all aspects of the environment in which older individuals function. These include personal living space and long-term-care residencies. Specific attention should be given to architectural barriers found in physical therapy departments and on stairs and escalators. Because driving is a skill that allows access to other activities of daily living, special consideration must also be given to this function. Special consideration should be given to apply appropriate design principles to maximize quality of life and enhance safety for individuals with dementia.

The roles of physical therapists as teacher and consultant should be emphasized. Physical therapists have unique knowledge of the needs of aging individuals, and they should be encouraged to share this knowledge with architects, designers, administrators, and others who deal with facilities and products used by older individuals.

Finally, physical therapists should recognize that there is a critical need for further research on age-related sensory changes and on the relationship between these changes and the use of environmental adaptations, assistive technology, and adaptive devices. A limited number of studies have been done to address these considerations, and the majority of the recommendations are based more on theory than controlled studies. Furthermore, many of these recommendations are based on assumptions about the older individual's perceptions related to aging, the environment, and the motivation to preserve maximum function within the environment through appropriate modifications. Qualitative studies are needed to support such assumptions. Physical therapists should be willing to participate in or support such research efforts in order to further this science, and benefit the older individuals that they serve.

REFERENCES

To enhance this text and add value for the reader, all references are included on the companion Evolve site that accompanies this text book. The reader can view the reference source and access it online whenever possible. There are a total of 38 cited references and other general references for this chapter.

Cognition in the Aging Adult

Dale Avers, PT, DPT, PhD, Ann K. Williams, PT, PhD

Successful achievement of physical therapy goals requires consideration of the mental health status of the patient. For older persons, two common mental health problems are depression and cognitive impairment. This chapter will first review the characteristics, assessment, and therapeutic management of the older person with depression. The second half of the chapter discusses the normal cognitive changes of aging, cognitive impairment, dementia, assessment of dementia, and therapeutic management of older persons with dementia. Case studies for both depression and dementia are also included.

DEPRESSION IN OLDER PERSONS

Depression is the most common psychological mood problem in the older person,[1,2] and is a significant problem encountered by health professionals working with older persons who are ill. For example, 40% of hospitalized older adults are clinically depressed.[3] Depression is often neglected in the older person, possibly because mental health issues are overshadowed by physical problems, especially in older patients who are frail.[4] Despite this problem, depression is actually quite treatable.[5]

Rates of depression in the older person are quite variable because of differences in diagnostic criteria. Major depression occurs in older adults at rates ranging from 1% to 4%, whereas rates of sub–major depression, including adjustment disorders and dysthymia, range from 15% to 30%.[6,7] In medically ill older adults, rates of clinically significant depression range from 10% to 43%.[6]

One factor that is commonly associated with depression in the older person is loss of health.[6] The stress of physical illness that may be associated with physical disability, pain, and lifestyle changes can result in the psychological response of depression. The relationship of depression and rehabilitation are significant, as depression can commonly and dramatically affect the response to rehabilitation. The hopelessness, apathy, and withdrawal of the person with depression can make rehabilitation a challenge. This section reviews the characteristics of depression in older adults, factors associated with late-life depression, common treatment approaches, and modifications of the physical therapist's treatment plan.

Characteristics and Assessment of the Older Person with Depression

Most people think of the predominant characteristic of depression as depressed mood, that is, feelings of sadness, hopelessness, and loss of interest and pleasure in previously pleasurable activities. Although these emotions are a key feature of depression, experts agree that for depression to be a psychopathology or a "clinical depression," other characteristics must also be present. These characteristics include cognitive problems such as difficulty concentrating, memory complaints, slowed thinking, indecisiveness, and perceived lack of competence and control. Individuals may have feelings of low self-esteem, worthlessness, apathy, and excessive guilt. The person with depression has difficulties with interpersonal interactions, including withdrawal from family and friends and neglect of previously pleasurable activities. Finally, depression includes somatic symptoms such as problems with appetite, sleep, and psychomotor function. The disturbances of appetite usually involve loss of weight but may involve excessive eating. Insomnia and early morning wakening are the most common sleep disturbances, but hypersomnia may also be demonstrated. Psychomotor functioning or motor activity is usually decreased or slowed but may also be hyperactive.[8]

To help standardize the diagnosis of depression and the terminology associated with it, the *Diagnostic and Statistical Manual of Mental Disorders TR*, ed. 4 (*DSM-IV*), of the American Psychiatric Association describes generally accepted and specific criteria for various diagnoses of mood disorders.[9] The two diagnoses that are important to this discussion of depression in the older person are Major Depressive Episode and Adjustment Disorder With Depressed Mood. According to the *DSM-IV*, the criteria for major depressive episode are either depressed mood or loss of pleasure in all activities and associated symptoms for a period of at least 2 weeks (Box 8-1). These symptoms must be relatively persistent and a change from previous functioning. The associated symptoms for major depressive episode include significant weight loss when not dieting or weight gain, insomnia or hypersomnia, decreased or hyperactive motor activity, fatigue or loss of energy, feelings of worthlessness or excessive or inappropriate guilt, diminished ability to think or concentrate, and recurrent thoughts of death, suicide ideation, or a suicide attempt. The person must exhibit at least five of all these symptoms to be diagnosed as having a major depression and the symptoms must cause significant distress or impairment in social, occupational, or other important areas of functioning. Box 8-1 lists common characteristics of depression.

Adjustment disorder with depressed mood is a subcategory of adjustment disorders in the *DSM-IV*.[9,10] Adjustment disorders are maladaptive reactions to an identifiable psychosocial stressor that occur within 3 months of the onset of the stressor. The clinical significance of the reaction is evidenced by impairment of social or occupational functioning or by marked distress that is in excess of a normal and expected reaction. In an adjustment disorder with depressed mood the predominant symptoms in addition to depressed mood are tearfulness and feelings of hopelessness. For example, a divorce may cause a person to have a depressed mood. This response would be classified as an adjustment disorder with depressed mood if the person's social relationships or job were affected. The depression response must be considered excessive to qualify as an adjustment disorder with depressed mood. The disturbance is considered acute if the depressive symptoms are less than 6 months old and chronic if the disturbance has persisted for 6 months or more.

Physical therapists may encounter two other classifications within the *DSM-IV*: Mood Disorder Due to a Medical Condition With Depressive Features and Dysthymic Disorder.[9,10] In a mood disorder due to a medical condition, there must be a prominent and persistent disturbance in mood that causes significant distress or impairment in social, occupational, or other functioning as well as evidence that the disturbance is the *direct physiological* consequence of a general medical condition. An example would be a patient classified as having Mood Disorder due to Hypothyroidism, with Depressive Features. Dysthymic disorder requires a depressed mood for most of the day, for more days than not, over a period of at least 2 years. At least two of the associated symptoms of a major depressive episode must also be present, for example, poor appetite, insomnia, low energy, low self-esteem, poor concentration, or hopelessness.

When reading the numerous books and articles available on depression, the reader may become confused by the varied terminology that may differ from the *DSM-IV TR*[9] just outlined. For example, some authors will use the term *endogenous depression*, which is similar to a major depressive episode. Similarly, the term *reactive*, or *secondary*, depression is similar to an adjustment disorder with depressed mood. Finally, the term *dysphoria* is sometimes used to describe a milder depression characterized only by depressed mood or unhappiness. The term *depression* may be used to represent any point on this continuum from unhappiness to a clinical depression.[8]

Assessment of Depression

Self-report tools are frequently used to screen for depression in the clinical setting. Using a printed form, the respondents will check off whether they have experienced any of the symptoms of depression. These self-report tools are generally accepted as good screening devices to indicate individuals who are at risk for depression and who may need further professional evaluation. However, the U.S. Preventive Services Task Force has found that an affirmative response to the following two questions may be as effective as using longer screening measures or may indicate the need for the use of more in-depth diagnostic

---

BOX 8-1	Characteristics of Depression

Major Depressive Episode*
1. Depressed (sad) mood
2. Markedly diminished interest or pleasure in all, or almost all, activities
3. Weight loss or weight gain when not dieting or decrease or increase in appetite
4. Insomnia or hypersomnia
5. Psychomotor agitation or retardation
6. Fatigue or loss of energy
7. Feelings of worthlessness or excessive or inappropriate guilt
8. Diminished ability to think or concentrate, or indecisiveness
9. Recurrent thoughts of death, recurrent suicidal ideation, a suicide attempt, or a specific plan for committing suicide

Adjustment Disorder with Depressed Mood
1. Emotional or behavioral symptoms in response to an identifiable stressor(s) occurring within 3 months of the onset of the stressor(s).
2. Clinically significant symptoms or behaviors as evidenced by:
   a. Marked distress that is in excess of what would be expected from exposure to the stressor
   b. Significant impairment in social or occupational functioning

*Criteria: At least five of the following symptoms present during a 2-week period and represent a change from previous functioning. One of the symptoms must be either (1) depressed mood or (2) loss of interest or pleasure.

(Adapted from American Psychiatric Association: Diagnostic and Statistical Manual of Mental Disorders TR, ed. 4. Washington DC, American Psychiatric Association, 2000.)

tools: (1) "Over the past two weeks, have you ever felt down, depressed, or hopeless?" and (2) "Have you felt little interest or pleasure in doing things?"[3,11] It is important to note that these screening tools indicate the severity of symptoms and do not diagnose depression. Physical therapists can administer these tools as screens for depression and then refer clients as appropriate to mental health or other medical practitioner. A physical therapist cannot make the diagnosis of depression.

Depression Scales. Depression scales are widely used for the screening of dementia and several are listed in Table 8-1. Four of the most commonly used depression scales for older adults are the Beck Depression Inventory (BDI),[12] the Center for Epidemiological Studies Depression Scale (CES-D),[13] the Geriatric Depression Scale (GDS),[14] and the Zung Self-Rating Depression Scale (SDS).[15] Shorter versions of the CES-D and the GDS are available and demonstrate similar sensitivity and specificity to the original versions.[16] Generally, the scales make statements about feelings or situations, and the respondent indicates how frequently each item occurs. Scales that deemphasize somatic signs of depression such as the GDS and the CES-D, are generally considered more valid for the older person. Although each measure has a unique scoring system, higher scores consistently reflect more severe symptoms. All measures have a statistically predetermined cutoff score at which depression symptoms are considered significant and demand further referral.

Models of Depression. Numerous authors have speculated about the causes of depression, and various models have emerged. Models of depression are useful in that they may indicate an approach to treatment. Five of the most frequently cited models for explaining depression with relevance to older adults are the cognitive model, the learned-helplessness model, the interpersonal model, the neurobiological model, and the integrative model.

The *cognitive model* of depression was proposed by Aaron Beck and is based on his empirical observation of depressed patients.[17] This model emphasizes the cognitive structure underlying depression, including the negative views of the self, the environment, and the future. In this model, the negative schemata are primary and the focus of treatment while the depressed affect is secondary. The Beck Depression Inventory was developed from this model, demonstrating the correlation between negative feelings of self and depression. Interestingly, a strategy to avoid negative feelings is to develop focused goals. It has been found that individuals who developed focused goals were able to avoid negative feelings more so than those with less focus, an important implication for physical therapists.

In the *learned-helplessness model* of Seligman, uncontrollable negative events can result in passive behaviors.[18] According to this theory, people who have an explanatory schema of pessimism are more prone to learned helplessness and depression than those with an explanatory schema of optimism. Cognitive theory approaches are then used to help affect the individual's explanatory schema.

The learned-helplessness theory has physical health implications. People with a pessimistic outlook may neglect healthful behaviors such as good diet, exercise, and wellness behaviors, which then places them at risk for poor health. Subsequent poor health and chronic diseases may contribute to learned helplessness as these individuals interpret their poor health as beyond their control and unexplained. The result may be excessively passive behavior, poor problem solving, weaker immune system, and depression.[19]

The *interpersonal model* for depression emphasizes overdependent personality traits that predispose the individual who has had a loss or negative life event to depression.[20] This model focuses on interpersonal relationships and personality rather than external causes for depression. For example, depression may result in the patient who may have been in a long-term abusive or demeaning relationship with a spouse who is now needed for caregiving. Treatment would be directed at the patient's relationship with her spouse and changing her perceptions about herself and/or the relationship.

The *neurobiological model* of depression suggests that the somatic symptoms of depression, such as the psychomotor retardation (characterized by changes in speech, motility, and cognition) and temporal variation, indicate a biological basis for the illness.[21] Clinical observations that some drugs produced depressive symptoms, whereas other drugs relieved them, pointed to decreased neurotransmission or a disturbance of catecholamine transmission as the cause of depression. Deficient brain serotonergic transmission has been suggested because of the sleep disturbances that occur with depression. Many drugs have been developed on the basis of the neurobiological model.

Many of these explanations of depression are combined in the integrative model first described by Lewinsohn et al.[22] The integrative model describes several individual predisposing characteristics that combine with environmental variables to result in depression. Individual characteristics include low self-reinforcement, negative self-evaluation, pessimism, global attribution, low coping skills, preoccupation with negative experiences, interpersonal dependency, withdrawal, and low self-esteem. Environmental issues include low socioeconomic status, low personal and social support, and stressful life events. Factors that provide immunity to depression were positive coping skills and good social support. In a study of adults with chronic musculoskeletal pain, stress, pain, catastrophizing, and activity interferences were related to increased depression.[23] Positive pain coping along with social and family supports were related to decreased depression.

TABLE 8-1	Common Depression Scales				
Scale	No. of Items	Total Score	Diagnostic Accuracy	How Scored	Sample Item
Zung Self-Rating Depression Scale	20	100	Not available	Scored for frequency: e.g, some of the time, most of the time, etc. 25-49, Normal range 50-59, Mildly depressed 60-69, Moderately depressed 70 and above, Severely depressed	"I feel downhearted and blue."
Beck Depression Inventory (BDI)	21	63	Cutoff score of 10 gave a sensitivity of 80.0 and specificity of 61.4[a]	Subject chooses one of four choices	"I do not feel sad." "I feel sad." "I am sad all the time and can't snap out of it." "I am so sad or unhappy that I can't stand it."
Center for Epidemiological Studies Depression Scale (CES-D)	10 or 20	60	The CES-D revealed a sensitivity of 40% and specificity of 82% for detecting minor depression[b] Sensitivity, 97%-100%[c] with a cutoff score of 16 Specificity, 84%-93%	Scored for frequency A cutoff score of 16 has been suggested to differentiate patients with mild depression from normal subjects, with a score of 23 and higher indicating significant depression.	"I felt that I could not shake off the blues even with help from my friends and family."
Geriatric Depression Scale (GDS)	15 (short) or 30 (long)	30	GDS-30 produced a sensitivity of 84% and specificity of 95% with a cutoff score of 11/12; a cutoff of 14/15 decreased the sensitivity rate to 80% but increased specificity to 100%.[d] In a sample of age >85 years and a cutoff point of 3 to 4 of 15, the sensitivity and specificity of the GDS-15 were 88% and 76%, respectively.[e]	Scored yes/no	"Do you feel that your life is empty?"
Patient Health Questionnaire (PHQ)-9	9-item	27	A PHQ-9 score ≥10 had 91% sensitivity and 89% specificity for major depression 78% sensitivity and 96% specificity for any depression diagnosis[f]		

[a] Aben I, Verhey F, Lousberg R, et al. (2002). Validity of the Beck depression inventory, hospital anxiety and depression scale, SCL-90, and Hamilton Depression Rating Scale as screening instruments for depression in stroke patients. Psychosomatics, 43(5), 386-393.

[b] Lyness JM, Noel TK, Cox C, et al. (1997). Screening for depression in elderly primary care patients. A comparison of the Center for Epidemiologic Studies-Depression Scale and the Geriatric Depression Scale. Arch Intern Med, 157(4), 449-454.

[c] Radloff, LS. (1977). The Center for Epidemiological Studies—Depression Scale. A self-report depression scale for research in the general population. Appl Psychol Meas, 3, 385-401.

[d] Yesavage JA, Brink TL, Rose TL, et al. (1982). Development and validation of a geriatric depression screening scale: a preliminary report. J Psychiatr Res 17:37-49.

[e] de Craen AJ, Heeren TJ, Gussekloo, J (2003). Accuracy of the 15-item geriatric depression scale (GDS-15) in a community sample of the oldest old. Int J Geriatr Psychiatry, 18(1), 63-66.

[f] Williams LS, Brizendine EJ, Plue L, et al. (2005). Performance of the PHQ-9 as a screening tool for depression after stroke. Stroke, 36(3), 635-638.

Unique Features of Depression in the Older Adult

Because health professionals and older individuals themselves may misinterpret prolonged depression as a natural and acceptable part of aging in reaction to the many physical, social, and economic losses that occur, help may not be offered or sought out as readily as in the young. Unfortunately, suicide occurs more often in the aging population at a rate of 16% as compared to 14% in the teenage population. Interestingly, up to 75% of older individuals who took their own lives saw their physician within 1 month before their suicide.[24] Because depression can mask itself in physical symptoms and yet is commonly related to suicide, recognition of depression is important. Many older adults complain about physical ailments, rather than emotional distress and many health professionals feel more comfortable dealing with physical symptoms. Older adults may deny feeling sad but complain about feeling tired or having low energy or low motivation. They may also show increased signs of anxiety, irritability, weight loss, and insomnia. The over-60 population, born in a time when mental illness was stigmatized and emotions were deemphasized ("big boys don't cry") contribute to the difficulty in recognizing depression. Some signs that indicate an older adult may be depressed are listed in Box 8-2.

Pseudodementia, an older term used for behavior such as depression that appeared similar to dementia,[25] is rarely used now, in favor of an accurate diagnosis. Several of the symptoms of depression relate to changes in thinking or cognition, creating a risk that the person may be diagnosed with dementia rather than depression. Knowing whether the main problem is depression or dementia is often difficult. Depression can imitate dementia, and both depression and dementia can have depressive symptoms. Depression can also be superimposed on dementia. In the early stages of dementia, the person knows his or her memory is declining and this loss can lead to depression. The apathy, decreased ability to concentrate, and memory complaints of the depressed older person may be misinterpreted as symptoms of dementia. Table 8-2 provides some distinguishing features between depression and dementia.

As geriatric psychiatrists have noted, the distinction between depression and dementia is complicated by the fact that each condition can coexist in the same person. If there is a clear psychosocial stressor that could lead to depression, geriatric psychiatrists recommend that treatment should be first initiated for depression because depression can be reversed. A thorough interview with family members becomes essential to help distinguish between the two diagnoses. Dementia should be a diagnosis of exclusion that is only given after other possible diagnoses have been eliminated. Instruments available to measure depression in persons with high levels of cognitive deficit include the Cornell Scale for Depression in Dementia, the Dementia Mood Assessment Scale, and the Depressive Signs Scale.[173]

Physical Illness, Function, and Depression

One factor consistently associated with depression in older persons is physical illness.[6,26-31] This is clearly of import to health care professionals. Numerous studies demonstrate an increased risk of depression in physically ill persons. There is mounting evidence that cerebrovascular disease is an important risk factor for late life depression. Other types of physical illnesses that can cause depression in old age include cancer, thyroid disease, vitamin deficiencies, and infections. Older persons with stroke and Parkinson's disease also have shown increased risk for depression.[29,32] In addition to studies of persons with specific diseases, studies that include persons with many comorbidities also demonstrate an increased risk for depression.

Many physical illnesses in old age result in permanent disabilities, which can restrict a person's mobility and often require assistance with self-care. This enforced dependency may cause a loss of dignity, a sense of being a burden on others, and a fear of institutionalization. Mood disorders are often left untreated in these circumstances, as being "down" is seen as a normal response to the situation. Medications that are required to treat many of these problems can also cause depression, particularly drugs used to treat high blood pressure, steroids, painkillers, and tranquilizers.

Some psychologists theorize that all persons with a physical illness or injury will experience a "stage" of depression similar to the stages of grief.[33] This traditional stage theory proposes that depression is a necessary and adaptive part of rehabilitation.[34] However, although physically ill persons have higher rates of depression, clearly not all physically ill persons develop *clinical* depression. At some point, dysphoric feelings may become excessive and maladaptive, which result in the cognitive,

---

BOX 8-2	Clues for Identifying Depression in Older Adults

- Unexplained or aggravated aches and pains
- Hopelessness
- Helplessness
- Anxiety and worries
- Memory problems
- Weight loss
- Loss of feeling of pleasure
- Slowed movement
- Irritability
- Lack of interest in personal care (skipping meals, forgetting medications, neglecting personal hygiene)
- Tiredness, listlessness

(Adapted from Gallo JJ, Rabins PV: Depression without sadness: alternative presentations of depression in late life. Am Fam Physician 60(3): 820-826, 1999.)

TABLE 8-2	Comparative Features of Delirium, Dementia, and Depression		
	Delirium	**Dementia**	**Major Depression**
Definition	Impaired sensorium (reduced level of consciousness)	Global decline in cognitive capacity in clear consciousness	Disturbance in mood, with associated low vital sense and low self-attitude
Core symptoms	Inattention, distractibility, drowsiness, befuddlement; signs of illness	Initially is alert, attentive. Gradually develops amnesia, aphasia, agnosia, apraxia, disturbed executive functioning No signs of illness	Sadness, anhedonia (inability to perceive pleasure), crying
Common associated symptoms	Cognitive impairment, hallucinations common, mood lability	Depression, delusions, hallucinations relatively uncommon, irritability	Fatigue, insomnia, anorexia, guilt, self-blame, hopelessness, helplessness
Language	Slurred speech	Normal speech in early stages	Normal speech
Temporal features	Sudden onset over hours or days	Slow onset over months or years	Episodic subacute onset
Memory	Memory loss	Memory loss	No memory loss
Diurnal features	Usually worse in the evening and night	No clear pattern	Usually worse in the morning

(*Adapted from Lyketosos CG: Diagnosis and management of delirium in the older person. JCOM 5(4): 54, 1998.*)

psychological, and somatic symptoms of a major depression. The severity and number of symptoms as well as a previous history of depression are suggestive of a major depressive episode.[35] Patients with an adjustment disorder with depressed mood will tend to have a recent history of higher function than currently demonstrated, less severe psychological symptoms and rather severe physical and psychological stressors.[34] Studies indicate the rate of severe depression in the physically ill older person somewhere between 20% and 35%.[36] The strong association of physical illness to depression has several factors. In a study of older medical clinic outpatients, Williamson and Schulz found that health status and psychosocial factors were about equally important in explaining depression.[37] Important health variables included physician and self-rated severity of symptoms, pain medications, and activity restrictions. Key psychosocial factors included worry about transportation, need for future services, satisfaction with social support, worry about becoming a burden, and loneliness. Box 8-3 lists other possible factors in the relationship between physical illness and depression.

The increased risk of depression in physically ill older persons makes it critical to identify factors of an illness that increase this risk. Several studies have indicated higher levels of functional incapacity and disability to be associated with higher levels of depression.[38] However, the relationship is not absolute. Many older adults have high rates of physical dependency without correspondingly high rates of depression. The very old may have different expectations regarding disability and are therefore more likely to accept it. Cummings et al found that functional deficits in performing instrumental activities of daily living (IADLs) was a significant predictor of depression. Results suggested that older adults become at risk for depression when physical/cognitive impairment threatens their independent operation in the community and their management of typical household tasks.[39]

Baltes and Lindenberger found differences in depressive symptoms between functionally impaired persons in the age groups 55 to 64 years, 65 to 74 years, and 75 years and older and observed that despite their objectively poor physical and functional health status, those in the 75 years and older age group may have better perceptions of their own health than those in the 55 to 64 years age group.[40] Adaptation to the difficulties of old age is gradual. Its problems are often most worrying and least acceptable in the earlier phases of aging. Such an explanation could raise important new issues for the professional approach to prevention and treatment of depression at different stages of the aging process.[41]

Effects of Depression on Function in the Older Person.
Because of the nature of depression, older persons with depression may have a reduced functional capacity.[42] The apathy, loss of pleasure in activities, and psychomotor retardation reduce the aging individual's capacity to participate in everyday activities and even perform

BOX 8-3	Factors Contributing to the Increased Risk of Depression in Physical Illness

Biological
Hormonal, nutritional, electrolyte, or endocrine abnormalities
Effects of medication
Physical consequences of systemic and/or intracerebral disease

Psychological
Sense of loss associated with serious medical illness
Effects on body image, self-esteem, sense of identity
Impaired capacity to work and maintain relationships

activities of daily living (ADLs). The deconditioning effects of age and illness combine with depression to result in a greater perceived effort for minor, everyday tasks. The depressed older person may perceive that even simple tasks require excessive amounts of energy, and therefore these tasks become extremely difficult. This decreased function is usually most evident in the morning.

For the physically ill older person with depression, this loss of functional capacity becomes even more problematic. Long-term goals may appear unattainable. In a study of patients with hip fracture, Mossey et al found increased depression to be associated with reduced functional recovery and reduced response to rehabilitation.[43] However, depression did not limit their rehabilitation outcomes.[44] In a study of inpatient rehabilitation patients, Berod et al found that depressed persons had a greater length of stay than nondepressed persons.[45] Depressed affect in older persons is also linked to decreased functional ability, higher disability, and increased utilization of health care services.[45] In a prospective study, Hays et al found that depression at baseline predicted increased loss of function 1 year later,[42] and Clark et al found that depression predicted an increase in limitations in performing ADLs over a 2-year period.[46] Depression and functional status and recovery are probably interactive, so that the depressed patient functions at a lower level, and this decreased function also reinforces the depression.

An additional factor with implications for physical therapists is that depression increases the risk of developing new illnesses, mortality, and the use of health care resources.[39] Significantly, depressed older adults have 50% higher health care costs. Because evidence exists for the role of physical activity in decreasing the symptoms of depression, exercise interventions for the functional deficits may mediate the symptoms of depression and lower health care costs.

Pain and Depression. Pain is linked to higher levels of depression.[47-49] However, the relationship between depression and pain across the life span is unclear. Some studies have shown no relationship of age to depression and pain,[49] whereas others indicate a strong relationship between pain and depression in older persons.[50] For example, Turk et al[51] found that there was a stronger relationship of severity of pain to depression in older persons with chronic pain when compared to younger persons. In contrast, in a study of persons with cancer, Williamson and Schulz[37] found that older persons were less distressed and depressed possibly because of lower expectations and more experiences with illness and disability. Few studies have combined physical disability and pain when assessing depression in the older person. Williams and Schulz found that when control for other variables is added to the analysis, pain becomes a more important factor than physical disability in level of depression.[52] This association between pain

and depression has also been shown in institutionalized older persons.[50]

Depression and Gender. Although more women than men become seriously depressed, this trend reverses itself in later years, especially after menopause.[53] After the age of 80, rates of depression among men and women become about equal. Several issues put older women at risk for depression. Biological factors like hormonal changes may make older women more vulnerable. Unmarried and widowed individuals as well as those who lack a supportive social network also have elevated rates of depression. In advanced old age, support networks may decline, resulting in more social isolation, especially with institutionalization.

The stresses of maintaining relationships or caring for an ill loved one and children typically fall more heavily on women, which could contribute to higher rates of depression. The responsibilities of caregiving are known to increase stress and depression, although not always. Whereas some people are natural caregivers and view caregiving as a preferred role, others experience more stress. The chapter on caregiving in this text explores the relationship between depression and caregiving.

One would expect that a high degree of social support from family and friends would buffer the negative effects of an illness and result in a lower risk for depression. Although research has generally supported this hypothesis,[42] some studies have shown higher levels of anxiety and dependency in patients with more social support.[54] Perceived adequacy of social support and presence of a confidant may be especially important in the ability of social support to moderate the negative effects of life's stressors.[42] Social support may only be important for persons who highly value social interaction. Social support, depression, and physical illness may form a complex web of interrelationships in which persons who are ill and in pain become depressed and have difficulty mobilizing the social support that is available to them.[42] Also, older persons with chronic physical illness may require support over long periods of time. This can stress any support system, so that expected support is not available, and this may contribute to or exacerbate depression.

Depression and Institutionalization. Depression occurs among residents of nursing homes at a rate of 15% to 25%, higher than the 15% among community-dwelling older adults.[55] Studies indicate that rates of major depression in this group range from 12% to 15% and rates of minor depression from 28% to 50%. Factors linked to depression among nursing home residents include pain, poor health, and cognitive decline.[56,57] A significant finding is the relationship between pain and depression among nursing home residents. Although this may be an issue of depression manifesting as somatic complaints, the relationship is not clear.[58] Moreover, although depression can respond to antipsychotic drugs, too often these drugs are linked to falls. Depression can also increase the risk of nursing home placement.[59] The rates of new cases of depression in nursing homes are striking, with a 14% incidence of major depression over a 6-month period. Those at highest risk for major depression are the cognitively intact nursing home patients who are sickest, most disabled, and most dependent, compared to cognitively impaired residents (24% vs. 10%, respectively).[174]

Suicide. Official suicide statistics identify older adults as a high-risk group.[60] In 1998 it was reported that older adults comprised about 13% of the U.S. population, yet accounted for 19% of its suicides; in contrast, young people, ages 15 to 24 years, comprised about 14% of the population and accounted for 15% of the suicides.[61] Among older persons, there are between two to four suicide attempts for every completed attempt.[61] However, the suicide completion rate of older adults is 50% higher than the population as a whole. This is because older adults who attempt suicide die from the attempt more often than any other age group. Not only do older adults kill themselves at a greater rate than any other group in society but they tend to be more determined and purposeful.[62] Firearms (71%), overdose (liquids, pills, or gas) (11%), and suffocation (11%) were the three most common methods of suicide used by persons aged 65 years or older. In 1998, firearms were the most common method of suicide by both males and females, accounting for 78% of male and 35% of female suicides in that age group. The highest suicide rates in the United States for any group are found in persons aged 65 years and older. Men accounted for 84% of these suicides.[175]

Risk factors for suicide among older persons differ from those among the young. In addition to a higher prevalence of depression, older persons are more socially isolated and more frequently use highly lethal methods.[1,175] They also make fewer attempts per completed suicide, have a higher male-to-female ratio than other groups, have often visited a health care provider before their suicide, and have more physical illnesses. It has also been found in one population-based case-control study that visual impairment, neurologic disorders, and malignant disease were associated with suicide in older people, along with cardiovascular disease, and musculoskeletal disorders.[63] Unbearable pain is also a factor in suicide.

MANAGEMENT OF DEPRESSION IN THE OLDER PERSON

The management of depression in the older person has many aspects. Two of the most common treatment approaches are pharmacotherapy and psychotherapy. Although psychotherapy has demonstrated positive results with older persons, pharmaceutical treatment is more commonly used.[28] Reasons for this bias may include resistance to and misunderstanding of psychotherapy on the part of the older person, older persons' preference for medical intervention as opposed to the mental health intervention, cost and transportation problems to receive psychotherapy, some psychotherapists' ageist attitudes, reimbursed pharmaceutical costs giving the appearance of lower cost, lack of access to mental health specialists and easy access to pharmaceuticals, and a preference toward drug treatment in the medical community, especially among general practitioners. Some experts have suggested that psychotherapy may be more effective for adjustment disorder with depressed mood, whereas drug treatment may be more effective for a major depressive episode. Nevertheless, drug treatment remains the most common approach in managing older adults with depression.

Pharmacotherapy

Pharmacologic treatment is the primary therapy for major depressive episodes in the older person.[64] Although there are many pharmacologic treatments for depression, medications used to treat major depression can be divided into five major categories: selective serotonin reuptake inhibitors (SSRIs), tricyclic or tetracyclic antidepressants (TCAs), heterocyclic antidepressants, serotonin/norepinephrine reuptake inhibitors, and monoamine oxidase inhibitors.[64] Table 8-3 indicates the common drug names in these categories.

The SSRIs are the mainstay of pharmaceutical treatment for depression in the older person. SSRIs have fewer adverse side effects, especially the anticholinergic and hypotensive effects that are characteristic of the TCAs.[64] The anticholinergic side effects of the TCAs include dizziness, tachycardia, constipation, blurred vision, urinary retention, postural hypotension, and mild tremor.[64] Of particular concern to physical therapists are the side effects of dizziness and postural hypotension. Patients taking tricyclic antidepressants may have poorer balance, particularly after moving from supine to sitting or sitting to standing. These effects are more pronounced in the period immediately after the medication is taken. Although there are numerous drugs in the category of tricyclics, the differences between them are primarily in the degree of side effects produced.[64] Several meta-analyses have found that adverse effects were more likely to lead to discontinuation in subjects treated with TCAs than in those treated with SSRIs.[65] The serotonin/norepinephrine inhibitors have potential side effects that are intermediate between SSRIs and TCAs.[65] The monoamine oxidase inhibitors also have major side effects similar to the tricyclics but are less commonly used in the older person.[64]

The choice of an antidepressant for a particular person is dependent on many factors, including prior response, concurrent medical illnesses, and other medications used by the patient.[64] Generally, the use of SSRIs and heterocyclic antidepressants are preferred in the

TABLE 8-3	Drugs Used in Depression	
Nonproprietary Name	**Trade Name**	**Common Side Effects**
Selective Serotonin Reuptake Inhibitors (SSRIS)		Nervousness, palpitations, nausea, anorexia, myalgias, arthralgias, blurred vision
Sertraline	Zoloft	
Fluoxetine	Prozac	
Paroxetine	Paxil	
Heterocyclic Antidepressants		Drowsiness, dizziness, hypotension, skeletal aches and pains, palpitations
Bupropion	Wellbutrin	
Trazodone	Desyrel	
Tricyclic or Tetracyclic Antidepressants (TCAs)		Drowsiness, dizziness, extrapyramidal symptoms, orthostatic hypotension, palpitations
Amitriptyline	Amitril, Elavil	
Nortriptyline	Aventyl, Pamelor	
Serotonin/ Norepinephrine Reuptake Inhibitors		Increased blood pressure, dizziness, nausea
Venlafaxine	Effexor	
Monoamine Oxidase Inhibitors		Dizziness, vertigo, orthostatic hypotension, drowsiness, confusion, nausea, blurred vision
Phenelzine	Nardil	
Tranylcypromine	Parnate	

(Adapted from Steinman LE, Frederick JT, Prohaska T, et al. Recommendations for treating depression in community-based older adults. Am J Prev Med 33(3):175-181, 2007; and Unutzer J: Clinical practice. Late-life depression. N Engl J Med 357(22): 2269-2276, 2007.)

older person.[64] It is estimated that 60% to 80% of older person clients with depression respond to medications, but only half of these respond to the first medication tried.[65] Medication is needed for at least 6 months to 2 years.[64]

Psychotherapy

Older patients less frequently receive psychotherapy and are not commonly included in studies of the effectiveness of psychotherapy in depression.[66] Older patients may be less likely to seek psychotherapy, but, moreover, health professionals may be biased against older persons in that they believe that older persons will not benefit from psychotherapy.[6] However, evidence-based reviews indicate that psychotherapy is an effective treatment for depression in the older person.[67,68] Psychotherapy treatments for the older person include behavioral, cognitive, problem-solving, interpersonal, and brief psychodynamic therapies.[67,68] Cognitive behavioral therapy (CBT) combines elements of behavioral and cognitive approaches. It challenges pessimistic or self-critical thoughts and emphasizes rewarding activities and decreasing behaviors that reinforce depression. Clients learn to recognize their faulty thoughts and behaviors and then modify them.

Problem-solving therapy teaches clients to address problems by identifying the smaller elements of larger problems and specific steps toward solutions.[6] Interpersonal therapy is a combination of psychodynamic therapy and cognitive therapies to address interpersonal difficulties and role transitions.[6] Psychodynamic therapies focus on the personality characteristics common in depression.[6] A recent panel of mental health experts recommends CBT with review of treatment effectiveness by care managers.[6] Taylor et al demonstrated that older persons with milder depression and excellent remission following drug and psychotherapy were well maintained on psychotherapy alone.[69]

Exercise/Physical Activity

Although a review of the effect of activity on mood in the older population is beyond the scope of this chapter, the following section will review studies of the influence of exercise/activity on depression in older persons. Numerous studies indicate an effect of exercise/activity on the reduction of depressive symptoms in older persons.[70-74] Both psychological and physiological effects have been suggested as causes for this reduction. Exercise may increase self-mastery and self-efficacy beliefs; it may also provide distraction from negative thoughts. Increases in endorphin and monoamine transmitters in the brain as a result of exercise may also reduce depression.[74] Exercise/activity has been shown to have a comparable reduction in depression compared to antidepressant medication.[75] Barriers to participation in exercise programs by older persons with depression include transportation and medication problems.[76]

The type of exercise that reduces depressive symptoms is not wholly clear. Blumenthal et al found a reduction of depression symptoms in patients aged 50 to 77 years after a program of aerobic exercise.[75] Progressive resistance training has also been shown to decrease depression and pain as well as increase quality of life and social functioning in older persons with depression.[73,77] It appears that either resistance or aerobic exercise is beneficial. Further research is also needed on the ideal dose of a therapeutic effect of exercise for depression. Most studies are of short duration (12 weeks) without follow-up. However, there is sufficient evidence to recommend high dose and frequency consistent with physical activity recommendations of 150 to 300 minutes of moderately intense exercise per week.[78,79] It is not known whether group or individual exercise is more effective. Other recommendations for exercise/activity programs for older persons with depression include the following:

- Screen for possible medical conditions that might limit exercise participation
- Provide multiple choices for exercise/activity so that the individual can pick enjoyable activities for himself or herself
- Recognize possible barriers such as medication and transportation problems and provide appropriate support[74,76]

Working with the Depressed Older Patient. Depression can affect many aspects of physical therapy treatment. The person with depression may have more difficulty with fatigue and may express negative or self-critical thoughts. The course of therapy would be expected to be longer, because the apathy and extra energy required necessitates more time to accomplish goals. More time may need to be spent on ADLs, because these tasks will seem more difficult for the patient. Goal setting may be more difficult with the older adult who is depressed but may help the patient recognize progress. Chapter 10, Motivation and Patient Education, provides some valuable suggestions of how to involve the patient in goal setting.

Physical therapists may need to consider their approach when working with an older person who is depressed. Experts agree that a matter-of-fact approach that emphasizes the patient's feelings of mastery is a more effective approach. The patient's negative self-perception should be discouraged and emphasis should be placed on achievement and appropriate perceptions of self-worth.[80] Encouragement and acknowledgment of

the great degree of effort required by the person with depression to accomplish even everyday tasks should be frequent. The person with depression may have difficulty visualizing goals far into the future, so goals should be discussed in small, easily achievable steps. Achievement of short-term goals will enhance the person's sense of mastery and improve motivation. Key support persons may also require extra assistance in dealing with the depressed patient.[42] Furthermore, persons with depression may need assistance and training to improve their interactive skills in order to maximize the effectiveness of their support networks.[26]

Some professionals may believe that being overly cheerful will "jolly" the patient out of feelings of sadness and low self-esteem. Generally this is not the case, and the effect may, in fact, be the opposite. The cheerfulness of the therapist may only emphasize the separateness and depression of the patient and increase negative feelings. Anyone who remembers a time when feeling quite depressed will recall that cheerfulness of others did not improve one's mood and often accentuated one's own sad feelings. Projecting a genuine regard for the person that comes from respect and valuing will be more effective than an insincere attitude or demeanor.

Dealing with the patient with depression may be psychologically difficult for the therapist. Research has shown that most people respond negatively and interact less with persons who exhibit depressed behaviors.[26] Health care professionals are not immune from these natural responses. Depressed patients are not "fun" and may appear unmotivated. It is important to remember that these people are not lazy. For them, large amounts of energy are required to accomplish even simple tasks. Working with these patients also has its rewards. Persons with depression almost always get better and will achieve therapeutic goals. Most of us have experienced depression to some extent. Remembering our own sad times can help to develop empathy for the depressed patient.

Case Study. Mr. Clark is 84 years old. Before his present hospitalization, he lived alone in his suburban home; his wife of 45 years had died 6 months previously. He has two sons, one of whom lives in the same city. He was hospitalized because he fell in his home and fractured the subcapital area of his right femur. A hemiarthroplasty was performed, and Mr. Clark was referred to physical therapy. Laboratory tests also indicated a high blood glucose level, and he is being evaluated for possible diabetes. Mr. Clark also has a history of mild congestive heart failure. The physical therapist working with Mr. Clark notes that he appears quite sad, has cried several times during treatment, and has expressed hopelessness about his future. He also has difficulty remembering the precautions regarding his hip that have been repeatedly explained to him. He is apathetic, shows little interest in participating in physical therapy, frequently complains of fatigue, expresses negative feelings about his progress, has a poor appetite, and has difficulty sleeping. The nursing and medical staff have noted similar problems. As his son indicated that these problems had been steadily getting worse since the death of Mrs. Clark, a psychiatric consult was requested. Although Mr. Clark's memory problems could have been due to early dementia, the consult indicated that the first treatment should be for depression, with later reevaluation. Antidepressant medication (SSRIs) and short-term cognitive therapy for depression were initiated. Mr. Clark was also prescribed blood glucose–lowering drugs and transferred to the rehabilitation unit.

Mr. Clark's progress in physical therapy was slower than expected, although he made steady improvement. His therapist established small short-term goals that could be accomplished in 2 to 3 days. Emphasis was placed on the mastery of these short-term goals rather than long-term goals. For example, Mr. Clark was given the goal of increasing his walking distance from 20 to 40 feet, rather than being given the long-term goal of independent ambulation. He was asked to be able to repeat one more precaution every other day, rather than learn all the precautions in 1 day. The extra effort required by Mr. Clark was acknowledged, but his negative expressions of low self-esteem and guilt were countered with more positive statements about his progress and his past and present accomplishments. The psychologist also worked with Mr. Clark to improve his personal interaction skills in order to mobilize his support network for his return home. These new skills were reinforced in physical therapy. Mr. Clark's depression gradually lifted, and he was discharged to his home. A home health agency continued his physical therapy and monitored the progress of his diabetes treatment. Antidepressant treatment was discontinued after 6 months. Mr. Clark's recovery was about the usual 1-year period required for major losses.

COGNITIVE DECLINE AND DEMENTIA

The dramatic aging of the U.S. population creates the reality of an increased incidence of all types of dementia. In fact, in 2009 there were up to 5.3 million Americans living with Alzheimer's disease (AD), the most common type of dementia, with a half-million new cases expected each year.[81] By 2050, there will be nearly a million new cases annually.[176] Approximately 13% of individuals older than age 65 years have AD.[81] The prevalence of dementia and how dementia affects the lives of older adults, their caregivers, and the rehabilitation process requires knowledge of the continuum and classification of cognitive change, as well as the etiology of dementia, its prevention, treatment, and rehabilitation impact.

Continuum of Cognitive Change

Neuroscientists generally view the cognitive changes occurring with age as a continuum from normal aging changes to mild cognitive impairment (MCI) to stages of

dementia.[82] Not all older individuals will move through this continuum; therefore, MCI and dementia are considered pathologic changes.

Normal Cognitive Aging. The interest in how the brain ages, how aging affects cognitive function, and why certain people develop pathologic changes that evolve into dementia has peaked the interest of researchers over the past 20 years, increasing our understanding of normal cognitive aging and its relationship to cognitive diseases. There is no clear line between a completely healthy brain and a diseased brain. However, the way we think changes gradually, becoming more noticeable after the age of 50 years. Changes in cognition are usually mild and affect visual and verbal memory, visuospatial abilities, immediate memory, or the ability to name objects. Changes in cognitive performance reflect an aging brain and nervous system.[82]

Aging Brain. The average adult male human brain weighs 1400 g, containing some 20 billion neurons with synaptic connections. Although neurons cannot divide after birth, their ability to remodel synaptic connections occurs throughout life, the anatomic basis for memory and learning. Loss of these synaptic connections is the neuroanatomic cause of normal age-related memory impairment. Pathologic loss of these synaptic connections is the basis of dementia.[83] Synaptic connections permit the flow of information from one neuron to another or to the end organ via neurotransmitters (acetylcholine). Synaptic connections are the crucial messaging exchange center between neurons. Suppression or enhancement of neurotransmission is the pharmacologic basis of most neuroactive compounds.[84]

Growth factors comprise a varied family of proteins and hormones that regulate and control cellular growth and differentiation (cell division). In the brain, nerve growth factors (neurotrophins) play a vital role in neuronal growth, development, and survival. Neurotrophins are important signaling molecules that regulate the synapse and lead to learning and memory. One particular neurotrophin, brain-derived neurotrophic factor (BDNF) has been linked to AD and other neurologic disorders. The inhibition of BDNF and another neurotrophic factor, neural growth factor (NGF), stimulates the molecular events typical of the AD process.[85] Amyloid beta (Aβ), the protein that accumulates and aggregates into the plaque lesions of AD, is increased in a deprived BDNF and NGF neural environment. The interruption of the BDNF and NGF signaling sets up the toxic mechanisms that induce the death and loss of neurons, which in turn cause brain tissue atrophy.[85]

Plaques and tangles, present in both healthy and diseased brains, are the waste products that fill up the spaces between neurons (plaques) and form inside the neuron (tangles). Although some normal, healthy aging is associated with no identifiable neuropathologic changes such as cortical atrophy, cell loss, and presence of senile neuritic plaques or neurofibrillary tangles, most older adults will show some pathologic changes. Both senile neuritic plaques and neurofibrillary tangles may be seen in cognitively intact aged individuals but are generally less extensive than seen in individuals with dementia of the same age. Senile neuritic plaques are considered to have no pathologic significance until the plaque matures and is filled with neurofibrillary tangles and other abnormal proteins. Although the distribution and frequency of mature neuritic plaques do not consistently correlate with cognitive function, neurofibrillary tangle frequency and distribution does predict cognitive status.

Normal Cognition. Cognitive abilities include memory, language, perception, reasoning, perceptual speed, spatial manipulation, and executive skills.[86,87] These abilities collectively form the concept of intelligence. Intelligence has been traditionally categorized into two broad types referred to as crystallized and fluid intelligence, as described in Table 8-4. Both fluid and crystallized intelligence increase during childhood and into adolescence. However, fluid intelligence tends to reach its peak during adolescence and decline rapidly during adulthood—affected by neurologic insult, genetics, and biological aging processes.[86] Crystallized intelligence, on the other hand, continues to increase gradually throughout adulthood, even until the ninth decade.[86] Cunningham, Clayton, and Overton found that when untimed tests were given to individuals, crystallized intelligence scores were the same or higher in the fifties as in the twenties.[88] Figure 8-1 illustrates the relationship of fluid and crystallized intelligence patterns with age. The observation that older adults have an intact long-term memory but poor short-term memory reflects the different effects of age on crystallized and fluid intelligence.

Intelligence is generally measured by IQ tests. The most accurate scores to discern cognitive decline are those achieved through comparison with suitable controls, comprising healthy older adults of similar age.[89] Typically IQ scores should remain steady throughout adulthood, with some decrease in later years. Starr et al compared healthy older adults with those with known hypertension, diabetes, dementia, and other cardiovascular disease to describe the changes in the Mini-Mental State Examination (MMSE) and an IQ test. They maintain that no more than 0.1 decline in MMSE points/year should be expected for healthy people into their seventies and eighties,[89] although the MMSE may not be appropriate (specific) to measure age-associated cognitive decline.[89]

In recent years, the view of intelligence has been expanded to include expertise, creativity, and wisdom. The broadened view of intelligence recognizes the importance of culture and acquired knowledge rather than only genetic intelligence that largely makes up fluid intelligence. Table 8-4 describes these other kinds of intelligence.[90] Although expertise, creativity, and wisdom can be found at any age when extensive experience with the hypothetical situation is present, wisdom is most frequently associated with age.

Executive Functioning. Executive functioning, or executive abilities, involves complex behavior that combines memory, intellectual capacity, and cognitive planning. Activities of executive functioning include planning, active problem solving, working memory, anticipating possible consequences of an intended course of action, initiating an activity, inhibiting irrelevant behavior, and being able to monitor the effectiveness of one's behavior.[91] These behaviors are often at the core of rehabilitative efforts. Working memory is the center of executive functioning and incorporates complex attention, strategy formation, and interference control. There is evidence of a mild decline of executive functioning with normal aging; however, this decline is greater when a neurologic disorder, such as a cerebrovascular accident or dementia, is also present. Decline in executive functioning is characterized by a decrease in planning ability, working memory, inductive reasoning, and ability to modify and update working memory.[92]

The interesting aspect of executive functioning is its relationship to motor function. Executive functioning is an important factor for self-reported and observed performance of complex, independent ADLs, such as managing money and medications.[93,94] Intact executive functioning can actually serve as a fall prevention measure by minimizing behavior that jeopardizes safety despite motor or sensory impairment.[95] Conversely, executive dysfunction should trigger the therapist's awareness of the risk for falls.[95]

Memory. Memory loss is the most common cognitive component associated with aging. When the process of remembering is slowed but still intact, this is considered normal aging. Although lapses in memory are common, memory loss does not mean an individual is becoming demented. In healthy individuals, memory loss usually does not interfere with social or personal activities.

There are four types of memory. Working memory is the memory that allows us to "hold on" to bits of information such as a phone number before we dial it. Another example is remembering how many putts we took on a hole of golf before writing down our score. Working memory is limited, allowing us to only hold onto a few bits of information at a time. To remember these bits of information, the information must be encoded into episodic memory. The second type, episodic memory, is the memory of an event or episode. Examples include remembering where the car was parked or recalling the day's events. Encoding is an effortful process and includes memorization. Memorizing is enhanced through repetitions and practice. Working memory must be encoded into episodic memory. Once information is encoded, information must be retrieved, again an effortful process. The hippocampus is critical for encoding, and because it is so often involved in AD, episodic memory, especially

TABLE 8-4	Categories of Intelligence	
Intelligence	**Characteristics**	**How Assessed**
Crystallized	Acquired knowledge and expertise such as numerical abilities, verbal comprehension, and inductive reasoning Occupational knowledge Relies on long-term memory	Tests of vocabulary Word knowledge General knowledge Understanding proverbs Measures of occupational expertise
Fluid	Novel problem solving Spatial manipulation Mental speed Identification of complex relations among stimulus patterns Relies on short-term memory storage while processing information.	Identify the next in a series of abstract patterns, matrices, or series of numbers Rote memory Word analogies Verbal reasoning Wechsler Adult Intelligence Scale (WAIS)
Expertise	Development of advanced skills and knowledge in a particularly well-practiced activity (task specific, not transferable) Requires intense practice over many years and appears immune to aging effects	Compare novices to experts. Knowledge is better organized, more accessible, can use more effective problem-solving strategies, performance is faster, more efficient, more accurate
Creativity	Ability to produce novel ideas that are high in quality and task-appropriate	Some studies have shown that scholars, scientists, and artists are most productive during their 60s. (Table 8-5) However, for what we might call everyday, "ordinary" creativity, this appears to peak at around age 30 years and to decline thereafter. Since the incentives for being creative for ordinary, everyday tasks may not be as powerful as those for creativity in scholarly, scientific, or artistic pursuits, it is important to consider the contexts in which creativity occurs.
Wisdom	Expert knowledge system applied to the fundamental pragmatics of life and that permits exceptional insight, judgment, and advice involving the conduct and meaning of life (Baltes PB)[40] • addresses important and difficult questions and the conduct and meaning of life • includes knowledge about the limits of knowledge and the uncertainties of life • represents a superior level of knowledge, judgment, and advice • involves an orchestration of knowledge and virtue • represents knowledge used for the good or well-being of self and others • is easily recognized when manifested, but difficult to achieve or to specify	Assessed through responses to hypothetical situations Participants in Baltes' wisdom research are given hypothetical dilemmas (e.g, "A 15-year-old girl wants to marry. What should she consider and do?") and asked to respond to the problem scenarios that are presented. Although there are no correct answers, the responses are scored on the basis of five wisdom-related criteria: • rich factual knowledge about fundamental matters of life • rich procedural knowledge about strategies useful in managing life events • a view of people and events that considers their multiple life contexts—family, school, work • an explicit concern with universal values such as virtue and the common good that is balanced by relativism of values and life goals • recognition of the uncertainties of life and the means to deal with uncertainty The latter three criteria are considered to be unique to wisdom. Examples of answers with low and high score Low wisdom: "A 15-year-old girl wants to get married? No, no way, marrying at age 15 would be utterly wrong. One has to tell the girl that marriage is not possible. . . . It would be irresponsible to support such an idea. No, this is just a crazy idea." High wisdom: "Well, on the surface, this seems like an easy problem. On average, marriage for 15-year-old girls is not a good thing. But there are situations where the average case does not fit. Perhaps in this instance, special life circumstances are involved such that the girl has a terminal illness. Or the girl has just lost her parents. And also, this girl may live in another culture or historical period. Perhaps she was raised with a value system different from ours."

(Data from Anstey KJ, Low, LF: Normal cognitive changes in aging. Aust Fam Physician 33(10): 783-787, 2004.)

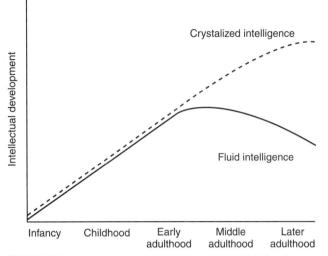

FIGURE 8-1 Relationship between crystallized and fluid intelligence with age.

retrieval, is frequently affected. Semantic memory, the third type, is strongly language-based and describes memory for facts and words. The fourth type of memory is remote memory, or memory for remote or past events. Semantic memory and remote memory can become independent of the hippocampus and thus may not always be impaired in pathologic cognitive dysfunction.[177]

In addition to normal aging, health issues can also affect memory. For example, medication side effects, vitamin B_{12} deficiency, chronic alcoholism, brain tumors, infections, or blood clots can cause memory loss or even reversible dementia. Some thyroid, kidney, or liver disorders can also lead to memory loss. Emotional problems such as stress, anxiety, or depression can make a person more forgetful and can be mistaken for dementia. For example, a person managing the day-to-day care of a terminally ill spouse may experience stress and anxiety and appear to be confused or forgetful.

Personality. Stereotypical beliefs about personality development, such as theories about stages of personality and an aged personality profile, are generally inaccurate. The best available evidence suggests that personality types remain fairly stable throughout life.[96] Therefore, younger individuals who are characterized by an internal locus of control or who believe they have the ability to control the events in their lives will continue to react accordingly as they age. Those who experience a severe mid- to late-life crisis tend to react similarly to the way they reacted to situations throughout life. Activity level also follows this model: with age, people who were active stay active. Any changes that do occur are promoted as a continuation of individuality of the person. Traits that have been predominant will continue to be influential as a person ages. Clinically, this means patients who display a negative outlook about therapy have probably always had a negative attitude about a variety of situations.[97]

The ability of the brain to change and keep itself vital is called "plasticity."[98] When a person is challenged, either by environmental conditions or by activities, neurons form new dendritic branches creating more synapses that enhance the brain and provide better capacities to resist insults from neurologic conditions such as delirium and dementia.[98] As knowledge of brain plasticity increases, old assumptions about cognitive aging are being dismissed. Scientists are discovering that when the mind is challenged, the brain responds positively, in physical and chemical ways, regardless of age. Increasingly, aging adults who expand their experiences and environment develop new intellectual pursuits, oftentimes accomplishing extraordinary things as seen by the examples of creative effort listed in Table 8-5.

Cognitive Reserve. The question of why pathologic changes in the brain are poorly correlated with cognitive function has driven researchers to look at the role of activity, stimulation, and health on cognitive function. Emerging from this work has come the concept of cognitive reserve. According to the cognitive reserve perspective, cognitive impairments become apparent only when cognitive or neurologic resources become depleted beyond a certain threshold. Those individuals with less initial cognitive reserve are more likely to demonstrate clinical signs of cognitive disease because they have fewer resources to sustain them in the face of normal and disease-related changes.[99]

Although a lower baseline self-assessment of school performance and IQ tests in adolescence demonstrate an increased risk for AD, other factors can provide protection.[100] Reserve is generally thought of as a dynamic property that is influenced by genetics, learning, education, experience, stimulation, social engagement, and others.[101] Therefore, reserve can be influenced throughout life, positively by activity or negatively by sedentary behavior. The disuse perspective emphasizes that sedentary activity (passive) patterns result in atrophy of cognitive skills and processes.[102] The disuse perspective has been commonly captured by the familiar "use it or lose it" phrase. Television watching is an example of passive activity. Lindstrom et al examined the relationship between television watching in midlife (ages 40 to 59 years) and the risk of developing AD. They found that each hour increase in television viewing in middle adulthood corresponded to a 1.3 times risk of developing AD.[103] The individuals studied who were at most risk devoted nearly 27% of all daily leisure-time activity to television viewing as compared with 18% of all leisure time activity in case-matched controls. They also found that increased daily social and intellectual activity hours, higher income, higher levels of education, and being female were all associated with decreased risk of developing AD.[103] Although the study's methods used case-control methodology and thus were of a lower level of evidence, this novel study reinforces the need for intellectually stimulating activity.

TABLE 8-5	Some Creative Accomplishments of Older Adults	
Name	**Creative Effort**	**Age**
George Burns	Academy Award winner	80
Gandhi	Indian Independence movement	72
Nelson Mandela	Nobel Peace Prize	75
Anna Mary Robertson "Grandma" Moses	Began painting in her 70s, becoming one of the most famous American folk artists of the 20th century, and continued painting in her 90s	100
G.B. Shaw	Writing plays	93
Strom Thurmond	U.S. Senator	100
Jesse Orosco	Major League Baseball pitcher	45
Julia Child	When she was just months shy of her 50th birthday, Julia Child collaborated on her first French cooking book, a two-volume set titled *Mastering the Art of French Cooking*. Soon after, she promoted her book on television and that catapulted her to overnight sensation in the culinary world.	>50
Col. Sanders	Colonel Sanders of "finger lickin' good chicken" fame had a difficult start in life but early on realized he had a creative cooking talent. However, it was not until he was in his 60s that he started KFC and became a millionaire.	>60
Charles Darwin	Charles Darwin was 50 years old when he published his complete theory of evolution in *On the Origin of Species*, which sold out the first day it was released and subsequently had six editions. He continued to write for at least 10 more years (e.g, *The Descent of Man*).	>50
John Glenn	Astronaut, senator, and oldest man to enter space	77
Robert Byrd	U.S. Senator	92

Preservation of Normal Cognition and Prevention of Cognitive Disease

Most epidemiologic studies that have examined cognitive stimulation as a lifestyle variable have found that the more engaged and mentally stimulated an individual, the less likely cognitive decline and disease will result.[104] Although most studies reporting the association between participation in cognitively stimulating activities and risk of cognitive disease are observational, some researchers have used sophisticated statistical modeling and long-term follow-up to explore this relationship.[105,106] These authors' findings strengthen the possibility that cognitively inactive lifestyles are an important risk factor for MCI and AD.

Just as muscle atrophy does not occur overnight, it is known that the plaques and tangles associated with AD occur over many years, prior to any indication of cognitive decline. This preclinical phase may indicate that intervention of cognitive stimulation prior to disease may delay the onset of significant symptoms.[87] This hypothesis is reinforced by the poor clinical correlation of imaging scans with clinical symptoms of disease. Therefore, cognitive disease, such as AD, may be thought of as a chronic disease that, like so many other chronic diseases, is not curable but is modifiable at some point in the continuum of the disease. Figure 8-2 illustrates the slippery slope of cognition that may remind the reader of the slippery slope of physical function.

Wilson et al found a 63% increase in developing AD in individuals in the 10th percentile of cognitive activity as compared with those in the 90th percentile, corresponding to daily engagement of cognitive activity as

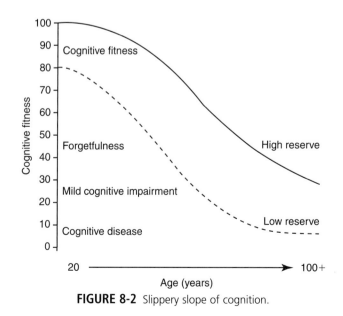

FIGURE 8-2 Slippery slope of cognition.

compared with several times a month.[104] Similar to physically inactive lifestyles and the risk of chronic disease, those individuals with cognitively inactive lifestyles had the greatest risk for developing AD. Interestingly enough, Boyle et al found that physically frail individuals had a similar risk for developing mild cognitive impairment (MCI), emphasizing the relationship between physical activity and cognitive health.[106a]

A physically active lifestyle is generally regarded as important in the prevention of cognitive decline; however, the evidence to date is from observational studies that demonstrate an association between active lifestyles, exercise, and decreased risk of AD. It is not yet known how physical activity protects the brain, but several hypotheses exist that have derived from animal model research. In one study focusing on aerobic exercise, cerebral blood flow in the dentate gyrus was found that correlated with enhanced performance on memory tasks.[107] Another study found that mandatory treadmill running altered the brain chemistries of middle-aged animals toward an environment that is favorable to neural stem cell proliferation, survival, and maturation.[108]

Lifestyles that combine cognitively stimulating activities with physical activities and rich social networks may provide the best odds of preserving cognitive function in old age.[87] In a 9-year follow-up of a healthy aging sample in Sweden, individuals who were active in *any* of the key dimensions of health (cognitive, physical, or social) had lowered dementia risk, and those who were active in two or all three dimensions had the lowest risk of all.[109] Although research has not definitively answered the question about which activities increase the odds of healthy cognitive aging, La Rue has developed and published recommendations for a cognitively active lifestyle, which are listed in Table 8-6.

To summarize, there is a great deal of evidence that older adults retain the ability to learn new things, especially those engaged in a cognitive and physically active lifestyle. Although some aspects of intelligence may decline in later years, these changes should not affect function in the noncognitively diseased individual. Although neuroanatomic changes are present in nearly all aging brains, the degree in which they occur and subsequently affect cognition is quite variable, representing the continuum of normal cognition to disease. Some

TABLE 8-6	Recommendations for a Cognitively Active Lifestyle
Recommendation	**Rationale**
Be physically active.	Regular *activity*, not necessarily planned exercise, seems to relate to brain fitness. Activities like gardening, dancing, and even cleaning, among others, could increase and maintain brain health.
Make time for cognitively stimulating activities that have always been enjoyed.	Continuing favorite activities can ensure sustainability of cognitive stimulation. Long-term exposure to cognitive stimulation may be needed for practical functional benefits.
Add some new cognitive challenges, as time and enjoyment permit.	Trying new activities may enhance brain plasticity by requiring new learning or development of new cognitive strategies. Calculate. Perform word-search games and crossword puzzles. Attend lectures, concerts, and museums. May benefit from performing mental gymnastics and mind challenges.
Aim to engage in cognitively stimulating activities several times/week or more; generate some mental sweat.	Current knowledge does not permit a prescription for how often or how long individuals should engage in cognitively stimulating activities. However, epidemiologic studies suggest that more is better, within clinically reasonable limits.
Be aware that there is no one cognitive activity or combination of activities that is uniquely good for decreasing AD risk.	Many different kinds of cognitively stimulating activities have been associated with preserved cognitive skill.
Social interactions can be a great way to stimulate the mind.	Group training of cognitive skills has been shown to be effective in sharpening specific cognitive skills, and broader social networks have been associated with reduced AD risk.

(Data from La Rue A: Healthy brain aging: role of cognitive reserve, cognitive stimulation, and cognitive exercises. Clin Geriatr Med 26(1): 99-111, 2010.)

mild memory loss and cognitive slowing is expected with age, but no functional loss should be apparent. Increasingly, researchers and the public are embracing the concept of brain fitness. Just as an individual can impact physical fitness, one may be able to affect cognitive fitness.[87]

MILD COGNITIVE IMPAIRMENT

Mild cognitive impairment (MCI) is a condition that lies between normal aging and dementia. The prevalence of MCI is approximately 15% of the nondemented population with a 2:1 ratio of amnestic MCI (aMCI) to nonamnestic MCI (naMCI) in one population-based study of a random sample of 3000 participants ages 70 to 85 years.[110] MCI prevalence increases as a function of age, with 1% at age 60 years, 6% at age 65 years, 12% at age 70 years, 20% at age 75 years, 30% at age 80 years, and 42% at age 85 years.[111] MCI is inversely related to years of education and is more prevalent among African Americans, experiencing aMCI type most commonly.[112]

Individuals with MCI have heightened risk for developing dementia (2% to 31% with a calculated mean conversion rate of 10.24% over 4 to 5 years).[111] Because of this association, there has been an explosion of research about MCI and its relationship to AD. In one large Italian population study, of those people with MCI that progressed to dementia, 66% progressed to AD and 33% progressed to vascular dementia.[113] In this study, MCI did not progress to dementia. Only MCI associated with memory seems to progress, generally at a rate of 3:1.[114] The best single predictors of likelihood to progress were measures of recent verbal/visuospatial learning and memory, especially from tests of delayed recall.[111] Other predictors frequently identified include assessments of language function and motor/psychomotor integration.[111,115] Table 8-7 lists the motor measures that are sensitive to MCI or early AD. The usefulness in motor tests is that motor tests do not seem to be correlated with education, as are cognitive tests. Box 8-4 lists the factors influencing rates of progression of MCI to dementia.

MCI was originally characterized by four criteria, which included (1) memory complaints, (2) normal ADLs, (3) normal general cognitive functioning, and (4) abnormal cognitive measures using age- and education-adjusted norms.[116] The diagnosis of MCI is made exclusively on clinical grounds and rests on the judgment of the clinician. The diagnosis of MCI begins with the subjective complaint of memory impairment. Current criteria include subjective, gradual cognitive decline for at least 6 months and objective criteria as measured by performance at 1 standard deviation below age and education norms by neuropsychological testing. All domains of cognitive performance are considered, including memory and learning, attention and concentration, thinking, language, and visuospatial functioning. Current criteria

TABLE 8-7	Motor Measures Sensitive to MCI or Early AD (Relative to Performance in Normal Aging)	
Measure	**Decline Found in:**	
	MCI	**Early AD**
Complex Motor		
Head tracking (with and without video feedback)	Yes	Yes
Purdue pegboard assembly	Yes	Yes
Digit symbol substitution test	Yes	Yes
Alternating hand movements	Yes	Yes
Fine Motor		
Grooved pegboard	Yes	Yes
Purdue unilateral and bilateral	Yes	Yes
Gross Motor		
Finger tapping speed (maximum no. of taps in five consecutive trials of 10 s each)	No	Yes
Foot tapping speed (maximum no. of taps in two alternating 15-s trials per foot)	No	No
Head steadiness	No	No
Hand steadiness (multihole)	Yes	Yes
Hand strength–dominant (hand dynamometer)	No	No
Hand strength–nondominant	No	No
Balance and Weight Transfer		
Force sensitive platform	Yes	Yes
Gait Function		
Composite of computerized and noncomputerized tests	Yes	Yes

(Adapted from Kluger A, Gianutsos JG, Golomb J, et al: Patterns of motor impairment in normal aging, mild cognitive decline, and early Alzheimer's disease. J Gerontol B Psychol Sci Soc Sci 52(1), P28-P39, 1997; and Kluger A, Gianutsos JG, Golomb J, et al: Clinical features of MCI: motor changes. Int Psychogeriatr 20(1): 32-39, 2008.)

MCI, mild cognitive disorder; AD, Alzheimer's disease.

BOX 8-4	Factors Influencing Rates of Progression of Mild Cognitive Impairment to Dementia

Clinical severity
APOE ε4 carrier status
Atrophy on magnetic resonance imaging
Fludeoxyglucose ^{18}F-positron emission tomography pattern of Alzheimer's disease
Cerebrospinal fluid markers compatible with Alzheimer's disease
Positive amyloid imaging scan

(Adapted from Petersen RC, Roberts RO, Knopman DS, et al: Mild cognitive impairment: ten years later. Arch Neurol 66(12): 1447-1455, 2009.)

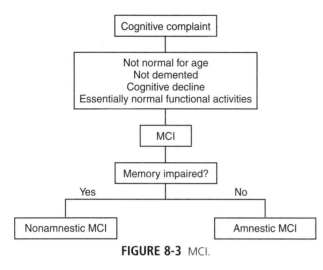

FIGURE 8-3 MCI.

are diagrammed in Figure 8-3 and differentiates between aMCI and naMCI. aMCI involves memory and naMCI involves attention.

Treatment of MCI

As of January 2011, there were no pharmacologic treatments of proven efficacy or regulatory approval for MCI in cumulative trials of 4000 to 5000 subjects.[116] A trial of donepezil in the Alzheimer's Disease Cooperative Study initially suggested a therapeutic effect for the first 12 months in subjects with MCI, but the results were not replicated in a 48-week trial with donepezil alone; thus no treatments have been approved for MCI.[116]

The classification of MCI, though more refined than 20 years ago, is still quite heterogeneous with respect to outcome and underlying pathology. Because pharmacologic treatment is relatively unsuccessful in preventing the decline into dementia, the usefulness of the diagnosis MCI is questionable and may cause unnecessary anxiety, especially since at least a third of cases of aMCI do not convert to dementia. However, regardless of the uncertainty of the MCI label, MCI will have great relevance in research on the causes, early diagnosis, and early treatment of AD.[111]

DELIRIUM

Delirium and dementia share some common characteristics that make them difficult to tell apart, but the hallmark of delirium is the sudden, and sometimes rapid change in mental function and should not be confused with dementia. Table 8-2 lists the characteristics of delirium contrasted with dementia.

Delirium is one of the most common complications of medical illness or recovery from surgery among older adults. It is also the most common complication of hospital admission for older people,[117] occurring in 11% to 42% of older adults admitted to the hospital.[118]

Delirium develops in up to a half of older adults postoperatively, especially following hip fracture and vascular surgery. In the intensive care unit, delirium occurs in 70% to 87% of older adults.[118] Box 8-5 lists the most common risk factors for the development of delirium.

Delirium has adverse consequences, including an average increase of 8 days in the hospital, worse physical and cognitive recovery at 6 and 12 months, and increased time in institutional care. Patients diagnosed with delirium in the hospital have an overall high morbidity because of a high risk of dehydration, malnutrition, falls, continence problems, and pressure sores. They also have higher 1-year mortality rates (35% to 40%) and higher readmission rates.[118] Although delirium is considered a short-term, temporary problem, evidence indicates it may persist in about one third of individuals.[119] Very old people with preexisting mental difficulties seem to be at the highest risk of long-term delirium.

The type, number, and severity of symptoms of delirium vary. About one quarter of people with delirium are agitated. Most people with delirium have "quiet" delirium, or delirium with a mix of symptoms (e.g., agitated at times and quiet at times). Agitated delirium is most often associated with adverse effects of anticholinergic drugs, drug intoxication, and withdrawal states. Older adults may exhibit disruptive behaviors such as shouting or resisting, may refuse to cooperate with medical care, and may sustain injuries from falling, combativeness, or pulling out catheters and intravascular lines. For these reasons, agitated delirium is more often treated than quiet or hypoactive delirium.[118] Prognosis for quiet and agitated delirium is the same.

Hypoactive or quiet delirium is often confused with dementia. Patients with hypoactive delirium may appear apathetic, sluggish, and lethargic or low in mood and confused—although the confusion may not be apparent in superficial conversation.[118] Although delirium may be hypoactive or agitated, many individuals experience a

BOX 8-5	Common Risk Factors for Delirium

Old age (older than 65 years)
Admission to hospital with infection or dehydration
Physical frailty
Visual impairment
Severe illness
Deafness
Multiple diseases
Polypharmacy
Dementia
Renal impairment
Alcohol excess
Malnutrition

(Adapted from Young J, Inouye SK: Delirium in older people. BMJ 334(7598), 842-846, 2007.)

fluctuating course, experiencing a mixture of the hyper- and hypoactive variants.

The causes of delirium are varied and not completely understood. The pathophysiology of dementia is thought to include neurotransmitter disturbances (especially acetylcholine deficiency and dopamine excess), illness-related stress with overactivity of the hypothalamic–pituitary–adrenal axis, and the effects of increased cytokine production on cerebral function.[117] Although the cause is unknown, patient vulnerability because of various risk factors in relation to stressor events has proved a practical approach to understanding delirium. Older people with multiple comorbidities are especially prone to delirium.

Prevention and Treatment of Delirium

Prevention of delirium is directly related to the risk factors for delirium. The most common risk factors are listed in Box 8-5. Immediate identification of the cause of the delirium should be ascertained and appropriate steps taken to remediate the cause. Drugs are an important risk factor and may be the sole factor in 12% to 39% of cases of delirium.[120] The management of hypoxia, hydration, and nutrition, minimizing the time spent lying in bed, and walking are also important steps to preventing and treating delirium. Physical restraints should be avoided because they tend to increase agitation and may cause injury.

The most common drugs associated with delirium are psychoactive agents such as benzodiazepines, narcotic analgesics such as morphine, and drugs with anticholinergic effects. Many drugs have anticholinergic effects and, whenever possible, should be discontinued in patients who are at risk for developing delirium.[117] Drug treatment should be used as a last resort, for those patients at risk to themselves or others. Ketamine is an intravenous anesthetic agent and has been associated with excitability, vivid unpleasant dreams, and delirium. The incidence of postoperative delirium varies from 10% to 26% and has been associated with inhalational anesthetics.[120] Low-dose haloperidol is the best studied agent with the least side effects for short-term use.[121]

Although the evidence for prevention of delirium is not high-level, there are some positive signs that delirium can be mediated. Delirium was reduced by one third in one study of specific interventions following hip fracture surgery.[122] In this study, a geriatrician made daily visits following surgery and then recommended individualized interventions that addressed specific problems. The most often-made recommendations (more than 60% of the time) with the best adherence (more than 75%) included early mobilization (postoperative day 1); use of dentures; discontinuance of benzodiazepines, anticholinergics, and antihistamines; bowel and bladder care; and transfusion to keep hematocrit higher than 30%.

Other effective strategies for preventing delirium include orienting communication, therapeutic activities, early mobilization and walking, nonpharmacologic approaches to sleep and anxiety, maintaining nutrition and hydration, adaptive equipment for vision and hearing impairment, and pain management.[117] Sensory deprivation, especially in the intensive care unit, can be a factor in delirium; therefore any stimulation, such as familiar objects, a family member's presence, the patient's favorite pillow or blanket, and familiar music and sounds may help. Finally, because of the inherent risk factors of hospitalization, early discharge to home-based medical management is associated with significantly reduced incidence of delirium.[123]

DEMENTIA

Dementia is not a disease but rather a group of disorders that affect the brain and present as symptoms that most commonly affect memory and language. The essential feature of dementia is the development of multiple cognitive deficits that include memory impairment and at least one of the following cognitive disturbances: aphasia, apraxia, agnosia, or a disturbance of executive functioning.[124] Many conditions can confound the diagnosis of dementia such as depression and delirium. Because of the stigma attached to dementia, the presence of ageism and the associated psychological effects of the diagnosis, an individual should not be assumed to have dementia until a thorough medical assessment has been made. A systematic approach to the assessment of any suspected dementia should be undertaken with an emphasis on *both* medical problems as sources of the cognitive symptoms *and* how the patient's cognition, mood, and home situation are affecting the patient and caregiver(s). Specific features of delirium, depression, and dementia are described in Table 8-2.[125,126]

Besides senile dementia, terms often used to describe dementia include senility and organic brain syndrome. Senility and senile dementia are outdated terms that reflect the formerly widespread belief that dementia was a normal part of aging. Organic brain syndrome is a general term that refers to physical disorders (not psychiatric in origin) that impair mental functions. Cognitive disorders can be classified many different ways and attempt to group disorders that have particular features in common, such as whether they are progressive or what parts of the brain are affected (Table 8-8). Two key parts of dementia are the characteristics of being *acquired* and *persistent*. "Acquired" means that the impairment represents a change from previous functional abilities to dysfunctional ones. "Persistent" differentiates dementia from delirium, which produces a fluctuating state of dysfunction. Cortical dementia tends to cause problems with memory, language, thinking, and social behavior and primarily affects the cortex. Subcortical dementia affects parts of the brain below the cortex and tends to cause changes in emotions and movement in addition to problems with memory.

TABLE 8-8	Types of Dementia and Clinical Features	
Classification	**Name**	**Clinical Features**
Cortical, progressive, primary	Alzheimer's disease	Memory, language, visual-spatial disturbances, indifference, delusions, agitation
Cortical	Frontotemporal dementia (Pick disease is one type)	Relative preservation of memory and visual-spatial skills, personality change, executive dysfunction, excessive eating and drinking, loss of language skills
Subcortical, progressive	Lewy body dementia	Visual hallucinations, delusions, extrapyramidal symptoms, fluctuating mental status, sensitivity to antipsychotic medications
Cortical and subcortical (depending on where the infarct(s) occur)	Vascular dementia	Abrupt onset, stepwise deterioration, executive dysfunction, gait changes

(Data from American Geriatrics Society: Dementia diagnosis. Available at: http://dementia.americangeriatrics. org/. Accessed May 15, 2010.)

Some types of dementia fit into more than one of these classifications. For example, AD is considered both a progressive and a cortical dementia.

The U.S. Congress Office of Technology Assessment estimates that as many as 6.8 million people in the United States have dementia, and at least 1.8 million of those are severely affected. Dementia increases with age, affecting only 5% of people aged 71 to 79 years, but 24.2% among people aged 80 to 89 years and 37.4% of those aged 90 years and older, with men and women having about the same dementia risk.[127] African Americans had a higher frequency of dementia and AD,[128] possibly because of overrepresentation in the lower socioeconomic, disadvantaged classes but also because of the increased incidence of vascular disease, hypertension, and hyperlipidemia and generally lower education level.[81] Although some researchers controlled for education, sex, and genotype and found the difference was no longer statistically significant, there is underdiagnosis among African Americans, which may negate this control.[81] Although dementia is common in very old individuals, dementia is not a normal part of the aging process. Many people live into their nineties and even past 100 without any symptoms of dementia.[129]

The most common cause of dementia is AD. Other frequent forms include vascular dementia and dementia resulting from other neurodegenerative processes such as Lewy body dementia (including dementia due to Parkinson's disease) and frontotemporal dementia (including Pick disease). Table 8-8 summarizes the clinical presentation of these different forms of dementia. Other causes are less common and include normal-pressure hydrocephalus, Huntington disease, traumatic brain injury, brain tumors, anoxia, infectious disorders (e.g., human immunodeficiency virus [HIV], syphilis), prion diseases (Creutzfeldt-Jakob disease), metabolic problems and endocrine abnormalities (hypothyroidism, hypercalcemia, hypoglycemia), vitamin deficiencies such as deficiencies of thiamine or niacin, immune disorders (e.g., temporal arteries, systemic lupus erythematosus), hepatic conditions, metabolic conditions (e.g., Kufs disease, adrenoleukodystrophy, metachromatic leukodystrophy, and other storage diseases of adulthood), and other neurologic conditions such as multiple sclerosis.[124]

Alzheimer's Disease

AD is the most common type of dementia accounting for 60% to 80% of those with dementia.[9] An estimated 5.3 million Americans of all ages have AD. This figure includes 5.1 million people aged 65 years and older and 200,000 individuals younger than age 65 years who have younger-onset AD. One in eight people aged 65 years and older (13%) have AD.[81] On average, patients with AD live for 8 to 10 years after they are diagnosed. However, some people can live as long as 20 years. Patients with AD often die of aspiration pneumonia, because they lose the ability to swallow late in the course of the disease.

AD is associated with advancing age and develops over a period of several years. AD typically progresses from mild memory problems to problems in recognizing friends and family and even self. AD is characterized by three pathologic changes in the brain. The first, amyloid plaques, are protein fragments known as β-amyloid peptides mixed with additional proteins, remnants of neurons, and bits and pieces of other nerve cells. The second pathologic change is the formation of neurofibrillary tangles that are found inside neurons. Neurofibrillary tangles are abnormal collections of a protein called tau. Although tau is required for healthy neurons, in AD, tau clumps together, causing neurons to fail and die. The third pathologic change is the loss of connections between neurons that are responsible for memory and learning. Because neurons cannot survive without connections to other neurons, they die, causing atrophy and shrinkage of brain tissue. AD has two types, early-onset and late-onset, both of which have genetic links.

Early-onset AD is rare, affecting only 5% of all people with AD. Early-onset AD develops in people between the ages of 30 and 60. Some cases of early-onset AD are inherited. This form, called familial AD, is caused by gene mutations on chromosomes 21, 14, and 1. Each mutation causes abnormal proteins to be formed. Even if only one of these mutated genes is inherited from a parent, the person will almost always develop early-onset AD.[130]

Late-onset AD makes up most of the cases of AD. Although specific genes have not been identified as a cause of late-onset AD, one predisposing genetic risk factor does appear to increase a person's risk of developing the disease. This increased risk is related to the apolipoprotein E *(APOE)* gene found on chromosome 19. *(APOE)* contains the instructions needed to make a protein that helps carry cholesterol in the bloodstream, and everyone inherits an *APOE* gene from at least one parent. *APOE* comes in several different forms or alleles. Three forms—APOE ε2, APOE ε3, and APOE ε4—occur most frequently and are described further in Box 8-6. Although a blood test is available that can identify which APOE alleles a person has, it is not yet possible to predict who will or will not develop AD.[10]

Much research is underway to identify the cause or causes of AD. Although the cause of AD has not been discovered as yet, research has identified several risk factors for the development of AD. Advancing age is the single most important risk factor. Prevalence increases from approximately 2% in those aged 65 to 69 years, to 4% in those aged 70 to 74 years, to 8% in those aged 75 to 79 years, to 16% in those aged 80 to 85 years, and

to approximately 35% to 40% in those older than age 85 years.

The second most important risk factor is a positive family history as discussed earlier. A three- to fourfold risk is present when there is a first-degree positive familial history. In families with early onset (ages 40 to 60 years), AD is generally inherited in an autosomal dominant manner, but these constitute only 5% of all cases of AD. Interestingly, the *APOE* gene does not explain the African Americans' increased genetic predisposition.[81]

African Americans and Hispanics are at higher risk for developing AD. African Americans are about 2 times more likely to have AD than whites, and Hispanics are about 1.5 times more likely than whites to develop the disease. Although there appears to be no known genetic factor for these differences, health conditions like high blood pressure and diabetes, conditions that are prevalent in the African American and Hispanic communities, may contribute and increase AD risk.[81] Whether head injury sufficient to produce loss of consciousness is a significant risk factor for AD remains unclear.

Although women are more likely than men to have AD, the larger proportion of older women who have AD is believed to be explained by the fact that women live longer.[81] Many studies of the age-specific incidence of AD show no significant difference for women and men.[81] Thus, it appears that gender is not a risk factor for AD and other dementias once age is taken into account.

Clinical Presentation. In the early stages of AD, memory impairment, lapses of judgment, and subtle changes in personality may be evident. Awareness of cognitive decline is often accompanied by depression. As AD progresses, memory and language problems worsen and patients begin to have difficulty performing independent ADLs, such as balancing a checkbook or remembering to take medications. They also may have visual-spatial problems, such as getting lost on formerly familiar routes. Patients may become disoriented to time and place, may suffer delusions (such as thinking someone is stealing from them or their spouse is being unfaithful) and may become short-tempered and hostile. During the late stages of the disease, patients begin to lose the ability to control motor functions. They may have difficulty swallowing and lose bowel and bladder control. Eventually, patients fail to recognize family members and to speak.

As AD progresses, the disease affects emotions, behavior, and personality. In one study of 55 caregivers from a list of 22 behaviors, more than half the caregivers described four problems: memory disturbance, catastrophic reactions, suspiciousness, and making accusations.[131] Decreased activity, loss of interest, tension, apathy, depression, and bodily preoccupation of the patient were the next most common problems reported by more than 20% of the caregivers. Many caregivers report repetitive physical behaviors as the most common behavioral problem. These behaviors included pacing, repeated folding, and repeated emptying and filling purses.[132]

BOX 8-6	**Alleles in Alzheimer's Disease**

APOE ε2 is relatively rare and may provide some protection against Alzheimer's disease (AD). If AD does develop in a person with this allele, it develops later in life than it would with the APOE ε4 gene.

APOE ε3 is the most common allele. Researchers think it plays a neutral role in AD—neither decreasing or increasing risk.

APOE ε4 occurs in about 40% of all people who develop late-onset AD and is present in about 25% to 30% of the population. Those who inherit one APOE ε4 gene have increased risk of developing AD. Those who inherit two APOE ε4 genes have an even higher risk. However, inheriting one or two copies of the gene does not guarantee that the individual will develop AD. Many people with AD do not have an APOE ε4 allele.

(Data from Alzheimer's disease genetics fact sheet. http://www.nia.nih.gov/Alzheimers/Publications/geneticsfs.htm. Accessed May 11, 2010.)

Vascular Dementia

Vascular dementia[81] represents the second most common type of dementia, representing 20% of all dementias and affecting more men than women. The *DSM-IV TR* classifies vascular dementia as an organic mental disorder, with the essential feature being cerebrovascular disease. Risk factors for vascular dementia include hypertension, smoking, hypercholesterolemia, diabetes mellitus, and cardiovascular and cerebrovascular disease. Brain damage and cognitive loss result from the cerebrovascular disease, usually stroke(s). Multi-infarct dementia is a type of vascular dementia and is the result of the additive effects of small and large infarcts that produce a loss of brain tissue. Deterioration is select, with some functions left completely intact. Predicting the exact course of the mental dysfunction based on site is often misleading. This may be in part because multiple strokes have occurred, obstructing a clear attribution of the deficit to a particular lesion. Three forms of vascular dementia are most common: large vessel disease, strokes, and multiple microcerebral infarcts.[6]

Clinical Presentation. Common disturbances include problems with memory, abstract thinking, judgment, impulse control, and personality. Although the clinical presentation may resemble some features of AD, the signs of abrupt onset, step-by-step deterioration, fluctuating course, and emotional lability are specific to vascular dementia.[9] Imaging and medical history information is necessary as cognitive tests alone cannot distinguish between vascular dementia and AD.[133] Focal neurologic signs such as exaggeration of deep tendon reflexes, extensor plantar response, and laboratory evidence of vascular disease are diagnostic criteria.[124] Vascular dementia has a higher mortality than AD, with a 5-year survival of 39% compared with 75% of age-matched controls.[134]

Treatment for vascular dementia focuses on the cause of the damage such as hypertension, hyperlipidemia, and uncontrolled blood glucose level. Vascular dementia may or may not improve with time, depending on the degree of control of the causative factors and further strokes. Sometimes, vascular dementia coexists with AD.

Some experts call for a designation of mixed dementia, which is a combination of AD and multi-infarct dementia that occurs simultaneously. Mixed dementia may be more common than previously thought and should be suspected when dementia symptoms and presence of cardiovascular disease are present together and symptom progression is slow.[135] The combination of the two types of dementia may have a greater impact on the brain and so is clinically important.

Lewy Body Dementia

Lewy body dementia (LBD) is one of the most common progressive types of dementia. Recent studies have indicated that up to 20% of persons with dementia have Lewy bodies on autopsy.[133,136] The central feature of LBD is progressive cognitive decline, combined with three additional defining features: (1) pronounced "fluctuations" in alertness and attention, such as frequent drowsiness, lethargy, lengthy periods of time spent staring into space, or disorganized speech; (2) recurrent visual hallucinations; and (3) parkinsonian motor symptoms, such as rigidity and the loss of spontaneous movement.

The symptoms of LBD are caused by the buildup of Lewy bodies—accumulated bits of α-synuclein protein—inside the nuclei of neurons in areas of the brain that control particular aspects of memory and motor control. Researchers do not know exactly why α-synuclein accumulates into Lewy bodies or how Lewy bodies cause the symptoms of LBD, but they do know that α-synuclein accumulation is also linked to Parkinson's disease, multiple system atrophy, and several other disorders, which are referred to as the "synucleinopathies." The similarity of symptoms between LBD and Parkinson's disease, and between LBD and AD, can often make it difficult for a physician to make a definitive diagnosis, especially since Lewy bodies are often also found in the brains of individuals with Parkinson's disease and AD. These findings suggest that either LBD is related to these other causes of dementia or that an individual can have both diseases at the same time. LBD usually occurs sporadically, in people with no known family history of the disease. However, rare familial cases have occasionally been reported.[178]

Clinical Presentation. People with LBD demonstrate gait and balance disorders, visual hallucinations, delusions, extrapyramidal symptoms, visual-spatial dysfunction, poor executive functioning, increased sensitivity to antipsychotics, and fluctuation in alertness. Individuals may also have clinical depression.[4,136-138] There is no cure for LBD and treatments are aimed at controlling the parkinsonian and psychiatric symptoms.

Assessment

Individuals with dementia have significantly impaired intellectual functioning that interferes with normal activities and relationships. They also lose their ability to solve problems and maintain emotional control, and they may experience personality changes and behavioral problems, such as agitation, delusions, and hallucinations. Although memory loss is a common symptom of dementia, memory loss by itself does not mean that a person has dementia. Dementia is only diagnosed if two or more brain functions—such as memory and language skills—are significantly impaired without loss of consciousness. A diagnosis of dementia is applicable only when there is demonstrable evidence of memory impairment and other features to the degree there is interference with social or occupational function. One characteristic of dementia is the decline in intellectual functioning from a previous level; therefore, knowing a person's baseline cognitive ability is essential. Unfortunately, clinical assessment of premorbid cognitive function is not always possible and is complicated in the older person when family input is unavailable. Consideration of educational, occupational, and socioeconomic levels can provide information in determining a previous level, but often the clinician must piece together a picture of the individual's prior status.

The diagnosis of dementia is primarily made on clinical grounds. The assessment of cognitive disorder begins with a medical history to determine the precise features of cognitive loss. The medical history should include the patient and the patient's caregiver and/or family members to form an accurate picture of the complaint. Questions about past medical history such as falls, head trauma, hypertension, heart disease, diabetes, vitamin deficiencies or thyroid disorder, and alcohol use and substance exposure should be asked to identify reversible causes of cognitive changes. Medications should be reviewed including alcohol use. Questions such as how the patient is taking medications and why may inform whether all medications are necessary and/or being taken appropriately.[139] A comprehensive physical and neurologic examination performed by the physician should include a check for focal weakness, gait impairment, language impairment, and extrapyramidal signs (rigidity, tremor, bradykinesia) to aid in the differential diagnosis. A gross assessment of functional status includes questions about bathing, dressing, toileting, transferring, as well as intermediate activities (e.g., managing finances, medications, cooking, shopping) to determine the degree of loss. Finally, an evaluation of mental status for attention, immediate and delayed recall, remote memory, executive function, and depression should be conducted.

Mental status examinations and neuropsychological testing reveal abnormalities in cognitive and memory functioning. Neuroimaging may aid in the differential diagnosis of dementia. Computed tomography (CT) or magnetic resonance imaging (MRI) may reveal cerebral atrophy, focal brain lesions (cortical strokes, tumors, subdural hematomas), hydrocephalus, or periventricular ischemic brain injury. Functional imaging such as positron-emission tomography (PET) or single-photon emission computed tomography (SPECT) are not routinely used in the evaluation of dementia but may provide useful differential diagnostic information such as parietal lobe changes in AD or frontal lobe alterations in frontal lobe degenerations.[124]

Most cognition screens have poor accuracy in detecting early dementia. Studies suffer from methodological errors, and few tests have been studied extensively. Useful screening tests are the Mini-Cog, number of animals named in 1 minute, Mini Mental Screening Exam (Folstein Mini Mental Exam), Geriatric Depression Scale, and Patient Health Questionnaire–9. These tests are further detailed in Tables 8-1 and 8-9.

Management

Approximately 20% of individuals with AD experience psychotic behaviors such as hallucinations or paranoia. Nearly 80% of individuals with AD exhibit agitation or aggressive behaviors and can be a leading reason for nursing home admission. Management of these challenging behaviors consists of pharmacologic, behavioral, and environmental strategies. Medication is used both for delay of the progression of dementia and for management of behavioral problems. Recently more attention has been focused on psychosocial management of dementia to include both behavioral and environmental modifications, but first we will briefly discuss pharmacologic management. Box 8-7 lists the American Geriatrics Society recommendations for comprehensive management of the individual with dementia.[139]

Pharmacologic Management. The pharmacologic management for individuals with dementia of any type is largely to manage behavior. Medications for behavioral control might include antidepressants (SSRIs), antipsychotics (such as risperidone or olanzapine), mood stabilizers, or anxiolytics. Mood stabilizers include carbamazepine and depakote, and a common anxiolytic is temazepam. Table 8-10 lists the most common nonproprietary drugs and their side effects that affect rehabilitation.

Much recent research and attention has gone to slowing the process of cognitive decline in individuals with

---

BOX 8-7 Management of Dementia

Primary goals are to improve quality of life and maximize functional performance by enhancing cognition and addressing mood and behavior.

General Treatment Principles
- Identify and treat comorbid physical illnesses (e.g, hypertension, diabetes mellitus).
- Institute stroke prophylaxis for vascular and mixed dementias.
- Avoid anticholinergic medications, e.g, benztropine, diphenhydramine, hydroxyzine, oxybutynin, tricyclic antidepressants, clozapine, thioridazine.
- Limit prescription psychotropic medication use.
- Promote brain health by exercise, balanced diet, and stress reduction.
- Maximize activities of daily living and exercise (e.g, walking).
- Set realistic goals.
- Specify and quantify target behaviors.
- Assess and monitor cognition, mood, and behavior.
- Intervene to decrease hazards of wandering.
- Monitor physical environment for safety (e.g, stairs).
- Establish and maintain relationship with patient and family.
- Advise patient and family about driving, sources of support, financial and legal issues, and advance directives, including establishing surrogate decision maker.
- Consider referral to hospice.

(Adapted from American Geriatrics Society: Dementia diagnosis. Available at: http://dementia.americangeriatrics.org/. Accessed May 15, 2010.)

TABLE 8-9	Screening Tests for Detection of Dementia or Need for Further Screening		
Test	**Instructions**	**Scoring**	**Notes**
Mini-Mental Status Exam (MMSE)[a]	10 questions with a total score of 30	Education[b]　　60-64　80-84 5-8 years[b]　　24　　22 9-12 years[b]　　27　　23 Some college[b]　28　　26	Influenced by education, ethnicity and age; requiring different cut points; copyrighted. Scores on specific elements may provide a better picture of the decline than the composite score. Does not test for executive control
St. Louis University Mental Screen (SLUMS)[c]	1. Day of the week 2. Year 3. State 4. Remember five objects 5. Calculation 6. Name as many animals in 1 min 7. Recall of five objects 8. Recite list of numbers backwards 9. Clock drawing test 10. Place an X in the triangle and determine which figure is largest 11. Recall of facts in a story read to patient	High school education: 27-30, Normal 21-26, Mild neurocognitive disorder 1-20, Dementia Less than high school education: 25-30, Normal 20-24, Mild neurocognitive disorder 1-19, Dementia	Has not been studied extensively Freely available at http://medschool. slu.edu/agingsuccessfully/ pdfsurveys/slumsexam_05.pdf
Mini-Cog[d]	Executive function. The clock drawing is a recall distractor	1 point for each recalled word after performing the Clock Drawing Test (CDT) 2 points for a normal CDT 0-2 (positive screen for dementia) 3-5 (negative score for dementia)	Takes 3 minutes to administer, requires no special equipment and is less influenced by education
Short Blessed Test[e]	Have patient answer 6 questions 1. Year 2. Month Then have patient repeat following name and address "John Brown, 42 Market Street, Chicago." Have patient remember name and address given in question for later recall. 3. Without looking at watch or clock, tell approximate time 4. Count aloud backwards from 20 to 1 5. Say the months of the year in reverse order. 6. Repeat the name and address asked earlier.	0-4, Normal cognition 5-9, Questionable impairment (evaluate for early dementing disorder) 10 or more, Impairment consistent with dementia (evaluate for dementing disorder)	Counting backward, spelling a word backward and forward, or listing the months of the year backward are tests of working memory and attention.
Clock Drawing Test (CDT)[f]	Instruct the patient to draw face of a clock, and then to draw the hands of the clock to read a specific time (11:10 or 8:20 are most commonly used and more sensitive than some others). These instructions can be repeated, but no additional instructions should be given. Typically 3 minutes is given to complete the task.	The CDT score is considered normal if all numbers are depicted, once each, in the correct sequence and position, and the hands readably display the requested time. Do not count equal hand length as an error. The more distorted and inaccurate the drawings, the more likely the person is to have dementia.	

Continued

TABLE 8-9	Screening Tests for Detection of Dementia or Need for Further Screening—cont'd		
Test	**Instructions**	**Scoring**	**Notes**
Time and change test[g,h]	The patient is given 60 seconds to read the time on a clock that is set to 11:10 The patient must make a dollar from three quarters, seven dimes, and seven nickels	Two attempts to get it right. The change test has a 3-minute limit, and two attempts are allowed. Incorrect responses on either or both tasks are scored as a positive result, indicating dementia. A correct response on both tasks is scored as a negative result, indicating no dementia.	To achieve a negative score, indicating no dementia, the patient must correctly complete the Telling Time task in one try within 3 seconds, and correctly complete the Making Change task in one try within 10 seconds. Use of timed cut points increases sensitivity of the test, but decreases specificity.
Sniff test[i]	10-item sniff test with odors of lemon, strawberry, pineapple, lilac, clove, menthol, smoke, natural gas, soap, and leather	Misidentification of two odors is predicative of a 5 times more likely change to progress to Alzheimer's disease.	Original test was of 40 odors, with <34 odors correctly identified increasing the likelihood of progressing to Alzheimer's disease.
Naming[j]	Name as many items as possible in a given category such as fruits or animals	Naming fewer than ten items in 1 minute suggests slowed mental functioning.	Tests language ability
Describe similarities between two items such as an apple and an orange[j]			Ability to reason and plan

[a]From Wind AW, Schellevis FG, Van Staveren G, et al. (1997). Limitations of the Mini-Mental State Examination in diagnosing dementia in general practice. Int J Geriatr Psychiatry, 12(1), 101-108.

[b]From Crum RM, Anthony JC, Bassett SS, Folstein MF. (1993). Population-based norms for the mini-mental state examination by age and educational level. JAMA, 269(18), 2386-2391.

[c]From Tariq S, Tumosa N, Chibnall JT, et al. (2006). Comparison of the Saint Louis University mental status examination and the mini-mental state examination for detecting dementia and mild neurocognitive disorder—a pilot study. Am J Geriatr Psychiatry, 14(11), 900-910.

[d]From Borson S, Scanlan J, Brush M, et al. (2000). The mini-cog: a cognitive "vital signs" measure for dementia screening in multi-lingual elderly. Int J Geriatr Psychiatry, 15(11), 1021-1027.

[e]From Brooke P, Bullock R. (1999). Validation of a 6 item cognitive impairment test with a view to primary care usage. Int J Geriatr Psychiatry,14(11), 936-940.

[f]From Watson YI, Arfken CL, Birge SJ. (1993). Clock completion: an objective screening test for dementia. J Am Geriatr Soc, 41(11), 1235-1240.

[g]From Froehlich TE, Robison JT, Inouye SK. (1998). Screening for dementia in the outpatient setting: the time and change test. J Am Geriatr Soc, 46(12), 1506-1511.

[h]From Inouye SK, Robison JT, Froehlich TE, Richardson ED. (1998). The time and change test: a simple screening test for dementia. J Gerontol A Biol Sci Med Sci, 53(4), M281-M286.

[i]From Devanand DP, Michaels-Marston KS, Liu X, et al. (2000). Olfactory deficits in patients with mild cognitive impairment predict Alzheimer's disease at follow-up. Am J Psychiatry, 157, 1399-1405.

[j]From John Hopkins. Memory on dementia screening tests. http://www.johnshopkinshealthalerts.com/reports/memory/1918-1.html. Accessed May 15, 2010.

MCI and AD. Cholinesterase inhibitors and neuropeptide-modifying agent receptor antagonists are the two medications used to reduce the progression of dementia.[140] Cholinesterase inhibitors (donepezil, galantamine, and rivastigmine) were developed to slow the breakdown of acetylcholine to make it more available for cellular use and are prescribed in mild to moderate AD. They have modest benefit for cognition, mood, behavioral symptoms, and daily function for approximately 1 to 3 years, especially when evaluated by caregiver impression.[140] Neuropeptide-modifying agents (memantine) regulate glutamate availability but have not been shown to be particularly effective in improving functional abilities. Neuropeptide-modifying agents are the only available drugs for severe AD but have not been shown to be particularly effective in slowing the progression of dementia.

However, a combination of memantine and Aricept appear more effective together than either alone.[140] Antidepressants have some effectiveness in treating depression in dementia.[140] Atypical antipsychotics are used to manage behavioral disturbances but because of their side effects, are discouraged for long-term use.[139]

Behavioral and Environmental Management. Evidence-based studies support psychosocial interventions in dementia both in the community and residential facilities. These interventions are designed to manage undesired behaviors through progressively lowering the stress threshold management. Triggers or antecedents for disruptive behaviors are identified and prevented through modification of the environment and schedules. One way to approach challenging behaviors is using Antecedent-Behavioral-Consequences (ABC) strategies. [12,141]

TABLE 8-10	Drugs Used for Dementia	
Nonproprietary Name	**Trade Name**	**Common Side Effects**
Cholinesterase Inhibitors		Fatigue, dizziness, ataxia, syncope, nausea, dyspnea, muscle cramps
Donepezil	Aricept	Abnormal dreams; diarrhea; dizziness; loss of appetite; muscle cramps, nausea; tiredness; trouble sleeping; vomiting; weight loss, fainting
Galantamine	Reminyl	Dizziness, fatigue, headache, inability to sleep, indigestion, loss of appetite, nausea, runny nose, sleepiness, tremor, urinary tract infection, vomiting, weight loss
Rivastigmine	Exelon	Dizziness, drowsiness, fainting, fatigue, flu-like symptoms, hallucinations, high blood pressure, increased sweating, tremor, unwell feeling, weakness, weight loss
Neuropeptide-Modifying Agent		Fatigue, dizziness, back pain, confusion
Memantine	Namenda	Dizziness; pain; change in behavior, such as aggressiveness, depression, or anxiety; chest pain or tightness; fainting; hallucinations; one-sided weakness; severe tiredness; speech changes; sudden severe headache; vision changes
Antipsychotics		Initial orthostatic hypotension, fatigue, sedation, nausea
Aripiprazole	Abilify	Dizziness; drowsiness; headache; nausea; vomiting; confusion; fainting; fast, slow, or irregular heartbeat; fever, chills, sore throat; increased sweating; involuntary movements of the tongue, face, mouth, jaw, arms, legs, or back (e.g, chewing movements, puckering of mouth, puffing of cheeks); loss of control over urination; loss of coordination; muscle tremor, jerking, or stiffness; new or worsening mental or mood problems (e.g, anxiety, depression, agitation, panic attacks, aggressiveness, impulsiveness, irritability, hostility, exaggerated feeling of well-being, inability to sit still); one-sided weakness; seizures; severe or persistent restlessness; shortness of breath; suicidal thoughts or attempts; swelling of the hands, ankles, or feet; symptoms of high blood sugar (e.g, increased thirst, urination, or appetite; unusual weakness); trouble swallowing; trouble walking; unusual bruising; unusual tiredness or weakness; vision or speech changes.
Risperidone	Risperdal	Orthostatic hypotension, arrhythmias, sedation, anxiety, dry mouth, constipation, sexual dysfunction, leukopenia
Olanzapine	Zyprexa	Peripheral edema, headache, orthostatic hypotension, somnolence, seizures, dystonic reactions, constipation, rash, dry mouth
Quetiapine	Seroquel	Headache, somnolence, dizziness, orthostatic hypotension, tachycardia, bradycardia, irregular pulse, A-V block, prolonged P-T interval, constipation, dry mouth, cataracts
Mood Stabilizers		Myalgia, arthralgia, cardiac arrhythmias, nausea, dizziness, vertigo, drowsiness
Carbamazepine	Tegretol	Sedation, dizziness, Stevens-Johnson syndrome, leukopenia, neutropenia, aplastic anemia, SIADH, nausea, gastrointestinal distress, diplopia, nystagmus, dyspnea
Divalproex	Depakote	Peripheral edema, drowsiness, ataxia, alopecia, nausea, vomiting, diarrhea, anorexia, abdominal cramps, thrombocytopenia, asterixis, diplopia, spots before the eyes
Anxiolytics		
Busiprone	BuSpar	Drowsiness, dizziness, palpitations
Temazepam	Restoril	Daytime drowsiness with repeated dosing

SIADH, syndrome of inappropriate antidiuretic hormone secretion.

The ABC method is based on social cognitive theory. The theoretical premise advocates that changing what happens directly before or after a problem behavior can be used to alter or decrease the frequency of problem behavior. Recognition that consequences can "reinforce" behavior, both positively and negatively, forms a basis for management. Behavior that is desired should be rewarded or encouraged and behavior that is undesirable should be negatively reinforced. The first step is to collect as much information about challenging behaviors to detect patterns about why the challenging behaviors occur or what function they might serve for the person with dementia. After the behavior has been observed for a week or so, the triggers or antecedents usually become obvious. The three elements that comprise the ABC chain are detailed in Box 8-8.

Behavior is also managed through consistency and providing a secure and safe environment.[142] Often, the individual with dementia is looking for some measure of control and may react to overchallenging tasks or too much stimulation, similar to what can occur in a physical therapy gym. These behaviors are referred to as provoked behaviors and are most often triggered by event-related factors such as the physical environment, physiologic needs, or the social environment. Once the provoked or antecedent behavior is understood, the triggers can be changed to decrease the challenging behavior. Table 8-11 lists the most commonly used behavioral

BOX 8-8	A-B-C Behavior Chain
Antecedent	Anything that happens prior to a challenging behavior or sets the stage for it to happen. Antecedents can be internal (thoughts or physical sensations) or external (environmental characteristics). Some examples of antecedents are loud noises, hunger, pain, frustration, busy environment, unfamiliar people or surroundings, or overwhelming tasks.
Behavior	Problematic or challenging behavior. Examples include agitation (restlessness, anxious, upset), aggression (shouting, cornering someone, raising a hand to someone or actually pushing or hitting), repetition (repeating a word, question, or action over and over), hallucinations, suspicion, apathy, confusion, sundowning, and wandering.
Consequences	Anything that happens right after the behavior occurs. Providing calm reassurance, offering a person a desirable item like food or a photo album, yelling, taking something away from the person or removing the person from the situation.

(Data from Teri L, Logsdon RG, McCurry, SM: Nonpharmacologic treatment of behavioral disturbance in dementia. Med Clin North Am 86(3): 641-656, viii, 2002.)

therapies and the strength of the evidence as reported by the American Academy of Neurologists.

Depression and Dementia. A study by Pearson et al examined the relationship between depressive diagnosis and cognitive and functional limitations in patients with AD.[143] They found that depression did affect functional status beyond the effects of cognitive impairment. Therefore, if depression is an overlying condition, functional status may improve with successful treatment of the depressive episode. A trial regimen of antidepressants may provide information for a clear diagnosis. If the mood improves as the depression is resolved, cognitive function will return to predepressive level. Should the individual continue to display characteristics of decline in mental ability, investigation for dementia would be initiated. The Patient Health Questionnaire–9 may be useful to differentiate dementia and depression.[144]

Exercise. Cohort and associational studies indicate that physical activity is associated with better cognitive function and less cognitive decline in later life.[145] In a large epidemiological study in Canada, high aerobic exercisers (at least three times per week) had stable or improved cognition over a 5-year period. This was especially true for those who started with high cognitive levels.[74] A recent randomized controlled trial demonstrated that a 6-month aerobic exercise program for older adults with memory decline resulted in modest improvements in cognition.[145]

Exercise may have several beneficial effects for persons with dementia. These positive effects may

TABLE 8-11	Strength of the Evidence for Strategies to Improve Function and Modify Behavior	
Goal	**Strategy**	**Strength of Evidence**
Reduce urinary incontinence	Behavior modification, scheduled toileting, prompted voiding	Strong
Increase functional independence	Graded assistance, practice and positive reinforcement	Good
Improve eating behaviors	Low lighting levels, music and simulated nature sounds	Weak
Improve ADLs	Intensive multimodality group training	Weak
Reduce problem behaviors	Music, particularly during meals and bathing	Good
	Walking or other forms of light exercise	Good
	Simulated presence therapy, such as use of videotapes of family	Weak
	Massage	Weak
	Comprehensive psychosocial care programs	Weak
	Pet therapy	Weak
	Cognitive remediation	Weak
	Bright light, white noise	Weak
	Using commands at the patient's comprehension level	Weak

(Adapted from Dementia_guideline.pdf (application/pdf object) http://www.aan.com/professionals/practice/pdfs/dementia_guideline.pdf. Accessed May 26, 2010.)
ADLs, activities of daily living.

include increased strength and endurance, increased ADL function, improved sleep, increased balance and decreased falls, improved mood, decreased anxiety, and decreased use of medications. The Seattle protocols[146] are an evidence-based program of exercise designed for older adults with dementia that includes encouraging pleasurable and easily achievable activities and work with caregivers to provide supports, work on problem solving for barriers, and establishing goals with very small steps. Because of the evidence that exercise effects may be task-specific and exercise with less cognitive demand has more effect, the Seattle protocols limit the cognitive component of exercise. Activities included in the Seattle protocol were dancing with simple steps, tandem walking on an imaginary tight rope, walking, stationary bicycle, and Tai Chi (sticky-hands technique). Results showed decreased depression, fewer restricted-activity days, increased physical functioning, decreased institutionalization due to behavioral disturbances, and less awake time at night.

The effects of resistance exercise have received less attention but shows promise in a limited number of studies. Chang and Etnier studied the acute effects of a 30-minute bout of high (100% 10 RM), moderate (70% 10 RM), and low (40% 10 RM) loads of resistance exercise on cognition as measured by the Stroop test (a colors naming test) and found a dose response with more effect from the high-intensity group on simple speed of information processing and on executive functions.[147]

Studies of activity and exercise with institutionalized persons with dementia also indicate positive effects of exercise. Volicer et al demonstrated decreased use of psychotropic medication, increased nutrition intake, decreased agitation and improved sleep with a program of continuous activity.[148] Edwards et al demonstrated decreased immediate and long-term (12 weeks) anxiety and depression following a 30-minute chair-based, moderate-intensity exercise program performed three times a week for 12 weeks.[149] Improved ADL activity and increased strength, endurance, balance, and flexibility was shown by Kwak et al in a 3-week program of exercise.[150] These studies indicate that given proper cueing, a supportive environment and appropriate exercises, individuals with dementia can participate and benefit from many different kinds and form of exercise.

Physical Therapy Management. The role of the physical therapist in the presence of dementia is threefold. First, the physical therapist needs to assist the patient, family, and caregivers with activities that will maximize the individual's functional abilities and slow down physical declines. For example, maintaining muscle strength, balance, and mobility can prevent falls, contractures, and pressure sore formation as well as enhance the individual's well-being and mobility. Second, the therapist can assist in changing and simplifying the environment to maintain function. Lastly, the physical therapist

should assist the caregiver(s) in providing functional, meaningful, pleasant, and safe activities.[179]

The features of dementia that most influence the rehabilitation process are memory decline and the difficulty or inability to learn new material. Because therapy is viewed as a teaching process, these features of dementia may be perceived as major obstacles to successful outcome. However, research now demonstrates that the presence and severity of cognitive status should not be a factor that denies rehabilitation.[151] Therapists should modify treatment methods and goals to accommodate the limitations of the patient's cognitive disability. Therapy should not be denied on the basis of cognitive dysfunction.

Function should be assessed to provide a baseline and to identify problematic areas. Simple tools such as the Timed Up and Go, gait speed, and the sit to stand test can be used to assess mobility.[152] Tests to evaluate ADLs include the Barthel Index, The Structured Assessment of Independent Living Skills (SAILS),[153] and the Erlangen test of ADLs.[154] The focus of these tests is on ADLs that are commonly affected in individuals with a dementia diagnosis. Task instructions are straightforward and can be demonstrated, thereby accounting for problems encountered with batteries designed for a general population. However, currently, no tests to measure ADLs in individuals with dementia have strong clinimetric properties.[155]

Traditional physical therapy interventions need to focus on task-specific and relevant activities. As Teri et al have shown, individuals with dementia can meaningfully participate in individual and group exercise if certain modifications are made.[146,156] These modifications include simple, one-step consistent commands or providing cues based on the individual's needs and abilities, making activities pleasurable (avoiding pain or discomfort), and establishing simple, immediate, and relevant goals.[146,156] Emphasis is on positive reinforcement while avoiding criticism. The use of consistent, simple commands, providing sensory cues, demonstration, provision of rest periods, and avoidance of environments with overwhelming stimuli are additional strategies to maximize the individual's success in a physical therapy session.[157] Learning should be approached in a simple, repetitious manner, often requiring cooperation from the family or nursing staff for consistency in the approach and directions for the individual. Whenever possible, the same personnel should work with the client to help establish a trusting and consistent relationship with the individual. Caregivers can help provide further reinforcement of the instructions and functional gains.

The physical therapy examination may need to be modified to accommodate the individual's cognitive abilities and to provide an accurate picture of the individual's abilities. For example, manual muscle testing may not be valid with an individual who is inconsistent in following directions. Modification to accommodate the cognitive limitation may result in a generalized assessment of strength documented as "voluntary motion noted in extremities; unable to grade specifically secondary to inconsistency in following directions." Muscle testing procedures are not familiar tasks to most people, necessitating learning that can be difficult for a person with dementia. Although strength can be assessed and reported, the approach is modified in relation to the limitations of the cognitive symptoms. Adults learn better when the information is relevant to their activities, and this may be even more relevant for older adults with cognitive deficits. For example, sit to stand could be a more appropriate functional measure of strength and balance. In addition, strengthening activities may be best accomplished using functional activities such as sit to stand activities and weighted ADL activities (weighted clothes or hair brush).

Hip Fracture. Individuals with AD sustain hip fractures more often than individuals with normal cognition, and their hospital and rehabilitation course is typically longer. However, several studies indicate that many of these individuals benefit greatly from short- and long-term rehabilitation, especially when a multidisciplinary approach is used.[158-162]

Modifications in the treatment plan may be necessary to achieve optimal benefits for the patient. For example, a surgeon-directed limitation of partial weight bearing poses challenges for the physical therapist or physical therapist assistant. Given the memory limitations caused by dementia, the patient may not understand or remember the weight-bearing status nor conceptualize the mechanics of using a walker, if unfamiliar with a walker. The surgeon must be consulted to determine the purpose of the limitation and the integrity of the repair if full weight bearing occurs. Many times, the surgeon may mean weight bearing as tolerated, assuming pain will inhibit full weight bearing until the repair is healed satisfactorily to safely allow full weight bearing. Other aids to encourage limited weight bearing might be the use of an elevated shoe on the nonaffected side, no shoe on the affected side, or a shoe with bumps that would provide negative sensory sensations with full weight bearing. One study demonstrated that treadmill training was more effective than over-the-ground training.[161] Extensive gait training may need to be postponed beyond transfer activity, until the repair is sufficiently healed to allow full weight bearing. The therapist should be aware of the adverse consequences of prolonged immobility and promote and advocate for mobility within the imposed constraints.

An additional issue with regard to hip fracture and dementia deserves to be mentioned. Individuals with dementia may not be able to express their physical discomfort in recognized ways. In one study whereby pain was evaluated on cognitively intact individuals following hip fracture, 50% of the individuals reporting severe pain did not receive adequate control. The authors also discovered that cognitively intact individuals received three times the pain management that individuals with dementia received for the same procedure.[163] Although surgery for a hip fracture is recognized as one of the most painful orthopedic procedures, pain medication is often delivered on a request-only basis. Current recommendations are to deliver pain medications on a regular and ongoing schedule to help manage pain and prevent delirium.[159]

Working with persons with dementia requires a careful balance of simple instructions and repetition without treating the person as a child. It is important to avoid debate or conflict with the person; rather, change the subject or task if it is too stressful. Finding a connection with the person, perhaps through their hobbies or past employment, can help create a more trusting and less stressful therapy session. Manipulating the patient's environment is often more successful than attempting to teach the person techniques to compensate for cognitive loss. Items and surroundings that are familiar minimize the impact of memory deficit, allowing the person to perform routine daily activities by rote without having to problem-solve. The emphasis on the environment includes safety as a valid factor in the therapeutic program. Failure to recognize and react to hazards becomes a major consideration in the person's ability to remain in an unsupervised situation. Because disorientation is often an issue, protection of the patient is part of the treatment program.

Because control of the environment seems to help with the person's disorientation and agitation, many facilities have developed dementia units that emphasize a structured, low-key environment with consistent staffing.[179] The focus in these units is on safety, specially trained staff, admission criteria, physical design, and activity schedules.[141] Management of behavior is facilitated by reinforcing the environment with constant reminders to orient individuals to time, place, and caregiver identity. Keeping the treatment environment consistent and avoiding multiple distractions during treatment sessions can be effective. Sloan and Gleason[164] suggest learning to recognize triggers to behavior problems such as room temperature, hunger, and toileting needs. Anxiety can be reduced by a consistent schedule and providing appropriate activities.[164] Environmental adaptations for the home include the following:

- Use of visual pictures for key rooms such as the kitchen and bathroom
- Storage of medications and harmful materials out of reach of the person
- Provision of adequate lighting, especially if the individual wanders
- Installation of a shut-off switch on the stove
- Limitation of clutter and mirrors
- Lower water temperature to avoid burns

Finally, therapists may benefit from the Common Mistakes in Working with a Patient/Client with Dementia (Box 8-9), constructed by Ellen Somers, an Alzheimer's

BOX 8-9	Common Mistakes in Working with a Patient with Dementia

1. Don't assume everything is the result of the person's dementia. Instead, anticipate the level of cognitive or functional impairment that would be expected for the disease process and assess if this level exceeds your expectations and experience. Also,
   - Rule out hearing problems, pain, vision, medication side effects, etc.
   - Address these issues (is the person wearing eye glasses? Hearing aid? Receiving pain management before physical therapy?)
   - Other medical problems (urinary tract infection, side effects of medications, sleep deprivation?)
2. Don't discount the person's opinion or preferences. Instead:
   - Assess how consistent this is with the person's prior history (did she or he like to exercise in the past? Did she or he aggressively pursue treatments? Was she or he compliant with medical treatment?)
   - Work with the family to respect what is most consistent with how the person would likely have responded if she or he didn't have dementia.
3. Don't use childish/infantile, "Elderspeak" language. Instead:
   - Use simpler, but adult, language
   - Use same voice, one you would use with other older adults
4. Don't talk in front of the person as if she or he isn't there or can't understand. Instead
   - Assume the person can understand
   - Include the person in the discussion
   - Have the discussion away from the person and out of eyesight.
5. Don't rely only on verbal communication. Instead:
   - Use written communication
   - Use visual cues
   - Use modeling, gestures, and physical prompts
6. Don't assume new learning can't occur. Instead recognize that people with dementia do learn new information, especially if it's:
   - Salient
   - Meaningful
   - Presented properly (e.g, build on current strengths)
   - Practiced in a way that facilitates development of a new habit (i.e., in the proper environment, with appropriate equipment, with lots of opportunity to practice but spaced over increasing intervals of time)
7. Don't conduct therapy in a noisy, distracting environment. Instead:
   - Reduce conversations between therapists or with other patients while working with one person
   - Use music judiciously (not as background)
   - Find quieter areas if possible
8. Don't give too much information. Instead:
   - Provide step-by-step directions
   - Focus on one step you want to work on and ignore or use nonverbal cues for other steps
   - Use as few words as possible
   - Repeat using same words if necessary
   - Allow enough time to process the information (spaces between sentences, not words)
9. Don't focus on the task. Instead:
   - Focus on the person
   - Build your relationship with the person first
   - Find out about the person's interests, family
   - Incorporate what you know about the person into the exercises you give her or him and how you communicate with the person
10. Don't conduct therapy only in the therapy environment. Instead:
    - Whenever possible, conduct therapy in the environment where the person will need to use the skill
    - Use materials/equipment that the person will be using upon discharge

And finally, if it's not working, systematically alter what you are doing, reassess and continue to make changes, and remember, what works today may not work tomorrow.

(From Ellen Somers, MA, LMAC, Alzheimer's Service Cooridinator at St. Camillus Health and Rehabilitation Hospital, Syracuse, NY.)

services coordinator who has observed physical therapists working with individuals with dementia for several years.

CAREGIVER ISSUES

The health professional must address not only the patient's environment but also available support systems and family situation in order to implement an individual plan of care. Education and training for the caregiver are essential because management of the patient is heavily dependent on the family support and coping resources.

Psychological health of the caregiver is a concern to the therapists and is often related to the function of the patient. Although the health care provider is with the patient for a few hours, the caregiver may be with the person every day, all day. Depression, anxiety, and caregiver burden are reported to be much higher among caregivers caring for an individual with dementia compared with caregivers of persons with physical frailty.[166] The increase in these symptoms is due to the changes in personality, disruptive behaviors, lack of spare time, isolation, and progressive deterioration associated with dementia.[166] The relationship was strongest for spouse caregivers, followed by children caregivers. Further investigation of spouse involvement reveals wife caregivers experiencing greater degree of negative psychological well-being than husband caregivers.[167] Only modest effects of caregiving for persons with dementia with respect to physical illnesses have been demonstrated.[168,169] Interestingly, positive effects of caregiving for persons with dementia have also been demonstrated. These include feeling useful, important, and competent as well as increased satisfaction in their role and the ability to provide a good quality of life to a loved one.[170]

The therapist's awareness of the potential for caregiver mental health problems is the first step. Identification of warning signs such as caregiver denial, anger, depression, exhaustion, or health problems should be a call for action by the therapist to avoid a complex situation. Studies of the REACH (Resources for Enhancing Alzheimer Caregiver Health) indicate that keys to decreasing caregiving stress include the following:

- Extensive education regarding strategies to deal with behavioral problems, including role-playing
- Enhance ADL abilities with strategies to reinforce
- Reinforcement with practice, home visits, and phone calls
- Encourage self-care with pleasurable activities and health-promoting behaviors.[171]

Some stress can be avoided by educating the caregiver on the limitations of the patient. This should minimize unrealistic goals that are translated into demands on the patients, resulting in failure, frustration, and sometimes behavior problems. The therapist can assist in identifying patient activities that can be performed successfully without failure. Identification of community support groups for the caregiver should be part of the treatment plan, offering an opportunity for education and emotional assistance. Numerous sources of information are also available on the Internet from the Alzheimer's Association, American Geriatric Society, and the National Institute on Aging. Respite care either in the home or at long-term care facilities can provide the caregiver needed time for self-care and enjoyable activities. The reader is also referred to Chapter 11 on family dynamics.

CASE STUDY

Mr. Martin was an 84-year-old male living at home with his 72-year-old companion. Also living in the home was the patient's 17-year-old nephew. According to the family, Mr. Martin had been fine until he fell and fractured his left hip. After a total hip replacement, Mr. Martin was admitted to a skilled nursing facility for rehabilitation. The physician referral for physical therapy included a specific request for partial weight bearing on the left. On initial evaluation, the therapist found the patient to be very confused. He was unable to identify family members and was not able to tell the therapist where he lived or where he was, with minimal awareness of sustaining a hip fracture and the restrictions of his injury. Consultation with the family revealed that Mr. Martin was fine before the fall, with some signs of "getting old" but much more aware than what he was presently displaying. The therapist modified the treatment program to accommodate Mr. Martin's cognitive status, including utilization of an adductor cushion to prevent dislocation and allowing no weight bearing until the physician was contacted regarding danger of nonadherence to non–weight bearing status. The therapist considered that postsurgical confusion could be a possible reason for the cognitive dysfunction. Possible sources of the postsurgical confusion could have been infection, metabolic abnormalities, or medication effects. Consultation with the physician resulted in medical intervention to modify metabolic abnormalities and reduce medications. When the mental function only slightly improved in the next few days, the therapist scheduled an interview with the individuals living with Mr. Martin in his home.

As an introduction for the family, the therapist explained that she was interested in Mr. Martin's ability to perform daily activities before the accident. She indicated that "just getting old" is usually not the reason for individuals to change the way they function, and that most people who experience normal aging have minimal changes in their memory, personality, or intelligence. With questioning, those interviewed recalled that Mr. Martin had become more forgetful about 2 years ago. He began to get lost while driving, only to be returned by a neighbor in the small farming community. The animals were neglected, as Mr. Martin either fed them five times a day or not at all for several days. When he forgot repeatedly to milk the cow, the nephew moved in to help out with the chores. In the past 6 months, the family reported that they had to answer the phone, because people outside the family were unable to understand Mr. Martin when he talked. Mr. Martin had also become very suspicious of the neighbors, accusing them of taking down his fence. After the interview, the therapist conducted a Mini-Cog.[172] Mr. Martin scored 0 out of 5. Based on the presenting cognitive function, history as revealed by the family, and the Mini-Cog score, Mr. Martin was referred to a psychologist for testing to rule out dementia of the Alzheimer type.

To maximize the benefit of the therapy sessions, Mr. Martin's treatment program was modified to accommodate the cognitive dysfunction. The physician was consulted regarding the difficulty of maintaining partial weight-bearing status and agreed to allow the patient to bear weight to tolerance if a wheeled walker was used. This allowed the patient to transfer with a modified standing pivot method and to begin gait training. Mr. Martin was treated in a quiet and consistent environment. Commands and instructions were stated in one-step progressions. The family was involved in therapy, as Mr. Martin continued to respond to instructions when a familiar person was present. They also were instructed in simple mobility exercises that they encouraged Mr. Martin to do whenever they visited. This modification in the treatment plan compensated for Mr. Martin's inability to perform exercises independently. As the family was vested in Mr. Martin's returning to his prior living situation, a home assessment was conducted with suggestions on safety, precautions for danger when wandering, and cues to minimize the effects of the memory loss. Family concerns were also addressed by explaining the characteristics and course of AD, which had been confirmed by the consultant, and the effects on the living situation and the family members. Resources were shared with the family to help with their coping and support of Mr. Martin. As Mr. Martin's confusion gradually improved, he reached treatment goals of independent ambulation and transfers that permitted him to return home. A home maintenance program of general exercise and balance was also developed.

CONCLUSION

Much progress in understanding the pathology and management of older adults with depression, delirium, and dementia has been made in the past 10 years. The idea that the brain is plastic and responds favorably to physical and cognitive challenges and less favorably to a lack of challenges similarly to the way the physical body responds has many implications for the physical thera-pist. Older adults can be creative, productive, and intelligent throughout their later years. Depression is now considered a pathology that should be treated aggressively with the expectation that older adults will respond similarly to younger adults. Depression does not have to adversely affect the process or outcomes of rehabilitation. Clear identification of the clinical presentation of depression is necessary so as not to misdiagnose an older adult with dementia.

Although the pharmaceutical management of dementia is still in its infancy, the evidence is strong for the role of exercise before, during, and after the development of dementia. In addition, research about behavioral management is creating the expectation that undesirable behaviors, once thought to be barriers to rehabilitation, can be managed with best practices. Depression, delirium, and dementia as well as normal cognitive changes in the older adult have significant implications for the physical therapists' care. Avoidance of ageist attitudes, awareness of current research, and compassionate care are keys to effective physical therapy management of the cognitively impaired older adult. Research indicates that older adults with dementia can be rehabilitated similarly to older adults without dementia and that the presence of dementia should never be used as the sole reason for the termination of physical therapy. Cognition in the aging adult is in its infancy with exciting discoveries on the horizon.

REFERENCES

To enhance this text and add value for the reader, all references are included on the companion Evolve site that accompanies this text book. The reader can view the reference source and access it online whenever possible. There are a total of 179 cited references and other general references for this chapter.

Evaluation of the Acute and Medically Complex Patient

Chris L. Wells, PhD, PT, CCS, ATC,
Martha Walker, PT, DPT

INTRODUCTION

The population of older adults is the fastest growing age group within the United States and represents a substantial segment of health care expenditures. Physical inactivity and a sedentary lifestyle are major contributors to disease and disability in this population subgroup.[1] Data from 2006 reveal that there was a 17% increase, from 21% to 38%, in hospital admissions in patients who were older than age 65 years, and a 22% increase in patients who were older than age 75 years, whereas there is a decline in admissions for patients younger than age 45 years.[2] Some of the increase in admissions among older adults is related to the increase in surgical options for individuals with cardiac problems. More than half of older adults, approximately 566,000, were admitted for fracture management.[2] From the Census Bureau, the most common discharge diagnoses for patients older than age 65 years include congestive heart failure, which is the leading diagnosis, coronary heart disease, pneumonia, and septicemia.[3]

When considering working with this population, the physical therapist must recognize the need to address a complex medical history and be aware of the interplay between each body system. Psychological and mood states as well as cognitive and social factors can also influence the presentation of the patient and the outcome of therapy. It is important to examine each system in order to identify the complexity of the problem, determine a proper diagnosis and prognosis, and develop a comprehensive plan of care that incorporates an understanding of the impact of medical comorbidity on function. The plan of care will be based upon a thorough evaluation and may address multiple impairments and medical deficits in order to improve the patient's functional mobility, health and well-being, and ultimately quality of life.

There are many reasons that have led to the need for the physical therapist to acquire the necessary skills to recognize, examine, and determine the proper plan of care when working within the health care system today

(Box 9-1). As a result of advances in medical management, people are living longer. As our population ages, mortality rates and medical complexity also increase substantially. A study conducted by the National Institute of Aging on postmenopausal women who have been diagnosed with breast cancer is a good example of the increasing amount of comorbidities. Of the 1800 women involved in this study, only 7% did not have any other documented disease. Forty-nine percent had 1 to 3 comorbidities, 34% had 4 to 6 comorbidities, and 9% had 7 to 13 comorbidities at the time of the cancer diagnosis.[4]

Regardless of the clinical setting, it is vital that the physical therapist be able to recognize signs and symptoms that do not fit within the authorized scope of practice and recognize "yellow flags" and "red flags" in order to make appropriate referrals with the ultimate goal to improve the well-being and health of the client. The purpose of this chapter is to summarize the knowledge and skills a physical therapist needs to demonstrate in order to complete a thorough screening to provide proper care for the older adult patient in an acute care setting, work effectively with an older individual in an acute phase of illness in other settings such as the outpatient primary care clinic, and respond appropriately to the individual with medical comorbidity in any setting. The goals of examination and evaluation are to develop a proper plan of care, make appropriate discharge recommendations, and to facilitate discharge. This is done by completing a thorough examination of the patient, putting primary and secondary diagnoses in proper perspective for the impact on function, establishing a prognosis, and formulating a comprehensive intervention plan. This process begins with gathering information in a thorough and systematic fashion from medical and health records and through communication with other health care members and caregivers as well as a comprehensive interview of the patient. Implementation of the plan of care will depend on the particular setting and the time frame for implementing the proposed plan of care and discharge recommendations if the patient will be going to another facility or type of residence.

BOX 9-1	The Impact of Comorbidity

It is commonplace for clinicians to focus their attention on the primary diagnosis or obvious impairments and functional limitations. Many fail to consider the other systems of the body, how they interact and affect the primary complaint and thus affect the rehabilitation outcome. Even with a healthy, aging individual, the multiple systems of the body are declining in function. This decline may not be substantial enough to cause an overt dysfunction or failure until another stressor is added.

Consider the following case: Suppose an 88-year-old healthy, very physically active woman undergoes an aortic valve replacement. The operation goes well except the patient experiences a slight decline in contractility of the myocardium in the first 24 hours postoperation. The physical therapist may tend to only be concerned with the heart when performing the examination initially after surgery.

However, her decrease in cardiac output leads to hypotension. The consequences of hypotension are a decrease in perfusion to the brain and kidneys. The patient's body cannot tolerate this deviation from homeostasis and the result is a clinically significant decline in mental status and acute renal failure. Along with the fluid retention from the renal failure and cardiac impairment, the patient becomes more agitated and is sedated.

These complications prolong the time her respiratory system is supported by a mechanical ventilator. She experiences a ventilator-acquired pneumonia and a partial bowel obstruction due to immobility. The stress and trauma contribute to temporary insulin glucose dysfunction, which in turn delays wound healing. Weakness and multiple joint pains develop that further complicate the ability to mobilize this patient and successfully wean her from the ventilator. The end result of this cascade of events after weeks in the intensive care unit is that the patient undergoes a tracheotomy and percutaneous endoscopic jejunostomy and will be discharged to a subacute skilled nursing facility for ventilator-weaning and rehabilitation.

CHART REVIEW

The information-gathering process typically is initiated when the physical therapist receives a request for consultation. This request may be very generic or may include pertinent information about the reason for the consult and indicate any restrictions or precautions. If the consult is generic, the therapist should determine if there are any restrictions to care, such as out-of-bed status or weight-bearing precautions.

Admission or Reason for Visit

Patients with acute conditions are not always in a hospital. Increasingly, physical therapists are part of primary care teams in the outpatient setting, or providing acute care services in the patient's own home or other residential setting. If a medical or health record is available prior to the initial clinical encounter, the admission or intake section of the record may contain several important documents that can be reviewed prior to

the physical therapist's initial examination. These documents may include the method of admission, information from any emergency medical service field treatment, emergency room evaluations and initial testing procedures, the referring physician's evaluation for planned admissions to an inpatient setting, or the patient's reason for the primary care or outpatient visit. An emergency department report typically concludes with a working differential diagnosis list and a medical problem list. The primary history and physical (H&P) that is usually completed by the admitting service may also be found among these documents. It is extremely helpful to review this data source to the degree it is available because it commonly contains the admitting diagnosis and summary of what led up to the admission, the patient's chief complaint, and past medical/surgical history. The H&P also typically contains social history, risk factors, a medication list, allergies, medical summary, and plan of care. The working medical problem list for an older adult may be extensive due to multiple comorbidities and, therefore, it is important to review all available information in order to fully understand the patient's medical status to prepare the appropriate physical therapy evaluation.

The therapist should review the medical or health record not only to glean information pertaining to physical therapy but also to understand what other services have been or should be consulted, what diagnostic tests have been requested, and what medications or other treatments have been prescribed. All services typically enter a contact note that describes their contribution to the patient's care. It is important to keep up to date as to who has been treating the patient, any changes in medical status, operative notes, tests that may have been done, and updates on the medical plan. The physical therapist needs to ensure that the physical therapy plan of care is consistent with the medical plan, which can be very complex when the patient has multiple comorbidities. There may also be reports from other health professionals, social workers, psychologists, and case managers that may be important to assist the therapist during formulation of a plan of care or discharge recommendations.

Laboratory Values

The analysis of blood work is critical to full appreciation of the medical status of the patient. Serum enzymes can be examined to determine cellular damage including myocardial injury and infarct. Blood lipids can determine the patient's risks for vascular disease, and the coagulation profile reveals the body's ability to clot. The complete blood count (CBC) examines such factors as hemoglobin (cells that contain iron used for oxygen transport), hematocrit (the proportion of blood that is red blood cells [RBCs]), RBCs, white blood cells (WBCs), and platelet counts. The body's ability to regulate the cellular pH through respiratory and renal function can be determined by examining the arterial blood gases (ABGs). Finally, electrolyte levels can be examined through blood analysis. See Table 9-1 for clinical laboratory studies.[5-9]

Serum Enzymes and Markers. Serum enzymes and markers are used to assist in the diagnosis of disease such as cancer or medical events like myocardial infarction, congestive heart failure, or liver dysfunction. Serum enzymes can also show muscle tissue breakdown in the event of trauma or rhabdomyolysis. The therapist can review these lab values to obtain an appreciation of the extent of tissue involvement or dysfunction as well as the

TABLE 9-1   Clinical Laboratory Studies[5-9]

Chemistry		
	Reference	**Function**
Sodium (Na)	136-146 mmol/L	Regulates water balance, regulates acid–base balance, membrane integrity, nerve impulse
Potassium (K)	3.5-5.1 mmol/L	Intracellular fluid osmolality, maintenance of resting membrane potential, glucose deposition in liver and skeletal muscles
Chloride (Cl)	98-107 mmol/L	Resting membrane potential, osmotic pressure regulation, extracellular enzymatic reactions
Carbon dioxide (CO_2)	21-30 mmol/dL	Acid–base balance
Anion gap	8-14 mEq/L	Measurement of the acid–base balance
Blood urea nitrogen (BUN)	6-20 mg/dL	Byproduct of protein breakdown, reflection of kidney function: glomerular filtration and urine concentration capacity
Creatinine (Cr)	0.64-1.25 mg/dL	Waste product of body's protein metabolism, reflects long-term glomerular function
Glucose	70-99 mg/dL	Reflects carbohydrate metabolism
Calcium (Ca)	8.8-10.2 mg/dL	Bone and teeth health, enzymatic cofactor for blood clotting, plasma membrane stability and permeability
Ionized calcium	1.15-1.29 mmol/L	Free flowing calcium that is not attached to protein
Magnesium (Mg)	1.6-2.6 mg/dL	Intracellular enzymatic reactions, protein synthesis, neuromuscular excitability
Phosphate (Ph)	2.3-3.7 mg/dL	Intra- and extracellular anion buffer, energy substrate
Total protein	6.1-7.9 g/dL	Rough measurement of albumin and globulin proteins
Albumin	3.5-5.2 g/dL	Protein synthesized by liver, protein found in blood
Prealbumin	20-90 mg/dL	Protein synthesized by liver that is source for amino acids for other protein production. Short-term measure of nutritional status
Bilirubin total	0.4-1.5 mg/dL	Yellowish pigment from heme (RBC) metabolism found in liver bile, test of liver/gallbladder function
Bilirubin (direct)	0.1-0.5 mg/dL	Is bilirubin attached to another molecule before being released in bile
Aspartate transaminase (serum glutamine-oxaloacetic transaminase)	10-41 units/L	Enzyme from liver or muscle cells released upon injury
Alanine transaminase (serum glutamic pyruvic transaminase)	14-54 units/L	Enzyme from liver or muscle cells released upon injury
Cortisol	7-9 a.m.: 4.2-38.4 μg/dL 4-6 p.m.: 1.7-16.6 μg/dL	Hormone produced by adrenal cortex that increases blood glucose and liver stores of glycogen in response to stress
Lipase	10-140 units/L	Enzyme that metabolizes dietary lipids
Amylase	27-131 units/L	Enzyme that metabolizes dietary carbohydrates
Lactate dehydrogenase	100-190 units/L	Five enzymes in various organs that are responsible for conversion of pyruvate and lactate. Specific enzyme markers can identify type of cellular damage.

Complete Blood Count

	Reference	**Function**
White blood cell (WBC) count	4.5-11.0 K/μL	Leukocytes, cells of the immune system
Red blood cell (RBC) count	4.0-5.7 K/μL	Erythrocytes, cells that have gas-carrying capacity
Hemoglobin (Hgb)	12.6-17.4 g/dL	O_2/CO_2-carrying capacity protein of the RBC
Hematocrit	37%-50%	Percentage of a given volume of blood that is occupied with erythrocytes
Mean corpuscular volume	80-96 fL	Average RBC volume

Continued

TABLE 9-1 | **Clinical Laboratory Studies[5-9]—cont'd**

Chemistry		
Complete Blood Count		
	Reference	Function
Mean corpuscular hemoglobin concentration	32-36 g/dL	Average concentration of Hgb in the RBC
Platelet	153-367 K/μL	Small cell that contributes to clotting
Blood Gases		
	Reference	
Arterial		
pH	7.35-7.45	
PaCO$_2$	32-48 mmHg	
PaO$_2$	83-100 mmHg	
Bicarbonate (HCO$_3^-$)	22-26 mEq/L	
Oxygen saturation	94%-99%	
Venous		
pH	7.32-7.44	
PvCO$_2$	38-54 mmHg	
PvO$_2$	35-45 mmHg	
HCO$_3^-$	22-26 mEq/L	
Oxygen saturation	60%-80%	
Urinalysis		
	Function	
Urine specific gravity	1.002-1.030	
pH	4.5-8.0	
WBC	0-5/hpf	
RBC	0-2/hpf	
Urine is also examined for presence of color, blood, protein, ketones, glucose, and nitrates		
Coagulation		
	Reference	
Prothrombin time	12.8-14.6 s	
Partial thromboplastin time	25-38 s	
International Normalized Ratio	0.8-1.2	
Blood Lipid Profile		
	Reference	
Total cholesterol	<200 mg/dL	
High-density lipoproteins	M: >43 mg/dL	
	F: >33 mg/dL	
Low-density lipoproteins	<100 mg/dL	
Triglycerides	<140 mg/dL	

phase of the event such as the evolution of a myocardial infarction by monitoring the enzymes and marker values and whether these numbers are trending up or down based upon serial analysis. See Table 9-2 for cardiac enzymes and diagnosis for myocardial cellular injury.[5-7,9]

Blood Lipids. The examination of the patient's blood lipid profile helps to risk-stratify the patient for cardiovascular disease. This finding can be helpful in determining how to focus part of the interview process (i.e., toward the signs, symptoms, and functional impacts of cardiovascular disease), particularly the review of systems as well as what specific tests and measures the therapist should consider, including more inclusive

cognitive testing beyond the gross screening, and peripheral perfusion testing.[10] Vital signs should be monitored at rest as well as during exertion to determine if the patient has hypertension that should be further medically addressed. Because cardiovascular disease is a multisystem disease, patients with abnormal blood profiles are at risk for further declines in cerebral function as well as risk of cerebral vascular events.[11] Further screening may include such brief testing as the Trails A and B test, counting backwards by 7, or the Stroop test[12] may give the therapist further documentation that cerebral function is impaired or has changed from previous admissions. Data on peripheral perfusion testing and skin

TABLE 9-2	Cardiac Enzymes[5-7,9]				
Cardiac Enzymes					
Enzyme	**Normal**	**Rise**	**Peak**	**Return**	**Abnormal**
Creatine phosphokinase (CPK)	5-75 mU/mL	2-8 h	12-36 h	3-4 h	Total ≥ 200
Lactate dehydrogenase (LDH)	100-225 units/mL	12-48 h	3-6 days	8-14 days	Total ≥170, ≥ 100 LDH + 40% CPK
CPK-MB	0%-3%	4 h	18-24 h		Total ≥ 200 with MB ≥ 4% or total <200 with MB ≥10 units
Troponin	< 0.2 μg/mL	4-6 h	24 h	>10 days	>1.5

inspection as well as tolerance to exertion may help to characterize any clinical hypothesis that a functional limitation is related to peripheral arterial disease.[13] Finally, by the therapist appreciating the patient's blood profile along with evaluating for other risk factors, the therapist can determine the patient's risk level for a cardiovascular event, how to safely prescribe an exercise program, initiate patient education on risk reduction and prevention, and make appropriate referrals.[14]

Coagulation Profile. The coagulation profile of the patient will indicate the ability of the patient's blood to clot, particularly important for the individual receiving anticoagulation therapy as a treatment for conditions such as atrial fibrillation, mechanical heart valves or devices, deep vein thrombosis (DVT), pulmonary embolism (PE), or trauma. Anticoagulation levels that are considered therapeutic will vary depending upon reason for coagulation, previous medical history, physician preferences, and institutional policies. The therapist needs to know the therapeutic level, medical goal, and any functional mobility precautions or restrictions. An increased risk of thrombus formation also increases risk for stroke, pulmonary emboli, and other embolic activity. Patients whose coagulation levels are too high are at risk for bleeding, so the therapist should monitor these patients for edema, ecchymosis, drops in hemoglobin and hematocrit, limitations in limb range of position, pain, and neurologic changes if there is a cerebral bleed. Patients on anticoagulation therapy in the presence of infection or other causes of physiological stress may develop a coagulopathy and be at risk for bleeding.

Prior to starting coagulation therapy and until the patient's titer is therapeutic, meaning the hematocrit levels are within a certain designated range, the patient may be placed on temporary bed rest or restricted to limited mobility. It will be important to look for signs and symptoms of clotting. For DVT, the signs and symptoms may include peripheral edema (typically unilateral), venous distention, and pain; for PE, the patient may present with shortness of breath, abnormal breath sounds, and oxygen desaturation. In those cases where the PE is of a clinically significant size, the patient can suffer from respiratory failure. The patient may also be at risk for all or a portion of the thrombosis to break away and become an embolus in the systemic circulation, which

may lead to a peripheral cellular injury or necrosis, including limb loss as well as an embolic stroke. Guidance for mobilizing a patient with a lower extremity DVT is conflicting and may vary dependent on how clinicians weigh the site and duration of the DVT as well as time since anticoagulation therapy was started.

Complete Blood Count. The CBC is one of the most common laboratory studies performed and can be used to aid in the formulation of a diagnosis, to assess medical treatment response, and to monitor recovery. The physical therapist can obtain a wealth of information from examining the CBC and should check daily to adjust the intervention accordingly.

The first group within the CBC is RBC count and differentiation. The count examines the number of actual RBCs. This information is valuable since the RBCs reflect the oxygen-carrying capacity of the blood that supports cellular activity. If the RBC count is too high, known as polycythemia vera, there is a significant risk of blood clot formation and a subsequent loss of perfusion to tissues. If the RBC count is too low, also known as anemia, then there are insufficient RBCs to adequately supply tissue with oxygen, particularly in the presence of cardiac or pulmonary dysfunction.

Part of the RBC study is the quantification of hemoglobin and hematocrit. Hemoglobin is the oxygen-carrying component of the RBC and reflects the ability of the body to sufficiently promote gas exchange to regulate pH. Hematocrit is the measure of the number of RBCs within the blood compared to the total volume of blood, represented as a percentage. These two numbers are very important to monitor when working with patients in general and especially when working with the older patient. The incidence of anemia is high within the older adult population, with the primary cause commonly related to gastrointestinal bleeding. Rockey et al reported that 62 of 100 subjects had anemia from gastrointestinal bleeding.[15] Anemia can be the underlying cause and a contributing factor to fatigue, disability, change in cognitive function, and activity intolerance. Patients with anemia in the presence of coronary artery disease (CAD) may experience angina, particularly with exertion, and if the coronary disease is extensive, the anemia may lead to heart failure (HF).[16]

Ten percent of people older than age 65 years suffer from anemia.[17] However, gastrointestinal bleeding is not the only cause of anemia and it is important to determine the actual cause to ensure proper medical treatment. Other causes of anemia, for example, iron, folate, and vitamin B_{12} deficiencies; renal insufficiency; anemia of chronic inflammation; and unexplained anemia, can be further worked up by analyzing the differentiation of RBCs or indices.[17] This set of tests looks at the size of the average RBC, otherwise known as the mean corpuscular volume (MCV). The mean corpuscular hemoglobin (MCH) and mean corpuscular hemoglobin concentration (MCHC) examine the amount and concentration of hemoglobin in an average RBC, respectively. These tests can aid in the diagnosis of what type of anemia the patient has and, therefore, allow the medical team to prescribe the best intervention.

The CBC also contains the analysis of WBCs with respect to both total number and differentiation of cells that will provide the therapist with information about the body's response to an infectious disease. An elevation in total WBCs, which is referred to as leukocytosis, may be due to a bacterial infection, with urinary tract and pulmonary infections leading the incidence of infections in older adults. This is significant, because with age, the chance of these infections progressing to bacteremia increases, as does mortality.[18] Leukocytosis can also be evidence of leukemia or stress related to trauma and inflammation. Leukopenia, or low WBC levels, may be caused by bone marrow depression, acute viral infections, or alcohol abuse. Differentiation of WBCs can further determine the underlying problem: neutrophils will be elevated in the presence of bacterial or fungal infections, eosinophils are elevated in allergic responses, and lymphocytes are elevated in viral infections.

Platelets, which are small cells that aid in clotting and the release of growth factors, are also measured when a CBC is ordered. When the endothelium is damaged, collagen is released into the bloodstream. When the platelets come in contact with the collagen, the platelets are then activated to form a clot to repair the injured area. Platelets also release platelet-derived growth factor and tissue growth factor-β, which contribute to cellular repair and regeneration. A reduction in platelets, otherwise known as thrombocytopenia, can be caused by chemotherapy, a large blood transfusion, or implantation of mechanical heart valves among many other reasons. Also, heparin-induced thrombocytopenia can result from the use of heparin postsurgically. Thrombocytosis, elevation of platelet count, is less common but is associated with iron-deficient or hemolytic anemia, cancer, or inflammatory or infectious processes such as inflammatory bowel syndrome and tuberculosis.

Electrolytes. The study of electrolytes, specifically creatinine, blood urea nitrogen (BUN), calcium, magnesium, sodium, potassium, and chloride reveals the state of the cellular function. Sodium and potassium are key to maintaining cellular membrane potential, and carbon dioxide is used to assist in the analysis of the body's acid–base balance. Chloride level is used for further analysis of acid–base balance through the calculation of the anion gap. Creatinine and BUN reflect renal function and reflect the efficiency of glomerular function. BUN is commonly elevated in the presence of heart or renal failure, and low levels of BUN are associated with starvation, dehydration, and liver failure. Electrolyte analysis is very important because the risk of death from chronic kidney disease increases with age, especially in patients with concurrent cardiovascular disease.[19]

Calcium levels can also be analyzed to identify parathyroid dysfunction, malnutrition, and chronic renal disease. Abnormalities in calcium level are related to hyperparathyroidism, malignancy such as metastatic breast, lung, or renal cancer, as well as immobility. Magnesium contributes to various cellular activities such as muscle and nerve function, assisting in the maintenance of normal cardiac rhythm, bone strength, and health status of the immune system. Abnormally low magnesium levels, hypomagnesemia, can be related to alcoholism, chronic diarrhea, hemodialysis, and cirrhosis. Renal failure, adrenal disease, and dehydration can cause hypermagnesemia.

Electrolyte abnormalities are common, and corrections for a toxic or deficient state are important in order to restore normal cellular function. See Table 9-3 for causes and signs and symptoms of electrolyte abnormalities.[5-9] In older adults, malnutrition, dehydration, adverse effects of medications, decline in organ function, and increased risk of infections and cancers increase their risk for electrolyte imbalances. A study by Oliveira et al reported that 29.1% of the 240 hospitalized older adult patients they studied were considered malnourished. Of those, 13.7% had hypertension, 15.7% had diabetes, 3.9% presented with osteoarticular issues, 12.8% had some form of cancer, and 15.7% had the sequelae of stroke.[20]

Special Tests. Serum glucose levels examine the body's ability to utilize glucose for cellular activity through the production of ATP. Hyperglycemia, elevated blood sugar, is generally associated with diabetes mellitus (DM); however, patients without a history of DM could present with elevated glucose levels in the acute care setting that may be related to physiological stress from trauma or surgery, or alterations in medications. Hypoglycemia, low blood sugar, is associated with alcoholism, adverse medication reactions, treatment for hyperglycemia, and critical illnesses related to liver or pancreatic disease.

Serum glucose, glycosylated hemoglobin (HbA_{1c}), and routine blood glucose testing are very important for the therapist to examine prior to intervention. If the patient's glucose is elevated, greater than 250 mg/dL, or low, below 70 mg/dL, the body does not have the ability to utilize glucose as an energy substrate for exercise. Modifications in therapy will need to be implemented to

TABLE 9-3	Causes and Clinical Signs and Symptoms of Electrolyte Abnormalities[5-9]	
Electrolyte	**Causes**	**Clinical Symptoms**
Calcium	Increased: Hyperparathyroidism, large consumption of calcium and vitamin D, cancer, immobilization, Paget disease	Asymptomatic, constipation, nausea, vomiting, abdominal pain, loss of appetite, thirst, and dehydration
	Decreased: Hypoparathyroidism; osteomalacia; decreased intake of dairy products; decreased vitamin D intake	Nonspecific central nervous system signs (e.g., mild diffuse brain disease mimicking depression, dementia, or psychosis), tetany or latent neuromuscular irritability; cardiac arrhythmias and heart block; osteoporosis; hypertension
Magnesium	Increased: Mg consumption in presence of renal failure, antacids, or laxative overdose	Weakness, low blood pressure, respiratory distress, asystole
	Decreased: Dietary depletion; renal loss; gastrointestinal (GI) disorders, including vomiting, diarrhea, and malabsorption syndrome; alcoholism; primary defect in renal tubular reabsorption; GI disorders that impair absorption, such as Crohn disease	Nonspecific, neuromuscular irritability and muscle weakness; arrhythmias; increased sensitivity to cardiac glycosides; hypertension; atherosclerosis; loss of appetite; nausea; vomiting; numbness; tingling; muscle contractions and cramps; seizures (sudden changes in behavior caused by excessive electrical activity in the brain; personality changes; abnormal heart rhythms; coronary spasms
Potassium	Increased: Renal failure, use of potassium-sparing diuretics, acidosis, cell damage, dehydration, uncontrolled diabetes, Addison disease, syndrome of inappropriate antidiuretic hormone (SIADH), pneumonia, sepsis, shock, potassium supplements in presence of renal failure	Asymptomatic, bradyarrhythmias
	Decreased: Decreased intake of potassium during acute illness, nausea, and vomiting; increased renal loss; hypomagnesemia; hematologic disorders; certain antibiotics or diuretics; diarrhea (including the use of too many laxatives, which can cause diarrhea; diseases that affect the kidney's ability to retain potassium (e.g., Liddle syndrome, Cushing syndrome, hyperaldosteronism, Bartter syndrome, Fanconi syndrome), eating disorders (such as bulimia); sweating	Fatigue; confusion; muscle weakness and cramps; frank paralysis; breakdown of muscle fibers (rhabdomyolysis); atrial and ventricular ectopic beats; atrial and ventricular tachycardia; ventricular fibrillation; sudden death; atrioventricular conduction disturbances
Phosphorus	Increased: Rare unless in presence of renal dysfunction, hypoparathyroidism. Diabetic ketoacidosis, crush injuries, rhabdomyolysis, severe infections, ingestion of large amounts	Asymptomatic, severe arteriosclerosis (angina, poor peripheral perfusion, changes in multiple sclerosis), increased risk of myocardial infarction, stroke and peripheral artery disease, severe itching
	Decreased: Deficiency rare because it is so readily available in the food supply; decreased intake and impaired intestinal absorption of phosphate; vomiting; acidosis; alcoholic ketoacidosis	Anorexia; muscle weakness; osteomalacia; rhabdomyolysis; hemolytic anemia; impaired leukocyte and platelet function; progressive encephalopathy; coma; death
Chloride	Increased: Dehydration, multiple myeloma, kidney dysfunction, metabolic acidosis, hyperparathyroidism, pancreatitis, anemia, prolonged diarrhea, respiratory alkalosis, salicylate toxicity, alcohol abuse, congestive heart failure (CHF)	Rare, changes in mental status, confusion, malaise, bradyarrhythmias, hyperventilation, stupor, muscle twitching, weakness, nausea, vomiting, diarrhea
	Decreased: Fluid loss (e.g., excessive sweating, vomiting, or diarrhea); diuretics	Dehydration; loss of potassium in the urine; alkalosis
Sodium	Increased: Dehydration, hyperaldosteronism, CHF, hepatic failure, severe vomiting/diarrhea, steroid administration, intake or use of high-protein and nutrient-dense products without enough fluid, diabetes insipidus, Cushing disease, glycosuria, hypervolemia	Hypertension, mental status changes, confusion, thirsty, seizures, coma
	Decreased: Use of low-sodium nutritional supplements; vomiting; diarrhea; GI suction; renal disorders; diuretic therapy; burns; CHF; use of diuretics; kidney diseases; liver cirrhosis; sweating	Delirium and confusion; hallucinations; depressed sensorium; depressed deep tendon reflexes; hypothermia; Cheyne-Stokes respiration; pathologic reflexes; convulsions; fatigue; headache; irritability; loss of appetite; muscle spasms or cramps; muscle weakness; nausea and vomiting

shorten the duration of functional activities to avoid adverse effects of immobility and further metabolic stress.

Other tests such as serum total protein, including albumin and globulin levels, contribute information about acid–base balance, clotting, immune response, and blood and tissue osmotic pressure. Albumin is very important to maintaining vascular pressure, with low albumin related to significant edema, poor functional outcomes, and high mortality. The prealbumin level reflects current nutritional status and can be helpful in examining the effectiveness of nutritional interventions or to document further progression of the catabolic state.[21] For the acute care therapist, attending to albumin, total protein, and prealbumin levels will reveal the level of protein stores, state of malnutrition, or responsiveness to nutritional intervention. This factor may greatly influence the patient's ability to make gains in therapy and may directly impact functional outcomes.[22,23]

Cardiac enzyme studies are used to make the diagnosis of myocardial injury or myocardial infarction. There are several specific cardiac enzyme studies that can be analyzed: creatinine phosphokinase–MB isoenzymes, lactic dehydrogenase, troponin, and myoglobin. These enzymes are released at variable rates, so serial studies are needed to determine the peak level, extent of cellular injury and necrosis, and recovery rate.

Arterial Blood Gases. The sampling of arterial blood is used to determine the oxygenation state and the acid–base balance, specifically the concentration of hydrogen ions of the body. The pulmonary and renal systems regulate acids, such as carbonic and lactic acids, respectively. The renal system is also the principal regulator of bicarbonate (HCO_3^-), which is the major base of the body.

The partial pressure of oxygen (PaO_2) declines with age. This is due to the combination of a reduction in the elasticity of the musculoskeletal system, a decrease in muscle fibers, a decrease in the alveolar gas exchange surface area, and a decrease in the responsiveness of the central nervous system. These natural changes lead to a decline in PaO_2, which normally ranges from 80 to 100 mmHg from childhood to middle adulthood, by approximately 1 mmHg per year after the age of 60 years, or can be calculated by $PaO_2 = 109 - 0.43 \times age$.[24] It is important to keep this information close, because physical therapists commonly participate in the pulmonary care of patients and supplemental oxygen prescriptions. For a patient who is 75 years old, it would be perfectly normal to have a PaO_2 of 73 to 77 mmHg and show no signs of desaturation or respiratory decompensation.

To examine the acid–base balance, the physical therapist should first look at the pH using 7.4 as the normal level. If the pH is below 7.4, the patient is in an acidotic state, and any level greater than 7.4 is considered an alkalotic state. The physical therapist should next examine the partial pressure of carbon dioxide ($PaCO_2$), with 40 mmHg as the reference point, and a value higher or lower being acidotic and alkalotic, respectively. Finally, the therapist also needs to look at the HCO_3^- level, with a value greater than 24 being alkalotic and below 24 being acidotic. To determine whether the disorder is respiratory or metabolic, it is as simple as determining if the $PaCO_2$ or the HCO_3^- matchces the same state as the pH. If $PaCO_2$ is consistent with the pH, meaning if both $PaCO_2$ and pH are acidotic or alkalotic, then the patient is suffering from a *respiratory* acidotic or alkalotic state. However, if HCO_3^- matches the pH, then there is a *metabolic* acidosis or alkalosis. See Table 9-4 for causes and signs and symptoms of acid–base disorders.[5-7,9] See Table 9-5 for an example of respiratory acidosis and Table 9-6 for an example of metabolic alkalosis.

Arterial blood gases further quantify the body's response to acid–base imbalance. The renal and pulmonary systems compensate for these imbalances by altering $PaCO_2$ (lungs) for metabolic disorders and HCO_3^- (kidneys) for respiratory disorders. In the case of a respiratory disorder where the HCO_3^- is still within the normal range, the body has not begun to compensate, and therefore it is referred to as an absent compensation. If the pH and HCO_3^- are both outside the normal ranges, this is referred to as a partial compensation. Finally, if the pH has been brought back into the normal range, the acid–base balance would be referred to as a compensated condition. The compensatory description is the same for metabolic disorders as well. In the example in Box 9-1 earlier, there is an uncompensated respiratory acidosis because the pH has not been brought back to normal levels.

Understanding at least the basics of ABG analysis is important for the acute care therapist for several reasons. First, understanding what diseases or disorders may lead to a disruption of pH should guide the physical therapist to tailor the evaluation process, particularly due to the pulmonary system compensation. Knowing the associated signs and symptoms of the four basic categories of acid–base imbalance will aid the physical therapist in detecting medical changes and will alter the other health care team members' concerns. Finally, the degree of compensation should be considered when developing a current treatment plan or deciding if there is a need to hold therapy for the day.

Electrocardiogram (ECG)

Abnormalities in the electrical cardiac cycle can lead to various significant medical problems for the older adult patient, including falls, stroke, and HF. There are several changes to the conduction system of the heart with aging, including a reduction in conduction cells within the sinoatrial node and delay in the depolarization of the atria and ventricles.[20]

Even if the physical therapist is not familiar with reading an ECG, there are a few things to keep in mind

TABLE 9-4	Causes and Signs and Symptoms of Acid–Base Imbalances[5-7,9]	
	Cause	Signs/Symptoms
Respiratory acidosis	Central nervous system (CNS) injury to respiratory center (traumatic brain injury [TBI], tumor, cerebrovascular accident), airway obstruction, pulmonary disease, respiratory muscle weakness (Guillain-Barré syndrome, myasthenia gravis , spinal cord injury), flail chest, ↑ metabolism (sepsis, burns), CNS depressant drugs (barbiturates, sedatives, narcotics, anesthesia)	Hypoventilation, hypercapnia, headache, visual disturbances, coma, confusion, anxiety, restlessness, drowsiness, ↓ deep tendon reflex, hyperkalemia, ventricular fibrillation
Metabolic acidosis	Uncontrolled diabetes mellitus, starvation, renal failure, acetylsalicylic acid (ASA) overdose, prolonged stress or physical stress, hypoxia, severe diarrhea, ethanol abuse, metabolic/ethanol ketoacidosis, lactic acidosis	HCO_3^- deficit, headache, hyperventilation, mental dullness, deep respiration, stupor, coma, hyperkalemia, arrhythmias, muscle twitching/weakness, nausea/vomiting/diarrhea, malaise
Respiratory alkalosis	Hypoxemia (emphysema, pneumonia, acute respiratory distress syndrome), stimulation of CNS (sepsis, ammonia, ASA overdose, TBI, tumor, excessive exercise, or stress, severe pain), hyperventilation, hepatic encephalopathy, congestive heart failure, pulmonary embolism, impaired lung disease (internal pancreatic fistulae, ascites, scoliosis, pregnancy)	Hypocapnia, tachypnea, lightheadedness, numbness/peripheral tingling, tetany, convulsions, diaphoresis, muscle twitching, hypokalemia, arrhythmias
Metabolic alkalosis	Loss of hydrochloric acid, loss of potassium, diarrhea, exercise, ingestion of alkaline substances, steroids, diuresis, nasogastric suctioning, peptic ulcer disease (PUD), massive blood transfusion	HCO_3^- excess, hypoventilation, mental confusion and agitation, dizziness, peripheral numbness, muscle twitching, tetany, convulsions, hypokalemia, arrhythmias

TABLE 9-5	Example of Respiratory Acidosis			
	Patient	Normal Range	Reference	Acidotic/Alkalotic
pH	7.24	7.35-7.45	7.4	Acidotic
PaO_2	74 mmHg	80-100 mmHg		
$PaCO_2$	67 mmHg	35-45 mmHg	40 mmHg	Acidotic
HCO_3^-	27 mEq/L	22-26 mEq/L	24 mEq/L	Alkalotic

TABLE 9-6	Example of Metabolic Alkalosis			
	Patient	Normal Range	Reference	Acidotic/Alkalotic
pH	7.5	7.35-7.45	7.4	Alkalotic
PaO_2	77 mmHg	80-100 mmHg		
$PaCO_2$	48 mmHg	35-45 mmHg	40 mmHg	Acidotic
HCO_3^-	37 mEq/L	22-26 mEq/L	24 mEq/L	Alkalotic

when working with patients. First, when looking at an ECG strip, immediately after the QRS complex, the large vertical spike that represents ventricular depolarization, the ventricles should contract, which is followed by a pulsatile flow of blood that should be felt at the peripheral pulses. It is useful to make sure that the rate of contraction heard when the physical therapist auscultates over the left chest wall is equal to the peripheral pulse. If some of the contractions eject a small amount of blood, the peripheral pulse may not be felt.

It is also important to remember that the time the heart contracts is the period of the highest myocardial oxygen consumption or demand. If the patient's heart rate is high, then there is a possibility that the coronary blood flow cannot keep up with demand and the patient may experience dysrhythmias and angina. Angina is defined as a discomfort that is experienced above the waist that is not associated with any musculoskeletal or neuromuscular dysfunction. Angina is commonly experienced substernally with or without radiation down the left upper extremity, but it is extremely important that the physical therapist does not forget that there are many patients who do not present with classic symptoms. Others may report discomfort of the jaw, back, right upper extremity or gastrointestinal discomfort.

Another point to remember about the ECG is that the time between QRS complexes is the time that the ventricles fill to send blood into the coronary arteries for myocardial perfusion. When the heart rate is high, there is a reduction in ventricular filling time that can reduce the forward flow of blood, particularly when the myocardial tissue is not able to compensate. There is also a reduction in myocardial perfusion time that may lead to angina.

There are other dysrhythmias that are associated with diseases such as hypertension and coronary disease. Hypertension is associated with myocardial left ventricular hypertrophy.[25] Over time, this may lead to enlargement of the left atrium because more blood is being held in the cardiac chambers at the end of contraction. The enlargement of the left atrium is associated with irritability of the atrial tissue and an abnormal control of rhythm, atrial fibrillation (Figure 9-1). The classic presentation of atrial fibrillation is an unpredictable, irregular heart rate. The patient may become symptomatic if the rate becomes too fast and the heart cannot meet the oxygen demand or the myocardium cannot compensate for the lower volume of blood delivered to the ventricles for circulation throughout the body. The patient may report angina, fatigue, shortness of breath, and dizziness, and changes in mentation may be noted.

Arrhythmias generated from the ventricles, premature ventricular contractions (PVCs), are also common with aging, but are benign when the dysrhythmia is less than 8 beats per minute (bpm) and the patient's heart is able to compensate for the premature contractions. Another ventricular dysrhythmia with an increased incidence among older adults is referred to as a bundle branch block (BBB) (Figure 9-2) which, again, may also be benign, but in the presence of depressed myocardial

dysfunction may lead to signs and symptoms including fatigue, decreased activity tolerance, and shortness of breath.

It is important to know the patient's history of dysrhythmias and current ECG rhythm. If equipment permits, monitoring the rate, rhythm, and regularity during activities will allow the therapist to document any changes along with any signs and symptoms during activity. Patients with a history of dysrhythmias may have a temporary or permanent pacemaker or an automatic implantable coronary defibrillator. For the patient with a temporary pacemaker, the physical therapist should understand what the underlying rhythm is and the patient's heart function (myocardial perfusion and contractility function). The physical therapist should make sure that the temporary pacer wires are secured, to reduce risk of disconnection during mobilization. For the patients with an internal defibrillator, it is important to know at what heart rate level the device will deliver a shock to the patient. The physical therapist needs to monitor these patients and avoid exercising beyond this heart rate level to avoid unwarranted shocks.

Operative Reports

After understanding the inpatient or outpatient operative procedures a patient may have undergone, the therapist may alter the examination process and identify precautions and restrictions. This information may also assist the physical therapist in working with the primary care or specialty service team in establishing mobility guidelines with the goal of protecting the surgical site to promote healing and allow the patient to achieve the highest level of function and possibly permit the avoidance of complications related to immobility such as pressure sores, pneumonia, and DVT.

The chart review, when possible, is an extremely important step in initiating the examination as it provides vital information about the patient's past and present medical status. There is typically a differential diagnosis list and a working medical diagnosis that can help to guide the physical therapist to develop and prioritize the examination. The presenting signs and symptoms associated with a chronic disease such as HF and obstructive lung disease may be helpful for the physical therapist to document and understand. This information may lead the physical therapist to educate the patient on proper self-monitoring with the goal that the patient will seek medical assistance prior to the need for admission to the emergency department. At the end of the chart review process, the physical therapist should be able to formulate a clinical picture of the patient in preparation for the examination process, determine the need for possible referrals, and probable discharge recommendations.

Beyond the chart review, the physical therapist should discuss the patient's situation with other members of

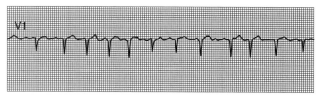

FIGURE 9-1 Example of atrial fibrillation.

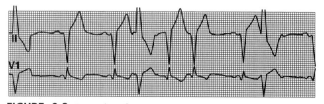

FIGURE 9-2 Example of premature ventricular contractions and bundle branch blocks in leads II and V1.

the medical team. The members of the team will have information that may not be contained within the chart at the time of the physical therapist consult. The therapist should also extend the information gathering to include the family or caregiver and patient.

Review of Systems. Beyond the chart review and standard interview, the physical therapist should also complete a review of systems. The review of systems is a method of screening the major organ systems in order to determine if the patient has certain symptoms that may lead the therapist to make a medical referral for further testing. In the acute care setting, this process is shared by the medical team, but the physical therapist should be aware of the process and may be able to add to this review to improve medical care and outcomes. The reader is referred to Table 9-7 for an example of a review of symptoms form that shows as an example of what may possibly be included in the medical review and places where the physical therapist may contribute to the screening process based upon the facility's practice, particular medical services, and type of clientele. The physical therapist should recognize the necessity of including in the questioning symptoms in the 3, 6, and 12 months prior to admission. Box 9-2 represents the implications of the review of symptoms.

Beyond the review of systems, the physical therapist should examine the patient for specific factors based upon age, occupation, and other behaviors. The most well-established risk factor screening is for CAD. Risk factors include the causative factors of smoking, diabetes, and hypertension; predisposing factors include obesity, inactivity, abnormal lipid profile, and family history. Other factors to consider include age, gender, and stress (see Box 9-3 for risk factors for CAD).[14] After establishing how many risk factors the patient exhibits, the physical therapist should determine if the patient is experiencing pain or discomfort above the waist that cannot be attributed to a musculoskeletal or neuromuscular dysfunction, shortness of breath at rest or with mild exertion, dizziness or syncope, orthopnea or paroxysmal nocturnal dyspnea, lower extremity edema, palpitations or tachycardia, claudication, known heart murmur, and/or unusual fatigue.[14] Finally, once all the risk factors are determined, the physical therapist can determine the risk level of a cardiac event during exertion. Box 9-4 lists the American College of Sports Medicine's (ACSM) risk stratification categories.[14]

The process of risk-stratifying patients for heart disease and other diseases, even in the acute care setting, can aid the therapist in determining what components of the examination should be completed and up to what

TABLE 9-7	Example of a Review of Symptoms	
Please place an X on any statement or condition that you have been feeling in the last 1 month, and 3 months		
1 month	**3 months**	
		Cognitive/Mood State
		Decreased ability to recall current events
		Decreased ability to remember past events
		Decrease in short-term memory
		Decreased ability to concentrate
		Decreased ability to focus in a busy room
		Decreased ability to complete a task
		Increase in tripping or falling
		Increase in making mistakes
		Difficulty falling asleep
		Difficulty staying asleep
		Wakes up coughing
		Wakes up short of breath
		Wakes up anxious
		Wakes up with pain
		Feeling depressed
		Feeling anxious
		Stopped participating in usual activities
		Stopped traveling out into the community
		Prefer to stay at home
		Prefer to be alone
		More irritable or quicker to being angry
		Feeling of forgetfulness

Continued

TABLE 9-7	Example of a Review of Symptoms—cont'd	
1 month	**3 months**	

1 month	3 months	
		General
		Increased fatigue
		Experiencing fever or chills
		Unplanned weight loss
		Change in voice or prolonged sore throat
		Increase in thirst or appetite
		Decreased appetite
		Body aches or malaise
		Dizziness or lightheadedness
		Changes in smell
		Changes in hearing, ringing in ears
		Dental pain, mouth sores
		Sweet odor to breath
		Brittle hair or nails
		Any lumps or masses
		Temperature intolerance (heat or cold)
		Muscles and Nerves
		Joint pain, swelling, or redness
		Increase in incidence of headaches
		Change in vision or hearing
		Difficulty finding words or speaking clearly
		Muscle soreness, weakness
		Numbness, tingling
		Dizziness or vertigo
		Decrease in coordination, feeling clumsy
		Pain radiating into arms or legs
		Restlessness, or tremors
		Decreased memory
		Loss of consciousness
		Muscle cramps
		Bones and Skin
		Joint swelling or stiffness
		Muscle pain or weakness
		Significant loss of body height
		White and painful fingers or toes
		Change in appearance of nails
		Skin discoloration
		Open wounds
		Skin rashes or itching
		Moles or skin marks that have changed in size or color
		Changes in hair (loss, additional growth, brittle)
		Heart and Blood Vessels
		Chest pain, pressure, heaviness, or tightness
		Irregular pulse (heart rate speeds up, slows down, and skips beats)
		Legs ache with walking or stair climbing
		Edema in feet or legs
		Weight gain despite loss of muscle
		Fatigue
		Shortness of breath at rest or during activity
		Avoidance of usual activities
		Discoloration or painful feet or legs
		Swelling in one leg or arm
		Any pain that goes away when you rest
		Changes in heart rate or blood pressure
		Persistent cough
		Bleeding

Continued

TABLE 9-7	Example of a Review of Symptoms—cont'd	
1 month	**3 months**	
		Pulmonary
		Shortness of breath
		Persistent cough
		Chest wall pain
		Clubbing of finger and toe nails
		Productive cough, increase in sputum production
		Abdomen
		Changes in appetite or taste
		Difficulty swallowing
		Abdominal pain
		Sense of bloating, gas
		Changes in bowel behavior
		Incontinence of bowel or bladder
		Changes in color or consistency of stool
		Indigestion or heartburn
		Nausea, vomiting, diarrhea
		Changes in urination pattern, stream, or color
		Pain or burning with urination
		Needing to urinate at night
		Hesitation or urgency to urinate
		Gender
		Decrease in sexual interest or activity
		Pain with sexual activity
		Female
		Changes in menstrual cycle
		Vaginal discharge
		Possibility of pregnancy
		Spotting or bleeding
		Irregular moods
		Changes in breast shapes, lumps or masses, painfulness
		Male
		Impotence
		Testicular pain
		Penile discharge
		Genital lesion

intensity level of exercise the patient can safely participate in, as well as guiding the follow-up interventions, home exercise program, and education. Depending upon the type of patient risk factors, the evaluation should be completed by the physical therapist in order to determine if the patient is at risk for other pathologies such as pulmonary disease, osteoporosis, cancer, or diabetes. Box 9-5 demonstrates some of the risk factors for type 2 diabetes, cancer, and osteoporosis.[26-28]

Risk factor stratification is a very important process for the therapist to complete for each patient. After the physical therapist has stratified a patient for the likelihood of having cardiovascular or pulmonary disease, or the likelihood of the patient experiencing medical difficulty during exercise, this information can be used to direct the examination and patient education and give appropriate referrals to physicians, program centers, or other health care professionals.

SYSTEMS REVIEW

Mental Status

Assessing the mental status of a patient can be difficult in the presence of acute and chronic medical conditions, and in the older adult population, this can be more of a challenge because of the increased incidence of dementia and Alzheimer's disease. Changes in mental state may be associated with a variety of factors, including metabolic disturbances, coexisting comorbidities, medications, and environmental conditions.[29] From a metabolic state, the therapist must recognize that hypoxemia, anemia, hyperglycemia, electrolyte imbalances, malnutrition, and dehydration are contributing factors to changes in mental status. Polypharmaceutical use in the older adult population is very common and has been associated not only with increased risk of falls[30] but also altered mental

BOX 9-2	The Implications of Review of Systems

Consider a patient with CAD. It is very common for patients to self-limit themselves to avoid symptoms, so their answers to questions such as "Are you presently experiencing chest discomfort with exertion or excessive fatigue after exertion?" may be negative but follow that up to include "Over the past year have you noticed a decrease in the activities you are willing to do, such as going on community outings, vacuuming, etc., or an increase in the time it takes for you to complete regular daily activities?"

Case: a 72-year-old man presents with excessive fatigue, clumsiness, and a recent fall. On the review of systems, the patient reports an increase in fatigue, inability to mow his lawn without taking rest breaks, and a decreased frequency in urination. He reports being treated for hypertension and has been experiencing this clumsiness for about 2 months. Fatigue is such a nondescript symptom and can be caused by multiple pathologies. The physical therapist puts forth other questions to determine if the fatigue is related to pathologies such as cardiac or renal disease, diabetes, or cancer. The patient revealed that he has been limiting his activity level to avoid shortness of breath with exertion. He reported tightness in the waist of his pants and that he is more comfortable sleeping in his recliner chair. With this information, the therapist knew to complete a thorough examination of the cardiovascular system, including heart and lung sounds, inspection for pitted edema, and jugular vein distention. With the findings of these tests, the therapist discussed with the medical team concerns for uncompensated heart failure.

These types of time-based questions are important to ask when screening for cardiovascular, metabolic, and oncologic conditions. The review of systems should lead the therapist to formulate and prioritize the examination to eventually determine a plan of care that may include recommendations for further medical evaluation and interventions.

BOX 9-4	ACSM Risk Stratification Categories[14]
Low risk	Men younger than age 45 years and women younger than age 55 years who are asymptomatic and meet no more than one risk factor
Moderate risk	Men age 45 years or older and women age 55 years or older or those who meet two or more risk factors
High risk	Individuals with one or more signs and symptoms or known cardiovascular, pulmonary, or metabolic disease

surgery, as well as the patient's environment, and use of restraints and medical equipment, such as Foley catheters, as contributing factors to a decline in mental status.

Delirium, also referred to as an acute organic brain syndrome, acute organic mental disorder, or acute confusional state, is a syndrome defined as an acute decline in mental status associated with transient changes that, in many cases, are reversible. The patient typically presents with fluctuations in levels of alertness, inability to attend to a task, perceptual disturbance, visual hallucinations, and a decline in cognitive skills such as learning, processing, and problem solving. Delirium may also be associated with changes in mood state such as withdrawal or agitation and combativeness.[29,32,33] There are three states of delirium: the hyperactive state in which the patient is restless and agitated; the hypoactive state where the patient is lethargic and withdrawn; and a mixed state where the patient's behavior fluctuates between the hyperactive and hypoactive states.[33] Delirium is often misdiagnosed as dementia in the older adult patient, which can lead to high mortality rates, longer lengths of stay in medical facilities, and poorer functional outcomes. Of note, there is a higher incidence of delirium in patients who have a baseline of dementia.[32]

Delirium is a significant issue when working with the older adult, particularly those in an institutional setting

status.[31] The therapist should not overlook the use of alcohol and over-the-counter or illicit drug use when gathering information during the evaluation. Finally, besides the past medical history of the patient, the therapist needs to recognize the effects of surgery, of general anesthesia and the physical stress associated with

BOX 9-3	Risk Factors for Coronary Artery Disease[14]	
Positive Risk Factors	**Defining Criteria**	
Family history	Myocardial infarction, coronary revascularization, or sudden death before 55 years of age in father or other male first-degree relative or before 65 years of age in mother or other female first-degree relative	
Smoking	Current cigarette smoker or those who quit within the previous 6 months	
Hypertension	Systolic BP ≥140 mmHg, or diastolic BP ≥90 mmHg, confirmed on at least two consecutive occasions, or on hypertensive medication	
Dyslipidemia	Low-density lipoprotein >130 mg/dL, high-density lipoprotein <40 mg/dL, on lipid-lowering medications, total cholesterol >200 mg/dL	
Impaired fasting glucose	Fasting blood glucose ≥100 mg/dL confirmed by measurements on at least two separate occasions	
Obesity	Body mass index >30 kg/m², or waist girth >102 cm for men and 88 cm for women, or waist/hip ratio ≥0.95 for men and ≥0.86 for women.	
Sedentary lifestyle	Not participating in a regular exercise program or not meeting the minimal physical activity recommendations from the U.S. Surgeon General's Report	

Modified from ACSM.

BOX 9-5	Common Risk Factors Associated with Three Common Medical Issues in the Older Adult[26-28]		
Type 2 Diabetes	**Cancer**	**Osteoporosis**	
Obesity	Tobacco use	Age	
Hypertension	Excessive alcohol use	Family history	
Hypercholesterolemia	Excessive sun exposure	Low body weight	
Race (African American)	Inactivity	Race (Caucasian, Asian)	
Genetics	Being overweight or obese	Menopause	
Inactive lifestyle	Others specific to each cancer	History of fractures	
Glucose intolerance		Diet	

(acute care hospital, subacute hospital, or a long-term-care facility), because of its high incidence and its impact on medical and functional outcomes. The therapist should be aware of the features of delirium. This syndrome has a typically acute onset of inattention, disorganized thinking, a change in the level of consciousness, disorientation, decreased memory, perceptual disturbances, and altered sleep–wake cycles.[34] It has been reported that as many as 25% of older adult patients admitted to the hospital will exhibit a delirious state, and an additional 30% will develop delirium. In the intensive care units, the incidence of delirium can reach as high as 90% and there is a higher discharge rate to long-term-care facilities for those with delirium.[32,34] In long-term-care facilities, delirium cases are reported in approximately 45% of the residents.[29] Consequently, the therapist should have the ability to contribute to the team by reporting delirium to improve morbidity and mortality and decrease health care costs associated with delirium.

Dementia may sometimes be separate or intertwined with delirium, which can complicate the evaluation and intervention process and significantly affect outcomes. Dementia is a syndrome of gradual onset and progressive decline of cognitive function. It is a common disorder in older adults that progresses with each decade of life. Alzheimer's disease and cerebral vascular insufficiency are the two more common causes of dementia, with Alzheimer's disease accounting for 50% to 60% of all cases.[35] There are a variety of standardized instruments that are used to screen and evaluate for dementia, such as the Folstein Mini Mental Status Exam. See Chapter 8, Cognition in the Aging Adult, for specific details related to evaluation of delirium and dementia.

Vital Signs

Every therapist, regardless of the practice setting and type of patient population treated, should be evaluating the patient's resting vital signs and response to exertion. Even in the acute care setting where the patient's vitals are routinely monitored, the therapist can provide valuable information about the patient's tolerance to upright postures, functional mobility, and activity tolerance. This information can assist in medical decision making,

including medication prescription as well as surgical management.

Heart Rate. The therapist should begin with an assessment of resting heart rate (HR). It is helpful if the patient can give you an estimate of what their HR and blood pressure (BP) typically run to establish a baseline. In the assessment of the pulse and heart rate, the therapist should appreciate the rate, regularity, and quality. When assessing regularity, the therapist is assessing the equal and consistent beat of the pulse. Regularity is defined as having less than six interruptions in the rhythm in 1 minute. If the pulse is regular, the rate can be calculated by counting the number of beats within 15 seconds and then multiplying that number by 4 to calculate the heart rate per minute. If the rate is irregular, the therapist should count the number of beats throughout the entire minute. For some patients who have an irregular pulse and those patients with a history of left ventricular dysfunction, the therapist should verify the palpatory rate with the auscultatory rate. The auscultatory rate can be taken over the left anterior chest wall, around the second intercostal space where the closure of the aortic valve can clearly be heard. Finally, the therapist should appreciate the quality, or how well the pulse is felt upon palpation. A pulse that is described as bounding is very difficult to obstruct, whereas a thready pulse is weak and easily obstructed and is, at times, rapid. Possible causes of a bounding pulse include exercise, fever, anxiety, arrhythmia, volume overload, and hypertension. A thready pulse is associated with dehydration, arrhythmias, aortic stenosis, ketoacidosis, and shock.

The therapist should also consider what is referred to as heart rate reserve (HRR), how much the heart can increase its rate from the resting value to respond to demand and it reflects the heart's ability to increase cardiac output. The physical therapist may infer how much activity the patient can tolerate from this calculation (Box 9-6). Heart rate reserve can be calculated by subtracting the resting HR from the maximal (predicted or actual) HR. Predicted HR is commonly estimated by 220 minus age, which has a standard deviation of 14 bpm. Actual maximal HR would be available if the patient had undergone some form of exercise test.

BOX 9-6	Application of Heart Rate Reserve

There are two patients who are 70 years of age with similar medical histories and functional abilities. They are admitted to the hospital with pneumonia. They both have a predicted maximal HR of 150 bpm. The first patient's resting HR is 70 bpm, which gives him an HRR of 80 bpm. The second patient has a resting HR of 120 bpm and therefore an HRR of 30 bpm. The physical therapist should expect the first patient to have a higher activity tolerance than the second patient because the first patient's heart rate is more able to compensate during exertion before reaching maximum HR.

Blood Pressure and Hypertension

Pulse Pressure. Pulse pressure can be easily assessed by the clinician and has significant predictive value in cardiovascular disease. Pulse pressure examines cardiovascular compliance—the ability of the arteries to vasoconstrict and vasodilate in order to circulate blood to properly meet activity demands. Pulse pressure is calculated by subtracting diastolic blood pressure from systolic pressure. With age there is a decrease in compliance of the aorta and small arteries, which leads to an elevation of systolic pressure and a decline in diastolic pressure, causing an increase in pulse pressure. Pulse pressure can also be elevated with exercise, aortic insufficiency, atherosclerosis, and when a patient has an elevated intracranial pressure, whereas it will narrow in the presence of aortic stenosis, HF, and pericarditis. As pulse pressure widens, there is an increase in the incidence of cardiovascular disease. Generally, a normal pulse pressure at rest is approximately 40 mmHg. A study conducted by Weiss et al found that an increased pulse pressure in the very old hospitalized patients was a predictor of higher mortality[36] and, therefore, when pulse pressure exceeds 60 mmHg, a medical referral should promptly be made.

Orthostatic Hypotension. Orthostatic hypotension is defined as a decrease in systolic BP by 20 mmHg or a drop by 10 mmHg with a reflexive increase in HR with transitional movements, such as moving from supine-to-sit or sit-to-stand. The incidence of orthostasis increases 20% in community-dwelling people older than age 65 years and has been reported to be as high as 50% in frail older adults living in nursing homes.[37] There are many causes of orthostatic hypotension, including adverse effects of medications, dehydration, anemia, arrhythmias, immobility, sepsis, adrenal insufficiency, and autonomic dysfunction related to diseases like diabetes, Parkinson's disease and central nervous system impairments.[38]

The patient may or may not be symptomatic with orthostatic hypotension and regardless of whether the patient demonstrates symptoms they are at risk for sustaining injuries, including falls, fractures, myocardial infarction, and cerebral injuries. The most common symptoms experienced are lightheadedness, dizziness, weakness, syncope, and angina. Some clients may experience visual and speech deficits, confusion, and changes in cognitive function. It is difficult to utilize symptoms as an indication of orthostasis, because the complexity of the older adult patient's medical history and presentation may be related to various issues. Therefore, it is critical that the therapist screen the patient's BP with position changes to rule out orthostatic hypotension. To thoroughly rule out orthostasis, the client should be monitored before and after medications, before breakfast, after meals, and before bed.[37]

Response to Exertion. Blood pressure assessment at rest and during exertion is a key examination that a physical therapist can provide toward assessing tolerance during exertion that can assist in medication prescription. The incidence of hypertension (HTN) rises with age, so it is very important to screen BP with every patient. Hypertension is an independent risk factor for cardiovascular and renal disease. The Joint National Committee on Prevention, Detection, Evaluation, and Treatment of High Blood Pressure is urging the health care field to focus not only on treating HTN, defined as a BP of 140/90 mmHg, but to also address pre-HTN, BP of 120/80 to 139/89 mmHg, with the goal being to decrease the incidence of CAD, stroke, and renal disease.[39] Not only can the therapist document the presence of HTN and make the proper referral for medical management but they can also assess the effectiveness of antihypertensive medications. Evaluation for HTN should be assessed on at least two to three consecutive sessions,[14] and if the patient is found to have either resting or exercise HTN, he or she should be referred for medical management.[39] See Table 9-8 for the classification of HTN. A physical therapist can have a major impact on a person's health care by assessing the patient's blood pressure during exertion, which few other practitioners do, so that a hypertensive blood pressure response to activity can be documented and appropriately treated.

During the examination process, the therapist should monitor the patient's vital signs with activity to determine if the client is having an appropriate HR and BP response to a given workload. It can be helpful to examine physiological response during common activities of daily living (ADLs) and instrumental activities of daily living (IADLs), as well as during a more formal exercise test. It should be noted that patients taking β-blocker medications will have some HR and BP response, although blunted, to an increase in workload. In these situations, it can be helpful to look at an activity chart to determine the patient's estimated metabolic equivalent level (MET level) to examine the relationship between vital signs and workload.[40] There should be an expectation that HR and BP and perception of work should rise with demand. In general, HR should increase 10 to 12 bpm and systolic BP should increase 10 to 12 mmHg per MET level in the absence of medications that will lead to a blunted response.

TABLE 9-8	Classification of Hypertension[14]		
	Systolic Blood Pressure (mmHg)		Diastolic Blood Pressure (mmHg)
Optimal	<120	and	<80
Pre-hypertension	120-139	or	80-89
Hypertension			
Stage 1	140-159	or	90-99
Stage 2	160-179	or	100-109
Stage 3	≥ 180	or	≥110

To complete the assessment of response to exertion, the therapist should take note of the vital sign response during the recovery phase. There should not be any immediate increase in HR upon stopping exercise, which would suggest that the patient is experiencing a reflexive cardiac response to venous pooling or orthostasis. However, within the first minute of recovery, there should be a significant decrease in systolic BP and HR. The rate of HR recovery has been linked to mortality and morbidity related to cardiovascular disease. Heart rate recovery of less than 12 beats in 1 minute walking recovery is associated with poor prognosis and a rate of HR recovery less than 42 beats at 2 minutes into recovery after a submaximal exercise test in older adults is associated with increased mortality rate from a cardiovascular event.[14,41]

Rate Pressure Product. Rate pressure product (RPP) represents an estimate of myocardial oxygen consumption and should increase as workload increases. Using the HR and BP data that were recorded at rest and during the various activities performed, the therapist can calculate the RPP by multiplying the HR with the systolic blood pressure. This can be valuable when working with a patient who has a history of coronary disease and the therapist wants to assess for myocardial limitations to exertion. Rate pressure product is also known as the anginal threshold because once the oxygen demand during exertion exceeds the coronary artery's ability to carry sufficient blood and oxygen to the myocardium, ischemia begins and the client will most likely become symptomatic. The point of imbalance between oxygen supply and demand can be predicted by examining the RPP. The therapist can use this information to document symptoms, the MET level where symptoms appear, monitor the progression of the disease, and progress the rehabilitation plan in a patient with known disease. This information can also be helpful in making a referral for medical workup and to design a safe exercise program below the anginal threshold.

Pulmonary Function

During the interview and examination process the therapist should also note the respiratory rate and breathing pattern. The average resting adult respiratory rate ranges from 12 to 20 breaths per minute.

The inspiratory-to-expiratory ratio should be 1:2. When the ratio becomes closer to 1:1, it may indicate hyperventilation, possibly associated with anxiety or a metabolic problem such as uncontrolled diabetes, alcohol abuse, or a restrictive pulmonary disease. A ratio that reaches 1:3 or greater can be associated with obstructive lung diseases like asthma, chronic bronchitis, and emphysema. The therapist should document the patient's ability to increase the depth and rate of breathing with an increase in exertion. There should be an expansion of the chest wall in all cardinal planes and the therapist should see initiation and expansion of the upper abdominal wall during inspiration, indicating diaphragmatic function. The patient should also be able to speak approximately 12 to 15 syllables per breath at rest. If the therapist has access to a pulse oximeter, oxygen saturation at rest and during exercise should be documented. For people with light complexion, a value greater than 92% at rest is normal and these values should not decrease with exercise, whereas that number increases to 95% for darker-skinned people.[42] It should be noted that pulse oximeter accuracy decreases significantly in darker-pigmented patients, especially with saturation values of less than 80%.[43] A value of less than 90% at rest or during exercise is abnormal and a value less than 88% indicates the need for supplemental oxygen.[44] If the therapist notes deviations in these respiratory factors, further investigation of the cardiopulmonary system is warranted. The physical therapist must recognize the limits of the pulse oximeter, which include inaccuracies in the reading and the fact that the device is measuring the percentage of existing hemoglobin to carry oxygen. Depending on the quality of the device, there may be as much as a 5% to 6% error rate, which becomes more inaccurate for patients who have atrial fibrillation or other highly irregular dysrhythmias, or when the oxygen saturation rates drop below 90%.[45]

Auscultation

As part of the assessment, the therapist should listen to the heart and lungs, both at rest and during exercise. Many therapists are unfamiliar and feel very uncomfortable with their auscultation skills, but the only way to begin to feel more confident is to listen to the chest walls of many patients. Not only is auscultation an important examination skill in order to rule out cardiopulmonary disease or dysfunction but it is also important to assess the heart and lungs during exercise prescription as it may reveal a reason for exercise intolerance. The authors encourage every therapist to listen to everyone's chest wall to build his or her skills. There are multiple heart and lung sounds posted on the Internet to provide examples of various sounds for independent learning.

When listening to basic heart sounds, the therapist should first assess the quality of valvular closure. If the valves are functioning properly, there should be a nice crisp and definitive sound. The best place to listen to the atrioventricular valves (tricuspid and mitral) is in the right fifth intercostal space, midclavicular line. Then the therapist should place the diaphragm over the second intercostal space just right of the sternum to hear the aortic valve the loudest. If the therapist does not hear a crisp, strong closure at rest or a sound that appears or worsens with exercise, the medical team should be notified. Next the therapist should place the bell of the stethoscope back over the mitral valve area. The therapist should vary the pressure between the bell and chest wall in order to hear low-pitched sounds. When the therapist presses the bell lightly on the chest wall, low-pitched sounds can be heard and when the therapist then presses the bell firmly, the low-pitched sound disappears. The appearance of an additional sound may indicate an atrial or ventricular gallop. If a harsh straining, a lush sound, or a low-pitched sound is heard at rest, worsens with exercise, or appears with exercise, the therapist should seek further assessment for the patient. Murmurs may be appreciated either during the systolic or diastolic phase of the cardiac cycle. Systolic murmurs can be heard between S1 and S2 and are associated with semilunar valve stenosis or atrioventricular valve incompetence. Diastolic murmurs are associated with atrioventricular valve stenosis or semilunar valve incompetence. See Figure 9-3 for a diagram of the heart sounds. A stenotic valve sounds harsh or strained, whereas an incompetent valve has a lush or swish-like sound. Some abnormal sounds may be benign, but most sounds are associated with a valvular problem or a dysfunction of the myocardium and must be further investigated.[46] Finally, a leathery rubbing sound heard over the chest wall that persists when the patient holds his or her breath, could possibly be a pericardial friction rub and should be further worked up. A pericardial rub is associated with friction between the pericardium and myocardium and is associated with inflammation or fluid within the pericardium. It is very helpful if the therapist is able to inform the physician if the sound worsens or appears with exertion, because many times the patient is examined at rest by the medical team.

The therapist should then listen to each major section of the lung, anteriorly, laterally, and posteriorly. At rest, the patient should be instructed to breathe slightly deeper than normal, in and out through the mouth. Refer to Figure 9-4 for general guidelines for auscultation sites and Table 9-9 for a brief description of types of lung sounds and associated causes.[47-49] The therapist should appreciate a gentle rustling sound that is louder the closer the therapist places the stethoscope to the main bronchus.[50] The therapist should not normally hear any wheezing or crackling sounds, as this can be indicative of lung disease. Lung sounds should be assessed at rest and during exercise to once again assess for cardiopulmonary disease and exercise intolerance.

Nutritional Status and Physical Appearance

The therapist needs to recognize the association between proper nutrition, body composition, and activity tolerance in order to progress in rehabilitation.[51,52] The therapist can refer to the Tufts University website for basic dietary recommendations for older adults.[53] In the acute care setting, the nutritional status is addressed and closely monitored by clinical dieticians and physicians, but the physical therapist needs to be aware of the plan and can contribute valuable information to the dietary plan of care.

There are many reasons why the older individual is susceptible to malnutrition and this type of screening should be part of the physical therapist evaluation, even in the acute care setting, because unless a complication arises, or the patient has diverted from the expected medical pathway, the patient's nutritional status may not be assessed or addressed during the hospital stay. Common factors that adversely influence nutritional status may include poor dentition, limited income, depression, cognitive impairments, chronic diseases, decreased ability to smell, and altered taste, particularly from medications.

In general, a decrease in activity level and decline in muscle mass likely account for the decrease in basal metabolic rate and a need for a lower caloric intake, but if the individual was active prior to admission, their dietary needs may be equal to that of a young adult's.[54] There are many reasons why the older adult requires an increase in dietary requirements, such as an increase in protein and total calories at times, such as in the presence of an infection, wounds, or stress. See Table 9-10 for general dietary recommendations for the older adult.

Energy requirements for the older adult can be difficult to determine because of complex medical histories, including HF, renal dysfunction, and different types of cancer. A specialized diet recommendation from a registered clinical dietician may be warranted. It is important to discuss with the referring physician and the patient about a clinical dietary referral to ensure the best health and wellness results and to account for the calories spent during rehabilitation (www.health.gov/dietaryguidelines/dga2005/document/default.htm).

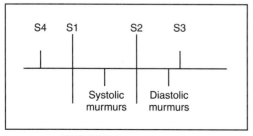

FIGURE 9-3 Heart sounds.

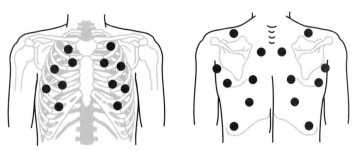

FIGURE 9-4 Lung auscultation sites. *(Redrawn from Buckingham EB: A primer of clinical diagnosis, ed 2, New York, 1979, Harper & Row.)*

TABLE 9-9	Lung Sounds[47-49]	
Normal Breath Sounds		
	Description	**Location**
Bronchial	Loud, high-pitched sound with a shorter inspiratory than expiratory duration with a pause between each phase of ventilation	Heard normally adjacent to the sternum.
Bronchovesicular	Softer version of bronchial sounds, except are continuous throughout ventilation	Normally heard between the scapulae from T3 to T6 and at the costosternal border of ICS 2 and 3
Vesicular	Low-pitched, muffled sound. Inspiratory sound is louder, longer, and higher in pitch than expiration	Normally heard in the peripheral lung fields
Adventitious Sounds		
	Description	**Dysfunction**
Crackles (rales): inspiratory	May be heard throughout respiratory cycle Heard in the early inspiratory phase Heard in the late inspiratory phase	Associated with fluid or secretion retention Associated with opening of proximal airways Atelectasis, pulmonary edema, fibrosis, or compression of lung tissue from a pleural effusion
Crackles (rales): expiratory	A rhythmic sound Nonrhythmic sound	Associated with opening of more proximal airways Associated with fluid and secretions in large airways
Wheezes: High pitched	A continuous, constant pitch of varying durations Inspiratory Expiratory	 Suggestive of rigid airways, bronchospasm, foreign-body partial obstruction, or stenosis Reflects unstable airways that have collapsed. It is associated with airway obstruction
Wheezes: Low pitched (rhonchus)	Low-pitched, continuous sound Expiratory	Associated with obstruction of airway, commonly thick secretions Reflects unstable airways, airway obstruction
Pleural friction rub	Course, grating, leathery sound from the pulmonary system	Inflammation

Observing the client's appearance can generally provide the clinician with valuable information of general health and well-being. The appearance of the patient's skin and fingernails can reveal the presence of pathology. The detection of body or oral odors can suggest diseases such as uncontrolled diabetes, dental abscesses, or pulmonary infections. Body odors and appearance may also suggest alcohol and tobacco abuse, incontinence, and organ dysfunction. Appearance may also suggest the need for a social work consult for referral to community resources and services. See Table 9-11 for signs of nutrient deficiencies that may affect body

appearance[53,55-57] and refer to the American Dietary Association (www.eatright.org) or the U.S. Department of Health and Human Services (www.hhs.org) for further information and dietary recommendations.

Older adults are at an increased risk of wound development and complications because of the age-related changes in skin, decreased arteriovenous health, decreased activity, cardiovascular disease, and an increase in incidence of malnutrition. Szewczyk et al described a study that examined the nutritional status in older adults with or without venous wounds and reported that 48% of the participants were malnourished or at risk for malnutrition.[21]

TABLE 9-10	General Dietary Recommendations for the Older Adult[53,55-57]	
	Recommendations	Cellular Function
Carbohy-drates	45%-65% of total daily caloric intake* 35-40 kcal/kg/day Using complex carbohydrates, not simple sugars 55%-65% of total caloric intake 35-40 kcal/kg/day Presence of infections, wounds, catabolic stress: additional 25-30 kcal/kg/day	Supports cell division, leukocyte function, and fibroblast activation
Protein	15% of total caloric intake 0.8-1.0 kcal/kg/day May need to be increased 1.25 g/kg in the healthy active adult Presence of infections, wounds, catabolic stress: 1.2-1.5 kcal/kg/day	Supports new protein synthesis, cell proliferation, tissue regeneration, inflammatory and immune function
Fats	20% of total daily caloric intake* Adjust to make food palatable to avoid deficiencies or anorexia, but should not exceed 35% of total caloric intake	Builds new cell membranes
Saturated fats	<10%	
Cholesterol	<300 mg/day	
Trans fats	Minimal to none	

*May need to be higher to support hormone and bile production.

TABLE 9-11	Signs and Symptoms of Nutritional Deficiency[53,55,56]	
	Signs and Symptoms	Abnormalities
Hair	Dull, dry lack of natural shine Thin, sparse, loss of curl	Protein deficiency, essential fatty acid deficiency Zinc deficiency
Eyes	White ring around eyes Pale eye membrane Night blindness, dry membranes, dull cornea Redness and fissures of eyelid corners	Hyperlipidemia Vitamin B_{12} deficiency, folic acid and/or iron deficiency Vitamin A deficiency, zinc deficiencies
Lips	Redness and swollen Soreness, swollen, bleeding	Niacin, riboflavin, or iron deficiencies Riboflavin deficiency
Tongue	Sores, swollen Soreness, burning	Folic acid and niacin deficiency Riboflavin deficiency
Taste	Diminished taste	Zinc deficiency
Face	Loss of skin color, dark cheeks and eyes, scaling of skin around nostrils Hyperpigmentation	Protein energy deficiency, niacin, riboflavin deficiencies Niacin deficiency
Neck	Thyroid enlargement	Iron deficiency
Nails	Fragile, banding Spoon-shaped	Protein deficiency Iron deficiency
Skin	Slow wound healing Scaliness Dryness, rough Lack of subcutaneous fat, bilateral edema	Zinc deficiency Biotin deficiency Abnormal vitamin A levels Protein energy deficiency
Muscles	Weakness Wasted appearance Calf tenderness, absent patella reflex Peripheral neuropathies Muscle twitch Muscle cramps	Phosphorus and potassium deficiency Protein energy deficiency Thiamine deficiency Folic acid and thiamine deficiencies Abnormal magnesium levels Decreased chloride, sodium deficiency
Bones	Demineralization	Calcium, phosphorus, and vitamin D deficiency
Nerves	Listlessness Decreased sensation, proprioception, depression, and decrease in cognitive function Seizures, behavioral disruption, memory loss	Protein deficiency Thiamine, vitamin B_{12} deficiency Magnesium and zinc deficiencies

Each phase of wound healing requires the proper nutrition in a sufficient nutrient distribution to promote healing. Even a short period of malnutrition, reflected in prealbumin levels, may occur early on in a hospital stay and can delay granulation tissue and collagen formation.[57] It has been reported that as high as 62% of hospitalized older individuals are protein deficient with low prealbumin and albumin levels. Malnutrition doubles the risk of developing pressure ulcers and increases mortality in the older adult.[21] The therapist should keep in mind that many obese patients have low albumin and prealbumin levels and are equally or more at risk for ulcers and other associated complications from malnutrition than their normal-weight counterparts.

Prealbumin level reflects the current nutritional status of a patient and for patients in the acute or subacute recovery phase of an illness. Monitoring these levels is critical to adjusting nutritional and fluid needs. There are many reasons why a patient may not be making the expected gains with rehabilitation, and the physical therapist must consider that malnutrition can be one of those causes and work with clinical dietary staff to ensure that sufficient nutrition and calories are being provided to account for the rehabilitation process.

Body Weight/Body Composition

As part of the patient's nutritional status, the therapist must consider the patient's body composition. The relationship between body weight and composition and function in older adults is a very complex matter. More research is needed to further understand how factors such as body mass index (BMI), fat mass, and lean muscle mass contribute to function, mortality, and morbidity.

The research is inconsistent depending upon the subjects, medical status, and variables measured. One finding that appears to be consistent is that a BMI lower than 19 is associated with an increase in mortality in hospitalized patients as well as older adult community dwellers. It has been suggested that under health stress, such as infections, hip fractures, or cancer, the older adult patient has less energy stores to combat the catabolic state that the patient's body is experiencing.[58-60] It also appears that patients older than age 60 years, and more significantly in patients older than age 75 years, with a BMI between 30 and 38 have an equal mortality rate when compared to age-matched subjects with normal BMI (20 to 25).[52,59] BMI, however, provides limited information for the clinician to truly assess the patient's body composition as well as mortality and morbidity rate. BMI does not speak to the percentage of body weight that is fat versus lean muscle that can contribute to function.

Protein deficiency, common among older adults, along with a reduction in activity can lead to sarcopenia, which is defined as a loss of muscle mass, strength, and function,[61] and it is associated with an increase in disability and mortality.[51] Sarcopenia is also commonly associated with a low BMI, but it has been documented that there is a group of older, obese individuals that also have been diagnosed with sarcopenia. These individuals have a lower muscle mass of the lower extremities and pelvic girdle than individuals with obesity or individuals of normal weight without sarcopenia. Patients with the combination of obesity and sarcopenia have a decrease in physical function when compared to individuals with sarcopenia and normal BMI.[52] With this in mind, it is important to obtain objective data on strength and function such as grip strength, standardized muscle strength, endurance and functional tests, for example, the timed up and go, physical performance test, Tinetti and Berg balance tests.

Another factor the therapist needs to consider when working with older adults is body fat deposition. With aging, there is a reduction in subcutaneous fat and an increase in visceral fat accumulation. There is also a reduction in muscle mass along with an increase in total fat mass.[62] This change in body fat deposition and composition is associated with an increase in mortality and morbidity. Skin-fold measurements may also be useful in assessing body composition, but the therapist needs to fully examine the formula so that it is an appropriate calculation for older adults. Because changes in body fat deposition may lead to an underestimation of percentage body fat, it is recommended to use a formula that includes at least one skin-fold measurement on the torso.[62,63]

Waist circumference can also show areas of fat deposition and is associated with cardiac disease. Women and men with a waist circumference greater than 35.5 inches (88 cm) and 39.5 inches (99 cm), respectively, have an increased risk of cardiovascular disease. BMI and waist circumference can be used to assist the therapist in stratifying the risk of diseases such as diabetes, hypertension, and cardiovascular disease.[63]

The authors suspect that nutritional status and body composition are not commonly assessed or considered in working with the older adult patient, but these factors have significant consequences to the rehabilitation process. It has been documented that older adults have a significant reduction in neuromuscular recruitment and muscle mass that was not recovered with rehabilitation after a 2-week period of immobility when compared to a young group of subjects with a similar prior level of activity.[51] For the patient who is medically compromised, the therapist needs to consider the level of protein stores and current nutritional impact to focus on regaining muscle strength to positively affect functional outcomes.[64]

According to the National Health Statistics reports, the five main causes of hospitalization among the older adults are CAD, HF, pneumonia, urinary tract infections (UTIs)/sepsis, and dizziness/falls.[2,65] Of late, the hospital admissions for adults older than age 65 years continue to rise, despite the downward trend among those younger than age 65 years.[66] With heart disease being the leading cause of death in the United States, it is important to evaluate and educate our patients to optimize health. Although the other main causes for admission are also prevalent, they may also be the sequelae to heart disease once an older adult is admitted to the hospital. The following section will cover all these topics in more detail.

Coronary Artery Disease (CAD)

Coronary artery disease is the leading cause of morbidity and mortality in the older adult, with the highest incidence between the ages of 65 and 84 years. Eighty percent of all deaths related to CAD are individuals older than age 65 years.[67,68]

There is a wealth of research linking risk factors to the development of atherosclerosis, but recent research is beginning to document the difference in the degree of risk of CAD for the older individual and differences between the genders. Cardiac risk factors in the young-old (age 75 years or younger) appear similar to those of middle-aged adults and include diabetes and smoking. Elevated low-density lipoproteins (LDL) and total cholesterol are independent risk factors associated with CAD for individuals younger than age 75 years; however, this risk is lower after the age of 85 years. A low level of high-density lipoproteins (HDL) along with elevated total cholesterol carries a higher risk for CAD in women than men.[67] The incidence of systolic hypertension increases with age along with the various changes that affect arterial function. With age, there is an increase in arterial stiffness and wall thickness that leads to a decrease in the compliance of the arteries and arterioles. There is also endothelial dysfunction that leads to an increase in substances that cause vascular constriction as well as the increase in leukocytes and platelet adherence and migration.[69,70] Untreated HTN leads to left ventricle hypertrophy, which happens to be an independent factor of CAD in the older adult. Left ventricular hypertrophy then results in a decrease in the compliance of the heart to allow for proper filling and ejection, and a subsequent increase in oxygen demand of the myocardium.[70] These changes increase the risk of myocardial ischemia and cellular loss, potentially evolving into HF.

Aging is also associated with an increase in inactivity and obesity, which are also clear risk factors for CAD, but there is a decreased link to mortality for the older adult in comparison to the younger adult.[52,71] The increase in obesity with aging is due to a reduction in activity level, excessive caloric intake, a decrease in muscle mass, and lower basal metabolic rates. Obesity is linked to chronic diseases such as diabetes, cancer, and atherosclerosis and is associated with an increase in functional impairments and disability but not directly associated with mortality.[71] Besides inactivity being linked to obesity, inactivity is also associated with a reduction in muscle mass, activity intolerance, and functional limitations.[66] The reduction in muscle mass is independently a predictor of higher mortality rates in older adults.[51]

Coronary artery disease compromises the blood flow to the myocardium. An imbalance between oxygen supply and demand initially results in myocardial ischemia and may lead to myocardial necrosis if the imbalance is not resolved. Angina in the older adult typically does not present itself with the normal symptoms. After the age of 74 years, patients commonly report signs and symptoms including general weakness, dyspnea, fatigue, syncope, and decrease in mental status and there is no gender difference in presentation and common reports.[72] Angina can be classified as stable or unstable. Stable angina refers to typical or predicted symptoms upon exertion over time for patients with a diagnosis of CAD. Unstable angina means there is a progression in symptoms with exertion or the patient is experiencing angina at rest.

If CAD progresses to the point where blood flow to the myocardium becomes significantly compromised, the patient is at risk for acute coronary syndrome (ACS) or a myocardial event. The risk of ACS can be from a severe imbalance of oxygen demand and supply during exertion or a further decrease in perfusion. Acute coronary syndrome refers to unstable angina, non-ST elevation myocardial infarction (NSTEMI), or ST-elevation myocardial infarction (STEMI). With ACS in the older adult, there is a reduction in incidence of ST-segment elevation from 85% of patients younger than age 65 years to less than 35% in patients older than age 84 years. There is also an increase in respiratory failure, syncope, and stroke associated with myocardial infarction and increase in mortality rates for the older adult.[72,73]

Exercise testing and cardiac catheterization are the principal procedures used to diagnose CAD. During the graded exercise testing, the clinician attempts to induce myocardial ischemia and observe the onset of angina along with changes in the 12-lead ECG for diagnostic testing purposes. The pattern of ECG changes on the 12-lead ECG can determine the wall that is underperfused. (For example, ECG changes in leads II, III, and the augmented AVF leads suggest inferior wall impairment.) Box 9-7 lists the signs and symptoms of CAD. The gold standard for CAD diagnosis is cardiac catheterization that examines the patency of the coronary arteries. Cardiac enzymes will be very important for diagnostic purposes and determine extent of injury. Clinical findings upon examination will vary depending upon the degree of CAD and its stability.

BOX 9-7	Signs and Symptoms of Coronary Artery Disease
Vitals	• Varies; dependent on degree and stability of coronary artery disease/acute coronary syndrome (ACS)
	• Heart rate and blood pressure will typically be elevated at time of ACS
	• Pulse rate may become irregular
	• Tachypnea associated with pulmonary edema, anxiety, and pain
Auscultation	• Rales associated with pulmonary edema
	• S3 and S4 cardiac sounds associated with contractility dysfunction
Palpation	• Apical pulse will shift to left with left ventricular hypertrophy
	• Peripheral edema, jugular vein dysfunction with heart failure
Arterial blood gases	• Varies
Observation	• ↑Work of breathing
	• Facial distress
Exercise tolerance	• Reduction in tolerance
	• Reports of angina
	• ST-segment depression with ischemia
	• ST-segment elevation with cell injury

Heart Failure

Heart failure (HF) develops when cardiac output cannot meet the metabolic needs of the body. Heart failure typically is associated with a functional or structural defect such as valvular disease, CAD, or hypertrophic cardiomyopathy.[74] There are approximately 5 million individuals in the United States who have been diagnosed with HF and more than a half million people are diagnosed annually. The prevalence of HF increases with age, with 10.3% of individuals ages 65 to 74 years versus 20.7% of those age 85 years and older. Approximately 300,000 individuals die annually with the primary diagnosis of HF.[74,75]

The most common cause of HF is ischemic left ventricular dysfunction secondary to CAD, with hypertension as the second leading cause.[76] Heart failure can also be associated with depressed left ventricular dysfunction, low ejection fraction (EF), and systolic or diastolic dysfunction, but may also be associated with normal left ventricular function. Heart failure can also be classified as right ventricular or left ventricular failure. In most cases, individuals have components of both ventricular dysfunction or both phases of cardiac cycle (systolic and diastolic) dysfunction

In systolic dysfunction, the left ventricular wall, which typically begins in a hypertrophic state, dilates, enlarging the chamber. This dilated state does not permit the myocardium to effectively contract and eject sufficient blood into systemic circulation. The ejection fraction, percentage of end-diastolic volume ejected per beat, normally

50% to 70%, is depressed to less than 40% with systolic dysfunction. In diastolic dysfunction, the left ventricle EF is normal, although it accounts for at least 50% of HF in the older adults.[77] However, with diastolic dysfunction, the ventricle walls thicken with normal or slightly smaller chamber size and reduce the myocardium's ability to relax to allow sufficient filling. Heart failure with normal EF is commonly associated with chronic HTN with left ventricle hypertrophy.[72,77]

Clinically, the signs and symptoms of HF are associated with the type of dysfunction: Either the myocardium is causing insufficient filling of the ventricles leading to an increase in venous blood volume or the ventricular contraction is unable to sufficiently eject the blood forward into the arterial circulation. See Box 9-8 for a list of the signs and symptoms of HF. In general, the most common symptoms related to HF are fatigue, shortness of breath, and decreased physical capacity.

To clinically assess diastolic dysfunction of the right ventricle, the physical therapist should inspect for pitted edema, commonly of the lower extremities. It is important not only to document the score but the degree of edema. In the pitted edema scale, a zero means no pitted edema noted and goes up to a 4, which means the pitted impression remains for longer than 30 seconds. Venous engorgement can also be assessed by examining jugular vein distention. The external jugular vein should rarely be noticeable while the patient breathes comfortably in the sitting position. If the vein is very prominent while the patient is sitting or is distended more than 3 cm above the horizontal line level to the sternal angle with the patient reclined to 45 degrees, it is positive for right ventricle dysfunction. The clinical findings for diastolic

BOX 9-8	Signs and Symptoms Associated with Heart Failure
Right Ventricle	**Left Ventricle**
Diastolic Dysfunction	***Diastolic Dysfunction***
Jugular vein distension	Dyspnea
Liver engorgement	Tachypnea
Peripheral edema	Cough
	Wheezing
	Rales
	S3 abnormal heart sound
	Systolic murmur
	Hypoxemia
	Orthopnea
Systolic Dysfunction	***Systolic Dysfunction***
Dyspnea	Fatigue
Desaturation	Angina
Cyanosis	Activity intolerance
Tachypnea	Exertional dyspnea
Hypoxia	Narrow pulse pressure
	Decreased mental status
	Decreased urination
	Cool, pale, diaphoresis

dysfunction of the left ventricle are commonly found upon assessment of the pulmonary system with dependent rales consistent with interstitial edema, and a nonproductive cough with high-pitched wheezing. Often, there is an additional low-pitched heart sound, S3, which can be heard over the left chest wall using light contact of the bell of the stethoscope. The patient may also report orthopnea, or the need to have the upper body elevated while in the supine position secondary to an inability to lay completely flat without progressive shortness of breath. This is most commonly experienced at night.

Systolic dysfunction is associated with fatigue and a decrease in activity tolerance, and therefore it is important that the physical therapist complete an assessment of muscular, cardiovascular, and pulmonary endurance and monitor vitals including pulse rate and regularity during activity and at the peak exercise stage as well as during the recovery phase.

Pneumonia

Pneumonia is an acute inflammation of the lungs caused by a bacterial, viral, or fungal pathogen. The normal defense mechanism of the respiratory system, a mucociliary blanket of macrophages, fails to keep the lower respiratory tract sterile, causing an accumulation of exudate in the small bronchioles and alveoli. The inflammatory process is then activated, along with the immune response, causing localized edema. A vicious cycle develops between the immune response and the infectious growth. With an increase in alveolar edema, the immune cells' ability to phagocytize the invader will be impaired. The collection of edema, RBCs, and WBCs will consolidate, leaving the lung tissue unable to perform ventilation and perfusion. This infection can also spread to other segments of the lungs as well as to the pleural space and pericardium.[78] Pneumonia is the third leading discharge diagnosis for individuals between the ages of 64 and 85 years, and the second leading diagnosis for individuals older than age 85 years.[79] Pneumonia can be classified by the infectious agent or by the environment in which the patient became infected with the agent that produces the pneumonia. The type of classification directs the pharmacologic intervention. Pneumonia can also be classified as the environment in which the individual contracted the infection. This system allows health care professionals to identify specific interventions to treat, minimize, and prevent the common characteristics of the environmental setting.

Community-acquired pneumonia (CAP) is an infection that occurs while the patient is living out in the community or the infection manifests itself within the first 72 hours after hospitalization. CAP has an incidence rate of 8.4 cases per 1000 for individuals between age 60 and 69 years and 48.5 cases per 1000 for individuals older than age 90 years.[80] Health care–acquired pneumonia

(HCAP) as defined by the American Thoracic Society is pneumonia that is acquired while the individual is in the hospital or a resident of some other type of institutional care facility, or an individual who has been exposed to a family member with a multidrug resistance.[81] The incidence of HCAP has been reported to be as high as 55 cases per 1000 for the older adult, accounting for more than 2 million acute care hospital admissions and more than 26,000 pneumonia-related deaths.[82]

There are multiple factors about the age-related changes to the pulmonary system that explain the higher incidence in pneumonia with advanced age. In the upper airway, there is a natural reduction in mucociliary function and oropharyngeal clearance, increasing the risk of aspiration. In the lower airways, there is also a decrease in the cellular and humoral immune response and phagocytosis.[81] These changes reduce the ability of the bronchial system to immobilize pathogens and clear the airways. Older adults also are more susceptible to pneumonia after surgery secondary to the depressive effects of anesthesia and the number and severity of comorbidities.[80]

Aspiration has been clearly identified as a common contributing factor to the development of pneumonia. Aspiration is associated with malnutrition, tube feeding, contracture of cervical extensor muscles, and use of depressant medications.[78] Other events have also been linked to aspiration, including dysphagia due to loss of dentition and poor hygiene, decreased saliva production, and weakening of muscles of mastication. Aging is associated with a delay in the neural processing needed to perform the proper swallowing sequence and decreased sensation of the oral cavity. Finally, there is an increased incidence of aspiration in the presence of Parkinson's disease, cerebral vascular accident, gastroesophageal reflux disease, connective tissue disorders, and Alzheimer's disease.[78,80]

The typical clinical presentation for pneumonia includes a fever and a productive cough with sputum production that is usually yellowish green or rust colored. There is also an elevation in the WBC count and, in most cases, a positive sputum culture identifying the infectious agent. Diagnosis is made based upon symptoms and a positive finding of infiltrates or consolidation on chest x-ray. There may be reports of chest wall pain, pleuritis, hemoptysis, or dyspnea, and if sufficient lung tissue is affected by the pneumonia with or without an underlying pulmonary disease, the patient may desaturate at rest or with exertion. The older adult, however, may present with more atypical signs and symptoms, including a change in mental status, anorexia, decrease in function and activity tolerance, and an elevated HR.[80] Once the patient has been treated for acute pneumonia, it is important for the physical therapist to objectively assess activity tolerance through some form of exercise test (e.g., the 6-minute walk test, or a bike or treadmill test). These data can be used to ensure stable vitals with exertion, rule out desaturation, and document activity tolerance so the rehabilitation plan can be appropriately prescribed. See Box 9-9 for clinical evaluation findings associated with pneumonia in the older adult.

Urinary Tract Infections

Urinary tract infections are the most common infections among older adults and have become a major clinical issue regardless of current health and mobility status, place of residence (home or nursing home), or amount of comorbidities.[83] With age, there are a multitude of reasons that can put a person at risk of developing a UTI including comorbidities that affect the bladder's nerve supply (diabetes, multiple sclerosis, and spinal cord injuries), urinary flow obstructions from kidney stones and tumors, prolonged catheter use, and weakened pelvic floor musculature from pregnancy in women and enlarged prostate in men.[84] Patients with Alzheimer's disease, Parkinson's disease, patients who have a stroke history, or have neurogenic bladders may also not fully empty their bladder and are prone to UTIs.[85] Box 9-10 lists common comorbidities that increase the older adult's susceptibility for a UTI.[82,85,86]

The urinary tract is usually sterile, except for the most distal portion of the urethra.[86] The urinary tract is designed to prevent the spread of bacteria with the outflow of urine; however, with age, physical and functional changes increase the risk of bacteria in the urinary tract to cause an infection. Urinary tract infections primarily start in the lower portion of the urethra. If untreated,

BOX 9-10	Reasons Patients Have an Increased Risk of UTI[82,85,86]
Female sex	Urinary obstruction
Prolonged catheterization	Kidney stones
Errors in catheter care	Enlarged prostate
Weakened pelvic floor musculature	Alzheimer's disease
	Parkinson's disease
Diabetes	History of neurogenic bladder
Multiple sclerosis	History of stroke
Spinal cord injuries	

an infection of the urethra can affect other structures of the urinary system such as the bladder, ureters, or the kidneys.

According to Liang, urinary stasis is the primary contributor to UTIs in the older adult.[85] In older women, there is a decrease in the strength of the pelvic floor musculature from prior pregnancies and a change in estrogen levels that contribute to urinary stasis and incontinence. Older men, on the other hand, have decreased bladder emptying due to obstruction secondary to benign prostatic hypertrophy.[86] Regardless of the reason for decreased urine flow, bacterial colonization is the result of urinary stasis. Also, the change in the normal vagina flora in women and bacterial prostatitis in men contributes to recurrent infections.

Having an indwelling catheter is another risk factor in the development of a UTI. Hazelett et al,[87] in a retrospective study, determined that 73% of patients who received an indwelling catheter in the emergency department were 65+ years old. Of those patients, 28% were diagnosed with a UTI during their hospital stay; however, 59% of those were diagnosed in the emergency department and therefore prior to receiving the catheter. This study suggests that many of the older patients with catheters who are diagnosed with a UTI may, in fact, have had the UTI prior to receiving the indwelling catheter. This is somewhat contrary to common belief, but it demonstrates that older adults do not present in the same manner as their younger counterparts.[87] There are many types of bacteria that can cause UTIs, including *Staphylococcus aureus*, *Proteus*, *Klebsiella*, and *Enterococcus*. However, they are mostly caused by *Escherichia coli*, a normal intestinal bacteria.[84,85]

Symptoms such as pain with urination, increased frequency, persistent urge to urinate, and hematuria, which are typically used to diagnose a UTI in the younger population, cannot necessarily be used with the older adult because of the changes mentioned above. For example, an older male with prostatic hypertrophy may have difficulty urinating, strong and sudden urges to urinate, pain, and hematuria. These are all symptoms of a UTI; therefore, it is difficult to determine the diagnosis of UTI in the presence of other genitourinary comorbities.[88]

BOX 9-9	Clinical Evaluation Findings Associated with Pneumonia
Vitals	Tachycardia
	Tachypnea
	Hypotension
	Dyspnea
	Desaturation
Auscultation	Diminished normal breath sounds
	Rales
	Low-pitched wheezes in presence of thick secretions
	High-pitched wheezes (associated with aspiration)
	Bronchial breath sounds (associated with consolidated pneumonia)
Palpation	Increased tactile fremitus
	Dull percussion over consolidation
	Possible ↓ chest wall excursion
Arterial blood gases	↓ PaO_2
	Possible altered $PaCO_2$
Observation	↑ Work of breathing
	Facial distress
	Cyanosis
Temperature	Fever

Diagnosis of a UTI in the younger population requires 10^5 colony-forming units (CFUs)/mL with associated symptoms as described earlier.[86] Diagnosis can be made in the older adult with a bacterial colony count of 10^2 or 10^3 CFUs if they are also symptomatic.[85] However, with the older patient, diagnosis is not that easy as they frequently present without symptoms or have UTI symptoms such as decreased urine flow, which can be a symptom of prostatic hypertrophy. Frequently, the first symptom that is noted is acute confusion. Other symptoms are a sudden functional decline and delirium. It is important to diagnose a UTI early in the older patient because it can quickly spread to the kidneys and to the blood, causing sepsis. Juthani-Mehta reports that diagnostic criteria for nursing home residents who do not have a catheter include having three of the following clinical signs or symptoms: (1) a fever of 100.4°F or greater; (2) new or change in burning of urination, frequency, or urgency; (3) new flank or suprapubic pain; (4) change in color, consistency, or cloudiness of urine; and (5) change in mental or functional status. For nursing home residents who have catheters, two of the following characteristics must be present: (1) fever as noted earlier; (2) new flank or suprapubic pain; (3) change in presence of urine; and (4) change in mentation or functional status.[86]

The physical therapist needs to consider the effects of the UTI during the evaluation and treatment process because for the older patient with a UTI, the acute confusion and decline in functional mobility may be transient and not appropriately represent the patient's true status. The therapist will need to constantly reassess function and needs to make the most appropriate discharge recommendations as the infection is medically treated.

Sepsis

Sepsis is a term used to describe systemic bacteremia with or without organ dysfunction. Basically, sepsis is an immunologic response to bacteria and can easily attack any organ system. Those that are most affected are the pulmonary and renal systems. Diagnosis and treatment of the cause of sepsis are of utmost importance because it is related to increased mortality.[89]

Twenty percent of all in-hospital deaths are related to sepsis, and the incidence of sepsis increases with age. Overall, 3 of 1000 patients are diagnosed with sepsis; however, 26 of 1000 patients older than age 85 years are diagnosed.[90] The function of the immune system changes with age and ultimately puts the older patient at increased risk for developing sepsis.

There are many reasons a patient in the hospital can become septic. Some sources of infection are intravenous lines, central lines, intra-abdominal or pelvic infections, abdominal surgery, and patients with UTIs, diabetes, lupus, or alcoholism.

Many older adults have multiple comorbidities making diagnosis of sepsis difficult as the clinical picture may represent infections of other systems.[89] Diagnosis of sepsis is important as there are many conditions that can mimic sepsis, including hemorrhage, PE, myocardial infarction, pancreatitis, diabetic ketoacidosis, and diuretic-induced hypovolemia, just to name a few. It is important to get a blood culture that might determine the underlying bacterial infection that needs to be treated. However, a CBC is not always helpful because results may mimic the above conditions, which are not technically sepsis. Along with urinalysis, intravenous lines should also be cultured to fully rule out the source. A chest x-ray is important to rule out pneumonia and PE.[91]

Patients who become septic usually present with a fever higher than 101.3°F, have an elevated heart rate greater than 90 bpm, a respiratory rate greater than 20 breaths per minute, and a probable or confirmed infection from cultures. If sepsis is not diagnosed and the source of the infection not identified, it can progress to severe sepsis or septic shock. Box 9-11 lists the signs and symptoms of sepsis, severe sepsis, and septic shock.[89,91,92]

Medical care and treatment of sepsis is aimed at maintaining all organ perfusion and a ventilator may be necessary for respiratory support. Refer back to previous sections in this chapter for guidelines on appropriate evaluation and treatment of patients. Evaluation and treatment may need to be deferred until the patient is stabilized.

OTHER MEDICAL ISSUES

There are a multitude of reasons why an older adult might present with a decline in function and health. The previous section addressed the most common diagnoses from acute care admissions. Following is a brief description of medical issues that may compromise the older adult's health, result in a decline in function, or lead to further medical complications contributing to increased morbidity and mortality rates.

BOX 9-11	Signs and Symptoms of Sepsis, Severe Sepsis, and Septic Shock[89,91,92]		
Sepsis	**Severe Sepsis**	**Septic Shock**
• Fever above 101.3°F • Heart rate > 90 beats per minute • Respiratory rate > 20 breaths per minute • Probable or confirmed infection	• Mottled skin • ↓ Urine output • Mental status change • ↓ Platelet count • Respiratory difficulties • Changes in cardiac function	• All signs of severe sepsis • Extremely low blood pressure

Dizziness

Dizziness is a common complaint of the older adult and it is difficult to determine the root cause because it can be caused by multiple etiologies, including vestibular, visual, or proprioceptive system dysfunctions.[93] It is very important to determine the cause because treatment varies greatly depending on the system involved. A study by Uneri and Polat determined that the most common causes of dizziness in older adults are benign paroxysmal positional vertigo, vestibulopathy (an abnormality of the vestibular apparatus), migraine vestibulopathy, and migraines.[94]

The incidence of patient presentation with dizziness to the emergency department is alarming. In the 10-year period from 1995 to 2004, 29% of emergency visits were secondary to dizziness in the 65+ age group.[95] To ensure proper diagnosis, appropriate screening and testing is of utmost importance. There are many diagnostic procedures that can be performed, including a thorough physical examination, provocation studies, and neurologic, visual, vestibular, cardiac, and psychiatric examination. The patient report will assist in ascertaining a clear picture of the symptoms and precipitating events.

Vertigo, the most common cause of dizziness among the older adult population, is defined as the abnormal sensation of movement that is brought on by certain positions. There are many causes of vertigo, including trauma, idiopathic, and inner ear diseases. Box 9-12 lists some of the common causes of vertigo. Diagnosis of vertigo can be easily made, as nystagmus is commonly seen in the eyes.[94,96,97] The direction of eye movement is indicative of the part of the inner ear that is affected.[96] Vertigo can be a symptom of basilar artery migraine, so migraines also need to be ruled out as the cause.[97] Patients with vertigo will often report a "spinning" sensation. Balance is dependent on sensory cues and vestibular function, both central and peripheral. Therefore, inner ear problems and gait disturbances affect balance and increase the risk of falls.

Near-syncope, or fainting, is often related to cardiovascular disease rather than to a peripheral or central nervous system disorder. If syncope is present, a search for a cardiac etiology should be initiated. An ECG and a Holter ambulatory cardiac monitor are obtained to evaluate for rhythm disturbances. Syncope also requires a careful physical examination and an echocardiogram to determine if there are blood flow abnormalities. Faintness during standing or bowel movements may relate to orthostatic hypotension or to a Valsalva maneuver, respectively.

Inability to describe symptoms may be related to dementia or psychiatric disorders. Individuals with dementia may be trying to describe the confusion they experience and not true dizziness. An evaluation for depression, anxiety, and dementia may be included in the differential diagnosis, if symptoms are difficult to describe. Finally, iatrogenic postural hypotension that causes positional dizziness is more common in older adults than in younger adults because of the increased prevalence of polypharmacy. Medications are always implicated initially as causative agents, until proven otherwise. These include antihypertensives, diuretics, and drugs that cause sedation.

With age, there are many changes that happen to balance, perception, as well as the changes in sensation, and neurologic and skeletal functioning. Chronic illnesses like diabetes can also contribute to sensory deficits.[94] Polypharmacy and orthostatic hypotension are also common causes and can be differential diagnoses for dizziness. Whatever the cause, dizziness is a precursor to falls, which can be life threatening for the older adult. Proper examination and treatment of dizziness can aid in reducing the incidence of falls and the morbidity and mortality from them.

Dehydration

Dehydration is a common problem in the older adult and directly increases rates of morbidity and mortality. Dehydration is a costly societal as well as individual problem. Nearly 40% of all hospitalization admissions in older adults is associated with dehydration.[98]

There are three primary reasons why the older adult is susceptible to dehydration. First, there is a blunted thirst mechanism. Second, there is a reduction in total body fluid with the reduction in muscle mass and an increase in body fat. Finally, a decrease in renal function that concentrates the urine prevents the body from retaining enough fluid to avert dehydration.[98] These changes along with a variety of comorbidities lead to the increased risk of dehydration.

Dehydration is categorized by the relationship between free water and sodium and can be caused by many factors. Hypertonic dehydration occurs when there is a greater loss of water when compared to sodium loss. This type of dehydration is more common in the presence of infection or exposure to hot environmental temperatures. In isotonic dehydration, there is an equal loss of water and sodium, and vomiting and diarrhea are the two most common causes. Hypotonic dehydration is caused by a greater loss of sodium than water. The use of diuretics is the most common cause of hypotonic dehydration. Hypotonic

BOX 9-12	Common Causes of Vertigo[94,96,97]
Idiopathic	Otosclerosis
Trauma	Sudden sensorineural hearing loss
Ear diseases	Central nervous system disease
Chronic otitis media	Vertebrobasilar insufficiency
Vestibular neuronitis	Acoustic neuroma
Meniere disease	Cervical vertigo

dehydration is the most common cause of dehydration in the older adult.[99] The most significant laboratory abnormality is sodium imbalance and should be carefully monitored.

There are multiple risk factors associated with dehydration, including advanced age; being of the female gender, because of the higher percentage body fat; and a BMI lower than 21 and greater than 27. Individuals with dementia, history of stroke, urinary incontinence, infections, use of steroids, polypharmaceutical use, and a decrease in functional independence also increase the risk of dehydration.[98]

Presenting symptoms of dehydration may include confusion, lethargy, rapid weight loss, and functional decline, all of which will interfere with rehabilitation goals. Therefore, the physical therapist is in a good position to monitor for dehydration and alert the medical team to the emergence of this syndrome. See Box 9-13 for the signs and symptoms of dehydration.

Metabolic Syndrome

Metabolic syndrome is characterized as a cluster of no fewer than three cardiovascular risk factors that are strongly associated with myocardial infarction. Risk factors from the National Cholesterol Education Program Adult Treatment Panel III Report include increased abdominal fat, high levels of triglycerides, low levels of high-density lipoproteins (HDLs), HTN, and an elevated level of fasting plasma glucose.[100] The International Diabetes Foundation definition criteria is slightly different, with abdominal circumference being more than 94 cm for men and more than 80 cm for women, and fasting glucose level greater than 100 mg/dL.[100,101] See Box 9-14 for specific criteria which may differ according to source.[100-102]

It is estimated that around one-quarter of the world's adult population has metabolic syndrome, which increases their morbidity and mortality from a cardiovascular event including stroke and myocardial infarction and HF. Metabolic syndrome was also referred to as syndrome X, but the term *insulin resistance*

BOX 9-14	Clinical Criteria for Metabolic Syndrome[100-102]
Risk Factors	**Criteria**
Abdominal obesity	
Men	>102 cm
Women	>88 cm
Triglycerides	≥150 mg/dL (1.69 mmol/L)
High-density lipoprotein (HDL)	
Men	>40 mg/dL (1.04 mmol/L)
Women	>50 mg/dL (1.30 mmol/L)
Blood pressure	
Systolic	>130 mmHg
Diastolic	>85 mmHg
Fasting glucose	>110 mg/dL

syndrome (IRS) is more recently used to label this clinical issue.[100,102]

Aging is associated with an increased incidence of obesity due to a reduction in activity level, a decrease in muscle mass, and an increase in visceral fat mass.[63] The link between obesity and metabolic syndrome, or IRS, is not fully understood but obesity is associated with increases in free fatty acids and triglycerides and an increase in inflammatory cytokines that is also linked to IRS.[102] Visceral adipocytes produce resistin, proinflammatory substances, interleukin-6, tumor necrosis factor, and plasminogen activator inhibitor-1, which promotes the development of insulin resistance as well as HTN and dyslipidemia.[101,103]

Insulin resistance and abdominal obesity appear to be predictors for the development of metabolic syndrome. Insulin resistance occurs when the cells become less sensitive and eventually resistant to insulin that leads to the inability of glucose to be absorbed by the cells. A vicious cycle develops with higher levels of glucose that leads to the release of more insulin. With the elevated release of free fatty acids, there is a reduction of glucose oxidation and glucose transport inducing liver production of LDLs that elevates triglycerides and lowers HDL levels.[100] With the increase in free fatty acids, the liver is stimulated to produce more LDLs, release more triglycerides, and lowers HDL levels.[100,101]

With obesity and the normal effects of aging, there is an increase in HTN. There is a further increase in the incidence of HTN with a BMI greater than 27 in people older than 40 years.[104] Older adults are among one of the high-risk groups for a cardiovascular event along with African Americans.[105]

Finally, there is an increase in incidence of type 2 diabetes and cardiovascular events in older adults with IRS. It is estimated that 29 million older adults will be diagnosed with type 2 diabetes by 2050.[103] Diabetes itself is defined as a fasting glucose level greater than 126 mg/dL, or a 2-hour postprandial glucose level greater than 200 mg/dL after a 75-g glucose load, or symptoms of diabetes plus casual plasma glucose concentration of

BOX 9-13	Signs and Symptoms of Dehydration
Examination	**Clinical Signs and Symptoms**
Interview	• ↓ Cognitive function and mental status
Observation	• Dry mucosa
Palpation	• ↓ Skin turgor
Vitals	• Tachycardia
	• ↓ Blood pressure
	• Orthostatic hypotension
	• Weight loss in short time, <1 kg/day
Jugular vein distention	• In supine, nonappreciable external jugular vein
Function	• ↓ Muscle strength, balance, and function

200 mg/dL.[100] Prediabetes is defined as having a fasting plasma glucose level between 100 and 125 mg/dL and a 2-hour postprandial glucose between 140 and 199 mg/dL. Diabetes is an independent risk factor for the older adult suffering a serious cardiovascular event and increases mortality and morbidity rates.[14] The reader is directed to review the sections on Coronary Artery Disease and Heart Failure within this chapter for the consequences of the cardiovascular risk factors including obesity, HTN, dyslipidemia, and glucose–insulin dysfunction.

PREVENTION

The stratification process is also an important step in disease prevention and in assessing the risk of experiencing a medical event during exercise or exertion. Every physical therapy plan should address prevention, starting with the initial examination and evaluation regardless of clinical setting. It is important that the therapist completes a thorough interview in order to determine the level of prevention the therapist should address for the primary and secondary diagnoses.

The ultimate goal of prevention is to optimize health and decrease functional limitations and impairments. All members of the team should address prevention and that, ultimately, should lead to the reduction in health care utilization and costs. The three levels of prevention are primary, secondary, and tertiary.

- Primary: focuses on instilling healthy behaviors and reducing risk factors by intervening prior to the biological signs of a disease. An example of primary prevention for CAD would be to instruct your client to eat well, avoid smoking, exercise routinely to control blood pressure, and control weight to minimize risk of diabetes. Another example may be the initiation of a weight training program for an older adult patient to improve muscle strength for the prevention of osteoporosis.
- Secondary: the pathology or disease is present, but intervention is focused on behavior modification to manage the disease. The goal is to control progression of the disease, improve strength, avoid loss of function, and minimize or eliminate pain. In treating a client already diagnosed with CAD, the physical therapist would educate them on the reduction or elimination of risk factors (see Box 9-3), activities to reduce blood pressure and cholesterol levels, importance of monitoring for diabetes, as well as management of the disease by percutaneous coronary intervention.
- Tertiary: the patient has a disease and is also afflicted with dysfunction associated with that disease including a decrease in activity tolerance and function. The focus of tertiary prevention is on functional mobility and education of signs of symptoms of the disease

and the prevention of further deterioration.[106] An example of tertiary prevention while caring for a patient with HF due to CAD would be to manage the cardiac dysfunction, protect renal function, medicate to improve cardiac function, control food and fluid intake, and introduce job simplification and energy conservation techniques.

If we consider CAD the leading cause of deaths in the United States, United Kingdom, and Europe, 83% of deaths related to ischemic heart disease involve patients older than age 65 years and the mortality rates continue to rise substantially after 75 years of age. In the geriatric population, there is a shift in the significance of typical risk factors with a reduction in the incidence of smoking and diabetes and an increase in hypertension, sedentary lifestyle, and obesity.[107]

It should be very common for physical therapists in all settings to address risk factor modifications for patients with known cardiac disease or HF, with the goal to minimize functional limitations and decrease hospitalizations. An example of prevention across the spectrum: primary prevention could focus on prevention of osteoporosis and diet to maintain proper weight and maintain muscle mass. Secondary prevention may include strength, aerobic exercise, and functional training to minimize skeletal muscle atrophy, promote airway clearance to minimize the effects of atelectasis, and proper nutrition to promote general health to avoid exacerbation of HF. Tertiary prevention may focus on functional training and education about signs and symptoms of HF, including progressive exercise intolerance, fatigue, and shortness of breath. Prevention in the young older adult, ages 65 to 75 years, may focus on primary or secondary prevention, including fitness, weight management, smoking cessation, and encouragement for routine lipid profiles and fasting glucose testing. In the older-old, age 85 years or older, prevention may focus on fitness and function, hypertension control, and weight management. In any prevention program, the therapist will need to consider the age of the patient, as advanced age is associated with an increase in comorbidities.

SUMMARY

Clinical management of the health and function of the older adult is complex. It should be the common goal of all professional practitioners in geriatric health care to treat illnesses and promote optimal health. There have been two shifts in geriatric health care: an increasing attention to wellness and prevention for the older adult, and the acutely ill patients are being seen by the physical therapist outside the traditional acute care hospital. The physical therapist needs a basic understanding of the common medical diagnoses that lead the older adults to seek medical care and how these diagnoses affect function and quality of life. Physical therapy intervention should consist of constant screening for signs and symptoms that suggest medical concerns, adjusting rehabilitation goals to minimize functional limitations and physical impairments, education, and healthy lifestyles. Finally, the therapist needs to be an active member of the older adult's health care team to maximize health care services and ultimately maximize quality of health and outcomes.

REFERENCES

To enhance this text and add value for the reader, all references are included on the companion Evolve site that accompanies this text book. The reader can view the reference source and access it online whenever possible. There are a total of 107 cited references and other general references for this chapter.

CHAPTER 10

Motivation and Patient Education:
Implications for Physical Therapist Practice

Barbara Resnick, PhD, CRNP, FAAN, FAANP,
Dale Avers, PT, DPT, PhD

MOTIVATION AND COMPLIANCE

Motivation is an important factor in the older adult's ability and willingness to participate in functional activities and engage in healthy behaviors such as exercise. By definition, motivation is the inner urge that moves or prompts a person to action. Motivation refers to the need, drive, or desire to act in a certain way to achieve a certain end. In contrast, compliance refers to doing what others want or ask rather than being driven by an inner desire. Ideally, health care providers want older adults to be motivated to comply with behaviors that are known to be effective in preventing disease and disability and improving overall health and quality of life.

Unfortunately, motivation to engage in behaviors such as physical therapy, going to exercise class, or adhering to a special diet are not often addressed nor are interventions utilized to improve motivation with regard to these activities. Rather, we consider motivation only when the older individual is not doing the desired behavior. It is at this time that he or she is labeled as unwilling to participate, unmotivated, and noncompliant. To help motivate older adults to comply with health-promoting behaviors, it is important to comprehensively consider the factors that influence motivation and implement appropriate interventions to ensure the desired behavior.

Age Changes in Motivation

Self-Regulation. Self-regulation is the process by which people control or alter their thoughts, emotions, and behaviors. Behaviors around self-regulation include such things as self-monitoring, reinforcements, goal setting, and corrective self-reactions. Older adults may have greater self-regulatory capacity simply from the experience of engaging in self-regulation activities over the course of a lifetime.[1,2]

Changes in Motivational Strategies: Focus on the Positive. There is a tendency to use motivational strategies that focus on losses; for example, if you do not go to therapy you will not be able to get back home, independently ambulate, or be able to walk without an assistive device. Older adults, however, respond better to emphasizing the positive outcomes of engaging in a behavior, avoiding regret, and maximizing satisfaction associated with a behavior.[3-9] Specifically, older individuals are interested in the immediate benefits of behaviors such as improved functional ability, improved mood, and overall sense of well-being, or improved strength and ability to carry grocery bags or laundry. In contrast, they do not respond well to long-term benefits such as the possibility of decreased evidence of cardiovascular disease. In addition, older individuals tend to be more focused on positive rather than negative emotions.[65] Therefore, disappointments following behavior change (e.g., slower improvements in strength) are less likely to undermine the new behavior than they are for younger people.

Stronger Adherence to Behavior Change. Older adults tend to be slower to initiate changes in behavior. Once initiated, however, they are more likely to adhere to the new behavior. The difficulty of initiating change, as well as the ease of maintenance, may be related to the stability of contextual cues in late adulthood.[10] Although older individuals are known to avoid novelty and lean toward what is familiar, with regard to physical activity they have indicated that new and different exercise activities are motivating.[11] Thus, new activities, such as incorporating Wii activities into therapy sessions, should not be totally ignored for the comfortable and routine activities for which older adults may be familiar.

Positive Self-Concept. It has been repeatedly noted that individuals, including older adults, who feel personally deficient are most likely to break their diets, stop exercise, spend excessively, or binge drink.[12,13] Fortunately, older adults tend to have positive self-concept[14] rather than conceptualizing themselves as personally deficient. Consequently, older adults succeed at self-regulation more often than younger adults because they do not experience as much dissatisfaction.

Social Supports. The impact of social support on behavior change around activities such as physical activity has been quite variable in older individuals.[15-20] Generally, African American older adults seem to be more influenced by social supports,[11] although overall these external forces seem to be less influential on engaging in physical activity than noted in younger individuals.

Providing social support to others is also an important motivator to older adult patients. Specifically, older adults who are caregivers of spouses, friends, or children are often highly motivated to engage in physical therapy to be able to fully resume caregiving activities.

Information-Seeking Behavior. Older adults tend to seek less information when making a decision[21] than do younger individuals. Without extensive information about an activity and the pros and cons of engaging in the activity, older individuals rely on their intuitions, gut feelings, and simple heuristics to form attitudes and make choices (e.g., if an expert said it, it must be true).[22-24] This process may be more efficient and thus decrease the time required for the individual to decide about making a change. It also means they are less likely to be influenced by negative input from others.

Normal Physical Changes with Age

When working with older adults, it is important to remember there are a number of changes that occur as a result of the process of aging itself. The changes that occur are normal for all people but take place at different rates. Table 10-1 lists the normal physiological changes that occur with age in the major body systems. The changes that occur in the sensory system can indirectly influence motivation and learning. Specifically, the following changes can occur: (1) there is an increase in the threshold needed for each sensory modality to be stimulated; (2) the activation of the corresponding receptors requires stimuli of increased intensity, and therefore a greater stimulus is needed for the sensation to occur; and (3) it is more difficult for the older individual to differentiate between different stimuli.

Factors That Influence Motivation

To consider the many factors that influence motivation in older adults, it is helpful to use a model of motivation based on social cognitive theory as well as empirical findings.[25-31] Social cognitive theory is based on reciprocal

TABLE 10-1	Normal Physiological Changes Associated with Aging That Can Influence Motivation
System	**Age-Associated Changes**
Skin	Decreased flexibility due to decreased collagen
	Increased wrinkles
	Increased dryness
	Decreased turgor
Lungs	Decreased compliance due to changes in collagen
	Decreased FEV$_1$
	Decreased total lung volume
Brain	Changes in vascular system, neurons, glial cells
	Hypoperfusion
	Atrophy
Heart/Vascular	Decreased response to beta-adrenergic stimulation
	Decreased cardiac output
	Decreased cardiac index
	Decreased compliance of ventricles/arteries
	Calcification of valves
	Increased systolic hypertension
Kidney	Decreased ability to concentrate urine, resulting in loss of free water and increased sensitivity to salt
	Decreased glomerular filtration rate
	Decreased blood flow
Stomach	Decreased digestive secretion enzymes
	Increased gastric pH
	Decreased absorptive surface
	Decreased motility
	Decreased blood flow
Immune system	Decreased memory of previous antigenic stimuli
	Decreased responsiveness to immunization
	Increased energy
	Decreased T-cell proliferation and function

determinism in which behavior, cognition, and other personal factors and environmental influences all operate interactively as determinants of each other. According to social cognitive theory,[2] human motivation and action are regulated by forethought. This cognitive control of behavior is based on two types of expectations: (1) self-efficacy expectations, which are the individuals' beliefs in their capabilities to perform a course of action to attain a desired outcome, and (2) outcome expectancies, which are the beliefs that a certain consequence will be produced by personal action.

Self-efficacy and outcome expectations are dynamic and are both appraised and enhanced by four sources of information[2]: (1) enactive mastery experience, or successful performance of the activity of interest; (2) verbal persuasion, or verbal encouragement given by a credible source that the individual is capable of performing the activity of interest; (3) vicarious experience, or seeing like individuals perform a specific activity; and (4) physiological and affective states such as pain, fatigue, or anxiety associated with a given activity. The theory of self-efficacy suggests that the stronger the individual's self-efficacy and outcome expectations, the more likely he or she will initiate and persist with a given activity.

Beliefs, both in relationship to outcomes (outcome expectations) and with regard to what older adults believe they are capable of doing (self-efficacy expectations), have been noted to influence motivation to engage in health-promoting behaviors.[32-35] Physical sensations associated with a treatment plan, such as pain, fear of falling or exacerbating underlying medical problems, or medication side effects, influence beliefs and actual behavior. Some older adults believe, for example, that exercise will exacerbate arthritis pain and therefore will not engage in a regular exercise program. These unpleasant sensations and their beliefs about them must be addressed and eliminated to facilitate motivation.

Individualized care and demonstrating caring have an important influence on the older adults' motivation to perform a given activity. Individualized care includes recognizing individual differences and needs, using kindness and humor, empowering older adults to take an active part in their care, providing gentle verbal persuasion to perform an activity, and positive reinforcement after performance of an activity.[11,30,36] An essential component of individualized care is letting the individual know *exactly* what it is that you recommend they perform. This may be simple written instructions about what exercise program to engage in or what medication to take, why it is important, and exactly how the activity should be done or the medication be taken. At each care interaction, it is critical to reevaluate how the individual is doing with the behavior of interest as it demonstrates caring and remembering. Individualized care is, in part, effective because the older adult simply wants to reciprocate for the care given to him or her by doing what the therapist requests (e.g., doing a certain exercise or a home revision such as getting a grab bar). Once the behavior is initiated, however, it is likely that the older individual will experience the benefit(s) associated with the behavior and thus continue to adhere for reasons beyond initial reciprocity for care received.

Social support networks including family, friends, peers, and health care providers are important determinants of behavior.[37-40] Repeatedly, motivation to exercise has been found to be influenced by the social milieu of the individual and/or the care setting. These social interactions can alter recovery trajectories by disrupting the progression of functional limitations to disability. The influence of any member of the individual's social network can be positive or negative depending on his or her philosophy and beliefs related to exercise. Social supports can directly serve as powerful external motivators by (1) providing encouragement, (2) helping the older adult feel cared for and cared about, and (3) helping to establish goals such as regaining self-care abilities and being able to return home alone. Social supports can also indirectly affect motivation by strengthening the individual's beliefs in his or her ability to participate in rehabilitation activities, for example, or engaging in a regular exercise program.

The ability to develop personal goals and evaluate one's performance toward that goal can influence motivation to engage in a given behavior.[2] Articulated goals give older adults something to work toward, and help motivate them to adhere to a specific health-promoting activity. In addition, input from therapists is important to goal development and motivation as the goal delineates for the individual what others believe he or she is capable of doing in a particular functional area, for example. Articulated goals should be short- and long-term. Short-term goals should provide the older individual with exactly what he or she should do on a daily basis (e.g., walk for 20 minutes; do ten sit-to-stands). Long-term goals should focus more on ultimate goals that the individual wants to achieve, such as being able to ambulate without an assistive device, care for oneself, walk to the grocery store, or to go on a trip. Goals are most effective when they are (1) related to a specific behavior, (2) challenging but realistically attainable, and (3) achievable in the near future.[2] Goals will be further explored later in this chapter.

Lastly, the individual's personality, self-determination, and resilience have an important influence on motivation. Older adults report that it is their own personality, that is, determination, and their own firm resolutions and adherence to those resolutions, that motivates them to perform specific tasks.[5,115] Resilience is a psychosocial factor that is defined as an individual's capacity to make a "psycho-social comeback in adversity."[41] Resilient individuals tend to manifest adaptive behavior, especially with regard to social functioning, morale, and somatic health,[42] and are less likely to succumb to illness.[43,44] Resilience, though a component of the individual's personality, develops and changes over time through ongoing experiences with the physical and social environment.[45-47] Resilience, unlike basic personality factors, may be more of a dynamic process that is influenced by life events and challenges.[48-50] Thus, there is the opportunity to influence personality, in a sense, by strengthening resilience.

Older adults are a heterogeneous group with very rich and diverse life experiences. Consequently, the factors that facilitate motivation in one may not work as effectively for another individual. As noted previously, the model of motivation can be used to explore the many factors that influence motivation and behavior in older adults. In so doing, interventions can be developed to specifically address identified areas, which may be negatively influencing the individual's motivation to engage in a certain activity.

Instruments to Measure Motivation

Conceptually, motivation can be considered as intrinsic to the individual and as part of his or her personality (i.e., a trait) as well as extrinsic to the individual and influenced by the many factors addressed above. Measurement of motivation, therefore, should ideally address all of these components. A list of tools to measure motivation, directly and indirectly by considering such things as their beliefs about a behavior, is provided in Table 10-2. Measures of self-efficacy, which focus on the individual's confidence in his or her ability to engage in the behavior of interest, and outcome expectations, which are the beliefs that doing the behavior will result in a specific outcome, are behavior specific. Table 10-2, therefore, provides some examples of different measures of self-efficacy and outcome expectations that can be used to focus on the beliefs associated with a given behavior of interest (e.g., exercise, functional activities, diet, and medication adherence). Measures of pain and fear of falling are important to consider, as they are known external factors that influence motivation. Likewise, social support for exercise, specifically related to social support from friends, family, and experts is also known to have an important impact on motivation in specific behavioral areas such as exercise.

Theoretically Driven Interventions to Improve Motivation and Behavior

Both self-efficacy and outcome expectations play an influential role in the performance of functional activities[51-54] and the adoption and maintenance of physical activity.[55-60] Self-efficacy expectations were associated with recovery following stroke,[61] cardiac,[62] and orthopedic events.[63] Outcome expectations are particularly relevant to older adults.[35] Older adults may have high self-efficacy expectations but if they do not believe in the outcomes associated with the behavior such as the benefits from specific exercises done during therapy, then it is unlikely that they will be willing to perform the activity.[51,53,64] The interventions that have been developed using a self-efficacy approach have generally included the following components to address motivation: verbal encouragement, goal setting, role modeling, mastery experiences, and decreasing unpleasant sensations. Alternatively, technologically focused interventions have included the use of hand-held computers to increase physical activity among middle-aged and older adults.

Social Ecological Model Based Interventions. The social ecological model provides an overarching framework for understanding the interrelations among diverse personal and environmental factors in human health and illness. There is increasing recognition that this type of multilevel perspective is needed to address health behavior change and facilitate changes in current care philosophies and care practices as has been done with regard to use of physical restraints,[67] promoting healthy behaviors,[68,69] and understanding caregivers' expectations and care receivers' competence.[70] The social ecological model addresses intraindividual factors such as cognitive status, physical condition, mood, and underlying diseases such as anemia. Interpersonal interactions are addressed using social cognitive theory and the interventions delineated above that strengthen self-efficacy and outcome expectations. Environmental issues focus on making changes in the physical environment that will optimize the individual's access to opportunities for physical activity or facilitate function by altering the person–environment fit (e.g., altering the height of a chair). Lastly, organizational, state, and national policy issues attempt to influence or alter policies in the event they inhibit or prevent participation in functional or physical activities. Alternatively, policies can be developed, or appropriate policies used, to encourage older adults to engage in physical and functional activity. The current public health guideline for physical activity for older adults established by the American College of Sports Medicine and the American Heart Association is a good example of this type of policy.[71]

The Res-Care-Assisted Living (Res-Care-AL) Intervention was revised using the social ecological model. Interventions for the participants in this study were focused at both the individual and facility level. At the intraindividual level, a number of factors that can lead to functional limitation, disability, and sedentary behavior in older adults were considered, including anemia, vitamin D deficiency, cognitive impairment, comorbid and acute medical problems, depression, and fear of falling. Individualized interventions were implemented such as replacement of vitamin D if

TABLE 10-2	Tools to Measure Motivation and Factors That Influence Motivation
Aspect of Motivation Being Measured	**Source for the Measure Identified**
Self-efficacy expectations	Functional performance[6]
	Exercise[102]
	Health-related diet[103]
	Medication adherence[104]
Outcome expectations	Exercise[102]
	Functional performance[6]
	Diet[105]
	Medication adherence[104]
Physical sensations	Pain: McGill Word Scale[106]
	Fear: 0 to 4 Fear of Falling Scale[107]
Social supports	The Norbeck Social Support Questionnaire[108]
	The Social Support for Exercise Habits Scale[109]
Self-determination	Apathy Evaluation Scale[110]
	Self-Motivation Inventory[111]

appropriate for the participant. At the interpersonal level, using social cognitive theory, the following four interpersonal interactions were implemented to engage the resident in physical activity and functional tasks: (1) enactive mastery experience, or helping the individual to successfully perform the activity (e.g., breaking down the task into simple steps that could be successfully performed, or starting with a sitting exercise and increasing the difficulty); (2) verbal persuasion, or providing verbal encouragement so that the individual believed that he or she was capable of performing the activity of interest and setting goals to reinforce that; (3) vicarious experience or exposing the individual to like others exercising; and (4) implementing interventions to decrease any unpleasant sensations associated with an activity (e.g., pain or anxiety with exercise) and increasing the benefits from exercise and other associated positive feelings (e.g., the sense of enjoyment or accomplishment associated with going to an exercise class). These techniques were taught to the caregivers who were encouraged to use them in all care interactions with residents.

Environmental interventions focused on evaluation of the person–environment fit using the Housing Enabler,[72] making appropriate changes to improve the fit and optimize physical activity and function (e.g., improving outdoor access, assuring that there are flat and smooth walking paths, placing chairs or benches at strategic locations to allow for brief rest periods during a walk), and increasing access to opportunities for physical activity, such as providing more exercise activities as part of the general activity programs offered in the facility. Lastly, policy/organizational factors included an evaluation of the marketing materials within the facility to ensure they focused on optimizing function and physical activity among residents, and review of the resident's plan of care (required by the State) so that it focused on what the resident would do with regard to function and physical activity and not what the caregivers would do for the resident.

Effective Strategies to Help Motivate the Older Adult

The theoretical guidance for motivational interventions with older adults is extremely important for ensuring a successful outcome for any intervention geared toward increasing physical or functional activity. Appreciating the techniques that can be used in the development of theory-based interventions is likewise helpful. Table 10-3 describes specific interventions that have been used

TABLE 10-3	Interventions to Strengthen Motivation	
Components of Motivation	**Specific Interventions to Improve Motivation**
Beliefs	Interventions to strengthen efficacy beliefs: 1. Verbal encouragement of capability to perform 2. Expose older adult to role models (similar others who successfully perform the activity) 3. Decrease unpleasant sensations associated with the activity 4. Encourage actual performance/practice of the activity 5. Educate about the benefits of the behavior and reinforce and underline those benefits

Unpleasant physical sensations (pain, fear)	1. Facilitate appropriate use of pain medications to relieve discomfort.
	2. Use alternative measures such as heat/ice to relieve pain associated with the activity
	3. Cognitive–behavioral therapy:
	  • Explore thoughts and feelings related to sensations
	  • Help patient develop a more realistic attitude to the pain—i.e. pain will not cause further bone damage
	  • Relaxation and distraction techniques
	  • Graded exposure to overcome fear of falling

Individualized care	1. Demonstrating kindness and caring to the patient 2. Use of humor 3. Positive reinforcement following a desired behavior 4. Recognition of individual needs and differences, such as setting a rest period or providing a favorite snack 5. Clearly and simply write out/inform patient of what activity is recommended
Social support	1. Evaluate the presence and adequacy of social network 2. Teach significant other(s) to verbally encourage/reinforce the desired behavior 3. Use social supports as a source of goal identification
Goal identification	1. Develop appropriate realistic goals with the older adult 2. Set goals that can be met in a short time frame—daily or weekly—as well as a long-range goal to work toward 3. Set goals that are challenging but attainable 4. Set goals that are clear and specific

successfully in the past and can be considered useful building blocks for more comprehensive motivational interventions. First and foremost, it is critical to establish whose motives are being addressed in the motivational interaction. If goals are established without the input of the older individual, it is not likely he or she will be willing to participate in the activities needed to achieve the goal. For individuals who are cognitively impaired and cannot articulate goals, it is useful to review old records and speak with families, friends, and caregivers who have known the individual previously. Goals can then be developed based on their prior life and accomplishments.[73,74] Further, it is important that the goals established be realistic and achievable so as to ensure feelings of success.

Demonstrations of caring and confidence in the skills necessary to help the individual (e.g., providing assistance with transfers) are central to motivating older adults in this area. Care can be demonstrated by behaviors and activities perceived by the individual as expressions of love, attention, concern, respect, and support.[75] Another important aspect of caring is setting some guidelines or limits with regard to behaviors. This does not relate to punishment or threats. Rather, it is focused on being firm and informing the individual of the activity they need to do and why they need to do it. For example, an older individual may need to get up and walk to the bathroom to prevent skin breakdown, optimize continence, and regain strength and function. In addition, individualized care includes recognizing individual differences and needs, using kindness and humor, empowering older adults to take an active part in their care, providing gentle verbal persuasion to perform an activity, and positive reinforcement after performance, or even attempts at performance.[4,5,66] Examining the setting in which motivational interventions are occurring, although basic, is important to ensuring successful interactions. If the older adults cannot see or hear what a therapist is telling him or her to do, for example, he or she will not perform the activity and thus be labeled noncompliant or unmotivated. Simple interventions such as eliminating background noise and speaking slow, low, and loud can greatly help these situations. For profound hearing loss, or if the therapist is soft spoken, an external device that amplifies sound can be used. In addition, establish an environment in which the older individual does not feel stressed that he or she has to move quickly. If stressed in this manner, it is likely the individual will freeze and not be able to perform at all.

Lastly, recognizing and appreciating the heterogeneity of older adults and the fact that what is effective in motivating one individual may or may not be useful when working with a different individual is important. Moreover, multiple interventions (e.g., individualized care, setting goals, providing verbal encouragement, and ensuring mastery experiences) may be necessary to optimally motivate the older individual.

Complex Motivational Challenges

Overcoming Fear. Fear of falling is common among older adults and occurs in 42% to 73% of those who have fallen.[76-78] Fear of falling is associated with reduced physical activity,[78-82] decreased participation in functional activities,[83,84] lower perceived physical health status,[85,86] and lower quality of life and life satisfaction.[87,88] When trying to increase participation in functional activities and time spent in physical activity, it is important to decrease or eliminate fear of falling. Most of the research that has been done to address fear has focused on fear of back pain. The interventions utilized for fear of experiencing back pain, however, are theoretically based and may be effective if translated to fear of falling.

Interventions to decrease fear of back pain are based on cognitive–behavioral therapy and include either Graded Activity or Graded Exposure treatment.[89-91] Graded Activity starts by finding out how much activity each patient can do before pain occurs. Then the patient is enrolled in a program that starts with that level of exercise or activity. The therapist guides the patient in building tolerance by slowly increasing duration, intensity, and frequency of the exercise or activity that was noted to cause pain. Educational strategies are incorporated into the intervention to teach the patient that pain is not harmful in terms of his or her underlying back problems and that the exercise/activity recommended is beneficial in spite of the pain that may occur. Positive reinforcement is provided as the individual works toward achieving success and overcoming fear associated with the activity.

In contrast, Graded Exposure treatment involves presenting the participant with anxiety-producing material (e.g., having him or her engage in an activity that causes pain) for a long enough time to decrease the intensity of their emotional reaction. Ultimately, the feared situation no longer results in the individual becoming anxious, or avoiding the activity. Exposure treatment can be carried out in real-life situations, which is called in vivo exposure; or it can be done through imagination, which is called imaginal exposure. The Graded Exposure intervention starts by looking at which activities cause fear (e.g., walking, stair climbing, twisting) and then having the individual engage in that activity repeatedly. As fear associated with the activity decreases, the frequency, intensity, and duration of the activity is increased.

Other interventions to decrease fear of falling have included exercise activities (walking, strengthening, balance activities, Tai Chi), educational programs, and use of hip protectors. There was some, albeit limited, evidence for the effectiveness of these interventions on decreasing fear of falling.[92-94] Outcomes are better when interventions are combined, such as when an educational program is combined with an exercise program.

Giving In and Giving Up: Dealing with Apathy. Apathy, or a lack of interest, concern, or emotion, has been conceptualized as the opposite of motivation.[95] Although apathy is commonly noted in those with dementia and depression,[96] it can occur independent of either of those two conditions.[95] Unfortunately, the presence of apathy is associated with a decrease in functional and physical activities in older adults.[97] Numerous pharmacologic interventions have been used to decrease apathy and improve participation in rehabilitation activities. These include amantadine, amphetamine, bromocriptine, bupropion, methylphenidate, and selegiline,[98] and more recently the cholinesterase inhibitors,[99] as well as the selective serotonin reuptake inhibitors.[100,101]

Medication management for apathy may be a useful, even necessary, first step in engaging the older adults with apathy. Behavioral interventions, however, should likewise be initiated. Behavioral interventions focus on structure and stimulation such that the individual is encouraged to engage in activities that he or she can easily do successfully. New and different activities such as participating in a visiting pet program or a Tai Chi class generally tend to be good sources of stimulation and motivation. Individuals with apathy will likely say "no!" to participating in any of the activities that are recommended or that he or she is invited to attend. In situations in which the apathy is profound and persistent, it may be necessary to ignore the "no" and engage the individual—if only for a short period of time—in the activity. This can sometimes be done by walking with the individual to the activity and sitting with him or her for a period of time. Persistent and regular encouragement to participate in activities in the community or within a facility, or encouragement to participate in simple bathing and dressing activities, is critical. All too often, health care providers and lay caregivers stop asking apathetic older individuals to engage in activities and thus propagate the disease.

The Comprehensive Approach to Motivation. Motivation in older adults is a complex multidimensional factor that must be evaluated on an individual basis. The evaluation should include intrapersonal, interpersonal, environmental, and larger social policy implications of motivation. Interventions can then be individualized based on where challenges are identified. Assessing motivation and intervening is an ongoing process, and persistence and determination to overcome motivational problems is needed on the part of the health care providers and lay caregivers. Working together, motivation can be treated and improved with regard to function and physical activity. In so doing, the individual will be able to obtain and maintain his or her highest level of function and optimal quality of life.

PATIENT EDUCATION

Introduction

Imparting information to a patient is one of the most common interventions a physical therapist uses. However, patient education is often the least addressed topic in physical therapy schools, with effective techniques the least understood. Physical therapists often do not perceive themselves as educators despite the fact that the therapist spends much of any treatment session instructing patients in new techniques or home programs or facilitating relearning of motor skills. Using appropriate education strategies grounded in sound theory and research may make the difference between the patient's success and failure in achieving rehabilitation goals. In the second half of this chapter, patient education and the physical therapist's role as a patient educator are emphasized in terms of a practical yet philosophically based experience that can influence the older patients' direction in prescribed interventions. A review of learning theories is presented, followed by a philosophical approach to learning and patient education. Characteristics of older adult learners and some common barriers to their learning also are summarized. The role of the caregiver and teaching strategies to enhance this role are discussed, and selected assessment methods are presented. The chapter concludes with three typical patient education scenarios that illustrate some of the concepts presented relative to patient education as an intervention.

Learning Theories

Learning by its very nature defies easy definition and simple theorizing. The concepts of behavioral change and experience are central to learning theories. *Learning* is defined as the capacity to behave in a given fashion, which results from practice or other forms of experience that causes an enduring change in behavior.[112] Learning as a process, rather than an end product, focuses on what happens as learning takes place. Explanations of this process are called *learning theories*. It is necessary to understand the components of how learning occurs to effectively address specific learning situations.

Behaviorist Orientation. Behaviorism focuses on observable behavior shaped by environmental forces. Learning occurs when there is a change in the form or frequency of observable performance.[113] The key elements in learning under behaviorist principles are the stimulus, the response, and the association between the two. The environment plays the most important role in the behaviorist theoretical approach. Behavioral theorists believe that the teacher's role is to design an environment that elicits desired behavior and to extinguish behavior that is not desirable. An example in physical therapy patient education would be the therapist verbally reinforcing a correct transfer technique as it is being performed while ignoring the behavior when the transfer technique is done incorrectly. Another example might be when the therapist instructs a patient in stair climbing and consistently reinforces the "correct technique," such as a particular foot advancing first. The patient eventually performs according to the therapist's instructions but may not know why, so when encountering unfamiliar situations, may have difficulty adapting his or her behavior to the new situation. The systematic design of instruction, behavioral objectives, notions of the instructor's accountability, programmed instruction, computer-assisted instruction, and competency-based education are strongly grounded in behavioral learning theory. The behaviorist orientation is thought to be ideal for learning that requires rote responses and recall of facts. Behaviorist principles are less appropriate for higher order thinking skills, such as problem solving.[113]

Cognitive Orientation. Cognitive processes such as thinking, problem solving, language, and concept formation are stressed in the cognitive approach. Learning is equated with discrete changes between states of knowledge rather than in the probability of response. Cognitive theories focus on the conceptualization of students' learning processes and address the issues of how information is received, organized, stored, and retrieved by the mind.[113] An example of applied cognitive theory in geriatric physical therapy would be demonstrated in how the therapist organizes a treatment session with the goal of instructing the patient how to weight shift prior to ambulation. In such an example, the therapist would build on the simple tasks of supine weight shifting, moving to more complex tasks such as sitting weight shifting and then standing weight shifting. Progression would then advance from bipedal weight shifting to unilateral weight shifting to advancing a foot forward. Concern for the proper pacing of instruction would be addressed throughout the treatment session.

Humanist Orientation. Humanist theories consider learning from the perspective of the human potential for growth. From a learning theory perspective, humanism emphasizes that a person's perceptions are centered in experience, as well as the freedom and responsibility to become what one is capable of becoming. These tenets underlie much of adult learning theory that stresses the self-directedness of adults and the value of experience in the learning process.

Social Learning Theory. Social learning theory is a system of thought based on imitation or modeling. Bandura postulated that one can learn from observation without having to imitate what was observed.[2] He further explored self-directed behaviors. In order for people to regulate their own behavior, well-defined objectives or goals are selected; contractual agreements are negotiated to further increase goal commitment; objective records of behavioral changes are used as additional sources of reinforcement for their self-controlling behavior; and the stimulus condition under which the behavior customarily occurs is altered. For example, for the older adult who has difficulty adhering to his or her diabetic diet, removing the source of temptation or storing the forbidden food in a different place would alter stimulus conditions. The progressive narrowing of stimulus control, for

example, may initiate change over a period of time instead of creating a total change at one time. A commitment to monitor food intake would also be important from the social learning viewpoint.

The term *locus of control* is used to explain which behavior in the individual's repertoire will occur in a given situation. Typically, people with an internal locus of control will adhere more consistently and longer than those with an external locus of control, which requires external motivation such as praise and material rewards. Social learning theories provide an additional factor in how adults learn by acknowledging the importance of context and the learner's interaction with the environment to explain behavior.

Adult Learning Orientation. *Andragogy* is a term popularized by Knowles to explain a philosophical orientation for adult education.[114] His four main assumptions of changes in self-concept, role of experience, readiness to learn, and orientation to learning lay the foundation for the instruction of older adults.

Changes in self-concept occur as individuals grow and mature. Their self-concept moves from one of total dependency (as is the reality of an infant) to one of increasing self-directedness. Any experience that adults perceive as putting them in a position of being treated as a child will interfere with their learning, commonly resulting in expressions of resentment and resistance. As mentioned earlier, older adults tend to have a positive self-concept.

Role of experience defines the role of lifetime experiences. As individuals mature, they accumulate an expanding reservoir of experience, producing an older adult who has a *rich* and varied background to facilitate new learning and knowledge. If older adults perceive their experiences to be devalued or ignored, they may then perceive this as rejecting their experience and even their person.

The concept of *readiness to learn* explains the shift from an external stimulus to an internal stimulus. As individuals mature, their readiness to learn is decreasingly the product of biological development and academic pressure and is increasingly the product of the developmental tasks required for the performance of evolving social roles. Learning experiences must be timed to coincide with the learners' developmental tasks. For example, an older patient may need to attempt ambulation and find that it is difficult before comprehending the importance of general strengthening or balance activities.

Orientation to learning reflects the adult's purpose for learning. Adults tend to have a problem-centered orientation to learning. Real-life problems are the purpose for seeking educational opportunities. The immediate application of information is a primary need of the adult learner.[114]

Transtheoretical Model. The transtheoretical model (TTM) of behavior change was developed in the early

1980s by Prochaska and DiClemente[115] to describe how people changed their behavior. The model suggests that people go through change as a process over time and that receptivity to information is dependent on the stage of change in which the person is in. Table 10-4 describes the stages and the appropriate types of information for each stage. The TTM has been used to promote adaptation of healthy behaviors such as engaging in exercise.[116] The key feature is the stage approach in that different strategies and interventions are used for individuals at different stages of readiness to change or adopt behavior.[116]

In conclusion, the following principles developed by Darkenwald and Merriam summarize the principles applicable to patient education as intervention[117]:

- Adults' readiness to learn depends on their previous learning.
- Intrinsic motivation produces more pervasive and permanent learning.
- Positive reinforcement is effective.
- Material to be learned should be presented in an organized fashion.
- Learning is enhanced by repetition.
- Tasks and materials that are meaningful are more fully and more easily learned.

- Active participation in learning improves retention.
- Environmental factors affect learning.
- Adults learn throughout their lifetime.
- Adults exhibit learning styles that illustrate various learning theories, such as the following:
  - Having personal strategies for organizing information.
  - Perceiving in different ways—cognitive procedures.
  - Perceiving learning activities to be problem-centered and relevant to life.
  - Desiring some immediate appreciation.
  - Having a concept of themselves as learners.
  - Being self-directed.

The learning theories and principles presented in this section are diverse but can also complement each other. The effective health care provider will use a variety of patient education interventions based on the outcomes desired.

Psychological Factors of the Learning Situation

To develop a philosophical approach to patient education, physical therapists must understand their own motivations and biases toward their role as the helper,

TABLE 10-4	Transtheoretical Model of Behavior Change		
Stage	Description*	Learner Characteristics	Type of Information Useful†
Precontemplation	Not engaged in the targeted activity with no intention to do so	Resistant to change, if thinking about change at all May fear failure May lack information May be overwhelmed with barriers	Personalized information about benefits of targeted activity, feedback about risks of current behavior
Contemplation	Intend to engage in the targeted activity in the next 6 months	May be open to information about benefits of new behavior May be curious about results that could be obtained from changing Ambivalence is common	Information about how to reduce barriers to targeted activity Identify role models Continue to provide education about personal risks and benefits Help to make a definite commitment to change
Preparation	Intend to engage in the targeted activity in next 30 days	May take small steps toward change	Identify alternatives to targeted activity that will accomplish same goal and make a plan Make a public commitment Involve others
Action	Begins the targeted activity for at least 1 day up to 6 months	Requires commitment and energy to make it work May be looking for reinforcement and encouragement	Frequent positive reinforcement Log of activity Provide support networks
Maintenance	Engaged in targeted activity for at least 6 months	Challenge is to sustain behavior and overcoming barriers that can cause relapse	Meaningful reward Long-term goals Support groups and networks

*Data from Lach HW, Everard KM, Highstein G, Brownson CA: Application of the transtheoretical model to health education for older adults. Health Promot Pract 5(1):88-93, 2004.
†Data from Burbank PM, Reibe D, Padula CA, Nigg C: Exercise and older adults: changing behavior with the transtheoretical model. Orthop Nurs 21(4): 51-61; quiz 61-3, 2002.

their attitudes toward their patients, and their attitude toward the information they are sharing. Understanding the older adult's perceptions of self and of learning is also important. This section discusses factors that contribute to the therapists' and patients' attitudes toward teaching and learning.

Therapist's Perception of the Patient Educator. One motivation for entering the health care field is to help people. People become helpers because they really enjoy helping others and want to affect their lives positively. Although the motive to help others focuses on the needs of the patient, the desire to control may also be present. The desire to exert control, to be in charge, and to have some noticeable impact on the world is particularly relevant when attempting to "teach" a patient. This attitude of control can make the physical therapist the authority of the learning situation, perhaps inhibiting the learning situation. The authority role may be in direct conflict with the stronger self-perception of the older adult as a critical consumer of health care and thus make the learning situation less effective.

Another common but deeper and less obvious thought that can interfere with the physical therapist's role as an educator is the fear of being in a similar situation someday when the patient becomes a disturbing mirror image of the physical therapist's real or potential suffering. Asserting authority or avoiding the person through minimal and superficial involvement are ways the physical therapist defends against this phenomenon.

The cure model of health care still is prevalent in today's health care environment. Paternalism places the health care provider in the role of decision maker about the type and amount of information the patient receives. Paternalism is most often associated with the traditional medical model, which uses authority, power, and superior knowledge to act on the patient's behalf. Paternalism tends to reinforce the passiveness of the patient and communicates expectations of compliance and unquestioning obedience. The role of the health care provider is a "father" figure, that is, authoritarian and all-knowing. If paternalism is supported by the environment, the older adult may view the physical therapist as overbearing. The physical therapist may not consider the patient's needs, concerns, and choices and therefore may act incompletely or inappropriately.[118]

An alternative to the cure model of health care is the care model. The care model values patient autonomy and mutual collaboration between the patient and the physical therapist. In the care model, the role of the physical therapy provider is one of consultant and enabler, peer, and adviser, facilitating the patient's needs and desires. In this model, the type and amount of information are determined by the patient with a commitment from the physical therapist to be honest and forthcoming. Individualized care, compassion, warm personal regard, and open communication are additional values. Limitations of the care model involve the need for

patients to make decisions for themselves. A patient may not be able to make his or her own decisions in times of grief or extreme stress or with certain medical conditions. This approach also takes longer, making it less efficient. Finally, the health care provider may not use his or her extensive knowledge as overtly as in the cure model, perhaps putting the patient at a slight disadvantage.[127]

Older Adults' Perception of Self. Multiple internal and external forces affect older adults' behavior, attitudes, and conditioning. Any number of these forces can affect how older patients respond to medical situations and their attitudes toward the learning situation. Interestingly, older individuals, over the age of 60 years, ranked their role as learners significantly below other age groups.[119] This section briefly presents several of the forces that affect the older patient related to learning.

Sensitivity to Failure. Many therapists treating older adults will be significantly younger than their patients. An older adult's sensitivity to failure may be affected by the age difference and by the perceived ease with which the younger therapist performs complicated tasks and physical movement. The therapist also must realize the patient may be comparing current performance with previous normal performance, which can enhance the perception of failure. A negative self-concept and the older adult's view of his or her own personal crisis, for example, disability, illness, or personal loss, also may accentuate the sensitivity to failure.

Resistance to Change. Resistance can be a normal coping strategy to change and fear and should not be viewed as rigidity of attitude or behavior and thus result in a person being less amenable to change. Rogers stated that resistance may be observed when the individual feels threatened. The older patient also may express total hopelessness for improved function and exhibit a resignation to accepting the present limitations. This attitude may be manifested in resistance to suggestions, change, or help. Skepticism and even some degree of fear may underlie resistance.

In summary, the older patient in treatment sessions is an individual with a complex psychosocial profile that will influence the degree of willingness to learn. The therapist also has complex attitudes and beliefs regarding the role of the health care professional that affect the tone, manner, and flexibility of the therapist in the teaching/learning situation. The initial step in becoming an effective patient educator is to recognize underlying attitudes affecting the learning situation.

Education can be viewed as the process of facilitating the learner's problem-solving skills with the goal that the learner will gain control over any specific problem.[120,121] Teaching does not imply learning. Teaching in the traditional sense is one-sided and asks nothing of the patient except that the patient be present. The "teacher" should place the responsibility for learning on the learner, the patient. An example of this concept is seen in motor learning. Motor learning uses the strategy of the patient's internal feedback to provide stimulus for learning, rather than the therapist's stimulus of telling the patient his or her movement is "right or wrong." For instance, while assisting a patient with the task of stair climbing, instead of directing the patient in a certain "technique" of stair climbing, the therapist may instead suggest that the patient begin to climb the stairs and then to facilitate the patient's internal feedback mechanism by asking questions such as "how did that feel" when the patient starts to lose his or her balance or "did you notice the difference" when the patient tries a technique that was more complex.[122,123]

Payton et al assert that only the patient can make the decision that a goal is worth working for.[124] Lindgren states that older patients should be viewed as individuals who are capable of making their own decisions.[125] These two statements clearly convey the important message that older adults can and do exercise choice in whether they will participate in treatment sessions. Rogers believes that it is impossible to "teach" anyone anything unless the learner wants to learn.[120] Think of the patient who sits through a detailed exercise program. A strong feeling is transmitted that the patient really is not listening to the therapist and is, in fact, in a hurry to leave. No matter how great a "facilitator of learning" the therapist is, if the patient does not want to learn, he or she will not.

Basically, one learns what one wants to learn. When one wants to learn, one is described as being "motivated," an internal phenomenon. Bille relates Maslow's needs hierarchy to patient motivation in an interesting and relevant manner.[126] Maslow theorized that one's basic physiological needs (air, food, water, movement, sex, avoidance of pain) and safety and security needs (assurance that the world is regular and predictable; that death, destruction, or physical/social/emotional/economic harm is not imminent) must be met before affiliation and esteem needs can be met.

Bille applies this concept to the patient who has experienced physical trauma and whose current needs basically are physiological and safety oriented. The patient may find it difficult to focus on adjusting to the trauma and the necessary rehabilitation and may not be able to envision managing the changes that may result from that trauma. Motivation will be enhanced, therefore, when instruction is centered on procedures that are, in the patient's perspective, physiological and safety oriented, such as strength, mobility, ambulation, or activities of daily living (ADLs). When these needs are met, self-esteem increases as progress is made.

Bille relates the need for esteem to the motivation to learn and states that as self-esteem increases, motivation to learn will increase. The therapist can foster the patient's self-esteem, and therefore motivation, which promotes two-way communication. The patient needs to feel free and unthreatened to tell the therapist what has affected or lowered his or her self-esteem. The basic characteristics a teacher needs to exhibit to facilitate this open communication as described by Rogers are realness or genuineness, prizing the learner, acceptance, trust, and empathic understanding.[121] When the health care professional exhibits realness or genuineness, the facade is lifted, and the therapist comes into a direct personal encounter with the learner and meets the learner on a person-to-person basis, as peers or equals. There is no hiding behind an authoritarian role; there is no sterile facade. The physical therapist can express emotions and attitudes and becomes, to the patient, a real person with convictions and feelings.

Rogers describes prizing the learner as valuing the learner's feelings, opinions, and the person as a whole. Prizing is caring for the learner, accepting the learner as a separate person, appreciating the learner's differences, and exhibiting a belief that the learner is fundamentally trustworthy. The physical therapist who exhibits this attitude can fully accept the fear and hesitation of the older adult as the patient approaches his or her own personal crisis. This attitude allows the therapist to accept the "poor motivation" of the older adult and to make attempts to understand the factors contributing to the motivational problem. Empathic understanding is the therapist's ability to appreciate the patient's reactions from the patient's perspective and to have a sensitive awareness of the way the processes of education and learning seem to the patient. The likelihood of significant learning is increased when these characteristics are exhibited by the therapist.[120]

To increase the patient's self-directedness, the therapist should provide opportunities for the patient to make decisions about treatment and to identify what is to be learned. The next section explores a specific model that encourages full patient participation in goal setting and intervention.

PATIENT PARTICIPATION IN GOAL SETTING

Facilitating the patient's full participation in each therapeutic interaction should be a primary goal of the therapist, and especially in the goal-setting process. Increasing patient participation in goal setting and treatment planning improves clinical outcomes and patient satisfaction and is recommended or required in regulatory and practice guidelines.[127-131] Although the vast majority of clinicians believe that they attempt to involve patients in a goal-setting process, the literature demonstrates that most clinicians involve patients at far less than optimal levels.[132-136] Tripicchio et al.[137] identified two areas where therapists failed patients when eliciting goals. First, therapists often confused goals with means. Means are the ways in which goals are accomplished, whereas goals are the patient's outcomes; that is what the patient is ultimately trying to achieve. Goals are highly personal and can serve as a significant motivation. Second, if therapists did correctly solicit a goal, they oftentimes failed to specify *exactly* what the patient wanted to be able to do. This specificity (i.e., what, when, where, degree) helps eliminate any confusion about what the goal is, ensures the goal is functional, and gives all parties involved a clear idea of what is to be achieved. A goal of "gait of 100 feet without an assistive device" is not a functional goal, whereas a goal of "walking to the bus stop (800 feet) in 4 minutes using the uneven city sidewalk without assistance" is a functional goal.

There are many reasons why therapists may not involve patients to the fullest extent in a goal setting process. These are listed in Box 10-1. However, few guidelines exist as to how therapists should elicit patient goals.[135,136] One process is the Ozer-Payton-Nelson (OPN) method.[138] Ozer, a physician; Payton, a physical therapist; and Nelson, an occupational therapist, collaborated to develop a systematic, cyclical method to involve patients in setting functional goals and evaluating functional outcomes to their maximal degree possible.[138,139] The therapist leads the patient to explore the range of individual concerns and then to identify the primary concern. Goal setting by the patient becomes a motivator because a greater degree of choice is exercised.

Individual concerns are elicited and explored in the OPN model through the use of four questions posed at different stages of treatment planning and three processes for each question (Table 10-5). A key to the OPN method is concerns clarification. Concerns clarification is a multifaceted process that includes the patient identifying personal functional, disabling problems caused by his or her pathology and impairment; ranking those problems as to importance and specifying (i.e., addressing what, when, where, how, degree) to bridge the gap to setting goals.

The OPN model uses hierarchical levels of patient participation to elicit and clarify patient concerns. Physical therapists trained in this method begin by initially asking patients open-ended questions and thus giving the patients control while not attempting to influence responses. If a patient is unable to answer an open-ended question at the free-choice level, the therapists can proceed to posing questions at three other levels (i.e., multiple choice, confirmed choice, and forced choice). Therapists ask for the patient's permission before moving to a lower level, never skip a level, and return to the level of free choice for further questioning whenever possible. Movement from open-ended questions to these lower three levels means that planning and evaluating are becoming less patient-centered and more therapist-centered. The goal is to cooperatively plan and evaluate with the patient at the highest level what the patient is capable of or desires; prescribing to the patient is to be avoided. The following example demonstrates how the OPN method can be used to elicit and clarify patient-centered goals.

A 70-year-old female elementary school teacher was receiving skilled occupational and physical therapy in a skilled nursing facility following cardiac surgery. She described her condition upon entering the skilled nursing facility as "I couldn't do anything, no confidence, I had fallen at the hospital, I couldn't walk at all."

Therapist	What are your present concerns about functionally getting you to move from where you are now to your baseline?
Patient	My feet are swollen.
Therapist	How does that interfere with your functioning?
Patient	It interferes with walking.
Therapist	People have to walk for different reasons. What about walking is important for you?
Patient	Walking to the classroom from the parking lot. Walking in the grocery store. Taking children to special classes like PE and library; we have many steps in our school that would be a challenge but we also have an elevator that I could use, but I would have to send children up on their own.
Therapist	What is your greatest concern of those listed?
Patient	Actually, none of those—just being able to walk.
Therapist	Being able to walk to do what?
Patient	Being able to walk even without a walker from physical therapy down the hallway where I have to go on my own or just with a cane.
Therapist	What do you see as a first step?

BOX 10-1	**Reasons for Therapist Control of Goal-Setting Process**

- Perceived time limitations
- Lack of preparation at the professional level of education
- Inexperience dealing with unrealistic and irrelevant patient goals (e.g., those related to other disciplines)
- Use of vague and inconsistently applied informal interview methods
- Professional versus patient role beliefs (e.g., control, expectations, paternalism)
- Limited or no awareness of patient-centered care standards and regulations

(Adapted from Tripicchio B, Bykerk K, Wegner C, Wegner J: Increasing patient participation: the effects of training physical and occupational therapists to involve geriatric patients in the concerns-clarification and goal-setting processes. J Phys Ther Educ 23(1): 55-63, 2009.)

TABLE 10-5	Features of the OPN Method Levels of Patient Participation		
Clinician	**Patient**	**Degree or Level**	**Patient's Involvement**
Asks open-ended questions (does not suggest answers)	**Free Choice** Explores	A	100%
Asks questions and offers suggestions	**Multiple Choice** Selects	B	75%
Asks questions, provides an answer (recommendation), and asks for agreement and confirmation	**Confirmed Choice** Puts into own words what has been selected	C	50%
Asks question, provides an answer (recommendation), and asks for agreement	**Forced Choice** Agrees or disagrees with what has been selected	D	25%
Does not ask, tells what to do. Prescribes.	**No Choice** Compliant or noncompliant	E	0%

These five patient participation levels, starting from Level A, Free Choice, are used to explore, select, and specify patients' concerns, goals, results achieved, and actions taken. The farther down you move from Level A, planning and evaluating are becoming more therapist-centered and less patient-centered.
(Adapted from Ozer MN, Payton OD, Nelson CE: Treatment planning for rehabilitation: a patient-centered approach. New York, NY: McGraw-Hill, 2000.)

Patient   Being able to walk without a wheelchair with a walker from the physical therapy room to the windows where you can see ice sculptures and deer. And without a wheelchair I would have to walk back and that would be a bigger accomplishment.

Therapist   Walking to the windows would be a short-term goal and to and from a long-term goal.

The therapist then pointed out how the patient herself had progressed from discussing concerns to the question of goals. She had also identified short-term and long-term goals. The therapist then continued with further exploration of concerns or goals.

Therapist   Do you have any other questions or anything else to add?

Patient   Walking into my house, a tri-level with one step in, that would precede walking into school, that's a biggie!

Patient   Completely getting myself out of bed.

This example demonstrates how the therapist elicited seven concerns/goals that were on a continuum from short-term to long-term, which took less than 10 minutes. Interestingly, the patient's initial stated concern was not her greatest concern. With the addition of the OPN processes of selection, specification, and the development of a plan (i.e., means and timeline) the framework was established for a treatment plan with her maximal involvement.

Only two studies have investigated the effectiveness of the OPN model. Tripicchio et al found there was a positive effect 1 to 3 weeks after training in the method on

10 of the critical skills dimensions those therapists need to effectively involve older patients to a higher level of participation in their treatment planning.[137] Holliday and colleagues[140] investigated the effectiveness of a process similar to the OPN method with neurologic patients. One of their measures was the Patient Participation Scale used in the OPN method. Findings showed that those patients involved in a structured goal-setting process had greater perceived autonomy, and greater perceived relevance of goals than patients whose goals were established by their therapist. The OPN model may provide a way to increase involvement of the patient, provide more autonomy for the patient, and establish more functional, personal goals. In turn, this process has the potential of increasing outcomes self-efficacy through the care model of interaction and thus enhancing motivation.

Older adults may exhibit some resistance to becoming partners in treatment decisions and sessions. Anderson suggests that this reluctance may be based on their perceptions of health care professionals as authorities whose wisdom is all-encompassing and whose decisions are not to be discussed or questioned.[141] In the traditional patriarchal and authoritarian health care model, the patient has a more passive role in treatment sessions, whereas the therapist is the activist. In contrast, in the helping process, the patient is more active in identifying the problem, setting goals, exploring alternative solutions, and assessing the results. When the patient is active in the helping process, the patient's resilience is strengthened.[141]

In summary, the helping process appears to be more congruent with the older patient's need for self-esteem, autonomy, the exercise of choice, and the partnership that Payton advocates. To be an effective patient educator requires an approach of empowering the patient rather than assuming an authoritarian role. An effective patient educator facilitates the learner's learning, appreciates the learner's differences, and helps the learner establish goals and responsibility for learning. A patient whose ideas, interests, concerns, and feelings have been heard and responded to by others is much more likely to enter into active, cooperative planning for necessary treatment. A patient who is actively involved in treatment planning is more likely to adhere to those cooperative plans and guarantee the success of treatment. The importance of self-esteem and choice relates closely to the older patient's motivational level. Lasting gains are possible when the older patient perceives the therapist as a supportive partner in treatment sessions. The therapist's degree of success when working with an older patient is related to the perception of that patient as a person against a background of cognitive and psychosocial characteristics.

Strategies to Affect Learning

The therapist's actions and behaviors are keys in working with an older patient whose negative self-concept presents a significant obstacle to treatment progress. To attempt to counter these doubts and to modify the patient's perception of self to a more positive view, the therapist should emphasize the successful experiences the patient has had as an adult in overcoming other difficult experiences. Other techniques include guiding the patient to identify the reason(s) for any past failures and assisting the patient to recognize that the reason(s) for failure may not be a factor in treatment. If, however, the reason(s) for past failure may be present in the therapeutic environment, the therapist should help the patient identify the factors that can be controlled at this time.[142] For example, consider the patient with previously treated low back pain who starts physical therapy. The patient's behavior indicates a reluctance to try the exercises. As the therapist explores this reluctance, the patient indicates, "No one really explained the previous exercises." The therapist indicates that doing an exercise incorrectly can cause increased pain. Extra care and a thorough explanation of the exercises are indicated to address the patient's history of perceived failure.

Creating a successful instructional environment and providing opportunities for successes, no matter how small they may be, are valuable tools. Any contributions the patient may make should be recognized, and establishing a partnership in the treatment goals and sessions is helpful.[142] However, psychological counseling is best done by counseling professionals.

During the treatment session, the therapist should provide tasks that the patient can do successfully. Focusing on relevant information in an organized, clear manner and providing adequate time for skill practice can enhance successful performance. The therapist should sensitively give adequate, honest feedback and encouragement for correct responses and performance to diminish the chances for and perception of failure.

The patient's positive contributions and correct performance of any tasks[142] should be stressed; be aware that patients who are depressed may demonstrate an increased sensitivity to failure and heightened self-criticism.

Accepting the patient's existing attitudes and recognizing that new attitudes, behaviors, and values cannot be forced on the older patient may help temper any resistance to change of treatment. Creating constructive dialogue and reasoning instead of participating in arguments that tend to further entrench negative attitudes may help prevent these natural reactions of resistance and resignation. Discovering elements that affect patient motivation is paramount.

Educational and Cultural Background

The number of years between earlier instructional activities and present instructional activities, previous level of education, and past experiences with learning are components of the older patient's psychosocial profile. Instruction related to job and profession or participation in adult education and community education courses may be factors that will influence the patient's positive predisposition toward learning new tasks. However, if the patient primarily remembers negative experiences in earlier educational situations, these unpleasant memories may make it more difficult for the older patient to be a cooperative and a willing participant in treatment sessions. The therapist should make every effort to ensure that the older patient experiences success in the initial treatment sessions and to assist in the differentiation of any earlier negative experiences from present therapeutic procedures.

Low literacy skills may be a barrier to successful learning and should be recognized by the physical therapist. Some older adults have deficient learning skills and can be proficient at hiding them because of embarrassment. Using a variety of teaching methods, simple vocabulary, and repetition of key points can enhance the learning opportunities of the older adult with low literacy skills.

Many ethnic populations reside across the United States—with African Americans, Native Americans, Asian Americans and Pacific Islanders, and Hispanics being the standard four major groups. The therapist must remember that in addition to the patients having lived many years, their ethnic environment will influence their predisposition toward, perception of, cooperation with, and follow-up of treatment. Traditional tribal and home treatment methods are influential in all four ethnic populations. Illness is not a word in some Pacific/Asian languages, and in others, illness is synonymous with acute conditions and death, and hospitals may be viewed with fear.[143]

Another consideration with ethnic older patients is level of English proficiency and education. Using translators if the therapist—or another member of an interdisciplinary team—does not have bilingual–bicultural skills is very helpful. Although family members and friends may appear to be the most logical choice for this important task, the recommended choice is an interpreter who has a background in medical terminology as well as in language and cultural expertise. Cultural differences must be translated in culturally appropriate terms and what may appear to be a single ethnic or racial group, for example, Pacific Islander or Hispanic older adults, may, in fact, represent multiple ethnicities and races with very different languages and customs. When working with an African American older adult, the therapist must remember the earlier segregation of health care facilities and must respect the black older person as a survivor of a health care system that was not accessible and perhaps was even hostile.[152] Figure 10-1 lists general health care characteristics of many cultures, compiled by South Miami Hospital.

Patient education materials for older patients of ethnic groups must be designed with cultural diversity as one of several important considerations. The translator should examine the text carefully for any words or phrases that might be incorrectly interpreted. Illustrations should reflect ethnic customs when possible. Software exercise programs are available that depict different ethnicities in exercise illustrations. Any number of reliable methods to test for appropriate reading level can be used. Field testing patient education materials using a sample of the intended audience before final production is recommended to determine the effectiveness of the material.

The extended family as caregivers to older adults is common among certain cultures. A lack of familiarity with health care resources and the bureaucratic processes for access often results in underutilization by minorities. Among Hispanics, the use of formal health care services can be viewed as the family's failure to take care of its own. The health care an individual family member is allowed to receive may be subject to the approval or disapproval by the older-adult dominant family member.[143] Building a level of trust through demonstration of sensitivity to the history and cultural view of illness and health care specific to the individual's culture in order to negotiate successful treatment regimens with ethnic older persons is effective.[143] The therapist should regard this interaction as an opportunity for learning and increasing cultural sensitivity and awareness.

The Older Adult as a Learner

This section relates patient education as an intervention to the knowledge of the process by which older patients "learn." The belief that "you can't teach old dogs new tricks" can be a negative influence on therapists who fail to recognize the fallacy of such a generalization. Older adults can and do learn. To work with older adults successfully, a therapist must develop a dual role as a caring

and competent therapist and as a skillful facilitative instructor.

Cognitive Aspects. Cognition refers to intellectual processes, whereas learning generally is considered the acquisition of knowledge or skills achieved by study, instruction, practice, and experience. An individual's performance becomes the basis for inferring the level of learning that has been achieved. Two aspects must be considered in discussing cognitive learning—the end product and the process. Many research studies focus only on the end product. Therefore, when a person's performance improves in an intellectual or physical task, the inference is that learning has occurred. Failure in performance, however, does not infer that learning has not occurred or has been lost. Many factors affect an older adult's performance, including motivation and physical and emotional states. The physical therapist must be sensitive to the fact that multiple variables affect the learning situation and avoid concluding that the older adult cannot learn.

Intelligence as measured by standard testing procedures has been shown to decline in later years. Traditional intelligence tests examine fluid intelligence, which is composed of factual knowledge. Disease, neurologic insults, genetics, and biological aging affect fluid intelligence. On the other hand, crystallized intelligence, knowledge that comes from experience, occupation, and a sense of the world, increases with age.[144]

Research generally concludes that memory does decline with age, especially short-term memory. However, evidence suggests that memory involving skills and tasks used frequently does not decline to the degree that infrequently used information decreases. The adage "if you don't use it, you lose it" can be appropriately applied to cognition and is referred to as the disuse theory of cognition. Other research shows that when new information can be related to older adults' existing knowledge, their new learning is facilitated. Some factors involved in the cognition or intellectual processes can be accommodated by the physical therapist. These factors are assessment of learning level, learning readiness, and learning styles.

There is a great deal of evidence that older adults retain the ability to learn new things, especially those engaged in a cognitive and physically active lifestyle.[144] Although some aspects of intelligence may decline in later years, these changes should not affect function in the normal, noncognitively diseased individual. Although neuroanatomic changes are present in nearly all aging brains, the degree in which they occur and subsequently affect cognition is quite variable, representing the continuum of normal cognition to disease. Some mild memory loss and cognitive slowing is expected with age, but no functional loss should be apparent.

Health Literacy. The educational level of the older population is increasing. Between 1970 and 2008, the percentage of older persons who had completed high school rose from 28% to 77.4%. About 20.5% in

The Culture Tool

Culture Group and Language	Belief Practices	Communication Awareness	Patient Care/ Handling of Death
AMERICAN English	Christian and Jewish beliefs are prominent; many others exist in smaller numbers. Family-oriented.	Talkative, shake hands, not much touching during conversation. Prefer to gather information for decision making. Some hugging and kissing, mainly between women.	Family members and friends visit in small groups. Expect high-quality care.
ARGENTINIAN Spanish	90% Catholic, some Protestant and Jewish. Strong belief in saints, purgatory, and heaven. People from rural areas may be more superstitious.	Talkative, very expressive, direct, and to the point. Extroverted. Good eye contact. Like personal and physical contact such as holding hands, hugging, and kissing.	Educated, yet reluctant to get medical attention or accept new medical advancements. Independent, often deny disability. Believe in natural and holistic remedies: herbal teas, pure aloe, natural oils, poultices. Family gets involved with caring for the ill family member.
BRAZILIAN Portuguese; diverse cultural backgrounds, including European, African, Indian	Mostly Catholic; some Spiritism. Growing Evangelical representation. Candomble and Macumba—similar to Santeria.	Very sociable. Will stand close to each other. Social kissing, hugging, and touching. Good eye contact.	Emphasis on family unity—will want to be actively involved. Tend to trust medical personnel, place great faith in doctors and nurses. Some believe in herbal treatments, teas, and balsams.
CANADIAN English, French, and Inuit (Eskimo)	Protestant, Catholic, and Jewish	May prefer no touching or kissing. Take things at face value.	Follow nurses' instructions. Accustomed to socialized medicine, less litigation. Take physicians at their word. Willing to wait for treatment.
CAYMAN English with some changes in accent and verbs	People are very religious. Majority of the island is Baptist or Church of God. Voodoo and psychics are outlawed.	Like to be acknowledged. Good eye contact. Prefer no touching or kissing. Very talkative and known for their friendliness. Everyone on the island knows each other.	Like to be told what is going on by doctor. Would rather talk to doctors than nurses. Prefer one-to-one care.
CHINESE Many dialects spoken; one written language.	Religions: Taoism, Buddhism, Islam, Christianity. Harmonious relationship with nature and others; loyalty to family, friends, and government. Public debate of conflicting views is unacceptable. Accommodating, not confrontational. Modesty, self-control, self-reliance, self-restraint. Hierarchical structure for interpersonal and family interactions.	Quiet, polite, unassertive. Suppress feelings of anxiety, fear, depression, and pain. Eye contact and touching sometimes seen as offensive or impolite. Emphasize loyalty and tradition. Self-expression and individualism are discouraged.	Women uncomfortable with exams by male physicians. May not adhere to fixed schedule. May fear medical institutions. Use a combination of herbal and Western medicine. Traditional: acupuncture, herbal medicine, massage, skin scraping, and cupping. Alcohol may cause flushing.
CUBAN Spanish	Catholic with Protestant minority. Santeria, which can include animal sacrifice.	Some may have a tendency to be loud when having a discussion. Use their hands for emphasis and credibility, and prefer strong eye contact.	Culture requires visiting the sick. The extended family supports the immediate family. It is an insult to the patient if there is not a large family/friend presence.
ECUADORIAN Spanish, Quechua-Indian	Primarily Catholic. Increase in Protestant, Baptist, and Jehovah Witness. Very respectful toward religious leaders. Small percentage of population is wealthy, with much political control. Family size is usually large.	Extremely polite. Reserved. Respectful. Especially helpful.	Prefer pampering ill family members; stay overnight with patient. Not stoic when it comes to pain. Very private, modest. Embarrassed if they do not look their best. Extremely protective of family; often parents live with grown children.

FIGURE 10-1 The culture tool. *(Adapted from Baptist Health South Florida, South Miami Hospital, South Miami, Florida.)*

Culture Group and Language	Belief Practices	Communication Awareness	Patient Care/ Handling of Death
FILIPINO English, Spanish, Tagalog (80 dialects)	Catholic. Seek both faith healer and Western physician when ill. Belief that many diseases are the will of God.	Value and respect elders. Loving, family-oriented. Set aside time just for family.	Family decision important. Ignore health-related issues; often non-compliant. In spite of Western medicine, they often leave things in hands of God, with occasional folk medicine. Home remedies: herbal tea, massage, sleep. May subscribe to supernatural cause of diseases.
GUATEMALAN Spanish, Mayan heritage, European influence	Primarily Catholic. Increase in Protestants. Very respectful toward elders. European heritage; strong family ties.	Quiet, reserved, and respectful. Will not question for fear of insulting professional.	Modest, private, and stoic. Believe in alternative methods of healing.
HAITIAN Creole; French is taught in schools.	Catholic and Protestant. Voodoo is practiced. Large social gap exists between wealthy and poor citizens.	Quiet, polite. Value touch and eye contact.	Obedient to doctor and nurse but hesitant to ask questions. View use of oxygen as indication of severe illness. Occasionally share prescriptions and home remedies.
HINDU Hindi	The belief of cyclic birth and reincarnation lies at the center of Hinduism. The status, condition, and caste of each life is determined by behavior in the last life.	Limit eye contact. Do not touch while talking.	Do not try to force foods when religiously forbidden. Death—the priest may tie a thread around the neck or wrist to signify a blessing. This thread should not be removed. The priest will pour water into the mouth of the body. Family will request to wash the body. Eldest son is responsible for the funeral rites.
JAMAICAN English, Patois (broken English)	Christian beliefs dominate (Catholic, Baptist, Anglican). Strong Rastafarian influence.	Respect for elders is encouraged. Reserved; avoid hugging and showing affection in public. Curious and tend to ask a lot of questions.	Will try some home remedies before seeking medical help. Like to be completely informed before procedures. Respectful of doctor's opinion. May be reluctant to admit that they are in pain. May not adhere to a fixed schedule.
JAPANESE Japanese	Self-praise or the acceptance of praise is considered poor manners. Family is extremely important. Behavior and communication are defined by role and status. Religion includes a combination of Buddhism and Shinto.	Use attitude, actions, and feelings to communicate. Talkative people are considered show-offs or insincere. Openness considered sign of immaturity, lack of self-control. Implicit nonverbal messages are of central importance. Use concept of hierarchy and status. Avoid conflict. Avoid eye contact and touch.	Family role for support is important. Insulted when addressed by first name. Confidentiality is very important for honor. Information about illness kept in immediate family. Prone to keloid formation. Cleft lip or palate not uncommon. Alcohol may cause flushing. Tendency to control anger. May be reluctant to admit they are in pain.
JEWISH Many from East European countries. English, Hebrew, Yiddish. Three basic groups: Orthodox (most strict), Conservative, Reform (least strict).	Israel is the holy land. Sabbath is from sundown on Friday to sundown on Saturday. It is customary to invite other families in for Friday evening Sabbath dinner.	Orthodox men do not touch women, except their wives. Touch only for hands-on care. Very talkative and known for their friendliness.	Stoic and authoritative; respect health care workers who show self-confidence. Appreciate family accommodation. Jewish law demands that they seek complete medical care. Donor transplants are not acceptable to Orthodox Jews, but are to Conservative and Reform. Death: Cremation is discouraged. Autopsy is permitted in less strict groups. Orthodox believe that entire body, tissues, organs, amputated limbs, and blood sponges need to be available to family for burial. Do not cross hands in postmortem care.

FIGURE 10-1, cont'd.

Continued

Culture Group and Language	Belief Practices	Communication Awareness	Patient Care/ Handling of Death
KOREAN Hangul	Family-oriented. Believe in reincarnation. Religions include Shammanism, Taoism, Buddhism, Confucianism, Christianity. Belief in balance of two forces: hot and cold.	Reserved with strangers. Will use eye contact with familiar individuals. Etiquette is important. First names used only for family members. Proud, independent. Children should not be used as translators due to reversal of parent/child relationship.	Family needs to be included in plan of care. Prefer non-contact. Respond to sincerity.
MEXICAN Spanish; people of Indian heritage may speak one of more than 50 dialects.	Predominantly Roman Catholic. Pray, say rosary, have priest in time of crisis. Limited belief in "brujeria" as a magical, supernatural, or emotional illness precipitated by evil forces.	Tend to describe emotions by using dramatic body language. Very dramatic with grief but otherwise diplomatic and tactful. Direct confrontation is rude.	May believe that outcome of circumstances is controlled by external force; this can influence patient's compliance with health care. Women do not expose their bodies to men or other women.
MUSLIM Language of the country and some English	Believe in one God "Allah" and Mohammed, his prophet. Five daily prayers. Zakat, a compulsory giving of alms to the poor. Fasting during the month of Ramadan. Pilgrimage to Mecca is the goal of the faithful.	Limit eye contact. Do not touch while talking. Women cover entire body except face and hands.	Do not force foods when it is religiously forbidden. Before death, confession of sins with family present. After death, only relatives or priest may touch the body. Koran, the holy book, is recited near the dying person. The body is bathed and clothed in white and buried within 24 hours.
NORTHERN EUROPEAN Language of the country and some English	Very similar to American customs. Protestant with large Catholic population. Multiethnic groups.	Courtesy is of utmost importance. Address by surname and maintain personal space and good eye contact.	Maintain modesty at all times. Stoic regarding pain tolerance. Death is taken quietly with little emotional expression. Patients/family tend not to question medical authority.
SOUTHERN EUROPEAN Language of the country and some English	Roman Catholic, Protestant, Greek Orthodox, and some Jewish.	Talkative, very expressive. Direct and to the point. Extroverted. Good eye contact. Like personal and physical contact: holding hands, patting on the back, kissing.	Educated, yet reluctant to get medical attention. Very independent. Birth control and abortion are accepted in some countries and not in others. Family gets involved with caring for ill family member.
VIETNAMESE Vietnamese language has several dialects; also French, English, Chinese	Family loyalty is very important. Religions include Buddhism, Confucianism, Taoism, Cao Di, Hoa Hoa, Catholicism, occasional ancestral worship. General respect and harmony. Supernatural is sometimes used as an explanation for disease.	Communication—formal, polite manner; limit use of touch. Respect conveyed by nonverbal communication. Use both hands to give something to an adult. To beckon someone, place palm downward and wave. Don't snap your fingers to gain attention. Person's name used with title, i.e. "Mr. Bill," "Director James." "Ya" indicates respect (not agreement).	Negative emotions conveyed by silence and reluctant smile; will smile even if angry. Head is sacred—avoid touching. Back rub—uneasy experience. Common folk practices—skin rubbing, pinching, herbs in hot water, balms, string tying. Misunderstanding about illness—drawing blood seen as loss of body tissue; organ donation causes suffering in next life. Hospitalization is last resort. Flowers only for the dead.

FIGURE 10-1, cont'd.

2008 had a bachelor's degree or higher. The percentage who had completed high school varied considerably by race and ethnic origin in 2008: 82.3% of whites, 73.9% of Asians and Pacific Islanders, 59.8% of African Americans, and 45.9% of Hispanics.[145] In spite of the fact that the educational level of older adults has risen, only 12% of U.S. adults are health literate. Health literacy—the ability to obtain, process, and understand health information needed to make informed health decisions—is associated with poor health and lack of compliance with health information.[146] Because many patients may not possess health literacy and therefore be more prone to poorer health, more frequent use of health care services, and less able to manage chronic medical conditions,[147] it behooves the physical therapist to improve the usability of health information.

Best practices in health communication can aid in improving health literacy. These best practices, described in Box 10-2, have been developed from work with

- Identify the intended users of the health information and services
  - Who is affected (consider culture, age, literacy, economic context, etc.)
  - Communication capacities
- Evaluate users' understanding before, during, and after the introduction of information and services
  - Talk to members of targeted group
  - Pretest materials
  - Assess material's effectiveness after use
- Acknowledge cultural differences and practice respect
  - Cultural factors include race, ethnicity, language, nationality, age, gender, sexual orientation, income level, and occupation.
  - Consider biases toward
    - Accepted roles of men and women
    - Value of traditional medicine versus Western medicine
    - Manner of dress
    - Body language
- Make written communication look easy to read
  - Minimum of 12-point font, avoid using all capital letters, fancy script, etc.
  - Keep line length between 40 and 50 characters.
  - Use headings and bullets to break up text.
  - Leave plenty of white space around margins and between sections.

(From Quick guide to health literacy; fact sheet. U.S. Department of Health and Human Services Office of Disease Prevention and Health Promotion. Available at: http://www.health.gov/communication/literacy/quickguide/factsbasic.htm.)

people with cancer and chronic disease and apply to written and oral communication. Some general guidelines include using simple language, defining medical and technical terms, providing culturally appropriate information, using clear pictures, and focusing on action.

Learning Readiness. Learning readiness means that until basic skills are mastered, the mastery of more complex behavior is not possible. A number of factors can affect the patient's readiness to learn, some of which are closely related to the patient's motivational intensity discussed earlier. Studies have indicated that extensive practice is necessary for older adults to develop learning readiness.[148] Learning appears less effective if practice is discontinued before the learner gains sufficient competence and confidence in the task. For older adults to process information into their first or primary memory store, application, practice, and rehearsal are essential.

To assess the patient's learning readiness for psychomotor activities, the therapist must determine the existing level of physical strength and skills and build from those points. To assess the patient's understanding of the reasons and need for therapy, the therapist would determine the patient's level of understanding of the particular physical condition and prescribed treatment. The therapist should sequence instruction from simple skills and concepts to the more complex ones, with sufficient supervised practice to ensure the correctness of performance and to develop the patient's learning readiness to progress to more difficult and complex tasks.

Learning Styles and Information Processing. Learning style refers to how information is processed and is unique to each individual. An individual's learning style determines the consistent way the individual receives, retains, and retrieves information. Learning style also includes how an individual feels about and behaves in instructional experiences. An individual's learning style often is identified at one extreme or the other of any given learning style continuum—a classification that is probably too rigid to be realistic.

An individual's typical mode of perceiving, thinking, problem solving, remembering, selecting, and organizing information and educational experiences defines how that individual processes information. McLagan describes three primary dimensions of information processing as continua: content, initiative, and tactics—each of which has its own continuum.[149] She also emphasizes that a profile that responds to specific functions is more descriptive and realistic than labeling an individual at a fixed point on any of the three continua. These three continua are described next.

Content, the first dimension, ranges from a detail learner to a main-idea learner. The detail learner will be attentive to the step-by-step explanation of a procedure but is less attentive to the overall goals of the therapy. The main-idea learner will be eager to hear about the overall goals but may be less attentive to specific instructions and details.[149] For example, a detail learner will be more interested in the number of repetitions and appropriate time of day to perform the exercise, whereas a main-idea learner will want to know the purposes and possible outcomes of the exercises.

Initiative, the second dimension, ranges from an active/aggressive/energetic learner to one who is passive in instructional sessions. The active/aggressive/energetic learner exerts a high degree of initiative and questions many aspects of the treatments, causes, and effects. However, conclusions may be reached erroneously. At the other extreme, the passive learner is one who exhibits little initiative and who must be encouraged to participate actively in treatment sessions.[149] A passive learner is a greater challenge to the instructor and does not necessarily indicate an unwillingness to learn.

The third dimension, tactics, refers to how information is processed in terms of organization and structure. The analytic learner processes best when structure is present and when step-by-step explanations and demonstrations are presented sequentially. The intuitive/creative learner, on the other hand, responds best to instruction that is less structured and more open-ended. Problem solving and shared decision making in treatment sessions are more productive with the intuitive/creative information processor.[149]

In summary, Cassata condensed a number of findings related to cognitive aspects of the older adult learner[150]:

- Patients forget much of what the doctor tells them.
- Instructions and advice are more likely to be forgotten than other information.
- The more patients are told, the greater the proportion they will forget.
- Patients will remember (a) what they are told first and (b) what they consider most important.
- Intelligent patients do not remember more than less intelligent patients.
- Older patients remember just as much as younger ones.
- Moderately anxious patients recall more of what they are told than highly anxious patients or patients who are not anxious.
- The more medical knowledge patients have, the more they will recall.
- If patients write down what the health provider says, they will remember it just as well as if they only hear it.

Physiological Aspects. A number of changes occur with aging that can be accommodated by the therapist to facilitate the older patient's learning. These changes, similar to the ones that can affect motivation, may involve neurologic functions, vision and hearing impairment, and diminished motor dexterity. Worcester[151] relates these physiological changes to patient education.

Neurologic Changes. Neurologic changes that may affect learning are slower nerve transmission, which affects pacing; decreased short-term memory; and a larger store of existing information that must be integrated into the treatment setting. Slower nerve transmission can slow the reception of information and reaction times of the patient and therefore create the need for more time in the treatment session. Implications for instruction include sensitivity to the pacing of instruction and speech and frequent assessment of the patient's level of understanding.[151]

Decreased short-term memory can cause difficulty in retaining new material and necessitates repetition and adequate practice time. Short-term memory can be enhanced through multisensory approaches, that is, visuals, models, demonstrations, and patient education materials. The volume of information accumulated over a lifetime can interfere with learning when the new information is not congruent with prior information and experiences. Cognitive overload—too much information—also is a potential factor. Strategies for effective instruction can be used to assess the patient's knowledge base about the particular physical condition, make connections between prior knowledge and new knowledge, clarify any misconceptions, and present less material in each treatment session.[151]

Visual Changes. Decreases in acuity, accommodation to dim lighting, and lens transparency are significant visual changes that may affect the patient's ability to learn effectively. The decreased sharpness of vision, or acuity, implies that details in print materials and illustrations are more difficult for the older patient to see clearly. Therefore, illustrations in patient education materials need bold lines, a minimum of detail, and a plain print style. In the same manner, decreased accommodation creates difficulty in the lens adjusting to different light intensities and to color differentiation. Bright overhead lights in the clinic may create accommodation difficulties for the older patient, just as dim lights may make visual perception more difficult. The patient should not be placed in a position that faces any source of glare. For patient education materials, black ink on nonglare yellow paper for optimum acuity and accommodation should be used. Decreased lens transparency may be due to external as well as to internal causes. The therapist should make certain the patient's glasses are clean and should provide magnifying aids, if needed, when referring to patient education materials.[151]

Hearing Changes. High frequencies, such as the *c*, *ch*, *f*, *s*, *sh*, *t*, and *z* sounds, are more difficult for older adults to distinguish clearly. By asking the patient to repeat what was heard, the therapist can detect problems and correct errors. The therapist's pace of speech and clear enunciation are more important than volume because slow or loud speech does not necessarily increase reception. Background noises need to be controlled because the older patient may have difficulty screening sounds. Patient education materials that have illustrations and audio/videotapes with individual headsets can assist the hearing-impaired patient.[151]

Motor Changes. A number of changes in the musculoskeletal condition of the older patient may affect his or her ability to respond to treatment. Adequate time must be provided to accommodate slower movement and responses, and adaptive equipment, as appropriate, should be available. The therapist should plan to have the patient begin with simple tasks that can be accomplished, then build to more complex tasks.[151]

Implications for Patient Education Materials. This discussion of the cognitive aspects, physical changes, and health literacy has particular implications for patient education materials. The vocabulary level, sentence length, complexity, and organization of content should be examined carefully for comprehension. Reading level for print materials should approximate fourth- to sixth-grade level for maximum patient comprehension. Visual changes experienced by older adults dictate using clear, simple print styles. Black ink on nonglare paper and distinctly contrasting colors are recommended. Patient education materials should be tested with a representative sample of the audience for whom they are designed for clarity, comprehension, cultural accuracy and sensitivity, and readability before production—an instructional and cost-effective strategy.

In summary, the therapist ideally facilitates the older patient's move toward self-direction, adherence, independent problem solving, and error detection. Therefore, consideration should be given to the positive impact that occurs when learning style and information processing are investigated, assessed, and used. Awareness of the physical changes that occur in the older patient can enhance the learning experience when appropriate techniques are applied. Time spent in careful assessment of the many cognitive aspects of learning and the physical changes can create a more productive instructional time for each patient. Older patients in treatment sessions will exhibit characteristics of older adult learners. The therapist who is aware of the cognitive and physiological aspects discussed in this section is better prepared to work more effectively and efficiently with older patients and to facilitate their progress in treatment sessions.

Assessment of Learning

Patient education is only as effective as the results of the education and learning experiences. Because instruction has occurred, it cannot be assumed that learning has been accomplished. Without evaluation, the instructor has no information on the success of the instructional activity. The effectiveness of the educational experience can be evaluated in many ways that vary from traditional tests. Variations of the question-and-answer format include learning contracts,[114] self-report,[152] interview, diaries, checklists, and return demonstration.

Self-Assessment Questions for the Therapist. The following questions, identified by Freedman and adapted by Gardner et al., may be helpful in a self-assessment of instruction and interaction[153]:

1. *Have I correctly assessed what my patient knows?* What has been taught before, and how much does my patient remember? What technical terminology needs to be reviewed or clarified?
2. *Am I certain that I know what needs to be taught and what my patient should be able to do as a result of my instruction?* Do the objectives reflect our negotiated goals? Are they in the appropriate sequence?
3. *Have I planned an introduction to the instruction?* Have I planned how to communicate clearly what will be taught and what my expectations are in this session?
4. *Did I present the information clearly and give pertinent examples?* Did I confuse my patient in my instruction? Was my instruction in logical sequence, with pauses for my patient to assimilate the information and to ask questions? Were my directions clear? Were there clear-cut guidelines for my patient to follow?

5. *Did I present information and examples that were relevant to my patient?* Did I keep the instruction focused on the main points without cluttering my patient's information-processing mode with extraneous material? Were my examples clear and to the point?
6. *Did I prevent or avoid an information overload for my patient?* Did I present information appropriate for the time I had with my patient? Did I limit my instructional aids or handouts to those that emphasized the major points?
7. *Were my handouts and other instructional aids appropriate?* Were my handouts organized, clear, simple, and legible? Was the reading level appropriate for my patient? Did they accommodate any vision impairment?
8. *Did my patient have enough practice time?* Did I remember that older learners do not respond well under pressure or on timed tasks? Did I help my patient develop a sense of confidence in the task? Were my verbal and nonverbal feedback reinforcing?
9. *Did I help my patient by providing cues to proper performance?* Did I coach my patient during the practice period? Did I point out any specifics that my patient could monitor to determine correct or incorrect performance?
10. *Was I sensitive to my patient?* Was I aware of my patient's reaction to the information I presented? Did I try to see things from the patient's perspective?

The effectiveness of instruction is greatly enhanced by clear, concise, and direct verbal expression. The therapist's nonverbal communication through body language, voice tone, and eye contact should inspire confidence in the therapist without limiting interaction or intimidating the patient. The therapist's verbal and nonverbal behaviors can contribute significantly to creating a positive learning environment that is conducive to positive and productive interaction between the patient and the therapist.

CASE STUDIES

The following three scenarios illustrate selected principles that have been presented in this chapter. As the reader reviews "The Incident" and "The Dialogue" sections, significant points that relate to the chapter's content should be noted. The reader should also check to see whether these points are included in the "Discussion" and "Summary" sections. The reader should identify more points than are included in those sections.

Scenario 1: The Inattentive Learner

The Incident. Mr. Smith, a 75-year-old African American male, was admitted to a rehabilitation facility 2 weeks ago for stroke. Although he has been willing to work toward his goals in all previous sessions, today he is inattentive to the therapist, as observed by his lack of eye contact, fidgeting, head movement, and other body language indicators. The therapist has to repeat instructions and questions, and basically no progress is being made.

The Dialogue

Therapist:	Mr. Smith, you seem to be preoccupied today. What's on your mind?
Patient:	Well, as a matter of fact, I've got a problem I need to take care of at the bank, and I don't know how or when I can take care of it.
Therapist:	I can understand why you are preoccupied. Anytime my bank calls me, I get worried, too! What could we do to help you with this problem?
Patient:	Well, I really need to personally talk with my banker as soon as possible. But I just don't see how I can do it. (*Pause*) Do you really mean that you would help?
Therapist:	The best we can do is to at least try. What do you need?
Patient:	I need a ride because I have to take care of this in person. But I don't know if I can get in and out of the car!
Therapist:	If I can arrange a car and driver for this afternoon, would you be willing this morning to work on how to get in and out of a car?
Patient:	Do you really think I can learn how to do that this morning?
Therapist:	Yes, I think you can with some hard work. You already have worked hard on improving your balance, and besides, you've been getting in and out of cars all your life. Let's go do it.

Discussion. The therapist recognized that the patient was distracted and preoccupied and that there was an obvious obstacle to a productive treatment session. The therapist provided an opportunity for the patient to communicate the factors that were creating interference with this treatment session by asking an open-ended question that gave the patient the opportunity to state his need. The therapist further demonstrated authenticity and empathy to the patient's concern in agreeing that a call from his banker also would concern this therapist.

With encouragement and another open-ended question, the therapist facilitated the patient's problem-solving skills. The patient was allowed to maintain autonomy and empowerment and was allowed to determine how specific needs could be met. The therapist also demonstrated valuing (prizing) of the patient by addressing the patient's need and by referencing the patient's accomplishments in therapy as well as past experiences.

Scenario Summary. The therapist recognized that the patient's problem was primary to the patient and that the therapy was low on his priority list. Therefore, the patient was not ready to learn. By having the patient identify the reason for inattentiveness and then using those needs and concerns, the therapist was able to negotiate the activity for this treatment session. Therefore, the patient's goals were accommodated and progress toward the discharge goals was made.

Scenario 2: Learned Helplessness

The Incident. Mrs. Aziz, a 69-year-old Arabian female, has an above-knee amputation and has been referred to physical therapy for prosthetic training. Her husband, who appears impatient and unwilling to let his wife attempt any task, accompanies her. She appears passive and willing for, if not expectant of, his assistance. During the evaluation, her passiveness and helplessness also appear to be her pattern of behavior in the home setting.

The Dialogue

Therapist:	Mrs. Aziz, what would you like to be able to do at home that you aren't doing now?
Patient:	Well, I'd like to be able to do things in my kitchen.
Therapist:	What kind of things do you want to do?
Patient:	I want to be able to cook dinner and do the dishes.
Therapist:	Is your husband doing those things now?
Husband:	Yes. I cook and do the dishes because my wife can't stand up.
Therapist:	What would you like for your wife to be able to do?
Husband:	I'd like for her to be able to stay by herself so I can get out and do my work. But that would mean I'd have to leave her alone, and I just can't do that.
Therapist:	Mrs. Aziz, do you think that you could be able to stay by yourself?
Patient:	Well, my husband does everything for me now. I don't know if I can or not.

Therapist:	Mr. Aziz, it is important to realize that your wife *can* learn to do a number of things for herself if she is given the opportunity. However, it means that you have to allow her enough time to perform a task in her way without interfering or taking over.
Husband:	That's really hard to do. It is easier and quicker for me to do it for her. Besides, she was so sick that she really needed my help.
Therapist:	I understand that. You obviously have done a terrific job, and lots of husbands would not have done as well as you have. However, she's progressing so well that she is ready to learn to walk on her artificial leg. For both of you to regain the independence you both want, she needs the opportunity, the time, and the encouragement to begin practicing those things that together we decide are the next steps in her treatment program.

Discussion. The therapist recognized that some social barriers prevented Mrs. Aziz's willingness to participate fully in a treatment program designed to promote her independence. Chief among these barriers was her husband's overt willingness to assist in her every movement. The therapist was sensitive that this level of caregiving was required initially and positively acknowledged the husband's caregiving.

The therapist recognized that in order to achieve the level of independence that both the Azizs desired, less assistance would be required from the husband and more initiative from Mrs. Aziz. The therapist achieved this in a supportive manner by focusing on both of their goals while describing the process in achieving those goals. In this way, goal negotiation is a mutual agreement rather than a unilateral decision by the therapist.

Scenario Summary. The therapist recognized the husband's caregiving in a positive manner and then literally gave the husband permission to decrease the level of caregiving as part of the treatment program, thus avoiding the exclusion the husband might feel as his wife worked toward greater independence. The therapist also made the wife aware that her physical condition now will safely accommodate increased activity and encouraged the patient's initiative by focusing on the patient's goal of being able to work in her kitchen.

Scenario 3: The Dominant Hurried Therapist

The Incident. Mrs. Miranda, an 80-year-old Hispanic female, checks in for her scheduled appointment at an outpatient clinic. She tells the receptionist in a thick accent that her granddaughter insisted she come and see about the pains in her right shoulder but that her granddaughter couldn't come with her. After a considerable period in the waiting room, she was shown to a treatment cubicle by the receptionist and was told to wait for the therapist. The therapist eventually rushed into the cubicle and, without introduction, told the patient that he was here to "fix her shoulder."

The Dialogue

Therapist:	So, honey, the receptionist tells me your left shoulder hurts. I think we can fix you up in a jiffy if you'll just do what I tell you to do.
Patient:	(*Hesitantly with accent.*) Well, really, it's my—
Therapist:	(*Interprets.*) What? Here, let's look at your shoulder. (*Therapist proceeds to examine left shoulder.*) I'm going to get a hot pack to put on your shoulder. Wait here.
Patient:	Si, si.
Therapist:	What?
Patient:	Si.
Therapist:	Oh, well, whatever. (*Therapist returns with the hot pack and places it on left shoulder.*) While the heat's on your shoulder, here's a sheet of exercises I want you to do. Eyeball these, and I'll be back in a flash.
Patient:	(*Looks at the sheet, but her lack of proficiency in English impedes her understanding. Folds sheet and puts it in her lap.*)
Therapist:	(*Returns and removes heat.*) Well, I know your little shoulder feels lots better now. Like I told you, honey, you just do these exercises like it says, and I'll see you next week.

Discussion. Mrs. Miranda's ethnicity may imply a low health literacy and lack of knowledge of the U.S. health care system. Her granddaughter, on the other hand, as a third-generation Hispanic, has become enculturated and recognized that her grandmother's traditional home remedies could be supplemented by professional care. Mrs. Miranda has some suspicion about people caring for her in an unfamiliar environment, but to please her granddaughter, she agreed to go to the clinic. In addition, Mrs. Miranda is aware of her limited English proficiency and her thick accent and is reluctant to speak when away from her community environment.

Often an older person has a greater comfort level with a nonauthoritarian person than with one who represents power and expertise. Mrs. Miranda told the receptionist and her granddaughter about her right shoulder pain; however, she did not persist in her attempt to correct the therapist when he placed the heat pack on the wrong shoulder. Further, she did not tell the therapist that she could not read the exercises on the paper that he gave her. No effort was made to determine her understanding or to demonstrate and practice the exercises.

This lack of communication occurred not only because of Mrs. Miranda's natural reluctance but also because of the therapist's dominant behaviors. The lack of an introduction, the ageist remarks, and no elicitation of the patient's needs or reasons for being at the clinic are examples of these behaviors. The therapist's body language also communicated to the patient that time was not available for attention to her situation. The numerous slang words used in the therapist's hurried speech only confounded Mrs. Miranda's difficulty with English. No directions were given concerning how she would make an appointment for next week.

Scenario Summary. This scenario attempts to present a negative role model for patient interaction that could result in, at the very least, ineffective treatment perhaps even to the wrong shoulder, and at the very most, the patient could actually be harmed if she didn't understand safety instructions. When communicating with an older person without fluent English, care must be given to adequately assess the level of English proficiency. The possibility that cultural perceptions of health care delivery can impede treatment necessitates the therapist's increased sensitivity. A willingness to assess the patient's understanding, the rate of speech, diction, attention to the patient's nonverbal reactions, and courtesy demonstrate this sensitivity.

SUMMARY

Even the most competent therapist can be successful with older patients only to the degree that the patient chooses to participate fully in the treatment regimen for the necessary time period. Given a therapist with the appropriate knowledge and skills in treatment techniques and modalities, the degree of success with a majority of older patients will depend (1) on the patient's physical condition, level of motivation, caregivers, and support systems and (2) on the therapist's skill as a patient educator.

A therapist who is a successful older patient educator has developed the following:

- A philosophy of patient education based on (a) some knowledge of learning theories from which a dominant orientation has evolved and (b) clarification of the therapist's approach as one of patient empowerment instead of authoritarian
- An awareness of the characteristics of and sensitivity to the older patient as an older adult learner
- The ability to develop negotiated goals with patients
- The ability to facilitate patients' learning
- A willingness to regularly and honestly assess the quality and results of the instruction provided

Patient education as an intervention has a solid base in educational psychology and instructional theories as well as in everyday experience and practice. Older patients need and deserve therapists who recognize the importance of this intervention and who will work to develop and enhance their competency as patient educators.

REFERENCES

To enhance this text and add value for the reader, all references are included on the companion Evolve site that accompanies this text book. The reader can view the reference source and access it online whenever possible. There are a total of 153 cited references and other general references for this chapter.

Older Adults
and Their Families

Michelle M. Lusardi, PT, DPT, PhD

INTRODUCTION

Physical therapists and other health professionals caring for aging adults routinely inquire about the availability of a spouse or adult children for assistance with home exercise programs or with basic and instrumental activities of daily living.[1] We seek to involve family members as informants during examination, as participants in goal setting and the rehabilitation process, and contributors to discharge planning. We believe that such inclusion enhances both outcomes of and satisfaction with rehabilitation and wellness care.[2] Although we would like to think that having a spouse or adult child available as caregiver is a resource that can be counted upon, we quickly learn that there are a variety of additional dimensions that influence availability, quality, and effectiveness of caregiving and support.[3] We work with some older patients and family members facing incredible challenges who do amazingly well in very difficult circumstances. We also encounter families who perceive any degree of challenge as a major crisis or disaster, making them unable to accommodate even small additional needs from their older family member. What accounts for these differences? How do health professionals facilitate "healthy" solutions when there is a need for caregiving and support of an older family member?[4] Framing the family as a dynamic system helps us to understand the perspectives from which the family operates, the ground rules and assumptions that influence decision making and interaction, and the family's ability to face stressors and adapt to changes.

In this chapter, readers will explore family as a dynamic system and a context for individual development from a life span perspective, as well as models of family interaction that may provide insights that enhance the efficacy of our care. Readers will explore the dimensions of caregiving and care-sharing roles, as well as factors that influence the physical and mental health of both care provider and care recipient. Finally, we will apply these concepts to one of the difficult transitions that aging adults and their families are often confronted with in later life: decisions about continuing to drive an automobile.

DEFINING THE FAMILY

To understand how families function in later life, we must first define the term. Few families currently "fit" the post–War World II view of the American family as a succession of relatively independent nuclear sets of parents and their children.[5] Family has changed in many ways. In the early 20th century, many family members lived in relative proximity to their family of origin and had frequent "in person" interaction. In contemporary society, however, families tend to be scattered geographically, as younger members move away to pursue job opportunities, and retirement-aged family members move to locations where quality of life and cost of living are perceived as more attractive.[6-8]

Geographically scattered families use communication technology (i.e., phone, e-mail, text messaging, social networking, etc.) to stay emotionally and socially engaged. For some families, in-person contact has become a special event rather than a routine occurrence.[9] Given this mobility within families, a substantial number of older adults are "aging in place" far from their adult children and other family members.[10] When this is coupled with the American cultural value of independence and self-determination, many older adults coping with chronic illness and associated functional limitations do not call upon their extended family networks for instrumental care until a crisis situation occurs.[11] At these times, health professionals are challenged to assist the older patient in their care, as well as family members who may be threatened and overwhelmed by the acuity of the situation they are facing. Some older family members opt to relocate from their distant retirement living residence to a location nearer to adult children when they have been widowed, become physically challenged, or need assistance with management of chronic health conditions.[12] This reverse migration requires flexibility and adaptation for all members of the family, and it can be quite stressful to the family as a system.

The complexity of today's family structure, with the majority of American families "blended" as a result of divorce and remarriage, also influences how families are able to respond to individual member needs.[13] The number of nontraditional households is on the rise, where individuals who are not related or legally bound, live together as family.[14] Given these trends, health professionals may best define family as the group of individuals who are most connected to our older patient by affection, knowledge, and care, whether this be a result of marriage or by choice.[15] In looking at family as a complex system, scholars in the field of family studies describe family as a set of interdependent individuals, across generations, who share history, are linked by emotional bonds, and who do their best to meet the needs of each member and of the family as a whole.[16] In this chapter, we will use the word *spouse* somewhat broadly to describe the individual, whether a married partner or significant other, who has the primary emotional relationship with the older person needing care. We must also note that, in an increasingly diverse society, the meaning of being "old" and the roles of and expectations for care of the oldest generation in a family vary by culture, as well as across generations.[17]

LIFE SPAN DEVELOPMENT

Theorists from the fields of life span development and family studies provide models to describe the interacting influences on health professionals for the care they provide to aging adults in the context of the patient's family system. Figure 11-1 depicts Bronfenbrenner's model of *ecological development*, which proposes a series of increasingly complex nested systems, with the individual patient at the center and broad societal influences at the periphery.[18-20] The individual patient has a unique set of inherent attributes shaped by relationships and activities of the individual within the immediate environments (microsystem): immediate family and friends, leisure activities, organizations or church groups, etc. The direct relationship of a health professional and an older adult in the role of the "patient" represents a *microsystem*-level activity. Interaction across multiple microsystems, such as family conferences, takes place at the *mesosystem* level. The next layer, the *exosystem*, includes other social structures or organizations that may not include the individual himself or herself but influences what happens to the individual. This might include the adult child's work demands that limit availability to provide care; hospital policies; rules and regulations of health insurances; mass media that deliver information; and the local or national government agencies that set health care policy. The final layer of the model is the *macrosystem*: the overall cultural, economic, legal, and political systems that influence the ideology and action of the layers that preceded it. For aging adults, the political debate about how health care and insurance systems should be structured and financed, what care should be routinely available, and eligibility criteria for care, all occur at the macrosystem level.

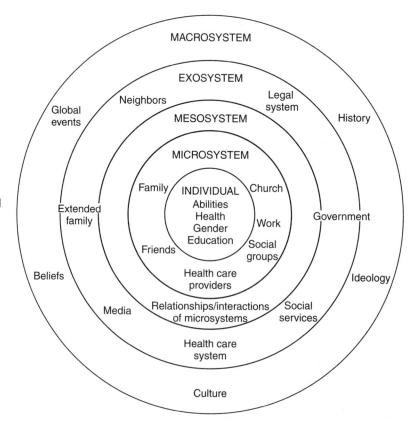

FIGURE 11-1 Bronfenbrenner's model of ecological development.

Health professionals build relationships with their older patients at the microsystem level. At the mesosystem level, we exchange information and ideas with other health professionals as part of the health care team, as well as provide education and counsel to family caregivers as decisions are made about priorities and anticipated outcomes. We provide care in the context of the agencies and organizations of which we are a part, incorporating both the affordances and constraints inherent in those systems (exosystem). We are influenced as well by societal perspectives on aging and later life (both positive and ageist), rights of the individual, and the "good" of the collective whole (macrosystem). This chapter emphasizes effective interactions at the mesosystem level and challenges us to be knowledgeable about the affordances and constraints in the exosystems and macrosystems in which we provide care.

THE FAMILY AS A COMPLEX SYSTEM

Each family has its own unique and complex structure, composition, governance process, organization, and underlying culture, beliefs, and themes.[16] A family's *composition* includes the number of generations that make up the family and each person's assortment of roles within and outside the family system. The *governance process* includes both the overt and the implicit rules for communication, relationships and behaviors, distribution of decision-making power, and patterns of interaction within the family. *Organization* refers to the family's interdependent subsystems (spouses, parent–child, sibling connections, grandparent–child, and relationships with the extended family) as well as the individual development status of each family member (their position within his or her life span and in the life span of the family system). Variability in structural relationships emerge with the blending of cultural and ethnic backgrounds and differing expectations and relationship rules as members are added to the family through marriage or partnership, or lost to divorce and death. Historical events and sociocultural change also shape expectations and experiences within and across generations of the family, subtly or significantly influencing family structure, organization, and rules.

FAMILY THEMES AND BOUNDARIES

The family provides context for the development of individual family members over time, as well as for the growth and continuity of family as a whole. This is accomplished in three ways: (1) by defining and implementing family "themes" about what is important for its members to believe, think, and do; (2) by socializing new, incoming, or potentially wayward members about "rules" of behavior necessary to ensure continuity of the family and the society in which they live; and (3) by shaping and supporting individual identities within the family system.[21-23]

Family themes serve as the organizing framework for the family's daily life and function, are the foundation for both family and individual identity, direct thoughts and behaviors of family members, influence distribution of resources (time, energy, emotional support, money) within the family, and determine the emotional climate in which the family operates.[16] To develop the most effective plan of care, health professionals caring for aging adults must consider explicit and implicit themes (i.e., attitude, values, and beliefs) about health and illness; ability/impairment, activity/functional limitation, and participation/disability; as well as about aging, death, and bereavement.[24,25] A family with a central theme of stoicism may respond to health-related problems very differently than families with a central theme of physical perfection or "suffering is part of life." Families that strongly value independence of members may respond to caregiving needs very differently than would families who strongly value nurturance. A family with themes of respecting authority may be difficult to engage in health care decision making, instead waiting for health care providers, as experts, to determine what should be done.

Family themes are greatly influenced by cultural context.[26] Some ethnic or cultural groups may consider illness or disability penance for past wrongdoing; others may perceive ill health as tragedy, as blessing, or as challenge to be overcome.[27] To deliver culturally competent care, health care providers must incorporate the cultural themes (while taking care to avoid stereotyping) in communication, goal setting, care delivery, and planning for future health care needs.[28]

Each family has a set of rules and strategies for managing both internal and external interactional boundaries.[16] External boundaries, as depicted in Figure 11-2,

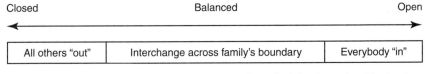

PERMEABILITY OF A FAMILY'S EXTERNAL BOUNDARIES

Closed   Balanced   Open

| All others "out" | Interchange across family's boundary | Everybody "in" |

Rigid membership structure   Loosely defined membership structure
High value for privacy   Physical/emotional "space" open to others
Limited communication across boundary   Easy flow of information across boundary
Well-defined rules for interaction with others   Changeable rules for interaction with others
Limited trust outside of the family   Comfortable interaction with others

FIGURE 11-2 Continuum of permeability and characteristics of open and closed external boundaries.

can be thought of on a continuum from closed to open. The permeability of a family's external boundaries influences communication with persons outside of the family, ability to accept recommendations and assistance from others, and the depth of relationships and level of trust extended to others, including health care providers.[29] Families of aging adults who have strongly "closed" boundaries may be reluctant to share information with health professionals or ask for assistance during times of stress. They may perceive a recommendation for home care following an acute care stay as invasion of their privacy, wanting instead to manage on their own using resources within the family for assistance. At the other end of the continuum are families with very open boundaries who may "adopt" health care providers as central members of the family, wanting to include these caregivers in family events and rituals long beyond the period of care. The majority of families are able to strike a functional balance between these extremes, maintaining enough closure to facilitate family identity and enough openness to allow members to have friendships and relationships outside the family system, and to access external resources when necessary.

There are additional rules and strategies for *internal boundaries* of the relational subsystems and individuals within the family. These rules relate to how the family tolerates individuality and autonomy, and the way that distances are regulated between members within the family.[16,23] Some families have rules that strongly encourage dependency of members on the family system. In such families, individuals may have little privacy, and what impacts on the individual member affects the whole. Other families encourage members to keep to themselves, such that interaction and resource sharing among members is limited. Optimally, families achieve a functional balance between autonomy and connectedness, such that the family can be responsive to the changing needs of aging family members.[30] Problems arise when the goals of the individual are different enough from the goals of the family; this creates tension within the family system. A frail aging parent's determination to remain independent and at home may be at odds with his or her spouse's or adult children's need for safety when such determination increases risk of falls, accident,

or injury. A related construct, *cohesion*, the strength of emotional attachment between family members, is discussed below under the heading of adaptability and responsiveness to change.[30]

MANAGING ESSENTIAL FAMILY DAILY FUNCTIONS AND TASKS

Families have in common the instrumental activities that ensure that each member's needs for food, clothing, shelter, education, and development are met. These include setting and managing schedules, housekeeping and cooking, shopping for clothes and doing laundry, dealing with bills and other financial concerns, providing personal care, and accessing resources within and outside the family. The family system must determine "who does what" for the family and for each of its members. It must have rules and strategies in place to face challenges and solve problems resulting from competing demands inherent in a multigenerational system.[31] The system must also manage the health care needs and routines of members, often most pressing for the youngest and the oldest generations.[32] The resources that a family brings to bear in managing daily tasks include time, energy, and money as well as the individual strengths and abilities of family members. Each family sets priorities about resource distribution and use based on the family's governing values, beliefs, and attitudes. Observation of a family's decision-making process about resource use reveals a great deal about power structure within the family system.

The continuum of management strategies used by a family system to make decisions about and manage daily tasks is illustrated in Figure 11-3. One extreme along the continuum represents underorganization and the opposite extreme represents overorganization. Although most families achieve a degree of balance between these extremes in management of resources, those at the extremes of the continuum often experience a great deal of stress. Lack of advanced planning and insufficient clarity about caregiving needs following an older family member's discharge from an acute hospital stay, although often automatically labeled as "not caring" by health care providers, may actually be evidence of an

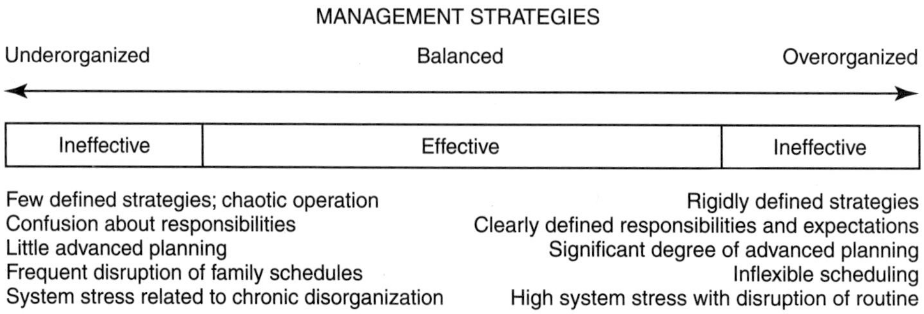

MANAGEMENT STRATEGIES

Underorganized	Balanced	Overorganized
Ineffective	Effective	Ineffective

Few defined strategies; chaotic operation	Rigidly defined strategies
Confusion about responsibilities	Clearly defined responsibilities and expectations
Little advanced planning	Significant degree of advanced planning
Frequent disruption of family schedules	Inflexible scheduling
System stress related to chronic disorganization	High system stress with disruption of routine

FIGURE 11-3 Continuum of strategies for management of a family's daily tasks and activities, and their related characteristics.

underorganized family system, operating without clear rules and expectations.[33] Overorganized systems, on the other hand, work well when things are routine but may be substantially disrupted when illness or some unanticipated event occurs.[34] Such families may insist that previous routine take priority when adaptation of routine would better serve individual members. Whatever the decision-making processes and level of organization, families tend to use resources in a manner consistent with the identity themes and rules that define them as a unique family.[16] As a family moves through its life cycle, developmental changes influence the needs of members and availability of resources, priorities and decision-making power shift, and the responsibility for maintenance tasks has to be redistributed.

In older person care, it may become evident that an adult child and his or her spouse have different perceptions and expectations about caring for aging parents, based on the rules about relationships (internal boundaries) in their individual families of origin.[35] This adds to family system stress as adult children attempt to meet the needs of aging parents while simultaneously nurturing their marriage, launching their own children, and being involved in the lives of their grandchildren.[36] Health professionals caring for senior members of the family may need to facilitate negotiation about use of the family's available resources when differences in expectations create system stress. In situations where conflict is problematic, referral to a family therapist or counselor may be necessary.[37]

MANAGING FAMILY STRESSORS

In family systems models, stressors are defined as events or situations that pressure the family system to change their structure or function, or to alter the way the family typically manages its primary tasks.[16,38] Normative stressors (typical stressors anticipated at specific times across the life cycle) may be positive or negative. Positive stressors include such things as the addition of a new family member by marriage, birth of a child or grandchild, "empty nesting" after successfully launching one's children, or retirement from a long-held job with the anticipation of enjoying the "golden years." Negative normative stressors include physical decline and death in the very old. Nonnormative stressors, such as sudden job loss or economic downturn that affects family financial resources, sudden illness or injury experienced by a family member, chronic unpredictable illness, or the unexpected death of a member of the family, often place a family in crisis.

Stressors, whether positive or negative, require the family to (1) adapt their self-definition, themes, and associated rules and patterns of internal interaction; (2) reevaluate internal and external boundaries and adjust the family system's permeability; (3) consider and reprioritize the distribution of their collective resources

for daily management of family tasks and needs; and (4) renegotiate rules and strategies for management of the family's emotional climate.[16,38]

The difference in the experience of these stressors lies in the family's ability to prepare for necessary changes. Stress management may be complicated by family legacy: the myths, values, and unresolved conflicts that are carried across generations.[38] In addition, it is not uncommon for multigenerational families to experience multiple normative and nonnormative stressors either simultaneously or within a short time period. The need to manage overlapping stressors exponentially increases pressure for adaptation of the family system, and demands greater flexibility in the roles and responsibilities of the members of the family.

Adaptability and Change

Families vary in their ability to tolerate differences among members, to meet challenges placed on the system by developmentally anticipated events (e.g., marriage, birth of a child, graduations, relocation to different geographic areas, retirement) as well as to unpredictable events (e.g., sudden or chronic illness, trauma, job loss, being victim of crime, natural disaster, historical event, or death of a family member) that potentially change family structure. The ability to effectively adapt both structure/organization and roles/responsibilities in carrying out essential family tasks in response to such challenges to the system can be thought of as a resource for the family.[39] The ability to adapt is related to the family's cohesion, flexibility, and ways of communicating.[30]

The family *cohesion* continuum, illustrated in Figure 11-4, refers to the family's ability to balance member individuality with family togetherness. The level of cohesion within a family is determined by the strength of emotional bonds between family members. When there is a healthy level of cohesion, family members are interdependent and emotionally close while, at the same time, able to respect each other's unique characteristics and interests.[40] Families at the enmeshed end of the cohesion continuum tend to experience an event affecting one of their members as an emotional whole; decisions about health care include the entire family system, and assistance or support may be provided in a way that challenges goals of independence for the individual member receiving rehabilitation care. At the opposite end of the continuum, families who are disengaged may be very difficult to involve in decision making or caregiving, as the connectedness between members is tenuous. Families at the center of the continuum are thought to have achieved a functional "balance" between the family as a whole and individual members. Such families are more likely to be adaptive in the face of challenges faced by aging members.

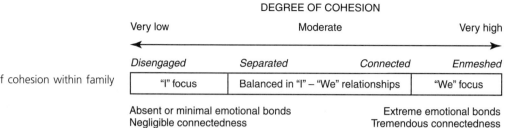

FIGURE 11-4 The continuum of cohesion within family systems.

DEGREE OF COHESION

Very low	Moderate	Very high

Disengaged	*Separated*	*Connected*	*Enmeshed*
"I" focus	Balanced in "I" – "We" relationships		"We" focus

Absent or minimal emotional bonds	Extreme emotional bonds
Negligible connectedness	Tremendous connectedness
Primary focus on individual needs	Importance placed on family needs
Low affiliation with family	Total affiliation with family
Indifference	Strong loyalty
Members independent in thought/action	Members dependent in thought/action

As long as all members of the family are satisfied and accepting of relationship rules shaped by the family's underlying culture or ethnicity, the family system will function effectively.

Although it is not the role of rehabilitation professionals to "fix" dysfunctional families, recognizing that families are operating at the enmeshed end of the continuum might prompt referral to a family therapist or social worker better prepared to help families sort through options and facilitate adaptation. Recognizing a family with characteristics of disengagement would prompt referral to formal systems of support (e.g., geriatric care managers, home health agencies, community- and nonprofit-based senior services) to augment caregiving resources for an aging family member.

Flexibility, described along the continuum outlined in Figure 11-5, refers to the family's responsiveness to factors that might alter or change family organization or leadership, roles and relationships of family members, or rules of family operation.[41] To be optimally functional, there is a need for both a sense of stability and the possibility of change within the family system. An effectively flexible family allows individuality of its members while concurrently maintaining a sense of connectedness. Families who are structured or flexible in orientation are able to negotiate changes in roles, rules, and organization, although at times this requires effort. Families who are rigid tend to resist any change, focusing instead on maintaining existing roles and their corresponding relationship rules. Those whose systems are chaotic lack rules of interaction among members and behave impulsively and inconsistently in their decision making.

Families at either extreme of the flexibility continuum are likely to have significant difficulty addressing changes in the role and needs of an older adult family member when disease or disability alters the capabilities of an aging family member.

Communication is a key modifier of the operation and structure of the family; it is the facilitating mechanism when change within the family system is necessary or when the family system is under stress.[40] Components of effective communication include each member's ability to listen to others (degree of attentiveness and empathy for other family members), to effectively interpret what is being said (remain "on target"), to effectively express thoughts (degree of engagement and acceptance of other's thoughts and feelings vs. being confrontational), and ability to accurately self-disclose, and respect and regard for other members during interchange. Communication within the family is influenced not only by the content being discussed or exchanged, but also by the individual family member's tone of voice, style of delivery, nonverbal behaviors, and underlying or implicit messages. Culture and ethnicity are also powerful influences on nonverbal (eye contact, touch, personal space, posture, among others) and spoken (directness of statements, ability to ask questions, among others) communication. Health professionals who are able to fit their communication style and strategies to those of a family will be more effective in gathering and sharing information and in assessing the effectiveness of such exchanges. Communication skills and strategies, to some extent, can be learned. When rehabilitation professionals determine that communication to and within the

DEGREE OF FLEXIBILITY

Very low	Moderate	Very high

FIGURE 11-5 Continuum of flexibility within family systems.

Rigid	*Structured*	*Flexible*	*Chaotic*
Resistant to change	Balanced relationships		Excessively changeable

Authoritative	Minimal leadership
Highly disciplinary	Erratic/inconsistent discipline
Inflexible roles/responsibilities	Dramatic shifts of roles/responsibilities
Intolerant of change	Ever-changing

family is somewhat problematic, we can model more effective communication strategies. When communication is significantly impaired, a referral to a family therapist for intervention focused on enhancing communication within the family system may be necessary.

Coping Resources, Strategy, and Efficacy

One of the ways that families immediately respond to stressors is to enact various coping strategies to minimize stress, thus allowing the family to continue with

essential family functions. Most stress-induced coping strategies aim to manage emotional responses and solve the immediate problems presented by the stressors. Box 11-1 summarizes the common coping strategies used by individuals and families, on both the cognitive–perceptual–emotional level and on the behavioral level. The degree and duration of stressors are one of the determinants of whether a family's coping responses will be effective. Other determinants of coping efficacy include emotional, financial, and intellectual resources available to the family; spirituality and cultural values

BOX 11-1	Examples of Cognitive–Emotional and Behavioral Coping Strategies Used by Individuals and Families Described in the Psychology and Family Studies Literature
Cognitive–Perceptual–Emotional Coping Strategies	
Positive reframing	Reinterpreting or redefining the stressor as a challenge to be overcome, a vehicle for growth or positive change, a means to bring the family together, or other positive outcome consistent with family beliefs and values.
Reflection	Examining and working through emotional responses to the stressor to gain understanding of self, others, and the stressor situation.
Minimization or denial	Temporarily or permanently reducing level of stress experienced by refusing to acknowledge the importance or effect of the stressor and the thoughts and feelings associated with the stressor.
Withdrawal	A response to being overwhelmed by the stressor event, associated with passiveness or reluctance to engage in dealing with problems associated with the stressor. Often associated with problems with motivation, adherence to intervention plans, and depression.
Expressing anger	Expressing frustration and pain resulting from the stressor by verbally or physically "acting out" in anger. This may be aimed at the situation, at the family member who is ill or impaired, at other family members, or at the health professionals involved in providing care.
Crying	Using the emotional release that follows a period of crying to release pressure associated with the stressor event. Acknowledges the grief process when the stressor event may lead to loss of function, role, personal meaning, or death.
Bargaining	Constructing an "if I/we do ____, then the desired outcome ____ will occur" framework as a way to provide a sense of control or mastery during a stressful situation.
Cognitive rehearsal	Imagining and preparing for a variety of potential outcomes for the stressful situation, in an effort to determine the most appropriate response to the stressor.
Prayer and spirituality	Turning to religious tradition or exploring one's spirituality in order to understand or interpret stressors, and enhance emotional health when faced with unpredictable, threatening, or potentially life-altering situations.
Humor	Defusing negative thoughts and emotions associated with the stressor by recognizing absurdity of the situation, jesting or joking, or using wit, satire, sarcasm, or self-depreciation.
Behavioral Coping Strategies	
Seeking emotional support	Ability to actively engage in acquiring emotional support from friends, relatives, and neighbors (informal support systems).
Seeking knowledge	Ability to actively engage in learning about contributors to the stressful situation (especially health issues) from professionals, experts, and Web-based resources.
Seeking instrumental help	Willingness to request and receive assistance from friends, neighbors (informal support systems), or from community resources, agencies, support groups, or professionals (formal support systems).
Active problem solving	Identifying immediate problems and needs associated with the stressor, as well as organizing, delegating, and mobilizing resources necessary to manage and meet the needs of the family during periods of stress.
Deferring other demands	Adapting priorities within the family to meet the most pressing challenges of a stressful situation; postponing events or activities that compete for resources or interfere with the family's ability to react effectively to the present stressor.
Distraction or avoidance	Engaging in other activities to avoid directly dealing with problems associated with the stressor event.
Engaging in leisure activities	Continuing with meaningful and pleasurable activities as a means of respite, an emotional outlet, for interaction with others, or to support self-esteem ("recharging") in the midst of a stressful situation.
Pacing	Building opportunity for rest, entertainment, or other activities into the family's or individuals' activities related to managing the stressor.
Relaxation techniques	Using activities such as meditation, massage, listening to quiet music, and other activities to reduce the amount of physical and psychological stress during a crisis or an ongoing stressor.
Use of alcohol or drugs	Substance use or abuse as self-medication to relieve or escape from the stressor situation.

and beliefs of the family; and availability of informal and formal support systems.[42]

Cognitive–perceptual–emotional coping strategies include appraisal of the event and determining its significance, consistent with family themes and beliefs, so that the family can understand the nature and potential impact of the stressor.[43] Families will try to define the immediate problems that need attention, framing them so that priorities and needs of family members can continue to be met, or be temporarily put aside, until the stress is resolved.[44] They will try to minimize the immediate emotional aspects of the situation to avoid becoming entirely overwhelmed.[45]

Consider, for example, an older woman living alone in the family homestead who falls and sustains a hip fracture. One family may cognitively reframe the event, saying, "We were worried about Mom's ability to be safe alone in the house. She was so determined to be on her own. One good thing that might come out of this situation is that now she'll consider moving in with us, or moving to assisted living once she finishes rehabilitation." Another family may understand the situation quite differently: "This is the beginning of the end. No one ever gets completely well after a hip fracture. She is going to pass away soon, probably from pneumonia. She'll never get home now; we'd better start looking at nursing homes, and make sure her affairs are in order." Whereas the first family reframes things in a positive light, and the other with a more negative connotation, both have interpreted the situation in a way that allows them to move forward in managing the situation. The difference in emotional interpretation is likely to affect family resources and functioning. The anticipation of loss and grief implied in the second family's interpretation is likely to use some of the family's emotional resources, making these resources less available for immediate actions.

Behavioral coping strategies are the actions that the family takes in response to the immediate stressor.[46] The specific strategies put into place vary from family to family but are consistent with the family's identity, rules and themes, and boundaries.[47] Some families may mobilize, coming together to be in the same place to provide support to their aging family member. Others, less organized in structure, may wait for one of their group to step to the front to take charge. Some, comfortable with seeking information and assistance, reach out to professionals to learn and prepare for the outcomes of the stressor event. Others, more enmeshed in structure, may be reluctant to consider recommendations made by the health professionals providing care to their aging family member. Families and individuals call on a variety of coping strategies, depending on the type of stressor and the intensity of the stressor that they are facing. Health professionals must be aware that coping strategies with negative connotations, such as denial, are not always associated with negative outcomes; temporary employment of such strategies may be a necessary component of the ongoing process of coping when facing stressful situations.[45,48]

Resilience is a term used to describe the outcome or efficacy of coping within the family system.[49] Resilient families are able to develop, enrich, and enact skills and resources that enhance their ability to cope. Resilient families are able to[40] (1) commit to working through problems together; (2) sacrifice for the benefit of the family and its members in times of crisis; (3) preserve a sense of emotional closeness while embracing individuality of members; (4) remain open, clear, honest, and reflective in their communication; (5) share purpose and values that go beyond self-interest; (6) contribute as well as receive assistance from others; and (7) effectively negotiate and use family resources of time, money, and energy when the family is under stress.

It is important for health professionals to recognize that, because resilience is not an innate characteristic, it can be facilitated and developed by individuals as well as by their family system.[50] To effectively facilitate such resilience in families facing stressful health-related situations when an aging family member is ill, health professionals can[51-53] (1) express empathy and concern for the individuals and the family in the stressful situation they are experiencing; (2) identify and celebrate strengths and successes of the coping strategies that the family is using; (3) suggest ways to reframe or redefine the meaning of or beliefs about the situation, to empower the individual and family, and provide a sense of potential mastery; (4) help the family develop more effective communication skills; and (5) provide instrumental assistance and education so that the family can better address the problems associated with the stressor they are facing.

Although these strategies are drawn from the family systems and family therapy literature, they are remarkably similar to the values and skills of the collaborative reasoning process that enhance patient outcomes in expert practice in physical therapy[54-56] and in geriatric and community health nursing.[57-59] Box 11-2 provides a selected list of key questions health professionals should consider asking to develop a sense of a family's patterns and dynamics of interaction, their perceptions of illness and health care, and the ways their unique family system responds to stress and accomplishes change.

The Family in Later Life

There are a number of "normative" or developmental events that families face as leading generations of the family age: redefining the older parent–adult child relationship, grandparenthood, retirement, and adjusting to physiological and functional changes associated with the aging of the oldest generation. Each of these requires the family to reexamine and adapt its organization and patterns of interaction. Such adaptation is a dynamic process that potentially causes conflict and strain, upsetting

BOX 11-2	Examples of Key Information-Seeking Questions Health Professionals May Ask to Recognize and Respond to the Patterns and Dynamics within a Family System Experiencing a Health-Related Crisis

Membership and Roles within the Family System
- Who are the members of the family and what are their typical roles within the family?
- Who will be involved in the patient's care and decision making?
- What are the resources, strengths, weaknesses, or concerns of each family member?
- What roles and responsibilities do key family members have, that are competing with caregiving?
- How will the patient's health issue affect roles and responsibilities within the family?
- Is there someone who can assist with these roles and responsibilities, and the daily tasks of the family?

The Family's Knowledge, Beliefs, Expectations, and Interpretation of the Health Event
- What are the family's views of illness, disability, and of death?
- What do family members understand about the disease process, future expectations and needs, and probable outcome of care?
- How do family members make sense of or define the meaning of this health crisis?

Rules and Regulations of the Family System
- What are the family's overall priorities?
- How are decisions made within the family? How is change negotiated?
- How willing is the family to seek and accept support and assistance from informal and formal sources? What does the family perceive as consequences of receiving such support?

Communication within the Family
- How do family members share their concerns, fears, issues, problems, hopes, and dreams?
- How effectively do family members listen and reflect on what they hear?
- How clear and direct are information exchanges within the family?
- How do family members express concern, caring, affection, and love (physically, verbally, by providing services, etc.)? How do they express worry, frustration, or fear?
- What additional skills might assist family members to communicate effectively during this health care encounter? How might these additional skills best be facilitated?
- What words and expressions are acceptable to the family system? What words or expressions are "red flags" that disrupt the process of communication?

Understanding of the Health Care System
- What does the family perceive as the role of each member of the health care team?
- What interaction approach do family members expect of health professionals (e.g., paternalistic decision makers and directors of care, experts who provide guidance to the family but do not make decisions, external authorities who are a threat to the family system, honorary members of the family during the period of care and beyond)?

Level of Stress, Coping Strategies, Coping Efficacy, and Resilience
- How do family members rate their level of stress as a result of this family health event?
- What coping strategies are being used by family members during this stressful time?
- Are their coping strategies effective in helping the family manage its level of stress?
- Would the family benefit from referral to pastoral counseling, a family therapist or psychologist, social service professionals, a community support group, or other formal resource?

the operation of the family system until a new level of equilibrium can be reached.

OLDER PARENT–ADULT CHILD RELATIONSHIPS

Older parent–adult child relationships continue to evolve over time and, hopefully, reach the level of a peer adult-to-adult relationship. There is no ideal or norm for a parent–child relationship in later life. The nature and quality of older parent–adult child relationship dyads is influenced by factors including family history and culture, prior degree of emotional closeness, power distribution within the relationship and how it has evolved over time, and any role strain (competing demands)

experienced by either member of the relationship.[60] Family studies and individual development theorists and researchers have examined this relationship in terms of reciprocity and exchange; degree of attachment, connectedness, or intimacy; filial responsibility, obligation, or altruism; family solidarity; and social norms.[61-63] In fact, many older parents and adult children experience ambivalence and mixed emotions, recognizing both positive and negative aspects of their evolving relationships.[64] Should physical or emotional frailty or illness of an older parent occur, this parent–offspring relationship often transitions into caregiving, where the older parent becomes the recipient of care and the adult child plays a more central role in decision making about parent and family needs and activities.[65,66]

Each adult child in the family negotiates and navigates the evolution of his or her relationship with aging parents; these changing relationships also affect the nature and quality of relationships between siblings.[67] When there are multiple adult children, there may be significant tension about what options should be considered and how decisions will be made regarding an aging parent's future, often reminiscent of patterns of interaction from earlier points in the family life cycle.[68] The degree to which the family is open to discussing aging and the eventuality of death is an important influence on whether aging parents and their adult children are able to plan for the future, in terms of providing instrumental assistance, organizing finances, making decisions about living situations and long-term care, and health care needs and advance directives.[69,70]

Grandparenthood

Although becoming a grandparent typically occurs in late midlife, the transition to grandparenthood is often a marker of shift in roles and power within the family system, in that the older generation of the family system relinquishes direct responsibility for rearing and launching of children to the next younger generation.[71] The contributions to and roles of grandparents (and great-grandparents) within the family system vary significantly across ethnic groups and are influenced by geographic location of generations of the family, as well as by the age, health status, and economic resources of the older generation.[72,73] Such contributions may include becoming the "kin-keeper" responsible for drawing the family together and preserving its history, being an extra pair of hands in the care of grandchildren, being a provider of advice and dispenser of wisdom when the family experiences stress, or sharing financial resources to assist younger generations with the cost of housing and education.[74] Relationships with grandchildren are often very important components of the lives of older adults, providing continuity of responsibility within the family, supporting their life's meaning, and their self-concept.[75]

Divorce and remarriage of adult children can have a profound impact on older adults who value their role as grandparents. Maternal grandparents are often called upon to assist with child care for newly single mothers. This is especially the case if one of the grandchildren has chronic illness, mental health or cognitive problems, or physical disability.[76] In addition to providing emotional support, grandparents may provide financial assistance or a place for their daughter and grandchildren to live.[77] In blended families, after remarriage of an adult child, step-grandparents must redefine and negotiate their roles and relationships with both grandchildren and newly added step-grandchildren.[78] In families with acrimonious outcomes following divorce, contact with grandchildren may be limited such that grandparents lose a role they valued significantly; this has significant impact on both mental and physical health of the grandparent.[79]

Almost 12% of grandparents in the United States are responsible for raising their grandchildren as a result of substance abuse, incarceration, illness, disability, or death of their adult child.[80,81] When grandparents take on this nonnormative expanded role, there are both positive and negative consequences for all members of the family, on social, economic, and legal levels.[82] Many of these households are considered to be fragile by social service and educational professionals because of low income, limited access to health care and other services, and physical or emotional problems of the grandchildren.[83] The off-time needed to assume the parenting role requires grandparents to redefine their expectations for their later years, often perceived as interruption of their own developmental path.[84] Age-related changes affect physical function, making the day-to-day activities associated with managing the household and caring for young children more challenging, although many grandparent caregivers take pride in their role.[85] The prevalence of depression, anxiety, and borderline health status is higher among grandparents raising grandchildren than among older adults who do not have to assume this role.[86,87] If a grandparent caregiver requires hospitalization or rehabilitation care, there may be few within-family resources to assist with child care and daily tasks; many of these families rely on church groups, nonprofit agencies, and formal social services to keep the family functioning when health-related stressors occur.[88,89]

RETIREMENT

The transition from an active working role into retirement typically occurs between 55 and 70 years of age. Because of this, with the lengthening of the life span, many aging adults can anticipate 10 to 25 years afterwork living. The level of transitional stress a newly retired person and his or her family experiences during adaptation from work to retirement varies considerably and is influenced by many factors, including the meaning of work for the retiring person,[90] voluntary versus involuntary nature of the retirement,[91] disruption of socially supportive peer relationships and work friendships, availability of meaningful substitute interests and activities,[92,93] and the perceived and actual physical and mental health and functional status of self and spouse.[94,95]

Retirement affects marital relationships, resources (time, energy, money), decision making, activity participation, and interaction with friends and family, especially if spouses have differing expectations of what life after retirement will be like.[96] For many couples in solid long-term marriages, retirement increases their ability to spend time together, strengthens their sense of companionship and closeness, and enhances marital satisfaction.[97] Similarly, couples unhappily married may experience more conflict and dissatisfaction in spending time together, and so may opt to lead emotionally separate, if parallel, lives after work roles end. Ongoing stressors over the retirement years include concern about income adequacy, sufficiency of financial resources for years yet to be lived,[98] and availability and adequacy of health insurance for future needs.[99] This is especially true for persons living on fixed incomes facing unexpected expenses when health insurance resources do not completely cover costs of health care for acute illness, injury, or chronic health conditions.

HEALTH AND PHYSICAL FUNCTION IN LATER LIFE

The aging process clearly affects physical ability. Gradual age-related changes in sensory, neuromuscular, musculoskeletal, information-processing, and learning/memory systems cumulatively alter an older adult's ability to accomplish physically demanding aspects of home maintenance and other instrumental activities of daily living.[100] Functional abilities among older adults vary greatly, as influenced by absolute age, physical activity and fitness over the lifetime, body weight and nutritional status, lifestyle (smoking, alcohol use), onset of chronic diseases, cognitive status, self-perception of ability, and fear of injury and falling.[101-104] The longer an older adult lives, the more likely he or she will accumulate chronic health conditions and age-related decrements in physiological systems that require adaptation or adjustment of activities, and increased risk of injury and falls.[105,106] Although health professionals and younger family members observing function might recommend assistance, the older adult family member may not perceive such a need and frame such suggestions as a threat to his or her competency, independence, and self-determination.[107] The tension between the aging adult's determination to continue to function independently and the family's desire to ensure safety can lead to significant conflict within the family system.

When a generally healthy 80-year-old man who climbs a ladder to paint a wall or clear gutters falls and sustains injury, family members and health professionals may immediately question his judgment and physical abilities. The patient may be angered by their concern, perceiving it as a threat to his independence and competence in activities he has done successfully all of his previous years. Acceptance of assistance requires the older family member to acknowledge changes in capacity, find alternative means of being self-directed or in control of his or her life, and adjust or adapt his or her self-concept and sense of worth to his or her actual abilities.[108] In cultures or traditions that value wisdom and experience of aged family members more than physical ability, acceptance of the need for assistance may be perceived as a privilege due to them, such that provision of assistance is the duty of younger generations of family.[109] In contrast, in popular American culture, where autonomy and self-direction are prominent themes, needing assistance may be interpreted as ineptitude and uselessness.[110]

As a result of the aging process, older adults (and their younger family members) must adapt the meanings of the physical self, in terms of appearances, functional abilities, health status, and the older person's eventual death.[111] In place of valuing their physical capabilities and appearance, many aging adults report components of successful aging as being able to live to an advanced age, having stable health, keeping a positive mental outlook and sufficient cognitive capabilities, and being able to be socially involved with family and friends who are important to them.[112] The viewpoint that aging is a process of *adaptation* in the face of physiological changes, rather than a state of being, contributes to a sense of well-being and self-worth, which in turn allows the older adult to continue to be a vital part of the family system.[113]

When an older adult requests assistance, however, family members and health professionals must be careful not to assume the need for help crosses multiple domains of function. An older family member who asks an adult child to accompany him or her to a physician's appointment may simply be requesting help in listening and gathering information. The adult child may incorrectly interpret the request as an aging parent's abdication of decision making and determination to manage his or her own care.[114] An astute health care provider will recognize situations in which a well-intentioned family member is overfunctioning for an aging adult.[114]

FAMILY CAREGIVING

In the geriatric health literature, caregiving is often described as a one-way flow of resources from a family member to an impaired or disabled aging adult. This theoretical orientation speaks to the difficulties and challenges that spouses, adult children, or formal caregivers encounter in providing such care. Studies framed by this perspective often focus on caregivers' depression or mental health, role strain, burden, conflict within the family, poorer health, and diminished quality of life.[115,116] Studies of caregiving in the gerontology and family studies literature, however, are more likely to define caregiving as an *exchange* of resources between the older adult who needs assistance and the caregiver who receives benefit or value.[117,118] In addition, being a caregiver affects roles and responsibilities beyond the relationship with the older adult needing care. The caregiver must balance time and energy across potentially competing family and work roles and responsibilities that in turn influence the efficacy of performance in these other dimensions of life.[119] These would be part of the exosystem of an aging patient's caregiver, per Bronfenbrenner's ecological model of development.

Reciprocity and Exchange

Social exchange theory, which has its roots in cost–benefit analysis, provides an informative perspective for health professionals interacting with aging patients and their caregiving family members.[120,121] In a balanced caregiving exchange, the value of the tangible/intangible resources and services being provided or received are perceived by both family caregiver and aging parent as relatively equal and reciprocal, such that expectations and needs of both are being met, and both are satisfied with the interaction. For many informal family caregivers, the act of caring is perceived as loving nurturance that protects their aging family member's sense of self-worth and enhances their quality of life.[118] The expressions of gratitude and appreciation they receive in return does much to counteract the stressors of providing care.[122]

In a less-ideal caregiving exchange, the aging parent may have more need or less resource to bring to the exchange, resulting in a growing sense of indebtedness and perception that the family caregiver has more power to influence the exchange process, and the exchange is less reciprocal. This exchange status is often stressful for both caregiver and aging parent. Physical therapists can often assist in reducing dependency and burden of care by facilitating function, providing assistive devices, and adapting the home environment to allow a more reciprocal caregiving exchange.

Developmental Transitions in Caregiving

Caregiving relationships within families do not automatically occur as soon as a need for care arises. Rather, the family proceeds through a series of transitions as the caregiving/receiving relationship evolves.[122] Initially, there must be *recognition that care is necessary* on the part of the aging adult as well as the potential care provider. In times of crisis, as when hip fracture or stroke drastically changes function and ability of the aging family member, the need for care is obvious. More often, however, early clues for the need for care are subtle, develop slowly over time, and may be masked by the aging adult who is intent on maintaining independence. The ability to admit the need for care and to discuss options is significantly influenced by the family's culture, expectations, and belief systems; the rules governing communication and role distributions; the degree of flexibility and cohesion in the family system; and the coping strategies the system and individuals typically employ.

Once the need for care is recognized and accepted, *caregiving and care-receiving roles* must be defined, type of assistance available from both formal and informal caregiver networks must be determined, and capabilities of caretakers must be established.[123] An aging family member in need of care must confront issues including possible loss of self-determination, independence, or control; threats to his or her sense of competence and capability; and a decreasing set of personal, emotional, or financial resources. For a family member, competence and efficacy as a caregiver often require development of a new set of skills in providing assistance for both basic and instrumental activities of daily living, in navigating the health care and insurance systems, and in coordinating an evolving system of informal and formal supporters who will contribute to care.[124] Family caregivers are challenged to manage competing responsibilities and stressors; meet the aging family member's needs across many dimensions of care; find, engage, and use resources within both informal and formal support networks; and recognize and respond to their own and their aging family member's emotional and physical responses to care.[125] Both caregiver and care recipient must recognize that needs will change over time and be ready to adapt their strategies for care as necessary.[126]

The need for care changes the nature of established relationships within the family. In addition to defining roles and responsibilities, *family relationships must be redefined* in response to shifting needs. Gender-based and generational roles and patterns of responsibility often must be modified, in turn altering perception of self and of spouse, parent, or caregiving adult child. Shifts in the power, nature, and meanings of relationships are also greatly influenced by the way that the family has been organized and has operated over the family's life span. The need for care and the provision of care reduces time and energy that both the older family member and caregiver have available to invest in relationships with extended family and with friends. Both are at risk of becoming socially isolated at a time where support, assistance, and understanding from their families and friends would be beneficial.[127]

An effective and healthy caregiving relationship emerges as both care provider and care recipient *accept and embrace the changes* that the need for care has triggered for self and for family. It is important to recognize that, in light of the progression of disease processes and age-related physiological change, the nature and amount of care necessary will continue to challenge the family system. As the level of challenge grows, strategies for care that had previously been effective may falter. The caregiving family may once again need to redefine roles and adjust relationships in an effort to reestablish equilibrium in meeting growing and changing needs.

Dimensions of Care

Family caregivers can be involved in a range of activities reflecting many dimensions of care for their older family member. Assistance with finances may range from balancing the checkbook and making sure bills are paid on time to making decisions and managing financial assets and investments. Assistance with care of home and property may range from the responsibility for the "heavy work" of seasonal duties (raking leaves, cutting lawn, clearing snow, etc.) to assisting with or performing routine household tasks (doing laundry, changing beds, cleaning bathroom, food shopping, etc.). Caregivers may also be called upon to provide transportation to stores, social events, and appointments; to manage the scheduling of activities and appointments; to organize, manage, or administer treatments and medications; and to provide meals in order to ensure adequate nutrition. The need for significant assistance with personal care, especially with bathing and toileting, can be distressing for both caregiver and their family member, because of the breach of privacy associated with assistance during these very intimate activities.[128] Caregivers, in addition to providing physical assistance, are often primary sources of emotional support for their older family member.[129]

The nature of the disease or condition that has created the need for care influences the stress experienced by caregiver as well as older-person care recipient. Caregiving is least stressful on the individuals involved in a caregiving dyad and on their relationship when the need for care is thought to be temporary and return to prior level of function is anticipated. When caregiving is perceived as an ongoing need, caregivers are faced with dealing with suffering of a family member, the need to be ready to respond if something unexpected occurs, being proactive to minimize or prevent potential problems, and carrying out routines and regimens required to manage the disease process.[130] Although the caregiving stress associated with a chronic illness such as diabetes, heart disease, or stroke can be significant, the psychological stress experienced by caregivers exponentially increases when the need for caregiving is a result of a terminal illness or of dementia.[129] In both latter situations, the family caregiver is confronted with the impending loss of their spouse or parent, and anticipatory grieving is a common experience. This is especially true when the underlying problem is dementia, where the caregiver must cope with difficult and unpredictable behaviors and emotional responses in their loved one who is, at the same time, losing the cognitive and emotional connection with the family member they are caring for.[131]

Caregiving for One's Spouse

Types and dimensions of caregiving and care-sharing vary based on the needs and abilities of the aging adult, and the gender and competing roles of the family caregiver. A spouse, when present, is the preferred caregiver for most aging adults, and nearly two-thirds of spousal caregivers are wives.[132] The relationship of many long-married couples becomes symbiotic over time. Together, the couple is able to accomplish much more and can more effectively respond to the challenges of aging and poor health beyond the sum of their individual resources and capacities. The development of physical or functional frailty or onset of disease requires the couple to adapt their long-held marital roles to the new demands of caregiving.[133]

The assumption of the caregiving role is influenced by a strong sense of duty, dedication, and commitment, rooted in deep emotional connection and long history of attachment and intimacy.[134] Spousal caregivers, especially husbands, employ a problem-solving strategy in adapting to increasingly more complex needs for care as the spouse's disease progresses.[135] In addition to providing personal care to their husband or wife, spousal caregivers strive to provide opportunity for socialization and interaction with others, manage daily tasks and the emotional climate within the home, maintain as safe and nurturing an environment as possible, and protect and preserve the self-esteem and dignity of their spouse.[133] One of the rewards that balances the stressors of caregiving is a sense of pride in their ability to fulfill a demanding and critical role in caring for their spouse.

Over time, as the caregiver is faced with his or her own health issues and aging process, he or she must reach out for additional assistance, especially if one or more adult children (most typically daughters) are within reasonable geographic distance, and so available to assist in the provision of care.[136] There is often tension between generations within a family; spousal caregivers may be frustrated at an apparent lack of interest, understanding, or assistance from their adult children. Adult children, as part of a different generation, may struggle reconciling the generational differences in structural and functional family expectations. Women caring for husbands with physical or cognitive decline are more likely to reach out to family for emotional support, whereas men caring for wives with illness or disability are often more stoic, keeping frustrations and doubts to themselves, reluctant to seek assistance for the emotional stressors associated with caregiving.[137]

Caregiving for a Spouse with Dementia. The physical and emotional costs of providing care can be high for the caregiver, especially if the spouse needing care has progressive cognitive impairment. The work of providing care for a spouse with dementia can contribute to loneliness and a sense of isolation, depression, and sleep deprivation.[137] Factors identified as contributing to caregiving stress include emotional lability and problem behaviors of the care receiver. Stress is moderated by the ability of the impaired spouse to express appreciation for care, to discuss their feelings and concerns, and to assist the caregiver in daily activities.[138,139] Caregiving spouses for persons with dementia experience significant anxiety about the progression of the disease over time, are distressed by feelings of anger and resentment toward their impaired spouse, have doubts about their ability to continue to provide the necessary care, and are concerned about the cumulative impact of caregiving on their own physical and mental health.[140] These concerns are realistic. The incidence of hypertension and risk of developing cardiovascular and cerebrovascular disease is three times higher in those caring for a spouse with dementia than in age- and gender-matched noncaregivers.[141] Likewise, the incidence of anxiety disorder and of depression is higher among caregiving spouses, especially wives, than among noncaregiving spouses.[142,143]

Caring for an Aging Parent

When a spouse is not able to provide necessary care, or if both aging parents require assistance, arrangements for provision of care often becomes the responsibility of one or more of the couple's adult children.[144] In the United States, sons (if available) tend to assume responsibility for maintenance of their parents' living environment and management of finances, whereas daughters (if available) tend to manage instrumental and basic activities of daily living and provision of emotional support.[145]

For many adult children, the need to provide assistance to aging parents occurs during or just after the "launching" of their young adult offspring, at a time when the effects of their own aging process are becoming more evident.[146,147] Their own emotional, physical, and financial resources may be further "strained" by competing demands associated with their jobs or professions.[148] Caring for aging parents, whether supporting modified independence in the aging parents' home, an assisted living community, or by joining the adult child's household, influences quality of life and marital satisfaction of the caregiver as well as his or her relationship with siblings.[148-150] It is not unusual for conflicts to arise between an aging parent's caregiver and his or her spouse or for underlying issues about family roles and dynamics to resurface among siblings. Caring for an aging parent significantly increases the complexity of daily life for caregiving adult children, affecting each component of the family systems that the care provider is a part of.[151]

The list of negative consequences for caregivers of aging parents is similar, in many respects, to those experienced by caregiving spouses: disruption of one's accustomed lifestyle; less time to interact with friends for social support; risk of developing anxiety and depression; sadness about the losses experienced by one's parent; having to cope with disappointment and anger as a parent's need for care increases; dealing with emotional, cognitive, and behavioral problems that the parent encounters; and risk of decline in health status. Daughters providing care experience such negative aspects of caregiving to a greater degree than sons.[151] These effects are lessened, to a degree, by factors including a strong sense of attachment and emotional closeness between aging parent and adult child,[152] deriving personal meaning or purpose from the caregiving role,[153] and providing care from a sense of wanting to help rather than being obligated to do so.[154]

Formal Caregiving Systems

Any care-related service that requires payment is considered to be part of the formal caregiving system. Efforts to control medical costs resulting from managed care has, in effect, shifted expectations away from the ongoing use of formal caregiving services toward increased dependence on informal family caregiving.[155,156] As aging adults are discharged from episodes of acute care or subacute care prior to full recovery from illness or surgery, health professionals place more emphasis on teaching family caregivers how to manage medical regimens begun in the hospital than on carrying out restorative services. However, families may be threatened or overwhelmed by these responsibilities.[157] One of the challenges for formal caregivers is to partner with family caregivers in decisions about what home-based skilled care is necessary, and how to provide that care safely and efficiently.[158]

The training and roles of "formal" caregivers vary greatly from home health aides and personal care attendants with high school education and several hours of instruction from the agency that employs them to health professionals with advanced degrees, credentials, and skills. Not all formal caregivers have formal education that prepares them to effectively interact with families and informal caretakers in managing an aging patient's chronic illness.[159-162] Financial resources and insurance coverage influence the type of formal care services available to the patient and the frequency and duration of access to available formal care.[163,164] The rules and regulations about eligibility, fragmentation of services, and documentation requirements within the existing health care system can further complicate a caregiving family's access to formal care and interaction with health professionals.[165] The network of formal care providers is loosely organized and challenging to understand for caregiving families new to the system.[166]

Most health care professionals, as members of the network of formal care providers, are motivated by a desire to help others and to lessen the burden for family caregivers.[167] Each discipline brings unique knowledge and special skills to interactions with older adults and family caregivers. Unfortunately, despite the genuine desire to help, providing care that is integrated and coordinated across all disciplines is often the exception rather than the rule. In interacting with health professionals providing formal care, family members have multiple roles: care coordinator/manager; advocate and watchdog to ensure necessary, safe, and effective care; provider of personal care and emotional support; companion; and surrogate decision maker.[165,168] When interacting with family caregivers, it is important for health professionals to consider potential differences in perspectives that hinder communication and collaboration.[165] All too often, family caregivers are labeled "dysfunctional" by health care professionals if they disagree among themselves regarding medical recommendations, are slow to make decisions about care when asked, are inconsistent in adhering to prescribed regimens (including home exercise programs), or respond emotionally rather than rationally during discussions.[169]

As well intended as the providers in the formal caregiving system may be, we operate outside the boundaries of the families of the aging adult patients that we care for. As much as families come to the formal health care system for assistance and guidance, they are faced with the challenge of allowing the health professional to breech the boundaries of the family system. In allowing this, family caregivers surrender to a nonfamily member a degree of control and decision making about the care of their loved one.[170] Without some sense of a family's themes about illness, sense of responsibility, level of cohesiveness, and rules about membership, health professionals cannot assume their interactions with the family will always have the desired outcomes.[171] The relationship between family caregivers and health professionals as formal caregivers is most likely to be successful if both frame the effort as a collaborative partnership.[172] When receiving services from members of the formal caregiving network, family caregivers value the support, relief, and respite that becomes available, as long as there is a sense of continuity in the health professionals providing care.[173] Older recipients of formal care are most concerned that health care professionals are trusted allies committed to helping them regain as much independence in function as possible.[162]

Supporting Caregivers

Effective communication is the foundation for health professionals to support family caregivers in their role. Health professionals strive to be clear in the delivery of patient and family education, respectful and empathic while listening to (and hearing) family caregiver and patient questions and concerns, and creative in adaptations of caregiving to best address their concerns.[174] Family caregiver–health professional relationships that are grounded in mutual input and shared decision making are perceived as supportive and empowering, as well as effective in reducing stress of spouses and adult children.[175]

Instead of assuming we know what is in an older patient's best interest, health professionals must discern the salience of the act of caregiving to the older patient and family caregiver, and what this means to their relationship. Subsequent discussions about who will provide which aspects of care, aimed at reducing stressors and minimizing risk of physical and psychological burnout and overburdening of the family caregiver will be much more effective.[176] When faced with progressive decline and terminal illness, family caregivers appreciate kindness and compassion, receiving key information and suggestions from health professionals about what to

expect, and being respected for their ability to use this information to make informed decisions.[177]

Physical therapists and other rehabilitation professionals working with aging adults have a responsibility to be alert for signs of distress, depression, overwhelming burden, and declining health status in their family caregivers.[178] As indicated, support can be provided in the form of referral to support groups, to colleagues in social work or mental health disciplines, or to the caregiver's primary care physician.[179,180] One simple but informative strategy to assess caregiver health is to ask three questions: (1) How would you rate your health right now: Is it excellent, very good, good, fair, or poor?[181,182] (2) Over the past 3 (or 6) months, has your health changed? Is it very much better, somewhat better, about the same, somewhat worse, or much worse than it was ____ months ago?[183] and (3) Rate your level of stress on a scale from 1 to 10.[184] Answers indicating fair or poor health, a decline in health, a decline in mood, or increased stress suggest a need for referral out to an appropriate medical or mental health provider and an appropriate support group. Poor health and high levels of emotional stress in family caregivers are predictive of institutionalization and of mortality of the aging adults they provide care for.[185]

There is strong evidence that programs that focus on stress management, effective problem solving, development of strategies and skills for more effective coping, peer mentoring and support, and positive self-care, among others, successfully empower family caregivers and improve the quality and efficacy of the care they provide.[157,186-188] Family caregivers may not understand that options such as adult day care or respite care programs are available; both create space within the caregiver's day or week for "time away" from the stressors of caregiving and opportunities to spend time with friends or to engage in activities that are meaningful and restoring for the caregiver.[189,190] Expressions of appreciation and affirmation of the importance and meaningfulness of the caregiver role by health professionals interacting with family caregivers not only build relationship but also positively affect caregiver self-efficacy.

What about the Health Insurance Portability and Accountability Act and Confidentiality?

The Health Insurance Portability and Accountability Act (HIPAA) is a law passed in 1996 intending to protect patient privacy and ensure confidentiality with respect to sensitive medical information. Originally, the law was designed to govern electronic transfer of information from the medical record between providers and payers (insurance). The law intends to limit access to sensitive patient information to those who "need to know" in order to provide necessary care. According to HIPAA language, family caregivers are *included* in the "need to know" group.[191] It is appropriate to ask an older adult for informal verbal consent about discussing care and sharing information with caregivers; written consent is not required.[192] HIPAA regulations do allow health professionals to use professional judgment in situations when an older adult is unable to provide consent because of acute or organic cognitive impairment, when the older patient would otherwise be at risk or in danger (including suspicion of abuse, neglect, or domestic violence), and when such disclosure is determined to be in the best interest of the patient.[192] HIPAA guidelines suggest that health professionals follow a policy of "minimum necessary information" when sensitive health information is shared.

What does this imply for rehabilitation professionals interacting with older adults and their families? To consider this question, it is informative to look carefully at how we gather key information during the examination/ evaluation process, as well as at how (and what) we share during intervention with our older patients and their families. As part of the examination process, we interview the patient and other relevant informants (family members, other health professionals), and review the patient's medical record (if available) to gather relevant information about current health status and chief complaint, comorbidities and past medical history, results of medical tests and measures, medication and substance use/abuse, health habits, living environment, preferred activities, and functional status.[1] If we are concerned that cognitive problems prevent the older adult from providing an accurate history, we routinely ask for additional information or clarification from a family member/caregiver as a surrogate historian. During the differential diagnosis process, we select appropriate examination strategies, explaining the purpose of the test and how results will inform our decision making. We clarify what the patient and/or family hopes will be the outcome of the care we provide, using this information to determine appropriate goals for our care. We generate a movement-dysfunction–based diagnosis, define an anticipated functional outcome as a prognosis, and determine the frequency, intensity, and duration of intervention in defining a patient-specific plan of care. Optimally, active participation by the patient and family during this process has established an effective team relationship so that formal care providers, informal caregivers, and older patients are collaborative and supportive in working toward the desired outcome. Along the way, each participant in the rehabilitation process monitors progression and contributes to modifications in the plan of care as needs arise and progress is made. All of this requires discussion, query, and interchange of information about health status, level of energy or fatigue, emotions and coping, and functional performance in key activities, such as activities of daily living, postural control, and ability to walk.

Interaction with family caregivers about functional status is not an exchange of sensitive health information; discussion of these issues with an older patient and their family caregivers is both practical and essential for effective physical therapy intervention. Interdisciplinary team meetings that include the patient and family caregivers provide opportunity for both family and health care providers to better understand the "big picture" and make informed decisions about what needs to be done in the situation that the patient and family find themselves facing.[193-195]

TO DRIVE OR NOT TO DRIVE

One of the most common challenges facing aging adults and their family caregivers concerns the question of driving. Is it safe to continue to drive? Or is it time to park the car and take away the keys? We will use this question to apply what we have learned about the family system in later life in a real-world situation.

Why Is Driving a Problem in Later Life?

The task of safely operating a vehicle in traffic is complex and demanding. In addition to being able to steer, brake, and accelerate, the driver must constantly scan the environment in which the car is moving for indications that surrounding cars are moving at similar speeds, slowing, changing lanes, or turning. Drivers must be able to read and interpret signs, traffic lights, and other directional information as they speed by them. They must be mindful of pedestrians, obstacles, and vehicles entering the road from driveways or cross-streets. They must be able to adapt their driving to weather, lighting, and road conditions. They must integrate and synthesize such information about the environment, speed/distance/direction of their car and others around them to maintain safe distances between vehicles, to brake or accelerate as appropriate, and to alter direction to avoid obstacles. Driving is the ultimate cognitive–motor multitasking activity!

Box 11-3 lists common age-related changes in sensory motor systems and frequently occurring medical conditions that can negatively affect driving ability in older adults. Chronological age alone is not a useful indicator of driving ability. Risk of accident increases with certain medical diagnoses including dementia, depression, and other psychological disorders, diabetes, sleep apnea, alcohol use/abuse, and cataracts.[196] A fall in the previous year as well as a diagnosis of orthostatic hypotension appear to increase risk of motor vehicle accidents for women older than age 65 years.[197] Any medication that affects efficacy of central nervous system function or level of consciousness may negatively influence attentiveness, decision making, and ability to respond to challenges encountered when driving. Aging drivers are less likely to be involved in motor vehicle accidents related to consuming alcohol than younger drivers.[198]

Accident rates of drivers age 75 years and older, though slightly higher than for adults age 30 to 74 years,

BOX 11-3 | Factors Affecting Driving Performance of Aging Adults

Age-related Changes	Possible Consequences during Driving
Sensorimotor systems	
Visual	• Decreased retinal luminance (impaired night vision)
	• Less effective distance accommodation (difficulty seeing dashboard)
	• Lower saccade and visual pursuit (difficulty tracking moving objects)
	• Less range of upward/downward gaze without movement of the head
	• Decreased sensitivity to light (diminished ability to see in dim/dark)
	• Greater glare recovery time (loss of vision due to oncoming headlights)
	• Less dynamic visual acuity (trouble reading signs while moving)
	• Impaired spatial contrast sensitivity (predictor of crash risk)
	• Diminished peripheral visual field (ability to discern nearby vehicles)
	• Smaller useful field of view in attentional tasks (predicts crash risk)
Visual-spatial perceptual	• Less precise depth and distance perception (stereopsis)
	• Less efficient space perception (risk of crash at intersection, left turns)
	• Less sensitivity to objects in motion in the environment
	• Less ability to judge depth/distance while moving
	• Difficulty judging relative speed of objects in environment
	• Accuracy judging absolute speed of their own vehicle
Cognitive	• Difficulty with tasks requiring divided attention
	• Less efficient selective attention (greater distractibility)
	• Slower and less efficient attention switching between key stimuli
	• Diminished capacity to retain/recall information in short-term memory
	• Less efficient information-processing speed (hesitant decision making)
	• Less efficient new long-term memory (e.g., changed traffic patterns)
	• Less efficient spatial/cognitive mapping (e.g., trouble using maps)
Motor systems	• Increased choice reaction time (responding to complex situations)
	• Impairment of range of motion and flexibility, especially neck rotation (affects ability to scan behind when backing up, changing lanes)
	• Less accurate control of precise continuous movement
	• Decrements in muscle performance, especially power
Medical conditions	
Sleep apnea	• Daytime drowsiness, risk of falling asleep while driving
	• Diminished vigilance and attention while driving
	• Impaired decision making and responsiveness to changing conditions
Repeated syncope	• Risk of loss of consciousness while driving
Previous stroke	• Homonymous hemianopsia (loss of left or right visual field)
	• Impaired visual–spatial perception/abilities (judging speed, distance)
	• Agnosia (inability to recognize key stimuli)
	• Apraxia (impaired motor planning ability)
	• Emotional lability
	• Deficits in attention and distractibility
Diabetes mellitus	• Visual deficits from retinopathy
	• Sensorimotor impairment/polyneuropathy (braking, acceleration)
Seizure disorders	• Risk of impairment/loss of consciousness
	• Risk of impaired motor control
Dementia (early to midstage)	• Getting lost while driving
	• Impaired judgment
	• Impulsiveness in lane changing and turning
	• Failure to use turn signals
	• Driving too slowly for the driving environment
	• Difficulty recognizing and responding to signs and signals
Parkinson's disease	• Rigidity (impaired ability to turn head to scan environment)
	• Bradykinesia (impaired timing: braking and acceleration)
	• Impaired postural control (stability/anticipatory balance while driving)
	• Drowsiness (adverse effect of medications)
Cataracts	• Sensitivity to glare, especially oncoming headlights in night driving
	• Impaired visual acuity for reading traffic signs and signals
Macular degeneration	• Impaired central (precise) vision

are similar to accident rates of drivers age 25 to 29 years, and lower by one third than are accident rates of drivers age 15 to 24 years.[199] The rate of fatalities, however, is exponentially higher for older drivers involved in automobile accidents, attributed to greater susceptibility to injury rather than high incidence of crashes.[200] Broad publicity about injuries and deaths of pedestrians hit by older adult drivers have raised public awareness about driving safety in later life, and calls for changes in driving laws, including more frequent assessment of driving and visual ability of adults age 65 years and older.[201] The legal requirements for reevaluation of driver fitness and for reporting potentially unsafe drivers vary from state to state. There is tension between protecting the needs of older drivers and ensuring the safety of the public. Although there are no well-established criteria for canceling driving licenses for older drivers, there are many easily accessible resources for older adults and their families, as well as for health care providers, who want more information about older adult driving safety and availability of older adult transportation options to driving. A variety of driving education programs are available (online and in person) that help older adult drivers self-assess and refresh driving skills as well as find adaptive driving strategies to enhance safety. Box 11-4 lists resources aimed at consumers and Box 11-5 lists resources aimed at health professionals.

The Meaning of Driving

Driving is not just for getting places. The ability to drive a car provides and supports an adult's sense of independence, autonomy, self-determination, and personal competence.[202] In many communities, especially in rural areas where public transportation is limited or unavailable, driving a car is necessary for individuals to be actively engaged in meaningful activities, to participate within their social networks, to access needed health care, and

BOX 11-5	Resources about Older Adult Driving Safety Aimed at Health Professionals
Resource Name and Description	**Contact Information**
National Highway Traffic Safety Administration Driving fitness assessment and educational tools	www.nhtsa.dot.gov: Traffic Safety tab, Older Drivers link
National Council on Safety (journal article links)	www.ncs.org/safety_road/ DriverSafety/Pages/ MatureDrivers.aspx

to fulfill important instrumental activities of daily living, such as grocery stores, pharmacies, or doctor's appointments. When contemplating "giving up the keys," an older adult and his or her family are faced with many questions about the emotional and practical aspects of driving cessation. It is important to note that older adults who stop driving are more likely to experience declines in health, depression, loss of social contact, and functional losses.[203-205]

As the task of driving becomes more challenging, many older adults recognize and appropriately respond by changing driving behavior, especially if they have concerns about the quality of their vision and visual perception.[206-208] The experience of repeated "near misses" of accidents because of driving errors is also a powerful stimulus to reevaluate driving ability.[209] Older adults may opt to avoid driving at night when glare from oncoming headlights is most problematic, when inadequate street illumination makes it difficult to scan the environment, or when weather conditions make driving dangerous.[210] They may avoid high-traffic highways, rush hour conditions, and unfamiliar areas.

The decision about driving safety is especially difficult when a loved one has been diagnosed with dementia.[211] In

BOX 11-4	Resources about Older Adult Driving Safety Available for Aging Drivers and Family Caregivers
Resource Name and Description	**Contact Information**
AARP Driver Safety Programs	888 687-2277 or www.aarp.org
AARP "We need to talk" Guide	www.thehartford.com/talkwitholderdrivers
AARP "We need to talk" Seminars	202 434-3919 or http://www.aarp.org/home-garden/transportation/we_need_to_talk/
AAA Senior Drivers	http://discover.aaa.com/PGA/SeniorMobility
AAA self-test, Drivesharp calculator, 55+ driving ability, Carfit, Safe driving for mature operators	www.seniordrivers.org/home/
NHTSA Older Drivers	http://www.nhtsa.gov/Senior-Drivers
Caring.com Guide to Driving: assessing driver fitness, safe senior driving, taking the keys, life without a car	www.caring.com/older-drivers
State Driving Laws	www.caring.com/calculators/state-driving-laws
Association for Driving Rehabilitation Specialists	www.driver-ed.org or 866-672-9466

this situation, families strive to preserve as much self-determination as safely possible in the midst of progressive cognitive impairment.[212] Because there is significant variability in types and severity of impairment in conditions such as Alzheimer's disease, performance on cognitive and memory tests alone are not strongly predictive of ability to drive safely and risk of a motor vehicle accident.[213] Neuropsychological testing of visual spatial skills and attention and reaction time are more strongly related to driving performance than cognitive status.[214,215] Persons with early- to midstage dementia who continue to drive, however, tend to overestimate their abilities and may become overwhelmed or confused when environmental conditions (construction areas, traffic congestion) increase and exceed their ability to process information and formulate appropriate responses.[216,217] For this reason, periodic on-road testing is recommended as an important determinant of capacity to continue to drive.[218]

Evaluation of Driving Ability and the Decision to Stop Driving

Two of the most important determinants of driving capacity are (1) the ability to see and to use vision effectively and (2) the ability to cognitively assess and respond to challenges encountered when operating a motor vehicle.[219] Many of the impairments that compromise the ability to drive develop and progress insidiously. Family caregivers and health professionals interacting with aging adults share the responsibility to screen for problems that may interfere with driving safety. Box 11-6 summarizes some of the key messages to discuss with patients and their families regarding driving capacity in older adults.

Ideally, conversations with an older family member about the eventual need to "give up the keys" when driving becomes unsafe will begin long before the need to stop driving occurs. Well-established and meaningful behaviors can be challenging to change. One of the first steps is to help the individual recognize that there is an issue or problem that needs to be addressed. Warning signs that the time to cease driving is approaching and that more careful assessment of driving ability may be

necessary are summarized in Box 11-7. The way that older adults and their families approach such discussion (and resulting efficacy of such discussion) is shaped by the family system's rules about communication, strategies for management of emotional climate and of daily tasks and responsibilities, boundaries and cohesion (i.e., willingness to seek and accept help from health professionals outside the family system), and flexibility. Strategies that are most likely to be effective in facilitating initial and subsequent discussion about driving ability include exploring the conditions under which driving may still be possible (daytime, low-complexity situations), being sensitive during discussions and anticipating an extended time period for final decision making, actively involving the older adult in the decision making, helping explore alternative transportation options, and involving others if driving is dangerous.

Health status considered alone is not a powerful indicator of the ability to drive; medical evaluation is only one component of a fitness-to-drive assessment.[220,221] When questions about the driving ability of an aging adult patient or parent arise, physicians and other providers can refer the older driver to a credentialed driver rehabilitation specialist (DRS) for evaluation[222,223] (see Box 11-4 for locating a DRS). Testing may include a clinical evaluation of overall health and medication use, examination of neuromusculoskeletal systems to identify impairments affecting the ability to drive, detailed examination of field of vision and visual perception, and additional neuropsychological and cognitive testing.[224,225] Driving simulation technology or on-road testing identifies the components of the driving task the patient can safely and effectively accomplish as well as components likely to improve with remediation or adaptation, and any components so unsafe that they should no longer be allowed.[226]

For older drivers who are found to be moderately to marginally safe, there are a number of remediation strategies that can facilitate safer performance. Computer-based activities that train cognitive processing speed (e.g., computer-based exercises stressing visual attention and speed of visual information processing) are particularly

---

BOX 11-6	Important Messages about Driving to Share With Aging Adults and Family Caregivers

- Age alone does not make someone a bad driver.
- Decisions about driving should focus on the older driver's functional driving ability.
- Driving ability typically declines gradually; modifications and interventions to sustain safe driving may be available in the early stages.
- Vision is the most important physical component of driving: 85% of driving ability is visual skill and 15% is motor skill.
- Most aging adults will "outlive" their capacity to drive: Acknowledge this and make plans to manage it.
- Driving is a privilege, not a right. Public safety must take priority over individual preference.
- Alternatives to driving are often available; ascertain options early.
- Resources are available to evaluate driving capacity and counsel about driving cessation (Boxes 11-4 and 11-5 provide resource contacts).

(Adapted from Driving Transitions Education: Tools, scripts, and practice exercises, National Highway Traffic Safety Administration & American Society on Aging, www.asaging.org/drivewell.)

BOX 11-7	Indicators That Driving May No Longer Be Safe for Aging Adults

- Almost crashing, with frequent "close calls"
- Becoming distracted or having difficulty concentrating while driving
- Changing lanes without signaling
- Difficulty moving foot between gas and brake pedal; confusing gas and brake pedals
- Difficulty turning around to check for cars or obstacles when backing up or changing lanes
- Experiencing road rage
- Finding dents and scrapes on the car, on fences, mailboxes, garage doors, curbs, etc. ·
- Frequently being "honked at" by other drivers
- Getting lost, especially in surroundings that were previously familiar
- Going through stop signs or red lights
- Going too fast or too slow for safety
- Having problems making turns at intersections, especially left turns
- Having trouble seeing or following traffic signals, road signs, and pavement markings
- Misjudging gaps in traffic at intersections and on highway entrance and exit ramps
- Receiving traffic tickets or "warnings" from traffic or law enforcement officers
- Responding more slowly to unexpected situations
- Straying into other lanes

(*Adapted from http://www.aarp.org/family/housing/driver_safety_program/resources/ warning_signs.*)

effective.[227] Opportunities to practice using driving simulation training also improve driving performance, especially in safety while turning (maneuvering the car into the correct lane and consistency in use of turn signals).[228] The efficacy of traditional driver education programs, although widely available at minimal cost, is not well supported by clinical studies.[229]

When an older family member who is unsafe refuses to stop driving, there are a number of strategies that caregivers may use. However, these strategies may be quite stressful to undertake. Although reporting regulations vary from state to state, families, health professionals, or law enforcement professionals can file a written report to the state motor vehicle department identifying the unsafe driver and describing the reason for concern and the problematic driving behavior.[230,231] In many states, this will prompt further evaluation, including a medical evaluation and an on-road driving test with an official from the motor vehicle department to determine fitness to drive; such evaluation often results in revocation of the older unsafe driver's license.[232] Many of the websites listed in Box 11-4 have links to state motor vehicle departments and their guidelines for reporting unsafe drivers.

Some older adults, especially those with cognitive impairment, may continue to drive even if their license has been revoked. As a last resort, family members may have to remove the keys from the person's possession, disable the car so that it cannot be driven (such as removing the battery), move the car to another location, or donate or sell the car so that the temptation and opportunity to drive is removed. Families who use these extreme strategies must be prepared to respond to behavioral, emotional, and practical consequences that are likely to result.

CONCLUSION

Early in the chapter, readers broadened their understanding of the family as a complex system that provides the environment for development of its members as they move forward over time in their life span. Bronfenbrenner's model of ecological development provided a framework to understand the interaction of formal care providers (health professionals) with older adult patients and members of their families during a time in which the health care system is in the midst of substantive change. We discovered that the organization, rules for interaction, permeability of boundaries, and strategies to accomplish necessary tasks vary greatly from family to family, and that assuming that families "work" much like our own can lead to miscommunication. We explored how acute and chronic illnesses of aging family members are nonnormative stressors that require families to use various coping strategies, and hopefully, adapt effectively to new situations. We discovered that taking the time to understand the family's operating system, the rules governing family interactions, and the family's beliefs about aging and health will enhance communication between health care providers, aging adults, and their family caregivers, ultimately improving quality of care and patient/family satisfaction with the outcomes of rehabilitation.

Next, we considered how the family responds to the need to provide older-patient care for ill, frail, disabled, or cognitively impaired members of its oldest generations. We discovered that the presence of a spouse or adult child does not always mean that the assistance needed will be available. We framed our view using a model of reciprocal exchange, considering the resources and the physical and psychological costs of a caregiving relationship for formal and informal care providers as well as the aging adult recipients of care. We reviewed the clinical research literature about caregiver stress and coping, and developed strategies to provide support to family caregivers so that they can be effective in their caregiving role.

Finally, we applied what we have learned about families in later life to a complex problem that many face: the determination of whether an aging family member should continue to drive. We discovered that the act of driving provides much more than transportation; it also affects an aging adult's self-image, sense of independence and self-determination, and sense of personal competence. Age and disease-related impairments of the visual system, visual perception, information-processing and problem-solving systems, and musculoskeletal systems interact to challenge or compromise an older adult's driving capability. Although discussion about driving cessation is in itself a stressor to the family system, beginning such a discussion before driving becomes unsafe allows the process of health behavior change to move forward, and the family can explore options and make plans rather than respond to a crisis situation. We also considered the roles and responsibilities of health professionals in screening for fitness to drive, counseling aging adults and their families, possibly making referrals to specialists in driving assessment and remediation, and, if necessary, reporting unsafe driving behavior to the state's department of motor vehicles.

The concepts and models explored in this chapter can be applied to many other situations and circumstances encountered by physical therapists and other health professionals who work with older adults and their families. This overview of family structure and function as a dynamic system, and discussion of the challenges and rewards of informal caregiving, will be a foundation for interaction with aging adults and their families across the health care settings in which physical therapists provide formal care, no matter what disease or injury has made such care necessary.

REFERENCES

To enhance this text and add value for the reader, all references are included on the companion Evolve site that accompanies this text book. The reader can view the reference source and access it online whenever possible. There are a total of 232 cited references and other general references for this chapter.

PART III

Evaluation, Diagnosis, and the Plan of Care

CHAPTER 12

Impaired Aerobic Capacity/Endurance

Tanya LaPier, PT, PhD, CCS

Impaired aerobic capacity, also known as impaired endurance, is a common patient impairment that can limit participation in functional, occupational, and recreational activities. Even functional tasks that require only a few minutes can be limited by aerobic capacity. Older adults are particularly vulnerable to impaired aerobic capacity due to anatomic and physiological changes that occur with aging, greater propensity for sedentary behaviors, and greater risk for disease processes that limit the oxygen transport system.[1] In addition, aerobic capacity is directly influenced by the habitual activity pattern of an individual, which may vary across individuals from total inactivity to frequent and intense activity. Any factors that limit habitual physical activity, such as illness, injury, and or travel, will cause adaptations that diminish aerobic capacity. Conversely, any factors that promote habitual physical activity, such as intentional exercise, yard work, and occupation-related physical tasks, will result in adaptations that improve aerobic capacity. In older adults, many physiological, pathological, and psychosocial factors can contribute to restricted physical activity. Figure 12-1 depicts the persistent vicious cycle that can be created when sedentary behaviors, chronic disease, and functional dependency interact.[2] This chapter will provide an overview of causes and factors contributing to impaired aerobic capacity in older adults and describes physical therapist patient management (examination, evaluation, diagnosis, and interventions) to address decreased endurance and its impact on function.

FACTORS INFLUENCING AEROBIC CAPACITY IN THE OLDER ADULT

In older adults, aerobic capacity impairments may be related to a number of issues, including deconditioning, age-related physiological changes, and specific pathology. Deconditioning, or decreased physical activity, is common in older adults and often associated with illness, functional limitations, restricted activity, and cognitive limitations. Many age-related physiological changes, such as reduced maximal oxygen consumption because of decreased cardiac performance and skeletal muscle endurance, directly impact aerobic capacity.[1] Also, conditions that affect functional mobility (stroke, Parkinson's disease, osteoarthritis, bone fractures, etc.) are more common in older than in younger adults, thus predisposing older adults to restricted physical activity. Lastly, older adults are also more likely to have cardiovascular, pulmonary, and metabolic pathologies that interfere with oxygen delivery and subsequently aerobic capacity. Physical therapists need to be able to identify and address any of these factors that may be contributing to impaired aerobic capacity in older adults.

Aerobic capacity limitations are associated with declining functional mobility, disability, and loss of independence in older adults. Long-term physical activity is related to postponed disability and longer independent living in older adults, including those with chronic disease.[3] Alexander et al[4] found that measures of submaximal oxygen uptake and maximal oxygen consumption were strongly predictive of functional mobility performance in older adults with and without impairments. An exercise training program of walking improved aerobic capacity and physical function in older adults with low socioeconomic status at risk for disability.[5] The evidence suggests that meeting recommended physical activity guidelines can improve physical function in older adults and help maintain independence and quality of life and reduce risk of frailty.[6,7] In addition, several studies have found that aerobic exercise training has a beneficial impact on locomotor function in older adults,[8] whereas multimodal exercise programs and group-based interventions can also minimize impaired mobility in older adults.[9,10]

PUBLIC HEALTH BENEFITS OF EXERCISE AND PHYSICAL ACTIVITY

The benefits of exercise, and particularly aerobic training, are numerous and extend beyond traditional physical therapy management of a single patient. Promotion

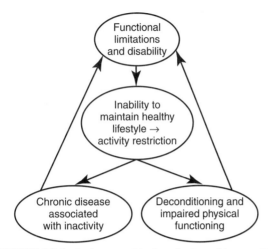

FIGURE 12-1 Cycle created by impaired aerobic capacity.

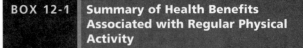

BOX 12-1	Summary of Health Benefits Associated with Regular Physical Activity

Adults and Older Adults
Strong evidence
- Lower risk of early death
- Lower risk of coronary heart disease
- Lower risk of stroke
- Lower risk of high blood pressure
- Lower risk of adverse blood lipid profile
- Lower risk of type 2 diabetes
- Lower risk of metabolic syndrome
- Lower risk of colon cancer
- Lower risk of breast cancer
- Prevention of weight gain
- Weight loss, particularly when combined with reduced calorie intake
- Improved cardiorespiratory and muscular fitness
- Prevention of falls
- Reduced depression
- Better cognitive function (for older adults)

Moderate to strong evidence
- Better functional health (for older adults)
- Reduced abdominal obesity

Moderate evidence
- Lower risk of hip fracture
- Lower risk of lung cancer
- Lower risk of endometrial cancer
- Weight maintenance after weight loss
- Increased bone density
- Improved sleep quality

(From US Department of Health and Human Services: 2008 Physical activity guidelines for Americans. ODPHP Publication #U0036 2008:1-76.)

of aerobic exercise in almost all patient populations has far-reaching effects on health promotion and disease prevention. Landmark studies by Blair et al[11,12] have demonstrated that the level of aerobic fitness is inversely related to risk of cardiovascular disease and all-cause mortality. Regular aerobic activity reduces the risk of many adverse health outcomes including those summarized in Box 12-1. Major research findings suggest that the health benefits of physical activity occur for all age, racial, and ethnic groups and that the benefits far outweigh the possibility of adverse outcomes.[13-15]

Numerous studies have demonstrated the benefits of aerobic exercise in populations of older adults. Recent studies have demonstrated the ability of older adults, both healthy and with pathology, to increase aerobic capacity with exercise training. Although masters athletes experience age-related decline in maximal aerobic capacity, their aerobic performance is better than that of sedentary older adults.[1] Aerobic exercise training is safe and beneficial even with significant chronic disease such as chronic obstructive pulmonary disease, chronic heart failure, peripheral artery disease, and stroke, which are common in older adults.[16-23] For example, in older patients with chronic obstructive pulmonary disease, 12 weeks of aerobic exercise training combined with resistance exercise training or recreational activities increased peak aerobic capacity and 6-minute walk test distance.[16] In older patients with stable chronic heart failure, a program of aerobic high-intensity interval training was well tolerated and improved aerobic capacity, functional status, and quality of life.[17] Interestingly, arm ergometry cycling and treadmill walking exercise training both increased maximal walking distance and pain-free walking distance in older patients with vascular claudication.[20] Exercise training with lower extremity cycling improved aerobic capacity and functional performance in patients with hemiparesis who were more than 5 months poststroke.[21]

Interestingly, aerobic exercise training has also been shown to improve cognitive function in adults, in addition to motor function, auditory attention, cognitive

speed, visual attention, and cognitive flexibility.[24,25] Even a single exercise bout of sufficient intensity may improve cognitive performance in older adults.[26] It has also been proposed that exercise may modify some of the psychological and physiological abnormalities associated with Alzheimer's disease.[27] Because cognitive decline is prevalent in older adults, ways to prevent or attenuate this are clinically relevant in this population.

PHYSIOLOGY OF AEROBIC CAPACITY AND EXERCISE

Aerobic capacity reflects the body's ability to take up, deliver, and use oxygen. Many processes are required to ensure that these three steps occur optimally, and dysfunction in any part of this oxygen transport system can interfere with a patient's aerobic capacity. Oxygen consumption ($\dot{V}O_2$) is a physiological measure of how much oxygen the body uses at rest or during activity. Oxygen consumption increases in proportion to intensity of exercise/physical activity and will plateau when maximal ability for oxygen delivery is reached, which is called maximal oxygen consumption ($\dot{V}O_2$ max). Maximal oxygen consumption is directly related to aerobic capacity. Increases in maximal oxygen consumption with exercise training reflect improvement in aerobic capacity. The Fick equation describes the relationship between oxygen consumption as being equivalent to the cardiac output (heart rate × stroke volume) × arteriovenous oxygen difference, as illustrated in Figure 12-2.[28-30] Dysfunction in one or more of these physiological processes can lead to impaired aerobic capacity. This chapter will briefly discuss how these key physiological variables respond acutely during a single aerobic exercise bout, can be altered by aging or pathology, and adapt chronically to a period of aerobic exercise training.

Heart Rate

During acute aerobic exercise, there is a linear relationship between heart rate and oxygen consumption, as shown in Figure 12-3. Heart rate increases with increasing workload via two mechanisms. At less than 100 beats per minute (bpm), heart rate increases via an inhibition of vagal (parasympathetic) tone. Conversely, as the rate approaches 100 bpm, heart rate increases primarily by stimulation of sympathetic tone. Maximal heart rate is related primarily to age and is estimated by subtracting age from 220.[28-31]

There is an age-related reduction in maximal heart rate that is thought to be due to attenuation of sympathetic drive or decreases in sensitivity and responsiveness of catecholamines.[1,32] Pathological processes that reduce the rise in heart rate with activity can limit aerobic capacity. Impaired function of the autonomic nervous system will decrease heart rate response to activity. Interestingly, autonomic nervous system activity (measured by heart rate variability) decreases with increasing age, especially in frail populations.[33] Disruption of the peripheral autonomic nervous system is a common finding in older adults with diabetes (autonomic peripheral neuropathy)[34,35] and also following heart transplantation ("denervated heart").[36] Interruption of the autonomic nervous system can also occur with lesions in the central nervous system, such as a stroke or cervical spinal cord injury. Chronotropic disorders in older adults are commonly caused by heart rhythm disturbances such as atrioventricular blocks and sick sinus syndrome.[37]

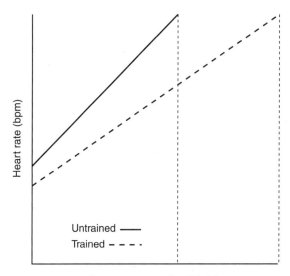

FIGURE 12-3 Heart rate (HR) response to an aerobic exercise bout and adaptation following aerobic exercise training. *bpm*, beats per minute.

With aerobic exercise training, heart rate is lower at rest and during submaximal exercise.[31,38] Heart rate at rest decreases following aerobic training because of increased parasympathetic activity while sympathetic activity declines. Exercise training results in a proportionally lower heart rate at specified submaximal workloads. Therefore, after a period of exercise training, more work can be performed at a lower heart rate. Maximal heart rate tends to be very stable within individuals and is not altered by exercise training. Following a period of aerobic training, the heart rate during recovery from exercise returns to resting levels more quickly.[28,31]

Stroke Volume

Stroke volume is the difference between the total amount of blood in the ventricles after completely filling (end-diastolic volume) and the amount of blood left behind after ventricular contraction (end-systolic volume). Stroke volume is often described clinically in terms of ejection fraction, which is stroke volume expressed as a percentage of end-diastolic volume. Stroke volume during acute aerobic exercise increases linearly up to intensities of 40% to 60% of maximal oxygen consumption and then plateaus, as illustrated in Figure 12-4. During aerobic exercise, dynamic skeletal muscle contraction and sympathetic-mediated vasoconstriction facilitate greater venous return and therefore ventricular filling. In addition, myocyte fiber stretching and sympathetic stimulation increase cardiac contractility and ventricular emptying. Both greater ventricular filling and emptying result in increased stroke volume during aerobic exercise.[28-31]

The evidence to determine whether or not stroke volume is reduced with aging is equivocal.[32] With

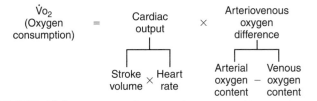

FIGURE 12-2 Parameters that contribute to aerobic capacity as described by the Fick equation.

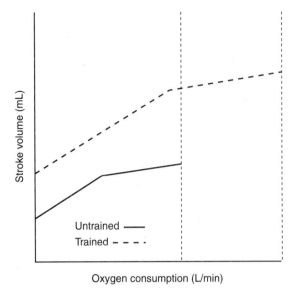

FIGURE 12-4 Stroke volume (SV) response to an aerobic exercise bout and adaptation following aerobic exercise training.

advanced age (>80 years), ejection fraction at maximal exercise does appear to decline.[1] Any pathological process that reduces ventricular filling or emptying will cause a reduction in stroke volume. With less volume of blood filling the ventricles, there is less volume available to pump out and a reduction in preload on the heart. Ventricular filling is reduced when there is a mechanical barrier present, such as cardiac valve dysfunction, heart fibrosis, or hypertrophic myopathy. All of these problems are associated with chronic heart failure, which is a major cause of disability in older adults. Ventricular filling is also impaired when venous return is reduced, commonly due to loss of active skeletal muscle pump (e.g., extremity paralysis) or impaired autonomic nervous system function (e.g., prolonged bed rest). Ventricular emptying is reduced when cardiac contractility is impaired (e.g., myocardial infarction) or the pressure that the heart has to pump against, or afterload, is elevated (e.g., hypertension). All of these cardiac problems are common in older adults and therefore often contribute to impaired aerobic capacity.

With aerobic exercise training, stroke volume increases at rest as well as during submaximal and maximal exercise. Following aerobic exercise training, ventricular filling (end-diastolic volume) increases due to an increase in plasma blood volume and also more compliant ventricular walls. In addition, ventricular emptying is greater (end-systolic volume) following aerobic exercise training. Ventricular emptying is facilitated by the greater cardiac contractility secondary to enhanced myocyte fiber stretching that occurs during ventricular filling and greater myocyte force production secondary to intrinsic changes and hypertrophy.[28-31]

Cardiac Output

At rest, cardiac output is approximately 5 L/min and with exercise can increase four- to eightfold up to approximately 20 to 40 L/min. The increase in cardiac output with increasing exercise intensity is linear, as illustrated in Figure 12-5. Increases in both stroke volume and heart rate contribute to greater cardiac output during acute aerobic exercise, because cardiac output is the product of heart rate and stroke volume. Oxygen demand is the ultimate stimulus for increasing cardiac output during exercise. With increasing skeletal muscle stimulation, more ATP is needed for cross-bridge cycling and force production. Oxygen is needed for mitochondrial oxidation to continue production of ATP. Greater cardiac output is needed to increase delivery of oxygen to the working muscles in order to meet the greater oxygen demand of heightened cellular energy metabolism.[28,31]

With aging, maximal cardiac output declines secondary to decreases in heart rate and stroke volume.[1] Any factor that diminishes heart rate or stroke volume response during activity can limit aerobic capacity. In older adults, there are a number of pathological processes that can contribute to impairments in cardiac output and therefore aerobic capacity.[39] In addition, deconditioning and bed rest can profoundly diminish cardiac output and aerobic capacity.[31]

With aerobic exercise training, cardiac output at rest and during submaximal exercise does not change significantly. Because cardiac output is directly related to metabolic demand, it remains similar under those conditions before and after exercise training. But at maximal workloads, cardiac output increases significantly following a

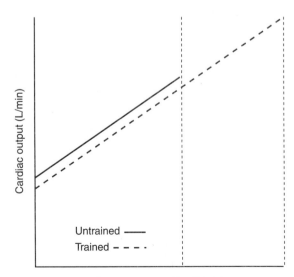

FIGURE 12-5 Cardiac output (CO) response to an aerobic exercise bout and adaptation following aerobic exercise training.

period of exercise training. This is the result of increases in stroke volume, because heart rate at maximal workloads remains relatively constant. After exercise training, metabolic work capacity (maximal oxygen consumption) is much greater primarily because of a greater cardiac output.[1,28-31]

Arterial Oxygen Content

Arterial oxygen content is determined by the oxygen-carrying capacity of the blood (hemoglobin concentration and red blood cell count) and oxygen loading in the lungs. Gas exchange at the alveolar–capillary interface is influenced by the time it takes a red blood cell to pass from one end of a capillary to the other end (transit time) and the time it takes for complete saturation of hemoglobin with oxygen in the pulmonary capillary (equilibrium time). Pulmonary capillary transit time at rest and during exercise normally exceeds equilibrium time, which allows for complete hemoglobin saturation. During aerobic exercise, transit time shortens because blood flow rate increases. The pulmonary arterioles normally vasodilate during exercise in order to accommodate the increased cardiac output and maintain adequate time for oxygen loading.[40]

Oxygen loading in the lungs is fairly well preserved during early aging but decreased oxygen saturation can be seen in the oldest-old (more than age 85 years).[1] With pathology, equilibrium time can become greater than transit time, leading to oxygen desaturation. This can be due to slowed oxygen diffusion (increased equilibrium time) or less time for oxygen loading (decreased transit time) across the alveolar–capillary interface.[41] This occurs in diseases that cause thickening of the alveolar–capillary membrane (e.g., chronic obstructive pulmonary disease) and low partial pressure of alveolar oxygen (e.g., restrictive pulmonary disease). Decreased transit time occurs when blood flow rate is elevated. This can occur when there is either inadequate vasodilation or an increase in cardiac output or both. Fast pulmonary arterial flow rates can be due to destruction of pulmonary capillaries (e.g., emphysema), a functional reduction in arterial conduits (e.g., pulmonary emboli), or increased cardiac output (e.g., renal failure).[28,41]

Aerobic exercise training does not normally change oxygen loading in the lungs, which is typically at full capacity. Some studies suggest that highly trained athletes have such a large cardiac output that oxygen saturation may drop during maximal exercise. This phenomenon has been attributed to an inability of the pulmonary vasculature to dilate enough to accommodate the increase in cardiac output resulting in a very high flow rate and decreased transit time[28,31]; however, this phenomenon is not likely to occur in most older adults or limit aerobic capacity, even in masters athletes.[1]

Venous Oxygen Content

Venous oxygen content is determined by oxygen delivery, uptake, and use in the peripheral tissues. Oxygen is required for continued regeneration of ATP through oxidative metabolism. Without adequate oxygen, energy production from glucose and fats is severely limited. When limited energy production occurs from inadequate oxygen, the energy for skeletal muscle cross-bridge cycling/muscle contraction must come primarily from anaerobic metabolism of glucose (glycolysis) and very limited use of fat as an energy substrate, leading to the rapid onset of fatigue and impaired aerobic capacity. During aerobic exercise, the lower venous oxygen content is primarily due to greater oxygen demand of the working skeletal muscle and diversion of blood to those capillaries. The other factor that reduces venous oxygen content during exercise is the shunting of blood flow away from nonmetabolically active tissues resulting in greater oxygen extraction from those capillary beds.[28,42]

Peripheral oxygen utilization with aging is often impaired by a variety of mechanisms. Pathology that interferes with blood flow, either on a macrovascular level (e.g., peripheral arterial disease) or a microvascular level (e.g., diabetes), can reduce oxygen utilization by peripheral tissues. Also, cellular changes, such as decreased myoglobin and mitochondrial density, can impair use of oxygen for energy production in skeletal muscle. Impaired aerobic capacity because of the loss of skeletal muscle oxidative capacity is common with decreased use, including deconditioning (e.g., bed rest), immobilization (e.g., extremity casting), peripheral nerve lesions (e.g., nerve entrapment syndromes), and central nervous system pathology (e.g., spinal cord injury).[42,43]

Following a period of aerobic exercise training, venous oxygen levels remain similar to levels measured at rest. At maximal exercise intensities, venous oxygen content may decrease slightly. Lower venous oxygen content with training is due to greater oxygen extraction at the tissue level and more effective distribution of cardiac output due to increased skeletal muscle capillary density. Skeletal muscle extraction and utilization of oxygen is facilitated by many adaptations such as increased skeletal muscle capillary density, mitochondrial proliferation, and increased skeletal muscle myoglobin concentrations.[42,43]

Arteriovenous Oxygen Difference

Gas exchange in the peripheral tissues is reflected in the arteriovenous oxygen difference, the difference between arterial and venous content of oxygen. Blood leaving the lungs normally has an oxygen content of 16 to 24 mL/100 mL blood and an oxygen saturation of approximately 95% to 98%. The arteriovenous oxygen difference at rest is approximately 5 mL/100 mL blood (25%). During acute aerobic exercise, oxygen extraction increases to approximately 15 to 20 mL/100 mL blood (75%-100%), as illustrated in Figure 12-6. The arteriovenous oxygen difference is greater during exercise, normally resulting from lower venous oxygen content in the presence of stable arterial oxygen content.[28-30]

With aging, sedentary people show a decline in arteriovenous oxygen difference during aerobic exercise.[42] A number of pathological processes can contribute to impairments in oxygen delivery and use (arteriovenous difference) and therefore aerobic capacity.[39] In addition, deconditioning and bed rest can profoundly diminish oxygen use in skeletal muscle and therefore aerobic capacity.[42,43]

Following a period of aerobic exercise training, the arteriovenous oxygen difference remains similar at rest. At maximal exercise intensities, the arteriovenous oxygen difference may increase slightly. This increase in arteriovenous oxygen difference is the result of lower venous oxygen content without a change in arterial oxygen content. Interestingly, older women show an increase in arteriovenous difference during exercise after aerobic training but older men do not.[44]

PHYSICAL THERAPY EXAMINATION

History

A comprehensive history of a patient with impaired aerobic capacity helps to elucidate contributory factors and to determine appropriate interventions. In addition, it is important to identify risk factors for cardiovascular disease and appropriate interventions based on risk and patient setting. Screening for cardiovascular risk factors,

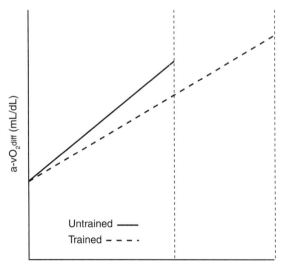

FIGURE 12-6 Arteriovenous oxygen difference (a-vO$_2$diff) response to an aerobic exercise bout and adaptation following aerobic exercise training.

defined in Table 12-1, serves many purposes, including determining need for referrals to other professionals, selecting specific tests and measures, establishing the prognosis, and developing a plan of care.[13] History and screening determine if a patient has experienced any signs or symptoms highly suggestive of significant cardiovascular or pulmonary disease. These signs and symptoms include shortness of breath at rest or with mild exertion, pain, discomfort (or other anginal equivalent) in the chest, neck, jaw, arms, or other areas that may result from cardiac ischemia, orthopnea, paroxysmal nocturnal dyspnea, bilateral ankle edema, palpitations, tachycardia, intermittent leg claudication, known heart murmur, and undue fatigue with usual activities.[13]

Systems Review

The examination of a patient with impaired aerobic capacity should include a systems review of the anatomic and physiological status of the four primary Practice Pattern systems, in addition to communication ability, affect, cognition, language, and learning style.[14] With aerobic capacity impairment, screening of the integumentary, musculoskeletal, and neuromuscular systems provides invaluable information for patient evaluation, diagnosis, prognosis, and intervention planning. Assessment of heart rate, respiratory rate, blood pressure, and edema is recommended for cardiovascular and pulmonary system screening. Integumentary system screening includes assessment of skin integrity, skin color, and presence of scar. Musculoskeletal system screening includes assessment of body symmetry, joint range of motion, muscle strength, height, and weight. Neuromuscular system screening includes assessment of balance, locomotion, transfers, and motor control.[14]

Tests and Measures

Signs and Symptoms in Response to Increased Oxygen Demand. Assessment of a patient's cardiovascular and pulmonary response to functional activity/aerobic exercise can provide important information about any aerobic capacity impairments, and factors contributing to it. Baseline measurement of resting vital signs, including heart rate, blood pressure, respiratory rate, and oxygen saturation provides valuable information regarding the patient's physiological state. Measuring these vital signs during aerobic exercise and comparing them to the patient's resting values can be used to evaluate aerobic capacity. As discussed in the first part of this chapter, aerobic exercise or activity stresses the oxygen delivery system and produces predictable changes in vital signs. Heart rate should increase proportionately to the metabolic demand placed on the body. Systolic blood pressure reflects cardiac output and therefore should also go up in proportion to the metabolic demand of the

TABLE 12-1	Cardiovascular Disease Risk Factors
Positive Risk Factors	**Defining Criteria**
Age	Men ages 45 years or older; women ages 55 years or older
Family history	Myocardial infarction, coronary revascularization, or sudden death before age 55 years in father or other male first-degree relative, or before age 65 years in mother or other female first-degree relative
Cigarette smoking	Current cigarette smoker or those who quit within the previous 6 months or exposure to environmental tobacco smoke
Sedentary lifestyle	Not participating in at least 30 minutes of moderate intensity (40% to 60% VO_2R) physical activity on at least 3 days of the week for at least 3 months
Obesity*	Body mass index $\geq$30 kg/m² *or* waist girth >102 cm (40 in.) for men and >88 cm (35 in.) for women
Hypertension	Systolic blood pressure (BP) $\geq$140 mmHg and/or diastolic BP $\geq$90 mmHg, confirmed by measurements on at least two separate occasions, *or* on antihypertensive medication
Dyslipidemia	Low-density lipoprotein (LDL-C) cholesterol $\geq$130 mg/dL (3.37 mmol/L) *or* high-density lipoprotein (HDL-C) cholesterol <40 mg/dL (1.04 mmol/L) *or* on lipid-lowering medication. If total serum cholesterol is all that is available, use $\geq$200 mg/dL (5.18 mmol/L)
Prediabetes	Impaired fasting glucose (IFG) = fasting plasma glucose $\geq$100 mg/dL (5.50 mmol/L) but <126 mg/dL (6.93 mmol/L) *or* impaired glucose tolerance (IGT) = 2-hour values in oral glucose tolerance test (OGTT) $\geq$140 mg/dL (7.70 mmol/L) but <200 mg/dL (11.00 mmol/L) confirmed by measurements on at least two separate occasions
Negative Risk Factors	**Defining Criteria**
High serum HDL cholesterol[†]	$\geq$60 mg/dL (1.55 mmol/L)

*Professional opinions vary regarding the most appropriate markers and thresholds for obesity; therefore, allied health professionals should use clinical judgment when evaluating this risk factor.
[†]Note: It is common to sum risk factors in making clinical judgments. If HDL is high, subtract one risk factor from the sum of positive risk factors, because high HDL decreases CVD risk.
(Adapted from Thompson WR, Gordon NF, Pescatello LS, editors: ACSM's guidelines for exercise testing and prescription. Philadelphia, PA, 2010, Wolters Kluwer/Lippincott Williams & Wilkins.)

exercise or activity. Diastolic blood pressure reflects total peripheral resistance, which remains relatively stable in most people during aerobic exercise. Respiratory rate increases with mild- to moderate-intensity aerobic exercise and then plateaus as exercise intensity continues to increase. Oxygen saturation should remain stable with aerobic exercise because arterial oxygen content should not change under normal conditions.

Patient symptoms can also be used to assess aerobic capacity. Onset of symptoms such as fatigue, shortness of breath, and weakness during exercise are often too ubiquitous and nonspecific to provide clinically useful information. However, several established symptom scales can be used to objectively ascertain patient symptoms such as dyspnea, angina, claudication, and perceived exertion (Box 12-2). In addition, assessment of pain can help to differentiate among competing hypotheses about the genesis of an activity limitation that might also be due to impaired aerobic capacity. Patient symptoms during aerobic exercise can also provide information regarding central perfusion (e.g., syncope, light-headedness, or change in mental status) and peripheral perfusion (e.g., extremity tingling, numbness, or coldness).

6-Minute Walk Test. Walk tests are commonly used clinically to measure aerobic capacity in older adults. Walk tests provide information about patient

endurance/aerobic capacity and functional activities that require household and community ambulation. Cooper originally described a 12-minute run test in 1968, which was subsequently modified to a 12-minute walk test and then to both 2- and 6-minute walk tests.[45,46] Walk tests are very inexpensive to administer because they require minimal equipment, facility space, expertise, and time. They can be used for a wide variety of patients and practice settings.[47-52] Walk tests are particularly useful for patients that require use of an assistive device for ambulation or that have very low exercise tolerance. In addition, walk tests pose very little risk to patients because the exercise intensity is completely controlled by the patient and rest intervals can be taken as necessary. Distance is the primary outcome measured with walk tests. Patients are instructed to walk as far as possible in the designated amount of time (2, 6, or 12 minutes) on an established, standardized pathway. It is important that the patients' self-selected walking speed not be altered by obstacles or traffic in the pathway, others walking alongside them, or the therapist guarding/assisting.[53,54] Standardization of walk test procedures is crucial for optimal reliability, sensitivity, and interpretation of results. It is important to provide consistent verbal encouragement during walk tests, choosing either no feedback or similar verbal phrases at each administration. Guyatt et al[55] found that verbal encouragement during a 6-minute

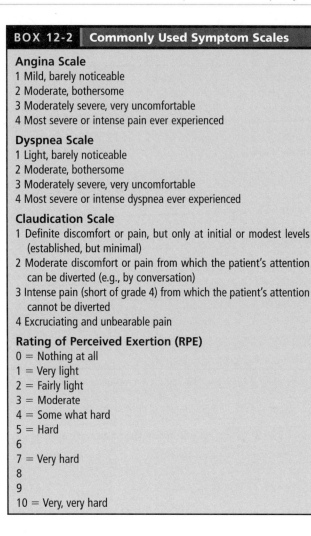

BOX 12-2 | Commonly Used Symptom Scales

Angina Scale
1 Mild, barely noticeable
2 Moderate, bothersome
3 Moderately severe, very uncomfortable
4 Most severe or intense pain ever experienced

Dyspnea Scale
1 Light, barely noticeable
2 Moderate, bothersome
3 Moderately severe, very uncomfortable
4 Most severe or intense dyspnea ever experienced

Claudication Scale
1 Definite discomfort or pain, but only at initial or modest levels (established, but minimal)
2 Moderate discomfort or pain from which the patient's attention can be diverted (e.g., by conversation)
3 Intense pain (short of grade 4) from which the patient's attention cannot be diverted
4 Excruciating and unbearable pain

Rating of Perceived Exertion (RPE)
0 = Nothing at all
1 = Very light
2 = Fairly light
3 = Moderate
4 = Some what hard
5 = Hard
6
7 = Very hard
8
9
10 = Very, very hard

walk test improved performance and increased within-person variability in patients with chronic airflow limitation and heart failure. Although multiple trials of a walk test are ideal to minimize the effects of learning,[54,56-59] this is often not feasible in a clinical setting, especially with older patients who have low aerobic capacity. Finally, the length and shape of the walking course influences distance covered on a walk; therefore, it is important to standardize the walking course for comparison of repeated measurements (i.e., initial and discharge tests). Shorter courses produce shorter walk test distances than longer courses, and linear courses produce shorter walk test distance than circular and rectangular courses.[53]

Walk test distance can be evaluated by comparing the patient's distance to reference values. When used as an outcome measure, change in walk test distance reflects change in aerobic capacity with intervention. Gibbons et al[60] reported 6-minute walk test distances for multiple repetitions in healthy subjects between the ages of 20 and 80 years. Their normative data for subjects between ages 60 and 80 years were 688.8 ± 89.3 m for men and 584 ± 53 m for women. Lusardi et al[61] identified normative distances for community-dwelling older adults when completing the 6-minute walk test once under typical clinical conditions, including use of an assistive device as needed.[61] She found that 60- to 69-year-old subjects (men and women combined) walked 420.4 m ± 105.4 m during the 6-minute walk test and 80- to 89-year-olds walked 292.1 ± 112.7 m. Steffen et al[62] evaluated community-dwelling older adults but eliminated subjects requiring use of assistive devices. She obtained scores more similar to Gibbons's for 60- to 69-year-olds (572 ± 92 m for males; 538 ± 92 m for females), and for 80- to 89-year-olds (417 ± 73 m for males; 392 ± 85 m for females).

Graded Exercise Testing. Graded exercise testing can be used to assess aerobic capacity objectively and has been used extensively in the past but is not as widely used now because of its time/cost burden and indirect relationship to functional ability. Briefly, graded exercise testing can be used to (1) diagnose cardiovascular and/or pulmonary disease, (2) determine disease severity/risk stratification, (3) evaluate functional ability, (4) establish baseline for exercise prescription or disease progress, and (5) evaluate intervention effectiveness. Data collection during graded exercise testing often includes measurement of heart rate, electrocardiographic (ECG) information, oxygen saturation, blood pressure, rating of perceived exertion (RPE), and signs and symptoms. Graded exercise test modes include treadmill walking/running, leg cycle ergometry, arm cycle ergometry, and stair stepping. Recently, Mendelsohn et al[63] described the validity of a graded exercise test as good to excellent using reciprocal upper and lower body forward and backward exercise using a NuStep in frail older adults. Graded exercise tests most often employ continuous protocols consisting of progressive preset stages of increasing work intensities with no rest intervals. Graded exercise tests can be submaximal (i.e., stopped at a preset exercise intensity), symptom limited (i.e., stopped when a specified contraindication presents), or maximal (i.e., patient exercises to volitional exhaustion). Outcomes of a graded exercise test include oxygen consumption, heart rate, RPE, and sign/symptom threshold. Oxygen consumption can be directly measured if metabolic instrumentation is available, but more commonly it is estimated using established equations.[13]

Graded exercise testing may be administered by a physical therapist in some circumstances, such as when trying to determine whether a patient's maximal aerobic capacity is limiting function. For example, when a patient wants to return to a specific occupational or recreational activity, it is often important to determine if the associated aerobic demands are safe. Graded exercise testing may also be used to determine symptom threshold. For example, in patients with claudication, treadmill walking at a specific speed and grade frequently will provoke leg pain. Graded exercise testing can also be used when a walk test is not feasible. For example, in patients with lower extremity paralysis testing with an upper body ergometer is most feasible.

Self-Report Measures. Self-report assessment measures can be useful in reflecting the functional impact of impaired aerobic capacity on physical activity level, participation, and health-related quality of life in older adults. Self-report assessments require patients to answer questions and rate statements regarding subjective perception of their functional ability. Self-report instruments are ideal for measuring patient perception of constructs, such as pain, difficulty, and depression, especially in home and community environments in addition to clinical settings. Functional ability is often measured using generic, self-report quality of life instruments. A primary disadvantage of generic health-related self-report instruments is they may not be as sensitive to change as disease-specific health-related self-report instruments.[64-66]

Generic health-related quality of life instruments, such as the Medical Outcomes Study Short Form 36 Health Survey (SF-36) or RAND 36-Items Health Survey, are commonly used in older adults. These instruments have been used extensively to study health-related quality of life in patients with impaired aerobic capacity secondary to cardiopulmonary problems since they have well-documented degrees of reliability, validity, and sensitivity.[64,67-69] Ten of the twelve items of the Physical Function subscale of this instrument reflect aerobic capacity (Table 12-2). To improve time efficiency and reduce response burden, this subscale can be used independent from the entire instrument.

Disease-specific self-report instruments also reflect patient aerobic capacity and often are more sensitive to change than generic self-report instruments. But many of the cardiovascular and pulmonary self-report instruments available rely on concurrent symptoms such as angina (Seattle Angina Questionnaire), dyspnea (Minnesota Living with Heart Failure Questionnaire, Kansas City Cardiomyopathy Questionnaire), or pain (Heart Surgery Symptom Inventory), which limits their use to specific populations of older patients.[70-73] The Duke Activity Status Index[74] is a self-report measure of aerobic capacity as it relates to functional activities. Although the Duke Activity Status Index is a disease-specific instrument, it was developed for patients with cardiovascular disease, which is very prevalent in older adults, affecting 73% of those between the ages of 60 and 79 years. The Duke Activity Status Index measures functional capacity using 12 questions regarding the ability to perform specific tasks. The questions are answered on a nominal scale (yes/no) and scores are weighted relative to the metabolic demand of the task (Table 12-3). The summary score generated from the Duke Activity Status Index reflects an estimation of the patient's maximal oxygen consumption; therefore, higher scores indicate better aerobic capacity than lower scores with a maximal possible score of 65.7.[75,76] The Duke Activity Status Index has been used in numerous populations of older patients to quantify aerobic capacity.[77-79]

The Physical Activity Scale for the Elderly (PASE) is a 10-item self-report questionnaire designed to assess leisure, household, and occupational activity in adults. This instrument measures physical activity participation involving tasks beyond activities of daily living. The PASE has been used to assess activity level in a variety of study designs ranging from retrospective to epidemiologic, and patient populations with chronic heart failure, pulmonary disease, and coronary heart disease.[80-82] In a study with 277 subjects, the PASE test–retest reliability coefficient was 0.75.[80] The PASE validity was examined

TABLE 12-2	Items in the Physical Function Subscale of the RAND-36 Item Health Survey and the SF-36		
The following items are about activities you might do during a typical day. Does your health now limit you in these activities? If so, how?			
	(Circle One Number on Each Line)		
	Yes, limited a lot	Yes, limited a little	No, not limited at all
3. Vigorous activities, such as running, lifting heavy objects, participating in strenuous sports	1	2	3
4. Moderate activities, such as moving a table, pushing a vacuum cleaner, bowling, or playing golf	1	2	3
5. Lifting or carrying groceries	1	2	3
6. Climbing several flights of stairs	1	2	3
7. Climbing one flight of stairs	1	2	3
8. Bending, kneeling, or stooping	1	2	3
9. Walking more than a mile	1	2	3
10. Walking several blocks	1	2	3
11. Walking one block	1	2	3
12. Bathing or dressing yourself	1	2	3

(From Hays RD, Sherbourne CD, Mazel RM: The RAND-36-Item health survey 1.0. Health Econ 2:217-227, 1993.)

TABLE 12-3	Duke Activity Status Index
Can you...	**Weighted score**
1. take care of yourself, that is, eating, dressing, bathing, or using the toilet?	2.75
2. walk indoors, such as around your house?	1.75
3. walk a block or two on level ground?	2.75
4. climb a flight of stairs or walk up a hill?	5.50
5. run a short distance?	8.00
6. do light work around the house, such as dusting or washing dishes?	2.70
7. do moderate work around the house, such as vacuuming, sweeping floors, or carrying groceries?	3.50
8. do heavy work around the house, such as scrubbing floors, or lifting or moving heavy furniture?	8.00
9. do yard work, such as raking leaves, weeding, or pushing a power mower?	4.50
10. have sexual relations?	5.25
11. participate in moderate-intensity recreational activities, such as golf, bowling, dancing, doubles tennis, or throwing a baseball or football?	6.00
12. participate in strenuous sports, such as swimming, single tennis, football, basketball, or skiing?	7.50
	Total

(Modified from Hlatky MA, Boineau RE, Higginbotham MB, et al: A brief self-administered questionnaire to determine functional capacity (The Duke Activity Status Index). Am J Cardiol 64:651-654, 1989.)

by comparison with accelerometry data ($r = 0.49$). The PASE was significantly correlated with strength, resting heart rate, systolic blood pressure, peak oxygen uptake, and quality of life ($P < 0.05$, $r = |0.13 – 0.42|$).[80] Although the PASE does not directly measure aerobic capacity, the level of daily physical activity parameters associated with aerobic capacity are directly related.

EVALUATION, DIAGNOSIS, AND PROGNOSIS

The evaluation, diagnosis, and prognosis of older adults with aerobic capacity impairment require integration of oxygen uptake, transport, delivery and utilization systems knowledge, physical therapy management strategies, and patient history and examination findings. Evaluation of older adults with aerobic capacity impairment should include screening for referral, identification of contributing pathologies with concomitant impairments, activity limitations, participation restrictions and disability, and differential diagnosis of cause(s). Lastly, anticipated prognosis related to improvement in aerobic capacity and the expected outcomes of remediating poor aerobic capacity should be determined.

Decisions to Refer

Evaluation of the older patient with an aerobic capacity impairment first requires that the physical therapist identify any history, signs, or symptoms suggestive of major medical issues that are undiagnosed or poorly managed. For example, if an older patient is referred to physical therapy with a diagnosis of bilateral knee osteoarthritis, but other examination findings highly suggest peripheral arterial disease

(skin atrophic changes, absent dorsal pedal and posterior tibial pulses, onset of calf pain with walking and relief with rest, etc.), it would be appropriate to refer the patient for medical follow-up. Also consider an older patient with known hypertension being treated with antihypertensive medication who presents to physical therapy with a blood pressure of 212/116 mmHg. This patient should be referred back to the physician before beginning physical therapy intervention that involves exercise or substantial physical activity. Next, screening for cardiovascular disease risk is completed by utilizing information obtained in the patient examination, including history of known disease, signs and symptoms, and presence of risk factors. This information can then be used to determine appropriate referral to a physician, if it has not already taken place (i.e., Direct-access), exercise testing, and exercise intervention. Physical therapists often detect currently undiagnosed abnormalities in the cardiovascular and pulmonary systems in older adults because assessment involves physical activity. Lastly, the presence of contraindications for exercise participation and indications for stopping exercise should be determined, as outlined in Box 12-3.[13]

Evaluation of Vital Signs

Evaluation of the patient's vital signs at rest can provide insight on factors contributing to aerobic impairment based on the oxygen delivery model. Resting bradycardia in older adults is most often due to medications (i.e., β-blockers) or a cardiac dysrhythmia such as atrioventricular block or sick sinus syndrome.[37] Resting tachycardia in older adults may be due to hypotension, atrial

BOX 12-3	Aerobic Exercise Contraindications and Stopping Points

Absolute Exercise Contraindications
- Unstable angina
- Uncontrolled cardiac dysrhythmias causing symptoms of hemodynamic compromise
- Uncontrolled symptomatic heart failure
- Acute or suspected major cardiovascular event (including severe aortic stenosis, pulmonary embolus or infarction, myocarditis, pericarditis, or dissecting aneurysm)
- Acute systemic infection, accompanied by fever, body aches, or swollen lymph glands
- A recent significant change in resting ECG suggestive of ischemia, myocardial infarction, or other acute cardiac event*

Relative† Exercise Contraindications
- Known significant cardiac disease (including left main coronary stenosis, moderate stenotic valvular disease, hypertrophic cardiomyopathy, high-degree atrioventricular block,* ventricular aneurysm)
- Severe arterial hypertension (systolic BP of >200 mmHg or a diastolic BP of >110 mmHg) at rest
- Tachydysrhythmia or bradydysrhythmia*
- Electrolyte abnormalities
- Uncontrolled metabolic disease
- Chronic infectious disease
- Mental or physical impairment leading to inability to exercise safely

Absolute Indications for Terminating Exercise
- Drop in systolic BP of >10 mmHg from baseline despite an increase in workload when accompanied by other evidence of ischemia
- Moderately severe angina (>2/4)
- Increasing nervous system symptoms
- Signs of poor perfusion
- Subject's desire to stop
- Technical difficulty with monitoring equipment
- Sustained ventricular tachycardia*
- ST elevation (+1.0 mm) in leads without diagnostic Q-waves*

Relative Indications for Terminating Exercise
- Drop in systolic BP of >10 mmHg from baseline despite an increase in workload in the absence of other evidence of ischemia
- Increasing chest pain
- Hypertensive response (systolic BP of >250 mmHg or diastolic BP of > 115 mmHg)
- Fatigue, shortness of breath/wheezing, leg cramps, or claudication
- ST or QRS changes such as excessive ST depression (>2 mm ST-segment depression)*
- Arrhythmias other than sustained ventricular tachycardia (including multifocal premature ventricular contractions (PVCs), triplets of PVCs, supraventricular tachycardia, heart blocks, or bradyarrhythmias)*
- Development of bundle-branch block or intraventricular conduction delay that cannot be distinguished from ventricular tachycardia*

*Assume that ECG monitoring is available.
†Relative contraindications can be superseded if there are benefits.
(Adapted from Thompson WR, Gordon NF, Pescatello LS, editors: ACSM's guidelines for exercise testing and prescription. Philadelphia, PA, 2010, Wolters Kluwer/ Lippincott Williams & Wilkins.)

fibrillation or flutter, cardiac autonomic disruption, or ventricular tachycardia. Systolic hypertension at rest in older adults is most often due to uncontrolled essential hypertension.[74] Systolic hypotension at rest occurs when cardiac output is low, such as with orthostatic hypotension, atrial fibrillation/flutter, heart failure, or volume depletion/dehydration. Oxygen desaturation at rest occurs when there is impaired oxygen diffusion between the alveolar capillary membrane. This phenomenon can occur when diffusion is slowed as a result of low oxygen concentrations in the alveoli or thickening of the interface. In addition, oxygen desaturation can also occur when blood flow through the pulmonary capillaries is increased, reducing time for oxygen exchange. Normal vital sign ranges at rest and implications are summarized in Table 12-4.

Vital sign response during aerobic activity can help to elucidate causes of aerobic capacity impairment. When physiological response to aerobic exercise is abnormal, the underlying cause of impaired oxygen delivery may be determined. Both a decrease in or a failure to increase heart rate or systolic blood pressure with exercise suggest that the heart is unable to respond to increased oxygen demand. A rise in diastolic blood pressure during aerobic exercise may indicate coronary artery disease and poses a dangerous threat to patient safety because it reduces coronary perfusion. Oxygen desaturation during exercise in older adults often occurs when increased pulmonary capillary flow reduces time for oxygen uptake in the presence of impaired diffusion. Oxygen desaturation during aerobic exercise does not reflect increased oxygen demand in the peripheral tissues, that is, skeletal muscles.

TABLE 12-4	Summary of Vital Sign Interpretation	
Vital Sign	**Normal Range (resting)**	**Implications**

Heart rate	60-100 bpm	<60 bpm →
		    no action if asymptomatic and normal ECG
		    refer to physician if symptomatic
		    refer to physician if no ECG available and there is no history of dys-
		        rhythmia or chronotropic medication use
		120-150 bpm →
		    precaution to initiating activity/exercise
		    refer to physician
		>150 bpm →
		    contraindication to initiating activity/exercise
		    refer to physician immediately
		With exercise/activity →
		    increases in proportion to workload
		    significant drop is an indication to stop exercise

dBP	70-90 mmHg	<70 mmHg →
		    no action if asymptomatic
		    refer to physician if symptomatic
		>115 mmHg →
		    contraindication to initiating activity/exercise
		    refer to physician
		With exercise/activity →
		    remains similar to resting or may drop slightly
		    increase >115 is an indication to stop exercise

sBP	100-140 mmHg	<100 mmHg →
		    no action if asymptomatic
		    refer to physician if symptomatic
		>200 mmHg →
		    contraindication to initiating activity/exercise
		    refer to physician
		With exercise/activity →
		    increases in proportion to workload
		    >250 mmHg is an indication to stop exercise

SpO_2	≥90%	86%-89% →
		    consider adding or increasing supplemental oxygen
		    refer to physician if previously undiagnosed
		≤85% →
		    add or increase supplemental oxygen
		    contraindication to initiating activity/exercise
		    refer to physician if remains <90%
		With exercise/activity →
		    should remain ≥90%
		    86%-89% relative indication to stop exercise
		    ≤85% absolute indication to stop exercise

Oxygen Consumption, Saturation and Energy Expenditure

In most adults, including older adults, maximal cardiac output is the physiological variable that limits maximal oxygen consumption and therefore aerobic capacity. During maximal aerobic exercise, the capacity for increasing ventilation is much greater than the capacity for increasing cardiac output.[28,31] Also there is a strong correlation between cardiac output and aerobic capacity measured by maximal oxygen consumption. Even during maximal exercise of older adults, oxygen saturation is maintained higher than 90%, suggesting no limitation in pulmonary gas exchange. But when pathology affects oxygen loading across the alveolar–capillary interface, exercise may cause oxygen desaturation and therefore be a limiting factor in maximal aerobic capacity. Limitations in skeletal muscle oxygen extraction/utilization are not thought to normally limit aerobic capacity but can be regarded as contributory factors. Sometimes a patient's apparent impaired aerobic capacity is not limited at all by oxygen delivery and utilization but rather by an adverse symptom such as pain or fear of falling.[83]

Sometimes older patients may present with what appears initially to be an impairment in aerobic capacity, but is actually a high energy expenditure for physical activity. One common clinical example of high energy expenditure during physical activity is the increased metabolic demand during movement associated with obesity. Another cause of high energy expenditure during activity, particularly walking, is decreased movement economy (i.e., greater oxygen consumption than normal is required for a particular workload). Reduced economy can occur whenever movement coordination is altered, for example, with hemiparesis or lower extremity amputation. Although aerobic capacity may not be significantly impaired under these conditions, older patients are performing functional activities at a higher percentage of their maximal aerobic capacity that can contribute to onset of fatigue.

Diagnostic Classification

The *Guide to Physical Therapist Practice* classifications used most often for patients with impaired aerobic capacity are the Cardiovascular/Pulmonary Preferred Practice Patterns. Pattern B: Impaired Aerobic Capacity/Endurance Associated with Deconditioning may include the following exam findings: decreased endurance, increased cardiovascular or pulmonary response to low-level workloads, increased perceived exertion with functional activities, and inability to perform routine work tasks as a result of shortness of breath. Pathologies that may be included under this practice pattern are acquired immune deficiency syndrome, cancer, cardiovascular disorders, chronic system failure, musculoskeletal disorders, neuromuscular disorders, and pulmonary disorders. Some of the anticipated outcomes of physical therapy intervention for older adults with impaired aerobic capacity include the following: (1) symptoms associated with increased oxygen demand are decreased; (2) tissue perfusion and oxygenation are enhanced; (3) endurance is increased; (4) energy expenditure per unit of work is decreased; (5) ability to perform physical tasks is improved; and (6) ability to resume roles in self-care, home management, work, community, and leisure is improved. Improvements in risk reduction/prevention and health status are anticipated outcomes for older patients with impaired aerobic capacity as well.[14]

Factors Affecting Prognosis

The prognosis for improving aerobic capacity in older adults is multifactorial and depends on the patient's prior level of physical inactivity, degree of pathology affecting the oxygen transport system, and activity restrictions that impede habitual activity level and participation in aerobic exercise. Factors that influence prognosis of a patient with impaired aerobic capacity are listed in Box 12-4. The physiological adaptations that occur

BOX 12-4	Factors That Influence Prognosis of a Patient with Impaired Aerobic Capacity

- Accessibility and availability of resources
- Adherence to the intervention program
- Age
- Anatomic and physiological changes related to growth and development
- Caregiver consistency or expertise
- Chronicity or severity of the current condition
- Cognitive status
- Comorbidities, complications, or secondary impairments
- Concurrent medical, surgical, and therapeutic interventions
- Decline in functional independence
- Level of impairment
- Level of physical function
- Living environment
- Multisite or multisystem involvement
- Nutritional status
- Overall health status
- Potential discharge destinations
- Premorbid conditions
- Probability of prolonged impairment, functional limitation, or disability
- Psychological and socioeconomic factors
- Psychomotor abilities
- Social support
- Stability of the condition

(*Data from American Physical Therapy Association: Guide to physical therapist practice, ed 2. Phys Ther, 81:9-744, 2001.*)

secondary to inactivity/bed rest and increased habitual activity level have a dose-response effect. The greater the change in activity level, the greater the degree of physiological adaptation that will occur. Consider the example of an older patient with New York Heart Association class III heart failure (dyspnea with ordinary activities). A prognosis for moderate improvement in aerobic capacity sufficient to increase household ambulation distances would be reasonable for this patient. In contrast, a reasonable prognosis for improvement in aerobic capacity for an older adult who was previously healthy but now diagnosed with pneumonia severe enough to require hospitalization and ventilatory support (e.g., bilevel positive-airway pressure) for 6 days, would be full return to previous activities.

PLAN OF CARE INTERVENTIONS

Therapeutic exercise, functional training, and prescription of assistive, adaptive, or supportive devices are the most frequently used interventions to improve aerobic capacity in older adults with aerobic capacity limitations. Other types of procedural interventions are appropriate when they address secondary issues that may be limiting aerobic capacity or ability to participate in therapeutic exercise or functional training. For example, use of airway clearance techniques would be appropriate to improve oxygen loading and therefore aerobic capacity for patients with pulmonary mucus retention.

Exercise

Therapeutic exercise is the cornerstone for treating older patients with impaired aerobic capacity. When prescribing exercise for older adults to improve aerobic capacity, the general principles of exercise should be considered. The overload principle of exercise training states that increases in habitual aerobic workload above that normally experienced will cause adaptations that improve maximal aerobic capacity. Conversely, the reversibility principle of training indicates that restrictions in habitual aerobic workload below that normally experienced will cause adaptations that impair maximal aerobic capacity. The greatest degree of improvement in aerobic capacity will occur during activities that are most similar to the training stimulus/activity (aka specificity of training). Conversely, some degree of improvement in aerobic capacity will occur even during activities that are dissimilar to the training stimulus/activity (aka generality of training principle).[13]

Traditionally, the four components of an aerobic exercise prescription are mode, intensity, duration, and frequency. The greatest improvements in aerobic capacity occur when the *mode* of exercise involves the use of large muscle groups contracting rhythmically over prolonged periods of time. Aerobic exercise modes can be categorized into weight-bearing (high- and low-impact) and non–weight-bearing activities. Examples of aerobic exercise modes in each category are provided in Box 12-5. When selecting a mode of aerobic exercise for a patient, physical therapists should also consider risk of injury, likelihood of adherence, and unique vocational/recreational objectives. It is important to select a mode of exercise that is not too metabolically demanding so that it can be continued for a period of time long enough to stimulate aerobic adaptation.

Aerobic exercise *intensity* can be based on heart rate (10 to 20 bpm below onset of adverse signs or symptoms or 60% to 90% of maximal heart rate) or on the individual's RPE (4 to 6 on a 10-point scale; or 12 to 16 on a 19-point scale).[13,14,84] Maximal heart rate (HR_{max}) can be predicted from age or determined by maximal graded exercise test. The most commonly used equation to predict maximal heart rate is the Karvonen, $HR_{max} = 220 - age$, but some studies have suggested that this overestimates in adults older than age 40 years and underestimates in adults age 40 years and younger.[13,85,86] As an alternative, maximal heart rate can be calculated using a formula developed by Gellish et al, $HR_{max} = 206.9 - (0.67 \times age)$.[13,87] Exercise intensity has also been defined qualitatively as moderate (physical activity that noticeably increases breathing, sweating, and heart rate) or vigorous (physical activity that substantially increases breathing, sweating, and heart rate).[88]

Aerobic exercise *duration* equal to 20 to 60 minutes of continuous activity is generally recommended for disease risk reduction. However, discontinuous activity can be used in very deconditioned patients when initiating aerobic exercise. Patients with functional capacities of less than 3 to 5 metabolic equivalents (METs) benefit from multiple (i.e., 2 to 4 times per day) and short (i.e., total sum of 20 to 30 minutes) exercise sessions. Recommended aerobic exercise *frequency* is "on most days," but even exercising with limited frequency is better than no exercise at all.[13,88] It is important to note that these recommended thresholds for aerobic exercise are based on epidemiologic evidence for obtaining health benefits.

Newer physical activity guidelines intertwine aspects of intensity, duration, and frequency. The *Physical Activity Guidelines for Americans* recommend that older adults participate in 150 minutes a week of moderate-intensity or 75 minutes a week of vigorous-intensity aerobic exercise.[88,89] Furthermore, aerobic exercise should preferably be performed in episodes of at least 10 minutes and spread throughout the week. It is also acknowledged that additional health benefits are provided by greater amounts of aerobic activity.[88,89] Moderate-intensity exercise is defined as increases in energy expenditure by 3.0 to 5.9 times more than the energy expended at rest (aka METs) or a perceived exertion of 5 to 6 of 10. Vigorous-intensity exercise is defined as increases in energy expenditure by 6.0 or greater times more than the energy expended at rest (METs) or a perceived exertion of 7 to 8 of 10.[88,89]

BOX 12-5	**Example Modes of Aerobic Exercise**	
Weight-Bearing, High Impact	**Weight-Bearing, Low Impact**	**Non–Weight-Bearing, Nonimpact**
Jogging	Walking	Swimming
Aerobic dancing (with jumping)	Leg cycle ergometry	Pool "cycling"/ "kicking"
Stepping (remove feet)	Aerobic dancing (without jumping)	Arm cycle ergometry
Jumping rope	Stepping (stationary feet)	Rowing
Calisthenics	Cross-country skiing	Chair aerobics
	Pool aerobics/walking	

Progression of aerobic exercise in older patients should be individualized and based on the patient's anticipated goals and expected outcomes. Often the initial phase of an aerobic exercise program progression is aimed at attaining the minimum intensity, duration, and frequency for a specific mode of exercise. The improvement phase of an aerobic exercise program progression utilizes a combination of adjustments in mode, intensity, duration, or frequency of exercise to reach a specific exercise capacity goal. For example, often to reach functional milestones, such as walking 150 feet without rest, it is more important to increase the duration rather than the intensity of aerobic capacity training. The exercise prescription parameters that optimally increase aerobic capacity have not been fully elucidated and most likely vary with patient characteristics. For example, Sisson et al[90] found that the volume of aerobic exercise was the most important predictor of improved aerobic capacity in sedentary, postmenopausal women. In addition, Bocalini et al[38] found greater improvement in aerobic capacity in older women participating in water-based versus land-based programs. Whereas both low- and high-intensity aerobic exercise training lowered systolic blood pressure in older adults, only high-intensity exercise training reduced weight and improved lipid profile.[91] Interestingly, Kruger et al[92] reported that often the prescribed dose of aerobic exercise used in research trials was lower than what is currently recommended.

The maintenance phase of an aerobic exercise program involves indefinite continuation of a specified exercise mode, intensity, duration, and frequency to preserve the existing aerobic exercise capacity. Many factors, such as lack of time, fear of injury, or level of importance placed on exercise may influence older patients' ability to engage in continued exercise.[93,94] Some studies suggest that older adults actually have greater self-efficacy (confidence) for symptom management, exercise participation, and physical activity than younger adults.[83,95] It is possible that age brings experience in coping with health problems, and in turn, these coping skills better prepare older adults to engage in physical activity. Over time, older adults may acquire self-management skills for exercise participation despite experiencing symptoms related to chronic conditions.[96,97]

Physical Activity

Another strategy for improving aerobic capacity and health is to increase total energy expended during daily physical activity. Physical activity includes both structured exercise and nonstructured lifestyle activities (physical activity not performed with the intention to constitute a structured period of exercise). Use of pedometers to promote increased physical activity through walking has gained popularity because they are inexpensive and easy to use. Research studies have supported the efficacy of using pedometers to increase physical activity and decrease body mass index and systolic blood pressure. Interestingly, this decrease in body mass index was associated with older age and having an identified step goal.[98] In addition, evidence suggests that there is an inverse relationship between body weight and physical activity. However, there is also a dose-response effect of physical activity on weight, with higher doses capable of providing greater weight loss. Guidelines for prevention of weight gain are 150 to 250 minutes per week of moderately vigorous physical activity with an energy equivalent of approximately 1200 to 2000 kcal/week.[99]

Functional Training

Functional training and physical activity can also be used for older patients with impaired aerobic capacity.[83] Improvement in functional ability often leads to more physical activity, which in turn further improves aerobic capacity. Improvements in balance ability may also contribute to increased aerobic capacity, because fear of falling is related to activity restriction and more sedentary behaviors. In some patients with impaired aerobic capacity (e.g., end-stage respiratory failure), improvement may not be possible, but using strategies that allow optimal function with a deficit in aerobic capacity can be employed. These energy conservation strategies minimize the energy demand of functional tasks by modification, organization, and prioritization. For example, tasks performed in sitting versus standing expend less energy (e.g., preparing food sitting at a table instead of standing at a counter). Another strategy is to plan daily activities to minimize redundancies in movement (e.g., organize a shopping list in the order that items are found in the store). Also, individuals should be encouraged to prioritize activities that are most important for them to do before the onset of fatigue (e.g., finish a woodworking project for a grandchild's birthday), or delegate tasks that are less important (e.g., ask someone else to fix a broken cabinet door). Box 12-6 provides examples of energy conservation techniques that patients with low aerobic capacity can employ.

Device Prescription

Prescription of a supportive or assistive device can help to improve aerobic capacity in some older patients. Oxygen therapy can help improve oxygen delivery in patients who have decreased arterial oxygen saturation. Although physical therapists do not prescribe supplemental oxygen, they often identify patients who would benefit from it and help patients optimize its use especially during activity. Many types of assistive devices may help to improve function and minimize disability in patients with impaired aerobic capacity. For example, four-wheeled walkers with a seat ("Rollators") are often used

---

BOX 12-6 | **Patient Instructional Sheet Highlighting Energy Conservation Techniques**

Strategies to conserve energy as you go about your daily activities
- Simplify tasks by planning in advance: get everything ready first, eliminate unnecessary work, and organize your working environment so that everything is handy.
- Break up large tasks into several parts or components.
- Prioritize daily activities to complete the most important tasks first or when you tend to have the most energy during the day.
- Avoid a lot of activity in the first hour after eating. Your body requires a good deal of energy to digest food after eating, and this means less energy available for other things.
- Pace yourself: slow, steady movements will accomplish more with less energy than fast, erratic movements. For example, when going upstairs take one step at a time, with brief rests as needed. Consider having a chair at the top of the stairs to rest, in case you need it.
- Maintain good posture and body mechanics during all activities. Poor posture and body mechanics contribute to fatigue.
- Use a small cart with wheels to transport items, whenever possible. Pushing objects in a cart requires much less energy and is safer than carrying them.
- Store frequently used items in convenient locations close to where they will be used and at shoulder to knee heights—not too high or too low.
- Keep a set of commonly used items on each level of your home.
- Avoid extreme temperatures during activity. Your heart, lungs, and muscles must use additional energy when your body is very hot or very cold.
- Sit during as many tasks as possible. Sitting requires less muscle activity than standing and therefore less energy.
- Complete tasks at waist level and close to your body, whenever possible. You expend more energy when bending down and reaching overhead during activity.
- Never hold your breath. Use pursed-lip breathing whenever you feel out of breath. Breathe out during the most demanding part of a task.
- Use supplemental oxygen during activity, if your doctor has prescribed it for you. Make sure that the flow rate is set correctly. If it is difficult for you to carry your portable oxygen tank, contact your oxygen supplier for alternative methods (many types of tanks and carrying cases are available).
- Get help when you need it! Family and friends are often more than happy to lend a helping hand. Many services may be available to you, such as Meals on Wheels or home health care.

---

by patients with impaired aerobic capacity to improve function by providing a seat for rest when needed, a basket to carry items, and upper extremity support which may facilitate respiratory muscle activity.[100] Other ambulatory aids can improve aerobic capacity by allowing mobility when weight-bearing is restricted or balance is impaired.

CASE EXAMPLE

History and Interview

Mr. C was a 76-year-old man who developed severe chest pain while lifting bales of hay. His wife took him to the nearest hospital, where his pain was resolved with nitroglycerin. He was diagnosed with acute myocardial infarction and then transferred to the nearest cardiac surgical center. Diagnostic cardiac catheterization was performed, which revealed 80% stenosis in the midportion of the left anterior descending artery, 90% stenosis in the circumflex artery, and 100% occlusion in the second diagonal and right coronary artery. Subsequently, Mr. C underwent emergent coronary artery bypass surgery of four vessels using the left internal mammary artery and left saphenous vein as conduit vessels. His surgery was performed without placing him on extracorporeal circulation (aka cardiopulmonary bypass machine) so his heart remained beating (aka off-pump or beating-heart surgery). Surgical access was via a median sternotomy. Mr. C was discharged from the hospital 6 days after surgery.

Mr. C was referred for outpatient rehabilitation and his initial physical therapy visit was 2 days after hospital discharge. His previous medical history included a right shoulder fracture, hypertension, and type 2 diabetes, but no major surgical procedures. His medications included aspirin, atorvastatin (Lipitor), lansoprazole (Prevacid), atenolol (Lopressor), ferrous sulfate, amlodipine besylate (Norvasc), rosiglitazone maleate (Avandia), insulin (Humulin), albuterol inhaler, hydrocodone/acetaminophen (Lortab), and furosemide (Lasix). Mr. C lived in a rural town (30 miles from a hospital) and with his wife in a two-level single-family home. He reported that he quit smoking 10 years ago, did not exercise regularly, and had a diet high in red meat products. Mr. C's family history was unremarkable for cardiovascular disease or other chronic diseases.

Prior to this episode of care, Mr. C worked the cattle farm that he owned, which required him to lift 70-lb bales of hay. The patient's goal was to return to all previous activities, including farming, but his family wanted him to "retire." Mr. C was independent with all activities of daily living (ADLs), instrumental ADLs (IADLs), and occupational tasks prior to the acute myocardial infarction and open heart surgery. At the initial physical therapy visit, he reported needing assistance with getting into and out of bed, standing up, walking, driving, and all work activities. His current symptoms included chest pain, shortness of breath/dyspnea, severe fatigue, and swelling in his hands and feet.

Systems Review and Examination

Mr. C was alert and oriented to person, place, time, and situation; responded appropriately to questions 80% of the time; and followed multistep directions. He reported that he learned best through demonstration. Mr. C had significant hearing loss, which was partially corrected by bilateral hearing aids, although he stated that he did not like to turn his hearing aids on very often "because it would wear out the batteries." Mr. C was a high school graduate and when questioned regarding his current learning needs, reported that he did not think that he had any. His wife accompanied him and stated that she would like to know what the family needs to do to help him recover.

Integumentary Screening. On integumentary inspection, he had sternal and left lower extremity incisions with staples still present and an abdominal chest tube site open with small amounts of clear serous drainage. He reported pain at the median sternotomy incision site with deep breathing. His dorsal pedal and posterior tibial pulses were right 1 of 3, left 0 of 3, and radial pulses bilaterally 2 of 3; his skin temperature was normal throughout the extremities and trunk.

Musculoskeletal Screening. Mr. C's chest wall motion was limited symmetrically in the upper and lower chest wall with deep breathing. Point tenderness was present in the anterior and posterior chest wall. His postural examination revealed forward head, rounded shoulders, and anterior pelvic tilt.

Active range of motion in his elbows, wrist, hand, lumbar spine, hips, and knees bilaterally were all within normal limits. Mr. C's cervical spine active range of motion was impaired, with all movements to ~50% of normal. His shoulder active range of motion was 110 degrees bilaterally and abduction was 90 degrees bilaterally. No overpressure was applied in the cervical spine and upper extremities because of his recent median sternotomy. Mr. C's ankle plantar flexion was 20 degrees and dorsiflexion was 5 degrees on the left with a tissue approximation end-feel. His right ankle active range of motion was within normal limits.

Mr. C's strength was at least 3 of 5 throughout the trunk and extremities but no resistance was applied in view of the fact that he was less than 2 weeks status post cardiac catheterization and median sternotomy.

Mr. C's height was 68 in. and weight was 229 lbs at the time of the initial physical therapy visit. Based on the body weight reported in his medical chart records, it appeared that his body weight had increased 20 lbs over the past week.

Neuromuscular Screening. Sensation to light touch was intact throughout the bilateral upper and lower extremities and intact on the plantar surface of both feet when tested with a 5.06 monofilament.

Deep tendon reflexes were normal bilaterally in the patellar and Achilles tendons. No clonus was detected with rapid wrist extension or dorsiflexion bilaterally. Mr. C's balance was normal in sitting and impaired in standing, with standing static balance subjectively rated good (4/5) and standing dynamic subjectively rated fair (3/5). Motor function was normal in his upper extremities, with rapid alternating forearm pronation and supination and normal in his lower extremities with heel to shin movement.

Mr. C had impaired functional mobility with limited weight bearing through his upper extremities secondary to the median sternotomy. He required verbal cues and moderate assistance from one person to go from supine to short sitting and back. He transitioned from short sitting to stand with assistance from one person and no upper extremity assist. Mr. C ambulated using a front-wheeled walker and contact guard assist. He was able to ascend and descend five steps using one railing and contact guard assist. His gait pattern was remarkable for decreased step length and heel strike bilaterally during swing.

Cardiovascular and Pulmonary Tests and Measures. Mr. C's general appearance revealed no jugular vein distension, digital cyanosis or clubbing, or signs/symptoms of acute distress. He had visible peripheral edema bilaterally in his feet and hands; the edema in his feet was so severe that he was unable to wear any of his shoes and was wearing slippers. Girth measurements were taken in his lower extremities to objectively assess the amount of edema.

Girth (cm)	Metatarsal heads	Malleoli	Lower leg
Right	28	27	42
Left	39.5	30.2	43

Lung auscultation revealed inspiratory crackles over the 8th to 10th intercostal spaces left posterior chest wall, which improved with activity. Mr. C's heart sounds were a normal S1 and S2 with no murmur, S3, S4, or pericardial friction rub. Mr. C's cough was infrequent, effective with splinting, and not productive. His phonation was normal and breathing pattern was shallow in depth with a regular rhythm.

Mr. C performed a 6-minute walk test during his initial physical therapy visit. During this test, he walked 330 feet using his front-wheeled walker and required one sitting rest period of 2 minutes as a result of overall fatigue. His vital signs were measured before, during, and after the walk test. He denied any adverse symptoms (chest pain, syncope, dyspnea, etc.) during ambulation.

Vital signs	Heart rate (bpm)	Blood pressure (mmHg)	Oxygen saturation (%)	Supplemental oxygen (L/min)
Resting (sitting in chair)	70	138/76	97	None – room air
Walking after 3 minutes	93	X	94	None – room air
Walking after 6 minutes	92	147/54	90	None – room air
Recovery after 5 minutes	74	136/56	97	None – room air

Additional self-report outcome measures that Mr. C completed included the RAND 36-Item Health Survey, a measure of generic quality of life, and the Duke Activity Status Index, a measure of disease-specific functional ability. Initial and discharge results from these outcome measures are presented in Table 12-5.

Evaluation

Given the amount of edema in Mr. C's hands and feet bilaterally and his apparent rapid weight gain, it seemed that the patient had significant fluid retention and volume overload. His cardiothoracic surgeon was contacted and Mr. C was seen in his office later that day for adjustment of his medications. Mr. C did not present with signs or symptoms of other postoperative complications, such as pneumonia, deep vein thrombosis/pulmonary emboli, incisional infection, or sternal dehiscence.

The patient's current level of knowledge regarding health-promoting behaviors including aerobic exercise was minimal. His readiness for learning was moderate or precontemplative, but his spouse was very supportive of his participation in cardiac rehabilitation and need for lifestyle modifications. Mr. C's only barrier to learning was a hearing impairment, which was not problematic when he wore and turned on his hearing aids. His coronary heart disease risk factors included age/gender, hypertension, dyslipidemia, diabetes, obesity, and physical inactivity.

Mr. C's aerobic capacity was significantly impaired, which was apparent in his scores on the outcome measures relative to age-matched norms (see Table 12-5). His physiological response to aerobic exercise was normal as reflected in his change in vital signs. Mr. C's heart rate and systolic blood pressure increased with activity and returned to baseline during recovery, indicating appropriate cardiac rate and contractility responses. His diastolic blood pressure went down slightly from rest to exercise, possibly indicating an orthostatic response to position change and vasodilation of skeletal muscle vasculature. Mr. C's oxygen saturation remained at or greater than 90% throughout the initial physical therapy visit, demonstrating that gas exchange in the lungs at rest and during exercise was normal.

In this patient, several factors likely contributed to aerobic capacity impairment. His cardiac function and therefore output may have been limited by the acute myocardial infarction, recent open heart surgery, and fluid overload. Despite being on a β-blocker, his heart rate at rest and during activity was within normal ranges, indicating that impairments in cardiac output were primarily related to stroke volume. He also most likely experienced both central and peripheral physiological changes from his recent bed rest and restricted activity level that resulted in a decline in aerobic capacity. Additional factors that may have limited Mr. C's 6-minute walk test distance/activity tolerance include fear of injury, illness, falling, or pain.

Diagnosis and Prognosis

Mr. C was categorized under Cardiopulmonary Preferred Practice Pattern D: Impaired Aerobic Capacity and Endurance Associated with Cardiac Pump Dysfunction. Box 12-4 lists factors that can influence the prognosis of a patient with impaired aerobic capacity. Many of these factors directly mediated the anticipated prognosis for Mr. C. For example, if we consider his age, severity of the current condition, and level of physical function, recovery prognosis would be somewhat guarded. But if we also consider his overall health, cognitive status, social support, and chronicity of his current condition, then his prognosis for return to previous activity level would be much better. Based on his previous and current functional status (physical, cognitive, and psychosocial), medical/surgical history, socioeconomic support system, and his desire to return to full activity, it was determined that Mr. C's prognosis for return to

TABLE 12-5	Patient Case Example Outcome Measure Scores		
Outcome Tool	**Normative Values**	**Initial Score**	**Discharge Score**
6-Minute walk test (feet)	2122	330	957
Duke Activity Status Index	48	4.5	41
RAND 36-Item Health Survey (%)	64	13	49
Physical functioning	70	5	75
Role limitation due to physical health	53	0	0
Role limitation due to emotional problems	66	0	0
Energy	52	0	65
Emotional well-being	70	3	48
Social functioning	79	25	38
Pain	71	0	78
General health	57	38	50

previous ADL/IADLs was good to excellent and prognosis for return to previous occupational activities was fair to good. Of particular concern for Mr. C was lifting heavy items, because after 2 months of median sternotomy precautions he would have significant disuse atrophy and weakness in the upper extremity and trunk muscles. In addition, high-intensity, static contractions of multiple muscle groups increase systolic and diastolic blood pressure, which in turn causes an elevation in myocardial work and oxygen demand.

Anticipated outcomes after 12 weeks included the following: (1) patient will be independent with all bed mobility and transfers, (2) patient will ambulate 1000 feet in 6 minutes with no assistive device, and (3) patient will lift 20 lbs from the floor to waist height 10 times.

Plan of Care Interventions

Anticipated episodes of care included three directly supervised visits per week for 12 weeks. Continuous ECG monitoring was used during each exercise session. Aerobic exercise training included treadmill walking, LE cycle ergometry, and eventually upper body cycle ergometry at an intensity of 1.5 METs (HR = 75 to 85, RPE = 4 to 5). Mr. C started with two 6-minute bouts of aerobic exercise that were lengthened progressively until he was able to participate in 30 minutes of continuous activity. Breathing strategies included deep breathing with a 3-second inspiratory hold and splinted coughing to prevent atelectasis and pneumonia. Flexibility exercises included heel cord, quadriceps, and hamstring stretches for five repetitions using a 10- to 20-second hold. Strengthening exercises included toe raises, sit-to-stand, unilateral hip abduction in standing starting with one set of five repetitions and progressing to three sets of ten repetitions. Functional training initially included bed mobility and transfer tasks and progressed to lifting a crate from floor to chair ten times with 10 to 20 lbs.

Outcomes

After a 12-week period of exercise training/rehabilitation, Mr. C demonstrated considerable improvement in aerobic capacity and functional status. As illustrated in Table 12-5, his distance on the 6-minute walk test and scores on the RAND 36-Item Health Survey and Duke Activity Status Index increased, indicating better aerobic capacity, quality of life, and functional capabilities. Mr. C's distance on the 6-minute walk test increased nearly threefold, indicating substantial improvement in his aerobic capacity. His increase in aerobic capacity most likely directly contributed to improvements in physical activity performance (as reflected by the Duke Activity Status Index) and functional activity performance (as reflected by the RAND 36-Item Health Survey), particularly physical functioning, energy, pain, and general health. Mr. C still had significant disability in role limitation as a result of physical and emotional health. This was most likely related to the fact that he had not been able to fully return to farming activities and this was an important part of his perceived self-identity and social role.

REFERENCES

To enhance this text and add value for the reader, all references are included on the companion Evolve site that accompanies this text book. The reader can view the reference source and access it online whenever possible. There are a total of 100 cited references and other general references for this chapter.

CHAPTER 13

Impaired Joint Mobility

Cory Christiansen, PT, PhD

INTRODUCTION

Joint mobility is a direct determinant of posture and movement, influencing activity and participation for all individuals. As a person ages, changes occur in joint mobility that can influence overall health and function. Thus, joint mobility is an important component of evaluation, diagnosis, and plan of care development for older adults. The purposes of this chapter are to (1) summarize current evidence of age-associated changes in joint mobility and (2) examine implications of impaired joint mobility for clinical management of older adult patients/clients.

As presented elsewhere, optimal aging is reflected by the capacity to participate in life with consideration of the interactions among many aspects of health. Isolating the influence of aging from other determinants of health, such as disease, environment, and other biopsychosocial characteristics of a person, is not possible. As a result, the unique health characteristics of each individual must be kept in mind as a context for considering the associations of aging and joint mobility. An understanding of typical age-associated changes in joint mobility will serve as one component of a larger knowledge base to guide physical therapists in optimizing health and function for older adults. A conceptual framework for interactions among the numerous factors for health and function in regard to age-related joint mobility impairment is presented in Figure 13-1.

The chapter consists of two primary sections. First presented are age-associated changes in joint mobility. Second, pertinent aspects of patient/client management are considered in view of the numerous interacting factors that contribute to impaired joint mobility in older adults.

JOINT MOBILITY WITH AGING

Operationally defined, joint mobility is the capacity of a joint to move passively, taking into account the joint surfaces and surrounding tissue.[1] Interactions between muscle, tendon, ligament, synovium, capsule, cartilage, and bone at a joint create the unique aspects of joint mobility. Because of the direct association between structure and function, joint mobility is directly influenced by changes in any of the related tissues. Distinct physiological change

occurs in joint structures and tissues over the life span. The result of the structural changes can include joint impairment, activity limitation, and participation restriction.

As will be seen, even for people who are aging successfully, changes in joint mobility occur. Although impairment of joint mobility is not concomitant with aging, the possibility of joint problems is a prominent consideration for physical therapists working with older adults. Illustrating the significance of impaired joint mobility in older adults is the increasing prevalence of reporting chronic joint symptoms that occurs as people age. For example, it has been reported by the Centers for Disease Control and Prevention that nearly 59% of individuals older than age 64 years self-report arthritis or chronic joint symptoms, compared with 42% of people aged 45 to 64 years (Table 13-1).[2]

Connective Tissue Changes

Connective tissue is the primary structural component of all joints, providing a mechanical framework dictating the structural and functional characteristics of individual joints. Changes in joint connective tissue occur as people age, independent of pathology. However, connective tissue aging is also influenced by factors unique to each individual, such as level of physical activity, pathology, segmental alignment, and prior injury.

All connective tissue structures of a joint (e.g., ligaments, joint capsule, and cartilage) consist of cellular, protein, and glycoconjugate components within an extracellular matrix. The unique configuration and composition of these components dictate the unique function of each structure. General age-associated changes in cellular and extracellular composition of connective tissue are presented in this chapter and summarized in Box 13-1. The majority of evidence for these changes is based on research on cartilage and bone in weight-bearing joints (e.g., knee, hip, and intervertebral), because of the comparatively large amount of study on those structures.

Cellular Level. Fibroblasts, the basic connective tissue cells, actively produce the extracellular matrix unique to each joint structure. For example, chondroblasts and osteoblasts are differentiated fibroblasts found in cartilage and bone, respectively. As people age, these cells

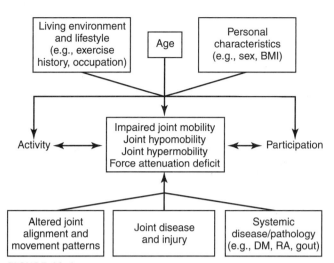

FIGURE 13-1 Interaction of factors contributing to impaired joint mobility.

demonstrate decreased proliferation (i.e., cellular senescence)[3,4] and altered control of apoptosis (i.e., programmed cell death).[5-8] The reduction in cell divisions appears to be related to a preset number of cell divisions (i.e., replicative senescence)[9] as well as altered responsiveness of tissue to exposure to stressful environmental agents over time (i.e., stress-induced premature senescence).[4] The result of decreased proliferation and altered regulation of apoptosis is a decrease in effective maintenance of tissue homeostasis.[3]

Another cellular change noted with age is decreased response to circulating growth factors, such as hormones and cytokines.[10-13] This change in cellular communication processes results in altered ability for repair and maintenance of connective tissue structures.[14] In addition, older connective tissue cells may be less responsive to adaptations with loading. In young individuals, cyclic physiological loading typically stimulates tissue synthesis. In contrast, Plumb et al[15] observed that cyclic loading of articular cartilage from older adults depressed, rather than stimulated, cartilage synthesis.

Molecular Level. Glycoconjugates are molecules of carbohydrate bonded to other compounds, such as protein and lipid. Forms of these molecules serve various functions in connective tissue, including cell-to-cell communication and cross-linkages between proteins. The presence of glycoconjugates in connective tissue is also critical for maintaining fluid content of the tissue, because of the highly negative charge of some of these molecules that serves to bind water.[16-18] The ability of connective tissue to retain water is diminished with aging as the content of glycoconjugates, particularly proteoglycan aggregates of the extracellular matrix, significantly decreases.[16,19] In addition, there is an increase in glycoconjugate degradation and decrease in synthesis that further contribute to decreased fluid content and connective tissue degeneration.[20-22]

Collagen, the primary structural protein of connective tissue, also changes across the life span. The unique structure of collagen molecules allows them to provide significant resistance to tensile load. Collagen molecules are arranged in fibrous strands with unique orientations that dictate the mechanical functions of the various joint structures. For example, obliquely oriented collagen

---

BOX 13-1	Generalized Age-Associated Changes in Connective Tissue

Molecular
Increased structural protein cross-linkages
Decreased proteoglycan size
Fragmentation of collagen

Cellular
Decreased proliferation
Altered control of apoptosis
Decreased response to growth factors
Altered response to loading

Connective Tissue Structures
Increased stiffness
Decreased water content
Decreased strength
Decreased cross-sectional area and volume

TABLE 13-1	Arthritis and Chronic Joint Symptom Prevalence in the United States					
	Self-Reported Arthritis/ Chronic Joint Symptoms*		**Doctor-Diagnosed Arthritis†**		**Arthritis-Attributable Activity Limitation†**	
Age (years)	Percent	(95% CI)	Percent	(95% CI)	Percent	(95% CI)
18-44	19.0	(±0.5)	7.9	(±0.3)	2.7	(±0.2)
45-64	42.1	(±0.7)	29.3	(±0.7)	11.8	(±0.4)
≥65	58.8	(±0.9)	50.0	(±0.9)	22.4	(±0.7)

CI, confidence interval.
*From Prevalence of self-reported arthritis or chronic joint symptoms among adults—United States, 2001. MMWR Morb Mortal Wkly Rep 51(42):948-950, 2002.
†From Prevalence of doctor-diagnosed arthritis and arthritis-attributable activity limitation—United States, 2003-2005. MMWR Morb Mort Wkly Rep 55(40):1089-1092, 2006.

fibers within the annulus fibrosus of the intervertebral disc are arranged in perpendicular directions for successive layers. This arrangement allows the disc to respond to compressive, tensile, and torsional loads between vertebrae through tension created in the collagen fibers.

Age-associated changes in collagen include fragmenting of collagen strands and a declining rate of collagen turnover.[3] Related to these changes is an increased formation of cross-links between collagen molecules. In part, the cross-links result from the formation of specific glycoconjugates, known as advanced glycation endproducts (AGEs). Interaction of the fragmented collagen and AGEs create intermolecular collagen cross-links.[23] Mechanically, increased cross-linkages alter the biomechanical function of the collagen structures by increasing stiffness and possibly decreasing the ability to absorb mechanical energy.[3] In addition, the cross-linkages may make structures more brittle, resulting in higher rates of structural damage in response to cyclic loading (i.e., decreased resistance to tissue fatigue).[24]

Another connective tissue protein is elastin, which typically functions in conjunction with collagen to return structures to their original shape after deformation.[25] Elastin also demonstrates age-associated cross-linkages related to AGE production.[25,26] The result, similar to collagen, is an increase in stiffness.

Change in Joint Structures

Joint structures can be categorized as chondroid, fibrous, and bony. Chondroid structures are of cartilaginous make-up and include articular cartilage, menisci, labra, and fibrocartilaginous discs. Fibrous structures include the ligaments and tendons that surround the joint (i.e., extraarticular) as well as ligaments within the joint boundaries (i.e., intraarticular). The other primary fibrous structure is the joint capsule of diarthroses, which defines the border between intra- and extraarticular structures. Bone creates the structural segments that move relative to one another at the articulations. The bones also disperse force and provide structure to the joints. Each of these categories of joint structures is directly influenced by the cellular and molecular changes described above.

Chondroid Structures. The majority of evidence for changes in chondroid structures with age comes from examination of articular cartilage and the intervertebral disc. The primary function of these structures is to disperse loads between segments and promote joint mobility by decreasing friction.[27,28] As with all joint structures, there is no clear distinction between typical aging and pathology of chondroid structures. One factor complicating this delineation is the influence of loading history.

Although it is known that moderate levels of intermittent joint loads promote articular cartilage health, excessive compression impacts and torsion loads are known to create damage.[28-30] Indication of the negative influence of excessive loading on articular cartilage is the increased incidence of osteoarthritis (OA) in individuals involved in sports[31] and occupations [32,33] with high levels of traumatic and static joint loading. Once articular cartilage becomes damaged, the capacity to heal is limited and initial injury may progress to the development of cartilage lesions (i.e., cartilage fibrillation).[28] The limited intrinsic healing response consists of lesion repair to the original hyaline cartilage with production of matrix molecules or fibrocartilage.[34] The result of increased matrix molecules and fibrocartilage is tissue with inferior load dispersion and friction-reducing characteristics.

A histologic change specific to articular cartilage is increased calcification over time. Calcification of articular cartilage has been shown to occur independent of osteoarthritic changes, indicating that it is a typical response to aging.[35] Calcification, along with cellular and molecular changes described in the previous section, leads to decreased osmotic pressure in articular cartilage.[36] Decreased hydration compromises the viscoelastic properties and load-absorbing capacity of the cartilage.[37-40]

Distinct changes specific to the intervertebral disc also occur over time. The nucleus becomes more fibrous and less gel-like and the annulus becomes less organized. As a result, delineation of annulus and nucleus is diminished in older adults.[41] Cracks may also develop in the annulus and nucleus.[41,42] Decreased water content is also noted in the intervertebral discs and is associated with shorter disc heights.[43] The loss of disc height can lead to the chronic pathological condition referred to as spinal stenosis, a major cause of pain and disability for older adults.[27] Change of the intervertebral disc also alters surrounding structures. For example, the diarthrodial facet joints may experience greater loads,[44] and elasticity of the ligamentum flavum may decrease because of decreasing tensile forces over time.[27,45]

Fibrous Structures. Information regarding the influence of aging on fibrous structures is relatively limited. As suggested earlier, the vast majority of evidence for age-associated changes of connective tissue structures is based on studies of cartilage and bone. In typical function, fibrous structures absorb and transfer some level of tensile load, based on collagen content. Although orientation and composition of tissue components vary between fibrous structures and between joints, the overarching similarities in response to aging are increased stiffness and reduced elasticity.[25,46] In addition, there is evidence in animal models that cross-sectional area and tensile strength of fibrous structures decrease with age.[47]

Bone

Bony change is both directly and indirectly related to joint mobility. Directly, changes in bone can influence the joint surfaces to alter joint mechanics. Indirectly, fractures and other bony structural change can alter joint alignment and function with possible secondary influences on joint mobility.

Subchondral bone is the layer of dense bone directly under the articular cartilage providing support to the articular surface. There is indication that the thickness and density of subchondral bone tends to decrease with advancing age, although this is not uniform at all joint surfaces.[48] For example, Yamada et al[48] examined 140 knee specimens from a wide age-range of donors (17 to 91 years) and found that thickness and density of the tibial subchondral bone declined with age, whereas no significant change was noted at the femoral condyles. The authors postulated that dispersion of loads during normal function may create differential response to subchondral bone structure between the femur and tibia.

It is well established that osteopenia is prevalent with aging, because of increased osteoclast and decreased osteoblast activity, leading to increased risk of osteoporosis.[49-53] Typically, bone acts along with cartilage to absorb and disperse forces transferred between body segments. As a result of osteopenia, the ability of bone to absorb loads is compromised. Corresponding to the problem of decreased load absorption by bone is decreased load dispersion in other joint structures and impaired neuromuscular function, both of which result in increased bone loading. The combination of lowered threshold for loading and increased load demand results in an increased risk of bone fracture with aging.

Fractures can alter joint mobility in a variety of ways, such as disrupting circulation to joint structures, altering loading patterns, and decreasing available range of motion. In addition, pain associated with fractures can be a major problem, interfering significantly with an individual's activity and participation. It is well documented that fractures are common and devastating injuries in older adult populations.[54] Common fracture locations that influence joint mobility in older adults are the proximal femur (i.e., hip fractures), pelvis, distal radius, and vertebrae.

Whole Joint Changes

Physiological and mechanical interactions between tissues create interdependence such that any change in one structure has direct consequences on the composition and function of other structures. At the level of the whole joint, changes include decreased joint space, increased laxity, altered dispersion of loads, and altered joint moments of force. Over time, the unloading of surrounding tissues and joint structures that provide tensile support, because of decreased joint space, may predispose the joint to decreased range of motion. However, change in mobility varies among joint complexes, with some joints having relatively little change in comparison to others.

Functionally, joint changes are reflected by age-associated changes seen in kinematics at both the segmental level (i.e., osteokinematics) and between joint surfaces (i.e., arthrokinematics). Motion of one

segment relative to another is considered osteokinematic motion and can be quantified with measurement of joint ranges of motion as well as angular velocities and accelerations. In comparison, arthrokinematics describes movement of joint surfaces in relation to one another. Research examining both osteokinematic and arthrokinematic motions of older adults compared to younger adults has revealed some general trends. This chapter provides information on individual joint kinematics without broader application in regard to functional task performance. Chapter 17, Ambulation, provides examples of changes in joint kinematics for the functional task of walking.

Range of Motion. Joint range of motion (ROM) decreases with increasing age, although nonuniformly among joints, and is often direction-specific within a given joint. Generally, active and passive motion both decrease, with active ROM tending to decline more than passive.[55] The differing response of active and passive motion indicates the influence of neuromuscular changes in addition to the structural changes of the joint. Also, passive ROM measures are typically independent of the individual's effort and motivation, whereas active ROM may be influenced by either of these variables.[55]

Motion of the axial skeleton has been examined relative to age in numerous studies. As an example, Figure 13-2 provides a graphic representation of data from a study by Malmstrom et al[56] that examined changes of cervical motion across the life span for a total of 120 participants. This figure illustrates the fact that change in movement with age is direction-specific. For the cervical spine, gradual decline in ROM is seen beyond the age of 30,[56-63] with extension and lateral flexion demonstrating the greatest decline.[58,63] Cervical transverse rotation and flexion are

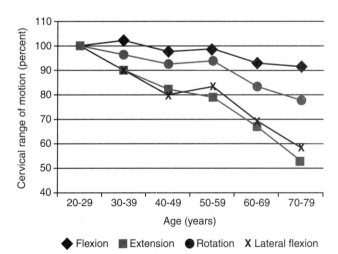

FIGURE 13-2 Cervical spine range of motion values across the life span. *(Data from Malmstrom EM, Karlberg M, Fransson PA, et al: Primary and coupled cervical movements: the effect of age, gender, and body mass index. A 3-dimensional movement analysis of a population without symptoms of neck disorders. Spine 31(2):E44-E50, 2006.)*

typically limited to a lesser extent than other planes, with some indication that upper cervical rotation may be less affected than lower segments.[57] Some investigators have suggested that limited lower cervical motion is possibly compensated for by increase of upper segment rotation.[57,59]

Examinations of thoracic and lumbar motion reveal extension to be most limited in older adults, with minimal or no age-dependent decline in rotation.[64-68] Bible et al[68] examined maximum sagittal lumbar motion using radiographic measures from 258 participants ranging in age from 18 to 50 years (some participants with and some without evidence of joint degenerative changes) and found age to be the most significant predictor of decreased ROM. In addition, statistical analysis indicated that declines in motion were seen independent of degenerative change.[68] Beyond 50 years of age, data indicate a continued trend for motion decline. For example, Troke et al[66] examined 400 participants ages 16 to 90 years and found a linear decline in trunk motion with approximate percentages of motion reduction across the span of ages, being 77% for extension, 50% for flexion, 44% for lateral flexion, and no change in rotation.

Research examining lower extremity ROM in older adults is common, with much consideration being directed toward the relationship between locomotor function and joint kinematics. Declines in joint motion occur at the hip[69,70] and foot/ankle[71-73] joint complexes, whereas knee motion, in the absence of pathology, remains relatively consistent across the life span.[74,75] At the hip, sagittal plane motion is primarily influenced. In this plane of motion, hip flexion is typically well maintained as people age.[75] However, extension ROM has been shown to decrease by more than 20% (decline from 22 to 17 degrees) when comparing individuals 25 to 39 and 60 to 74 years of age.[69] It has been postulated that reduced hip extension seen with aging may directly relate to decreased walking speed in older adults, especially those with sedentary lifestyles.[70,76] Decreased ankle sagittal plane motion is also seen with aging, particularly in the direction of dorsiflexion.[71,72,77,78] Although strength of ankle dorsiflexion is postulated to account for a major portion of decline in ankle motion during function,[71] the presence of progressive decreases in passive ROM indicates causes other than muscle strength alone.[72,78]

Compared to the lower extremity and trunk, there is relatively less influence of age on upper extremity joint ROM. The shoulder complex is most influenced, with flexion and external rotation being the primary motions affected.[63,79] Movement of the shoulder complex involves glenohumeral, scapulothoracic, and spinal segment interaction.[80,81] As such, the increased thoracic kyphosis typically seen with age can play a significant role on the amount of motion available at the shoulder. At the elbow and wrist, no age-associated declines in motion have been noted in absence of disease.[63,79,82]

Arthrokinematics. Arthrokinematic motions include glide, spin, roll, compression, and distraction of joint surfaces relative to one another. The connective tissue changes previously described can potentially alter arthrokinematics through such mechanisms as increased fibrous structure stiffness, decreased chondroid structure volume and viscoelasticity, and altered bone structure. Although isolated arthrokinematic motions cannot be performed volitionally, limitations can have a direct influence on joint mobility. For example, glenohumeral abduction includes inferior glide of the humeral head in relation to the glenoid fossa.[83] In the case of adhesive capsulitis, a disease more common with age progression, the joint capsule does not allow sufficient laxity. The increased tightness of the joint capsule alters arthrokinematics, reducing inferior glide during activities requiring glenohumeral abduction.[84] Reduced inferior glide may lead to symptoms of shoulder impingement. This example of joint capsule change demonstrates how impaired joint mobility can have direct consequence on arthrokinematics and osteokinematics, leading to activity limitation.

Force Transmission. Kinetic implications of joint mobility relate to force transmission within joint structures and between body segments. It has already been noted that connective tissue structures demonstrate altered capacity to transmit tensile and compressive loads in older adults. These alterations can result in increased demands on specific regions within joints, possibly leading to disease. For example, areas of articular cartilage breakdown are found in specific regions of joints.[85] These areas of breakdown may be correlated with areas of altered contact pressures and can lead to the degenerative changes in cartilage.[86] Additionally, age-related tissue changes can limit the ability of joint structures to heal and a cascade can ensue, leading to greater impairment.[85]

Joint structural changes can also indirectly influence the moment of force (i.e., torque) demands on joints. As discussed in Chapter 16, posture change is predictable over the life span. The changes in posture relate to alterations in joint alignment and mobility. As a consequence of alignment change, static and dynamic demands on joints are altered. A specific example is the typical increase in thoracic kyphosis seen even in successfully aging adults.[87] This change increases the moment arm between the line of action of gravity and mediolateral axes of rotation for the thoracic spine segments. As a result, increased kyphosis will create a larger flexion demand moment on the thoracic joints during daily standing and sitting activities (Figure 13-3). If these changes in joint mobility and alignment are not corrected, greater neuromuscular activation is needed to compensate or further joint impairment will occur.

Any joint structural change can influence the linear and angular effects of forces. A physical therapist, equipped with foundational knowledge in mechanics and joint anatomy, can determine how changes in joint structure will alter kinetic qualities of each specific joint.

Because joints work to produce motion in segmental systems, subtle changes at one joint can have significant alterations in demands at other joints.

Influence on Activity and Participation

Postural control during activities such as walking, position transfers, and reaching are known to decline with age. Among the multiple factors related to these alterations in activity is change in joint mobility. Changes in joint mobility have significant activity- and participation-related consequences for older adults, as evidenced by correlations such as cartilage thinning with patient-identified disability[88] and intervertebral disc degeneration with back pain.[89] A specific example of joint mobility association with activity is the relationship of ankle mobility and balance. Menz et al[90] have shown ankle dorsiflexion ROM to be significantly related to decrements in older adult postural control. Of the balance measures in their study, pelvic forward and backward displacements during leaning were most highly correlated with ankle dorsiflexion motion. Similar findings have been noted with correlations in ankle motion and functional forward reach.[91]

Impaired joint mobility has also been implicated as a factor in walking limitations. For example, Kerrigan et al[92] observed gait speed to be decreased between older adults who reported frequent falls compared to "non-fallers" of the same age. In addition, smaller hip extension displacements were observed for individuals reporting falls. The difference in hip motion during gait was the only variable noted to be significantly different between the groups, when analyzing any of the ten joint kinematic variables tested.

Age-associated activity limitation often culminates in decreased participation in life events. The relationship also works in the opposite direction, with changes in activity and participation leading to more sedentary lifestyles and secondary changes to joint structure and function (see Figure 13-1). Because of the interdependent nature of these factors, it is important that changes in joint mobility are identified and addressed in older adult patients/clients presenting with all types of diagnoses. The second section of this chapter focuses on the process of patient/client management with specific attention to the role of joint mobility.

JOINT EXAMINATION

All older adult patients/clients require consideration of joint mobility as a result of the integral role of joints in health and function. Beyond typical age-related changes,

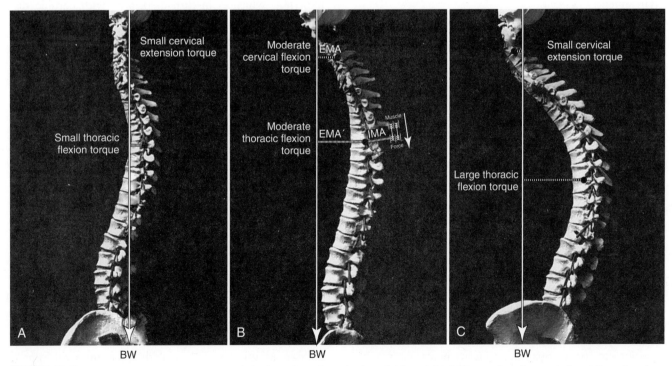

FIGURE 13-3 Model showing the orientation of the force line of gravity from body weight (BW, *arrow*) at the cervical and thoracic spines. **A** through **C** show a progression in severity of kyphosis. Each model demonstrates the mediolateral axis at the midpoint of the thoracic and cervical regions (*dark circles*) and the associated external moment arms (*hatched lines*). **A,** Patient with ideal standing posture and normal thoracic kyphosis. BW creates a small cervical extension torque and a small thoracic flexion torque. **B,** Patient with moderate thoracic kyphosis. BW creates a moderate cervical and thoracic flexion torque. EMA' = external moment arm at the thoracic spine midpoint; EMA = external moment arm at cervical spine midpoint; IMA = internal moment arm for back extensor muscular force. **C,** Patient with severe thoracic kyphosis. BW causes a small cervical extension torque and a large thoracic flexion torque.

there are many joint conditions with a higher prevalence in older adults, such as osteoarthritis, rheumatoid arthritis, polymyalgia rheumatica, and gout.[93,94] Examination of the patient/client allows the therapist to determine the relative influence of joint mobility on the presenting activity limitations.

Joint mobility examination is incorporated in the comprehensive examination and should not be viewed as an independent process. Specific lines of questions included in the history and observations from the systems review will determine the extent to which further examination of joint mobility is indicated. If evidence of joint impairment is provided by specific tests and measures, the impairment can be targeted through remediation, compensation, or prevention strategies. Throughout this process, joint mobility is considered in the context of complete patient/client management.

History

A thorough history interview is a key component in the examination of the patient/client. Knowledge gained from the history is critical in determining possible influence of impaired joint mobility on the presenting problems. Included in the history interview are questions regarding activity limitations, participation restrictions, symptom characteristics, activity history, previous joint impairments, family history of joint disease, and living environment.

Activity and Participation. It is important to begin the history interview by first identifying activity limitations and participation restrictions. This process clarifies the needs and functional goals of the patient/client. In addition, identifying problems with activity and participation focuses the examination by providing a context for determining how impaired joint mobility may be contributing to the presenting problems. Clear identification of these functional problems will also help in the process of determining appropriate outcomes measures.

It is possible for an older adult to have impaired joint mobility that does not influence the presenting functional problem. Although it is important to consider nonsymptomatic joint impairment for preventive reasons, focusing on impairments not related to the presenting problem can distract from the examination and care planning process. Determining the relative influence that impaired joint mobility has on functional problems can only be made if the activity limitations and participation restrictions are clear to the therapist.

Symptoms. If an individual relates chronic symptoms, development of compensatory movements over time should be suspected. In these cases, the original symptoms as well as the most recent symptoms are important to consider. Altered movement patterns in response to impaired joint mobility can eventually lead to secondary problems. Understanding compensation helps the

therapist to develop hypotheses for both original symptoms and symptom progression. It is also of interest to link routine activity change, such as new exercise participation, to symptoms. Knowledge of temporal onset of symptoms is necessary to make this determination.

Behavior of symptoms, such as timing and duration, can indicate the type of joint mobility problem. For example, symptoms of stiffness related to OA are often increased after periods of stationary postures (e.g., upon getting out of bed) and last for short periods (e.g., less than 30 minutes) after movement is initiated. In contrast, morning stiffness common with rheumatoid arthritis typically lasts for periods greater than 30 minutes.[95] In another example, a patient/client may indicate lower extremity pain during periods of standing and walking that resolves shortly after sitting. One reason for this type of symptom behavior can be neurogenic intermittent claudication related to lumbar spinal stenosis.[96]

Occupation/Activity. Information on joint loading and movement history is provided with knowledge of occupational and leisure activity. Loading history of joints is known to be an important influence on joint mobility in older age, often linked to impairment. For example, evidence indicates that occupations involving extensive periods of kneeling and squatting activity are associated with increased risk of OA,[33] especially in combination with heavy lifting.[32] Lack of activity is also of interest, as it has been shown that older age is associated with sedentary lifestyle,[97] which is in turn associated with chronic disease.[98] It is well accepted that joint structures, along with all other biological tissues, will adapt to the amount of physical stress applied to them.[99] Adaptive response of chronically low activity can decrease the tolerance of joint structures to loading. Combined with the typical age-associated joint changes, activity reductions play a key role in joint mobility impairment and threshold for joint injury.

Health Condition/Injury/Surgery. The importance of information regarding disease history cannot be overstated. For joint function, comorbid conditions are often significant factors. Endocrine, neuromuscular, cardiovascular, pulmonary, and musculoskeletal pathology can be linked to systemic conditions that significantly influence joint function. An example is the association of impaired joint mobility with diabetes mellitus, a common endocrine disease affecting older adults. The high glucose and insulin levels in patients with diabetes are associated with increased cross-linkage formation in connective tissue structures that can compound the age-associated changes discussed earlier in this chapter.[100] Joint mobility impairments that occur as complications of diabetes include adhesive capsulitis of the glenohumeral joint[101] and diabetic stiff-hand syndrome (also termed "limited joint mobility").[102]

Joint loading is also influenced by history of health condition, injury, and surgery. Perhaps the most common health condition associated with atypical joint loading is obesity. History of obesity is a known risk factor related to impairments of weight-bearing joints.[103,104] Additionally, injury and surgery are often closely related to joint loading through movement and posture compensations. Knowledge of the history of such factors related to joint loading also provides insight into the incidence of degenerative joint change later in life. Murphy et al[105] performed a longitudinal examination (mean time from baseline to follow-up of 6 years) for knee OA in 1739 people (mean age at baseline 61 years) and found the lifetime risk of symptomatic knee OA was 44.7%. The two factors found to significantly increase the risk of knee OA were the presence of obesity and history of knee injury, which increased the lifetime risk to 60.5% and 56.8%, respectively.

Family History. Studies have demonstrated increased likelihood of joint-specific diseases in older adults resulting from genetic predisposition.[106-108] OA,[106] gout,[108] rheumatoid arthritis,[109] and systemic lupus erythematosus[109] are all examples of joint pathologies linked to genetic influence. Knowledge of family disease history alerts the physical therapist to early signs of problems and potential relevant interventions. Even patients/clients presenting without joint impairment can benefit from preventive intervention if family history, in combination with other findings, indicates high potential for future joint mobility problems.

Living Environment. Discussion of living environment is integral when gathering information on activity limitations and participation restrictions. Living environments, including both home and community, are unique to each individual. Items such as stair height, chair types, and flooring determine the varying degrees of joint mobility necessary for routine activity. Even if the therapist does not perform a home visit, information regarding environmental aspects of living can be ascertained through the history interview. Identified environmental concerns can be directly assessed further in the home or simulated in clinical settings. Identification of environmental conditions also allows the potential of targeting environmental modification with intervention.

Systems Review

It is evident that joint mobility should be considered in the complete context of a person's health and function and not solely as a musculoskeletal issue. Joint mobility influences, and is influenced by, multisystem interactions. For example, pulmonary function can be altered by joint mobility of the thorax and spinal column. Study of sternocostal synarthroses reveals increased cartilage calcification and ossification with aging.[110] These sternocostal changes, in conjunction with decreased intervertebral disc height and elasticity, may lead to pulmonary dysfunction by creating increased work of breathing.[111] Such interactions between systems are a primary reason for performing a systems review, as recommended in the *Guide to Physical Therapist Practice.*[1]

Another benefit of the systems review is increased examination efficiency. Selection of focused tests and measures is generated by combining history information with findings of the review. For example, consider a 70-year-old man presenting with symptoms of pain at the posterolateral deltoid region of the shoulder. During the interview, he also reveals a history of chronic lateral elbow pain that has been treated ineffectively in the past as lateral epicondylitis. During the systems review, gross assessment of cervical motion reveals that extension and ipsilateral side flexion reproduce pain symptoms at both the elbow and shoulder. Based on this preliminary information, cervical spine joint mobility would be of primary interest for further examination.

Tests and Measures

Selection of appropriate tests and measures for an older adult with impaired joint mobility requires consideration of health and functional status of the individual, practicality of administration for a given clinical setting, and psychometric properties of the measure.[112] These considerations continually change because each patient has a unique presentation, methods for established tests and measures evolve, psychometric properties are defined with research over time, and new tests and measures emerge. Considering these dynamic aspects, a "cook-book" recipe approach with a specific list of tests and measures for all patients/clients is not reasonable. However, a categorical framework for the selection of tests and measures can be followed and applied to the current state of knowledge. In this section, a guide for a comprehensive approach to tests and measures, applicable to patients with impaired joint mobility, is provided.

The four primary types of tests and measure categories are listed in Box 13-2. Combining results of these four categories of measures allows for quantification of all levels of potential dysfunction: impairments, activity limitations, and participation restrictions (as defined by the International Classification of Functioning, Disability and Health[113,114]). Considering the intimate interaction between these levels of dysfunction, a comprehensive

---

BOX 13-2   Four Major Types of Tests and Measure Categories to Consider When Assessing Joint Mobility

- Observational task analysis
- Self-report measures of activity and participation
- Performance-based measures of activity
- Joint-specific mobility testing

battery of tests and measures is needed to fully quantify the impact of altered joint mobility.

Observational Task Analysis. A suggested first step in the implementation of tests and measures is observational analysis of the specific functional task(s) identified as problematic by the patient.[115,116] Observational task analysis can guide the formation of hypotheses, considering impaired joint mobility as a potential cause of activity limitation. In addition, observational task analysis may allow the physical therapist to identify appropriate quantitative tests and measures to further the examination. Procedures for observing and analyzing must be systematic in order for the process to be effective. Systematic analysis is improved if the therapist has a strong working knowledge of the movement mechanics required for the task, as well as sufficient practice observing and analyzing the given task.[117]

Methods for performing observational task analyses are outlined in various frameworks for patient/client examination.[115,116,118] Much of the published work on observational task analysis is rooted in the analysis of walking gait, particularly in relation to the practice of neuromuscular physical therapy. Although observational gait analysis procedures have been published and used in the clinic for many years, reliability for identifying altered joint movements is poor to moderate.[117,119,120] Considering this lack of established reliability, observational task analysis should be used cautiously, with emphasis on guiding selection of other tests and measures, rather than being used independently for diagnosing or quantifying impaired joint mobility. For example, impaired knee mobility ROM is a potential cause for lack of full knee extension at initial contact during gait. Observed absence of full knee extension, during task analysis, should suggest that valid and reliable measures of knee motion be performed.

Self-Report Measures of Activity and Participation. In addition to direct observation of task performance, patient self-report measures can be used to gather information during the examination. These measures document the patient's perspective of activity performance, which provides different information than direct observation.[121] Valid self-report measures inform the therapist regarding the influence of domains such as pain and psychological functioning on activity limitations. Many self-report measures also allow for gathering information regarding the patient's restrictions in regard to life participation.

Impaired mobility of a given joint will directly influence a specific region of the body: the spine, upper extremities, or lower extremities. Region specificity is a characteristic of a great number of standardized self-report measures. A benefit of having numerous region-specific self-report measures available is the ability to gather information to assess interaction between regional joint mobility impairment and perceived function. A practical problem of having numerous region-specific

measures is deciding which measure is most appropriate for a given patient. In order to provide assistance with the process of selecting self-report measures for the patient with impaired joint mobility, further discussion of these measures is provided in the Outcomes section of this chapter.

Performance-Based Measures of Activity. Observational task analysis and patient self-report measure(s) provide the physical therapist information that allows for selection of appropriate performance-based activity measures. In contrast to self-report, performance-based measures quantify activity while minimizing the patient/client's perception of the performance. An individual's perceptions of activity limitations and participation restrictions are important aspects in every examination. Supplementary to understanding the patient/client's perception in relation to health and function is the ability to directly quantify performance of specific activities. Quantification of actual tasks through performance-based measures provides unique information that will be used, in light of the other examination information, to further evaluate the interaction of impaired joint mobility and other presenting problems of the patient/client.

The quantification of activity, if based on valid and reliable measures, allows the therapist to describe patient/client progression over the course of intervention as well as document outcomes. Similar to self-report measurement, there are a large number of standardized performance-based measures available. Selection of appropriate performance-based measures is guided in part by determining the daily tasks most likely to be influenced by the joint impairment. As pointed out above, the tasks most influenced are determined by the patient/client history and results of the self-report measure(s). Once an activity category is determined, selection of specific performance-based measures can be made. Discussion of selecting activity measures is addressed in the Outcomes section of this chapter.

Joint-Specific Mobility Testing. Targeted examination of older adults with suspected impairment of joint mobility also includes joint-specific mobility testing. Joint-specific mobility is typically examined through measurement of joint range of motion (ROM), muscle–tendon unit (MTU) extensibility, and segmental mobility. These measures provide the final pieces of information needed to guide formation of the clinical hypotheses required to develop a plan of care.

Established goniometer and inclinometer measurement methods are utilized to clinically quantify joint ROM.[122-126] Quantification of joint ROM allows for comparison of a given individual's joint ROM with established normative values for people of similar age.[62,66,67,69,74,82,127] Joint ROM values can also be compared between the right and left sides to document the amount of asymmetry for a given patient/client.

Another aspect of joint mobility that can be quantified by measurement of joint ROM is MTU extensibility.

Extensibility refers to the ability of an MTU to lengthen. If an MTU crosses multiple joints, it may limit joint mobility when the position of the joints creates maximal lengthening of the muscle. To measure the maximal length of an MTU, standardized joint positioning has been established to account for all joints that are crossed by the MTU.[128] A few examples of multijoint MTU groups that have been linked to shortening with age are the ankle plantar flexors,[71,72] hamstrings,[70] and hip flexors.[69,76,129]

The final component commonly included in examination of joint-specific mobility is segmental mobility testing. Segmental mobility refers to the accessory joint movement that is not under volitional control. As stated previously, the amount of accessory movement at a joint is expected to change with age because of joint structure changes. The difficulty in implementing clinical tests of segmental mobility is the low level of reliability and lack of established validity for the tests. For example, poor levels of interrater reliability are seen with spine segmental mobility testing, regardless of specific advanced training of the therapist.[130-133] In addition, a consensus on the best rating scale to use and the validity of grading in relation to joint mobility is currently lacking. As a result, it is recommended that segmental mobility testing be used as a qualitative guide for selection of quantitative measures such as joint ROM, valid instrumented tests for mobility of specific joints, and other joint and region-specific special tests.

EVALUATION AND DIAGNOSIS

The evaluation process incorporates all examination results, including joint mobility tests and measures, into a complete clinical impression of the patient/client presentation. Arriving at the clinical impression requires critical analysis by the therapist to determine the potential causes of the patient/client's presenting problems. In assessing causes of the presenting problems, the suspected role of impaired joint mobility will be identified.

Once joint mobility has been identified as an impairment, determining an appropriate diagnostic classification is possible. Numerous physical therapy diagnostic classifications are outlined in the *Guide to Physical Therapist Practice*, which contains joint mobility impairment as a primary component (see Patterns D, E, G, H, and I).[1] In addition, impaired joint mobility may be a secondary component of other diagnoses. For example, consider an older adult presenting with impaired hip mobility that limits walking. If this individual seeks intervention after a proximal femur fracture, "Impaired joint mobility, muscle performance, and range of motion associated with fracture" is an appropriate diagnostic classification. In contrast, consider the patient who presents with hip mobility impairment in addition to several other ipsilateral symptom manifestations from a cerebral vascular accident. In this case, the musculoskeletal diagnostic classification of

the hip is secondary to a primary neuromuscular diagnosis. Such distinctions in diagnostic classification serve to clarify the therapist's clinical impression to the patient/client, other health care providers, and reimbursement sources.

Once the diagnosis is clarified, the influence of joint mobility impairment on patient/client prognosis can be determined, considering the expected time required to achieve an optimal outcome. In the absence of other impairments, the prognosis is favorable for remediating age-associated joint mobility impairment within a short (e.g., 4- to 6-week) time period. Basic factors common to older adults that often complicate prognosis include chronicity of impairment, level of physical activity, and high level of comorbidity. In patients with one or more of these additional factors, prognosis determination can be challenging.

The process of identifying diagnostic categories, previously performed to arrive at a clinical impression, can also be a significant help in forming the prognosis. The *Guide to Physical Therapist Practice* provides broad ranges for expected number of visits with each diagnostic category, based on input of numerous expert therapists.[1] These ranges provide the therapist with a starting point for determining time expectations. Even if the expected number of visits from the diagnostic categories is used and the multiple comorbidity categories are considered, the process of developing a prognosis for older adults with impaired joint mobility is not simple. Factors such as the patient/client goals and perceptions, medical management of disease processes, family support, financial considerations, and cognition must also be considered. Being able to effectively incorporate all factors related to prognosis requires practice and experience in working with older adults.

The plan of care should include considerations specifically related to the identified joint mobility impairment. Strategies for addressing joint mobility impairment should be outlined, including the general intervention categories. The intervention approach will also be reflected in the specific intervention goals. Although it is reasonable to have goals specific to impaired joint mobility, they should be written in terms of the activity limitations or participation restrictions identified in the examination (see Box 13-3). The activity- and participation-based goals will reflect the functional relevance of the joint mobility problem.

INTERVENTION

Three primary intervention approaches for older adults with problems related to joint mobility impairment are remediation, compensation, and prevention. Education, therapeutic exercise, and manual therapy techniques can be valuable remediation interventions for individuals with functional limitations related to joint mobility. For these same individuals, compensatory interventions such as use of assistive devices can also be of value. For individuals who have not yet developed symptoms or functional difficulties, the interventions mentioned may be

BOX 13-3	Writing Patient Goals to Include Activity Limitation or Participation Restriction

A. Incorrect: Incomplete patient goal statement
   The patient/client will increase hip extension ROM to 20 degrees within 4 weeks of intervention.
B. Correct: Inclusion of target activity in patient goal statement
   The patient/client will increase hip extension ROM to 20 degrees to enable walking with a symmetrical gait pattern within 4 weeks of intervention.

used to help prevent onset or progression of problems associated with joint impairment.

As will be presented below, favorable responses to remediation of impaired joint mobility have been seen in body structure and function, activity performance, and participation for older adults. In particular, exercise and increased physical activity can effectively reverse much of the detrimental influence of aging in regard to activity limitations and participation restriction.[134-138] However, age-associated changes in joint function are seen even in people who remain highly active.[139] As a result, compensation and prevention strategies must also be considered as approaches to intervention. In this section of the chapter, patient/client education, therapeutic exercise, manual intervention techniques, and assistive/adaptive devices and equipment will be discussed in relation to remediation, compensation, and prevention of joint mobility impairment for the older adult.

Patient/Client Education

One of the most beneficial interventions for addressing impaired joint mobility is patient/client education. Education for modifying lifestyle in terms of activity and exercise is known to be helpful for older adult populations and can be an important component of preventive, compensatory, and remediation intervention. For example, meta-analyses have revealed significant reduction of pain and improvement of function following education of patients/clients with OA and rheumatoid arthritis.[140]

An example of compensatory activity modification relates to patients/clients with lumbar spinal stenosis. The result of spinal stenosis is a decrease in the spinal canal space, often producing radiating symptoms (termed intermittent neurogenic claudication). Changing upright postures to increase lumbar flexion, such as walking uphill or using an assistive device to shift the upper body position anteriorly, can greatly reduce symptoms by increasing the spinal canal space. Education provided to make this activity change may make as large an impact on function as any other intervention for these patients/clients. In most cases, patient/client

daily activity will have the greatest impact on determining success of the intervention.

Therapeutic Exercise. There is evidence that targeted therapeutic exercise, such as stretching and strengthening, can improve joint mobility. However, many intervention studies with older adults include several simultaneous modes of exercise, predominantly combinations of stretching, strengthening, endurance training, and balance training. Joint mobility has been shown to improve with multiple-mode exercise programs, although the amount and location of improvement is program specific. In general, it is apparent that exercise can reverse the trend of age-associated decline in joint mobility.[87,141,142] The primary mode of exercise targeting impaired joint mobility is stretching.

Stretching Exercise. Researchers have demonstrated the usefulness of isolated stretching, static stretching particularly, for improving joint mobility of older adults.[129,143-146] Feland et al[144] examined stretch duration and found straight leg raise stretches held 15, 30, or 60 seconds were effective for increasing the combined motion of hip flexion and knee extension for older adults with initially impaired hamstring extensibility. The suggestion by these authors is that the longer the hold of stretch, up to 60 seconds, the greater the ROM benefit. In general, studies using greater than 15 seconds of stretch have identified improvements in joint mobility.[129,145]

Of particular importance in terms of stretching is that joint mobility increases are linked to improved activity performance. For example, walking performance is known to improve in older adults after stretching of the hip flexors and ankle plantar flexors.[129,145,146] Trends of improved gait speed and kinematics have been noted after static stretching even for community-dwelling, active older adults without participation restriction.[129,146]

Strengthening Exercise. Muscle strengthening influences joint mobility through indirect mechanisms. An indirect link between muscle strength and joint mobility has been demonstrated through the contribution of muscle to joint loading and control of motion.[147] Muscle–tendon units typically serve as a primary mechanism for attenuating load transmission across joints by absorbing energy in activities such as walking. Impaired muscle function associated with aging diminishes this capacity to absorb loads and may result in increased loading of other joint structures, possibly leading to negative changes. Some evidence to support the influence of muscle function on prevention of impaired joint mobility is the link seen between muscle weakness and onset of knee OA[148-150]; however, a causal relationship has not been definitively established.

Strengthening exercise has been shown to influence joint mobility in older adult populations. For example, Fatouros et al[151] demonstrated that individuals (mean age 70.6 years) not previously active in an exercise program gained shoulder, elbow, hip, and knee ROM after interventions including resistance and endurance training in the absence of stretching. This finding indicates that joint mobility improvement can be achieved partly as a result of improved muscle function.

Strengthening also influences joint mobility by loading the joint structures. Dynamic loading can stimulate growth of joint connective tissue structures, such as articular cartilage and bone.[152,153] For instance, Roos and Dahlberg[154] studied knee articular cartilage of patients/clients (mean age 45.8 years) who had previously undergone partial medial meniscectomy. After 4 months of progressive resistance training, there was noted improvement in glycoconjugate, specifically glucosaminoglycan, content in the articular cartilage of the postsurgical knees. Continued examination specific to the influence of resistance exercise on cartilage and other joint structures in older adults is needed.

Combined Exercise Interventions. Several studies that include older adult participants across various levels of fitness and health status, have examined the effect of combined exercise interventions (e.g., stretching, endurance exercise, resistance exercise, and functional activity) on joint mobility, with various results.[151,155-157] For example, Brown et al[157] examined sedentary men and women older than age 78 years and found an increase in trunk, hip, and ankle mobility following 3 months of combined resistance, endurance, and stretching exercise. In another study, Thompson and Osness,[155] using a program including resistance, flexibility, and functional training (3 times a week for 8 weeks) found no significant increases in hip motion for older adult golfers. It is obvious that findings from such studies are difficult to compare because of the multiple interventions and lack of targeted impairments. Although improvements in joint mobility result from such multimode exercise programs, it is not possible to determine which aspect of the program has the greatest influence on joint mobility.

Other Forms of Exercise Related to Joint Mobility. Other forms of exercise that influence joint mobility include stabilization, Tai Chi, and yoga. These forms of exercise can theoretically indirectly influence joint mobility by improving motor control. These exercises have limited evidence in relation to remediation or prevention of joint mobility impairment in older adults. Although evidence in research literature is limited, there are indications that all three of these exercise types may benefit joint mobility.

Stabilization exercises are designed to selectively target coactivation of muscles and provide joint stability.[158] Most of the research on stabilization exercises has been based on the spine. In relation to the lumbar spine, it has been concluded that stabilization exercises may improve pain and function in individuals with chronic low back pain, including older adults.[159]

Tai Chi, a Chinese form of mind–body exercise that has gained popularity in use among older adults across the world, has been linked to improving balance, muscle function, life participation, and reducing risk of falls.[160-163] In addition to these benefits, there has also been research indicating that older adults with impaired joint mobility can benefit from Tai Chi. For example, Tai Chi exercise has been shown to improve self-report of pain, stiffness, and physical function for older adults with diagnosed OA of the knee.[164,165]

Yoga is a traditional Indian form of exercise combining resistance, balance, and flexibility exercises. Initial studies have shown yoga to be an appropriate and simple-to-learn activity for older adults that can improve joint mobility.[166-168] For example, DiBenedetto et al[168] examined walking in older adults before and after 8 weeks of participation in a yoga exercise program. Participants in the yoga program demonstrated increased hip joint extension during walking along with increased stride length and a trend toward improved walking speed.[168]

Manual Intervention Techniques

Historically, use of manual joint mobilization and manipulation has been approached with much caution when working with older adults. The typical changes to joint connective tissue structures, leading to generalized weakening, has been the primary cause for concern. Although it is important to use caution when dealing with joint structures weakened with age, age is not a contraindication to joint mobilization and manipulation. Initial studies of joint mobilization and manipulation interventions for older adults indicate favorable results. Hoeksma et al[169] demonstrated specific joint mobilization and manipulation combined with stretching to be superior to exercise alone for remediation of joint impairment in individuals with hip OA. The improved outcome measures for the manual intervention group were patient subjective assessment, Visual Analog Scale reporting for pain, hip ROM, and Harris Hip Score.[169]

Joint mobilization has also been examined for people diagnosed with lumbar stenosis.[170] In this study, two groups of patients/clients (mean age of 69.5 years), with magnetic resonance imaging evidence of lumbar spinal stenosis, were treated for 6 weeks with one of two intervention regimens. One group received lumbar flexion exercise and treadmill walking and the other lumbar mobilization, hip mobilization, partial body weight–supported treadmill walking, stretching, and resistance exercise. Although both treatment groups demonstrated improvement, a significantly greater increase in Global Rating of Change Scale scores and walking tolerance was seen in the group receiving joint mobilization. However, the obvious differences in intervention beyond joint mobilization make it difficult to determine the direct influence of joint mobilization.

In relation to older adults with osteoporosis, the use of manual intervention techniques is controversial. For individuals with spinal osteoporosis, grade V mobilization (i.e., manipulation) has been contraindicated based on concerns for fracture risk.[171] In a survey of Canadian physical therapists by Sran and Khan,[172] 91% of the respondents reported concerns with using manual therapy for patients/clients with osteoporosis. For the same respondents, 45% have used manual therapy with this population. However, data to support the use of joint mobilization and manipulation for older adults with osteoporosis is insufficient. One published case report of a patient/client with osteoporosis, by the same authors, found that treatment including grade III and grade IV joint mobilization to thoracic and cervicothoracic regions, respectively, resulted in improvement in scores in pain level, quality of life, and function questionnaires.[173] In addition, it has been shown that anteroposterior mobilization forces are typically well below the level of force required to induce fracture in osteoporotic bones.[174] Substantially more research is needed before clear-cut recommendations can be made regarding the use of mobilization techniques for patients/clients with osteoporosis.

Assistive/Adaptive Devices and Equipment

Assistive and adaptive devices can be used as compensatory or preventive approaches to protect joint structure and assist with load transfer across joints. Devices such as canes and walkers are useful components to physical therapy intervention for individuals with joint mobility impairment. For example, Kemp et al[175] analyzed knee forces during walking in a group of 20 people (mean age 65 years) with medial knee osteoarthritis. Their finding was a mean decrease in peak knee adduction moment with cane use in the hand contralateral to the symptomatic knee. However, variability among patients/clients illustrated that technique in use of the cane is important. The suggestion is that proper training and evaluation of assistive device use is needed to ensure that patients/clients are benefiting. There is also evidence, in younger adults without joint impairment, that use of walking poles may enable people to walk with reduced vertical loads through the lower extremities, resulting in faster walking speeds.[176-178] Based on these findings, further examination of walking pole use with older adult populations is warranted.

Braces designed to alter joint alignment have also been used with older adults. Findings indicate that alignment can be altered and joint loading decreased across painful areas of osteoarthritic joints during gait function.[179-181] There is also evidence that use of unloading braces for older adults with knee osteoarthritis can result in improved functional outcomes (e.g., 6-minute walk test and stair climb testing) and patient/client reports of quality of life.[182]

Footwear can also influence loading of lower extremity joints in older adults during walking.[175,183] Selection of appropriate footwear, designed to strategically cushion and support, may be a simple way to provide immediate relief of symptoms by decreasing loads across lower extremity joints. Additionally, shoe orthotics may improve lower extremity alignment and bring about changes in joint loading.[184,185]

OUTCOMES

Observation of task performance, self-report measures of activity and participation, performance-based activity measures, and joint mobility measures from the initial examination guide the development of the patient/client's intervention goals. The design of the intervention, remediation, compensation, or prevention dictates which outcome measures are most appropriate. The outcome measures chosen can be focused at the level of impairment, activity limitation, or participation restriction. Often, self-report measures of activity and participation or performance-based measures of activity are most appropriate as the primary outcome measures because they can effectively quantify how function is influenced by the impairments. In cases of prevention intervention, direct joint mobility measures may be most appropriate for quantifying outcome.

As mentioned previously in the Tests and Measures section, selection of specific instruments is based on individual characteristics of the patient/client with joint impairment, practicality of administering the test/measure, and psychometric properties of the test/measure. The selection process is complicated by the large number of self-report and performance-based tests and measures available for use in the clinic. This section provides some recommendations of specific tests and measures appropriate for an older adult with impaired joint mobility that has negatively influenced activity or participation.

Self-Report Outcome Instruments

Self-report measures that are specific to a given region of the body, though not directly measuring joint mobility impairment, can be helpful to determine patient/client activity limitation and participation restrictions related to a given joint impairment. For example, a patient/client with impaired cervical joint mobility can be given a self-report measure designed specifically to measure their perception of function related to the cervical spine. Although there is limited research for established reliability and validity of cervical spine measures for older adults, there is some evidence that the Neck Disability Index (NDI)[186] and Neck Pain and Disability Scale (NPAD)[187] are useful for patients/clients in this age group. Chan Ci En et al[188] compared NDI and NPAD scores from

20 participants (mean age 64.5 years) who had nontraumatic neck pain, finding a high correlation between scales. In addition, the investigators concluded that there was good content validity of these two measures, based on commonality between the questionnaire items and self-identified problems by the individuals in the study.[188] Based on the relatively short time needed to complete these questionnaires, the practicality of scoring methods, and the initial evidence regarding their psychometric properties, the NDI and NPAD are relevant self-report measures to consider for use with the older adult with cervical joint impairment.

With respect to low back joint impairment, a great number of self-report measures have been developed.[189] Zanoli et al[190] identified 92 instruments designed to evaluate pain, function, disability, health status, and patient satisfaction in relation to low back impairment. In relation to older adult patients/clients with chronic low back problems, the Roland-Morris Disability Questionnaire (RMDQ)[191] and Oswestry Disability Index (ODI)[192] are two of the most established and commonly used measures. The RMDQ and ODI have established validity for measuring functional ability across wide ranges of age, including older adults.[193]

A variety of questionnaires are also available for assessing function of upper extremity joints.[194,195] Some of the most widely used instruments, with validity in measuring function in older adult populations, are the Western Ontario Osteoarthritis of the Shoulder Index (WOOS),[196] the Western Ontario Rotator Cuff Index (WORC),[197] the Rotator Cuff Quality of Life Questionnaire (RC-QOL),[198] Australian/Canadian Osteoarthritis Hand Index (AUSCAN),[199,200] and the Disabilities of the Arm, Shoulder, and Hand Questionnaire (DASH).[201] As indicated by the titles, elbow-specific measures have been generally less emphasized than shoulder and wrist. In addition, the specific type of impairment (e.g., rotator cuff injury) is a key determinant for questionnaire selection. Of these measures, the DASH is an attractive device for clinical use due to its applicability for any upper extremity joint.

Gummesson et al[202] selected 11 items from the 30-item DASH to determine if a shorter version would be valid and reliable for use with clinical populations. In their study of 105 participants (age range 18 to 83 years), they found outcomes of the 11-item scale to be highly similar to the full 30-item DASH. The conclusion is that the 11-item QuickDASH can replace the DASH while maintaining the established validity and reliability of the original questionnaire. Considering the practicality of time efficiency, the QuickDASH is recommended as a clinical tool for older adults with impaired mobility of upper extremity joints. For individuals with specific pathology, such as a rotator cuff tear or shoulder osteoarthritis, the pathology-specific questionnaires mentioned above may be more appropriate.

Functional status related to lower extremity joint impairments can also be captured using self-report measures. Various reviews have compared the psychometric properties and usefulness of lower extremity measures.[203-206] Common clinical measures with research evidence based on older adult populations are the Lower Limb Core Score,[207] Functional Ankle Disability Index (FADI),[208] Functional Ankle Ability Measure (FAAM),[209] Knee Injury and Osteoarthritis Outcome Score (KOOS),[210] Oxford Knee Score,[211] Western Ontario and McMaster Universities Osteoarthritis Index (WOMAC),[212] and Lower Extremity Functional Scale (LEFS).[213] As with the upper extremity measures, many lower extremity self-report measures are highly specific to joint and pathology. The Lower Limb Core Score and LEFS are recommended for clinical application in older adults with joint mobility impairment due to the usefulness across a variety of joints, similar to the QuickDASH for the upper extremity. Also, the therapist should consider the potential increased specificity that using a pathology-specific measure may provide to a patient/client with the given pathology.

Performance-Based Outcome Instruments

As stated previously, standardized quantitative measurement of common functional tasks adds to the information gained from self-report measures by providing information on functional performance without direct influence of the patient perceptions. The selection of an appropriate performance-based outcome instrument is based on the daily tasks that are problematic, in addition to the other considerations of appropriateness for a given patient/client, practicality, and psychometric properties. Tasks such as walking, reaching, and transitioning between postures are common targets for quantification with performance-based measures, based on the common need for these activities during daily living. The specific activities that will be measured as outcomes depend on the findings of the initial exam and the goals of the intervention.

Suggested performance-based measures of specific activities for older adults with impaired joint mobility include the functional reach test,[214] timed up and go test,[215] five times sit-to-stand test,[216] six-minute walk test,[217] stair climb test,[218] and gait speed.[219] These measures are recommended based on their appropriateness for use with older adult populations, clinical practicality, and established psychometric properties.[112,220,221] The measures must be able to capture the activity limitation that has been linked to impaired joint mobility. However, there is a need to further establish which measures are best for given impairments of joint mobility. For example, Terwee et al[222] reviewed the psychometric properties of 26 performance-based measures for individuals with hip or knee osteoarthritis. The conclusion of the authors, based on the need for establishing adequate validity and reliability, was that no consensus can yet be made on what activity measures are most appropriate for patients/clients with hip or knee osteoarthritis.[222]

There are numerous other performance-based measures that may be indirectly linked to joint mobility. A comprehensive review of all performance-based measures of activity is not in the scope of this chapter. For more information on performance-based measures related to specific activities, the reader is referred to Chapter 17 (Ambulation) and Chapter 18 (Balance and Falls) of this text.

This section of the chapter has provided some recommendations on specific outcome measures for patients with joint mobility impairment. It is important to keep in mind that joint mobility is only one part of the larger picture of a given patient/client's health and function. Perspective of the larger picture must be maintained in order to practically apply the appropriate tests and measures. An outcome measure that is appropriate, based on all impairments, limitations, and restrictions is ideal. However, it is impractical to capture the complete health and functional status of an individual with a single test or measure. Applying a reasoned approach to outcome selection will allow for a feasible number of tests and measures to be selected that can be performed in a reasonable time span to best capture the health and function of an older adult with impaired joint mobility.

SUMMARY

The health and function of older adults can be greatly influenced by impaired joint mobility. Age-associated decline in joint mobility can occur in the absence of disease or as a result of an interaction of disease processes. Any impairment of joint mobility can be linked to activity limitation and restricted participation, which often results in older adults presenting to a physical therapist for treatment. The therapist can effectively identify joint mobility impairments through systematic examination. Once identified, impaired joint mobility can be addressed as a component of the comprehensive patient/client plan of care. Therapists and patients/clients can be encouraged that an appropriate plan of care can effectively restore joint mobility and promote successful aging.

REFERENCES

To enhance this text and add value for the reader, all references are included on the companion Evolve site that accompanies this text book. The reader can view the reference source and access it online whenever possible. There are a total of 222 cited references and other general references for this chapter.

CHAPTER 14

Impaired Muscle Performance

Robin L. Marcus, PT, PhD, OCS, Karin Westlen-Boyer, PT, MPH,
Paul LaStayo, PT, PhD, CHT

INTRODUCTION

Hallmarks of aging include progressive and, in the very old, profound changes in health, body composition, and functional capacity. The age-related loss of muscle, coined *sarcopenia* in 1989,[1] is no longer simply considered another term to describe muscle atrophy associated with disuse and inactivity. The muscle wasting associated with sarcopenia can be a contributing factor to an older individual's deteriorating functional status and can manifest itself in deficits in mobility and metabolic function. With that, the definition of sarcopenia has expanded to include a loss of muscle strength (and power) and functional quality.[2] Because the relationship between the waning conditions of muscle and function is nonlinear, the clinical deficits in function may not manifest until a critical level of sarcopenia is reached. This does not, however, preclude the need for initiating muscle interventions early as a way to build muscle reserve and delay the older individual's eventual functional limitations and disabilities. Moreover, metabolic deficits stemming from sarcopenia have been linked to age-related hormonal changes that affect the muscle hypertrophic response and function, thus increasing the importance of optimizing muscle structure and function in all older individuals. Finally, the prevalence of sarcopenia is increasing in parallel with an increasing aging population, with best estimates ranging from 6% to 40% of those older than age 65 years, and this is coupled with a compounding impact as sarcopenia progresses at a rate of 1% to 3% per year after the age of 50 years.[2]

The purpose of this chapter is to review the consequences associated with sarcopenia in an aging population and collate the studies describing ways physical therapists can counter the associated adverse changes. It is not possible to assign the specific contribution to sarcopenia stemming from aging alone, decreased levels of physical activity, or the impact of comorbid conditions, but it is fair to characterize the adverse muscle and functional consequences as being compounded by all of these factors. With that, a primary focus of this chapter is placed on resistance exercises that have proven to be robust countermeasures in the face of all of these contributors to

sarcopenia; this is also supplemented with descriptions of the benefit of protein intake relative to exercise as an additional important consideration when attempting to combat sarcopenia.

CONSEQUENCES OF SARCOPENIA

The loss of skeletal muscle mass is accompanied by the loss of muscle strength, rate of force development, and muscle power. Sarcopenia contributes to deficits in mobility, a decline in functional capacity, and a reduction in skeletal muscle oxidative capacity. These muscle impairments, in combination with a greater fat mass, contribute to the greater risk of falling, frailty, and the development of comorbid conditions such as insulin resistance or type 2 diabetes that adversely impact health.

Because muscle mass represents the protein reserve of the body, sarcopenia is associated with a diminished ability to meet the extra demand of protein synthesis that is so often necessary with disease and injury in old age. As recently described by Muhlberg and Sieber,[3] sarcopenia leads to a decline in protein reserves that makes it more difficult to meet the increased protein synthesis demands that occur with disease or injury, which then leads to a worsening of the sarcopenia. Muhlberg and Sieber[3] suggest that frailty is the result of the convergence of the metabolic vicious loop of sarcopenia with neuromuscular and nutritional impairments. Figure 14-1 displays this metabolic vicious loop and a hypothesized path to frailty.

The following sections characterize the age-induced changes in muscle structure, function, and metabolism that typify sarcopenia.

Changes in Muscle Structure and Function Associated with Aging

Whole Muscle and Muscle Fiber Atrophy and Slowing. The loss of muscle mass and strength with aging is thought to be due to progressive atrophy and slowing of muscle. Lean muscle mass contributes up to 50% of total body weight in young adults, but with aging it diminishes

Path to frailty

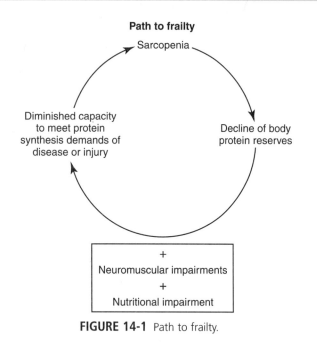

FIGURE 14-1 Path to frailty.

to 25% by age 75 to 80 years.[4,5] The cross-sectional area of the vastus lateralis is reduced by as much as 40% between the age of 20 and 80 years,[6] and the total number of muscle fibers decreases by 25%.[7,8] Box 14-1 summarizes the typical muscle changes observed in older adults. In general, the loss of muscle mass is exchanged by gains in fat mass, with the lower limb muscle groups undergoing the most atrophy. The muscle fiber is also characterized by specific type II atrophy, fiber necrosis, fiber type grouping, and a reduction in type II muscle fiber satellite cell content.[6,8-10] The more powerful myosin heavy chain (MHC) IIa (fast-twitch) muscle fibers undergo greater atrophy than the less powerful MHC I (slow twitch) muscle fibers.[6,7,11-13] The potential recovery of muscle mass following disuse is also more impaired in predominantly fast,

---

BOX 14-1 | **Typical Muscle Changes with Aging**

Whole Muscle Changes
- Decreased muscle mass, replaced by increased fat mass
- Decreased muscle strength (particularly lower extremities)
- Slowing of muscle contractile properties and rate of force development
  - Reduced rate of cross-bridge cycling
  - Alterations on excitation and contraction coupling
  - Increased compliance of muscle's tendinous attachment

Muscle Fiber Changes
- Type II (fast twitch) atrophy more than type I (slow twitch)
- Fiber necrosis
- Fiber type grouping
- Reduction in type II muscle fiber satellite cell content

Reversibility of These Changes
Exercises that overload atrophied and weak muscles can partially reverse "typical" age-related muscle changes.

---

compared to slow, muscles.[14] The slowing of muscle contractile properties can be ascribed to a reduced rate of cross-bridge cycling,[15,16] alterations on excitation and contraction coupling,[17,18] and an increased compliance of the muscle's tendinous attachment, which collectively can reduce the rate of force development.[19] When considering the clinical impact of these collective changes, physical therapists must recognize that although a complete reversal is unlikely, mitigation of these changes through interventions is very likely. Specifically, skeletal muscle is amenable to change if the correct stimuli are applied. For example, an exercise program that overloads atrophied and weak muscle should enhance muscle size, strength, and power (see section, Muscle Countermeasures for Older Individuals).

Impaired Regeneration of Muscle and the Progressive Denervation/Reinnervation Process. A primary mechanism attributed to the development of sarcopenia in those aged 60 to 65 years and older is a progressive denervation and reinnervation process involving the alpha motor neurons. A 50% decline in available motor neurons[6,20-22] and a diminished number and availability of satellite cells[23,24] that parallel the age-related temporal changes in muscle size and strength have been noted. Fiber type grouping also characterizes aging as remaining alpha motor neurons enlarge their own motor unit territory. When coupled with the reduction in alpha motor neurons and motor units, a reduced motor coordination and strength results,[6,20] which may underlie age-related mobility impairments. In addition, muscle fiber regeneration is impaired more in type II fibers than type I in large part due to the degradation of the myogenic satellite stem cells.[10] Compounding these age-related losses are reports of substantially lower basal mixed, myofibrillar, or mitochondrial muscle protein synthesis rates in older adults versus younger ones.[5,25-27] However, recent studies have failed to reproduce these findings and generally show little or no differences in basal muscle protein synthesis rates.[28-30] Likewise, the response to anabolic stimuli, that is, food intake and physical activity, may[31] or may not[32] be blunted in older adults.

Deficits in Absolute and Specific Force Generation. Consistent with the current interpretation of sarcopenia, older individuals become weaker over time. These strength deficits, however, do not necessarily match the magnitude of atrophy that has occurred. In part, this may be explained by the fact that muscle generally becomes weaker even if atrophy is avoided, which suggests that force production, separate from muscle atrophy, also is impaired with aging. Deficits in specific contractile force production (force normalized to muscle cross-sectional area) with aging has been described repeatedly in the literature.[33,34] That is, when the maximum isometric force (for aged mice and rats) is normalized to the smaller muscle fiber cross-sectional area, a significant deficit in specific force remains unexplained by atrophy.[35,36] The deficit in specific force has been shown to be a widespread phenomenon involving fast- and slow-twitch fibers in different muscles.[36] This has been reported in humans with significant differences noted in specific force in single-skinned muscle fibers between younger and older men.[37,38] Interestingly, however, a recent study demonstrated that single muscle fiber contractile function is preserved in older humans in the presence of significant alterations at the whole muscle level.[39] Currently, this discrepancy in the literature has not been resolved, but in general the consensus remains that both absolute and specific force production is adversely affected with aging. Mechanisms have been proposed that might explain the skeletal muscle weakness associated with aging; however, whether the loss of specific and absolute force share common mechanisms is not known at the present time. It appears that the age-related impairment in muscle force is only partially explained by the loss in muscle mass. Therefore, both the loss in specific and absolute forces contributes to the muscle weakness measured in older adult and in animal models of aging. This global weakness of muscle underscores the need for effective countermeasures that not only increase the size of the muscle but also the functional ability of muscle.

Muscle Activation Deficits. The declining force production abilities with aging occur at a faster rate than the decline in muscle mass; hence, neural alterations are also thought to contribute to muscle weakness by reducing central drive to the agonist muscles and by increasing coactivation of the antagonist muscles.[40-42] Researchers have attempted to quantify the contribution of impaired voluntary drive to the decline in muscle force using superimposed electrical stimulation during maximal voluntary contractions and by recording surface electromyographic activity. Although reduced voluntary activation of agonist muscles and increased coactivation of antagonist muscles have been reported with advancing age, such changes are not supported by all studies.[43] Clinically, when encountering an older patient with an apparent inhibition/cocontraction of their muscle(s), a detailed assessment of other potential contributors (e.g., pain and central or peripheral nervous system disorder) should be performed. After therapeutically addressing these other contributors, a cautious yet progressive resistance exercise program can be initiated, with or without supplemental neuromuscular electrical stimulation, in an attempt to reverse the muscle activation deficits.

Deteriorating Muscle Quality and Metabolism. A reduction in muscle "quality" due to infiltration of fat and other noncontractile material such as connective tissue,[44,45] coupled with changes in muscle metabolism, also contribute to the deteriorating muscle condition and advancing frailty with age.[46-48] In addition, oxidative damage accumulated over time is thought to lead to mitochondrial DNA mutations,[49] impaired mitochondrial function,[50] muscle proteolysis, and myonuclear apoptosis.[51] Collectively, these impairments are thought to play additional and prominent roles in the age-associated loss of function.

Changes in Metabolic Function Associated with Aging

Whole body resting metabolic rate (RMR) progressively declines at a rate of 1% to 2% per decade after 20 years of age.[52] This change is linked with age-associated decreases in metabolically active whole-body fat-free mass[53,54]; however, whether this change is due solely to loss of fat-free tissue is currently a topic of debate. Even after correcting for differences in body composition, RMR remains significantly lower in older than younger adults[55]; thus reductions in metabolically active mass (including muscle)[56] as well as declines in specific metabolic rates of tissues likely contribute to the overall age-related decline in RMR.[57]

Altered Endocrine Function and Its Consequences. Box 14-2 lists age-related hormone changes commonly linked to sarcopenia, including insulin, growth hormone, insulin-like growth hormone I (IGF-I), estrogens, testosterone, parathyroid hormone (PTH), and vitamin D. There is significant controversy as to the effects of these changes on skeletal muscle mass and strength, though the following synopsis reflects current thinking.

Insulin, the main postprandial hormone, is a critical regulator of protein metabolism in muscle, and its anabolic action is essential for protein gain and muscle growth.[58,59] Lack of insulin, such as that seen in individuals with type 1 diabetes, is associated with substantial muscle protein mass wasting.[60] Progressive resistance to the actions of insulin is commonly reported in the older adults. In addition, it is becoming increasingly well accepted that sarcopenia is accompanied by increased whole body, regional, and intramyocellular adipose stores and that this fatty infiltration is also accompanied by increased insulin resistance.[61] Considering the important role that insulin plays in stimulating skeletal muscle protein synthesis, and the evidence that this role may be impaired in aging muscle,[62-64] insulin treatment in older adults has now been suggested as an appropriate therapeutic strategy to enhance muscle protein gain and possibly to mitigate the development of sarcopenia.

BOX 14-2	Aging-Associated Changes in Endocrine Function Linked to Sarcopenia

- Increased insulin resistance
- Decreased growth hormone
- Decreased insulin-like growth hormone (IGF-I)
- Decreased estrogen and testosterone
- Vitamin D deficiency
- Increased parathyroid hormone (PTH)

Caution must be exercised with this strategy though, because in nondiabetic older individuals, insulin treatment could involve serious risk of hypoglycemia that would likely worsen during exercise.

Growth hormone (GH) and IGF-I have each been implicated as potential contributors to sarcopenia, and both are frequently deficient in older adults.[65] Although GH has been reported to lower fat mass, increase lean tissue mass, and improve lipid profiles, a recent systematic review of 31 studies representing 18 unique study populations that compared healthy older adults who were GH treated to a non–GH-treated control sample concluded that GH treatment in healthy older adults is not supported by a robust evidence base.[66] Further, this review revealed that GH supplementation is associated with substantial adverse events including joint pain and soft tissue edema in the healthy older adults and should not be recommended for use in this population. IGF-I, a growth factor that stimulates skeletal muscle protein synthesis and inhibits protein degradation, plays a critical role in signaling a hypertrophic response in aging skeletal muscle.[67] This role is recognized by activating satellite cell differentiation and proliferation, and increasing protein synthesis in existing fibers.[68,69] Although there appears to be consensus regarding the role of IGF-I in improving muscle mass, the effects on muscle strength and function are equivocal.[70-75] This suggests that IGF-I may increase noncontractile proteins and possibly fluid retention in muscle. When evaluating the impact of any intervention on muscle mass, caution must be advised when the method used to assess muscle mass (such as anthropometry, bioelectrical impedance analysis, or densitometry) is unable to differentiate aqueous from nonaqueous components.

Epidemiologic studies suggest that estrogens prevent muscle loss,[76,77] though clinical trials have not found a relationship between hormone replacement therapy (HRT)—sometimes referred to as estrogen replacement therapy (ERT)—and increased muscle mass.[78] Moreover, the data on the relationship between estrogens and muscle strength are equivocal, as HRT has been shown to be associated with increased muscle strength in some studies[78] but not in all.[79] The association of estrogen with strength improvements does not seem to be supported by an anabolic effect, as estrogens indirectly decrease the level of serum free testosterone[80] and this should have a negative impact on muscle mass.[81] Epidemiologic studies also suggest a relationship between low levels of testosterone and loss of lean muscle, strength, and function in older adults. Further, studies support the hypothesis that low levels of testosterone result in lower protein synthesis and loss of muscle mass.[82] Results of the effectiveness of testosterone therapy on muscle strength and function in community-dwelling older adults, however, are inconclusive.[83] Although in general the administration of testosterone to older subjects results in moderate improvements in muscle mass, there

have been few reports of concomitant improvements in muscle strength. This may in fact be due to the low levels of testosterone supplementation that are commonly employed in these studies, as there are concerns that testosterone replacement at higher levels may accelerate the usually slow progression of prostate cancer in older men.

Vitamin D deficiency is common in older adults.[84,85] Declining 25-hydroxyvitamin D (25-OHD) levels are also associated with low muscle mass,[86] low muscle strength,[87] poor physical performance,[88,89] and increased risk for falls in older individuals.[90,91] In ambulatory individuals older than age 65 years, a vitamin D deficiency (<10 ng/mL) indicates that individuals may be more than twice as likely to be sarcopenic than those at higher vitamin D levels (>20 ng/mL) based on both muscle weakness and on muscle mass loss. In a similar population, those with the lowest mean values of 25-OHD (14 ng/mL) performed worse (3.9%) on the sit-to-stand test and 8-meter walk test (5.6%) than those with higher mean levels (42 ng/mL), even after adjustment for age, sex, ethnicity, body mass index (BMI), number of comorbid conditions, use of an assistive device, or activity level. In addition, a recent meta-analysis concludes that vitamin D supplementation in older adults with stable health may reduce the risk of falls by more than 20%.[92] These associations may be explained by the observations that vitamin D may influence muscle protein turnover through reduced insulin secretion,[93] and low levels of vitamin D have been shown to decrease muscle anabolism.[94] Because of the strong associations between vitamin D and sarcopenia, it is recommended that older individuals be screened for vitamin D deficiency, and if found to be less than 30 ng/mL, vitamin D supplements should be considered.[95]

Consistent with the positive associations observed between low levels of vitamin D and age, elevated levels of PTH are also commonly seen in older adults both independently[96,97] and in combination with vitamin D deficiency.[98,99] Evidence linking elevated PTH to sarcopenia is found in the positive associations between higher PTH levels and falls in nursing home residents,[100] and between higher PTH levels and grip strength and muscle mass in community-dwelling older persons.[86] Further, studies of patients with hyperparathyroidism demonstrate not only impaired muscle function but also improved muscle function following treatment.[101,102] Despite these findings, the question of whether hyperparathyroidism is a primary cause of muscle structural and functional impairments remains unanswered as low vitamin D levels stimulate PTH production. PTH may influence muscle directly through impaired energy production, transfer and utilization,[103] muscle protein metabolism,[104] or altering calcium concentrations,[105] or indirectly through the production of proinflammatory cytokines.[106] Vitamin D supplementation, as well as an increased exposure to sunlight, will help to normalize vitamin D status and indirectly PTH levels as well.

Cytokines and Adiposity. Aging, as well as several chronic medical conditions (chronic obstructive pulmonary disease [COPD], heart disease, cancer, diabetes) that are prevalent with increasing age, is associated with a gradual increase in the production of proinflammatory cytokines (responsible for accelerating inflammation and regulating inflammatory reactions), chronic inflammation, and loss of lean body mass. Although it is currently unknown whether cytokines predict the occurrence of sarcopenia, sarcopenia has been suggested to be one of the outcomes of the cytokine-related aging process.[107] Associations between elevated levels of tumor necrosis factor–α (TNF-α), interleukin 6 (IL-6), C-reactive protein (CRP) muscle mass, and muscle strength have been reported,[108-110] though the role of these cytokines appears complex.

Several hypotheses have been put forward as potential explanations of how inflammation contributes to sarcopenia. One hypothesis is that increased proinflammatory cytokines contribute to an imbalance between muscle protein synthesis and breakdown, with the net result favoring protein breakdown.[111] A second hypothesis is that inflammation increases activation of the protein-degrading ubiquitin–protease pathway.[112] Finally, inflammation is accompanied by a decrease in IGF-I, and TNF-α in particular may stimulate muscle loss through the activation of the apoptosis pathway.[75]

Additional evidence implicating an inflammatory role in sarcopenia is found in the link between obesity and inflammation.[113,114] Sarcopenic obesity, a condition that combines excess adiposity with loss of lean tissue is defined as appendicular skeletal muscle mass adjusted for stature (ASM/Ht^2), or body mass (ASM/kg). Using the most conservative measure (ASM/Ht^2) reveals that sarcopenic obesity occurs in 2% of older adults up to age 70 years and up to 10% of those older than age 80 years.[115,116] Although not clearly established, the relationship between sarcopenic obesity and increased fatty infiltration of skeletal muscle has been reported.[117,118] This finding is especially interesting in light of the significant associations reported between fatty infiltration of muscle and decreased strength,[119,120] physical function,[121] and the future risk of a mobility limitation.[122] Motor unit recruitment is also reduced in the presence of muscle fatty infiltration,[121] and increased fatty acids in muscle fibers result in abnormal cellular signaling.[123] Taken together, the current evidence suggests a role for fat mass in the etiology and pathogenesis of sarcopenia. Alternatively, because sarcopenia occurs regardless of adiposity changes with aging, it may be that the associated chronic low-level inflammatory state that is associated with aging itself, and not just obesity, could lead to accelerated muscle loss in the older adults.

Mitochondrial Dysfunction. The role of mitochondrial dysfunction in sarcopenia is controversial. The aging-associated damage to muscle mitochondrial DNA (mtDNA) may reduce the rate of muscle cell protein synthesis, adenosine triphosphate (ATP) synthesis,[124] and ultimately may lead to the death of muscle fibers and loss of muscle mass.[125,126] Consistent with other metabolic changes that are seen with aging, because these mitochondrial abnormalities have also been shown to be at least partially reversible with exercise,[127,128] these abnormalities may also be the result of inactivity. However, recent evidence identifying mitochondrial abnormalities and dysfunction in older adults subjects across species[129,130] suggests that the mitochondrial changes seen in older humans[131,132] are not due to decreased physical activity alone. The clinical importance of the early reports of improved mitochondrial gene transcription[131] and function[127,128] as a result of exercise training suggests that this research area should be closely monitored by physical therapists.

Apoptosis. The role of apoptosis in sarcopenia is currently being investigated and although it remains uncertain, apoptosis may represent the link between mitochondria dysfunction and loss of muscle in older adults. Research on animal models strongly suggests that apoptosis plays a key role in age-related loss of muscle,[133-135] and that aged muscle has a different apoptotic response to disuse than younger muscle. Age-related loss of myocytes via apoptosis has been suggested to be a key mechanism behind the muscle loss associated with human aging[136] as well, though this evidence is preliminary. Recent data demonstrate that physical exercise can mitigate skeletal muscle apoptosis in aged animals.[137] These basic science considerations should prompt the clinician to consider exercise as not only a counter to loss of physical fitness and function, but perhaps also a mode of slowing down the apoptotic pathways underlying sarcopenia. Readers are referred to a recent review[138] on this topic.

Diseases and Conditions Associated with Skeletal Muscle Decline. Sarcopenia is specifically defined as the *age-related* loss of skeletal muscle mass and strength. Independent of age, however, muscle loss is also a primary impairment that is associated with a variety of disease states. Box 14-3 lists diseases and conditions common in older adults that are associated with skeletal muscle decline. Each of these diseases and conditions can potentially influence the progression of age-related skeletal muscle decline.[139] Cachexia is a hallmark impairment in cancer, COPD, and congestive heart failure (CHF); increased inflammatory levels are present in arthritis, cancer, COPD, CHF, diabetes, metabolic syndrome, kidney disease, and stroke; and all are often accompanied by a sedentary lifestyle. Disease-related inactivity in these individuals then becomes a secondary factor that contributes to the equation of muscle loss.

Influence of Genetics. Genetic epidemiologic studies suggest that between 36% and 65% of an individual's muscle strength and up to 57% of their lower extremity performance can be explained by heredity.[140-143] Moreover, several genetic factors have been identified that contribute

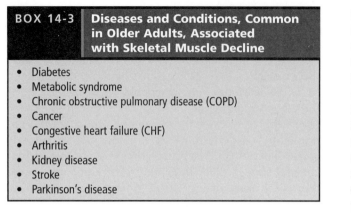

BOX 14-3 | Diseases and Conditions, Common in Older Adults, Associated with Skeletal Muscle Decline

- Diabetes
- Metabolic syndrome
- Chronic obstructive pulmonary disease (COPD)
- Cancer
- Congestive heart failure (CHF)
- Arthritis
- Kidney disease
- Stroke
- Parkinson's disease

to muscle mass and strength.[144,145] As more information concerning the gene expression patterns surrounding sarcopenia become available, future treatment strategies can be expected to be aimed at these gene targets.

MUSCLE COUNTERMEASURES FOR OLDER INDIVIDUALS

Resistance Exercise

The concept of resistance training in older adults is not unlike that in younger adults: providing muscles with an overload stimulus will lead to an improvement in the muscle's force-producing capability, thus helping to mitigate sarcopenia. Adaptive changes that result from resistance training include improved muscle strength and power, enhanced levels of mobility, a hypertrophic response, and improved muscle composition. The optimal magnitude of the overload stimulus that induces these changes in older adults, however, is not clear. Further, both increased habitual physical activity and nutritional supplementation are also alluring potential countermeasures for sarcopenia.

Resistance training for individuals age 65 years and older induces predictable increases in muscle strength, muscle power, and mobility function in community-dwelling older persons,[146-149] nursing home inhabitants,[150-154] and the hospitalized older adults.[155-157] Significant improvements in strength and mobility function have also been reported in individuals 80 years of age and older.[151,152,158-160] Several recent review papers on this topic[161-165] have successfully cataloged these beneficial adaptations and ingrained the notion that resistance exercise for older individuals is effective. Evidence of this has existed as early as 1998 in the American College of Sports Medicine Position Stand on Exercise and Physical Activity for Older Adults, where resistance training is recommended as an important component of an overall fitness program. Increases in muscle size, though in absolute terms less than that seen in younger individuals, are also a by-product of resistance training programs in older individuals. Regardless, the ability to increase muscle size with resistance training appears to remain intact, at least

through the seventh decade,[166,167] but may diminish after age 80 years.[151,160,168] Because the increases in muscle strength and power that occur in older adults oftentimes exceed that expected with the muscle size improvements, the variable of muscle quality or force produced per unit of muscle mass has gained recent interest. Increased muscle quality from resistance training is a common finding among older adults, and in men there appears to be no difference in young versus old[169] though there is some evidence that older women may have a blunted response relative to younger women.[170] Just as changes in muscle composition (increased fatty infiltration) have been shown to accompany aging, resistance training has also been recently found to be associated with maintenance or return of skeletal muscle, specifically in the legs, to a more youthful composition.[171,172] Box 14-4 highlights some of the key resistance exercise considerations discussed in the upcoming pages.

Dosage Considerations for Resistance Exercise. In order for these positive adaptations to take place, resistance exercise can be performed at different intensities, at different frequencies per week, and at different volumes per session. Resistance training with loads that range from 20% of the maximum weight that an individual can lift (1 RM), to greater than 80% 1 RM have resulted in significant gains in muscle strength, muscle power, and mobility in older individuals.[146-149,151,152,158,161,166,177-189] There is evidence that older individuals who train with loads at or below 50% of the 1 RM can improve their strength, stair-climbing ability, gait speed, and balance to a level equivalent to those exercising with higher-intensity exercise.[146,149,158,160,184,186,189] Despite this, recent guidelines from the American College of Sports Medicine recommend resistance training with a minimum of moderate (5 to 6 on a 1-to-10 scale) intensity.[190] Further, a recent systematic review by Liu[163] suggests that high-intensity strength training results in greater improvements in lower extremity strength compared to low-intensity exercise, based on the studies reviewed.[146,149,157,158,183,186,189,191,192] Although the literature lacks a clear distinction of what

BOX 14-4 | Evidence-Supported Suggestions for Resistance Training with Older Adults

- Resistance exercise—against sufficient load—can increase muscle strength and power, even in the very old
- Effective exercise options:
  - Intensities >50% of 1 RM, performed two to three times per week, with one to three sets per exercise session[161,162,164,165]
  - Intensities >60% 1 RM,[173] performed one to two times per week, with one to three sets per exercise session
- For individuals older than age 80 years, resistance exercise one time per week at high intensity (70% to 80% 1 RM) may add benefit[148]
- Eccentric resistance exercise at high intensity is particularly beneficial for older adults[159,174-176]

constitutes the ideal intensity dosage for resistance exercise in older adults, the findings that older individuals respond positively to a variety of different intensities suggests that aging muscle is responding to resistance training with both neural and structural adaptations.

Training frequencies of one, two, or three times per week have all resulted in strength improvements.[148] When older individuals train with greater loads (at or above 1 RM) there is evidence that training at a lower frequency (one time per week) at this higher intensity[148,193] induces improvements in strength and neuromuscular performance that are similar to those achieved with a two- and even three-times-per-week training frequency. As well, training at higher intensities may result in greater sustainability of the strength gains. Although exercise volume has not been studied extensively in older adults, it appears that gains in muscle power,[194] strength,[148,195,196] and physical functioning[189,197] in older adults may be achieved with less exercise volume (either lower frequency per week, or less overall volume per week, e.g., one set vs. three sets) than that required by younger adults.

Overall, it appears that maximum benefit relative to strength, power, and mobility function from resistance training in older adults can be achieved with intensities greater than 50% of 1 RM, performed two to three times per week, with one to three sets per exercise session.[161,162,164,165] The available literature suggests that maximizing volume is more important than frequency; hence, if frequencies of one or two times per week are used, intensity should be progressively increased to 60% to 80% 1 RM. As well, if muscle size improvements (hypertrophy) are the primary goal of a training program, higher overall intensities of greater than 60% 1 RM[173] and higher volume are recommended. When considering resistance training for individuals older than age 80 years, it may be particularly effective to exercise less frequently (one time per week), at higher relative intensities, in order to optimize the sustainability of strength gains, while not exhausting the older individual's energy reserves. Older individuals should be monitored closely for adverse reactions to resistance training. Although there are risks to participation in a resistance-training program, the evidence is strong that physical activity, of which resistance training can be considered a subset, significantly reduces the age-associated risk of chronic disease, with the benefits outweighing the risks of participation.[190]

Adaptations in Muscle Strength and Mobility Levels with Resistance Exercise. Without a doubt, older individuals who participate in at least 6 to 12 weeks of resistance training will improve their strength and mobility function.[161,162,164,165,190,198] A 2009 systematic review reporting on 73 exercise trials with 3059 participants revealed that progressive resistance training had a large positive effect on muscle strength; thus, there is overwhelming evidence that older adults can substantially increase strength following resistance training.[163] Strength improvements range from 25% to well over 100%. However, the influence of age on the capacity to increase strength is complex, as some studies report the same response in older versus younger individuals,[32,199-202] whereas others report a blunted response in the old.[203-206] There are also other variables that affect the strength response. The effects of age may be influenced by gender,[146,169,207] duration of training,[208] or muscle groups investigated.

A recent Cochrane review[163] confirms that resistance training improves not only strength but also functional abilities in older adults. This review revealed modest improvements in gait speed (24 trials, 1179 participants, mean difference [MD] = 0.08 m/s; 95% confidence interval [CI], 0.04 to 0.12) and a moderate to large improvement for getting out of a chair (11 trials, 384 participants, standardized mean difference [SMD] = −0.94; 95% CI, −1.49 to −0.38). Data from 12 trials that assessed the timed up-and-go test revealed that participants of resistance training programs took significantly less time to complete this task (MD = −0.69 second; 95% CI, −1.11 to −0.27). In addition, time to climb stairs, available from only eight trials, favored the resistance training groups, but was quite heterogeneous, and there were small but nonsignificant improvements for balance in the resistance-trained groups.

Adaptations in Muscle Power with Resistance Exercise. Resistance training that specifically targets muscle power (40% to 70% 1 RM, "as fast as possible") has a significant impact on physical functioning as well as muscle power production and muscle strength. Leg muscle power—the ability to generate force rapidly—is a strong predictor of both self-reported functional status[209] and falls[210] in older adults, and it accounts for a large percentage of the variance in physical functioning in older individuals.[11,211] Leg muscle power is especially important when considering that muscle power declines more sharply than strength in older individuals.[212-215] Previous literature suggests that 4 to 16 weeks of power training results in robust (100% to 150%) improvements in leg muscle power in both healthy[173,199,208,216,217] and impaired[152,190,218] older individuals. Although some authors have reported a dose–response relationship with power training,[218,219] more recent evidence[220] suggests that the gains in leg muscle power resulting from a three-times-per-week, 12-week high-velocity power training regimen were not only similar to more traditional slow-velocity strength training but also less than power improvements reported previously by other authors.[216,218] This may be because previous authors have studied healthier populations,[177,216] or self-reported performance measures only,[218] where the recent study measured actual performance in more disabled individuals. There may not be a clear advantage for power training over high-force slow-velocity resistance training with respect to physical function, power production, or strength enhancement.

However, it does appear that power training in older individuals is well tolerated and can counteract the age-related decline in neuromuscular function that is customarily observed with aging. Power training may be especially efficacious when considering that it may be performed in a shorter time per session and that fewer sessions per week may be necessary to capitalize on the associated improvements.[221]

Adaptations in Muscle Size and Composition with Resistance Exercise. The impact of resistance training on muscle hypertrophy, an expected outcome in the young, is less predictable in older individuals, especially those older than age 80 years. Early studies suggested that older muscle responded to resistance training with a robust hypertrophic effect, but more recently that assertion has been challenged. Slivka et al[168] recently reported limited muscle plasticity in men age 80 years or older after 12 weeks of resistance training at 70% 1 RM. Older women (mean age 85 years) have also been reported to have a blunted hypertrophy response at both the whole muscle and fiber level.[206] This limited hypertrophic response may or may not be important clinically as muscle size has been reported to be less influential than muscle power and strength on functional mobility.[11,211] However, considering that cross-sectional area is an important variable in the muscle power equation (force = mass × acceleration, power = force × velocity), it may be prudent to recommend individuals begin resistance training prior to age 80 in order to realize the maximal hypertrophic response.

Although sarcopenia is a well-accepted characteristic of normal aging, aging muscle is also associated with an increase in fat infiltration.[45,119,222] Increased fat infiltration has been associated with abnormal metabolic consequences[223-225] and, more recently, with both muscle strength[119] and mobility limitations in older adults[120,122] and those with diabetes.[226] A recent review paper suggests that muscle fat infiltration may in fact be more important than muscle lean when referring to mobility function.[227] The effects of resistance training on altering muscle composition in older individuals is only now beginning to be investigated.[172,174] Resistance training appears to be a promising modality to counter this fatty infiltration.

Both the total amount of muscle and its composition appear to be critical to overall health. Low body mass has been linked with sarcopenia, and sarcopenia with frailty. In some older individuals, resistance training that induces muscle hypertrophy may be critical for solely increasing muscle mass, or by combining increased muscle mass and muscle force-producing capabilities, resistance training may enhance muscle strength and power. This is especially important when taken in the context of older individuals with limited muscle energetic reserves secondary to comorbid conditions that often accompany aging. Further research should attempt to define the critical variables for

improving muscle mass in older adults, and specifically in those older than 80 years of age.

Resistance Exercise via Negative, Eccentrically Induced Work. Physical functioning requires muscle to function concentrically, isometrically, and eccentrically. Although direct comparisons of resistance training with the three modes of muscle contraction are not found in the literature, there is evidence suggesting that resistance training that exploits the high-force–producing capabilities of eccentric muscle activity are both feasible and effective for older individuals. Because eccentric resistance training can produce high forces at relatively low energetic costs,[228-231] eccentrically biased resistance training programs are especially useful in an older population. A recent systematic review and meta-analysis[232] compared the effects of eccentric and concentric resistance training on muscle strength and muscle mass in healthy adults. This review revealed that, compared to concentric resistance training, eccentric resistance training performed at high intensities was associated with greater improvements in total and eccentric strength, and that these strength gains were more pronounced when the velocity of testing and training was the same. The authors also concluded that eccentric resistance training was more effective at promoting overall increases in muscle mass. Finally, the superior gains in both strength and mass were thought to be mediated by the capacity to achieve higher forces during eccentric muscle actions. This review included adults up to age 65 years. Although there is limited evidence comparing the effectiveness of eccentric resistance training in older individuals, the available literature suggests findings similar to that found in younger adults.[159,174,175,233] Older adults with and without significant comorbidities can realize muscle strength, size, and functional mobility improvements from eccentric resistance training that are superior to those achieved in the concentrically trained comparison groups.

Nutritional Intake as a Countermeasure for Sarcopenia

In addition to decreased physical activity, inadequate protein intake may also contribute to sarcopenia. Inadequate protein intake in a malnourished older individual is a barrier to building muscle mass and strength even when the individual is participating in a resistance training program. Nutritional intake, like exercise, is a modifiable countermeasure that may help to minimize loss of lean muscle tissue and muscle strength in older adults, though there is significant controversy as to the amount, quality, and timing of protein supplementation in this population. There is general agreement that, in order for resistance exercise to stimulate muscle hypertrophy, there must be a positive energy balance and adequate protein intake.[176] In order to achieve a positive protein balance, muscle protein synthesis (MPS), stimulated by resistance exercise and by feeding, must be greater than muscle protein breakdown. The accumulation of these acute periods of positive protein balance will result in increased muscle fiber protein content and, finally, in increased muscle cross-sectional area. Several studies support the ability of dietary protein to acutely stimulate MPS in older adults.[29,234-236] However, there is no current consensus on the amount of protein intake that is necessary for the maintenance of muscle mass, strength, and metabolic function in older adults, or whether the current recommendations of 0.8 g/kg/day for all adults are adequate for older individuals.[237] Although very high protein diets (>45% energy) have been associated with adverse events,[238,239] diets containing a moderate amount of protein (20% to 35% energy) do not appear to be associated with poor health outcomes.[240,241] Current literature suggests that moderately increasing daily protein intake to 1.0 to 1.3 g/kg/day may enhance muscle protein anabolism and mitigate some of the loss of muscle mass associated with age.[242,243] Moderate protein intake (30 g) at any one meal need not exceed 113 g or about 4 ounces of lean meat. More information on adequate protein consumption and nutritional information for older adults can be found at http://fnic.nal.usda.gov. Although there is little evidence linking high protein intakes with impaired kidney function in healthy men and women, higher protein intake may be contraindicated in individuals with renal disease.[244]

The primary variable affected by resistance exercise appears to be MPS, which is stimulated 40% to 100% over resting rate with exercise.[245-247] There appears to be subtle differences in the ability of different protein sources to promote MPS. Recent research suggests that essential amino acids stimulate protein anabolism in older adults, in whom nonessential amino acids added to essential amino acids have no additive effect.[248,249] Currently, it is recommended that all meals for older adults contain a moderate amount of high-quality protein. Timing protein supplementation in association with a resistance-training program may also affect the anabolic response. Protein supplementation immediately before or immediately after a resistance training session has been reported to be more successful at enhancing muscle hypertrophy[250-254] than protein supplementation not closely associated with the exercise session.

SUMMARY

The muscle structural and functional changes associated with sarcopenia contribute to a greater risk of falling, frailty, and mobility impairment in older adults. Because muscle is critical to both mobility and metabolism, the development of muscle-related comorbid conditions, like insulin resistance and type 2 diabetes, amplify the clinical impairments associated with muscle loss. Coupled with a variety of other disease states, age-associated loss of muscle mass and strength is compounded by the primary muscle loss that is often associated with cancer, COPD, CHF, arthritis, diabetes, kidney disease, stroke, and Parkinson's disease as well as the secondary muscle loss that is accompanied by a disease-imposed sedentary lifestyle. Overarching all of these disease states is a progressive inflammatory and apoptotic milieu that accelerates these impairments and functional limitations. Although the specific mechanisms underlying the development and treatment of sarcopenia have yet to be elucidated, several candidate interventions have been suggested to both prevent and reverse muscle loss. Currently, resistance exercise is the most widely accepted countermeasure that has definitive evidence to mitigate muscle loss in older adults. Nutritional intervention is also a promising therapeutic approach to treating sarcopenia.

REFERENCES

To enhance this text and add value for the reader, all references are included on the companion Evolve site that accompanies this text book. The reader can view the reference source and access it online whenever possible. There are a total of 254 cited references and other general references for this chapter.

CHAPTER 15

Impaired Motor Control

Catherine E. Lang, PT, PhD

Human beings have the capacity to execute an enormous repertoire of movements. Our movement repertoire spans typical daily activities such as sitting, transfers, and walking as well as a multitude of specialized capabilities such as dancing, piano playing, and skiing. Compared to young children, adults and older adults typically use only a fraction of many possible movements. Each movement, regardless of its purpose, can be thought of as a concert of complex muscle actions. Like the notes and instruments in a musical concert, each muscle used in the movement must be turned on *just the right amount* and *at just the right time* to produce a coordinated movement. Some muscles provide the melody (agonist and antagonist muscles) while other muscles play on in the background (preparatory and/or supporting muscle activity). The brain and spinal cord are the instruments that play this beautiful concert of muscle actions. Impairments in motor control are the result of breakdowns within and between these instruments.

This chapter opens with a discussion of the most common motor control impairments seen in adults and their neural mechanisms. Next, examination and interpretation of findings related to impaired motor control are covered at the impairment and activity limitation levels. The chapter then discusses the issues relevant to making human movement system diagnoses and prognoses in adults with impaired motor control. The chapter concludes with information on outcome assessment and treatment for these impairments. Discussion and examples in this chapter often emphasize movement control in people with stroke because stroke is the most common cause of motor control impairments in older adults. Additionally, particular attention is placed on upper extremity movement control as several other chapters provide detailed discussion of lower extremity and trunk considerations related to postural control (Chapter 16), balance (Chapter 18), and mobility and gait (Chapter 17). Motor control impairments in adults are usually a result of a disease or health condition and not a result of the normal aging process. It is this author's bias that motor control impairments in older adults are not different from motor control impairments in younger adults. What may or may not differ with older adults are the movement goals a person wants to achieve and the health status of the body

with which they are trying to achieve them (e.g., other existing comorbidities).

COMMON MOTOR CONTROL IMPAIRMENTS

Motor control is the ability to regulate or direct movements.[1] The field of motor control is focused on studying movement and the neural control of movement. Neural control of movement involves the cooperation of numerous structures within the nervous system. Figure 15-1 provides a simplified overview of the critical neural structures associated with motor control. The motor cortical areas include the primary motor cortex and nonprimary cortical motor areas, such as the premotor and supplementary motor areas. These areas work together to plan and execute voluntary movements. They communicate with the spinal cord and muscles via the corticospinal tract. The corticospinal tract makes both direct (monosynaptic) and indirect (di- or polysynaptic) connections to spinal motoneurons controlling muscles of the trunk and limbs. The reticulospinal tract assists the corticospinal tract in communicating movement information from subcortical structures to the spinal cord. Spinal cord circuitry includes peripheral afferents (sensory neurons), interneurons, and motoneurons that work in concert with the descending motor commands to produce movement. The major role of the cerebellum is coordination and correction of movement. The basal ganglia focuses the selection of desired movements and inhibits competing movements. Sensory information about the body and environment is used in a feedforward manner to plan movements and as feedback about recent or ongoing movements. This overview provides a foundation from which to examine motor control impairments.

Motor control impairments in older adults result from medical conditions that preferentially affect this population, such as stroke or Parkinson's disease. Box 15-1 lists the major motor and sensory system impairments contributing to motor control deficits.

Figure 15-2 is a conceptual model of how motor control impairments contribute to activity limitations and participation restrictions in adults. More often than not,

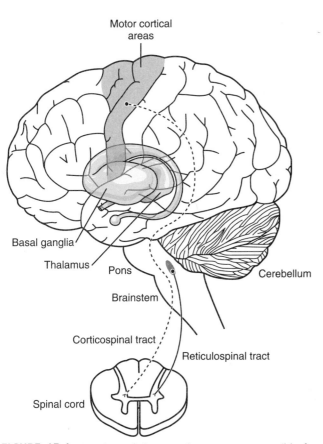

FIGURE 15-1 Overview of the neural structures responsible for control of movement. The corticospinal system is made up of the motor cortical areas, corticospinal tract, and spinal cord.

BOX 15-1	Major Motor Control Body Structure and Functional Impairments

Motor System Impairments
Paresis
Abnormal tone
Fractionated movement deficits
Ataxia
Hypokinesia

Sensory System Impairments
Somatosensory loss
Perceptual deficits

patients have multiple motor control impairments, as represented by gray, overlapping circles. The central nervous system (CNS) condition will determine the prognosis for recovery from the motor control impairments. Motor control impairments directly limit activities and restrict participation. The direct activity limitations associated with motor control impairments also lead to additional, secondary impairments that further affect activity and participation. For example, decreased endurance may develop in the presence of paresis when the patient has difficulty ambulating or participating in general exercise programs. Furthermore, the presence of

comorbid impairments can further compound an older adult's movement problems. The ovals representing secondary and comorbid impairments are large, representing the idea that these are the areas that may be most amenable to change with rehabilitation. The onset of motor control impairments together with preexisting comorbid impairments such as muscle weakness and pain in an older person can easily push them down the "slippery slope" to loss of independence with daily activities.

Paresis

The most common motor impairment is paresis. Paresis is the reduced ability to voluntarily activate the spinal motoneurons. Total paresis is called plegia, reflecting a complete inability to voluntarily activate the motoneurons. In the clinical examination, paresis manifests as weakness during movement in gravity-eliminated positions, against gravity, and/or against manual resistance. Paresis can result from a wide range of neurologic conditions, such as stroke, multiple sclerosis, cerebral palsy, amyotrophic lateral sclerosis, traumatic brain injury, Guillain–Barré syndrome, peripheral neuropathy, polio, postpolio syndrome, and spinal cord injury. The medical condition will determine the distribution of the paresis and other accompanying motor control impairments. A number of prefixes are used with the terms *paresis* or *plegia* to define their distribution. Although most of what we know about paresis comes from studies of stroke, the neural mechanisms underlying paresis are the same regardless of what causes it.

Paresis can be largely considered a problem of movement execution.[2] The primary mechanism underlying paresis is damage to the corticospinal system, that is, the motor cortical areas, the corticospinal tract, and the spinal cord (schematically drawn in Figure 15-1). Figure 15-3 illustrates how the disruption of corticospinal system input alters the activation of motor units,[3-9] the activation of muscles,[10-18] the activation of sets of muscles,[19,20] and the ability to move. Together, the changes in the ability to volitionally activate motor units, muscles, and sets of muscles can explain much of the observed alterations and compensatory movement patterns seen in people with paresis. For example, the diminished ability to sufficiently activate the hip and knee extensor muscles when moving from sit-to-stand often results in increased time to complete the transfer, multiple attempts, and the use of compensatory strategies. Likewise, the common observation in the person post stroke of hip circumduction on the affected side during the swing phase of gait is a compensatory action due to the failure to activate hip flexors and ankle dorsiflexors with sufficient speed and appropriate timing. For upper extremity movements, paresis results in slower, less accurate, and less efficient reaching and grasping movements.[21,22]

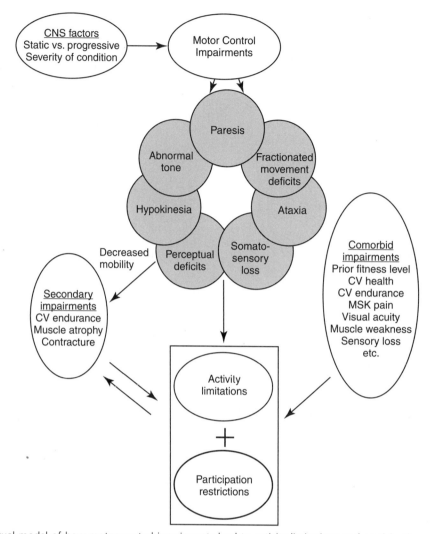

FIGURE 15-2 Conceptual model of how motor control impairments lead to activity limitations and participation restrictions of movement. Patients typically have multiple motor control impairments, represented by the gray, overlapping circles. The central nervous system (CNS) condition will determine the prognosis for recovery. Motor control impairments directly limit activities and restrict participation. Decreased mobility can lead to secondary impairments that further affect activity and participation. Comorbid impairments can further compound movement problems. The large ovals representing secondary and comorbid impairments indicate that these may be the areas most amenable to change with rehabilitation. *CV,* cardiovascular; *MSK,* musculoskeletal.

The distribution and severity of paresis will affect the ability to move. Individuals with more mild paresis will have movements that appear to be normal or near normal. Individuals with more severe paresis, or plegia, may not be able to move at all. Paresis of the upper extremities results in limitations with activities such as bathing, dressing, grooming, and feeding. Paresis of the trunk and lower extremities results in limitations with transfers, balance, gait, and stair climbing. Even mild paresis can limit an older athlete's ability to participate in sport and recreational activities. In the presence of other comorbidities that commonly occur with age, the manner in which paresis affects functional activity can often be magnified (see Figure 15-2). For example, an older adult with osteoarthritis may already have weakened quadriceps muscles due to pain that has led to decreased mobility. If this individual has a stroke, he or she may be less adept at generating sufficient forces at sufficient rates, even in the less affected lower limb (ipsilateral to the lesion), to successfully climb stairs.

Abnormal Tone

Abnormal muscle tone is another common motor control impairment. Muscle tone itself is the resistance of muscle to passive elongation or stretch. Muscle tone is a result of inertia, the intrinsic biomechanical stiffness of the muscle and connective tissue, and the residual muscle contraction.[23] There is a broad range of normal muscle tone seen in healthy individuals. Abnormal muscle tone can be divided into two major categories: hypotonicity and hypertonicity.

Hypotonicity is reduced muscle tone. Flaccidity is the extreme case of hypotonicity, where there is a complete

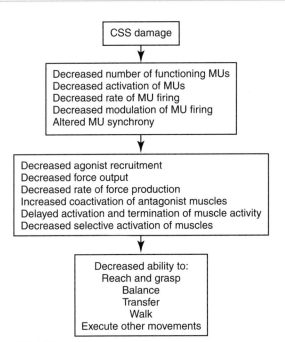

FIGURE 15-3 Schematic of relationships between corticospinal system (CSS) damage, motor unit (MU) activity, muscle activity, and movement. Damage to the CSS results in numerous impairments at the MU level (2nd box). MU impairments in turn lead to muscle activation impairments. Finally, the muscle activation impairments manifest as activity limitations in many movements of interest to physical therapists.

loss of muscle tone. Clinically, hypotonicity is apparent as a decreased resistance to passive movement and a decreased or absent stretch reflex response.[24] The limbs move easily and the joints are often hyperextensible. Hypotonicity is seen in a variety of conditions such as peripheral nerve damage, polio, degenerative neuromuscular diseases, and acutely after stroke affecting the corticospinal system or cerebellum. The mechanism underlying hypotonicity is a decreased or absent neural drive to the muscle.[25] In the case of peripheral nerve damage, the muscle may have lost its innervations or be only partially innervated. In the cases where hypotonicity is due to central nervous system damage, it is the spinal motoneurons that are damaged or have lost their major excitatory inputs (i.e., corticospinal connections).

Hypertonicity is increased muscle tone. Clinically, hypertonicity is apparent as increased resistance to passive movement and an increased stretch reflex response.[24] The limbs are harder to move and it may not be possible to move the limb through its full range of motion. Like paresis, hypertonicity is seen in a variety of conditions that cause damage to the central nervous system, such as stroke (typically, hypotonicity is seen first and then hypertonicity develops after the first few days or weeks), spinal cord injury, traumatic brain injury, multiple sclerosis, and cerebral palsy.

Hypertonicity is largely a result of loss of supraspinal inhibition to the spinal cord. An often forgotten fact about the corticospinal tract is that 40% of it arises from

the parietal lobe, and these fibers are primarily inhibitory.[26] When the parietal lobe and/or the corticospinal tract are damaged, then a major source of spinal inhibition is missing. Without this inhibition, the response to afferent input (e.g., input from muscle spindles, cutaneous receptors) is abnormally large. This manifests as increased resistance as a muscle is stretched and even greater increases when the muscle is stretched quickly.

Spasticity is a special type of hypertonicity that has been the subject of considerable attention by rehabilitation clinicians and researchers. Spasticity is defined as a velocity-dependent resistance to passive movement.[27] The resistance is often stronger in one direction than the other (e.g., greater during passive elbow extension vs. flexion). Spasticity is to be differentiated from rigidity by the fact that rigidity is not velocity dependent (e.g., resistance is the same regardless of the speed of passive movement) and is less likely to be directionally dependent (e.g., feels the same during flexion and extension). Unlike spasticity, which arises from corticospinal system damage, rigidity[28] is believed to stem from altered basal ganglia pathology. Rigidity is commonly seen in patients in the later stages of Parkinson's disease and in patients with dystonias. The clinical management of rigidity is generally part of the pharmacologic management of the underlying medical condition.

A particularly challenging aspect of spasticity is that it varies within individuals on a day-to-day basis and on a movement-by-movement basis.[28] Factors such as body position, temperature, and the recent history of movement at that segment influence the degree of spasticity. For example, when repeatedly stretching spastic muscles at a given joint, one often feels less resistance with later movements than with earlier ones. The variability in spasticity makes it hard to assess and manage clinically.

It is critical to appreciate that hypertonicity is rarely seen by itself (see Figure 15-2). It is typically part of a collection of impairments, paresis being one of them. The underlying health condition causing the corticospinal system damage will affect the severity and pattern of hypertonicity. For example, people with spinal cord injury often experience greater levels of spasticity than people with stroke. In stroke, the severity of the spasticity, matches reasonably well to the severity of paresis.[29] Patients with more severe paresis have more severe spasticity, whereas patients with mild paresis have minimal or no spasticity. From a neuroanatomical perspective, this is logical because both paresis and hypertonicity are a product of corticospinal system damage. Although hypertonicity (or spasticity) is often correlated with the degree of activity limitation, it is now generally agreed that it is not causal to the activity limitations. The best evidence for this comes from studies of botulinum toxin to treat spasticity. The major conclusion from this collection of studies is that botulinum toxin reduces spasticity in the injected muscles but does not improve functional capabilities.[30]

Fractionated Movement Deficits

Fractionation of movement is a critical part of our ability to use our limbs, particularly the upper extremities, for many different movements.[31] A reduced ability to isolate or fractionate movement will severely limit the ability to perform daily functional tasks. A variety of central nervous system pathologies affecting the corticospinal system result in fractionated movement deficits, including stroke, traumatic brain injury, spinal cord injury, multiple sclerosis, and cerebral palsy. Fractionated movement deficits can also result from less common movement disorders affecting the basal ganglia, such as dystonia (discussed separately later).

Clinically, the ability to fractionate movement can be seen when asking the patient to move one segment in isolation and keep other, adjacent segments still. Assessment of fractionation is most common at the fingers, where patients are asked to touch the tip of the thumb to the tip of each of the other fingertips. Loss of fractionated movement also occurs at more proximal segments. This can be assessed by asking patients to flex the shoulder alone or knee alone and observing what else moves. Fractionated movement deficits can be seen as they flex other joints distal and proximal to the target joint at the same time. This reduction in fractionated movement, particularly in patients with stroke, is the same as the abnormal movement synergies described many years ago by Brunnstrom.[32,33] Like hypertonicity, the degree of fractionated movement deficit is related to the degree of weakness. Patients with more severe paresis and hypertonicity have less ability to fractionate movement, and people with more mild paresis and minimal hypertonicity can make well-fractionated movements.[29]

The cause of fractionated movement deficits is damage to the corticospinal system resulting in a decreased ability to selectively activate muscles.[15,20] The corticospinal system is the neural substrate that affords humans the ability to execute their extensive repertoire of movements.[26,34] With damage to this system, the ability to turn on one muscle or a specific set of muscles at just the right time and just the right amount is altered. For example, when turning on the shoulder flexor muscles to reach for an object, the shoulder abductor, elbow flexor, and forearm pronator muscles turn on as well.[15,35] Likewise in the lower extremity, attempting to plantarflex the ankle may result in simultaneous extension at the knee and hip. As with paresis, fractionated movement deficits result in limitations with activities of daily living and mobility.

A different form of fractionated movement deficits is seen in people with dystonia. Dystonias appear as sustained, involuntary muscle contractions producing abnormal postures.[36] People with dystonia may have a primary dystonia or a secondary dystonia that results from an injury at birth, stroke, as side effect of antipsychotic medications, or other central nervous system pathology. This form of fractionated movement deficit is generally a result of pathology to the basal ganglia and its associated structures. The basal ganglia are a collection of large, functionally diverse nuclei located deep within the cerebral hemispheres (see Figure 15-1). With respect to movement control, the direct pathway through the basal ganglia is thought to focus the selection of the desired motor plan while the indirect pathway is thought to inhibit selection of undesired motor plans.[37] The general hypothesis is that dystonias are caused by an underactive indirect basal ganglia pathway, resulting in reduced inhibition of the thalamus, and the inability to suppress unwanted muscle activity. Thus, people with dystonia have fractionated movement deficits because many sets of muscle are turned on nearly all of the time.

Ataxia

Ataxia is a lack of coordination between movements and/or body parts.[38] The term *ataxia* has often been applied broadly to refer to any movement that is even somewhat uncoordinated. It is more correctly applied to specific movements (e.g., ataxic gait) that have the characteristic features of dysmetria. Dysmetria comes in two forms: hypermetria, or overshooting the intended target, and hypometria, or undershooting the intended target. People with ataxia tend to make hypermetric movements when trying to move quickly and hypometric movements when trying to move slowly.[39] Hyper- and hypometric movements are most easily seen in movements such as reaching and stepping. Overshooting or undershooting an intended posture with the trunk can also be seen when trying to control balance. When deciding if ataxia is present, it is important not to confuse ataxia with observed coordination problems that arise from paresis and/or fractionated movement deficits. When ataxia is present, the person will still have the capability to move quickly (although may not choose to) and the ataxia will typically look worse at faster movement speeds.

Ataxia results from damage to the cerebellar inputs, outputs, and/or cerebellar structures themselves (see Figure 15-1). The spinocerebellar atrophies are a group of degenerative, progressive disorders whose major symptom is ataxia.[40] People with other neurologic conditions such as stroke or multiple sclerosis can also have ataxia if the neurologic damage affected the cerebellum, its inputs, or its outputs. In rare cases, large-fiber peripheral neuropathies can result in a type of sensory ataxia that worsens when visual information is not available to assist in movement control.[41,42]

Moving at multiple joints is not merely the sum of all the movements of single joints. A major role of the cerebellum is to incorporate multisegmental movements together in a coordinated fashion. One way it does this is by controlling or exploiting interaction torques,[43] that is, rotational forces generated from the movement of one segment on another segment. People with ataxia have difficulty controlling movement-generated forces (interaction torques) such that movements are largely influenced by these rotational forces and not by the intended muscle actions.[38] For example, overshooting a target during fast reaching is largely due to the uncontrolled rotational forces generated at the shoulder and elbow.[43] Likewise, during walking, abnormal knee joint flexion during swing may be due to poorly controlled rotational forces generated by the movement of lower limb segments.[44] Many people with ataxia learn to compensate by moving slowly. Slower movements result in reduced interaction torques because the torques are velocity and acceleration dependent.[38] Many different activities can be limited by ataxia. The most salient of these, the ones that most often bring people to physical therapy, are limitations in gait and balance. It is the gait deficits that are most immediately obvious to clinicians and families, but interestingly, the gait deficits are often due to difficulties in controlling balance during gait.[45]

Hypokinesia

Hypokinesia is a primary motor control impairment associated with Parkinson's disease, other parkinsonian-like conditions, and sometimes dementia. It is characterized by slow movement (bradykinesia) or no movement (akinesia). In Parkinson's disease, hypokinesia co-occurs with tremor at rest and with rigidity. Hypokinesia is caused by basal ganglia damage and, in Parkinson's disease, with loss of the dopaminergic cells in the substantia nigra pars compacta. The general hypothesis underlying hypokinesia is that there is an overactive indirect basal ganglia pathway, resulting in nearly constant thalamic inhibition, and the inability to select the desired motor plan.[46] Clinically, hypokinesia appears as frequent muscle cocontraction where there is difficulty turning off the muscles that are not needed and turning on the muscles that are needed to execute a particular movement.[46] These muscle problems lead to a flexed-forward posture with instability and a slow, shuffling gait. People with hypokinesia have difficulty getting started with movement and can freeze during movement.[47] The major upper extremity movement complaint is tremor and small, sometimes illegible, handwriting (termed micrographia). Postural instability, gait deficits, tremor, and micrographia will worsen with disease progression and as pharmacologic management of the disease becomes less effective.

Somatosensory Loss

Somatosensory loss is a common impairment in older adults often resulting in altered motor control.[48] Beyond normal aging, abnormal somatosensory loss can occur in many of the same conditions named previously, such as stroke, spinal cord injury, traumatic brain injury, and multiple sclerosis. Abnormal somatosensory loss can be peripheral or central in origin. If it is from peripheral nerve damage, then the pattern of somatosensory loss will follow the distribution of the damaged nerve, root, or branch. If it is from central nervous system damage, then its distribution will be determined by the underlying condition. Somatosensory loss comes from damage anywhere along the pathways from the somatosensory receptors up through the somatosensory cortical areas in the cerebrum.

The major consequence of somatosensory loss on motor control is that ongoing monitoring of movement is less effective. The somatosensory system provides rapid, ongoing feedback about the consequences of movement.[49] For example, cutaneous receptors on the fingertips can provide feedback that a glass full of water is slipping. This information results in increased excitation of motoneurons at the spinal cord and cortical levels, resulting in an increased grip force that rapidly stops the glass from slipping. The visual system can partially, but not totally, compensate for the lack of somatosensation when planning movements.[42,50] In the glass-of-water example, somatosensory loss means that the person would detect that the glass was slipping only *if* visual attention was focused on the object. But by the time the slip was detected visually and acted upon, the glass might have dropped. Thus, people with somatosensory loss need to rely heavily on the visual system to plan and monitor movements. Their movements are slow, a compensatory response to adjust for the slower visual feedback, and are worse in poor vision or visually distracting conditions. Although somatosensory loss can occur in isolation, it is usually accompanied by other motor control impairments, especially paresis.

Perceptual Deficits

Perceptual deficits are another sensory impairment that often results in significant motor control problems. Pusher syndrome is a good example of a perceptual deficit commonly encountered and treated by physical therapists.[51] Medical conditions causing pusher syndrome include stroke, traumatic brain injury, and in some instances dementia or brain tumors.[51] People with pusher syndrome due to stroke or brain injury push with the unaffected extremities toward the affected side.[52] Although the specific mechanisms remain unclear, a current hypothesis explaining the pusher syndrome is that these patients have a distorted perception of body orientation with respect to gravity despite intact visual and vestibular inputs.[51,52] The pushing to the affected side and the resistance to correction may be a compensatory control strategy to correct for a sensory and perceptual mismatch. Fortunately, the brain seems to be able to adjust with experience (therapy), because pusher syndrome is less often seen 3 to 6 months after stroke.[52] If the pusher syndrome persists at 3 months post stroke, then the prognosis for functional independence is poor.

The three most common characteristics seen in patients with pusher syndrome are self-selected body posture that is tilted toward the paretic side, abducted and extended limbs on the unaffected side pushing toward the paretic side, and resistance to passive correction of the abnormal posture.[52] This behavioral phenomenon is distinctly different from other balance impairments seen in people with stroke or traumatic brain injury, where the presence of paresis and its accompanying reduction in the ability to activate muscles at the right time and right amount results in an inability to maintain the body in upright posture in sitting or standing. The pusher syndrome can occur in sitting, standing, walking, or even in supine (resistance to rolling to the nonparetic side). In more severe cases, the person will be unable to maintain independent sitting. In milder cases, the deficit will only appear during walking.

In stroke, the pusher syndrome is often accompanied by neglect (inattention) of the affected side of the body, aphasia, paresis, and somatosensory loss.[51,53] Interestingly, the pusher syndrome often co-occurs with perceptual deficits such as neglect if the right cerebrum is damaged, or with aphasia if the left cerebrum is damaged.[51,53] Additionally, the paresis in these patients is typically severe. From a physical therapy perspective, the salient feature in patients with pusher syndrome is that the pushing is the most significant impairment contributing to functional deficits. In other words, it does not matter if the arm and leg do not move much (paresis) when the patient resists sitting upright with support and resists postural corrections. Pusher syndrome used to be considered a result of right parietal lobe damage, but is now thought to arise from damage to the posterolateral thalamus on either side.[51-53]

EXAMINATION OF PATIENTS WITH IMPAIRED MOTOR CONTROL

The neurologic examination of motor control impairments requires a slightly different conceptual approach than examination for musculoskeletal problems. This is because motor control impairments most commonly appear in groups versus in isolation. For example, a person with stroke is more likely to have paresis, hypertonicity, and fractionated movement deficits than they are to have paresis alone. When performing a musculoskeletal examination, much of the effort is focused on muscle length, muscle strength, and specific mobility tests in order to determine the impairments contributing to the musculoskeletal problem.[54] When performing a neurologic evaluation, the impairment assessments are differently detailed (e.g., testing muscle groups vs. individual muscles) such that the focus is on determining which of the impairments present are contributing to the loss of movement activity.[55] Much of the examination is then devoted to observation and assessment of functional movements. In addition to judging the capability to execute a movement, observational analysis is needed to determine how impairments may be either associated with or contributing to the functional deficits.

Physical therapists have traditionally been trained to place a strong emphasis on assessment of impairments. As a result, many examination forms are filled with numerous impairment measures and fewer functional assessments. Evidence is beginning to accumulate that some of these impairment measures could be replaced with a quick screening or be removed entirely from the exam, at least in some patient populations. For example, clinical impairment measures of light touch sensation and joint position sense are not consistently related to upper extremity movement performance,[56,57] and are only minimally related to upper extremity function[29,58-61] in people with stroke. Somatosensory loss at one location on the affected limb is strongly correlated with somatosensory loss at other locations on the limb (Lang, CE, et al., unpublished observations). Furthermore, people with somatosensory loss in one modality such as light touch typically also have somatosensory loss in other modalities, such as proprioception.[60] It would therefore be reasonable to do only a quick screen of one somatosensory modality at one location. A logical choice would be light touch sensation at a fingertip, because it is easy to do and the fingertips are the location that people use to "feel" the world. Based on the evidence described earlier, the screening results would be most useful for providing patient and family education about the somatosensory loss and less useful for diagnosing the movement system problem. In contrast to the upper extremity, in the lower extremity, it might be more useful to screen for joint position sense. The rationale behind doing joint position sense is because of the importance of sensing foot placement during gait. As more data accumulate, evidence-based physical therapy examinations will be generated in a variety of patient populations. These shorter examinations will serve to reduce the testing burden on the patient and the therapist and permit more time to be devoted to education and treatment.

The physical therapy examination has two important goals: (1) to determine the underlying movement system problem, that is, diagnosis, and (2) to determine the initial level of impairment, activity, and participation so that future progress can be measured, that is, outcome assessment. Some items on the exam may serve one goal or the other, whereas other items might serve both goals. Table 15-1 lists and briefly describes each recommended test, specifies the motor impairment addressed by each test, and highlights salient issues related to each test. The first section of Table 15-1 describes the objective tests used to determine the presence and severity of motor control impairments. The second section of Table 15-1 provides a list of movements for observational analyses.

Paresis is one of the most important impairments and is the one most easily tested. Active range of motion (AROM) and manual muscle testing can be considered

TABLE 15-1 Recommended Tests to Assess the Presence, Severity, and Functional Consequences of Motor Control Impairment

Test	Description	Impairment Assessed	Comments, Interpretations, Judgments
Objective Tests of Motor Control Impairments			
Active range of motion[58,59] (AROM)	Goniometric measurement of voluntary movement against gravity. Two UE segments and one LE segment	Paresis	There is no need to measure all segments because the loss of active movement covaries across segments. For the upper extremity, the best choices are one proximal and one distal segment: shoulder flexion and either wrist or finger extension. For the lower extremity, the best choice is knee extension.
Motricity Index[62,63]	Test uses standard MMT of three specific UE and three specific LE segments to create UE and LE scores of overall paretic deficit. UE segments: shoulder abduction, elbow flexion, pinch grip. LE segments: hip flexion, knee extension, ankle dorsiflexion	Paresis	A benefit of this is that it yields both standard MMT scores that are useful in communicating with other professionals and an overall limb score that is useful in communicating with patients and families.
Modified Ashworth Scale[64]	Test uses passive range of motion of multiple UE and LE segments at varying speeds.	Spasticity	There is rarely a need to assess all segments because the degree of spasticity covaries across segments (Lang et al., unpublished observations). For the upper extremity, the best choice is the elbow because if spasticity is present, it will be most easily felt at the elbow.
Finger–thumb opposition	Patient is asked to touch the thumb to the tips of the each finger rapidly.	Fractionated movement deficits	This may be unnecessary because it is possible to determine the presence/absence of fractionated movement deficits by observation during AROM measurements.
Finger-to-nose[24]	Patient is asked to touch the examiner's finger then touch his or her own nose ~10 times rapidly.	Ataxia	Recommended that this test be skipped if AROM and/or Motricity Index measures indicate more than mild paresis. If given to people with moderate–severe paresis, then coordination deficits are secondary to the paresis.
Rapid alternating movements	Patient is asked to rapidly pronate and supinate the forearm for 10-20 sec.	Ataxia	Recommended that this test be skipped if AROM and/or Motricity Index measures indicate more than mild paresis. If given to people with moderate–severe paresis, then coordination deficits are secondary to the paresis.
Light touch sensation	Patient is lightly touched on fingertips/foot-ankle. If affected unilaterally, sensations can be compared to other side.	Somatosensation	Recommend scoring as present, impaired, or absent. See text for discussion of this item.

TABLE 15-1	Recommended Tests to Assess the Presence, Severity, and Functional Consequences of Motor Control Impairment—cont'd		
Test	**Description**	**Impairment Assessed**	**Comments, Interpretations, Judgments**
Observational Analyses of Movement to Detect Motor Impairments			
Observation of active range of motion	See above.	Fractionated movement deficits	Note the presence/absence if other segments in the same limb or segments in other limbs are moving when the target joint moves.
Observation of in-hand manipulation[55]	Place a pencil in the patient's palm. Ask him or her to manipulate it for writing.	Paresis Fractionated movement deficits	Recommended for higher level patients. Note if there is sufficient movement and if the finger movement is fractionated.
Observation of posture[55]	Patient is asked to sit (feet supported, no UE support) and stand quietly with eyes open.	Perceptual deficits	This is included as an assessment for perceptual deficits and is not intended as a formal assessment of postural control (see Chapter 16). Perceptual deficits are present if posture is not grossly at midline, pushes strongly to one side, and/or resists corrections to midline. Patients with just paresis and no perceptual deficits will not push or resist correction to midline.
Observation of sit-to-stand[55]	Patient is asked to come to standing from bedside or chair without UE support.	Paresis Hypokinesia Perceptual deficits	*Paresis:* cannot lift bottom out of chair, cannot extend hips/knees to stand, rapidly falls if support is removed, performance degrades with fatigue. *Hypokinesia:* limited or slow preparatory movements, falls slowly if support is removed, freezes during attempt. *Perceptual deficits:* shifts toward weaker side, pushes away from midline, resists correction to midline
Observation of gait[55]	Patient is asked to walk ~10 m, turn around, and come back. Assistance is provided as needed.	Paresis Fractionated movement deficits Ataxia Hypokinesia	*Paresis:* lateral trunk bending, hip/trunk flexion, knee hyperextension, leg circumduction, minimal dorsiflexion, performance degrades with fatigue. *Fractionated movement deficits:* stiff leg, movements of UE(s) when trying to step with LE. *Ataxia:* variable foot placement in both A-P and M-L directions, variable line of progression, limited change in performance with corrections or fatigue. *Hypokinesia:* limited or slow preparatory movements, slowness initiating stepping, freezes during attempt.

Note: The measures in the top half of the table are direct impairment assessments. Not all impairments have identified specific tests. The measures on the bottom half of the table are observations of activities where the specific impairments and their contribution to function can be identified.[55] The Comments, Interpretations, Judgments column is intended to highlight salient issues and is not intended as an exhaustive list.

A-P, anterior-posterior; *LE,* lower extremity; *M-L,* medial-lateral; *MMT,* manual muscle testing; *UE,* upper extremity.

indirect measures of the ability to volitionally activate the spinal motoneuron pools. AROM measures may be better able to capture deficits at the lower end of the severity spectrum, that is, can the muscles be activated enough to move the segment through the range. Manual muscle testing may be better able to capture deficits at the higher end of the severity spectrum, that is, can the muscles be activated sufficiently to produce force against externally imposed loads. For people with stroke, AROM measures of two upper extremity segments (one proximal and one distal) can determine both current and future upper extremity activity limitations.[58,59]

It is not yet clear how AROM at the lower extremity joints relates to gait function.[65] Given that gait requires greater force production capacity, it is likely that the relationships between how far segments can be moved against gravity and how well people walk are not as clear-cut as those in the upper extremity. Standard manual muscle testing in the context of the Motricity Index is a useful way to capture strength.[62,63] The Motricity Index is one of the preferred tools for patient assessments post stroke [66] and is used widely around the world in research and clinical practice.[67-70] The benefits of using the Motricity Index are that it allows one to test only three muscle groups per limb and not all of them, reducing the required testing time, and does not require equipment or difficult scoring criteria. The Motricity Index and the Fugl-Meyer Assessment[71] measure the same construct of global limb impairment; it is this author's bias that the Motricity Index is more useful because it takes less time to administer (5 vs. 30 minutes) and the manual muscle testing rating scale and definitions are familiar to most clinicians. An additional benefit of the Motricity Index is that the scores are easily understandable to patients and their families (e.g., "Your left leg strength is about 30% of your right leg").

A major debate in the physical therapy community over the years has been whether or not one can reliably test strength in the presence of fractionated movement deficits.[1] In people with stroke, these two impairments are highly correlated.[29] People who cannot move much cannot move in isolation, whereas people who can move a lot can make fractionated movements. Thus, an assessment of how much they can move, such as with AROM, can provide sufficient information about both of these motor control impairments. When making AROM measurements, appropriate goniometric alignment allows for measurement even if segments other than the targeted one move (e.g., it is possible to measure shoulder flexion AROM even if the elbow is also flexing).

A common observation in adults with motor control impairments is that movements are slow. Slowed movement is a consistent finding across patient populations for a variety of reasons. In patients with paresis, slowness is due to motor unit activation deficits. In patients with ataxia, slowness of movement may be a compensatory technique to avoid having to coordinate larger interaction torques.[38,43] In patients with somatosensory loss, slowness of movement may also be a compensatory technique, allowing time for accessing the slower visual feedback.[42,50] In patients with hypokinesia, slowness of movement may be the hallmark feature and a result of the inability to select the desired motor program and turn off other undesired programs.[37] Thus, it is probably most useful to note the consistencies and/or inconsistencies between observed movement slowness and specific movement impairments versus simply noting that movement slowness is present.

Table 15-2 provides a list of recommended tests used to assess outcomes. Outcome measures should be administered at the time of the initial evaluation and then periodically during the course of treatment to determine patient progress. Outcomes are most appropriately assessed at the activity and participation levels, but it may be useful to assess a few impairment level measures as well. Results from the impairment items can be compared to results from the activity items in order to confirm or refute the therapist's initial judgment about how the impairments contributed to the activity limitations. The measures in the table are recommended based on ease of use in a busy clinic and published psychometric properties. Interestingly, many of the common upper extremity outcome measures are highly related to each other, and their relationships are similar regardless of time post stroke.[93] Thus, if a patient scores well on one measure, he or she also scores well on other measures. This suggests that there may be no gold standard for measurement of upper extremity activity limitations, and that measures may be selected that are most useful for a particular patient or readily available in a particular clinic.

The main functions of the lower extremities are walking and transfers. Thus, the best measures to assess lower extremity outcomes in people with motor control impairments are the same as measures used for other patient populations: walking speed, the timed up and go, and the 6-minute walk test (see Table 15-2). Clinician reference tools, such as the book by Finch et al[94] provide an easy-to-read resource summarizing the key psychometric properties of many physical rehabilitation outcome measures.

Note that Tables 15-1 and 15-2 address motor control impairments and their typical functional movement problems. In addition to motor control impairments and function, the evaluation will need to cover other domains such as mental status (see Chapter 8, [Cognitive and Effective Impairment]) and assessment of the living situation (see Chapter 7, [Environmental Assessment]).

Lastly, it is important to evaluate secondary (indirect) impairments that may arise from the motor control impairments. The presence of motor control impairments will typically lead to decreased mobility (see Figure 15-2). Moving less results in secondary impairments such as

TABLE 15-2	Recommended Tests to Assess Outcomes at the Activity Level		
Measure	**Domain**	**Time to Complete**	**Comments**
Action Research Arm Test[72-81]	Activity: UE function	10 min	Performance on this test is highly correlated with performance on many other UE function tests. Instructions for making test kit and administering are found in Yozbatiran et al.[78]
Canadian Occupational Performance Measure[82]	Activity and participation: self-rating of UE function and its importance to daily life	20 min	Validated for general rehabilitation population Useful for identifying patient goals
Berg Balance Scale[83,84]	Activity: balance, risk of falling	20 min	
Timed Up and Go[85]	Activity: functional mobility, risk of falls	5 min	
FIM motor items[86]	Activity: functional mobility	10-20 min	Required for most inpatient rehabilitation facilities Can also be administered as questionnaire Most useful early after injury/lesion when have not yet attained independence
Walking speed[87,88,94]	Activity: walking ability	<5 min	Current gold standard for assessing walking ability
6-Minute Walk Test[88,94]	Activity: walking endurance	10 min	
Stroke Impact Scale[89,90]	Multiple domains	10 min	Contains useful subscales for UE function, ADLs, and mobility Can be administered as interview or questionnaire Stroke-specific
Reintegration to Normal Living Index[91,92]	Participation	10 min	

Note: Tests are recommended based on common usage, published psychometric properties, and ease of use in a busy clinic. It is intended that therapists may use this list to help in their selection of specific tests for specific patients, and that no one patient needs to be given all these tests.
ADLs, activities of daily living; *UE*, upper extremity.

contracture and muscle atrophy. Another huge secondary impairment in people with motor control deficits is cardiovascular deconditioning (see Chapter 12, Impaired Aerobic Capacity/Endurance). The presence and severity of secondary impairments will affect the process of selecting the most appropriate treatment and the success of the treatment for an individual patient.

DIAGNOSIS AND PROGNOSIS

The first goal of the physical therapy evaluation is to diagnose the movement system problem. Physical therapists are experts in understanding human movement because of their education in all of the systems that contribute to movement (e.g., musculoskeletal, neurologic, cardiovascular). It is outside the scope of physical therapy practice to diagnose the medical condition. It is within the scope of practice to diagnose the movement system problem,[95] that is, the impairments in body function and structure that lead to activity limitations of movement. The diagnosis, along with the prognosis, is used to determine a plan of care.

Motor control impairments are found in a variety of medical conditions and are not unique to any one condition. Furthermore, older adults typically have more than one medical condition, and even within the same medical condition, often have different mixes of motor control impairments. A patient example is shown in Figure 15-4A and illustrates how medical diagnoses and motor control impairments can occur together. The patient is a 72-year-old female with relapsing and remitting multiple sclerosis as well as diabetes and hypertension. As with many older adults, she has more than one medical condition. Two of her medical conditions result in motor control impairments, whereas the third does not. Similarly, two of her motor control impairments are caused by a single medical condition, whereas the third is a result of two medical conditions. One can imagine that as the number of medical conditions increases in any given patient, their map between conditions and motor control impairments becomes more complex. As the prognosis is strongly influenced by the underlying medical condition (see later), and as the prognosis and the movement system diagnosis will determine the treatment plan, the

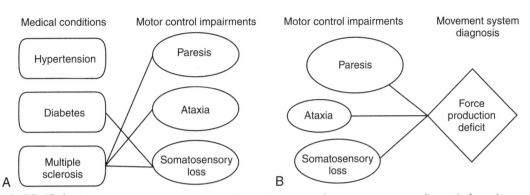

FIGURE 15-4 Medical conditions, motor control impairments, and movement system diagnosis for a hypothetical patient case. The patient is a 72-year-old female referred to physical therapy for evaluation and treatment of mobility problems associated with her multiple sclerosis. **A,** A map of the relationships between her medical conditions and her motor control impairments. **B,** A map of how her motor control impairments contribute to her movement system diagnosis. The size of the oval represents the severity of the impairment. The thickness of the line represents the therapist's observations and judgment as to how the impairments contribute to activity limitations and participation restrictions.

challenge to the physical therapist is to understand these relationships in individual patients and to determine the appropriate movement system diagnosis.

There is currently only one published set of movement system diagnoses for people with motor control impairments.[55,96] This system was developed from systematic clinical observation and has not been tested empirically. Within this system, there are eight distinct diagnoses related to motor control impairments. The names for the diagnoses (labels) are derived from the impairment believed to be the major contributor to the movement problems.[55] The eight diagnoses within this system and a brief description of each are provided in Table 15-3. A key component of this diagnostic system is that it recognizes that motor control impairments co-occur. Therapists determine a diagnosis based on the motor control impairment that is thought to be the biggest contributor to the movement dysfunction, instead of having to list diagnoses for all motor control impairments. As such, the diagnostic system provides a very useful framework to think about how motor control impairments present in adults. The more formal structure is particularly useful for novice clinicians, who are either new to physical therapy or new to treating patients with neurologic dysfunctions. The system supplies a framework for how to treat and manage people falling within each diagnostic category. The management ideas that underlie this framework are discussed later in the next sections. Additional research into movement system diagnosis is critically needed, both for patients with and without motor control impairments. Over the next decades, it is hoped that a variety of research approaches can be used to refine current systems or develop new ones. The challenging aspect of this type of research is that it requires large numbers of patients who are evaluated and treated in a standardized, systematic way.

The movement system diagnosis for the patient example is shown in Figure 15-4B. Here, the size of the oval represents the severity of the impairment and the thickness of the line represents the therapist's observations and judgment as to how the impairments contribute to activity limitations and participation restrictions. In this example, the paresis (termed "weakness" in the diagnostic system) is most severe and is judged to be the biggest contributing factor to limited mobility. The patient is diagnosed with "force production deficit," indicating that it is the reduced ability to generate sufficient forces at appropriate rates and times that is the major contributor to her limited mobility.

Prognosis in older adults with motor control impairments is largely a function of the underlying medical condition. It is useful to think about prognosis with regard to the medical condition *and* with regard to the likelihood of possible improvement with rehabilitation intervention. With respect to the medical prognosis, a critical piece of information is whether or not the underlying medical condition is progressive or nonprogressive. Nonprogressive conditions include stroke, spinal cord injury, and traumatic brain injury. Progressive conditions include Parkinson's disease, multiple sclerosis, and other degenerative neuromuscular diseases. In nonprogressive conditions, the impairments are more likely to improve early after injury than later after injury. In progressive conditions, the impairments are expected to worsen over time. The progressive or nonprogressive nature of the underlying medical condition is an important factor in selecting appropriate interventions for individual patients.

Epidemiologic data on prognoses are available for most medical conditions. After stroke, recovery of paresis occurs along a fairly predictable time course. Figure 15-5 illustrates the typical time course of recovery from paresis at the impairment and at the functional activity

TABLE 15-3	Movement System Diagnostic Categories for Motor Control Impairments[55]		
Movement System Diagnosis	Primary Movement System Impairment	Description	Relation to Impairments in This Chapter
Movement pattern coordination deficit	Coordination between segments and limbs	Altered timing and sequencing of tasks requiring movement at multiple segments or multiple body parts	No direct match for a specific impairment. The observed movement problems in this diagnostic category often result from very mild paresis, somatosensory loss, or other primary or secondary general immobility.
Force production deficit	Weakness	The origin of the weakness may be central (e.g., paresis) or peripheral (e.g., muscle, neuromuscular junction, nerve).	Paresis
Sensory detection deficit	Sensory loss	Lost sensations can be proprioceptive, visual, and/or vestibular. The lost sensation results in difficulty with movement control.	Somatosensory loss
Sensory selection and weighting deficit	Inability to attend to and weight sensory information	Difficulty with using/choosing incoming sensory information to plan and execute movements	No direct match with any one motor control deficit. The observed movement problems in this diagnostic category can result from sensory loss in one or more modalities. The movement problem is primarily with postural control.
Perceptual deficit	Altered perception of body orientation/posture	This is the pusher syndrome in stroke, where resistance to postural correction is medial/lateral. In a few conditions, pushing has been observed in the anterior/posterior direction.	Perceptual deficit
Fractionated movement deficit	Inability to make isolated movements	This diagnosis is always associated with central nervous system dysfunction.	Fractionated movement deficit
Hypermetria	Ataxia	This diagnosis is generally associated with damage to the cerebellum or its input/output structures.	Ataxia
Hypokinesia	Slowness of initiating and executing movement, paucity of movement	Most often associated with Parkinson's disease and/or dementia	Hypokinesia

Note: The diagnostic label identifies the major problem resulting in movement dysfunction; it does not mean that other problems are not present. Note that there are a few minor differences in terminology between this system and the way impairments are discussed in this chapter. These differences are detailed in the last column of the table.

level, as derived from epidemiologic data after stroke. Most epidemiologic data on stroke recovery are from samples of older adults, with average ages in most samples about 65 years. In general, most motor recovery will occur within the first 3 months.[97,98] The pattern of recovery is similar in older and younger adults with stroke, although older adults (in this study defined as older than age 75 years) are less likely to regain independence with basic activities of daily living and less likely to return to living at home.[99] The reason for limited independence may be the increased number of comorbid impairments present in older adults (see

Figure 15-2). Initial severity of the paretic impairments is the best predictor of eventual motor deficits and function.[100-102] Those with milder deficits recover more quickly and completely, whereas those with more severe deficits recover more slowly and to a much lesser extent (*inset*, Figure 15-5).[97] For the purpose of predicting recovery of individual patients, the therapist must appreciate that epidemiologic data provide the general pattern of recovery and that most, but not all, patients will follow a similar time course of changes. There are several consistent predictors of poor outcomes post stroke that are useful to look for when trying to

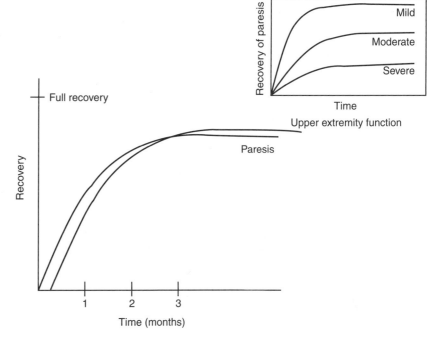

FIGURE 15-5 Schematic of the time course of recovery from paresis at the impairment and at the function level, as derived from epidemiologic data after stroke. Recovery of function typically lags recovery of motor deficits by about 1 to 2 weeks, where the shapes of the two recovery curves are very similar. The reason for the lag and the similar shape may be because as the motor ability emerges, movement practice is required to capitalize on the motor recovery and incorporate it into daily function. *Inset:* Those that are most mildly affected will recover more quickly and to a greater extent, whereas those that are more severely affected will recover more slowly and to a lesser extent.

determine prognosis in individuals. First, the more nonmotor impairments (e.g., somatosensory loss or visual field loss) there are that accompany the motor deficits (e.g., paresis, fractionated movement deficit), the less likely a person is to return to functional independence.[103] Second, earlier improvements in motor control impairments indicate that a person is more likely to reach higher levels of independence.[98,104] And third, the presence of any of the following at or after 1 month is associated with poor functional outcomes: no or minimal grip strength, no or minimal shoulder flexion, no or minimal hip flexion against gravity, and assistance needed for sitting.[59,102,105,106] Recovery of function typically lags recovery of motor deficits by about 1 to 2 weeks, where the shapes of the two recovery curves are very similar.[98] The reason for the lag and the similar shape may be that as the motor ability emerges, movement practice is required to capitalize on the motor recovery and incorporate it into daily function.

With respect to the rehabilitation prognosis, three important questions to consider with every patient are identified in Box 15-2. The first question reflects back on the medical condition. Motor control may worsen as in progressive conditions, may stay the same as in chronic nonprogressive conditions, or may improve as in acute/subacute nonprogressive conditions. The second question is partially, but not totally, independent from the first question. In many, many cases, motor control impairments will not change, but activity limitations and participation restrictions can be lessened. For example, ankle dorsiflexion strength may not change in someone who is 2 years post stroke, but a well-fitted ankle foot orthosis may allow return to community ambulation and volunteer activities. For older adults, there is high personal value placed on resuming participation in activities of interest. Assisting with improving participation can improve quality of life and help to foster optimal aging.

The third question is perhaps the most important and difficult to ponder. As physical therapists, one assumes that interventions will result in better outcomes. In reality though, this assumption is rarely tested in individual patients. For example, it is possible that a patient's gait improves over the course of therapy because he or she must walk to and from the parking lot to receive services and not because of the short time spent practicing gait during therapy.[107] The purpose of asking this third question is not to argue against the value of physical therapy services but to force ourselves to thoroughly examine the value of any possible intervention. Given limited services and busy patient lives, it behooves us to expend services wisely. Trying to answer these three questions about rehabilitation prognosis will allow one to make decisions about treatment goals and whether the

---

BOX 15-2   Key Questions to Guide Rehabilitation Prognosis and Treatment Decisions

1. What is the likelihood for motor control changes?
2. What is the likelihood of functional changes?
3. What is the likelihood that a specific intervention is going to change the expected outcome?

approach in reaching the goals should be remediation or compensation.

PLAN OF CARE AND REHABILITATION APPROACH

The first, critical decision when deciding on a plan of care to address motor control impairments in adults is to determine whether to use a remediation or a compensation approach to treatment. A remediation approach is aimed at restoring the previously lost motor ability and function. A compensatory approach is aimed at maximizing function within the confines of the limited motor abilities. This major decision is arrived at by careful consideration of prognosis. For example, in an older adult with Parkinson's disease, the compensatory approach is usually most appropriate, given that the individual's motor dysfunction is expected to worsen over time. In treating the upper extremity post stroke, a remediation approach would be chosen if the individual had a stroke less than 3 months earlier *and* there is voluntary fractionated movement against gravity at several upper extremity segments.[108] In contrast, a compensatory approach would be chosen for a patient with minimal or no voluntary fractionated movement, whether early or later post stroke.[108] In the case of the remediation approach with the upper extremity, the expectation is that therapy will restore the hand to a reasonable level of dexterity. In the case of the compensatory approach, the expectation is that therapy will teach the individual to maintain the health of the limb (i.e., minimize contracture development, edema, and potential hygiene problems) and will permit the hand to be used as an assist or support in daily activities.

Similar to the upper extremity, treatment for the lower extremity (primarily focused on gait) post stroke follows the same thought process. A remediation approach for gait, where the intent is to restore a relatively normal gait pattern, would be chosen if the individual had a stroke less than 3 months earlier *and* there is voluntary fractionated movement against gravity at multiple lower extremity segments. A compensatory approach for gait would be chosen to allow for safe ambulation in the patient with minimal or no voluntary fractionated movement, whether early or later post stroke. In the compensatory approach, therapists will be unconcerned with quality of movement (unless directly affecting safety) and may use assistive devices and/or bracing. By closely monitoring the motor capabilities of each patient, the therapist can determine if the appropriate approach was chosen and can be prepared to change approaches if needed.

Once the treatment approach has been decided upon, then specific interventions can be chosen. Interventions for impaired motor control should be targeted toward improving function and not targeted at improving impairments in isolation. Support for interventions targeting specific activities and not their underlying impairments comes from the mechanisms underlying motor learning and neuroplasticity, and from clinical rehabilitation research.[108-110]

Motor learning is the acquisition, modification, or reacquisition of movement.[1] *Neuroplasticity* is a term indicating that neurons, neural connections, and neural representations are modifiable.[111] Evidence from motor learning and neuroplasticity studies suggests that the experience-dependent changes to the nervous system are unique to the neural structure used during practice.[109,112] The cellular and neural network mechanisms that underlie learning and plasticity are illustrated in Figure 15-6. Figure 15-6A illustrates long-term potentiation, a prerequisite for neural changes associated with learning. With long-term potentiation, a neuron's response to input is enhanced by receiving repeated input, as through repeated practice.[113] If the repeated input is sustained, as through practice that is repeated over days and weeks, then the synapse between the presynaptic (input) neurons and the postsynaptic (output) neuron is remodeled (Figure 15-6B). The remodeling results in structural changes that allow more transmitter to be released from the presynaptic neurons and more transmitter to be picked up by the postsynaptic neurons.[109] This process does not only happen at one neuron or one pair of neurons but across the specific network of neurons used to execute that movement (Figure 15-6C). Thus, as a movement is practiced, connections within the network that are critical for its execution are enhanced and other connections are left alone or diminished. Lastly, the neural representation of the particular practiced movement is enhanced (Figure 15-6D), and neural representations of unused movements may be diminished.[109,112]

The specificity of the neural changes occurring as a result of practice/experience therefore support the importance of task-specific practice for optimizing function both in intact and damaged nervous systems. Practice of part of a movement in isolation, such as hip flexion in standing, is unlikely to activate the *exact* same network of neurons that are activated when trying to flex the hip during gait. Tracing the process in Figure 15-6, if a patient does not start with activating the specific network of neurons needed for the activity of interest, then the network needed for the desired activity will not be enhanced or strengthened. This is the scientific reason why basketball players practice free throws to improve their free throw percentage and do not practice extending their arms or flexing their wrist only.

Evidence from clinical studies also supports the idea that task-specific training is critical for function. In older adults, practice of balance improves balance but not gait, whereas practice of gait improves gait but not balance.[114] Although this study specifically investigated older adults, it is reasonable to generalize their results to all adults. In people with stroke, task-specific training is largely considered to be the best way to

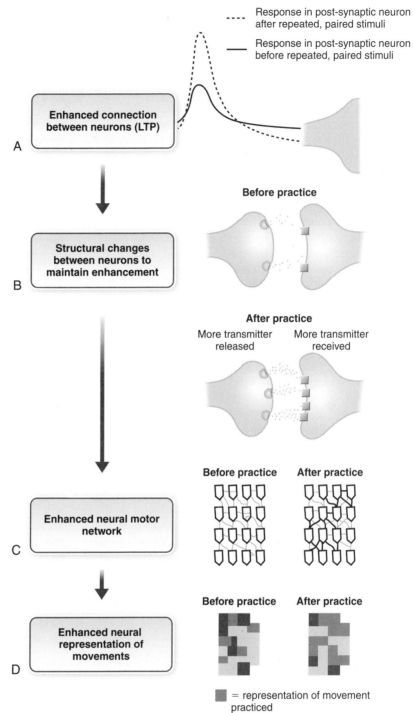

Response in post-synaptic neuron after repeated, paired stimuli

Response in post-synaptic neuron before repeated, paired stimuli

A   Enhanced connection between neurons (LTP)

B   Structural changes between neurons to maintain enhancement

Before practice

After practice
More transmitter released   More transmitter received

C   Enhanced neural motor network

Before practice   After practice

D   Enhanced neural representation of movements

Before practice   After practice

= representation of movement practiced

FIGURE 15-6 Schematic of neural mechanisms of motor learning/plasticity. **A,** As a new/challenging movement is practiced in a session, the connection between neurons that are fired together is enhanced. **B,** As the movement is practiced over time, structural changes between the two neurons make the enhancement more permanent. **C,** This happens with many neuron pairs across the motor system, such that some connections and combinations of neurons in the network are selectively enhanced via practice. **D,** Neural representations of specific movements (combinations of muscle actions) that are practiced become enhanced. *LTP,* long-term potentiation.

promote functional recovery.[110] Practice via circuit training of gait and stair climbing resulted in improvements in gait and stair climbing in people with stroke.[115] Further support for task-specific training over impairment-based training comes from a recent review of the efficacy of strength training and its effect on function post stroke.[65] Strength training results in improvements in strength but only results in improvement in function if the strength training is done within the context of the functional task.[65] An excellent practical example of this is practicing sit-to-stand transfers repeatedly and from surface heights that are increasingly difficult. In most individuals, this will lead to improved sit-to-stand transfers and to increased quadriceps strength,[116] whereas quadriceps strengthening in the standard seated, non–weight-bearing position may lead to increased quadriceps strength but with little carryover to functional mobility involving quadriceps. Thus, the skills of the physical therapist are needed to appropriately structure the task-specific training to address the movement dysfunction and its underlying impairments.

Taken all together, the above literature suggests that interventions should be most often at the activity level and even occasionally at the participation level. This is true whether the selected treatment approach is remediation or compensation. For example, the primary intervention to improve walking is with gait training and not with exercises to address weight-bearing, weight-shifting, and lower extremity strength.[117] If the approach is compensation, then the specific treatment will focus on walking safely with whatever gait pattern and assistive devices are deemed appropriate. If the approach is remediation, then the specific treatment will work on resuming a more normal gait pattern. The role of the skilled physical therapist is to design the gait-training activities to address the specific goals and to challenge the activity limitations and impairments of each patient.

It is often the case that there are different rationales for choosing the same intervention. An example of this is body-weight–supported treadmill training (BWSTT). An early rationale for the use of BWSTT for gait training in patients with central nervous system injury was to provide practice that mimicked the sensory inputs experienced during normal gait.[118] Upon further examination, BWSTT may be selected as an appropriate intervention for a variety of reasons. These reasons include the following: as a way to practice gait training sooner than if patients had to support their entire weight, as a way to stimulate the cardiovascular system, as a way to stimulate loading of the long bones, and as a way to facilitate a more normal gait pattern. For interventions having multiple rationales, the important aspect to appreciate is which rationale led to the selection of the intervention and how that rationale will affect how the intervention is delivered (e.g., BWSTT for cardiovascular fitness vs. BWSTT for improved motor control).

CURRENT EVIDENCE UNDERLYING IMPAIRED MOTOR CONTROL INTERVENTIONS

It is important to keep in mind that evidence is continually emerging and being refined. The major body of knowledge regarding treatment of motor control impairments comes from people with stroke. Because people with stroke have many of the same motor control impairments as people with other medical conditions, readers may consider the application of these results to others that may have similar motor control impairments but different medical conditions.

Sorting through all the available evidence supporting or not supporting a particular upper or lower extremity/gait treatment is burdensome for a practicing clinician. It is our great fortune that an outstanding and current synopsis to guide evidence-based treatment is provided free of charge by the Canadian Stroke Network. It is called Evidence-Based Review of Stroke Rehabilitation (EBRSR) and is available at www.ebrsr.com. The aim of the EBRSR is to provide an up-to-date review of stroke rehabilitation evidence in a clinician-friendly manner, where specific conclusions can be used to guide stroke rehabilitation care.[108] Each of the 23 sections can be downloaded separately in pdf format. The first section provides an introduction to EBRSR and its strong methodology. Each subsequent section deals with a specific area of stroke rehabilitation, including one section on mobility and lower extremity interventions and another on upper extremity interventions. Other sections focus on aphasia, perception, cognition, depression, etc. An important feature of the EBRSR is that it summarizes all the relevant studies, providing clinically relevant conclusions and the level of evidence from which the conclusions are derived. A new edition of EBRSR is available each year, so that recently published studies are quickly incorporated into the summaries and conclusions.

As with most rehabilitation evidence, conclusions regarding upper extremity and lower extremity/gait interventions are hampered by small sample sizes, mixed outcome measures, and differing "control" treatments. Nonetheless, there have been great gains in the available evidence for treating motor control impairments and function. More and stronger evidence will emerge in the next few decades.

Considerations for Upper Extremity Interventions

Given the limited therapy services and the general emphasis on task-specific training, clinicians are faced with the dilemma of determining what tasks to practice and in which contexts. There are a large number of tasks that are performed by the upper extremities. For example, people generally have a daily grooming routine, which may include five to six tasks, such as brushing teeth, washing the face, brushing hair, shaving, applying make-up, etc. If one multiplies the number of daily routines by the number of tasks within each routine, the result is an enormous number of tasks within specific contexts that need to be performed by any given individual on a daily basis. It is impossible to practice all tasks in their specific contexts.

There are four essential components of most upper extremity movement tasks: reach, grasp, move or manipulate, and release. Almost all functional tasks of the upper extremity involve some combination of these four components. What varies across the repertoire of upper extremity functional tasks is how the combinations of the components are strung together and the specifics of the component (e.g., direction of reach, type of grasp, manipulative forces required). For example, when eating, a person reaches for the fork, grasps it, manipulates the fork to pick up the food, moves the food and fork to the mouth, returns the fork to the table, and releases the fork. When opening a door, a person reaches forward, grasps the door knob, turns it, pushes the door, and releases the knob. It is not yet known how practice and improvement of one functional task (one string of components) might translate or generalize to improvement on other functional tasks. Based on limited generalization of movements in contrived, laboratory settings,[119-122] it is safest to assume that there is little generalization across tasks.

The job of the treating therapist is to select specific upper extremity tasks to practice that are functionally important to the patient receiving treatment and that challenge but do not overwhelm the patient's motor abilities. The easiest way to determine which tasks are important to the patient is to ask him or her directly. A more formal way to determine specific tasks for the upper extremity is with the Canadian Occupational Performance Measure (COPM; see Table 15-2).[82,94] Once the patient has identified the tasks he or she is most interested in improving, the therapist and patient can problem-solve together to make sure that the task and goal of being able to do the task are realistic given the patient's motor capacity. For example, consider a 70-year-old woman, with a 1-year history of right hemiparesis post stroke. Her motor capabilities include the ability to flex the right shoulder to 45 degrees, an upper extremity Motricity Index score of 48/100, and an Action Research Arm Test score of 9/57. Together, these results indicate she has limited use of her affected upper extremity. If she identifies that she wants to be able to regain normal, dexterous use with her (previously dominant) right hand, then it is critical to have a conversation that helps her identify goals that are more realistic given her prognosis and current motor capabilities. A more realistic set of functional goals for her would focus around learning to use the affected right side as an assist during bilateral tasks, such as securing the jar with the right hand while the left hand opens the jar.

Once a task of interest is identified, the therapist needs to creatively arrange the task to repeatedly challenge but not overwhelm the patient's current motor abilities. If the task is too easy, then practice will become rote. If the task is too hard, the patient may quickly become frustrated. A movement task that takes 1 to 2 seconds is probably too easy, whereas a task that takes 30 seconds or more may be too hard. Based on our clinical observations, a useful rule may be to grade the task so that it takes between 6 and 15 seconds to complete a repetition. In our experience, this allows the patient to easily judge success or failure and keeps the patient from getting too frustrated. An example of a task that is of interest to many patients and is easily graded is lifting cans to and from a shelf. This task incorporates the essential components of reach, grasp, move/manipulate, and release. In everyday life, it is similar to many movements needed to function in kitchens, bathrooms, and workshops. The difficulty of the task can be graded up or down by changing can size, can weight, starting location, ending location, and whether or not the patient is sitting or standing while performing the task. With multiple repetitions of a task like this, one can understand how impairments such as decreased AROM (change location), strength (change can weight), or endurance (increase the repetitions, have patient stand) can be addressed in a task-specific manner. As the patient improves, the task can be graded up to continually challenge and improve his or her motor capabilities.

In a busy clinic, it is not possible to have the set-up and equipment to practice every possible upper extremity task. One way to get around this is to have space and materials set aside to practice the most common tasks. For example, a basket or box could be filled with a variety of containers/bottles and their respective lids. Many individuals need to be able to open bottles and containers to prepare food, take medicine, or do self-care activities. The basket can be filled with containers used in daily life, such as medicine bottles, margarine containers, laundry detergent bottle, that are different sizes, shapes, and present various difficulties. The variety of containers will allow variability in how the patient practices, and thereby potentially improve the generalizability of the motor skill to other containers that may be encountered outside of therapy. This is only one example of a useful way to store and use materials for upper extremity task-specific practice. Baskets with other themes (e.g., crafts, office work) can be created in therapy clinics to address other common upper extremity tasks, based on the needs and interests of the older adults served by that clinic.

Most adults, regardless of age, are highly motivated to improve their function and are therefore interested in practicing outside of therapy sessions. This should be strongly encouraged. Similar to within therapy sessions, home programs for the upper extremity are most appropriately focused on functional task practice and not on traditional therapeutic exercise. Careful thought in choosing the specific tasks to be practiced at home will permit both impairments and function to be addressed with one or a few activities. If the goal of an older adult male is to use his workshop again, then standing or sitting at the workbench while practicing grasping and releasing specific tools may be highly engaging and motivating for him. Many of the materials and tasks created in the clinic can be easily and cheaply re-created in patients' homes (e.g., look in recycling bin, workshop, or game closet). As patients practice functional upper extremity tasks in their own environments, they often come up with creative and unique solutions to successfully executing activities that are important to them.

The EBRSR[108] section on upper extremity interventions reminds us that there are interventions, which are observed routinely in clinics,[123] that have moderate to strong evidence of *minimal or no* benefit. Three interventions that have moderate to strong evidence of no benefit are hand splinting for the reduction of contractures and/or improvement of function, general stretching and splinting for the reduction of spasticity, and intermittent pneumatic pressure for the reduction of hand edema. Two interventions for the upper extremity that have strong evidence showing that they are not superior to conventional physical therapy are neurodevelopmental techniques and electromyographic biofeedback techniques. Other interventions have strong evidence supporting their benefit, but often only for particular circumstances. There is strong evidence that constraint-induced movement therapy is beneficial in people with subacute and chronic stroke who have some active movement of the wrist and hand. There is conflicting evidence, however, that it is beneficial in people with acute stroke. In contrast, there is strong evidence that functional electrical stimulation is beneficial for lower-level patients at all time points post stroke. Additionally, there is strong evidence that injections of botulinum toxin (Botox) is temporarily beneficial in reducing spasticity but is not beneficial in improving upper extremity function. A final set of interventions are labeled as having uncertain evidence. These include enhanced therapy (additional minutes), sensorimotor training, mental practice, robotic training, and virtual reality. Many of the interventions on this last list are considered emerging interventions that are currently being or will be more thoroughly tested in the future.

Considerations for Lower Extremity and Gait Task-Specific Interventions

The Mobility and the Lower Extremity section of the EBRSR provides a summary of the evidence of many commonly used physical therapy interventions.[30] A key finding in their analysis is that task-specific gait training improves gait in adults with stroke. Likewise, certain types of balance training improve balance and functional outcomes in adults with stroke. Of importance to most patients with motor control impairments, cardiovascular training can improve physical fitness and function. Critical ingredients for effective cardiovascular treatment are to monitor vital signs and to ensure that cardiovascular training is of the appropriate intensity to stimulate improved fitness (see Chapter 12, Impaired Aerobic Capacity/Endurance, for further details). Improved cardiovascular fitness for a person with motor control impairments may provide the person with the endurance needed to make it through their day and to permit participation in meaningful sport or leisure activities. This is a way to lessen activity limitations and participation restrictions by addressing the secondary consequences of motor control impairments (see Figure 15-2). Other interventions for mobility and the lower extremity with strong evidence of benefit include ankle foot orthoses and functional electrical stimulation for those adults with moderate to severe paresis. Interventions with strong evidence of not being superior to conventional therapy include neurodevelopmental techniques, teaching/encouraging self-propulsion in a wheelchair, and robotic gait training. Interestingly, robotic gait training (with commercial devices such as the Lokomat and AutoAmbulator) have recently been shown to be less effective at improving gait post stroke compared to dose-matched traditional overground gait training.[124,125] This may be because the robotic device, not the patient, does the work during gait training.[126]

SUMMARY POINTS

1. The major motor control impairments in adults are: paresis, abnormal tone, fractionated movement deficits, ataxia, and hypokinesia. Two additional impairments, somatosensory loss and perceptual deficits, also have important consequences for motor control.

2. Similar motor control impairments can be seen across numerous medical conditions.

3. Most individuals present with multiple motor control impairments rather than just one.

4. A critical aspect of evaluating adults with motor control impairments is determining which of the motor control impairments are the chief contributors to the loss of activity and which ones make only minimal contributions. This step is critical in formulating a movement system diagnosis.

5. The prognosis of the underlying medical condition is a critical factor in determining the rehabilitation prognosis in adults with motor control impairments. A critical role of the therapist is to determine how to improve activity and participation in individuals whose motor control impairments will stay the same or may worsen.

6. Outcomes assessment for adults with motor control impairments should be done at the activity or participation levels. Currently available measurement tools are reliable, valid, and responsive to clinically meaningful change.

7. A key decision in the treatment of adults with motor control impairments is whether to choose a remedial or a compensatory approach.

8. Task-specific training is the treatment of choice for adults with motor control impairments. Support for interventions targeting specific activities rather than specific impairments comes from the mechanisms underlying motor learning and neuroplasticity, and from clinical rehabilitation research.

9. Determining which tasks to practice to improve upper extremity function can be challenging.

10. An excellent up-to-date synopsis of the current evidence for and against various treatments is Evidence-Based Review of Stroke Rehabilitation (EBRSR) and is freely available from the Canadian Stroke Network at www.ebrsr.com.

ACKNOWLEDGMENTS

My thanks to Drs. J.S. Stith and P.L. Scheets for their helpful insights and comments during the writing process, and to the editors, particularly Dr. R.A. Wong, for her feedback. Salary support was provided to CEL by NIH HD047669.

REFERENCES

To enhance this text and add value for the reader, all references are included on the companion Evolve site that accompanies this text book. The reader can view the reference source and access it online whenever possible. There are a total of 126 cited references and other general references for this chapter.

CHAPTER 16

Impaired Posture

Carleen Lindsey, PT, MScAH, GCS

INTRODUCTION

Optimal posture, which provides biomechanically well-balanced positioning of body parts, allows the upright position to be maintained with very efficient use of muscles, low energy expenditure, and little stress on joints. Postural dysfunction is generally considered an impairment[1] and as such may be a factor in pathology, such as osteoporosis and spinal stenosis, and in functional disability, such as the inability to walk efficiently, to lift, or even to stand without support. The chapter begins with a discussion of posture and the postural changes commonly occurring with advancing age, and of the interactive impact on posture of selected comorbid health conditions (osteoporosis, osteoarthritis, spinal stenosis) that commonly affect the biomechanics of postural alignment in older adults. The chapter then reviews the consequences of these postural changes on the functional activities of the older adult and provides insights into the evaluation, management, and outcome assessment of these patients.

NORMAL POSTURE

Posture is a result of static and dynamic components. Static posture is made up of the alignment of body segments to maintain a selected position in space. Dynamic posture emphasizes the ability to appropriately control and maintain a well-aligned upright posture while moving the body (or body parts) in space. Although static and dynamic posture are closely intertwined, this chapter focuses primarily on issues of static postural alignment from the perspective of aging-related changes and prolonged positioning. Chapter 15 on motor control and Chapter 18 on balance and falls each address issues of dynamic control of posture.

The American Physical Therapy Association's *Guide to Physical Therapist Practice*[1] (the *Guide*) defines posture as "the alignment and positioning of the body in relation to gravity, center of mass, and base of support." The Posture Committee of the American Academy of Orthopaedic Surgeons[2] provides the "classic" and still applicable description of optimal posture as "that state of muscular and skeletal balance which protects the

supporting structures of the body against injury or progressive deformity, irrespective of the attitude (erect, lying, squatting, or stooping) in which these structures are working or resting. Under such conditions muscles function most efficiently and optimum positions are afforded for thoracic and abdominal organs." This same group defines less than optimal posture as "a faulty relationship of the various parts of the body which produces increased strain on the supporting structures and in which there is less efficient balance of the body over its base of support."[2]

DEVIATIONS FROM OPTIMAL POSTURE

Frequently, individuals adopt less than optimal habitual postures that stress underlying structures, beginning either in early childhood or later in life. Their postural control system adapts to these chronic "malalignments" and provides the additional active muscular or passive ligamentous supports needed to maintain a safe and effective upright posture. Prolonged postural malalignments lead to stress and strain on supporting structures that gradually change these structures. Habitual and prolonged trunk and head flexed postures are rampant in societies whose members tend to spend many hours daily in flexion-biased activities such as sitting at a computer. A prolonged flexion moment results in the constant activation of the extensor muscles in a lengthened position and the gradual shortening of the flexor muscles held for prolonged time periods in a shortened position.[3] Habitual postures that overstretch extensor muscles and shorten flexor muscles can lead to structural changes with potentially permanent negative impact on physical functioning and quality of life.[4-9] Postural impairments with subsequent dysfunctions and activity limitations are not an inevitable part of aging; however, thoracic kyphosis, forward head posture (FHP), and decreased lumbar lordosis become more apparent in aging adults in part from the accumulation of remodeling in response to habitual postures.[4,7,10-12] Although associations between poor postures and functional limitations among older adults are frequently reported in studies, little is definitively known about the causal impact of postural abnormalities on function and participation of older adults, or on the ability to influence outcomes by changing postures.

Forward Head Posture

FHP is a common habitual postural malalignment often present since a young age and often observed in individuals who spend a lot of time sitting and reading or working at a computer. In the FHP there is shortening of the suboccipital muscles (cervical extensors) concurrent with lengthening of the prevertebral muscles (cervical flexors). In a FHP, the weight of the head is maintained in front of the line of gravity, increasing the flexion moment on the spine. FHP and hyperkyphosis are closely related mechanically and functionally,[13-15] although FHP can exist in older adults separate from hyperkyphosis. A linear relationship between age and FHP has been demonstrated in healthy community-dwelling older women, with an average FHP of 49 degrees for individuals in the 65 to 74 years age range, 41 degrees for those in the 75 to 84 years age range, and 36 degrees in the 85 and older age group.[16] The angle used to measure head posture, depicted in Figure 16-1, clarifies that a smaller angle represents a more pronounced FHP.

Thoracic Kyphosis

Thoracic kyphosis remains fairly constant in adult men and women until somewhere about age 40 years. After age 40 years, thoracic kyphosis begins to increase in both men and women, with a more marked increase in women across the remainder of the life span. Excessive thoracic kyphosis (hyperkyphosis) is a commonly

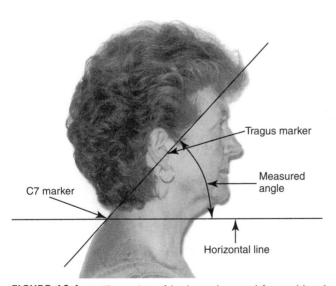

FIGURE 16-1 An illustration of body markers and forward head posture measurement on individual photo. *(From Nemmers TM, Miller JW, Hartman MD. Variability of the forward head posture in healthy community-dwelling older women. J Geriatr Phys Ther 32(1):10-14, 2009.)*

observed postural dysfunction in older adults, particularly older women. A thoracic kyphosis angle greater than 40 degrees exceeds the 95th percentile value of thoracic kyphosis angle in young adults[17,18] and, thus, may serve as a possible cutoff for hyperkyphosis. Multiple researchers[4,5,7,11,13,14,19-25] have associated clinically symptomatic hyperkyphosis with advancing age, often linking increasing kyphosis with increasing functional limitations,[4,7,11,18,23] decreased participation in outside activities,[4,18] and lower self-reported health and life satisfaction.[18] In addition, significant correlations have been demonstrated between fall risk and kyphosis.[15,26] Although clinical kyphosis alone is not linearly predictive of either osteoporosis or vertebral fractures, an association does exist, [7,11,14,26,26a] and has been demonstrated to be most prominent in women with multiple thoracic vertebral compression fractures (VCF).[7] It has also been demonstrated that a composite risk score using calcaneal qualitative ultrasonometry and kyphosis had better discriminatory power than low dual-energy x-ray absorptiometry bone mineral density to predict prevalent vertebral fractures in community-dwelling women.[26a]

Consequences of Less Than Optimal Posture

Long-standing repetitive stress on supporting structures such as excessive lordosis, rounded shoulders or a forward head position can produce wear and tear on supporting structures and lead to repair and remodeling in poor alignment, perpetuating the postural dysfunction. When habitual poor posture is combined with normal age-related changes in supporting structures, particularly in the presence of common chronic health conditions such as osteoporosis and osteoarthritis, considerable activity limitations and disability can result.

Low back pain is one of the most common musculoskeletal symptoms for which adults seek medical attention. The presence of severe disc pathology is associated with increased odds of having chronic low back pain (CLBP)[27] and hyperkyphosis.[25] In addition to serving as a potentiating factor for vertebral fracture, disc degeneration is associated with nerve root impingement and related stenosis in the central canal or the neural foramina.[25] Although no direct causal link exists between less than optimal posture and low back pain, excessive lumbar positions are frequently seen in patients with pain. Pain can reduce the desire to move into positions that produce pain and thus may lead to long-standing restrictions of motion. Pain can also reduce the incentives for a person to move, contributing to habitual postures, muscle weakness, disuse of postural control mechanisms, and increased disability.

Older adults with hyperkyphosis and substantial FHP can have difficulty with many tasks and actions important to daily activities, such as bending, lifting, climbing, and rising from a chair when compared to older adults with relatively normal head and thoracic alignment.[23] For example, hyperkyphosis puts the spine extensors in a lengthened, and thus weakened, position, making lifting more effortful. FHP is also associated with symptomatic head and neck pain in patients of all ages.[28,29] Excessive FHP may produce difficulties swallowing, breathing, and an inability to lie comfortably in supine or prone. A patient who sits in an excessively flexed position can compress the contents of the abdomen against the diaphragm, causing breathing to be restricted.

A reduced intervertebral space decreases the diameter of the intervertebral foramen, which may compromise nerve root integrity and cause the patient to flatten the lumbar spine. Symptoms of nerve root impingement, back pain, and even ischemia may result in conditions such as spinal stenosis. Reduced diameter of the spinal canal may make lumbar extension painful and produce symptoms of leg pain and ischemia. In turn, activity may be limited as standing and walking can be painful or uncomfortable. External support such as a cane or walker may be needed to accomplish mobility-related tasks.

The frequent clinical sign of a flattened lordotic curve is a tendency to lean forward when walking or standing.[30,31] Because a forward-leaning position requires more energy to maintain, the body will typically recruit low back, buttock, and posterior thigh muscles to help normalize posture by tilting the pelvis to achieve better alignment. Fatigue of these excessively recruited muscles can lead to muscle soreness and pain. A loss of the lumbar curve is an independent predictor of vertebral fractures.[32]

Age-Related Changes in Body Structure and Function That Influence Postural Spinal Alignment

Bone, Disc, and Cartilage Changes in the Spine. Changes in intervertebral discs, articular cartilage, and bone can contribute to postural alignment and an age-related loss in height. Height tends to decrease about 0.1% per year in women and 0.02% in men, beginning around 45 years of age (Figure 16-2).[33,34] These age-related changes in intervertebral height and in bone can lead to a 2-inch loss of height over a lifetime that is considered typical.

With aging the intervertebral discs become progressively more fibrous; the peripheral annulus widens and becomes densely fibrous and the nucleus loses its mostly proteogylcan content, becoming similar to a flat tire.[35] In this state, the individual disc, in concert with the facet joints, can no longer accept the considerable compressive, tensile, and shear stresses as when it is younger.[36] The neural arch becomes an increasingly load-bearing structure, bearing up to 40% of weight when standing, with compressive force concentrated anteriorly in forward bending, and posteriorly in erect posture.[37,38]

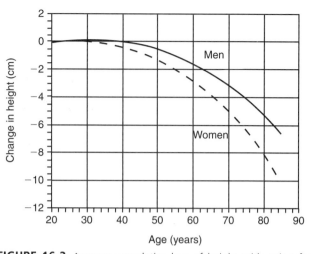

FIGURE 16-2 Average cumulative loss of height with aging for men and women from the Baltimore Longitudinal Study of Aging, Baltimore, Maryland, 1958-1993. *(Data from Galloway A, Stini WA, Fox SC, Stein P. Stature loss among an older United States population and its relation to bone mineral status. Am J Phys Anthropol 83(4):467-476, 1990.)*

Because annulus height determines the separation of adjacent neural arches, the collapse of the annulus probably explains why narrowed discs are associated with osteoarthritis in the apophyseal joints and with osteophytes around the margins of the vertebral bodies.[39]

Reduced thickness and resilience of articular cartilage with aging increases the possibility of articular cartilage microfractures or damage when forces such as those related to overuse, obesity, trauma, metabolic disease, or hereditary factors are applied. Over 90% of older adults demonstrate some level of disc degeneration, regardless of presence of clinical signs and symptoms.[37] Thus, "abnormal" imaging findings are very common in older adults. However, imaging studies are poorly correlated with symptoms.[40-42] Imaging findings must be combined with a careful clinical examination to determine the clinical impact of long-standing structural changes.

The ligaments of the spine are depicted in Figure 16-3. Spinal ligaments respond to tensile forces by becoming taut. The reverse is true when the spine is subjected to compressive loads; namely, the collagen fibers in ligaments buckle and become slack. In young adults, elastic fibers make up about 75% of the ligamentum flavum (LF).[43] With aging, the proportion of elastic fibers declines by nearly one half with the likely cause being the conversion of elastic fibers into cartilaginous tissue as the result of scarring. This scarred tissue becomes thickened. There is also an increase in type I collagen mRNA production with increasing age suggesting that increased thickness of both the collagen and the remaining elastin fibers are correlated with hypertrophy of the LF.[43] This ligamentous hypertrophy can cause symptomatic spinal stenosis in both the cervical and lumbar regions.

Loss of vertebral bone volume with age is associated with decreased vertebral body strength as the trabeculae

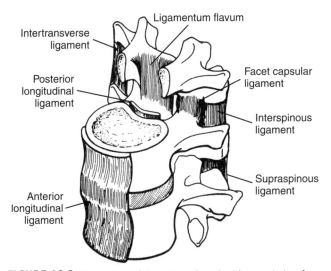

FIGURE 16-3 Ligaments of the spine. *(Used with permission from White AA, Panjabi MM: Clinical Biomechanics of the Spine, 2nd ed. Philadelphia, 1990, JB Lippincott.)*

Labels in figure:
- Intertransverse ligament
- Ligamentum flavum
- Posterior longitudinal ligament
- Facet capsular ligament
- Interspinous ligament
- Supraspinous ligament
- Anterior longitudinal ligament

gradually become thinner. These changes are particularly apparent in those over 40 years of age.[44] A 25% loss in bone tissue volume results in a greater than 50% decrease in vertebral body strength, which illustrates a mechanism for the increased risk of spinal deformities and fracture, even when bone tissue loss appears relatively small, and highlights the importance of intervening early to prevent or slow down osseous tissue loss. Flexion forces on the spine increase vertebral body fracture risk, making spinal posture training a key component of any spinal fragility fracture prevention program.[45-47]

Loss of height is greater in the presence of low bone mineral density (BMD) and progresses at a significantly faster rate than in individuals with normal BMD.[11,34] Changes in bone contribute to changes in body height. Even older adults without any evidence of osteoporosis or degenerative arthritis demonstrate wedging and increased kyphosis in the thoracic spine, increasing in severity with increasing age for both men and women; but, in the lumbar spine, demonstrated primarily in men.[48] Although loss of height is a normal age-related change, age only explains approximately one third of the variance in height. Greater loss in height is associated with a more pronounced hyperkyphosis, greater odds of having a vertebral fracture, and of having upper and middle back pain.[7,34]

Muscle and Soft Tissue Changes. Muscles, ligaments and tendons can profoundly affect posture. With age, these structures experience declines in water, elastin, and proteoglycan content combined with changes in amount, diameter, fibril size, and aggregation of collagen. The numbers of cross-links between adjacent tropocollagen molecules also contribute to increased stiffness, decreased distensibility, and ultimately decreased maximal length at

which tissue rupture occurs.[49-51] Another concern with muscle aging is muscle length and muscle strength capability. Optimal muscle strength capability occurs between 75% and 105% of a muscle's resting length. The number of sarcomeres in series is important in determining the distance through which the muscle can shorten during normal limb movement, and position at which the muscle exerts its maximum tension. Muscle is a very adaptable tissue and sarcomere number is not fixed. If a muscle is immobilized in the shortened position, sarcomeres are lost and the remaining sarcomeres are pulled to a length which enables the muscle to develop its maximum tension in this new shortened position.[52,53] Adult muscle immobilized in a shortened position undergoes a reduction in the maximum tension it can develop when called upon to function in a position other than the shortened position. Abnormal muscle elongation leads to an increase in the number of sarcomeres and the ability to develop maximum tension only in more lengthened positions.[3,54-56] A common geriatric patient example is that of kyphosis-related shortening of the pectoral muscles and lengthening of the paraspinal muscles. In this example, the paraspinal muscles have been held in a lengthened position for a prolonged time period with gradual adaptations that make these muscles less capable of producing strength and holding a contraction within the range most relevant to counter the flexor moment and maintain a more normal upright posture.

THE ROLE OF POSTURE IN COMMON SPINAL CONDITIONS

Some of the more common chronic conditions of the musculoskeletal system associated with postural malalignments are osteoporosis with or without related vertebral fracture; cervical and lumbar spinal stenosis; and degenerative osteoarthritis of the back, neck, and lower limbs.

Osteoporosis

Osteoporosis is defined by the World Health Organization as "a systemic skeletal disease characterized by a low bone mass and a microarchitectural deterioration of bone tissue, with a consequent increase in bone fragility and susceptibility to fracture"[57] with two commonly identified levels of bone fragility, defined in Box 16-1.

Osteoporosis-related fractures have a major impact on posture and on health. Given current projections about fragility fractures, it is likely that up to 50% of women and 20% of men who reach 50 years of age will have a fragility fracture in their remaining lifetime.[58] Anterior vertebral body fragility fractures are the most common spinal fragility fracture. These fractures may cause hyperkyphosis, pain, height loss, and are associated with functional loss and increased mortality.[12,13,21,23,52,59,60] Although the acute fragility fracture can be very painful,

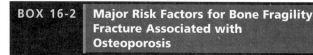

BOX 16-1	Criteria for Osteoporosis and Osteopenia[55]
Bone Density Category	**Key Characteristics of Each Category**
Osteoporosis	BMD more than 2.5 standard deviations less than the mean of BMD of young adult women (BMD T-score < −2.5)
Osteopenia (low bone mass)	BMD value between 1 and 2.5 standard deviations less than the mean BMD of young adult women (−2.5 < BMD T-score < −1).

BMD, bone mineral density.

it can also be asymptomatic so that it is only discovered when a person is evaluated radiographically for an unrelated condition or because of concerns over a progressively increasing hyperkyphosis.[53]

The most obvious postural concern for a person with osteoporosis and vertebral fragility fracture is the danger of additional fractures when performing any activity of daily living (ADL) in the increasingly trunk flexed position. Trunk twisting and lateral bending load the spine and trunk muscles substantially less than activities done in trunk flexion or holding weights in front of the body.[45] Risk of injury is also increased in the presence of intervertebral disc degeneration.[61] Box 16-2 summarizes the major risk factors for bone fragility fractures commonly associated with osteoporosis.

Spinal Osteoarthritis

Degenerative osteoarthritis (OA) of the lumbar and cervical spine is increasingly common with advancing age. Individuals with degenerative osteoarthritis (without any associated osteoporosis) have been found to have nearly

BOX 16-2	Major Risk Factors for Bone Fragility Fracture Associated with Osteoporosis

Primary Risk Factors
- Low bone mineral density
- Flexion-oriented body mechanics

Additional Contributing Factors
- Advanced age
- Low body height and weight
- History of previous fragility fracture or parent with osteoporosis
- Current smoking
- History of glucocorticoid use
- Certain medications (selective serotonin reuptake inhibitors anticoagulant or antiseizure medications)
- Rheumatoid arthritis
- Three or more glasses of alcohol daily
- Presence of risk factors for falls
- Sedentary lifestyle with inadequate bone-stimulating exercise

twice as much vertebral wedge deformity as similarly aged individuals with normal spines; nevertheless, the extent of the wedge deformity is less in those with osteoarthritis than in individuals with osteoporosis (13% vs. 21%, respectively).[19] Spinal osteoarthritis is a longstanding condition, developing throughout the adult years. Many individuals who have advanced osteoarthritic changes may have few to no symptoms, while others with relatively minor changes may have pronounced and disabling symptoms. Advanced spinal osteoarthritis that compromises the diameter of the spinal canal is one cause of spinal stenosis.

Spinal Stenosis

Lumbar spinal stenosis (LSS) and cervical spinal stenosis (CSS) are associated with hypertrophy of spinal ligaments, osteoarthritis, and disc degeneration. Decreased elasticity of the ligamentum flavum with age combined with an accumulation of fibrotic scarring (possibly inflammation-related), and with thickening of remaining elastin fibers are likely contributors to LF hypertrophy, particularly in its dorsal layer.[43] The effects of many years of stress and microtrauma to spinal structures resulting in such changes as loss of joint space, osteophyte development, protrusion of the annulus fibrosus, and hypertrophy of the LF may each contribute to decreased diameter of the intervertebral foramen that can progress sufficiently to cause symptomatic entrapment of spinal nerve roots.[62]

LSS increases the likelihood of low back pain (LBP) threefold, after adjusting for sex, age, and body mass index.[63] Symptomatic leg and back pain from LSS can progress to paresis from associated nerve compression. LSS is commonly associated with decreased lordosis and with complaints of pain with the lumbar spine in an extension posture, and pain relieved by assuming a flexed lumbar posture.[64] There is evidence from many studies that those with fixed cervical or lumbar flexion deformities have greater pain, decreased function, and do less well after surgical intervention than those who are able to assume a more normal lordotic alignment.[18,65,66]

PHYSICAL THERAPY MANAGEMENT OF THE PATIENT WITH POSTURE DYSFUNCTION

The physical therapists' role in optimizing posture is often limited to the management of postural impairments that have become symptomatic, resulting in activity limitations and secondary conditions. Physical therapists should also address the primary prevention role of optimizing postures to avoid symptomatic conditions. Because the factors contributing to postural impairment and dysfunction can be quite variable, particularly among older adults, an individualized posture evaluation is necessary.

Postural dysfunction can emerge from primary impairments associated with muscle imbalances or in association with comorbid conditions. Habitual poor posture can contribute to secondary conditions, and sedentary lifestyle can promote age-related decline across physiological systems.[67-70]

Patient management starts with a comprehensive patient examination, which includes assessment of the impairments, actions, and tasks affected by the postural dysfunction, and the body mechanics typically used during functional activities. Examination findings (history, systems review, and tests and measures) serve as the basis for hypothesizing the cause of the postural dysfunctions (or risks for dysfunction) and, thus, a diagnosis. The plan of care and specific interventions to implement the plan of care consider such factors as the medical prognosis of the patient, influence of comorbid and secondary conditions, personal and environmental enabling and disabling factors, best scientific evidence, and patient preferences.

History

The patient's medical and social history can contribute substantively to the patient's activity participation prognosis and toward the choice of intervention approach. Key factors that should be included in any history are summarized in Chapter 6, Figure 6-10. Many medications commonly taken by older adults have side effects or adverse reaction that can affect posture and mobility: sedation (decreased motivation), postural instability, fatigue and weakness, depression, and postural hypotension. Assessing medications as part of the patient history provides valuable information that contributes to the evaluative decisions regarding posture. Chapter 4 on pharmacology provides a detailed discussion of common reactions to medication(s) that affect functional mobility and movement.

Objective Testing

Pain. Measures of pain comprise two broad categories: self-perception of the amount, intensity, and location of pain and the impact of pain on activity. Common measures of the intensity of pain include the numerical index and the pain analog scale. These measures are explained in detail in Chapter 21 on pain management. Both the 12-item Oswestry Disability Index (ODI)[59,60,71,72] Box 16-3 and the Back Pain Functional Scale (BPFS)[73] Box 16-4 are valid, reliable, and responsive measures of the impact of pain on functional activities of patients with low back pain. Because both tools are sensitive to change over time in the areas of function- and posture-associated pain, they can be valuable for guiding the physical therapy plan of care and making decisions about the continuation of physical therapy services. A greater discussion of pain assessment tools, as well as the impact of pain on functional ability, is included in Chapter 21 on pain management.

Alignment

Total Body Alignment. Traditionally, postural alignment is assessed through a plumb line. The plumb line tests, as depicted in Figures 16-4 and 16-5, are used to determine whether the points of reference of the individual being tested are in optimal alignment for efficient and effective weight bearing. A plumb line or posture grid can provide a vertical reference line around a standard fixed point (either at a point equidistant between the heels for frontal view, or anterior to the lateral malleolus for the sagittal view). Deviations from the plumb alignment are usually described as slight, moderate, or marked,[3,74,75] but may also be measured in terms of centimeters or degrees with measurements derived from a photograph using a "graph paper" grid overlying a photograph of the patient. A photograph that uses a posture grid as a reference back drop (vertical and horizontal lines in a grid format) is likely to improve accuracy in the visualization of upright postural alignment against postural landmarks and lends itself to quantitative measurement of deviations from optimal alignment by assessing extent of deviations against posture grid lines. Photographic analysis also allows use of anatomical landmarks to draw angles[76] on the picture. Although clinical logic suggests that the closer a person's posture is to "optimal" the fewer posture-related symptoms he or she will experience, the reader is cautioned that the scientific evidence supporting this assumption is weak.

Spinal Curve Alignment. Spinal radiographs, if readily available, can provide direct visualization of spinal alignment and allow calculations of curves (e.g., Cobb angles). However, obtaining radiographs are often impractical and not required as a part of routine physical therapy examination of alignment, unless there is concern about conditions such as fractures or impingements. Clinical assessment of spinal curves can be measured with flexible curve rulers or inclinometers. There are strengths and weaknesses with each approach.

Flexible Curve Ruler. A surveyor's flexible curve ruler is a semirigid device composed of parallel lead strips encased in a plastic sheath that can efficiently and cost-effectively obtain reproducible measurements of kypholordosis. Any patient observed to have an abnormal kypholordosis during examination, or who has a history of a back-related health condition, is an appropriate patient for assessment with a flexible curve ruler. Figure 16-6 depicts the measurements and three major formulas used to calculate curvature scores. Thoracic to lumbar width ratio (TW/LW) compares the depth of the thoracic kyphosis to the depth of the lumbar lordosis, and thoracic to lumbar length ratio (TL/LL) compares the length of the thoracic kyphosis to the length of the lumbar lordosis. These two ratios quantify the relative percentage of the spine in kyphosis or lordosis. The third ratio, the Kyphosis Index (KI), is expressed by the equation ($100 \times$ TW/TL) and provides an approximation of

BOX 16-3	**Oswestry Disability Index (ODI) Version 2.0**

Please complete this questionnaire. It is designated to give us information on how your back or leg trouble has affected your ability to manage in everyday life. Please answer **every section**. Mark **one box only** in each section that most closely describes you **today**.

Section 1: Pain Intensity in Back and/or Legs
- ☐ I have no pain. (0 pts)
- ☐ The pain is very mild. (1 pt)
- ☐ The pain is moderate. (2 pts)
- ☐ The pain is fairly severe. (3 pts)
- ☐ The pain is very severe. (4 pts)
- ☐ The pain is the worse imaginable. (5 pts)

Section 2: Personal Care (e.g., washing, dressing)
- ☐ I can look after myself normally without causing extra pain. (0 pts)
- ☐ I can look after myself normally, but it is very painful. (1 pt)
- ☐ It is painful to look after myself, and I am slow and careful. (2 pts)
- ☐ I need some help, but manage most of my personal care. (3 pts)
- ☐ I need help every day in most aspects of self-care. (4 pts)
- ☐ I do not get dressed, wash with difficulty, and stay in bed. (5 pts)

Section 3: Lifting
- ☐ I can lift heavy weights without extra pain. (0 pts)
- ☐ I can lift heavy weights, but it gives extra pain. (1 pt)
- ☐ Pain prevents me from lifting heavy weights off the floor, but I can manage if they are conveniently positioned (e.g., on a table). (2 pts)
- ☐ Pain prevents me from lifting heavy weights, but I can manage light to medium weights if they are conveniently positioned. (3 pts)
- ☐ I can lift only very light weights. (4 pts)
- ☐ I cannot lift or carry anything at all. (5 pts)

Section 4: Walking
- ☐ Pain does not prevent me walking any distance. (0 pts)
- ☐ Pain prevents me walking more than 1 mile. (1 pt)
- ☐ Pain prevents me walking more than ½ mile. (2 pts)
- ☐ Pain prevents me walking more than 100 yards. (3 pts)
- ☐ I can walk only by using a stick or crutches. (4 pts)
- ☐ I am in bed most of the time and must crawl to the toilet. (5 pts)

Section 5: Sitting
- ☐ I can sit in any chair as long as I like. (0 pts)
- ☐ I can sit in my favorite chair as long as I like. (1 pt)
- ☐ Pain prevents me from sitting more than 1 h. (2 pts)
- ☐ Pain prevents me from sitting more than ½ h. (3 pts)
- ☐ Pain prevents me from sitting more than 10 min. (4 pts)
- ☐ Pain prevents me from sitting at all. (5 pts)

Section 6: Standing
- ☐ I can stand as long as I want without extra pain. (0 pts)
- ☐ I can stand as long as I want, but it gives me extra pain. (1 pt)
- ☐ Pain prevents me from standing more than 1 h. (2 pts)
- ☐ Pain prevents me from standing more than ½ h. (3 pts)
- ☐ Pain prevents me from standing more than 10 min. (4 pts)
- ☐ Pain prevents me from standing at all. (5 pts)

Section 7: Sleeping
- ☐ My sleep is never disturbed by pain. (0 pts)
- ☐ My sleep is occasionally disturbed by pain. (1 pt)
- ☐ Because of my pain, I have less than 6 h sleep. (2 pts)
- ☐ Because of my pain, I have less than 4 h sleep. (3 pts)
- ☐ Because of my pain, I have less than 2 h sleep. (4 pts)
- ☐ Pain prevents me from sleeping at all. (5 pts)

BOX 16-3	**Oswestry Disability Index (ODI) Version 2.0—cont'd**

Section 8: Sex Life (if applicable)
- ☐ My sex life is normal and causes me no extra pain. (0 pts)
- ☐ My sex life is normal, and causes me some extra pain. (1 pt)
- ☐ My sex life is nearly normal but it is very painful. (2 pts)
- ☐ My sex life is severely restricted by pain. (3 pts)
- ☐ My sex life is nearly absent because of pain. (4 pts)
- ☐ Pain prevents any sex life at all. (5 pts)

Section 9: Social Life
- ☐ My social life is normal and causes me no extra pain. (0 pts)
- ☐ My social life is normal but increases the degree of pain. (1 pt)
- ☐ Pain has no significant effect on my social life apart from limiting my more energetic interests (e.g., sports). (2 pts)
- ☐ Pain has restricted my social life, and I do not go out as often. (3 pts)
- ☐ Pain has restricted my social life to my home. (4 pts)
- ☐ I have no social life because of pain. (5 pts)

Section 10: Traveling
- ☐ I can travel anywhere without pain. (0 pts)
- ☐ I can travel anywhere, but it gives me pain. (1 pt)
- ☐ Pain is bad, but I can manage journeys exceeding 2 h. (2 pts)
- ☐ Pain restricts me to journeys of less than 1 h. (3 pts)
- ☐ Pain restricts me to short necessary journeys shorter than 30 min. (4 pts)
- ☐ Pain prevents me from traveling except to receive treatment. (5 pts)

Section 11: Previous Treatment: Over the Past 3 Months Have you Received Treatment, Tablets, or Medicines of any Kind for your Back or Leg Pain?
_____No _____Yes (specify treatment)_____

The first 10 sections relate to symptoms today. Section 11 does not contribute to the score. Patients often omit section 8. Each section is scored from 0 to 5. The final score equals total score for all sections completed/50 × 100 = percent of disability.
(Adapted from Baker D, Pynsent P, Fairbank J, The Oswestry Disability Index revisited. In Roland M, Jenner J, editors: Back pain: new approaches to rehabilitation and education. Manchester, 1989, Manchester University Press, pp. 174-186. Fairbank JCT, Pynsent PB. The Oswestry Disability Index. Spine 25: 2940-2953, 2000.)

the angular shape of the thoracic kyphosis. General procedures for molding the flexible curve ruler to the spinal curves and then transferring the model to graph paper are summarized in Figure 16-7. The KI can be used to assess changes in kyphosis over time.[18] However, no minimally detectable change score has been identified; thus interpretation is difficult.

Milne and Lauder[77] calculated the KI using the flexible curve tracings and compared these scores with the wedging index calculated from lateral radiographs performed the same day on 513 men and women between 62 and 90 years of age. These scores were highly correlated, supporting the validity of the flexible curve measure as an index for kyphosis.[77,78] The flexible curve ruler has good to excellent interrater and intrarater reliability when subjects are directed to stand in an erect posture.[15,79] Although both younger and older women demonstrated significantly different curve measurements

BOX 16-4	Back Pain Function Scale

On the questions listed below, we are interested in knowing whether you are having ANY DIFFICULTY at all with the activities because of your back problem for which you are currently seeking attention.

   Please provide an answer for each activity.

   Today, do you or would you have any DIFFICULTY at all with the following activities BECAUSE OF YOUR BACK PROBLEM?

(Circle one number on each line)

	Unable to Perform Activity	Extreme Difficulty	Quite a Bit of Difficulty	Moderate Difficulty	A Little Bit of Difficulty	No Difficulty
1. Any of your usual work, housework, or school activities	0	1	2	3	4	5
2. Your usual hobbies, recreational, or sporting activities	0	1	2	3	4	5
3. Performing heavy activities around your home	0	1	2	3	4	5
4. Bending or stooping	0	1	2	3	4	5
5. Putting on your shoes or socks (pantyhose)	0	1	2	3	4	5
6. Lifting a box of groceries from the floor	0	1	2	3	4	5
7. Sleeping	0	1	2	3	4	5
8. Standing for 1 h	0	1	2	3	4	5
9. Walking a mile	0	1	2	3	4	5
10. Going up or down two flights of stairs (about 20 stairs)	0	1	2	3	4	5
11. Sitting for 1 h	0	1	2	3	4	5
12. Driving for 1 h	0	1	2	3	4	5

Subtotals =

Total score = /60

The respondent is asked to rate ability to engage in the following activities on a scale of 0 to 5, where 0 = unable to perform activity; 1 = extreme difficulty; 2 = quite a bit of difficulty; 3 = moderate difficulty; 4 = a little bit of difficulty; and 5 = no difficulty.

Total score = /60 (The points are totaled and compared with a maximum possible score of 60, which represents no difficulty in performing any of the listed activities.)

(From: Stratford PW, Binkley JM, Riddle DL: Development and initial validation of the back pain functional scale. Spine 25(16):2095-2102, 2000.)

when standing in usual versus erect posture, younger women as compared to older women were able to achieve a greater degree of active reduction of their kyphosis when assuming an "erect posture."[13]

Inclinometer. The degree of thoracic and lumbar curvature can be measured in standing using either a mechanical[80-84] or a digital[85] inclinometer, as illustrated in Figure 16-8. Inclinometer readings reflect the angle formed by tangents to the curves created by alignment of the spinous processes. Patients are asked to stand up as straight as possible. Thoracic kyphosis is assessed by positioning the two inclinometer arms at T1 downward and T12 upward to capture the upper and lower thoracic slope, respectively. The intersecting angle of these two lines provides a thoracic kyphosis score. Similarly, lumbar lordosis can be assessed using the inclination from T12 downward and S1 upward and calculating the angle formed by the tangents to the spinal processes on each end of the thoracic and lumbar curves. Although the digital inclinometer is time efficient to use, it is expensive to purchase and does not capture the shape of the curve from the entire C7 to S1 span. The mechanical

inclinometer does not have the same degree of validity and reproducibility as either the digital inclinometer or flexible curve method.[18]

Head Alignment. Anyone who cannot touch their occiput to the wall when standing with buttocks and midback against the wall and eyes focused straight ahead is classified as having a flexed posture.[4,76,86-88] A meta-analysis concluded that a wall-to-occiput distance greater than zero yields a 4.6 likelihood ratio for occult vertebral fractures for all women age 65 years or older.[89] The occiput-to-wall test (or tragus-to-wall variation of the test) has been recommended as a screening tool to identify individuals with possible vertebral fracture for whom closer assessment is warranted.[88] As pictured in Figure 16-9, the extent of forward flexed posture can be easily and reliably assessed by measuring the distance from each tragus to the wall and recording the average of the two values. Tragus-to-wall is generally the measurement of choice as it also assesses rotational dysfunction, can be done in the standing position, and requires only a ruler for valid and reliable examination.[4,86,87] Forward-flexed posture can also be measured

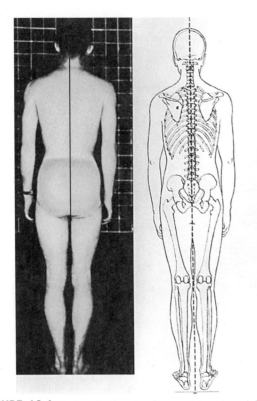

FIGURE 16-4 Posture in the standing position viewed from the posterior. *(Used with permission from Kendall EP, McCreary EK, Provance PG, et al: Muscles: testing and function. ed 5. Baltimore, 2005, Lippincott Williams & Wilkins).*

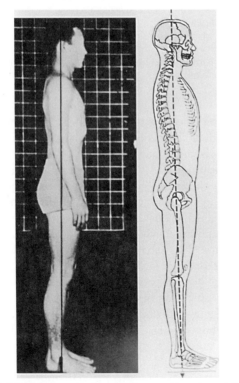

FIGURE 16-5 Posture in the standing position viewed from the side. *(Used with permission from Kendall EP, McCreary EK: Muscles: testing and function. Baltimore, Williams & Wilkins; and Kendall EP, McCreary EK, Provance PG, et al: Muscles: testing and function, ed. 5. Baltimore, 2005, Lippincott Williams & Wilkins.)*

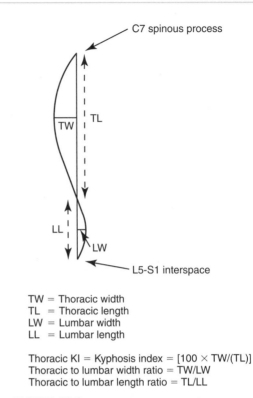

TW = Thoracic width
TL = Thoracic length
LW = Lumbar width
LL = Lumbar length

Thoracic KI = Kyphosis index = [100 × TW/(TL)]
Thoracic to lumbar width ratio = TW/LW
Thoracic to lumbar length ratio = TL/LL

FIGURE 16-6 Flexible curve tracing of spinal curves.

in the supine patient by determining the distance between occiput and mat that must be accommodated to achieve neutral head/neck positioning. This distance can be measured by using a series of thin supporting blocks to position the head and neck until neutral head/neck is achieved.[14,23,26]

Extremity Alignment. Even small malalignments of the lower extremity joints may have a major impact on both total body alignment as well as spinal alignment. The lower extremities distribute and dissipate compressive, tensile, shearing, and rotatory forces during the stance phase of gait. Continued weight bearing and ambulation with lower extremity joint malalignments may result in painful and weakened joint structure impairments, impaired balance, and inefficient functional movement. Lower extremity joint alignment should be assessed from all three planes of motion: frontal plane for valgus and varus alignments; sagittal plane for any flexion and extension abnormalities; and coronal plane as an assessment of rotational alignment.

It is also important to assess foot biomechanics. Proper arthrokinematic movement within the foot and ankle influences the ability of the lower limb to distribute and dissipate forces.[90-92] It is particularly important to assess arch sufficiency in the older adult. Arch sufficiency can be assessed by measuring the height of the navicular tubercle above the floor. Comparison measurements between sitting unsupported in subtalar neutral, and then in relaxed standing, yields the "navicular drop" score[93,94] illustrated in Figure 16-10.

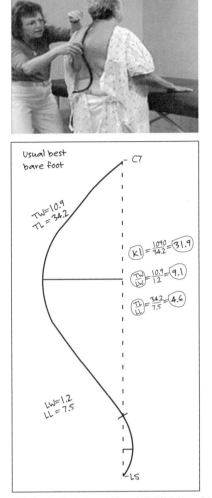

Thoracic kyphotic index: $100 \times (10.9/34.2) = 31.9$
TW to LW ratio: $10.9/1.2 = 9.1$
- TW is 9.1 times greater than LW
TL to LL ratio: $34.2/7.5 = 4.6$
- TL is 4.6 times greater than LL

FIGURE 16-7 Example of flexible curve spinal alignment measurement process. The patient stands in her "usual best posture," holding table lightly until the curve is molded to her shape from C7 to LS interspace, upon which time her hands are removed, and the contour of the curve is finalized, then traced onto graph paper. *LL,* lumbar length; *LW,* lumbar width; *TL,* thoracic length; *TW,* thoracic width. *(Used with permission from Lindsey C, Bookstein N: Kypholordosis measurement using a flexible curve [instructional CD]. American Physical Therapy Association Section on Geriatrics, 2007.)*

Range of Motion

A targeted examination of joint range of motion, muscle–tendon unit extensibility (two-joint extensibility), and segmental (accessory) movements of the spine should be performed for all patients being assessed for postural dysfunction. Initial observational analysis of posture and postural alignment during various movements provides clues to potential joint and muscle extensibility

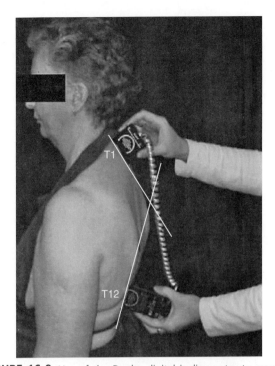

FIGURE 16-8 Use of the Dualer digital inclinometer to measure angle of thoracic kyphosis. Spinous processes of T1 and T12 were used as landmarks for positioning the inclinometer sensors. The angle of the intersection of the solid lines demonstrates the angle of thoracic kyphosis. *(Used with permission from Greig AM, Bennell KL, Briggs AM, Hodges PW: Postural taping decreases thoracic kyphosis but does not influence trunk muscle electromyographic activity or balance in women with osteoporosis. Man Ther 13(3):249-257, 2008.)*

limitations and narrows down the choice of movements needing ROM assessment.

Range of motion of extremity joints can be measured with a standard universal goniometer; overall spinal flexibility can be assessed with a set of two inclinometers or with a standard tape measure to document the distance between specified anatomical points.[83,95] However, unless a patient's goal is to improve spinal flexibility, measuring the full range of spinal flexibility as a baseline measure may be unnecessary; and for some patients, attaining full spine motion may be contraindicated. Attaining full spinal flexion for a patient with osteoporosis, or full spinal extension for a patient with spinal stenosis, is neither a desirable nor useful outcome.

Examining two-joint muscle flexibility is particularly important as many postural changes are associated with altered muscle length.[3,4,84,95-98] The important issue concerning muscle shortness is not the degree of loss at each joint but rather the percentage of loss of overall muscle excursion and the consequences of such losses on joint behavior during functional activities.

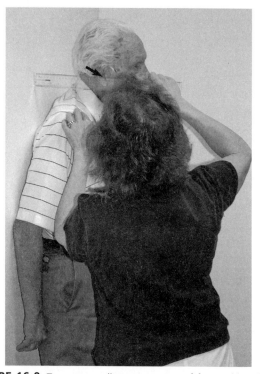

FIGURE 16-9 Tragus-to-wall measurement of forward head posture. Subject stands with heels, buttocks, and back against wall, head as close to the wall as possible while looking straight ahead. For accuracy, it is crucial to be sure that the cervical spine is *not* in extension (the most common error that reduces both validity and reliability of this test). *(Used with permission from Bones, Backs & Balance, LLC, New Hartford, CT.)*

Strength

Core muscle weakness and imbalances can have a major impact on postural alignment. Trunk strength can be difficult to test in frail older adults, particularly those with osteoporosis for whom forceful trunk flexion is contraindicated, and those with conditions such as spinal stenosis or spondylolisthesis for whom lumbar extension is problematic. However, there is a growing body of evidence about the extent of trunk muscle force required to maintain safe alignment of the spine during a variety of functional positions. This knowledge provides insights into the clinical value of providing progressively greater challenge to trunk muscles while avoiding potentially unsafe trunk movements. In trunk extension, an example of a low-challenge activity may be to have the standing patient positioned near a wall facing it with arms overhead and hands resting on the wall. The physical therapist palpates the back extensor muscles as the patient is directed to focus on contracting these muscles as they lift their arm away from the wall. In contrast, a highly challenging activity would be to have the patient lying prone with arms overhead and focus on contracting the back extensor muscles as they lift the back from this position. A weighted vest on the back can add further challenge to a prone position test. When testing trunk extension in the prone position, it is important to include a towel roll under the forehead to keep the cervical spine in neutral as well as a pillow under the abdomen to avoid additional lumbar extension in case of spinal stenosis or spondylolisthesis.[43]

Traditional abdominal strength testing that utilizes trunk flexed positions must be modified for individuals at risk for vertebral fragility fractures. A low-challenge activity for functional control of abdominal muscles is the ability to hold an "abdominal hollow position" for several seconds in the hook lying position. In comparison, a high-challenge activity is the ability to maintain a neutral lordosis with abdominal hollowing for

Arthrokinematic (joint play or accessory) motions should be assessed for all joints found to have limited or painful osteokinematic motions. Arthrokinematic motions are necessary for full and symptom-free osteokinematic motions. The careful examination of accessory motions helps to more specifically locate and treat the source of impaired osteokinematic motions.

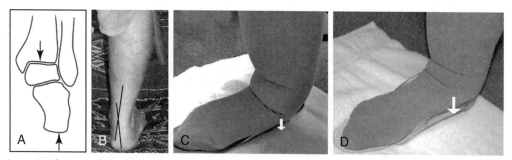

FIGURE 16-10 Pronation forces and clinical measurements. **A,** When the heel strikes the ground on the lateral aspect, a force comes vertically up the outside of the foot. *(Posterior view)* The force of body weight is acting down through the ankle joint. Because these two forces do not line up, the talus is driven medially, initiating and producing the pronation movement. **B,** Valgus angle between calcaneal midline and distal third of lower leg at midline. **C,** Navicular tuberosity to floor distance *(arrow)* should be measured non-weight-bearing, then compared to weight-bearing. Orthotic indicated if drop is 3.5 cm. **C, D,** Compare support offered by two different orthotics for severely pronated foot. *(**A,** Used with permission from Hamill J, Knutzen KM: Biomechanical basis of human movement, ed 3. Media, PA, 2009, Williams and Wilkins. **B, C, D,** Used with permission from Bones, Backs & Balance LLC, New Hartford, CT.)*

60 seconds while supine and performing various hip and knee flexion and extension movements.[99]

There are many approaches and philosophies to testing muscle strength that are beyond the scope of this chapter.

Respiratory Function

An initial systems review may suggest compromised respiratory function that requires further examination. Several studies show significant correlations between kyphosis associated with osteoporotic fractures and impaired pulmonary function.[82,100,101] A patient who sits in an excessively flexed position can compress the contents of the abdomen against the diaphragm, causing breathing to be restricted. History questions aimed at assessing respiratory compromise include the following: (1) Does the patient experience difficulty breathing when lying supine? (2) Does the thorax appear to move easily and comfortably during each breath when the patient is sitting? (3) Is the breathing rhythm regular? (4) Is the movement of the thorax excessively fast or too slow? (5) Does the patient sigh more often than is necessary? (6) Does the person execute a Valsalva maneuver when changing positions or when doing a task? Chapter 12 on impaired aerobic capacity discusses respiratory examination in more detail.

Balance

Although static positions are important to assess, it is equally important to assess posture in terms of dynamic balance and coordination by administering appropriate balance assessments. Chapter 18 on balance and falls outlines this aspect of the examination. While assessing body alignment, it is also necessary to determine the extent to which a person is able to maintain a posture (posture holding) or position of the body without extraneous movements (equilibrium or postural sway). Maintaining postural control in a static position decreases with age and is potentially problematic for the older adult, as the loss of postural control is well known to increase the risk of falling.

CHANGING FAULTY POSTURE: EVALUATION, DIAGNOSIS, PROGNOSIS, AND PLAN OF CARE

The patient who has impaired posture as the primary contributor to pain or activity limitation would be classified in the "Impaired Posture" preferred practice pattern (4B) according to the *Guide*.[1] This practice pattern provides a comprehensive framework of key elements to be considered in the assessment and management of patients with impaired posture. Alternatively, Practice Pattern 4A addresses primary prevention to reduce the risk of skeletal muscle demineralization and its associated postural dysfunction. For other patients, alternative

practice patterns may serve as the primary guide to management of the patient. However, if postural dysfunction is a substantive contributor to the need for physical therapy, elements of Practice Pattern 4A or 4B may be included as secondary practice patterns.

Physical therapist decisions about diagnosis, prognosis, plan of care, and interventions must be based on a thorough, accurate, and skillful patient examination; the incorporation of best available evidence to ground your clinical decisions; and a careful assessment and application of the preferences and goals of the patient.

Individual items from functional assessment tools such as the Oswestry Disability Index or the Back Pain Functional Scale can help identify specific activity limitations that can help guide the specific focus of the plan of care. It is also crucial that the therapist observe the patient's body mechanics during the activities that cause pain, gather subjective and objective data, and use these data to formulate a plan that includes both informative patient feedback and specific corrective exercises.

Interventions

Interventions for impaired posture are based on the evaluation of the history and examination data. Patient compliance with an exercise program is essential to improve impaired posture and reduce its functional sequelae. A partnership between physical therapist and patient must be established. The patient recognizes that they are responsible for consistent practice of component tasks (exercises) designed to maximize their ability to function in improved postural alignment. The physical therapist determines the exercise prescription, provides feedback and guidance on correct performance of the exercises, progresses the exercises as improvements are made, and offers instruction in good body mechanics and in risk factor reduction strategies.

All intervention approaches are designed to optimize the ability of the patient to function within their optimal postural alignment and thus achieve their goals of movement and function in a pain-free and physically competent manner. When exercise alone is insufficient to create the desired outcome, soft tissue impairments may need to be treated with manual therapy or modalities (thermal agents or electrotherapeutics) in order of the area of greatest restriction. If the patient is still unable to support himself or herself in good functional alignment, an external postural support may be indicated while the patient continues the exercise program. The treatment plan should be organized so that each identified problem is addressed in the order of greatest functional impact for the patient.

The following sections focus on therapeutic exercise approaches to correct faulty posture so that the patient can maintain good alignment during daily activities; selected manual therapy approaches to increase flexibility and decrease pain as a mechanism of achieving better posture; and use of external supports to assist in maintaining posture. The use of thermal and electrotherapeutic modalities will not be specifically discussed in this chapter.

Therapeutic Exercise to Correct Faulty Postural Muscle Imbalances

One of the most common postural problems is that caused by faulty patterns resulting from synergistic muscle imbalances.[102-106] When addressing postural alignment, it is vital that the therapist be certain that the patient understands and is able to execute the exercise in appropriate alignment. Sahrmann's work extensively describes faulty postural patterns and gives approaches for exercise intervention to treat these impairment syndromes.[3]

Her primary approach is to teach patients to perform motions correctly in the test position and thus reverse the compensatory pattern. Exercise in the test position, which is the position that represents movement patterns in optimal alignment, ensures that the motion is restricted to the segment that is supposed to move, and also that the segment is moving in the appropriate plane. Examples of exercise movements that use this approach are illustrated in Figure 16-11.

As Sahrmann stresses, a desired muscle action should be practiced under the specific conditions in which it is to be used (principle of specificity). Improving a muscle's function under one set of conditions does not automatically generalize to improved function in the same muscle under different conditions. Training is relatively specific, and improving the contractile ability of a muscle does

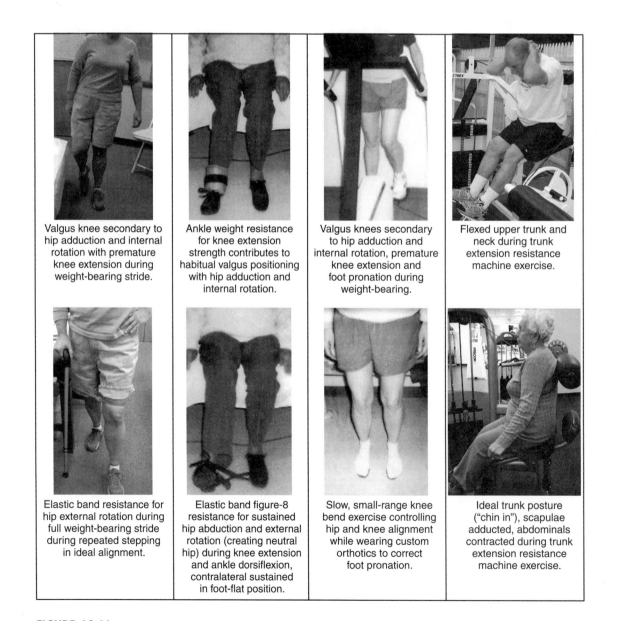

FIGURE 16-11 (*Top row*) Exercise in faulty alignment. (*Bottom row*) Exercise interventions for healthy alignment. (*Used with permission from Bones, Backs & Balance LLC, New Hartford, CT.*)

not ensure that its participation will become generalized to other activities. Because joints are arranged in series, when the joints are the site of compensatory movement, effective treatment requires simultaneous control of all the affected segments.[106]

Axial (Core) Strengthening Exercises. Approaches to abdominal and paraspinal muscle strengthening are many and varied. Those presented in this chapter are based on the principles of biomechanical safety and of training directed toward functional postural stabilization. The best available research evidence should be used as the basis for choosing specific exercise. Key considerations in core strengthening, particularly in individuals with low bone density, is to avoid forceful trunk flexion and to facilitate trunk extensor muscle contraction in positions that minimize flexion moments on the trunk.

Several randomized controlled trials have provided evidence that older adults with kyphosis can improve their spinal posture by using a battery of specific exercises. All of the studies used thoracic extension exercise as the cornerstone of their intervention protocols.[18,52,107-110] The classic study of Sinaki and Mikkelson identified a much higher incidence of vertebral compression fractures in patients with postmenopausal osteoporosis who either followed a flexion exercise program (FE) or did not engage in any trunk extension or abdominal exercises (NE) compared with patients who followed an extension exercise (EE) program (follow-up vertebral fracture rate of FE = 89%, NE = 67%, EE = 16%). Although a retrospective study without random assignment to group, the finding that there is a high association of fracture with flexion exercise led to the commonly accepted principle that flexion exercise is relatively contraindicated in the presence of osteoporosis. A prospective study by the same investigators demonstrated the long-term protective effect of stronger back muscles on the spine in 50 healthy white postmenopausal women, aged 58 to 75 years, which was still present 8 years after they had completed a 2-year randomized controlled trial of back extensor strengthening exercises.[46] The back extensor strengthening exercises utilized a weighted backpack to provide resistance to the subject positioned prone, beginning with 30% of maximal isometric strength and progressively increasing to a maximum of 50 pounds (10 repetitions; 1 time per day, 5 days per week). The relative risk for compression fracture was 2.7 times greater in the control group than in the back extensor exercise group. Mean vertebral bone density was also significantly greater for the exercise than the control group.

Extremity Postural Exercise. Control of frontal plane knee motion, especially in prevention or treatment of valgus deformity, is clinically important, as this impairment places stress on passive tissue restraints and, in combination with anterior tibial translation, increases stress on the anterior cruciate ligament.[111] Furthermore, abnormal stresses are transmitted both proximally and distally. As femoral adduction and internal rotation contribute to a knee valgus position, muscular control of hip joint alignment during activities may assist in frontal plane knee control. Progressive strengthening exercises for hip abductors, extensors, and external rotators are important. Elastic band resistance exercise can promote a neutral position at the knee during exercise to improve control across multiple planes of movement. Figure 16-11 provides examples. Exercises that emphasize rhythmic and integrated movements of the trunk and extremities in multiple planes improve automatic postural control.[112-114]

Specific Stretches for Trunk and Extremities. There are three key rules for prescribing stretching exercises: (1) Do not put any structure at postural risk (e.g., do not allow trunk flexion concurrently with hamstring stretch)[6,47,74,115]; (2) assure the movement isolates and stretches only the targeted tissue[75]; and (3) utilize a stretching time duration that is equal to or greater than 30 seconds.[96,116] The muscles most likely to need stretching exercises to either maintain or restore an older individual to optimal posture are the suboccipital muscles for the cervical spine, the shoulder protractors and downward rotators (pectoralis major and minor, latissimus dorsi), the hip and knee flexors, and the plantar flexors. When shortened, these muscle groups biomechanically bias the trunk toward a spine flexion and FHP.[52] In addition, movement becomes more difficult and less efficient.

Conditioning and Endurance Exercise. Regular strength and conditioning exercise are well-known to be an integral component of optimal aging, both in healthy and chronically ill older adults.[70,117,118] As people fatigue, posture deteriorates. Exercises that focus on fatigue resistance of postural muscles as well as overall cardiopulmonary endurance contribute to the ability of the patient to maintain good alignment.

Interventions Targeting ADLs

In the author's clinical experience, practicing selected components of ADL tasks in risk-free movement patterns daily for at least 2 weeks is critical for learning and implementing new patterns of behavior for patients who have been performing ADLs in poor postures for years, and often decades. For example (as depicted in Figure 16-12), patients with painful knee OA who have habitually used a movement pattern that places great demand on the knees when bending down, can be taught to use a hip-knee-ankle flexion strategy that places greater demand on the hip extensors than the knee extensors.[119]

Similar principles can be applied to body mechanics training for protection of the thoracic and lumbar spine during bending and lifting activities. During cyclical lifting, substantial changes with fatigue can alter the angular displacements at the knee, hip, trunk, and elbow.[120] Patients engaging in cyclical lifting activities should be educated in

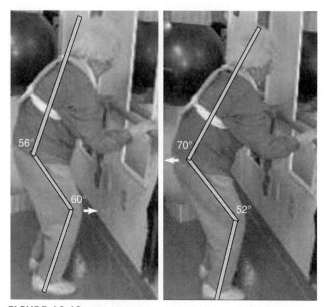

FIGURE 16-12 When training a patient with knee arthritis to use hip-knee-ankle flexion strategy, rather than spinal flexion strategies, it is crucial to teach the corrected action in such a manner that greater demand is placed on the hip extensors rather than the knee extensors. She is also wearing a clavicle support for kyphosis control. *(Data from Flanagan S, Salem GJ, Wang MY, et al: Squatting exercises in older adults: kinematic and kinetic comparisons. Med Sci Sports Exerc 35(4):635-643, 2003. Patient pictures used with permission, photos used with permission from Bones, Backs & Balance LLC, New Hartford, CT.)*

safe body mechanics and appropriate spacing of rest periods to avoid excessive fatigue and, as needed, engage in progressive exercises to enhance fatigue resistance.

Sitting activities while in poor posture can decrease spinal safety at all levels. Use of an appropriate lumbar backrest support can diminish lumbosacral and sacroiliac movement.[65] The choice of best lumbar support for each individual will need precise evaluation and patient education. Some examples of simple back rest support choices and the need for patient education are presented in Figure 16-13. Poor sitting posture has been implicated in the development and perpetuation of neck pain symptoms during tasks such as computer work, hand crafts, and reading. Falla et al[121] reported that people with chronic neck pain demonstrate a reduced ability to maintain an upright posture when distracted.

Exercise Instruction Resources

For postural ADL training, it is very helpful to use a handout with "Do's and Don'ts" and to devise safe individual home exercises based on the usual activities of the patient. An example of such a handout, illustrated in Figure 16-14, is Betz's "Prevent Fractures!" chart.[115] The use of mechanically sound exercise videos directed toward geriatric postural health can also be a valuable resource for either individual or class instruction.

Manual Therapy

Little has been published to help physical therapists use scientific evidence to guide decisions about the various manual therapy techniques applied to older adults with postural dysfunction. Most espoused techniques are based on interpretations of experienced clinicians who have reflectively examined various practice approaches and the responses of their patients to these approaches. There is a great need for high-quality studies to examine the relative effectiveness of these various approaches. Manual therapy is widely used to treat somatic pain syndromes and associated disabilities. Although there is a growing body of research supporting manual therapy,[122-130] few studies have included older adults among their subjects. There is no reason to suspect that the beneficial effects of manual therapy found in younger adults would not be also applicable to older adults.

Manual Joint Mobilization. Joint play movements based on joint arthrokinematics are necessary for full active range of motion at any given joint. Improvement in the form of pain relief may be attainable with very minimal forces (grade 1-2 mobilization), and thus these techniques are safe for all patients, including older adults.[131] For example, the actual change in position during a prone spinal posterior joint mobilization is at most 3 degrees.[132] Evidence supports the use of grade 2 mobilization to treat knee osteoarthritis,[133,134] as well as joint limitation symptoms 2 years after total hip arthroplasty.[135]

Spinal Mobilization Combined with Passive Motion. A randomized controlled trial of postmenopausal women with osteoporosis and kyphosis used gentle regional (whole thoracic spine) passive angular mobilizations toward thoracic extension combined with lateral flexion and/or rotation addressing asymmetrical dysfunctions concurrently. The interventions were performed in sitting with full passive support of the patients' trunk and repeated 10 to 15 times with a 5-second hold at the end. The intervention consisted of 18 treatments spread over 3 months and included postural exercise and taping in addition to the mobilization with passive motion. Thoracic kyphosis in the experimental group improved significantly more when compared to the individuals in the control group. The women who were adherent to the active postural exercises improved significantly more than those who were not adherent.[106]

Muscle Energy Treatment. Muscle energy treatment (MET) is a manual therapy technique that facilitates gentle postural change when vertebral, rib, or pelvic girdle malalignment is identified as the area of greatest restriction. MET utilizes voluntary muscle contraction in a precisely controlled direction, at varying levels of intensity, against a distinctly executed counterforce applied by the practitioner. The intensity of muscle effort may vary from a minimal muscle twitch to a maximal

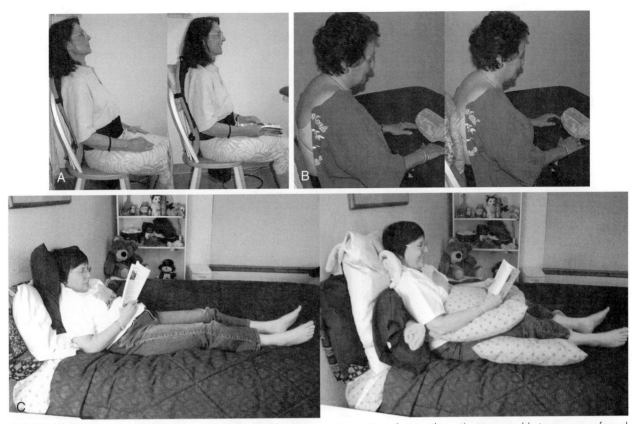

FIGURE 16-13 Teaching use of lumbar support for healthy sitting postures. In each case, the patient was unable to arrange safe and comfortable support until guided by the physical therapist. **A,** Patient cannot figure out how to use lumbar support in chair with moderately reclined back. A small pillow is strapped to superior end of device to correct angle for functional support. **B,** Simulated computer posture. Pillows are added behind waist and kyphosis, picture given to patient to use at home. **C,** Patient's usual position for TV or reading in bed, which she does for 3 to 4 hours per day. Towel rolls are used for cervical and lumbar support, pillow in "T" formation for graduated support behind the head and trunk, pillow under upper extremities for lap-desk support, pillow under knees for more neutral joint position and hips and knees. *(Patient pictures used with permission from Bones, Backs & Balance LLC, New Hartford, CT.)*

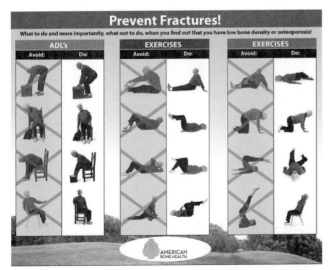

FIGURE 16-14 Body mechanics do's and don'ts for vertebral fracture prevention. *(From American Bone Health, Sherri Betz, PT, 2009. Used with permission.)*

muscle contraction according to the comfort and capability of the patient. The duration of the effort may vary from a fraction of a second to a sustained effort lasting several seconds.[126,127,136] Underlying mechanisms explaining the effects of MET have not been extensively researched, particularly in older adults.

Soft Tissue Mobilization Combined with Contract–Relax. Soft tissue mobilization (STM) is the application of specific and progressive manual forces with the intent of promoting changes in the myofascia, allowing for elongation of shortened structures.[137] STM procedures are often combined with proprioceptive neuromuscular facilitation (PNF) procedures because they are both used to effect changes in myofascial length. Contract-relax (CR) PNF procedures have been shown to be effective in increasing range of motion (ROM).[138,139] PNF techniques, particularly those involving reciprocal activation of the agonist and antagonist to the desired motion, are generally believed particularly effective in increasing joint ROM.[140,141] A combination of STM and PNF have been found to improve hip movement[137] as well as glenohumeral external rotation and overhead reach in patients with shoulder disorders.[125] Figure 16-15 provides a patient example of treating stiff kyphosis and protracted shoulders by alternating joint mobilization with CR.

External Supports

Lumbar supports are frequently recommended for treatment of postural dysfunction. However, current best evidence suggests lumbar supports without the use of concurrent strengthening exercises are ineffective in preventing low back pain, with weak and conflicting evidence about the benefit of lumbar support when combined with direct physical and educational interventions.[142] There is evidence that lumbar supports reduce trunk motion for flexion–extension and lateral bending, but not rotation; however, the functional implications of this are unknown.[143]

There is evidence for effective treatment of osteoporotic kyphosis with external supports. This is important, because greater thoracic kyphosis is associated with increased flexion loading of the spine, which is in turn associated with risk for osteoporotic vertebral fracture.[45,144,145] Greig et al[85] demonstrated that the application of postural therapeutic tape to women with osteoporotic vertebral fractures resulted in an immediate reduction in thoracic kyphosis. In the author's experience, "X" taping[85] from the upper trapezius to the lower rib is useful for patient education during postural interventions, particularly for patients with difficulty internalizing strategies to reduce habitual flexion posture. Figure 16-16 illustrates "X" taping plus a variety of supports that can be used periodically through the day to relieve pain and train for reduced flexed posture, both for patients with and for those without acute vertebral fracture. Figure 16-17 illustrates a variety of external

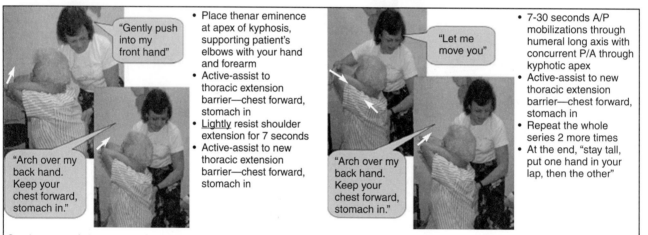

Gentle contract/relax against shoulder extension and trunk flexion

Thoracic P/A mobilization with humeral A/P long axis glide

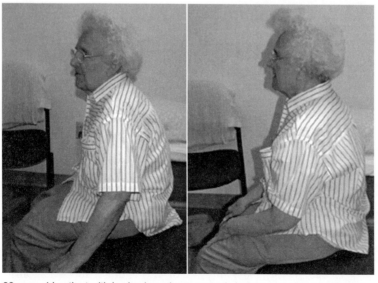

83-year-old patient with kyphosis and osteoporosis before and after mobilization with exercise (asked to "sit as straight and tall as you can").

FIGURE 16-15 Thoracic posterior/anterior joint mobilization and humeral anterior/posterior long axis glide alternated with contract/relax manual treatment for stiff kyphosis and shoulders. *(From Lindsey C: Manual therapy with contract/relax. Course presented at Geriatric Exercise—Principles and Practice for Optimal Function, 2009; Sacramento, CA. Used with permission from author.)*

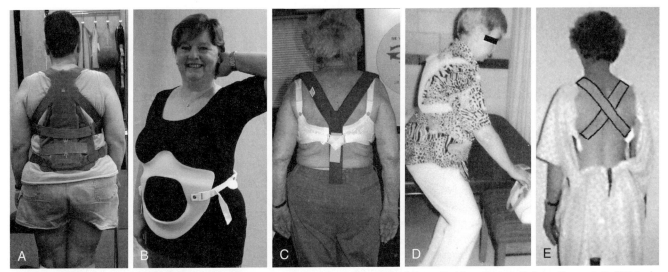

FIGURE 16-16 External postural supports. **A,** Spinomed. **B,** Physiologic. **C,** Universal Strap. **D,** Mayo Posture Training Support. **E,** "X" taping. *(**A,C-E** used with permission from Bones, Backs & Balance LLC, New Hartford, CT; **B** from Weiss HR, Dallmayer R, Stephan C: First results of pain treatment in scoliosis patients using a sagittal realignment brace. Stud Health Technol Inform 123:582-585, 2006.)*

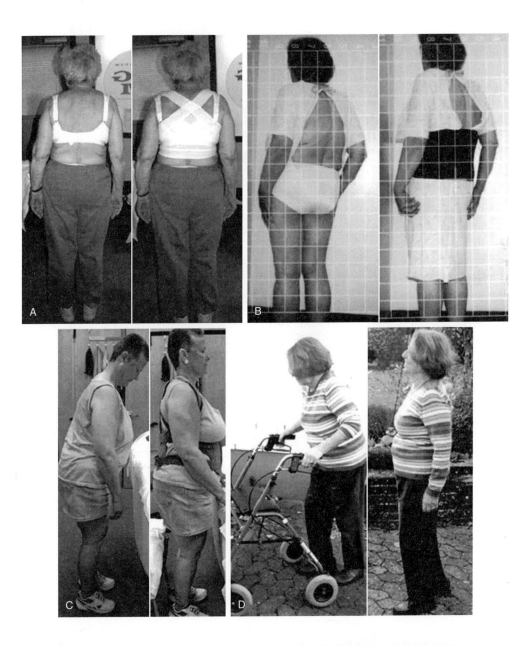

FIGURE 16-17 External postural supports for kyphosis and scoliosis control—comparison pictures of patients with and without support. **A,** Best posture with no support, DM Posture connector. **B,** Best posture with no support, Neoprene Professional's Choice lumbo-sacral corset. **C,** Best posture with no support, Spinomed. **D,** Walker dependent with no brace, Physiologic Brace. *(Patient pictures used with permission from Bones, Backs & Balance LLC, New Hartford, CT. **D** used with permission from Weiss HR, Dallmayer R, Stephan C: First results of pain treatment in scoliosis patients using a sagittal realignment brace. Stud Health Technol Inform 123:582-585, 2006.)*

supports used for kyphosis and scoliosis control. In patients with vertebral fractures caused by osteoporosis, wearing the Spinomed orthosis 2 hours per day for 6 months has been associated with decreased pain, increased trunk muscle strength, a small but statistically significant decrease in angle of kyphosis, improved vital capacity, increased sense of well-being, and greater ability to perform daily living activities.[146] The researchers hypothesized that the increased muscle strength may have been associated with the ongoing feedback about trunk position provided by the brace, as no trunk exercise program was included in the intervention.

Use of a four-wheeled braking walker, as illustrated in Figure 16-18, is a commonly advocated clinical approach to decrease discomfort and achieve improved posture in patients with osteoporotic vertebral fracture. Preliminary data suggest that interventions aimed at keeping the spine stable during transition movements and use of a four-wheeled walker can improve measures of pain and function in patients with osteoporotic vertebral compression fractures.[147]

Lower leg pathologies common in older adults such as heel spurs, hallux valgus, neuromas, hallux limitus, shin splints, and nonspecific knee pain can contribute to abnormal joint biomechanics resulting in abnormal postural alignment. The use of orthotics to reestablish the normal biomechanics of the foot and ankle have important clinical applications.[89,92] Although 4 to 6 degrees of triplanar subtalar joint (STJ) pronation is necessary to provide adequate shock absorption and accommodation to uneven ground terrain, persistent or recurrent abnormal pronation disrupts normal temporal sequencing of the gait cycle.[88-92,148] This disruption creates an unstable osseous and arthrokinematic situation that may lead to compensatory musculoskeletal pathology. A functional foot orthosis promotes structural integrity of the joints of the foot and lower limb by resisting the ground reaction forces that cause abnormal skeletal motion during the stance phase of gait.[92,149] Orthoses, as those illustrated in Figure 16-19, control abnormal skeletal motion during the stance phase by controlling excessive STJ and metatarsal joint motion, decelerating pronation, and allowing the STJ to function closer to its neutral position at mid-stance.[89,92,149,150] When plantar flexors are stretched, the effectiveness of the stretch is significantly greater when wearing arch supports. In the presence of pronation, the difference is greater than when a normal foot is fitted with an orthosis.[151]

SUMMARY

This chapter has reviewed normal posture and typical postural changes found in older adults. Throughout the chapter, we infer a complex interaction of factors influencing an individual's deviation from optimal posture: primary stressors, comorbid conditions that become (or influence) stressors, secondary conditions

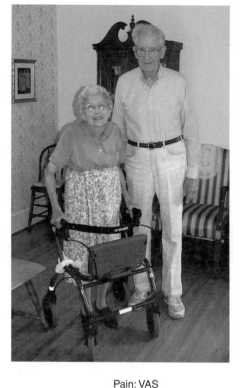

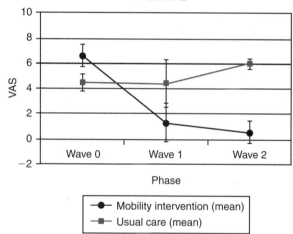

FIGURE 16-18 Physical therapy management of acute vertebral fracture. *(Used with permission From Shipp KM: Physical therapy management of acute vertebral fracture. American Physical Therapy Association Combined Sections Meeting. Las Vegas, NV: APTA; 2009.)*

that become stressors, and the decline of physiological systems with aging. How they all interact with each other is not always clear. A picture emerges of a struggle between stressors that negatively impact normal upright alignment and physiological systems tasked with maintaining optimal upright posture. If negative stressors overcome the physiological systems' effectiveness, then impaired posture results. Impaired posture begets additional stress and poorer posture as well as secondary conditions that again negatively impact posture. Comorbid conditions can increase the stressor or undermine our normal posture control. Evaluation and treatment of impaired posture is accomplished by using the generic

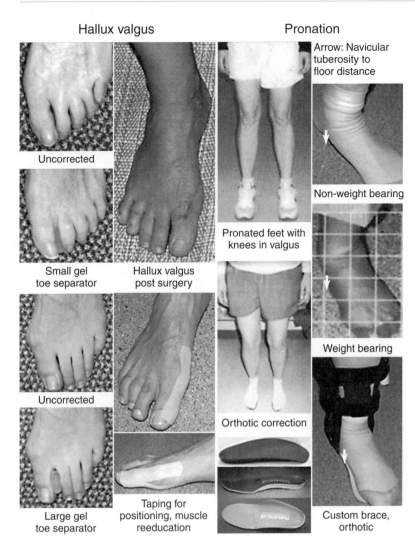

Hallux valgus

Uncorrected

Small gel
toe separator

Hallux valgus
post surgery

Uncorrected

Large gel
toe separator

Taping for
positioning, muscle
reeducation

Pronation

Arrow: Navicular
tuberosity to
floor distance

Non-weight bearing

Pronated feet with
knees in valgus

Weight bearing

Orthotic correction

Custom brace,
orthotic

FIGURE 16-19 External supports for correction of faulty foot postures. All are most effective when combined with corrective postural exercise training. *(Photos used with permission from Bones, Backs & Balance LLC, New Hartford, CT.)*

skills of the physical therapist and adapting them to the older patient. What is most important for the physical therapist to consider and remember is that older adults are exceptionally variable and that an individualized examination and plan of treatment directed toward postural change is required to maximize likelihood of success. It is important to view posture as an integration of multiple systems. With physical therapist guidance and skilled interventions, older adults can make changes in their posture that will enhance the aging process.

CASE EXAMPLE

The following case represents a typical patient with a postural disorder of primarily musculoskeletal origin. The case illustrates patient assessment and diagnosis as well as the development and implementation of a physical therapy plan of care, as presented in this chapter. The postural disorder discussed is common in older adults seen in an outpatient setting for back dysfunctions and represents the typical older patient with several secondary conditions in addition to the primary complaint.

Case: Osteoporosis with Vertebral Compression Fracture

Examination

History. S.Z. is a 68-year-old Caucasian woman with osteoporosis, a long history of steroid-dependent asthma, hypothyroidism, and a 60- to 70-pack-per-year history of smoking. Her current complaint is pain and disability secondary to a new-onset anterior 7th thoracic vertebral compression fracture. This is her fourth minimal trauma fracture over the past 10 years, with the first three being wrist, coccyx, and vertebral compression (mild anterior wedging at T7-T8). Patient reports that the mechanism of action for the first compression fracture was holding a heavy picture in front of her to hang it over her couch. According to the radiologist's report performed the day before this physical therapy visit, lateral spinal radiographs show marked osteopenia, an anterior compression fracture of T7, and mild anterior wedging at T8. S.Z.'s radiographs are illustrated in Figure 16-20.

Her medications include thyroid replacement, estrogen hormone replacement, steroid inhalers, calcium, and

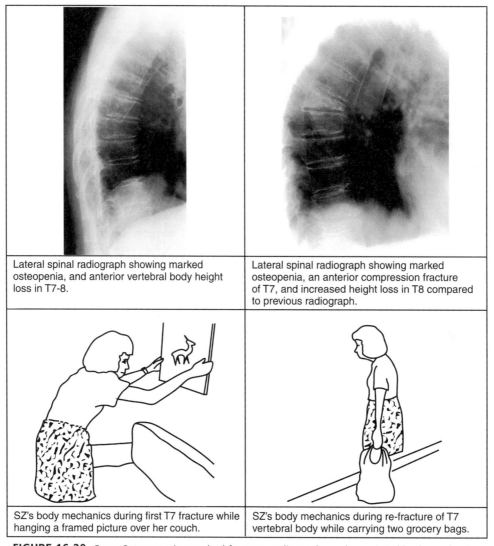

Lateral spinal radiograph showing marked osteopenia, and anterior vertebral body height loss in T7-8.

Lateral spinal radiograph showing marked osteopenia, an anterior compression fracture of T7, and increased height loss in T8 compared to previous radiograph.

SZ's body mechanics during first T7 fracture while hanging a framed picture over her couch.

SZ's body mechanics during re-fracture of T7 vertebral body while carrying two grocery bags.

FIGURE 16-20 Case: Osteoporotic vertebral fracture: radiographs and associated body mechanics.

vitamin D. She did little or no exercise until she was referred to physical therapy for osteoporosis intervention several years prior to her current injuries. She continued doing 20 minutes of postural and mild aerobic dance exercises daily until she was injured. She is married and lives in senior housing, has decreased smoking to one half of one pack per day. Two months prior to this visit, her bone density scores were as follows:

Lumbar (L2-L4): T score = −2.6
Proximal femoral: T score = −2.0

These bone density results together with her history of fragility fractures are consistent with the diagnosis of severe osteoporosis.

On the initial visit, S.Z. reported severe unrelenting thoracic and rib pain, centering in the midthoracic region with a numerical rating scale grade of 10/10. The pain began 3 days before the first visit after carrying plastic grocery bags in both hands. She reported that she had been doing better since the picture-hanging injury and thought she could "handle it." She was prescribed oxycodone/acetaminophen (Percocet), which afforded minimal relief. She reported that she had been unable to lie in bed since the fracture. Standing, deep breathing, coughing, and any movement all increased her back pain. She reported that all activities of daily living were severely limited because of extreme pain and weakness, which included inability to don socks and shoes.

Review of Systems. Heart rate, blood pressure, and pulse oximetry measures were within normal limits. Skin pliability, color, and integrity were grossly normal, and no edema was noted. Her communication abilities and orientation were age-appropriate and without any indication of dysfunction. Although she reported pain with every step and was observed to have a generally flexed trunk posture, her gait was symmetrical with no evidence of overt weakness or other neurologic deficits. Her lower extremity posture showed no notable malalignments. Musculoskeletal systems review was accomplished via observation of her extremely antalgic movement pattern with all postural changes including the need to use her arms to push herself up from sitting and also to help

CHAPTER 16 Impaired Posture 313

maintain upright during the flexible curve tracing test. She needed to sit down immediately on completion of the flexible curve tracing test (5 minutes of standing) because of back pain and fatigue. Hypotheses formed during task analysis were that her limitations appeared to be due to pain, poor posture, and trunk muscle weakness as a result of her T7 vertebral compression fracture.

Tests and Measures. Initial examination revealed generalized weakness secondary to the pain, evidenced by her great difficulty in changing positions. She leaned heavily on her upper extremities during sit to stand, and was unable to egress without use of her upper limbs. She was unwilling to transfer on and off the treatment table because of her level of pain. Her symptoms were too severe to allow for formal muscle testing. She was able to actively contract her thoracic paraspinal muscles in a gravity-assisted position by minimally decreasing her kyphosis while supporting her flexed upper extremities against a wall, but she was unable to decrease the kyphosis while standing unsupported, suggesting very low ability to actively contract her trunk extensors. The strength of her abdominals was not measurable because of her level of pain and the risk of further injury if conventional flexion-based muscle testing was employed. Gross standing trunk range of motion was notably limited because of acute thoracic pain with any attempt to move out of her usual standing position. She had severe tenderness to minimal palpation in the mid- and lower thoracic regions with associated paraspinal muscle spasm bilaterally from T5 through the lumbar region. Although her shoulder motion was not formally tested because of her pain, she was capable of performing only partial elevation with wall support. She had no focal pain on palpation of shoulder structures. Spinal posture was notable for marked observational thoracic kyphosis and loss of lumbar lordosis, which was confirmed when measured with a surveyor's flexible curve. Her kyphotic index (KI), depicted in Figure 16-21, was 18.6 on the initial exam, higher than 13.0 which is considered clinically kyphotic.[11,17] The Oswestry Disability Index v2.0 (ODI) was the patient-specific outcome measure chosen to assess S.Z.'s rating of the impact of her injury on her daily activities. Her score of 80% disability was consistent with her examination findings.

Evaluation/Diagnosis/Prognosis and Plan of Care. The diagnoses to guide the physical therapy plan of care were (1) impaired posture, joint mobility, muscle performance, and range of motion associated with an osteoporotic vertebral compression fracture, which falls within practice patterns 4A "Primary Prevention/Risk Reduction for Skeletal Demineralization," and (2) 4B "Impaired Posture" of the *Guide to Physical Therapist Practice.*[1] The patient goals were to (1) function independently and without pain during positional changes

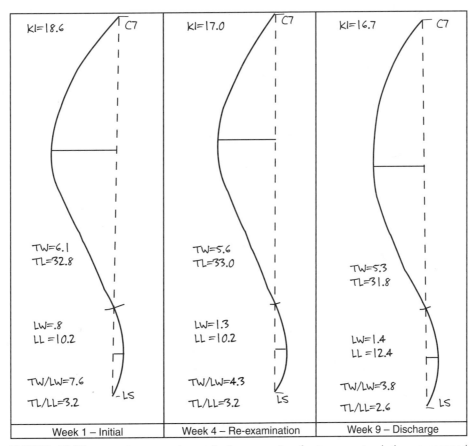

| Week 1 – Initial | Week 4 – Re-examination | Week 9 – Discharge |

FIGURE 16-21 Case: Osteoporotic vertebral compression fracture—postural change assessed with flexible curve kypholordosis tracing examinations. *(Used with permission from Bones, Backs & Balance LLC, New Hartford, CT.)*

and normal housekeeping ADLs; (2) maintain an optimal posture, with flexible curve KI value decreased to 13.0 or less; (3) gain trunk extension and abdominal strength equal to 3/5 or better; and (4) achieve pain reduction to 2/10 or less with all ADLs and exercise.

Interventions. S.Z. received 18 physical therapy treatments over a 9-week period. Treatment emphasis, as depicted in Figure 16-22, was placed on interventions designed to decrease pain and kyphosis, increase lordosis, and teach maintenance of safe spinal posture during all ADL and bone stimulating exercise. She was treated for soft tissue spasm and pain with gentle soft tissue mobilization, sensory level electrical nerve stimulation,[152] and ice massage. Muscle energy treatment techniques were used to increase her thoracic extension and rib mobility.[136,153,154]

With every treatment, she received instruction in body mechanics to eliminate trunk flexion and rotation. She was also instructed in progressive trunk strengthening with extension bias, lateral basal expansion and diaphragmatic respiratory exercise, and eventually overall conditioning and resistive limb exercises. A month after the fracture she started a walking and performing an "osteoporosis dance"[155] weight-bearing exercise program that focused on standing balance, coordination, and muscle endurance exercise while maintaining optimal posture. She started at 5 to 10 minutes per day and had reached 15 minutes' duration every other day at the conclusion of her therapy 9 weeks after the fracture diagnosis.

Initially, she was "X" taped from her upper trapezius to the contralateral 10th rib to help minimize her kyphosis, but her husband was not able to apply the tape at home. Therefore, she was fitted with a Spinomed brace to use during activities of daily living, particularly those involving lifting, bending, or reaching tasks. She was instructed to continue wearing the brace during these activities as a reminder to use safe body mechanics for a life-long prevention strategy in combination with purposeful safe postures and regular specific exercises.

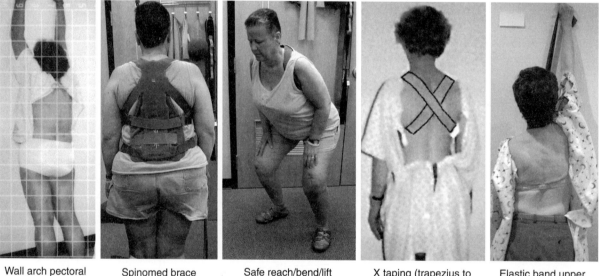

Wall arch pectoral stretch and trunk extension strength with transversus abdominis co-contraction | Spinomed brace | Safe reach/bend/lift practice | X taping (trapezius to rib 10) for kyphosis reduction via paraspinal extension/biofeedback | Elastic band upper extremity strengthening with abdominal and paraspinal control (at 6 weeks post fracture). Hands to contact with wall for spinal safety.

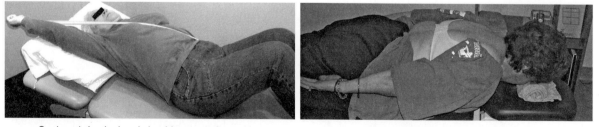

Supine abdominal and shoulder strength exercise | Prone paraspinal strength exercise

FIGURE 16-22 Case: Examples of types of exercise and support interventions appropriate for a patient following T7 osteoporotic vertebral compression fracture. *(Patient pictures used with permission, photos used with permission from Bones, Backs & Balance LLC, New Hartford, CT.)*

Outcomes. Over the course of treatment, flexible curve measurements reflected decreased kyphosis and increased lordosis as her strength increased and her pain decreased. TW decreased from 6.1 to 5.3 cm, TL decreased from 32.8 to 31.8 cm, LW increased from 0.8 to 1.4 cm, and LL increased from 10.2 to 12.4 cm at discharge. Her KI, depicted in Figure 16-21, decreased from 18.6 to 16.7. The KI did improve, but the importance of this improvement is unknown because of lack of established minimal clinically important change score. On discharge, she was able to perform a prone trunk lift with arms at her side, holding the lift for 5 seconds with a slight movement out of kyphosis (suggesting improvement from pretest). She rated her pain at 0 to 1 out of 10 for most of the day, and up to 2/10 by the end of the day (down from 10 out of 10 on initial examination), thus exceeding the 30% improvement necessary to signify minimally important change.[156] Her ODI disability score had decreased to 14% (down from 80%), also above levels representing minimally important change.[157] She understood and could demonstrate safe body mechanics with her tasks of everyday living, and agreed to wear the Spinomed brace while performing any lifting, bending, or reaching tasks. She could also attain standing from a chair without use of her upper extremities.

REFERENCES

To enhance this text and add value for the reader, all references are included on the companion Evolve site that accompanies this text book. The reader can view the reference source and access it online whenever possible. There are a total of 157 cited references and other general references for this chapter.

CHAPTER 17

Ambulation:
Impact of Age-Related Changes on Functional Mobility

Julie D. Ries, PT, PhD

INTRODUCTION

Physical therapists play a unique and important role when examining the older adult with gait dysfunction. Although "ambulation" training may sound like a simple and straightforward task, this is rarely the case with older adult clients. Bipedal locomotion is a uniquely human skill that requires multiple systems (neurologic, musculoskeletal, cardiopulmonary, cognition) to work in a congruent and sophisticated manner. Normal age-related decline across these systems, even in healthy individuals, has a predictable impact on gait in the older adult.

Often, health care professionals look to physical therapists to "clear" an older adult for safe discharge from the inpatient environment, or a patient or primary care physician requests a consultation from a physical therapist to assess mobility concerns. A high level of clinical skill is required to adequately analyze and identify specific dysfunctions in the complex task of functional ambulation, particularly in older adults who have multiple potential contributing factors to impaired mobility. Safe ambulation requires the ability to quickly accelerate and decelerate, engage proactive and reactive balance control mechanisms, and address a myriad of different environmental and specific task demands.[1-4] Before "clearing" a patient for discharge, a professional judgment that implies the individual is safe and independent in ambulation in various environments, or making suggestions that would restrict independent community mobility, a skilled assessment of ambulation capabilities and safety must be conducted.

To perform a comprehensive and accurate examination of ambulation capabilities of older adults followed by effective interventions for identified dysfunctions, a physical therapist should have (1) extensive knowledge of normal gait and of gait changes that occur with aging, (2) a clear understanding of the functional requirements of ambulation with and without assistive devices, (3) a repertoire of tests and measures appropriate for gait assessment, and (4) an ability to evaluate examination findings and create an appropriate and effective evidence-based plan of care.

This chapter begins with a discussion of locomotor functions, primary tasks of locomotion, and phases of the normal gait cycle. The chapter will then describe anticipated gait changes that occur with normal aging, and provide an analysis of the complex functional gait requirements of community ambulation related to speed, distance, and navigation of various terrains. The chapter then continues with a discussion of planning and justifying a comprehensive, yet efficient, examination of gait for a given older individual using appropriate tests and measures and ends with an analysis of evidence for various treatment interventions used in gait-training the older adult.

NORMAL GAIT

A solid understanding of the biomechanics of normal gait is a prerequisite of the highest quality care. Generally speaking, humans all walk similarly, striving to move forward keeping the center of gravity over the base of support in the most energy-efficient manner possible. Perry and Burnfield's[5] traditional framework for describing the gait cycle, organized from a biomechanical perspective around the sagittal plane, highlights the basic components of normal gait. This chapter assumes the reader is familiar with the basic principles of kinetics, kinematics, and muscle activity that are relevant to human walking. Only a brief review of the major tasks and phases of the gait cycle is provided. An understanding of normal gait is a necessary foundation for identifying and problem solving gait abnormalities.

Perry and Burnfield[5] present four locomotor functions: shock absorption, stance stability, propulsion, and energy conservation. Shock absorption is the result of muscle activity when loading the stance extremity. Eccentric dorsiflexor activity, eccentric knee extensor activity, and eccentric hip abductor activity all work to absorb shock as the limb is loaded.

Stance stability is determined by ground reaction force vectors (GRFVs), ligament and joint support, and muscle activity. Using GRFVs to determine the flexion or extension moment at each joint of the lower extremity, the static (joint and ligamentous structures) and dynamic (muscle activity) components required to control movement of the lower extremity segment during stance can be determined. It is accepted that GRFV is an imperfect and simplistic way of conceptualizing the physics of gait[6,7]; however, the principles underlying GRFV serve as a useful framework for examining basic principles of muscle and joint activity within the phases of gait.

Forward propulsion in gait is the result of the body's forward fall, rocker mechanisms that allow smooth translation of weight over the distal lower extremity, momentum created by the swing of the contralateral lower extremity, and active push-off of the stance lower extremity.

Energy conservation is thought to be maximized by selective muscle recruitment and the determinants of gait. Selective muscle recruitment is the efficiency achieved by using muscles strategically so as not to require excess or redundant muscle activity (e.g., short head of biceps femoris can flex the knee without unwanted extension of the hip during the swing phase; biarticular hamstrings can eccentrically slow both hip flexion and knee extension during late swing).

The determinants of gait are biomechanical adjustments that are purported to decrease the excursion of the body's center of mass in all planes, thereby decreasing the energy required to maintain stability over the base of support throughout the gait cycle. It should be noted, however, that the assumptions underlying this long-standing and well-accepted biomechanical theory have undergone very little empirical testing.[8]

The gait cycle is conceptualized as eight phases within three major tasks: (1) weight acceptance, (2) single limb support, and (3) limb advancement.[5,9] In normal gait, weight acceptance includes the phases of *initial contact* and *loading response,* during which the heel is the first to contact the support surface (during initial contact) and the limb absorbs shock as the weight of the individual is translated onto the stance lower extremity (loading response). Single limb support includes the phases *mid-stance* and *terminal stance.* during *mid-stance,* the individual is in single limb support while the other leg advances. The body begins posterior to the weight-bearing foot but moves anterior by the end of the phase, controlled primarily by eccentric soleus and gastrocnemius activity. In *terminal stance,* body weight moves anterior to the forefoot and the heel rises from the support surface. Perry and Burnfield identify this as

"roll off," suggesting that "push off" occurs later in the pre-swing phase of gait, but others consider that terminal stance offers a propulsive "push off" with concentric plantar flexor activity which aids in the forward momentum of the body during gait.[9] Limb advancement is successfully carried out by the combination of *pre-swing* (final unloading of the lower extremity), *initial swing* (preparing the swinging leg for foot clearance), *mid-swing* (assuring continued clearance), and *terminal swing* (slowing of the leg in preparation for stance).

An appreciation for the range of motion (ROM), muscle activity, and motor control requirements of the various phases of gait makes for easier problem solving related to gait deviations. Table 17-1 provides a general summary of the normal gait cycle, including the primary tasks of gait, the phases of gait, and some of the key events that occur within each of the phases.

Gait Characteristics: Typical Changes with Aging

Aging is accompanied by multiple changes in sensory, motor, and central nervous system integration of systems that interact to bring about predictable changes in gait performance. Common sensory (affector system) changes include decreased acuity of visual and auditory systems, and decreased somatosensory and proprioceptive status. These changes can lead to inaccurate appraisal of environmental demands or erroneous self-assessment of positioning and/or movement. Common motor (effector system) changes include decreased motor neuron conduction velocity, periarticular connective tissue stiffness, and decrease in numbers of motor fibers resulting in limitations in ROM and muscle strength. Central nervous system integrative changes might include loss of brain cells and altered level of neurotransmitter production resulting in slowed reaction time and decreased facility of movement presenting as motor control deficits.

Armed with an understanding of the specific requirements of normal gait, a physical therapist can anticipate how specific changes in ROM, strength, and motor control can lead to predictable gait changes. Take, for example, a subtle decrease in hip extension ROM in an older adult. Hip extension ROM is required late in the stance phase. If the trailing limb is not extended at the hip during terminal stance, this will affect efficiency of swing for that leg: the stretch usually applied to hip flexors in preparation for swing will not be effectively applied, and the leg also loses some of its swing preparation time, making foot clearance during swing more difficult. A loss of terminal knee extension ROM will affect the gait cycle during loading response, making shock absorption at the knee difficult or potentially ineffective because it eliminates the excursion of the range where the eccentric activity of the quadriceps works to load the limb in a controlled manner.

TABLE 17-1   Summary of the Normal Gait Cycle: Three Primary Tasks and Eight Embedded Gait Phases

	Weight Acceptance		Single Limb Support			Limb Advancement		
Eight Phases of Gait	**Initial Contact**	**Loading Response**	**Mid-Stance**	**Terminal Stance**	**Pre-Swing**	**Initial Swing**	**Mid-Swing**	**Terminal Swing**
Temporal location of each phase along the gait cycle	~0%-2%	~2%-10%	~10%-30%	~30%-50%	~50%-60%	~60%-75%	~75%-85%	~85%-100%
Objectives/Critical events within each phase	• Heel strike • Stable, upright trunk is key to *all* phases	• Shock absorption • Weight-bearing stability • Preservation of progression	• Progression over stationary foot (controlled tibial advancement) • Limb and trunk stability	• Push-off; heel rise • Progression of body beyond supporting foot (free forward fall)	• Transfer of body weight unloads limb • Knee flexion in preparation for foot clearance	• Foot clears floor (knee flexion essential) • Limb advances from its trailing position	• Ankle dorsiflexion to neutral key for foot clearance • Continued limb advancement	• Hip and knee deceleration, complete limb advancement • Limb prepares for stance with knee extension and ankle neutral
Rocker mechanism	Heel rocker	Heel rocker	Ankle rocker	Forefoot rocker	Forefoot rocker			
Selected muscle activity	• Firing of lower extremity extensors in preparation for weight bearing • Isometric dorsiflexor activity keeps ankle in neutral for heel contact	• Period of maximal muscle activity • Hip extensors help progress body • Eccentric knee extensors, hip abductors, and ankle dorsiflexors aid in shock absorption	• Hip abductors stabilize pelvis • Eccentric plantar-flexors allow controlled forward progression of tibia over fixed foot to dorsiflexion 10°	• Ankle plantar-flexor activity provides "push-off"	• Hip flexors and adductors assist in actively initiating hip flexion (passive hip and knee flexion are the result of the tibia rolling forward)	• Momentum carries limb to great extent • Some hip and knee flexion activity • Pretibials fire to begin to bring foot back into dorsiflexion	• Primarily momentum carrying limb • Pretibials bring ankle to neutral	• Eccentric hamstring activity to slow the swinging limb at both hip and knee • Isometric pretibials keep ankle in neutral

Alignment and arthrokinematic changes can *result from* or be *caused by* changes in strength and flexibility with aging. It is difficult to know which came first—the gait deviation or the ROM limitation—but they are clearly interrelated.[10] Consider the example above. A loss of hip extension ROM necessitates shorter step length on the contralateral limb, and shorter step length requires less hip extension ROM. One of the more common habitual postures of the older adult, especially the frail older adult, is a posture that is succumbing to gravity (kyphotic trunk, with or without flexion at the hips and knees).[11-13] This flexed posture changes the influence of GRFVs at each joint and alters the excursion of movement and the demand on muscle activity during the gait cycle. Anticipating the incompatibilities between a habitual posture and the requirements of normal gait prepare the physical therapist to conduct an efficient evaluation of gait.

Although patients are unique in their clinical presentation and impairments, there are some generalizations that can be made about typical gait changes that are associated with aging. Box 17-1 lists the most predictable gait changes in older adults, and Table 17-2 briefly describes some of the most notable research related to alterations of gait characteristics with aging. Although there does seem to be general agreement that the changes described are seen with the typical or usual aging process, there is some evidence to suggest that with "successful aging,"[23] it may be possible to have well-preserved gait, spared of these changes.[24,25]

Decrease in self-selected or "typical" gait speed with aging has been repeatedly demonstrated in the literature.[14,15,19-22,26] This is an extremely important finding as gait speed correlates well with, and is predictive of, functional dependence.[27-30] As evidenced in Box 17-1, older adult gait is not simply a slower version of younger adult gait. Older adults display a more conservative gait pattern (e.g., increased double-limb support phase, increased base of support) in an effort to be safer and more stable in upright.[20,22] The gait differences identified between younger and older individuals appear to be somewhat exaggerated when looking at older individuals prone to falls. Older individuals with a history of falls are slower than their age-matched peers without a fall history,[31] and they demonstrate an inability to increase speed on demand.[32] In a study examining treadmill walking at progressively faster speeds, Barak et al[32] demonstrated that nonfallers completed all trials up to the highest of speeds (1.52 m/sec), whereas 57% of fallers found the highest speeds to be incompatible with safe walking.

ROM excursions during the gait cycle are less in older adults when compared to younger adults, and there is evidence of more profound limitations in ROM when comparing older adult fallers with nonfallers.[1032] Decreases in hip extension and ankle plantar flexion during the late stance phase have been demonstrated in fallers as compared to nonfallers. The one exception to diminished ROM excursion in the context of gait is a demonstration of *increased* hip flexion angle in fallers as compared to nonfallers in swing phase (especially at faster speeds),[32] suggesting that these individuals might exaggerate the early swing movement perhaps to compensate for decreased push-off and assure clearance of the swinging limb.

Gait variability (with a variety of different operational definitions) has been the subject of much study in recent years,[16,17,33] as an increase in gait variability has been associated with an increased risk of falls.[32,34,35] Variability in gait characteristics is more pronounced in older adults than in young adults and also appears to be greater in fallers as compared to nonfallers.[32,34,35] In healthy older adults, variability is magnified at higher speeds, under the influence of postural threat or under dual task demands.[15,32,33,36,37] Many of the identified gait pattern changes in older adults represent an effort to increase stability and safety in gait (e.g., decreased speed, increased base of support, increased double-limb support time, decreased single-limb support time). Although one might expect gait variability to also decrease in an effort to increase stability, variability of many gait parameters increases with age. Variability within a movement pattern is not inherently detrimental. In fact, variability is typically associated with adaptability and flexibility of movement performance, which is critical to an adaptive control system. However, in the older adult, increasing gait variability seems to translate to increasing instability. Older adults adopt a more conservative gait pattern in an effort to increase stability and reduce the likelihood of falls, yet they demonstrate an increased variability in many gait parameters. Paradoxically, the increased gait variability that accompanies the more conservative gait pattern may actually increase falls risk.

PATHOLOGIC GAIT CHANGES

Although normal aging brings about predictable gait changes, clinicians need to be able to distinguish between normal age-related changes and those resulting from pathology. Verghese et al[38] studied the epidemiology of gait disorders in community-residing older adults ($n = 468$). Classifying subjects as "normal" and "abnormal," and further identifying "neurologic" and "nonneurologic"

BOX 17-1	Typical Gait Changes in Older Adults

- Decreased gait speed[14,15,19-22,26]
- Decreased step or stride length[19,20,22,26]
- Increased stance time and double-limb support time[19,22]
- Increased variability of gait (operationally defined as variability in step or stride time, length, width, frequency, or velocity)[15-17,20]
- Decreased excursion of movement at hip, knee, and ankle.[10,18,26]

TABLE 17-2	Summary of Notable Studies Demonstrating Typical Gait Changes with Aging	
Author & Year	**Key Study Characteristics**	**Key Clinically Important Findings**
Bohannon, 2008[14]	Retrospective study of gait speeds of 1923 subjects >50 years of age, stratified by decade, using 6-m walk.	↓ gait speed with each decade
Krishnamurthy & Verghese, 2006[19]	Compared 31 nondisabled "old old" (>90 years, mean age [SD] = 91.9 [2.4] years) with 170 "young old" (<85 years, mean age = 70.7 [15.8] years), using GaitRite walkway.	↓ gait speed in old-old ↓ step & stride length in old-old ↑ support base in old-old
Menz et al, 2003[20]	Compared 30 older adults with low fall risk (mean age [SD] = 79.0 [3.0] years) and 30 younger adults (29.0 [4.3] years) using three-dimensional motion analysis.	↓ gait speed in older adults ↓ step length in older adults ↑ step timing variability in older adults
Laufer, 2003[21]	Compared gait of 40 older adults (mean age [SD] = 77.68 [6.19] years) and 30 younger adults (24 [2.27] years) using GaitRite walkway.	↓ gait speed in older adults ↓ stride length in older adults ↓ cadence in older adults ↓ swing phase in older adults ↑ double-limb support time in older adults
Grabiner et al, 2001[16]	Compared gait of 15 older adults (mean age [SD] = 72.13 [3.96] years) and 18 younger adults (25.06 [4.02] years) using GaitRite walkway.	↑ stride width variability in older adults ↑ step length variability
Ostrosky et al, 1994[18]	Compared 30 older adults (60-80 years) and 30 young adults (20-40 years) using two-dimensional motion analysis system.	↓ stride length in older adults ↓ knee extension ROM in older adults
Winter et al, 1990[22]	Compared gait of 15 "fit & healthy" older (mean age = 68 years, range = 62-78) with 12 younger adults (mean age = 24.6 years, range = 21-28) using video digitized system & force platform.	↓ gait speed in older adults ↓ stride length in older adults ↑ double-limb support time in older adults ↓ power generation at push-off (terminal stance) in older adults ↓ power absorption at heel strike (initial contact-loading response) Author demonstrates statistical significance of the five gait parameters listed; cadence and toe clearance did not differ significantly between groups.

gait patterns, the authors demonstrated that the prevalence of abnormal gait was 35% in their study population. Nonneurologic abnormal gait characteristics were more common than neurologic, and mild abnormalities were more common than severe. The incidence of abnormal gait increased with advanced age and was associated with progressive risk of institutionalization and death. If these findings can be generalized to all older adults, clinicians might expect up to one third of their older adult patients to display gait changes beyond those demonstrated with typical aging.

Physical therapists should be especially astute in identifying individuals who are "transitioning to frailty." These individuals may not have a discrete diagnosis, but may demonstrate a pronounced decline in temporal and spatial parameters of gait as compared to healthy older adults.[39] Deterioration of performance within a transitionally frail group is not necessarily associated with age, suggesting that other factors (e.g., depression, muscle strength, fear of falling) may be more related to gait performance within this group than age alone.[39] Gill et al[40]

suggest that mobility disability is an extremely dynamic process involving transitions from no disability to intermittent disability to continuous disability, and back again. They concede that transitions from disability back to no disability are less common than trends in the direction of disability, but certainly improvement is possible for some individuals. They state a case for physical therapists to focus not only on prevention of mobility impairments but also restoration of mobility in those who become disabled, especially frail older women, as they are most susceptible to mobility disability.

An exhaustive listing and description of common gait deviations observed with different diagnostic groups is beyond the scope of this chapter; however, some generalizations can be made about gait characteristics associated with specific pathologies. For instance, older adults with hemiplegia present with significant asymmetries in gait that are often motivated by avoidance of weight bearing through the involved lower extremity, affecting both the hemiplegic and uninvolved side.[41,42] Given various compensatory strategies and the intricacies related to abnormal tone in individuals with hemiplegia, evaluating hemiplegic gait is a unique challenge. Parkinson's disease is associated with decreased speed, decreased step length, and increased variability of gait[43,44] and often presents with the classic festinating or shuffling gait. Difficulty with initiation and freezing episodes provide an added dimension to the management of parkinsonian gait. Individuals with dementias generally display amplified findings of the typical aging changes,[45] although there are sometimes subtle differences between different types of dementias.[46] Evaluating and working with individuals with cognitive impairment brings with it a whole new set of challenges.

Regardless of diagnosis, each client will require careful examination of his unique clinical presentation of gait. The underlying diagnosis may suggest certain gait characteristics but there is variability within each diagnostic group.

FUNCTIONAL AMBULATION REQUIREMENTS

If functional mobility in the real world were confined to the demands of walking on a level, cleared, well-lit pathway, then individuals walking a lap around the physical therapy clinic or a length of the facility hallway would easily demonstrate their readiness for safe discharge from physical therapy. Clearly, this is not the case. The International Classification of Functioning, Disability, and Health (ICF) model, described in Chapter 6, demonstrates the significant impact that environment and personal factors have on activity and participation of our older adult clients. Functional mobility in the real world depends upon what the individual brings to the encounter, as well as what the task and the environment demand (e.g., variations in speed, distance, and terrain; obstacle clearance/avoidance; dual- or multitasking while walking). Individual, task, and environmental constraints determine the ultimate movement strategies used within specific gait challenges.

Individual Constraints

At the level of the individual, potential constraints (disabling factors) to walking ability at home and in the community may be physiological and/or psychological. Physiological factors may include impairments in range of motion, strength, motor control, sensation, or endurance. Examination of impairments likely to affect the actions influencing walking ability is integral to the physical therapist's approach to the patient. Although an association is apparent, there is no direct formula to predict the strength of the correlation between each of these impairments and activity limitation in gait performance. Familiarity with the requirements for normal gait and common constraints to ambulation in older adults enhances the physical therapist's ability to organize the

patient examination to quickly uncover impairments that will affect gait.

Often overlooked is the enabling or disabling influence of an individual's psychological status on gait performance. There is some indication that depression may influence gait speed; however, this is not a completely replicated finding.[19,47] Perceptions about aging, personal abilities, and self-efficacy related to gait and balance are useful indicators for gait performance.[48-52] Self-selected gait speed has been found to correlate with self-perceived physical function in older adults.[53] Chapter 18, Balance and Falls, discusses commonly used self-efficacy tools related to gait and balance. Considering the multiple dimensions of environmental demands, it is not surprising that older individuals may avoid venturing out into their communities. A comprehensive patient interview will reveal patients' perceived risks for community ambulation, which are as important as patients' real risks.

Anxiety or fear related to community ambulation is fairly common in older adults and is highly correlated with measures of gait and indicative of whether individuals will venture into the community.[48,54-56] Alleviating individuals' fears and building confidence for community mobility is a potentially powerful and underutilized tool.[57] The most obvious perceived risks are general concerns associated with balance and the risk of falls. Delbaere et al demonstrated that individuals with excessive concerns about falling displayed maladaptive behaviors to enhance stability in threatening environments, and that these behaviors may paradoxically increase their falls risk.[48] Talkowski et al demonstrated that individuals who perceived their own health and balance to be good walked more than those who did not.[49] Although patients should not have a false confidence about their abilities in the community, unwarranted fears that limit community mobility or increase the risk of falls are also undesirable. Hausdorff et al demonstrated that exposing older adults to positive stereotyping about aging increased their gait speed, suggesting that therapists might be able to exploit the relationship between self-perception and function.[58]

Individuals may have other and less obvious perceived risks associated with community mobility that might include concern about self-image related to appearance while walking, inability to access public necessities easily (e.g., restrooms), and fear of physical harm at the hand of individuals in the environment. Neighborhood socioeconomics and perceived neighborhood safety have been found to correlate with community activities[59,60] and mobility disability in older adults.[61] Individuals are unlikely to venture into their communities if they feel threatened by the people or the environment, and this is sometimes the case in socioeconomically deprived neighborhoods.

A final consideration in interviewing older adults about community ambulation is that individuals may report that they are independent in the community, but upon further investigation, the therapist might discover that the individual has significantly modified their community outings and adjusted their community lifestyles to meet their decreased mobility level.[57,62] This could be an appropriate and realistic adjustment, or it could be a premature withdrawal from community activities that has a negative impact on quality of life (e.g., an individual may order grocery delivery to avoid outings to the grocery store, but also might forfeit enjoyable outings to the community center for weekly social events). A comprehensive assessment of individual capabilities and a realistic understanding of the demands of the community will help the therapist to identify the optimal goals related to community mobility. Therapists can survey their patients to determine what challenges they have encountered and which ones they have avoided in their recent outings.[63] Sometimes, the reality is that independent community ambulation is no longer safe for an older adult, and helping individuals to problem-solve ways in which they can continue community activities that are important to them in a safe manner becomes the focus of the physical therapist's attention. But sometimes, individuals may pull out of community activities prematurely, and physical therapy can positively affect quality of life by preparing patients for and reintroducing them to community ambulation. Accompanied ambulation in the community may be a useful intervention to facilitate patients' community mobility.[57] When an individual successfully performs community ambulation under the watchful eye of a health care professional, this achievement can be an excellent confidence builder.

Speed and Distance Requirements for Functional Ambulation

Physical therapists generally consider mobility on a continuum: nonfunctional ambulation, household ambulation, limited community ambulation, independent community ambulation.[3] However, universally accepted operational definitions of these terms are lacking. Oftentimes in the clinic environment, guidelines for community mobility are arbitrarily identified—the distance to lap a section of the hospital floor or the perimeter around the physical therapy gym becomes the distance to which physical therapists aspire to have their patients walk. Preserving community mobility in older adults has been the subject of several recent publications[2,63,64] as has the effort to understand the relationship between environmental demands and community ambulation.[3,57,65,66]

How does one define *mobility disability*? What does it mean to state that an individual is an "independent community ambulator"? The answer depends upon who is asked. Box 17-2 presents several different operational definitions for mobility disability and community ambulation from the published literature. Many physical therapy clinics use 150 feet (45.72 m) as the criterion for community ambulation. This may originate

---

> **BOX 17-2** | **Variations among Commonly Used Operational Definitions of Terms Related to Mobility**
>
> **Mobility Disability**
> - "The impaired ability to move independently from one location to another and reach the desired destination." (Patla and Shumway-Cook[3])
> - "The inability to walk one quarter mile or climb a flight of stairs without assistance." (Gill et al[40])
> - "The inability to walk one half mile or climb a flight of stairs without assistance." (Strawbridge et al[67])
>
> **Community Ambulation**
> - "Walking in the community to pursue recreational, social, or employment goals and to destinations significant for participation in activities that fulfill quality of life." (Corrigan and McBurney[57])
> - "The ability to walk with or without a gait aid to destinations important for participation in community life." (Corrigan and McBurney[65])
> - "Independent mobility outside the home which includes the ability to confidently negotiate uneven terrain, private venues, shopping centers and other public venues." (Lord et al[68])
> - The ability "to ambulate a distance sufficient to conduct business in a variety of locations, ... ascend and descend curbs, and cross a street within the time provided by a crossing signal." (Lerner-Frankiel et al[62])

from the widely used Functional Independence Measure (FIM), which defines the highest level of locomotion (FIM score 7) as the ability to walk 150 feet safely and without assistance in a reasonable time period.[69] When third-party payers read documentation that a patient is ambulating 150 feet, they may question the need for continued physical therapy, and they certainly will challenge the need for home health care. The reality, however, is that successful community mobility requires ambulation of distances well over 150 feet. In addition, although short-distance gait speed tests are valid and reliable in themselves, they do not generalize to community distances. For instance, gait speed during an 8-foot, or even a 20-foot, walk test may not accurately project how an older adult will fare when crossing a large intersection.

Lerner-Frankiel et al[62] suggested minimum standards for community ambulation to be the ability to walk 332 m, and to walk at a speed of 79 m/min for 27 m, for the purpose of crossing the street safely. Robinett and Vondran[70] noted how the distance and velocity requirements of a community vary between cities and rural towns. Being independently ambulatory in a highly populated city will require walking faster and further than being independently ambulatory in a rural, less-populated town. The authors make a case for knowing the disposition plan of a patient and objective distance and speed measurements specific to the individual to represent community requirements. They identify speed requirements varying from 30 m/min (rural) to 82.5 m/min (urban) for safe street crossing, and identify distance requirements in all communities that are generally greater than individuals are typically trained to walk in physical therapy (e.g., 480 m for an urban grocery store).[70] A recent study,[71] using methodology similar to Lerner-Frankiel's research,[62] presents ambulation distance requirements for the oversized stores that have become so popular. They identified mean walking distances of 380.6 m for grocery stores, 606.6 m for "super stores" (e.g., Target, WalMart), and 676.8 m for club warehouse stores (e.g., COSTCO, Sam's Club). Gait speed required to cross intersections with traffic lights ranged from 0.21 m/s to 0.89 m/s, with a mean crossing speed of 0.49 m/s required to safely cross with the light.

Task and Environment Demands

True independence in the community requires so much more than specific distance or speed requirements. Box 17-3 identifies some of the many environmental demands that characterize community mobility. A conceptual framework introduced by Patla and Shumway-Cook[3] provides a comprehensive way to analyze environmental factors or "dimensions" that can operationally define the complexity of a specific mobility task. They identify eight environmental dimensions that can be classified or measured to characterize the external demands an individual may face in an effort to be independently mobile within a specified community. The dimensions are minimum walking distance, time constraints, ambient (light, weather) conditions, terrain characteristics, external physical load, attentional demands, postural transitions, and traffic level. What is unique and intriguing about this model is that it informs mobility training such that it can meet the needs of a particular client. The interactions among the dimensions have yet to be determined. Although only some aspects of this framework have been systematically evaluated,[63,66] it is a paradigm that underscores the multifaceted nature of community mobility.

BOX 17-3 Examples of Environmental Demands Commonly Encountered during Community Ambulation

- Starts and stops
- Acceleration and deceleration
- Changing directions and turning around
- Obstacle clearance/avoidance
- Picking up/carrying/putting down objects
- Pushing/pulling doors
- Managing displacement forces
- Terrain changes
- Lighting changes
- Weather changes
- Stepping up and down curbs/stairs/ramps of different heights and grades
- Concurrent execution of other tasks (mental and physical)

Ambulation with Assistive Devices

The use of assistive devices can have a significant impact on the mobility of older individuals, providing much needed support and confidence that may enhance household and community locomotion. Mobility devices have been demonstrated to enhance the activity and participation of mobility-impaired individuals.[72] The U.S. Department of Health and Human Services, National Center for Health Statistics, reports an increased use of assistive devices for mobility with increasing age, as well as an increase in use of assistive devices in more recent years.[73] This is attributable, in part, to increased population size and increased representation of older adults within the population, but also to increased prescription and availability of assistive devices. The most commonly used assistive device in noninstitutionalized adults older than age 65 years is a cane. Of individuals older than age 65 years who use an assistive device, canes are used by 70% and walkers are used by 30%.[73] For those older than age 65 years, the prevalence of assistive device use is 146.5 per 1000 individuals.[73]

Physical therapists are responsible for optimal assistive device prescription. Finding the best possible location for each patient on the stability–mobility continuum is an ongoing challenge for therapists. The goal is to prescribe the least restrictive assistive device that provides the exact degree of stability and support required by the patient. Proper adjustment and maintenance of assistive devices is a key factor to safe mobility. Clear instruction as to the optimal use of an assistive device and assessment of patient understanding of assistive device use is an important component of a comprehensive physical therapy program. Although assistive devices are useful in aiding patients' stability, clinicians need to remember that these devices also require considerable attention for proper use, as an additional physical task (manipulation of assistive device) is superimposed on the primary functional task of walking.[74] This may require a good deal of practice and instruction. Energy consumption is greater for ambulation with an assistive device than without one.[75,76] This is a consideration in the prescription of an assistive device. Individuals using assistive devices ambulate more slowly than those without[77]; however, it is not known whether they are slower in an effort to preserve energy or to enhance their stability.

Finally, some older adults take pride in their ability to ambulate without a cane or walker and are resistant to the notion and the appearance of needing external support. Although the physical therapist will actively listen and acknowledge a person's concerns related to use of assistive devices, safety should be the driving force in assistive device prescription, followed closely by function. Convincing an older adult that an assistive device will afford the safest and most functional independent access to the community can be a difficult but necessary discussion.

Stair Negotiation

Successful stair negotiation requires greater ROM (hip and knee flexion, ankle dorsiflexion) and muscle strength (extensors of the lower extremity working concentrically in ascent and eccentrically in descent) than level ground walking. Individuals may identify difficulty with ascent or descent or both.[78] Speed for ascending stairs in older adults correlates with strength and power of the lower extremity extensors.[79-81] Self-efficacy on stairs relates to speed and safety precautions undertaken (e.g., use of rails).[81,82] Because stairs are one of the most common environmental obstacles that are encountered both at home and in the community, it is important to consider the prerequisite actions and tasks needed for this activity and prioritize stair training within the plan of care.

EXAMINATION AND EVALUATION OF GAIT

A comprehensive examination of gait will include gathering a patient history, reviewing all pertinent systems, and carrying out appropriate tests and measures[83] related to ambulation. A thorough gait assessment has significant redundancy with balance assessment, and the reader is directed to Chapter 18, Balance and Falls for complementary content.

A survey or interview of a patient's perception of difficulty with walking is a reasonable component of the physical therapy examination; however, it has been noted that patients frequently underreport gait difficulties.[84] Goals related to gait activities are pivotal in planning an intervention, as the intervention strategies will need to demonstrate specificity to goals. Prior level of function, and the duration of that level, is a key factor to appropriate intervention selection in a rehabilitation program. If an older adult was "nonambulatory" prior to admission to an inpatient setting, it is important to quantify the duration of this nonambulatory status (i.e., days, weeks, months, or years) as this information will significantly affect the goal setting for the rehabilitation program. An individual who has only recently stopped walking due to acuity of illness or a progressive condition that is now being medically managed might return to prior level of functioning very quickly. A careful evaluation of patient potential and an individualized plan of care might even lead to an individual exceeding their previous level of function. Individuals whose ambulation disability is long-standing (e.g., months or even years) are also deserving of careful evaluation even if the preexisting nonambulatory status might not be completely reversible.

Careful review of comorbidities and medications is another important component of the patient history. Some musculoskeletal and neurologic diagnoses affect gait in fairly predictable ways as previously noted. Many medications have systemic side effects that can affect a patient's tolerance for therapy or alter movement strategies. The reader is directed toward the in-depth discussion in Chapter 4, Geriatric Pharmacology.

Physical therapy tests and measures for an older adult with mobility issues would include a thorough assessment of ROM, strength, motor control and coordination, somatosensation and proprioception, and functional mobility (bed mobility and transfers). Observational gait analysis (OGA) is a reasonable place to initiate a gait assessment, but cannot be considered the sole "test" of gait within an examination. Although the reliability of observational gait analysis is poor,[85] it is very commonly used in the clinic. Its usefulness is to give the clinician a starting point to make some general observations about an individual's gait. It can be done without interrupting the flow of other parts of the examination, such as when the patient walks from the door back to the living room after letting the home care therapist into the house, or from the bed to the bathroom in the inpatient environment, or when the patient enters the outpatient clinic. The therapist can make general observations about speed, symmetry, stability, and efficiency of gait. The observations made during OGA, including any specific gait deviations, will help direct the appropriate selection of more objective outcome measures. There are many gait-specific outcome measures from which to choose, and the clinician should have a reasonable rationale for selecting and combining specific measures. Commonly used gait outcome assessment tools include gait speed, timed up and go (TUG), 6-minute walk test (6MW), modified gait abnormality rating scale (GARS-M), performance oriented mobility assessment (POMA), functional ambulation categories (FAC), and dynamic gait index (DGI).

Gait Speed

Using a timed walk of a specific distance is an easy, reliable, and efficient way to procure an objective measure of gait performance. The strong psychometric properties of walking speed, the clinical usefulness, and the potential modifiability of this measure have led to its identification as a "functional vital sign"[86] in the assessment of older adults. Self-selected or "comfortable" gait speed tends to be the most individually efficient gait speed.[87] It is often useful to collect both self-selected and fast gait speed capabilities, as there are environmental challenges that sometimes demand increased gait speeds (e.g., crossing streets). Collection of gait speed data is feasible and useful even in the home care environment[88] and can be collected using a 2.4-m (8-foot) versus 6-m (20-foot) walkway if necessary.[14]

Gait speed can be assessed with sophisticated equipment (e.g., portable computerized walkways, two- or three-dimensional motion analysis systems, triaxial accelerometer), but can be just as reliably assessed with a measured course and a stopwatch. The suggested method of data collection is a 20-m pathway, where the central 10 m are marked for timed testing.[86] This allows for appropriate acceleration and deceleration outside of the timed walking course, such that the measured distance represents a steady state of speed. In a typical clinical environment, a 20-m uninterrupted walkway may be unrealistic. Published protocols for gait speed calculation span distances from 2.4 m to total 6-minute walk distances, and many values in between.[89] Reliability of comfortable gait speed as assessed with a stopwatch and measured path has been consistently determined to be excellent, with repeated measure reliability intraclass correlations (ICCs) reported as 0.903 and 0.97[90,91] in representative studies.

Table 17-3 represents comfortable or self-selected gait speed norms of community-dwelling older adults by decade as presented by Bohannon,[14] Lusardi et al,[77] and Steffen et al.[91] Bohannon presented the retrospective data of 1923 subjects' performance on a 6-m measured walk, timed with a stopwatch. Lusardi et al presented the data of 76 subjects using a 3.7-m GaitRite walkway.[77] Steffen et al studied 96 subjects using a stopwatch to measure the time to traverse the central 6 m of a 10-m walkway.[91] These subjects were all healthy, independently living, self-reliant older adults.

The differences in norms in Table 17-3 may be explained to some extent by methodological differences in the studies cited. Steffen et al, who reported the fastest self-selected gait speeds, had the most stringent inclusion criteria, required that subjects were able to stand or walk for 6 minutes without complaints, and eliminated anyone using an assistive device.[91] Lusardi et al included individuals with assistive devices, as it was felt that this inclusion was representative of the population of study.[77] Bohannon presented times for walks that were initiated from a standing position, including acceleration within the recorded time, thereby accounting for why these scores may appear slower than the others.[14] Access to these norms and the idiosyncratic differences among these studies provides the clinician with reference values for particular clients and can give more meaning and perspective to data collected in the clinic environment.

Gait speed is often considered the most critical of the gait parameters, but there are ways in which other parameters of interest can be assessed in the clinic. The GaitRite walkway is a valid and reliable quantitative gait analysis system that uses imbedded sensors in a portable mat that are triggered when mechanical pressures (footfalls) are applied.[92,93] The software program provides a diagrammatic representation and mathematical profile of the subject's temporal and spatial gait parameters. This type of equipment is not often found in a typical clinic because of its expense. An inexpensive, but reliable, alternative for measuring step length, stride length, step width, and cadence is to ask the individual to perform a timed walk down a measured paper walkway (brown roll paper works well) with ink footprints, measure the appropriate distances between landmarks, and

TABLE 17-3	Comfortable Gait Speed Reference Values for Community-Dwelling Older Adults as Reported in Three Different Studies			
		Bohannon[14] Gait speed over 6 m using stopwatch mean (SD) (m/sec)	Lusardi et al[77] Gait speed over 3.7-m GaitRite walkway mean (SD) (m/sec)	Steffen et al[91] Gait speed over central 6 m of 10-m walkway using stopwatch mean (SD) (m/sec)
	Key subject characteristics	Subjects were patients receiving home care PT for varied diagnoses	Included subjects both with and without assistive devices	Able to walk 6 minutes without complaints or assistive device
Reference norms by gender and age in decades (years)				
Female	50-59	1.11 (0.22)	***	***
	60-69	1.01 (0.23)	1.24 (0.12)	1.44 (0.25)
	70-79	0.93 (0.23)	1.25 (0.18)	1.33 (0.22)
	≥80 (Bohannon)	0.78 (0.22)		
	80-89		0.80 (0.20)	1.15 (0.21)
	90-101	***	0.71 (0.23)	***
Male	50-59	1.12 (0.21)	***	***
	60-69	1.03 (0.21)	***	1.59 (0.24)
	70-79	0.96 (0.23)	1.25 (0.23)	1.38 (0.23)
	≥80 (Bohannon)	0.83 (0.22)		
	80-89		0.88 (0.24)	1.21 (0.18)
	90-101	***	0.72 (0.14)	***

***, not measured in these studies.

calculate mean values for the walk.[94] The patient can also walk with water footprints and the therapist can simply mark the point of heel strike on each footprint with a marker before the water dries to be measured later.

Identifying change scores that represent a clinically important difference in performance is a relatively new area of study in physical therapy.[95] Studies across a variety of older adults (community dwelling, sedentary, chronic stroke) have suggested that a change in gait speed of approximately 0.05 m/sec represents a small but clinically meaningful change, and a change greater than approximately 0.10 m/sec represents a substantial meaningful change in gait performance.[96,97]

Gait speed "norms" should also take into account the use of an assistive device, as assistive device use does correlate with slower self-selected and fast gait speeds.[77] Both age and use of assistive device are predictors of performance on functionally based tests such as gait speed, TUG, and 6-minute walk.[77]

Timed Up and Go

The TUG, developed by Podsiadlo and Richardson,[98] is a tool that has been extensively used with healthy and frail older adults as well as older adult fallers. The TUG correlates well with balance, gait speed, and functional capacity.[77,98,99] The test requires the subject to stand from a standard-height arm chair, walk forward 3 m to a target mark (or around a cone) and walk back to the chair and sit. The score is the time required for the task. The TUG has demonstrated excellent intra- and interrater reliability, with ICCs of 0.97 to 0.99.[91,98] Reference values for community-dwelling older individuals have been documented[77,91,99] and the results of a recent meta-analysis are presented in Table 17-4. Because of the large number of subjects represented through this meta-analysis ($N = 4395$), it is suggested that the upper level of the confidence interval can be used to identify poorer than average performance for the given age group on this test.[99] Recent publications have confirmed the general finding that age and gender affect TUG performance, with females consistently taking longer than males.[100,101]

Six-Minute Walk

The 6MW was initially introduced as a measure of endurance in patients with cardiac and pulmonary problems, but it has come to be considered a broader measure of mobility and function in older people rather than an assessment of cardiovascular fitness.[91,102] The subject walks as far as possible, at a safe speed, in 6 minutes, and the test score is the distance covered in meters. Several studies have demonstrated the degradation of performance on the 6MW with increasing age.[77,91,102-104] The 6MW has excellent test–retest reliability (ICCs = 0.95 to 0.97)[91,105] and correlates well with other measures of functional performance.[77,91,102,105] Six-minute walk reference values are identified in Table 17-5. The difference in values in the two studies cited may be a function of the study subjects. While Lusardi et al included participants with and without assistive devices,[77] Steffen et al included only individuals who were ambulatory without the use of an assistive device.[91] A change of 20 m in the 6MW represents a minimal clinically important change, and a change of 50 m represents a substantial change.[97]

Modified Gait Abnormality Rating Scale

The GARS-M[106] (a seven-item modification to the original GARS[107]) has been found to be a valid[108] and reliable gait assessment tool for use with older adults, with intra- and interrater ICCs ranging between 0.932 and 0.984.[106] It requires the videotaping of an individual walking roughly 8 m, turning and walking back. The videos are evaluated for gait variability, guardedness, staggering, foot contact, hip range of motion, shoulder extension, and arm–heel strike synchrony. Scoring criteria are operationally defined for each item. Video playback with slow motion and stop-action capabilities are used to score each item. A unique element of the GARS-M is that it does document variability of gait,[108] a gait

TABLE 17-4	Timed Up & Go (TUG) Reference Values for Community-Dwelling Older Adults[99]	
Decade (years)	Mean TUG (sec)	95% confidence interval*
60-69	8.1	7.1 – 9.0
70-79	9.2	8.2 – 10.2
80-99	11.3	10.0 – 12.7

*Upper limit of the confidence interval is the cutoff point for a normal TUG score.

TABLE 17-5	Reference Values for Six-Minute Walk Test for Community-Dwelling Older Adults as Reported in Two Different Studies		
Gender	Decade (years)	6MW[91] Mean (SD) (m)	6MW[77] Mean (SD) (m)
Female	60-69	538 (92)	405.0 (110.0)
	70-79	471 (75)	406.4 (94.8)
	80-89	392 (85)	281.8 (122.7)
	90-101	N/A	261.4 (81.1)
Male	60-69	572 (92)	497.7 (0)
	70-79	527 (85)	475.3 (93.0)
	80-89	417 (73)	319.6 (79.7)
	90-101	N/A	295.7 (14.6)

characteristic that is important in considering fall risk and an item that is not measured with the other tests identified, with the exception of the GaitRite walkway.

Performance Oriented Mobility Assessment

Tinetti's POMA is another observational test that, like the GARS-M, addresses some of the issues of quality of gait, including variability of gait in a very general sense.[109] The test has both balance and gait components, with the gait section including seven items: initiation, step length and height, step symmetry, step continuity, walking path, trunk sway, and walking stance (width). Each item is scored 0 to 1 or 0 to 2 based upon specific criteria. A recent review[110] cautions clinicians about the varied representation of this test in the literature, identifying that it is referred to by many titles, and that there are inconsistencies in the items and the scoring of the test in the literature. Because the balance component of the test is often used without the gait component, it is difficult to interpret reliability and validity reports related to the gait component of this tool.

Functional Ambulation Categories

The FAC was introduced by Holden et al for the purpose of categorizing the assistance needs of neurologic patients.[94] Temporal and spatial gait characteristics showed a significant linear relationship with FAC such that velocity, cadence, step, and stride length all increase linearly with increasing levels of FAC. The FAC, although rather general, can provide a useful categorization as to the amount of assistance required for ambulation. The ratings are as follows: 0 = nonfunctional ambulator, 1 = ambulates with significant and constant physical assistance of one, 2 = ambulates with light and/or intermittent physical assistance of one, 3 = ambulates with supervision for safety, 4 = ambulates independently on levels only, and 5 = ambulates independently on level and nonlevel surfaces.

Dynamic Gait Index

The DGI[111] consists of eight gait tasks: walking on level surfaces, changing speeds, head turns in horizontal and vertical directions, walking and turning 180 degrees to stop, stepping over and around obstacles, and stair climbing. Each component is scored 0 to 3 per item-specific scoring criteria. The DGI has primarily been used in assessment of individuals with vestibular disorders, for which the reliability has been only moderate.[112] The test encompasses items that are appropriate to everyday community activities for the older adult.

Choosing from the available tools may seem overwhelming, but careful history taking and keen observational gait analysis of the patient on walking into the clinic can help the physical therapist to focus the gait

examination and make appropriate decisions about which tool(s) to use. A gait speed measure is always a good starting point and can be quickly and easily assessed with a measured course (2.4, 6, 10, or 20 m) and a stopwatch. The TUG does not assess gait speed, per se, but rather gives the physical therapist an opportunity to assess more functional components of mobility: transitioning sit–stand and turning. This may be very important if the history or the observation of the individual reveal that these components of mobility are challenging. When a person presents with a history that implicates diminished endurance for walking activities (e.g., "I feel less steady after I have been walking for a while"), then the 6MW is an excellent tool for both an objective measure of distance covered and perhaps a more subjective observation of changes in gait quality from start to finish. Individuals who present with some obvious variability within their walking might be best assessed using the GARS-M or the POMA, as these tools have some ability to assess this parameter. For individuals with high level of function, but complaints of gait difficulty within challenging environments, the DGI may be a useful tool, as it provides some higher level challenges to the individual. With so many tests and measures to choose from, the physical therapist needs to consciously decide what data would be most useful for a given individual and focus the gait examination accordingly.

PLAN OF CARE AND INTERVENTIONS

Through thoughtful organization and prioritization of examination findings, the physical therapist considers the clinical presentation in terms of body structure and function and activity and participation limitations as related to ambulation, and determines how to orient the plan of care toward specific ambulation goals. A plan of care is developed that might include addressing impairments as well as activity limitations.

Treatment at the Impairment Level

Intuitively, it makes sense that specific impairments would have a significant effect on gait performance. Yet there is a dearth of evidence to draw the direct relationships between impairments at the body systems level and activity limitations at the functional level. Nevertheless, training to address impairments identified upon initial examination is an appropriate component of the plan of care.

Flexibility Training. Normal gait requires a considerable arc of motion at each of the lower extremity joints. According to Perry and Burnfield's[5] model,

- The hip moves from 30 degrees of flexion early in stance to 10 degrees of extension late in stance.
- The knee is nearly fully extended at initial contact and again in midstance and reaches its peak of 60 degrees of flexion by the end of initial swing.

- The ankle displays its maximal amount of dorsiflexion (10 degrees) when the tibia rolls over the foot at the end of midstance and its maximal amount of plantar flexion (20 degrees) during the transition from preswing to initial swing.

It is prudent to strive toward increasing ROM in older adults who have flexibility limitations. Decreased excursion of movement of the lower extremity joints during gait has been identified by several authors,[10,18,26] who suggest that flexibility training may improve gait parameters. It is important to recognize, however, that improvements in flexibility alone will not translate into functional gains.[113] Flexibility gains must be consciously integrated into gait and other functional tasks in order for gains to be appreciable and maintained. Flexibility training is one component of a comprehensive program, and it is often a component that the patient can independently work on in the context of a home exercise program.

Strength, Power, and Agility Training. Lower extremity muscle weakness has been associated with decreased speed of gait and decreased performance on functional measures by many authors.[20,114-116] There is some evidence to suggest that improved lower extremity strength, in particular, correlates with improved gait speed in older individuals.[117-120] Impaired lower extremity function in the context of balance and strength (sit to stand test) has been demonstrated to be predictive of functional disability.[27,28] Strength training appears to be an appropriate component of a gait intervention program. Speed and agility training is often overlooked in the older adult. Muscle power and agility deficits have also been related to changes in gait, balance, and mobility.[1,22,116,121] This highlights the potential need for power and agility training to maximize community mobility in older adults. Exercise that emphasizes fast and powerful muscle activity is likely the best way to train reactive balance control mechanisms.[1] It has been demonstrated that older women display a significantly slower reaction time in the context of balance recovery than young women.[121] Benefits from agility training on falls risk in older women has been demonstrated.[122,123] Brisk walking; lower extremity target identification; timed drills involving varied directional movements; video games with dance, stepping, and weight-shifting components or that challenge reaction time in an upright position are all examples of activities that might enhance agility. Power and agility training are extremely underutilized in rehabilitation of the older adult.

Cardiovascular Training. Certainly, cardiovascular training in the form of a walking or other aerobic program will enhance endurance for walking activities. Aerobic training has also demonstrated the added benefit of improving gait speed in older adults.[120,124] Yeom et al in a recent review article, identified walking and other aerobic activities as a primary component of successful mobility-enhancing programs in older adults.[125] Striving for general health and fitness in the older adult is a consistent emphasis of the physical therapist, and a simple walking program is an excellent mode of delivery for cardiovascular exercise.

Specific Interventions for Gait Training

Gait Training versus Assisted Ambulation. One thing to consider is that all individuals needing assistance with ambulation may not be appropriate for physical therapy. Sometimes physical therapists are consulted for individuals who may not benefit from skilled physical therapist intervention for various reasons. If an individual requires the assistance of another for ambulation activities, this need does not necessarily equate to the need for gait training. Educating physicians and other health professional staff about the roles and responsibilities of a physical therapist can be beneficial. If an older adult's long-standing ambulation status has required assistance of another for safety, or if an individual has no personal goals to increase or improve ambulation abilities, "assisted ambulation" is appropriate and can be carried out by any caregiver after appropriate training. "Gait training" is a skillfully applied intervention using the education, experience, and expertise of a physical therapist. It implies that an analysis of gait and an evaluation of what specific interventions might enhance gait performance precede the training.

Specificity of Training: Community Mobility. As detailed elsewhere in this text, general motor learning theory indicates that optimal learning occurs when the learner receives task-specific training, practice, and repetition and is also allowed to solve his or her own motor problems. If preservation or recovery of community walking function is a therapy goal, then community walking should be part of the treatment plan. Simonsick et al made a case for having older adults "just get out the door!" in a study that demonstrated that functionally limited older women who walked as little as eight blocks per week maintained their functional abilities better than women who walked less or not at all.[64] Encouraging individuals to push the limits of their ambulation mobility, under supervision for safety if necessary, is an integral part of rehabilitation. Gradually increasing ambulation challenges while always respecting the importance of "safety first" is an effective training tool. Individuals limited to their households may venture to the mailbox with guidance. Individuals who avoid community mobility may even agree to a supervised outing. The first step out the door is often the hardest.

It may be useful to monitor distance covered or time spent in outings in individuals who are working toward increasing their community mobility. Pedometers to measure distance covered in community outings over a set time period (e.g., 1 week) are a reasonable measure of community mobility, but require excellent compliance and recording by the patient. A global positioning satellite (GPS) system to measure the "mobility envelope" of an individual over a set period of time has been preliminarily studied.[2]

Training Speed. Working toward improvements in gait speed is a critical goal as gait speed correlates with many functional mobility skills and activities of daily living.[27-29] Although comfortable gait speed is known to decline with age,[14,15,19-22,26] there is some indication that older adults may be capable of faster gait speeds but are simply reluctant to use them. Improvement in gait speed has been demonstrated in a variety of different studies of older adults (both healthy and frail) as a result of strengthening, aerobic training, and exercise programs with mixed therapeutic activities.[120,126-129] Improvement in gait speed over time is predictive of a substantial reduction in mortality.[130] This alone should warrant consideration of training speed as a component of interventions to improve gait.

Progression of Tasks: Modification of Task or Environment. Frank and Patla have suggested a framework for structuring rehabilitation programs for older adults for enhancing adaptive locomotion.[2] They discuss the importance of reactive control (recovery from extrinsic destabilizing forces), predictive control (minimizing intrinsically derived destabilizing forces), and anticipatory control (adjusting walking pattern to avoid obstacles). They identify vision as the most critical sensory modality to community mobility and suggest that training include tasks that challenge the visual system. Training activities might include (1) step-by-step modifications to hitting targets and avoiding obstacles of varying heights, (2) ambulating while carrying an object that obscures view of legs, (3) training under challenging lighting conditions, and (4) scanning the environment prior to and during locomotion.[2]

Obstacle Courses. Newstead et al demonstrated that older fallers are not just slower than nonfallers in their ability to clear an obstacle but their approach and technique for obstacle clearance is distinctly different than nonfallers.[31] Whether this is due to impaired anticipatory control, limited strategies to respond to balance challenges, or difficulty with dual tasking (i.e., walking and avoiding obstacles) is unclear. Conservative strategies for walking and obstacle clearance are typical findings when individuals feel threatened (e.g., decreased single-limb support time, increased double-limb support time, and decreased speed). Obstacle course training is an excellent component of a physical therapist intervention aimed at improving mobility. Obstacles can include stepping up and over a step or stool, walking on different surfaces (e.g., foam, floor mat, ropes on floor) including rugged terrain (e.g., can put small items under a thin floor mat), walking around cones, picking up items, kicking balls, and carrying objects. Stair and ramp training can be part of a walking course, or can be practiced in isolation. Practicing strategies that encourage enhanced independence on stairs (e.g., working without the handrail, progressing step over step vs. step to step) might be appropriate for some higher level individuals.

Directional Training. Lateral stepping, turning 360 degrees, and backward walking have functional implications in high-level mobility activities and are all appropriate components of a gait training program. Improvements in speed of lateral stepping with metronome practice have been demonstrated in older adults.[131] The time required to turn in a circle has been associated with gait speed and chair rise time in older adults.[132] Backward walking in older adults, as compared to younger adults, is characterized by decreased speed, shorter stride length, increased double-limb support phase, and decreased swing time.[21,133] Physical therapists should be advised that older adults may be limited in their ability to increase backward walking speed,[133] but it is a functional and useful task for training.

Dual Tasking. Attention required for the control of gait in older individuals and the potential impact on fall risk has been heavily researched in recent years.[37,134-137] Gait was once considered to be an automatic motor activity that occurred entirely separate from cognitive processes. However, dual-task research suggests that gait and other postural control activities are more demanding of attention than previously thought, and that the demand is greater for older adults than for younger adults. When a secondary cognitive task is superimposed on a gait activity, older individuals show degradation of performance on the primary task of gait (e.g., decreased gait speed), with older individuals with a fall history showing even greater degradation of performance.[137] Although the mechanism underlying difficulty with dual tasking is not entirely understood, one hypothesis is that older adults may have more difficulty allocating attention appropriately to competing tasks than younger adults.[135,136]

Dual tasking is a relevant consideration for examination of gait and for treatment of gait impairment in older adults. The Stops Walking When Talking Test has been found to be an easy and inexpensive assessment of patients' dual-tasking abilities and is useful for predicting falls in older adults.[138] The test is as simple as its title: Does the individual stop walking when engaged in conversation by his or her walking companion? The ability for dual tasking can be screened with a variety of walking while talking tasks. Counting backward while walking,[134] responding to a sudden question while walking,[139] and walking while remembering numbers presented before the task[140] have all been suggested as reasonable screening tools to assess difficulty with dual tasking and prospective fallers.

Training older individuals using a dual-task paradigm is a relatively new area of research.[128,141,142] Training under dual-task conditions does improve performance and retention on those dual tasks[128,142] but does not transfer to novel dual-task conditions.[141] Training in dual-task conditions should therefore be purposefully planned to meet dual-task demands anticipated for each individual client.

SUMMARY

An understanding of the normal gait cycle allows the therapist to easily identify deviations from typical gait in older adults and make an informed hypothesis as to why an individual may present with a particular gait deviation. Older adults walk slower and with greater variability of gait parameters than young adults. Psychological and physiological factors may contribute to mobility disability in older adults and limit their community ambulation (a term that is not clearly defined). Physical therapists should train their patients to ambulate the distances required for patient-specific functional community ambulation. Mobility in the community requires great flexibility in gait skills to meet the varied distance, speed, and terrain demands as well as allow for management of ambient conditions and multitasking as the environment demands. An examination of an older adult with gait dysfunction may include the assessment of ROM, strength, and motor control as well as the use of a variety of different gait tests and measures that complement one another in terms of information gleaned. Physical therapists will be deliberate and creative in putting together the optimal intervention techniques for a given individual's deficits. There is some evidence to support a variety of different therapeutic interventions to enhance gait and mobility in the older adult. Treatment sessions should be engaging and challenging, with specific functional goals driving the intervention. The consistent observation that functional ambulation in the community requires walking distances of well over 300 m has been specifically emphasized so that training of such distances is warranted if community ambulation is a goal. Repeated use of outcome measures over the course of treatment and comparison to established norms for specific measures will aid the physical therapist in goal-setting and reevaluation of client performance. The ability to ambulate is key to an individual's sense of independence, self-reliance, general health and fitness, and overall function. Physical therapists play an important part in restoring or enhancing this ability in many older adult clients, thereby significantly influencing quality of life.

REFERENCES

To enhance this text and add value for the reader, all references are included on the companion Evolve site that accompanies this text book. The reader can view the reference source and access it online whenever possible. There are a total of 142 cited references and other general references for this chapter.

CHAPTER 18

Balance and Falls

Alia A. Alghwiri, PT, MS,
Susan L. Whitney, PT, DPT, PhD, NCS, ATC, FAPTA

INTRODUCTION

Falls are common throughout the life span, but the consequences of a fall event vary depending on the person's age. Young children fall frequently but rarely suffer consequences of a fall other than bumps and bruises. The incidence of falling increases with age. One study reported that approximately 18% of individuals younger than age 45 years fall each year compared to 25% of those between ages 45 and 65 years, and 35% of those older than age 65 years.[1] As people increase in age beyond 65 years, falling increases in frequency and can result in catastrophic loss of function.[2] Another study indicated that 30% of adults older than age 65 years and 40% older than age 75 years fall each year.[3,4]

We define a fall as "an unintentional loss of balance that leads to failure of postural stability"[5] or "a sudden and unexpected change in position which usually results in landing on the floor."[6] Recurrent fallers are those who have fallen two or more times in either 6 or 12 months.[7,8] The fall does not need to be accompanied by an injury to be categorized as a fall, that is, a fall without injury is still a fall. A challenge in examining studies focused on falls is the wide variety of operational definitions used to categorize someone as having "fallen" or, more commonly, the lack of any operational definition of a fall. Hauer et al,[9] in a recent systematic review of falls, reported that falls were not defined in 44 of 90 studies reviewed.

There are a variety of ways of classifying, and thus approaching the discussion of, fall incidents. Falls can be classified as accidental versus nonaccidental, syncopal versus nonsyncopal, intrinsically versus extrinsically driven, falls with injury versus falls without injury, and a single fall incident versus recurrent falling.

HOW SERIOUS IS THE PROBLEM OF FALLING

Falls represent the most common mechanism of injury,[10] and the leading cause of death from injury, in people older than age 65 years.[1] Approximately 30%

of community-living older adults in developed countries fall per year, with 10% to 20% falling more than once.[11] The Centers for Disease Control and Prevention reported that in 2004, nearly 15,800 people aged 65 years and older died from injuries related to unintentional falls, and another 1.8 million were treated in emergency departments for nonfatal injuries from falls.[12] Of those who fall, 10% have a serious injury (fracture, dislocation, or head injury).[11,13,14] In 2000, medical treatment for falls among people older than age 65 years cost the United States more than $19 billion, and the number is projected to increase to $43.8 billion by 2020. Shumway-Cook et al[15] recently reported increased costs to Medicare for individuals who fell in the previous year, with a greater cost increase associated with more reported falls.

In addition to the medical costs, there are also enormous societal and personal costs. Falls are associated with pain, loss of confidence, functional decline, and institutionalization.[13,14,16] Falls pose a health hazard and can seriously threaten the functional activities, participation, and well-being of older adults. The United States Congress has recently even enacted H.R. 3710, Safety of Seniors Act (2008), that focuses research efforts on methods to prevent falls in older adults.[17]

FALL RISK FACTORS

Identifying specific risk factors for falls in older adults and using these risk factors to predict who will fall is a very complex undertaking. Although the underlying "causes" of falls are typically divided into extrinsic (environmental) and intrinsic (postural control mechanisms),[18] falls often represent a complex interaction of environmental challenges (tripping, slipping, etc.) and compromises across multiple components of the postural control system (somatosensory inputs, central processing, musculoskeletal effectors) in responding to a postural challenge.[19-21] Intrinsic factors that place one at risk of falling could stem from an accumulation of multiple age-related changes in postural control structures, particularly in those older than age 80 or 85 years, or, more commonly, a combination of health/medical conditions that compromise the postural control system superimposed on age-related changes.

Identifying those at risk for falling, and the particular factors placing them at risk, can guide an intervention program to ameliorate or accommodate risk. In order to provide a more precise assessment of fall risk, most studies choose a relatively narrow category of older adult, chosen either by their current health status (community-dwelling, nursing home, acutely ill, frail, active, etc.) or because they have a specific disease (diabetes, stroke, hip fracture, etc.) likely to affect one or more specific components of the postural control system. Specific risk factors can vary widely across these groups. Similar themes do emerge, however. These include common age-related changes that when combined with health-related conditions across several body systems, serve as intrinsic factors contributing to falls. Figure 18-1 provides a summary of the many intrinsic factors that are commonly associated with falls in older adults.

The American Academy of Neurology (2008) fall guidelines suggested that people with the diagnoses of stroke, dementia, walking, and balance problems or a history of recent falls, plus people who use walking aids such as a cane or a walker, are at the highest risk of falling.[22] This group also identifies Parkinson's disease, peripheral neuropathy, lower extremity weakness or sensory loss, and substantial loss of vision as probable predictors of fall risk.[22]

Polypharmacy, and issues of drug interactions and drug adverse effects, can add substantially to impaired balance and risk of falls. Antidepressants, antianxiety drugs, sedatives, tranquilizers, diuretics, and sleep medications are all related to increasing the risk of falling in older adults.[23] Chapter 4 provides a detailed discussion of this issue. Environmental hazards such as a slippery walking surface, loose rug, poor lighting, and obstacles in the walking path can each increase risk of falling, particularly in individuals with already compromised balance. Chapter 7 provides an in-depth discussion of this topic.

Overall, the take-home message is that, as the number of risk factors increase, there is an associated increase in the chance of falling. Decreasing the number of risk factors can decrease the person's risk of falling, particularly for individuals at high risk. Yokoya et al[24] reported that, after participating in a weekly exercise class, the number of falls decreased in high-risk persons living in the community. There were no differences noted in the low- to moderate-risk groups.

BALANCE AND POSTURAL CONTROL

Postural control is achieved by continually positioning the body's center of gravity (COG) over the base of support (BOS) during both static and dynamic situations.[25] Physiologically, postural control depends on the integration and coordination of three body systems: sensory,

central nervous (CNS), and neuromuscular. The sensory system gathers essential information about the position and orientation of body segments in space; the CNS integrates, coordinates, and interprets the sensory inputs and then directs the execution of movements; and the neuromuscular system responds to the orders provided by the CNS. All postural control components undergo changes with aging. Deficits within any single component are not typically sufficient to cause postural instability, because compensatory mechanisms from other components prevent that from happening. However, accumulation of deficits across multiple components may lead to instability and eventually falls.

Sensory System

Sensory information plays a significant role in updating the CNS about the body's position and motion in space. Sensory inputs are gathered through the somatosensory, visual, and vestibular systems. Advancing age is accompanied by diverse structural and functional changes in most of the sensory components of postural control.

Somatosensory Input. Somatosensory information, gathered from receptors located in joints, muscles, and tendons, provide the CNS with crucial information regarding body segment position and movement in space relative to each other, as well as the amount of force generated for the movement. There are age-related declines in two-point discrimination, muscle spindle activity, proprioception, and cutaneous receptors in the lower extremities, plus changes in vibration sense. Vibration sense is decreased or diminished in 10% of people older than age 60 years and 50% of people older than age 75 years.[26] Kristinsdottir et al[27] compared postural control of younger adults (mean age of 37.5 years) and older adults (mean age of 74.6 years), some with intact and others with impaired vibration perception in their lower extremities. Vibration perception in lower extremities was found to be the main determinant for postural control in these older individuals. Older adults with intact vibration perception were found very similar to that of the younger adults, whereas older individuals with impaired vibration perception had increased high-frequency sway. Proprioceptive and cutaneous inputs have been identified as the primary sensory information used to maintain balance.[28-30] Judge et al[31] compared the contribution of proprioception and vision on balance in older adults by using the Equitest sensory organization test (SOT) (discussed in the examination and evaluation section of this chapter) of the computerized dynamic posturography (CDP). Reduction in vision with reduced proprioceptive inputs increased the odds ratio of a fall during testing by 5.7-fold.[31] Therefore, somatosensory sensation including vibration, proprioception, and cutaneous inputs are important to consider in the evaluation and intervention processes in older adults who have postural instability.

INTRINSIC FALL RISK FACTORS

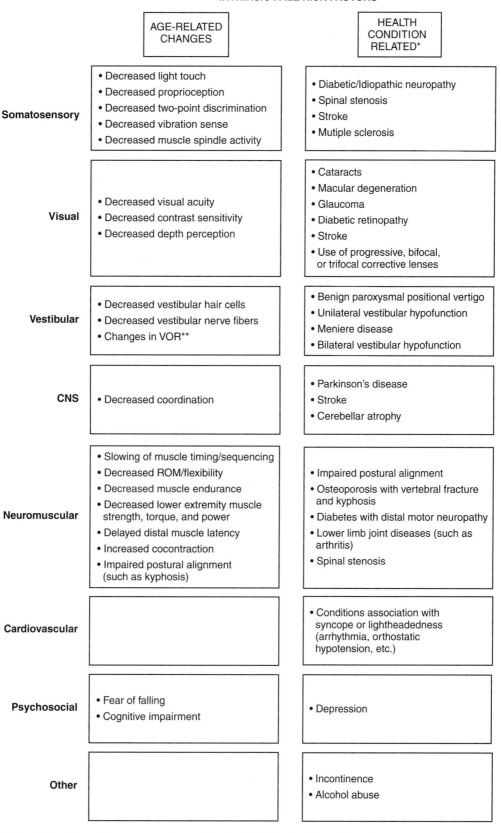

*Selected health conditions commonly associated with fall risk in older adults and responses to medications used to manage the condition
**Vestibular ocular reflex

FIGURE 18-1 Commonly identified factors associated with increased fall risk, organized by postural-control–related body systems.

Visual Input. Visual input provides the CNS with upright postural control information important in maintaining the body in a vertical position with the surrounding environment.[32] Visual acuity, contrast sensitivity, depth perception, and peripheral vision are all essential visual components that provide the CNS with the required information about objects in the surrounding environment. Visual acuity, contrast sensitivity, and depth perception diminish with advanced age.[33] Impairments of visual acuity and contrast sensitivity have been associated with a higher number of falls in older adults.[30] Therefore, examining visual capabilities and the use of the appropriate glasses can be very helpful for older adults who use their vision as a compensatory mechanism to control their balance when their other sensory modalities decline.

Vestibular. The vestibular system provides the CNS with information about angular acceleration of the head via the semicircular canals and linear acceleration via the otoliths. This information is considered key sensory data for postural control. The vestibular system regulates the head and neck position and movement through two outputs: the vestibular ocular reflex (VOR) and vestibular spinal reflex (VSR). The VOR is important for stabilizing visual images on the retina during head movements. The VSR allows for reflex control of the neck and lower extremity postural muscles so that the position of the head and trunk can be maintained accurately and correlated with eye movements. Information from sensory receptors in the vestibular apparatus interacts with visual and somatosensory information to produce proper body alignment and postural control.

Anatomic and physiological changes occur in the vestibular system of older adults. Anatomically, progressive loss of peripheral hair cells[34] and vestibular nerve fibers[35] have been reported in people older than 55 years of age. Physiologically, changes in the VOR and the VSR were attributed to the anatomic changes in the vestibular system. However, these changes do not cause vestibular disorders unless another insult happens to older individuals. For people with unilateral vestibular hypofunction, Norré et al[36] found that their central adaptive mechanisms become less effective with advancing age. Thus, the VSR becomes "dysregulated" and, as a result, postural sway disturbances and imbalance take place with any balance perturbation.[36] Older adults produce significantly more sway in SOT (2 to 6) conditions than younger adults, which contributes to loss of balance.[37-39]

Central Processing

Central processing is an important physiological component of the postural control system. The CNS receives sensory inputs, interprets and integrates these inputs, then coordinates and executes the orders for the neuromuscular system to provide corrective motor output. Multiple centers within the CNS are involved in the postural control processes including the cortex, thalamus, basal ganglia, vestibular nucleus, and cerebellum.

In real-life circumstances, postural responses are elicited in both feedback and feed-forward situations. However, researchers have primarily examined the automatic postural responses in feedback paradigms. Four main conditions have been studied to examine postural control: standing without any perturbations, standing with sudden perturbation using movable platforms, postural control during execution of voluntary movement, and sudden perturbation during voluntary movement execution.[40]

Movable platforms have been used to create perturbations in forward, backward, and rotational directions. Muscle responses then have been recorded using electromyography to determine muscle sequencing and timing. The latency and the sequence of muscle responses have been identified to define strategies of postural control in such perturbations.[41]

Response Strategies to Postural Perturbations. Five basic strategies, depicted in Figure 18-2, have been identified as responses to unexpected postural perturbations. The strategy elicited depends upon the amount of force created and the size of the BOS during the perturbation:

- An *ankle strategy* is the activation of muscles around the ankle joint after a small disturbance of BOS when standing on a "normal" support surface. The latency

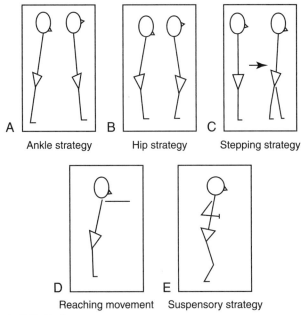

FIGURE 18-2 Five basic postural strategies used in response to postural perturbations. **A,** Ankle strategy: Activation of muscles around the ankle joint after a small disturbance of BOS when standing on a "normal" support surface. **B,** Hip strategy: Activation of muscles around the hip joint as a result of a sudden and forceful disturbance of BOS while standing in a narrow support surface. **C,** Stepping strategy: Taking a forward or backward step rapidly to regain equilibrium when the COG is displaced beyond the limits of the BOS. **D,** Reaching strategy: Moving the arm to grasp or touch an object for support. **E,** Suspensory strategy: Bending the knees during standing or ambulation to enhance stability.

is approximately 73 to 110 ms with a distal-to-proximal muscle sequence.[41] Horak and Nashner have suggested that one may be able to "train" people to execute an ankle or hip strategy based on training paradigms.[41]

A significant amount of ankle strength and mobility is a requisite for successful execution of an ankle strategy. One might use an ankle strategy in order to maintain balance with a slight perturbation of the trunk or center of mass such as reaching for objects in front of you off of a shelf without taking a step.

- A *hip strategy* is the activation of muscles around the hip joint as a result of a sudden and forceful disturbance of BOS while standing in a narrow support surface. The latency is the same as in the ankle strategy; however, the muscle sequence follows a proximal-to-distal pattern.[41] It has been suggested that older adults often utilize the hip strategy rather than an ankle strategy.

A combination of both ankle and hip strategies was reported while standing in an intermediate support surface.[41] In both ankle and hip strategies, muscle activity is generated to keep the COG within the BOS. However, if the disturbances are more forceful to put us at the edge of a fall, other movements must occur that change the BOS to prevent falling.[42]

- The *stepping strategy* has been defined as taking a forward or backward step rapidly to regain equilibrium when the COG is displaced beyond the limits of the BOS.[42] This can be observed clinically by resisting the patient enough at the hips to cause a significant loss of balance requiring one or more steps to maintain postural control.[43] It is very important to recognize when and if a patient can utilize a balance control strategy to optimize their postural control.
- The *reaching strategy* includes moving the arm to grasp or touch an object for support.[42] Arm movements play a significant role in maintaining stability by altering the COG or protecting against injury.

Stepping and reaching strategies are the only compensatory reactions to large perturbations; thus, they have a significant role in preventing falls.[42] In unexpected disturbances of balance, older adults tend to take multiple steps to recover, with the later steps usually directed toward recovering lateral stability.[42,44]

- The *suspensory strategy* includes bending knees during standing or ambulation for the purpose of maintaining a stable position during a perturbation. Bending of the knees usually lowers the COG to be closer to the BOS, thereby enhancing postural stability.

The sequencing and timing of muscle contraction appears to undergo changes with advanced age including delay in distal muscle latency and increases in the incidence of co-contraction in antagonist muscle groups.[45] Older adults with a history of falls demonstrate greater delay in muscle latency when compared to age-matched nonfallers.[46] In a recent study, older adults showed slower reaction times to change the direction of the whole body in response to an auditory stimulus compared to young individuals, and moved in more rigid patterns indicating altered postural coordination.[47] These changes make it harder for an older adult to respond quickly enough to "catch" themselves when challenged with a large unexpected perturbation.

Neuromuscular System

The neuromuscular system represents the biomechanical apparatus through which the CNS executes postural actions. Muscle strength, endurance, latency, torque and power, flexibility, range of motion (ROM), and postural alignment all affect the ability of a person to respond to balance perturbations effectively. Most of those factors change with advanced age in a way that decreases the capacity of the older adult to respond effectively to balance disturbances.

Muscle strength, especially for lower extremity muscles, plays a significant role in maintaining a balanced posture.[48] There is an average reduction of muscle strength of 30% to 40% over a lifetime,[49] which might be due to the loss of type I and type II muscle fibers. Marked reduction in muscle strength of the lower extremities has been noted among older adult fallers.[46,50] Muscle endurance is maintained with aging much more effectively than muscle strength.[51] Prolonged latency in lower extremity muscles, especially those around the ankle joint, was found to be related to frequent falling among older adults.[46] Studenski et al determined that older adult fallers produce significantly less distal lower extremity torque than healthy older adults.[46] Similarly, Whipple et al found that nursing home residents with a history of recurrent falls demonstrated diminished torque production of both the ankle and knee.[50]

Reduction of joint flexibility and ROM are the main consequences of joint diseases that affect postural stability and may contribute to falls. Stooped posture or kyphosis is one of the impaired postural alignment problems in older adults that interfere with balance and stability.[6]

EXAMINATION AND EVALUATION OF BALANCE AND RISK OF FALLS

Figure 18-3 provides an evidence-based, expert panel–approved conceptual framework for best-practice steps to reduce falls in vulnerable older adults. The framework is built around 12 quality indicators for fall risk reduction listed in Box 18-1. The conceptual framework is grounded in the work of Rubenstein et al[52] with a more recent update by Chang and Ganz.[53] The authors

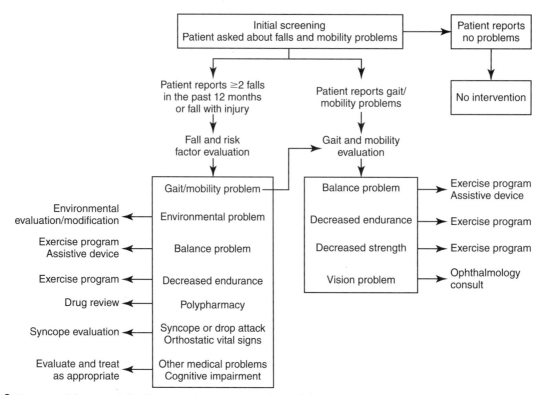

FIGURE 18-3 Conceptual framework for "best practice" steps to reducing falls in vulnerable older adults. *(From Rubenstein LZ, Powers CM, MacLean CH: Quality indicators for the management and prevention of falls and mobility problems in vulnerable elders. Ann Intern Med Oct 16;135(8 Pt 2):686-693,2001.*

intend the framework to be applicable across a variety of health profession fields. The basic framework can be expanded to provide additional specificity. For example, a physical therapist should perform the Dix-Hallpike test for any person whose balance problem appears to be associated with dizziness, with the canalith repositioning maneuver applied if a positive Dix-Hallpike test was obtained.

Determining the underlying cause of balance deficits and related fall risk is a complex undertaking. Most typically, balance dysfunctions gradually emerge from the accumulation of multiple impairments and limitations across many components of postural control, some associated with normal age-associated changes and others with acute and chronic health conditions. The redundancies built into the postural control system often

BOX 18-1	12 Evidence-Based Quality Indicators for Best Practice in Managing Older Adults at Risk for Falling[53]

For All Vulnerable Older Adults Regardless of History of Falls There Should be Documentation of:
1. Inquiry about falls within the past 12 months
2. Basic gait, balance, and muscle strength assessment for anyone expressing new or worsening gait difficulties
3. Assessment for possible assistive device prescription IF demonstrating poor balance, impairments of proprioception, or excessive postural sway
4. Participation in a structured or supervised exercise program IF found to have a problem with gait, balance, strength, or endurance

In Addition to the Above, All Older Adults Who Have Fallen Two Times or More in the Past Year, or Who Have Fallen Once With an Injury, There Should be Documentation That:
5. A basic fall history has been obtained
6. An assessment for orthostatic hypotension has been done
7. Visual acuity has been examined
8. Basic gait, balance, and muscle strength have been assessed
9. Home hazard assessment has been completed
10. Medication side effects have been assessed with special note if the person is taking a benzodiazepine
11. The appropriateness of the device has been assessed
12. Cognitive status has been assessed

(Adapted from Chang JT, Ganz DA: Quality indicators for falls and mobility problems in vulnerable elders. J Am Geriatr Soc 55 (Suppl 2):S327-S334, 2007.)

allow one system to compensate for deficiencies in another system, thus masking developing deficits. Once the extent of the deficits reaches a critical point or an acute illness incident exceeds the "deficit" threshold, the patient can no longer consistently manage challenges to their balance and begins to fall.

Ideally, the physical therapist would intervene at an early point in the process to remediate, compensate, or accommodate the impairment. Frequently, however, the physical therapist is only called upon following one or multiple falls, often for individuals at risk of frailty. A hypothetical functional progression along the "slippery slope" of aging, including critical thresholds for functional ability, is graphically depicted in Chapter 1. This slippery slope is partially modifiable: the physically fit and healthy older adult has less downward slope in the curve; the unfit or unhealthy individual has a sharper downward slope. Interventions to improve physiological factors contributing to functional ability can move the entire curve upward (and perhaps above key critical thresholds); illness and deconditioning can move the entire curve downward. Although the trajectory can be modified at all levels of the curve, it is much easier to modify the curve upward when the person is starting from the "fun" or "functional" levels than when they have reached the frailty level.

Although it is important to assess all physiological and anatomic factors likely to contribute to a given patient's fall risk, the physical therapist must develop strategies to narrow down the factors considered so as not to overwhelm the patient with tests and measures. Each test and measure should have a reasonable likelihood of revealing significant contributors underlying the balance dysfunction and to be of assistance in guiding a balance intervention program.

The examination and evaluation process includes taking the medical history and performing a review of systems. The data gathered from this preliminary step help guide our choice of tests and measures deemed important to understanding the postural control and functional performance issues of this patient as well as the impact of environmental factors and current health conditions on psychosocial status and participation.

There is no "one" best way to structure examination activities. For extremely frail individuals or individuals with marked balance deficits, the examiner may start with the simplest static postural tasks and move to more dynamic tasks as deemed appropriate. For the person who walks into your clinic independently with less obvious signs of balance deficits, beginning the examination by having the person complete one or two functional movement tests (TUG, BBS, DGI, etc.) allows you to observe movement under various postural challenge conditions while identifying a baseline score for fall risk based on norms for the tests. The physical therapist's observation of the quality of the individual's performance of specific items within these functional tests can provide invaluable clues

about possible impairments to guide subsequent examination activities.

Tools assessing functional balance typically aim to examine balance challenges across many conditions and situations. Functional balance tests can also examine activity across each of the multiple systems contributing to postural control. Horak et al have recently proposed a model that has promise as a treatment classification system to identify specific structures contributing to postural deficits, each of which suggests a specific direction for more specific examination, and likely leading to differential intervention approaches. More of these types of integrated frameworks are likely to emerge in the future. As described later, the wide variety of characteristics of patients to be assessed for falls requires a substantial "toolbox" on the part of the physical therapist, with functional assessment tools carefully linked to a given patient with consideration of floor and ceiling effects as well as amount of new information to be gleaned and the ability of the test findings to contribute to the decision about plan of care.

The physical therapist is uniquely qualified to assess the components of gait, mobility, and balance that contribute to fall risk, and then, in conjunction with information about environmental and personal factors, guide an intervention program to improve or accommodate many of these risk factors. The physical therapist will also screen for balance and fall risk conditions that may be outside the scope of physical therapy and refer to, or consult with, the appropriate practitioner (e.g., vision consult when significant undiagnosed visual issues are uncovered, medical consult when orthostatic hypotension is identified).

History

During the initial interview the physical therapist gathers medical history data and listens carefully to the patient's self-report of any gait and balance deficits or fall incidents. It is critical that the patient and the therapist have the same definition of a fall. Patients who have slid down to the floor or who have fallen onto their knees often incorrectly fail to define these incidents as a "fall." Other patients fail to perceive an incident as a fall unless they were injured.

Interview data can provide critical information about the etiology and the likely problems contributing to falling incidents and to the person's risk for future falls. A thorough exploration of the circumstances surrounding previous falls should be conducted in order to help guide the patient examination and inform the evaluation and diagnosis. One can much better manage and develop a plan of care for a patient when all of the facts about falling or near-falling episodes are available.

This exploration should start with open-ended questions. Then, the questions can become progressively narrowed. It is important to ask about the onset of falls, activities at the time of falls, symptoms at or prior to falls, direction of falls, medications, and environmental conditions at the time of the fall. Box 18-2 summarizes the key questions that should be addressed with every patient who has fallen. The causes of a fall can be as varied as syncope associated with an acute medical problem or inability to recover from a simple balance challenge as a consequence of gradual decline in postural control mechanisms. In general, a history of a recent fall (within 3 months to 2 years) is an important indicator for future falls, and recurrent fallers are at particularly high risk for additional fall events.[22] Determining an individual's activities at the time of a fall and symptoms prior to a fall event provide valuable clues toward identifying factors contributing to the fall. For example, symptoms of dizziness or vertigo at or prior to the fall can signal a circulatory or vestibular problem. Gathering information about the direction of a fall (forward, backward, or to the side) provides the therapist with ideas for additional patient education. Falling to the side is much more likely to result in a hip fracture than a fall forward or backward.[54]

The risk of falling increases with taking multiple medications and with use of specific medications such as antidepressants, tranquilizers, and benzodiazepines

---

BOX 18-2 | **Key Questions to Ask Someone about Falling**

1. Have you fallen?
   - If yes, in the past month how many times have you fallen?
   - How many times have you fallen in the past 6 months?
2. Can you tell me what happened to cause you to fall?
   - If the person cannot tell you why they fell, this clearly deserves more questions and is a "red flag" to question them more thoroughly. (Consider cardiovascular or neurologic causes carefully if they are cognitively intact and cannot tell you why they fell.)
3. Did someone see you fall? If yes, did you have a loss of consciousness (LOC)?
   - If they had an LOC, make sure that their primary care physician is aware of this finding.
   - Often with a hit to the head with an LOC, persons may develop benign paroxysmal positional vertigo (BPPV)
   - The Dix-Hallpike test is indicated to rule out BPPV after an LOC with a hit to the head.
4. Did you go to the doctor as a result of your fall or did you have to go to the emergency room?
5. Did you get hurt?
   - No injury
   - Bruises
   - Stitches
   - Fracture
   - Head injury
6. Which direction did you fall?
   - To the side
   - Backwards
   - Forwards
7. Did you recently change any of your medicines?
   - If yes, what was changed?

(see Chapter 4). Thus, the past and current medication history should be noted for possible contribution to unsteadiness. Lastly, it is important to examine any extrinsic or environmental factors likely to contribute to fall risk. Chapter 7 provides a detailed discussion of environmental risk factors and home modification strategies and summarizes some of the key environmental risk factors for falls. In general, it is useful to ask about the height of the bed, lighting, loose carpet, cords or other material on the floor, railings on steps, and the presence or absence of any supportive bars in the bathroom, any impediments in the entranceways (rough, uneven surfaces), and the lighting outside the home.

Cardiovascular changes with advanced age can increase risk of losing balance and falling.[6] Sudden blood pressure alterations can cause syncopal falls. Lower standing systolic blood pressure (128 vs. 137 systolic in standing) was found to predict falling among older adults.[55] Ooi et al found that if the subjects had falls in the past 6 months, those with orthostatic hypotension had an increased risk of a subsequent fall, especially if the orthostatic hypotension was seen two or more times.[56]

Cognitive changes complicate the taking of a fall history, as the patient may not be a reliable source of information about fall history or the conditions surrounding the given falling incident. Family members are a valuable resource while taking a history of a person with significant cognitive impairment. In addition, careful examination of the skin can help the therapist identify recent or new injuries from falls. Particular attention should be paid to the knees, elbows, back of the head, and hands.

SYSTEMS REVIEW AND TESTS AND MEASURES

The next step after history taking is to examine the components of postural control to determine the etiology of the imbalance problem. Systems review should always include an assessment of vital signs. Blood pressure should be assessed for signs of orthostatic hypotension with positional changes in older adults who have fallen, particularly those who complained of lightheadedness at the time of the fall or who are taking medication to control their blood pressure.

Sensory

Sensory changes may play an integral role in determining the etiology of falls. We know that abnormal or insufficient sensory input due to injury or disease in one of the sensory systems (vision, vestibular, or somatosensory) may predispose a person to falling.[57] Therefore, it is important to examine each of these sensory components contributing to postural control.[58]

Vision. Vision is an important sensory component of intrinsic postural control as well as an important mechanism for avoiding balance challenges from environmental hazards. Significantly impaired visual acuity as well as impaired contrast sensitivity and depth perception have been associated with falls, as well as health conditions resulting in central or peripheral visual field cuts.[59]

Visual Acuity. Visual acuity can be estimated clinically by having the patient read a Snellen chart with both eyes and then, as deemed appropriate, with each eye separately, both with and without the glasses the patient typically wears while walking. An extreme loss of visual acuity is associated with gait instability in older adults.[33] Bifocals, trifocals, and progressive lenses often used by older adults can increase the likelihood of a fall event, especially on steps.[60]

Contrast Sensitivity. Contrast sensitivity is the ability to detect subtle differences in shading and patterns. Contrast sensitivity is important in detecting objects without clear outlines and discriminating objects or details from their background, such as the ability to discriminate steps covered with a patterned carpet. Contrast sensitivity declines with increased age and with health conditions such as cataracts and diabetic retinopathy. Brannan et al[61] found that falls decreased from 37% prior to cataract surgery to 19% by 6 months following cataract surgery.[33] Contrast sensitivity can be measured clinically by using a contrast sensitivity chart such as the Hamilton-Veale contrast test chart[1] depicted in Figure 18-4. Persons are asked to read all of the letters they can see on the special visual chart.

The letters at the top of the chart are dark with a greater number of pixels and then gradually become lighter until they are almost impossible to visualize. The chart has eight lines of letters. Each line of letters has corresponding line numbers associated with the person's performance. Scoring is based on the ability to see the letters. Persons fail when they have guessed incorrectly two of the three letters out of a combination of three letters. The score is based on when the person has last guessed two of three correctly. Poor performance has been associated with persons requiring a low vision assessment and disease, that is, Parkinson's disease, glaucoma, and others.

Depth Perception. Depth perception is the ability to distinguish distances between objects. There are different ways to screen depth perception. One simple clinical test, depicted in Figure 18-5, is to hold your index fingers point upward in front of the patient at eye level, one finger closer to the patient than the other. Gradually move the index fingers toward each other (one forward, one back), until the patient identifies when the fingers are parallel or lined up. If the patient's perception of parallel is off by 3 in. or more, then depth perception may be a problem and referral to an ophthalmologist for additional investigation is warranted.

Visual Field Restrictions. Peripheral vision is the ability to see from the side while looking straight ahead. To test peripheral vision, the examiner brings his or her fingers from behind the patient's head at eye level while the patient looks straight ahead. The patient identifies when he or she first notices the examiner's finger in his or her side view. A significant field cut unilaterally or bilaterally would be important to notice. Loss of central vision, most typically seen with macular degeneration, has also been related to falling.

Vestibular. It has been suggested that persons with impaired vestibular function may be more likely to fall.[62] In adults older than age 40 years, those who reported vestibular symptoms had a 12-fold increase in the odds of falling.[63] Vestibular evaluation may be necessary if the patient is complaining of dizziness or significant postural instability. Vestibular assessment ranges from simple tests and measures to highly sophisticated examination tools. Visual impairments may reflect vestibular dysfunction as a result of the complex central connections between the vestibular system and eye movements.

For smooth pursuit, the examiner asks the patient to follow a moving target (18 in. from nose) across the full range of horizontal and vertical eye movements (30 degrees all directions) while keeping the head stationary. Abnormality in smooth pursuit is reported as a corrective saccade and indicates central (brain) abnormality. To examine saccadic eye movement, patients are asked to keep their head stationary while switching their gaze back and forth quickly between two targets, each positioned at a distance of 18 in. from the patient's nose and slightly (15 degrees) to the side of the nose horizontally, and then repeated with the targets similarly positioned but in a vertical midline position. Saccadic eye movements are very quick eye movements. It is important to note if the patient over- or undershoots the target and in what direction. Over- or undershooting the target may indicate a brain abnormality. A magnetic resonance image (MRI), computed tomographic (CT) scan, or other imaging may be needed to identify the central origin of the disorder.

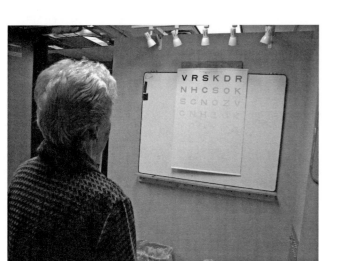

FIGURE 18-4 An older adult reading letters from a contrast sensitivity chart.

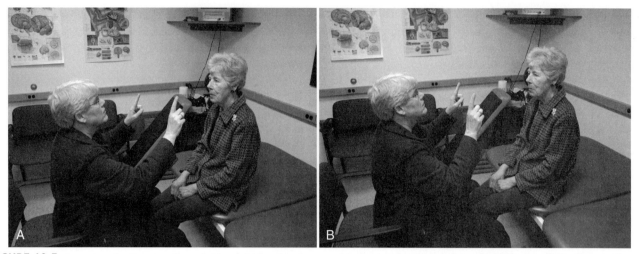

FIGURE 18-5 Assessing depth perception. **A,** The right hand is closer and is slowly moved away from the patient until the fingers align an equal distance from the patient's face. **B,** The patient reports that the fingers are of equal distance from their face.

Three clinical tests to assess VOR function, which controls gaze stability, are briefly described here. VOR can be tested clinically by asking the patient to focus on a fixed target and move the head to the right and left (horizontally) and then up and down (vertically) with various speeds. Normally, a person should be able to maintain gaze without blurring of the target. Inability to maintain gaze fixation on the target indicates abnormal VOR function as a result of peripheral or central vestibular lesion.[64] VOR function can also be tested clinically by assessing the patient's response to rapid head thrusts, with the patient seated.[65] Ask the patient to relax and allow you to move his or her head and check his or her cervical ROM. Then ask the patient to focus on a fixed target directly in front of him or her (usually your nose) while you move the patient's head rapidly over a small amplitude. Observe the patient's ability to sustain visual fixation on the target and look for corrective saccades plus note the head thrust direction if a saccade occurs. A positive head thrust test indicates an impaired VOR due to a peripheral lesion.

A third clinical test of VOR function is the assessment of static/dynamic visual acuity. This test is performed by asking the patient to read a visual acuity chart to the lowest possible line (until he or she cannot identify all the letters on a line) with the head held stationary. Then, the patient reads the chart again while the examiner moves the patient's head side to side at 2 Hz. A drop in visual acuity of three or more lines indicates an impaired VOR as a result of either peripheral or central lesion.[66]

Patients with an acute peripheral vestibular disorder will have positive test results with the head thrust test, have abnormalities with the VOR, and will have impairments of static and dynamic visual acuity. With a central vestibular disorder, one would expect to see impairments of saccades or smooth pursuit. Therefore, if the therapist is expecting a peripheral vestibular disorder then testing

the head thrust, the VOR, and the static and dynamic visual acuity will be a priority to perform. While inspecting abnormalities with saccadic eye movement or smooth pursuit, the therapist's attention should be directed to a central vestibular disorder.

The assessment of the VSR requires examination of gait, locomotion, and balance. Some examples of clinical tests that can examine VSR include walking with head rotation, the Dynamic Gait Index (DGI),[67] the Timed Up and Go (TUG),[68] and functional reach.[69]

Somatosensory

A somatosensory examination includes proprioception, vibration, and cutaneous sensation. Proprioception (sense of position and sense of movement) can be tested clinically by a joint position matching test beginning distally with a "toe up/down" test with eyes closed, and moving more proximally to the ankle and knee if impairments are noted in the toes. A patient with normal proprioception should be able to detect very subtle movements of the big toe. Vibratory sense can be tested by placing a tuning fork at the first metatarsal head. Proprioception testing, vibration testing, cutaneous pressure sensation, and two-point discrimination were together found to have reliable results in assessing sensory changes that affect balance.[70]

Sensory Integration Testing

The interaction between all sensory modalities (vision, vestibular, somatosensory) can be tested in different ways. The Clinical Test of Sensory Interaction and Balance (CTSIB) is a commonly used measure to examine the interaction between the vision, vestibular, and somatosensory systems.[71] Traditionally, the CTSIB has been performed by assessing a person's balance under six different standing conditions. The person stands on a solid surface with eyes open, eyes closed, and with altered visual feedback by wearing a visual conflict dome and then repeats each visual condition while standing on a foam surface. The magnitude of the sway (minimal, mild, or moderate) and fall occurrence are then reported or the performance can be timed with a stopwatch. The CTSIB was able to classify 63% of people at risk for falling.[72] More recently, based on studies finding little difference between the eyes closed and the visual conflict dome conditions, the visual conflict dome condition has been omitted in many tests.[73,74]

The sensory organization test (SOT) of computerized dynamic posturography, depicted in Figure 18-6, is a quantitative test that objectively identifies abnormalities in the sensory components that contribute to postural control during standing balance. The subject stands on a movable force plate with a movable surrounding wall. Visual and somatosensory elements are manipulated in various combinations to provide six different sensory conditions, described in Box 18-3. Functional responses of subjects and occurrence of falls are reported.

Patients who fall under conditions 5 and 6 are often assumed to have vestibular dysfunction, whereas patients who fall under conditions 4, 5, and 6 are considered to be surface dependent. The SOT is a very helpful tool in determining how to treat patients. Older adults have lower (less effective) SOT scores compared to younger individuals.[75] In young adults, a 10-point score or better on the composite SOT has been noted to have optimal sensitivity and specificity for improvement in postconcussed athletes,[76] and composite SOT has also been noted to change over time in older adults who have undergone rehabilitation.[77]

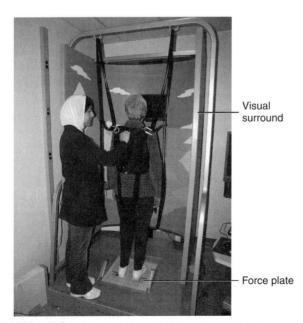

FIGURE 18-6 The sensory organization test (SOT) of computerized dynamic posturography. The physical therapist is guarding the patient but *not* touching them during the testing.

Neuromuscular Testing

Muscle strength, range of motion, and endurance should be assessed in all older adults. The neuromuscular system changes that occur with aging affect the ability of individuals to react quickly to postural perturbations and, thus, can become important risk factors of falling. A loss of muscle mass, strength, and endurance especially in the lower extremities has been found to increase the risk of falling by 4 to 5 times.[78] Small changes within multiple systems may reduce physiological reserve, resulting in challenges in the postural control system.

Strength. Muscle strength is known to be reduced in older adults and should be addressed when there is a history of falling. Testing strength in older adults provides essential information regarding the ability to generate enough muscle force to recover from balance disturbances. Manual muscle testing (MMT) is the traditional way of testing muscle strength. However, MMT is a subjective measure and may not provide the most useful information regarding balance control. Isokinetic testing of lower extremity (LE) muscles at both slow and moderate speeds provides a more accurate picture of patient's torque-generation capacity under different conditions. A patient who can produce sufficient torque at very slow speeds but has difficulty generating torque at faster speeds may have difficulty generating torque quickly enough to produce an effective postural response.[79] Toe flexor strength, ankle range of motion, and severe hallux valgus have all been related to increased risk of falling for seniors living in the community.[80]

The five times sit to stand test (FTSST)[81] and the 30-second chair rise time[82] are both functional performance tests that assess multiple components of neuromuscular effectors of balance, with both requiring good lower extremity muscle strength to complete at age-appropriate norms. For the FTSST, patients are asked to cross their arms on their chest and start by sitting at the back of the chair. Subjects then are asked to stand and sit five times as quickly as possible. The time is measured by a stopwatch from the word "go" until the subject sits completely in the chair after the fifth repetition.[81] Poor performance in rising from a chair is a strong predictor of fall risk in community-dwelling older adults when combined with other fall risk factors such as medications, comorbid disease, or at least one other fall risk factor.[83] A score of 13 seconds or higher on the FTSST demonstrates a modest ability to predict those at risk of falls, particularly for multiple fallers.[84] The FTSST has good test–retest reliability (intraclass correlation [ICC] was 0.89).[81] Normative data suggest that FTSST scores higher than 15 seconds are abnormal in healthy older adults.[81,85]

For the 30-second chair rise time,[82] patients are asked to cross their arms on their chest and start by sitting at the back of the chair. Subjects then move from

BOX 18-3	Six Testing Conditions of Sensory Organization Testing Using Posturography
Condition 1	Person stands on the force plate with eyes open, feet together. There is no movement of the force plate or the visual surround.
Condition 2	Person stands on the force plate with eyes closed, feet together. There is no movement of the force plate or the visual surround.
Condition 3	Person stands on the force plate with eyes open and the platform surface is sway referenced to visual surround (the floor moves commensurate with the person's sway).
Condition 4	Person stands on the force plate with eyes open while the force plate is sway referenced, and fixed visual surround
Condition 5	Person stands on the force plate with eyes closed while the force plate is sway referenced.
Condition 6	Person stands on the force plate with his or her eyes open while both the force plate and the visual surround are sway referenced

sit to stand for 30 seconds. The number of full standing positions in 30 seconds is recorded.

ROM and Flexibility. Assessing the ROM of the ankle, knee, hip, trunk, and cervical spine is particularly important in uncovering ROM impairments that can negatively affect balance. Assessment of ROM can be accomplished by using standard goniometric methods. Reduced ROM of the ankle or hip joints may affect the ability to use ankle or hip strategies, respectively, in recovering from external perturbations.

Aerobic Endurance

Endurance is another important factor that should be carefully determined. Assessing general endurance provides an idea about an older adults' ability to generate adequate force during tasks that require continued effort, such as walking for a long distance. The 6-minute walk test (described in Chapter 17) is a commonly used quantitative test to assess endurance. The 6-minute walk test can assess endurance in frail older adults.[86] In this test, the patient walks up and down a premeasured walkway, for example, a hospital corridor, at his or her normal pace for 6 minutes, resting as needed. The distance covered after 6 minutes is recorded as well as perceived exertion. Fatigue in older adults has been related to increased mortality rates.[87]

Functional Balance and Gait

Balance and gait are closely intertwined. Assessment of balance requires a variety of tests. Some tests emphasize one specific postural control system such as the ability to maintain balance during a static standing or sitting pos-

ture. Other tests assess balance across multiple systems during a variety of complex activities. Typically, these latter tests contribute to the assessment of overall upright functional ability, including gait and mobility under a variety of conditions and activities of daily living (ADLs).

The choice of the most appropriate functional balance and postural control measures to use to assess a specific older adult depends on many factors, including the main goal of the assessment, the mobility level of the person, history of falls, availability of required equipment, and time. Table 18-1 provides insights to help differentiate many of the commonly used balance tools discussed later.

Functional performance tests provide insights into balance capabilities that are critical to the management of balance deficits. It is during this part of the evaluation that the therapist must determine how specific deficits in the system affect the patient's overall function. In targeting tests and measures for balance capabilities, one often starts with simple static tests assessing one physiological system and progresses to more dynamic tests assessing across multiple systems.

The first static measure that the therapist can begin with is the Romberg test. Functionally, the Romberg test helps to determine if the patient can stand with feet together without falling and is purported to assess proprioception. Older adults less able to maintain the Romberg position were more likely to have had a previous fracture.[106] A "positive" Romberg occurs if the person demonstrates substantially more sway or loses balance when comparing standing in Romberg position with eyes open for 20 to 30 seconds to standing in Romberg with eyes closed. A positive Romberg test should make one suspect sensory loss distally and lead to testing distal lower limb sensation. The tandem (sharpened) Romberg test is very difficult for older adults and can separate those who are more capable from those who have minimal to significant balance impairment. It is performed by asking the subject to put one foot directly in front of the other and remain still.

Single-Leg Stance. Single-leg stance (SLS) is another difficult static test for older adults.[91] It requires good strength in the lower extremities. Single-leg stance provides the therapist with useful information about the strength of each leg individually and guides the intervention. Often it is timed for 30-second intervals. The SLS test has demonstrated a sensitivity of 95% and specificity of 58% in separating older adults who fell from those who did not.[92] This suggests that individuals who can stand on one leg for at least 30 seconds are at low risk of falling (high sensitivity). However, being unable to stand on one leg for at least 30 seconds does not provide much information about an individual's risk of falling (fairly low specificity).

Functional Reach. The functional reach test assesses a person's ability to reach forward with the right arm and recover without altering the BOS.[69] The excursion of the arm from the beginning to the end of reaching is

TABLE 18-1 | Functional Balance Measures

Balance Measure	Type of Balance Assessed (Sitting, Standing, Dynamic Standing, Gait)	Items Included	Equipment Required	Interpretation of Scores	Administration	The Main Uses of the Measure in Older Adult Population
The Romberg test[88]	Examines standing balance with feet together	Standing with feet together with eyes closed and hands crossed and touching the opposite shoulders for 30 seconds	Stopwatch	Substantial increase in sway or loss of balance (positive Romberg) indicates sensory loss distally, so clinician should test distal sensation	Easy to administer, simple, and safe	Used to detect distal sensory loss in older adults[88]
The Tandem (sharpened) Romberg test[89]	Examines standing with one foot in front of the other	Standing with one foot in front of the other with eyes closed and hands crossed and touching the opposite shoulders for 60 seconds[90]	Stopwatch	Difficult to perform for older adults	Easy to administer, simple, and safe	Used to detect distal sensory loss in older adults[89]
Single-leg stance (SLS)[91]	Examines standing balance on one leg	Standing on one leg with eyes open and hands crossed and touching the opposite shoulders for 30 seconds	Stopwatch	Sensitivity of 95% and specificity of 58% in separating older adults who fell from those who did not[92]	Easy to administer, simple, and safe	Used to examine lower extremity musculature strength
Functional reach[69]	Examines dynamic standing while reaching	Standing and reaching forward	Yardstick fixed on the wall	A reach <6 in. predicted the risk of falling within the next 6 months[93]	Easy to administer, simple, and safe	Used to assess the maximum forward reach to the edge of the base of support
The Multidirectional Reach Test (MDRT)[94]	Examines dynamic standing while reaching in four directions	Standing and reaching forward, backward, and laterally	Yardstick fixed to a telescoping tripod at the level of the acromion[94]	Fear of falling may prevent people from reaching further	Easy to administer, simple, and safe	Used to determine maximal reach in multiple directions, which provides insights into risk of falling.[94] It is a dynamic standing test with no gait included
Five times sit to stand test (FTSST)[81]	Examines dynamic sit to stand	The time required for an older adult to perform sit to stand five times as quickly as possible	Chair and stopwatch	Scores >15 seconds: abnormal in healthy older adults.[81] A score of >12 seconds had a sensitivity of 0.66 and a specificity of 0.55 and a likelihood ratio of 1.47 in the tool's ability to discriminate between nonmultiple fallers and multiple fallers[84]	Easy to administer, simple, and safe	Poor performance in rising from a chair was found to be a strong predictor of fall risk in community-dwelling older adults[83]

Continued

TABLE 18-1	Functional Balance Measures—cont'd				
Balance Measure	**Type of Balance Assessed (Sitting, Standing, Dynamic Standing, Gait)**	**Items Included**	**Equipment Required**	**Interpretation of Scores**	**Administration**	**The Main Uses of the Measure in Older Adult Population**
The four-square step test (FSST)[95]	Examines dynamic standing balance through measuring the ability to perform multidirectional movements	Stepping over canes forward, backward, and sideways	Four canes and a stopwatch	The cutoff score is >15 seconds.[95] Sensitivity score of 89%, and for nonmultiple fallers a specificity of 85% with a positive prediction value of 86%[95]	Easy to administer, takes approximately 5 minutes or less to complete	Used as a screening tool for older persons.[95] It can assist with helping the clinician to determine if the patient can change directions quickly. Backward stepping is particularly difficult
The Berg Balance Scale (BBS)[96]	Examines standing and dynamic standing	14 total items: sitting to standing, standing unsupported, sitting with back unsupported but feet supported on floor or on a stool, standing to sitting, transfers, standing unsupported with eyes closed, standing unsupported with feet together, reaching forward with outstretched arm while standing, pick up object from the floor from a standing position, turning to look behind over left and right shoulders while standing, turn 360 degrees, place alternate foot on step or stool while standing unsupported, standing unsupported one foot in front, standing on one leg	Chair, stool, yardstick, stopwatch	Score < 45: high risk for falls[97] Scores ≤ 36: 100% chance of falling in the next 6 months in older adults[98] However, it has been suggested that the BBS is best used as a score with no cutoff value ascribed to fall risk, as fall risk increases significantly as the score on the test decreases[99]	A skilled evaluator can complete the test in less than 15-20 minutes	Used for patients who exhibit a decline in function, self-report a loss of balance, or have unexplained falls Can predict fall risk of older adults. Good to use for persons of lower functional ability also because the tests incorporate sitting and standing but no locomotion. A person cannot use an assistive device

Test	Purpose/Focus	Description	Equipment	Interpretation	Administration	Use
The Physical Performance Test (PPT)[100]	Examines dynamic balance such as turning 360 degrees and picking up a penny from the floor	Nine total items: sentence writing, simulated eating, turning 360°, putting on and removing a jacket, lifting and then placing a book on a shelf, picking up a penny from the floor, a 50-foot walk test, and two measures of stair climbing (time to ascend one flight; number of flights climbed up and down)[100]	Pencil and paper, a jacket, a book, a penny, stopwatch, and stairs	Detect risk of falling	Easy to perform within 10 minutes	Used as a follow-up tool to monitor changes in physical frailty, quality of life, and increasing function following exercise training programs including strength training and treadmill walking[101]
The Short Physical Performance Battery (SPPB)[102]	Examines standing, dynamic standing, and gait	Three types of physical maneuvers: the balance tests (Romberg, semi-tandem Romberg, tandem Romberg), the gait speed test, and the chair stand test[102]	Chair and stopwatch	Scores ≤10: high risk of mobility disability[102]	Easy to administer and safe, takes 10-15 minuets	Used as a predictive measure for morbidity and mortality in older persons[102]
Dynamic Gait Index (DGI)[67]	Examines gait	Eight total items: gait level surface, change in gait speed, gait with horizontal head turns, gait with vertical turns, gait and pivot turn, step over obstacles, step around obstacles, and steps	Boxes, cones, and steps	A score ≤19 was found to be predictive of falls in older adults[98]	It takes 10 minutes or less to administer	Used to assess older adults' ability to modify gait and maintain normal pattern and pace in response to changing task demands[67]
Timed Up and Go (TUG)[68]	Examines gait	The therapist measures the time an older adult needs to stand from a chair with armrests, walk for 3 m, turn around, and return back to the chair and sit down at his or her normal, comfortable speed	Chair with armrests and stopwatch	Older adults who took ≥13.5 seconds were classified as fallers, with an overall correct prediction rate of 90%.[103] A score ≥30 seconds indicates that the patient will have significant difficulties in ADL.[103] It is a very reliable test with high sensitivity (87%) and specificity (87%).[103]	Very easy to administer	Used to measure the functional mobility in older adults that is important for ADL
Gait speed[104]	Examines gait	Timed walking over 3-4 m	Stopwatch	Predict hospitalization and mortality rate[105]; 0.1 m/second change is considered clinically significant[104]	Easy to administer	Used as a measure of functional exercise capacity in older adults

measured via a yardstick affixed to the wall. It is a useful measure for patients complaining of falling. A reach of less than 6 in. has been reported as a risk factor for falling within the next 6 months, with an adjusted odds ratio of 4.0.[93]

The multi-directional reach test (MDRT) was developed by Newton[94] to determine how well older adults could reach forward, to the side, and backward. A yardstick fixed to a telescoping tripod at the level of the acromion was used. Their instructions included "without moving your feet or taking a step, reach as far as you can to the (right, left, forward, or lean backwards)."[94] The test appears to be a reliable and valid measure of the "limits of stability."[94] Forward reach is less when done via Newton's test compared to the functional reach test. This difference is most likely because the tripod is not located next to a wall. Fear of falling may prevent people from reaching further.[94]

Reaching tests can serve as a quick and low-effort mechanism for gathering crucial information regarding the postural stability of older adults. Reaching tests provide an option for examining postural stability in frail older adults who cannot perform other tests that include ambulation and can be used as a quick screen for community testing of seniors.

Four-Square Step Test. The four-square step test (FSST) has also been used in older adults to assess fall risk. The FSST involves stepping over four standard canes at 90 degree angles to each other, whereby the tips all touch each other at the center to create the "four squares."[95] The patient is asked to stand in one square facing forward and then is asked to step clockwise over the canes by moving forward, to the right, backward, to the left, and then reversing the path in a counterclockwise direction. Both feet are to enter each designated spot. The patient is instructed to move as quickly as possible without touching the canes with both feet touching the floor in each square. They are also asked to face forward throughout the testing.[95] Interrater reliability has been reported to be $r = 0.99$.[95] Using a cutoff score of >15 seconds to predict individuals with two or more falls, the test has good sensitivity and specificity (89% and 85%, respectively).[95] The FSST is especially helpful in quantifying how well your patient can change directions and move backward quickly.

Berg Balance Test. The Berg Balance Scale (BBS) was developed by Katherine Berg in 1989 to measure balance ability (static and dynamic) among older adults.[96] The BBS is a qualitative measure that assesses balance via performing functional activities such as reaching, bending, transferring, and standing that incorporates most components of postural control: sitting and transferring safely between chairs; standing with feet apart, feet together, in single-leg stance, and feet in the tandem Romberg position with eyes open or closed; reaching and stooping down to pick something off the floor. Each item is scored along a 5-point scale, ranging from 0 to 4, each grade with well-established criteria. Zero indicates the lowest level of function and 4 the highest level of function. The total score ranges from 0 to 56. The BBS is reliable (both inter- and intratester) and has concurrent and construct validity.[107,108]

Although a cutoff score of greater than 45 has been traditionally identified as a useful cutoff to predict falls in those who scored below the cutoff score,[97] recent work by Muir and Berg[99] suggests an alternative scoring system as well as suggesting that the BBS is more effective in identifying those who will fall more than once than those who have fallen one time only. They suggest a cutoff score of 40 to predict those who will experience multiple falls (positive likelihood ratio of 5.19 with 95% confidence interval [CI] of 2.29 to 11.75) and injurious falls (positive likelihood ratio of 3.3 with 95% CI of 1.40 to 7.76). In the Shumway-Cook et al model for using the BBS to predict the likelihood of falling, a score of 36 or less indicated a nearly 100% chance of falling in the next 6 months in older adults.[98] The BBS is less useful in confirming someone is at low risk of falling. Even subjects who achieve a very high score (53 or 54 of 56) only have a moderate assurance that they are not at risk for a fall in the next few months. The BBS is particularly helpful in determining sitting and standing balance. No measures of gait are directly recorded within the scale.

Physical Performance Test. The physical performance test (PPT) was developed to assess function in community-dwelling older adults[100] and is a useful measure of early physical decline in older persons.[109] The PPT's relationship with recurrent reported falls demonstrated a sensitivity of 79% and a specificity of 71% in older men.[110] The PPT tool assesses multiple domains while observing the patient performing various tasks. The PPT includes nine items such as eating, putting on a sweater, writing, picking up a penny from the floor, turning while standing, walking, and stair climbing, with three degrees of difficulty. An ordinal scale is used based on the time that it takes the subject to complete the tasks, except for the last item, stair climbing, which is based on the number of flights that the person can ascend and descend.[100]

The Short Physical Performance Battery (SPPB) was developed to assess risk of falling in older adults.[102] The SPPB has three components: (1) the Romberg, semitandem Romberg, and tandem Romberg; (2) repeated sit to stand; and (3) gait speed. Scores range from 0 to 12, which has been norm-based on more than 10,000 older adults (higher scores indicate better function).[111]

Dynamic Gait Index. The Dynamic Gait Index (DGI) is particularly useful for individuals with suspected vestibular disorders because the test incorporates various head rotation actions that challenge vestibular responses to gait activities.[112] The DGI is an eight-item test with each item graded (0 to 3) as severely impaired, moderately impaired, mildly impaired, or normal, for a maximal score of 24.[67] Scores on the DGI provide only a modest contribution to falls risk prediction, with both sensitivity and specificity generally ranging between 55% and 65% when the "best" cutoff score of 19 or less is defined as a "positive" risk factor.[98] However, the ability to observe the interaction of visual and vestibular input when head movement is superimposed on forward walking may provide insights into specific impairments that can help direct decision making about interventions. Obviously, people must be able to ambulate with or without an assistive device and need to have the endurance to complete the eight gait tasks.

Timed Up and Go. The TUG (described in Chapter 17) is a gait-based functional mobility test that is easy to administer, reliable, and has high sensitivity (87%) and specificity (87%) for predicting falls.[103] Individuals taking 13.5 seconds or longer to perform the TUG were classified as fallers with an overall correct prediction rate of 90%. The TUG is advantageous because it includes people who use an assistive device, is not overly time burdensome, only requires that individuals be able to walk 6 m (20 feet) to be included, and provides opportunities to assess more complex balance activities such as moving sit to stand and turning around at the halfway point of the walk to return to the chair.

Gait. Gait speed is an essential component to include in the test battery for older adults with a history of falls. A change of 0.1 m/sec is considered clinically significant in older adults. During assessment of gait, the physical therapist should vary the conditions under which the patient performs the task.[113] For example, it is useful to see how the patient responds to changes in gait speed and direction, negotiates obstacles, manages with various competing attentional tasks,[114] and handles changing surfaces and other environmental distractions and conditions.

Environmental Assessment

Environmental factors can either facilitate or hinder the abilities to function within one's surroundings. The International Classification of Functioning, Disability and Health (ICF) recognizes the role of the environment, providing it a prominent role in the ICF model of disability.[115] The level of disability experienced by an individual depends not only on body functions and structures but also on the environmental support and personal factors.

Patients or their family members may complete a home safety checklist that assesses the home environment and highlights extrinsic factors that serve as fall hazards. These data are then incorporated into patient education interventions. An "in-home" safety check should be a routine part of the home-care physical therapist's role and is occasionally incorporated into discharge activities of a rehabilitation patient. A safety check examines things like lighting in the house, types of flooring, availability of grab bars in the tub or shower, and handrails for stairways. The physical therapist may

need to watch the patient's performance during routine activities within his or her home. The therapist may observe the patient getting in and out of bed and in and out of the shower or bath tub. In addition, it is important to assess the patient's access to light switches. Obstacles, cords, and clutter become particularly relevant to the patient with serious visual deficits or gait abnormality but need to be addressed only to the extent that they pose a threat to the patient's safe function. Environmental evaluation allows the physical therapist to determine the degree of environmental hazard and suggest modifications that aid in preventing falls.[116,117] Chapter 7 provides further details about environmental assessment.

Psychosocial Assessment

Social support and behavioral/cognitive function should be addressed in the comprehensive evaluation of patients experiencing recurrent falls. Impaired cognition has a strong relationship with falls[118-127] as it is often difficult for the cognitively impaired person to recognize "risky" situations and make prudent choices that would prevent a fall. Strong social support can help minimize fall risk by providing a safe and supportive environment that allows the cognitively impaired person to function maximally within their environment. Memory deficits, dementia, and depression are health conditions seen with greater prevalence in older adults and that have been associated with increased fall risk.[128]

Fear of Falling

Fear of falling is a potential behavioral outcome of previous falls that may limit older adult activities. One third of older adults who experience a fall develop a fear of falling.[129] Fear of falling may lead to more sedentary lifestyle with subsequent deconditioning that creates an ongoing downward spiral leading to frailty[130] and increased risk of future falls.[131] Fear of falling has been associated with the use of a walking device, balance impairment, depression, trait anxiety, female gender, and a previous history of a fall or falls.[132,133]

The Falls Efficacy Scale International (FES-I) is a short tool that records fear of falling and is growing in acceptance in Europe, with a recently developed short version. The FES-I consists of either seven[134] or sixteen[135] items that are very similar to the 16-item Activities-specific Balance Confidence Scale (ABC).[131,135] Box 18-4 displays the short-form FES-I. The additional factors on the 16-item version include cleaning the house, preparing simple meals, going shopping, walking outside, answering the telephone, walking on a slippery surface, visiting a friend or relative, walking in crowds, and walking on an uneven surface.

The ABC was developed for use with older adults to attempt to quantify fear of falling.[136] The test items,

BOX 18-4	The Short-Form Fall Efficacy Scale–International (FES-I): Patient Directions, Seven Items That Make Up the Scale, and Response Options

Introduction

Now we would like to ask some questions about how concerned you are about the possibility of falling. Please reply thinking about how you usually do the activity. If you currently do not do the activity, please answer to show whether you think you would be concerned about falling IF you did the activity. For each of the following activities, please put the number in the box which is closest to your own opinion to show how concerned you are that you might fall if you did this activity.

☐ 1. Getting dressed or undressed
☐ 2. Taking a bath or shower
☐ 3. Getting in or out of a chair
☐ 4. Going up or down stairs
☐ 5. Reaching for something above your head or on the ground
☐ 6. Walking up or down a slope
☐ 7. Going out to a social event (e.g., religious service, family gathering, or club meeting)

Answer options:

1 Not at all concerned
2 Somewhat concerned
3 Fairly concerned
4 Very concerned

Handling Short FES-I sum scores:

To obtain a total score for the Short FES-I, simply add the scores on all the items together, to give a total that will range from 7 (*no concern of falling*) to 28 (*severe concern about falling*).

Handling Short FES-I missing data:

If data are missing on more than one item then that questionnaire cannot be used. If data are missing on no more than one of the seven items, then calculate the sum score of the six items that have been completed (i.e., add together the response to each item on the scale), divide by six, and multiply by seven. The new sum score should be rounded up to the nearest whole number to give the score for an individual.

(From Kempen GI, Yardley L, van Haastregt JC, et al: The Short FES-I: a shortened version of the Falls Efficacy Scale-International to assess fear of falling. Age Ageing 37:45-50, 2008.)

with varying degrees of difficulty, were generated by clinicians and older adults. Each item is rated from 0% to 100% related to how confident the person is that he or she can perform the activity. Lower scores indicate greater fear of falling and higher scores greater confidence (less fear) of falling. ABC scores can help categorize the functional level across a wide range of capabilities: Scores less than 50 indicate low physical functioning; scores above 50 and below 80 indicate moderate levels of physical functioning; and scores above 80 indicate high-functioning older adults.[137] Lajoie et al[138] determined that scores on the ABC and the BBS were highly correlated, suggesting that fear of falling is related to falls in older persons.

The Falls Efficacy Scale (FES) is a ten-item test rated on a 10-point scale from not confident at all to completely confident.[139] It is correlated with difficulty getting up from a fall and level of anxiety. The test–retest reliability was 0.71.[139] The FES and fear of falling were correlated.[140]

Participation

The evaluation of participation in older adults at the societal level is another essential area to address. More than 50% of older adults (50 years and more) reported participation restriction in a population survey.[141] The International Classification of Functioning, Disability and Health emphasizes the term *participation* and defines it as "involvement in a life situation."[142] Assessing participation in older adults provides information about the level of concern an older adult has about his or her specific functional activities, regardless of actual observable impairment.[143] Activities and participation can be assessed by asking about difficulties in performing daily living activities (eating, dressing, bathing, reading, and sleeping) and outdoor activities (driving and working). In addition, the difficulty in performing recreation and leisure activities and relationship with family members should also be addressed.

The life habits (LIFE-H) questionnaire can be used to assess participation.[144] The LIFE-H was developed to assess the handicapping situations in people with disability based on the International Classification of Impairment, Disability and Handicap (ICIDH). The intrarater reliability of using the LIFE-H in the older adult population with disabilities was greater than 0.75 for seven of the ten life habits studied, and overall the interrater reliability (ICC) was 0.89 or higher.[145]

INTERVENTION

Comprehensive, and frequently multidisciplinary, examination and evaluation should guide the management of the older adult with substantial postural instability.[146,147]

The main goal of management is to maximize independence in mobility and function and prevent further falls. Physical therapists are the health professionals most uniquely prepared to analyze movement dysfunctions and provide interventions to address the physical functional impairments and limitations contributing to the movement dysfunctions.

The physical therapist may be working in an environment that allows them to be part of an existing interdisciplinary geriatric assessment or management team or may refer to and collaborate with other health professionals to achieve a team approach as needed. Other team members may include a physician, social worker, nutritionist, occupational therapist, nurse, and psychologist or counselor. Existing fall risk factors should be addressed and prevented first. Several preventive strategies have been used to reduce the rate of falling by eliminating factors contributing to falls and improving balance and gait. Table 18-2 provides a listing of the common fall risk factors and strategies used by physical therapists to decrease or eliminate these risk factors. Overall prevention and intervention management can be categorized into medical, rehabilitative, or environmental strategies.

Medical strategies include careful review and modification of medications used by older adults.[2,146] Four or more medications, or any psychotropic medications (neuroleptics, benzodiazepines, antidepressants), should be reviewed to see if all are needed.[146,148] In addition, any combination or interaction between drugs should be

TABLE 18-2	Fall Risk Factors, and Strategies a Physical Therapist Should Consider to Ameliorate the Risk Factor and Improve Patient Function
Fall Risk Factor	**Strategies to Ameliorate the Fall Risk Factor**
Weakness	• Individualized muscle strengthening program followed by • Community exercise program for continued participation in strength training
Loss of flexibility and range of motion	• Stretching program • Modifications if range of motion cannot be achieved
Low/high body mass index	• Refer patient for consultation with a physician • Refer patient for consultation with a nutritionist • Assess for depression
Impaired vision	• Determine when the patient received their most recent glasses • Refer patient for consultation with an ophthalmologist if any undiagnosed or changing visual impairments • Patient education on environmental strategies to minimize risk in the presence of impaired vision • (Be sure physical therapist's environment adequately accommodates low vision needs.)
Impaired recreation	• Careful listening to the patient's interests and desires for specific recreational activities, and strategize options to achieve participation (in typical or adaptive form) • Building a rehabilitative program to address the specific skills required to participate in the activities • Recommendations for local programs that provide recreational opportunities consistent with the individual's capabilities.

Impaired sensation	• Exercises to maintain or improve distal muscle strength
	• Tai Chi has been demonstrated to be successful at enhancing distal sensation
	• Patient education in skin checks to prevent injury to feet:
	  • Daily check of skin on feet
	  • Wearing cotton socks
	  • Checking shoe wear and condition frequently
	• Patient education in use of alternative balance systems (visual and vestibular) to maximize balance function.
	• Future direction could be subthreshold vibration in the shoe

Cognitive impairment	• Review of medication, with particular emphasis on medications with a sedative effect • Attempt to keep the environment consistent • Evaluate the environment for safety hazards • Family education on safety and monitoring in the home setting • Participation in exercise and physical activity programs appropriate to individuals with cognitive impairment • Referral to primary physician if cognitive impairment is new or has demonstrated substantial change recently

Continued

TABLE 18-2	Fall Risk Factors, and Strategies a Physical Therapist Should Consider to Ameliorate the Risk Factor and Improve Patient Function—cont'd
Fall Risk Factor	**Strategies to Ameliorate the Fall Risk Factor**
Incontinence	• Patient and caretaker education in establishing a regular toileting program • Patient and caretaker education about effects of caffeine and particular risks of excessive fluids late in the day requiring trips to the bathroom at night • Consultation with physician, as indicated, for medication management

Environmental hazards	• Provide an environmental assessment:
	  • Stability of furniture likely to be used to assist with ambulation in the home
	  • Need for grab bar, tub floor mat installation in the bathroom
	  • Recommend handrails on steps
	  • Adequacy of lighting and accessibility of light switches
	• Assess clothing and footwear

Postural hypotension	• Consult with the physician about a medication review or need for a cardiovascular referral
	• Patient assessment for, and education in, physiological maneuvers beneficial in decreasing an orthostatic event:
	  • Active movements of the lower extremities prior to moving from sit to stand
	  • Use of elastic pressure stockings or an abdominal binder
	  • Slowly move from supine to sit
	  • Ankle pumps or upper extremity movement prior to changing position

Osteoporosis	• Standing exercises/weight-bearing exercise • Consider hip pads • Patient education in the benefits of medications and vitamin D supplementation
Polypharmacy	• Review of medications: Consult with physician if signs that an adverse medication response may be affecting balance, particularly those causing postural hypotension or confusion • Attempt, with the help of the team, to determine if benzodiazepines are necessary
Impaired gait	• Determine factors contributing to the gait disturbance • Balance exercises • Establish a walking program • Assistive device use or modification
Impaired balance	• Exercises performed in standing • Attempts to increase the person's limits of stability in all directions
Joint pain	• Strengthening program • Physical agents as an adjunct

monitored carefully, especially drugs that contribute to fall risk, such as sedatives and hypnotics.[146,147]

Another medical strategy is to address visual problems that might be corrected simply by changing eyewear. Glasses with prisms can compensate for peripheral-field deficits, tinted glasses can increase contrast sensitivity, and different glasses for near and far vision can reduce problems caused by bifocals. Lord et al suggest that multifocal lenses impair both edge-contrast sensitivity and depth perception.[60] Significant visual restrictions from cataracts may require cataract surgery to improve vision and decrease fall risk. Maximizing vision in both eyes appears to be critical.[33] For macular degeneration in older adults, medication and careful observation by the ophthalmologist can slow the progression of macular degeneration. The physical therapist should determine if an older adult with a balance complaint has had an eye examination within the last year and, if not, to be even more vigilant to the possibility of an undetected eye impairment as a possible contributor to the balance deficits, with recommendations to the patient for obtaining an eye examination.

The use of vitamin D plus calcium in persons in long-term-care facilities has been found to decrease the number of falls over the intervention period.[149,150] Vitamin D and calcium together reduced the risk of falling by 49% compared to calcium alone.[150] There were associated improvements in musculoskeletal function by vitamin D and calcium intake. Vitamin D may be more useful in frail older adults than in healthy persons. A recent Cochrane review suggests that vitamin D reduced the rate of falls but not fall risk in 4512 subjects living in long-term-care environments.[151]

Physical therapy interventions may play a restorative, compensatory, or accommodating role in minimizing balance instability and decreasing risk of falls. Therapeutic exercise is a primary restorative approach[116,118,124]; footwear[6] that provides increased sensory cues in the presence of decreased position sense serves as a compensatory approach; and wearing hip protectors[152] or using an assistive device[148] serves an accommodating role. The physical therapist has a leading role in providing safe mobility training and in referral and collaboration with other health care providers to address all salient patient issues. Muscle strengthening, gait training, balance training, and flexibility or range of motion exercises are all key ingredients for a successful physical therapy program to address balance deficits.

Individuals who are frail are at high risk for falling and can often benefit greatly from a comprehensive fall risk assessment and subsequent targeted interventions that include physical therapy. Frail individuals have low physiological reserve and impairments across multiple physiological systems, thus making them particularly vulnerable to stressors.[153] Figure 18-7 provides examples of the many therapeutic interventions that should be considered for "frail" and "very frail" older adults.

The examination data regarding fear of falling needs to be considered when developing and implementing the plan of care. The exercise environment and exercise activities should be structured to minimize fear while ensuring adequate challenge to lead to improvements. Particular attention should be paid to home exercise programs, as exercises that are perceived as too challenging are less likely to be carried out because of fear of falling. For all except the extremely frail, it is essential that balance exercises be performed in upright stance in order to adequately challenge balance responses. Seated balance exercises do little to affect standing balance responses, and very few people fall from the seated position. It is also important to move the older adult beyond low-level elastic resistance exercise in order to use overload principles to increase muscle strength.[154] Often frail older adults will need more supervision to perform their exercise program and move about the physical therapy gym. Those older adults who are very frail in outpatient settings may initially need to be seen more frequently so that they can be closely supervised during their exercise program.

Balance Training

One aspect of balance training focuses on exercises that improve the speed and accuracy with which the patient responds to unexpected perturbations via ankle, hip, stepping, or reaching strategies. Simple weight shifts in a safe environment with the hips and knees straight while leaning forward and back may enable the person to more effectively choose an ankle strategy. Performing active leaning forward or back with resistance at the shoulders and then "letting go"[43] (done carefully to protect the patient from falling) may be used as an intervention aimed at having patients practice executing an optimal postural control strategy when required. An option to train hip strategy response is to ask the patient to practice leaning forward at the hips while maintaining foot position (touch their nose to the mat table), or pulling the patient off balance at the hip enough that they must lean at the trunk to control their balance.

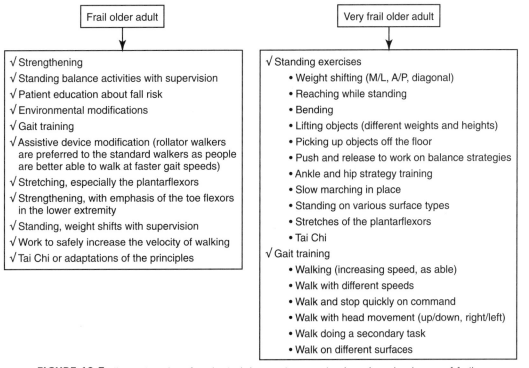

FIGURE 18-7 Illustrative ideas for physical therapy intervention based on the degree of frailty.

Standing, standing with fast and slow weight shifts in all directions, standing and reaching, standing with small pushes and then reaching for an object with a slight push would be an example of how to progress the patient's standing balance. During any weight shift, it is important to teach the patient to better recognize where their weight is under their feet. Activating distal sensation has been reported to be one of the possible reasons that Tai Chi may be successful in reducing falls in older persons.[155] Success is key when working with individuals with balance deficits. One can always incorporate the more difficult part of the exercise program in the middle, ending the session with exercises that are a little less challenging, thus boosting the patient's confidence and sense of success.

Any individual with a balance deficit can fall while performing a balance activity, so each patient must be carefully assessed while performing each new activity in order to determine the level of supervision necessary for adequate patient safety.

Tai Chi.   Tai Chi (TC) is considered a balance training program because it contains slow movements that stress postural control.[156] TC can be performed in groups and requires the person to move body parts gently and slowly while breathing deeply. TC has a positive effect on balance in older adults. Wolf et al demonstrated that the TC group had a reduction in fear of falling, a decrease in risk of falls by 47.5%, and lower blood pressure.[156] Hakim et al found that greater balance ability was achieved in both the TC group and structured exercise group in a randomized control trial.[157] However, the multi-directional reach test (MDRT) scores from sitting position were significantly better in the TC group. Richerson and Rosendale recorded distal sensation after TC exercise in older adults with diabetes and healthy older persons and found that both groups demonstrated improvements in their distal sensation.[158]

Vestibular Training.   Dizziness is never normal in older adults. Persons with vestibular deficits (dizziness, lightheadedness, or vertigo complaints) benefit from exercise and balance programs. Often older adults do not complain of spinning but may only report lightheadedness during movement. Other conditions that cause dizziness must be ruled out to ensure that you are treating a vestibular condition. Not all persons with vestibular disorders have both dizziness and balance problems. The exercise program should specifically address the impairments and functional deficits noted.

The most common intervention for older adults is the use of the canalith repositioning maneuver (Epley maneuver) for benign paroxysmal positional vertigo (BPPV).[159] Benign paroxysmal positional vertigo is extremely common in older persons and reports of dizziness in people older than age 40 years are related to reported falls.[63] The canalith repositioning maneuver is highly effective in resolving dizziness that is associated with a change of head position relative to gravity.[160]

Eye/head movements are often used with visual fixation in order to attempt to normalize the gain of the VOR in persons with vestibular dysfunction.[161-163] It is thought that retinal slip drives the adaptation of the VOR.[162]

Standing balance and gait exercises that are progressed in difficulty are provided to patients, including the following key concepts: (1) starting in more static and advancing toward more dynamic movements[164]; (2) considering subject learning style and key motor learning concepts such as knowledge of results and performance[165]; (3) increasing the difficulty of the environment (closed to open skills, quiet vs. busy environment)[165]; (4) varying from no head movement to complex head movement during standing and gait[165]; (5) adding secondary tasks to the balance or gait task (talking, holding/carrying, calculating)[67]; and (6) manipulation of the support surface (flat/stable surface progressing to a dynamic surface [towel, foam pad, gravel, grass]).[164]

Exercise Interventions: Strength, ROM, and Endurance

To the extent that muscle strength, ROM, and aerobic endurance contribute to a patient's instability, each needs to be addressed in the intervention program. Research indicates that lower extremity weakness is significantly associated with recurrent falls in older adults,[46,50] and that improved lower extremity strength is associated with improvements in static and dynamic balance.[166] Therefore, exercise therapy may be an effective strategy to increase lower extremity strength and endurance, improve functional balance, and reduce fall risk. A multidimensional training program that included stretching, flexibility, balance, coordination, and mild strengthening exercise has demonstrated improvements in physical functioning and oxygen uptake in community-dwelling older adults.[167] Similarly, a strength and balance training program improved muscle strength, functional performance, and balance in older adults with a history of recurrent or injurious falls.[168] Although it is clear that exercise is important to balance training, the optimal type, duration, and intensity of exercise programs are unclear.[2,148] In general, exercise programs should address static and dynamic balance, coordination, strength, endurance, and ROM. Most exercise/balance programs that have demonstrated effectiveness lasted for greater than 10 weeks.[2,148] Chapter 5 provides a detailed discussion of general exercise principles for the older adult.

Assistive and Accommodative Devices

Ambulation devices, such as different types of canes and walkers, may provide older fallers with greater stability and reduce risk of falling. These devices increase the BOS in standing and walking by increasing the ground contact. Ambulation devices may also help in reducing fear of falling by providing physical support and by adding tactile cues to enhance somatosensory contributions to postural control and sense of where the person is in space.[6,169] The proper ambulatory device can be prescribed according to older adults' needs based on a comprehensive balance assessment.

Hip pads are most commonly used with patients in nursing homes who are at very high risk for injury from a fall. Hip pads have been shown to reduce the fracture rate marginally in older adults.[6,152] Compliance is a concern as the hip pads are somewhat cumbersome and unattractive worn under clothing. However, wearing hip protectors may provide psychological support for some older adults who are fearful of falling.[6]

Properly fitting footwear with a low heel and high sole/surface contact area also decreases the risk of falling. Because decline in distal somatosensory function with advanced age can lead to instability and increased risk of falling, special insoles have been designed to enhance somatosensory input. A facilitatory insole, as depicted in Figure 18-8, was recently shown to improve lateral stability during gait and decrease the risk of falling in older adults.[170] Vibrating insoles have also been used to enhance sensory and motor function in older adults.[171,172] The use of vibrating insoles demonstrated a large reduction in older adults' sway during standing trials. Therefore, vibrating shoe insoles might contribute to enhancing the stability of older adults during dynamic balance activities.[173] Gait variability in the laboratory was reduced for older adults plus older fallers while wearing the subthreshold vibratory device during gait.[174]

Environmental Modifications

Environmental modifications may prevent falls and reduce the risk of falling significantly. They also can serve as important adaptive strategies to promote mobility. Environmental modifications at home may include changes in lighting, floor surfaces, handrails, bed, and the bathroom.[6] Certain locations at the home or in the hospital need extra lighting, especially at night such as the bedside area, the path to the bathroom, and in the bathroom. Lack of slip-resistant surfaces contributes to high fall rates.[128] Therefore, it is helpful to identify risky floors and to modify surfaces that can make them safer. In the bathroom, for example, a slip-resistant surface or nonslip

bathmat can be used to reduce the risk of falling. Removal of rugs in the home is recommended to avoid tripping and falling.[175] The absence of grab bars in the tub/shower of older adults was found to be a dangerous influence on the risk of falling.[176] Therefore, adding grab bars in the tub/shower may have a beneficial effect on reducing the number of falls. Handrails are also important to install to provide support for older adults. It is very important to consider the angle and the diameter of the bar so that the installation of the grab bar is customized for the person.

Other modifications can be added to the bed and its surrounding area to provide support and prevent falls. These modifications may include adjusting the height of the bed to be appropriate for the older adult, adding a slip-resistant footboard, and installing bedside rails.[6] The other area in the home that requires modifications for older adults with balance and mobility problems is the bathroom. Toilet seat modifications may include raising the seat or adding grab bars to help the older adult get on and off the seat safely.[6]

SUMMARY

Falls in older adults are a major concern and are a major cause of morbidity and mortality. Falls are multifaceted and a heterogeneous problem. A comprehensive evaluation of pathophysiological, functional, and environmental factors of falls is important for effective management. The goal of intervention should always be to maximize functional independence in a manner that moves the person up higher on the "slippery slope," away from the line that indicates frailty and closer to the line that indicates "fun," and to do this safely so that older persons can participate in their community.

REFERENCES

To enhance this text and add value for the reader, all references are included on the companion Evolve site that accompanies this text book. The reader can view the reference source and access it online whenever possible. There are a total of 176 cited references and other general references for this chapter.

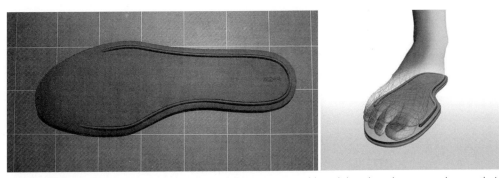

Figure 18-8 An insole that provides increased lateral cues to older adults when they move close to their limits of medial/lateral stability. *(From Perry S, Radtke A, McIlroy W, et al: Efficacy and effectiveness of a balance-enhancing insole. J Gerontol 63A:595-602, 2008.)*

PART IV

Special Problems and Interventions

CHAPTER 19

Impaired Integumentary Integrity

John Rabbia, PT, DPT, MS, GCS, CWS

INTRODUCTION

Skin and wound care is a dynamic, ever-evolving field particularly in relationship to the management of older adults. Physical therapists are vital members of the skin and wound care team. Physical therapists bring a specialized and unique body of knowledge and skills that contribute to the team's ability to benefit the older adult patient.

Advanced age, by itself, is not a risk factor for impaired integumentary integrity. However, several comorbid conditions more common in older adults are also commonly associated with integumentary impairments (e.g., diabetes and arterial insufficiency). These comorbid conditions put older adults at higher risk for integumentary impairments. With diligent care and effective prevention and educational interventions, most older adults with conditions that put them "at risk" for integumentary impairments can enjoy intact skin into oldest age.

This chapter begins with a discussion of normal age-related changes in skin and selected skin conditions prevalent in older adults. The chapter continues with an examination of normal wound healing in older adults and factors that can delay wound healing, followed by a discussion of the role of the physical therapist as a member of the wound care team.

Five distinctly different categories of wounds are presented, each with a distinct etiology and management approach: skin tear, pressure ulcer, venous insufficiency ulcer, arterial insufficiency ulcer, and diabetic ulcer. The steps of the physical therapist patient management process—examination, evaluation, diagnosis, prognosis, intervention, and outcome assessment—are applied to each wound category. The chapter ends with a detailed discussion of interventions used by physical therapists to manage patients with integumentary conditions.

NORMAL AGING-RELATED CHANGES IN THE SKIN

As with other organs in the body, the skin undergoes changes with aging. However, these changes do not typically cross the threshold of impairment. Integumentary-related impairments most typically occur when the demand of extrinsic stresses plus the presence of comorbid health conditions are added to normal aging.

The skin is composed of two main layers, the epidermis and the dermis, with a basement membrane separating the two layers (Figure 19-1). The epidermis is the thin outermost layer of the skin composed of five sublayers. From deep to superficial, the five sublayers of the epidermis are the stratum germinativum, stratum spinosum, stratum granulosum, stratum lucidum, and stratum corneum. The two main functions of the epidermis are moisture retention and protection of deeper structures. The epidermis regenerates every 4 to 6 weeks and does not have a blood supply. With normal aging, the epidermis thins and decreases in density of Langerhans cells. Langerhans cells initiate the immune response when foreign cells are present. Consequently, with decreased thickness and immune function, the epidermis becomes less effective at protecting the body from infection and dehydration.[1,2] The basement membrane is the interface between the epidermis and dermis. The basement membrane is composed of many projections of the dermis into the epidermis. These projections are known as rete pegs and they provide resistance to shearing forces between the epidermis and dermis. The basement membrane also thins with age because of a flattening of the rete pegs, and this increases vulnerability to shear-related insults to the skin.[2-4]

The dermis is the thick, deeper layer of the skin responsible for structural integrity of the integument. The dermis provides nutrition, hydration, and oxygen to the epidermis via diffusion. The dermis is primarily composed of the protein collagen, which provides tensile strength, and elastin, which allows the skin to stretch. Collagen and elastin are produced by fibroblasts. As fibroblasts decrease with age, so too does the rate of production of collagen and elastin. Elastin fibers become degraded while collagen bundles become disorganized.[2,3,5] The dermis also thins as a normal consequence of aging with fewer blood vessels and nerve endings. As the blood vessels in the skin become thinner, they are more prone to hemorrhages known as

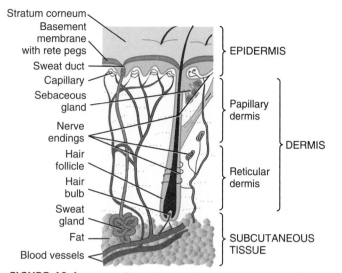

FIGURE 19-1 Layers of the skin and its underlying tissue. *(From Goodman CC: Pathology: implications for the physical therapist, ed 3, Saunders, Philadelphia, 2008.)*

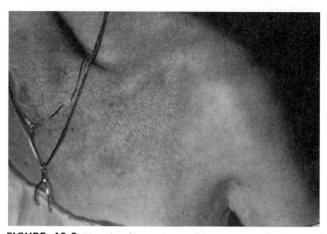

FIGURE 19-2 Xerosis. *(From Ignatavicius DD: Medical-surgical nursing: patient-centered collaborative care, ed 6, Saunders, Philadelphia, 2009.)*

senile purpura. Senile purpura are often the site of skin tears, possibly due to a decrease in pain perception in the area of the purpura.[1,6] Finally, pacinian and Meissner corpuscles found in the dermis degenerate with normal aging and contribute to decreased perception of light touch and pressure sensation.

Below the dermis is the subcutaneous layer, composed mainly of adipose tissue but also consisting of blood and lymphatic vessels as well as nerves. The subcutaneous layer facilitates regeneration of the dermis by providing blood supply and it also connects the dermis to underlying structures. As with the more superficial layers of the skin, the subcutaneous layer becomes thinner with age and diminishes in its ability to provide mechanical protection and thermal insulation.[1,2]

Lifestyle considerations, particularly sun exposure and cigarette smoking, have an aging effect on skin, including the formation of wrinkles, hyperpigmentation, and change in skin texture. The most significant extrinsic cause of skin degeneration is photoaging, that is, the effect of exposure of the skin to ultraviolet irradiation. The effects of photoaging are seen only in areas of the body exposed to the sun, primarily the face, neck, and hands.[1,7] Cigarette smoking has been shown to increase the incidence of skin wrinkling in smokers when compared to similarly aged nonsmokers. Although the exact cause for increased wrinkling is unknown, it is believed to be a consequence of the cigarette smoke's toxicity on microvasculature as well as a negative effect on oxidative and enzymatic activity in connective tissue in the dermis.[1,8]

Skin Conditions

Xerosis. The incidence of xerosis, or dryness of the skin, increases as people age. Xerosis, depicted in Figure 19-2, occurs when the moisture level of the stratum corneum is below 10%.[1,9] The precise cause of xerosis is not known; however, age-related changes as well as environmental and genetic factors contribute to the severity of this problem. Xerosis can negatively impact the quality of life for older adults by producing pruritus (itching), burning, or stinging, and an uncomfortable sensation of tightness in the skin. As xerosis becomes more severe, it can lead to redness or cracking of the skin.[1] Older adults should be encouraged to keep hydrated and to use a moisturizing lotion to prevent or manage dry skin.

Cellulitis. Cellulitis, illustrated in Figure 19-3, is a rapidly spreading infection of the dermis and subcutaneous layer most commonly seen in the face and extremities. Typically, cellulitis occurs at a site where the skin has been broken: cracks, cuts, blisters, insect bites, burns, injection sites,

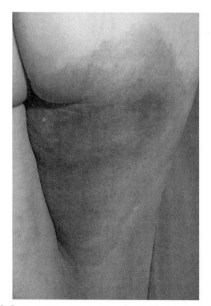

FIGURE 19-3 Cellulitis. *(From Gould BE: Pathophysiology for the health professions, ed 3, Saunders, Philadelphia, 2006.)*

surgical incisions, and catheter insertion sites. The infection can be caused by the normal flora of the skin but may also be caused by exogenous bacteria, most commonly, group A *Streptococcus* or *Staphylococcus*. Signs and symptoms of cellulitis include pain, increased warmth, erythema, and edema. Older adults are at higher risk for cellulitis in the presence of edema, obesity, and openings in the skin.[1,10] When edema is present anywhere in the body, there is a higher risk of cellulitis in that area, and obese people are at highest risk for cellulitis in the folds and rolls of the skin. The prevalence of cellulitis has been reported as high as 32% for people aged 65 or older who have been admitted to the hospital.[11] Cellulitis is most commonly treated with oral antibiotics but in severe cases, intravenous antibiotics may be considered.

Methicillin-Resistant *Staphylococcus aureus*. Methicillin-resistant *Staphylococcus aureus* (MRSA) is a strain of antibiotic-resistant bacteria growing more and more prevalent in the United States and around the world. Older adults are three times more likely to be hospitalized with MRSA infections than any other age group; hospitals and long-term-care settings are known as major locations where MRSA infections originate.[1,12] Although hospital-acquired MRSA typically results in systemic infections, community-acquired MRSA most often leads to infections of the skin and soft tissue. Patients with skin infections comprise the greatest percentage (19%) of MRSA cases.[1,13] Systemic MRSA infections are treated with oral or intravenous antibiotic medications to which MRSA is not yet resistant; localized infections of wounds can be treated with topical agents such as silver-containing dressings.

Herpes Zoster. Herpes zoster, also known as shingles, is illustrated in Figure 19-4. Herpes zoster results from the reactivation of the varicella zoster virus, which lies dormant in nerve ganglia after chickenpox. Age is one of the most significant risk factors for developing shingles, with reported prevalence of 6.9 cases per 1000 in people aged 60 to 69 and increasing to 10.9 cases per 1000 in people older than age 80 years.[14] Shingles can be identified by complaints of tingling or pain in a unilateral dermatome followed in 1 to 2 days by erythema and vesicles. The vesicles break down into crusted plaques, and patients remain contagious for chickenpox until all of the vesicles have crusted over. It typically takes 2 to 3 weeks from the initial onset of dermatomal pain to the resolution of the zoster plaques.[15] Shingles occurs most commonly in the thoracic, cranial, lumbar, and sacral dermatomes. Once identified, shingles are treated with oral antiviral agents such as valacyclovir and famciclovir to minimize the duration of the disease and incidence of postherpetic neuralgia (PHN).[1,16] Areas of skin affected by vesicles can be treated by topical application of emollients, and PHN symptoms are commonly managed through oral agents such as gabapentin and tricyclic antidepressants.[1] Physical therapists may be involved in the management of PHN.

Candida. Candida, illustrated in Figure 19-5, is a superficial yeast infection that most commonly affects older adults and the immunocompromised. Candida presents most often in the groin, axilla, or breast folds;

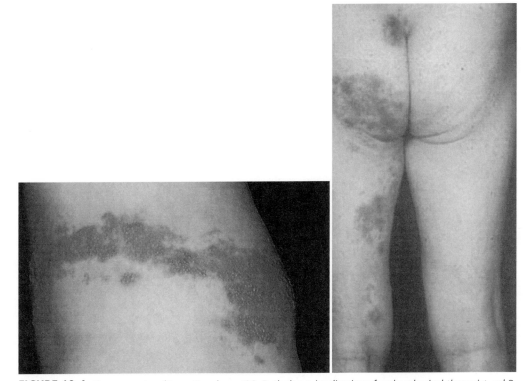

FIGURE 19-4 Herpes zoster. *(From Goodman CC: Pathology: implications for the physical therapist, ed 3, Saunders, Philadelphia, 2008.)*

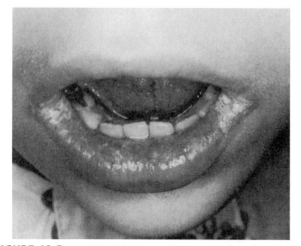

FIGURE 19-5 Candida. *(From Gould BE: Pathophysiology for the health professions, ed 3, Saunders, Philadelphia, 2006.)*

affected skin may appear macerated and erythematous with papules and pustules. Standard treatment for candida consists of topical antifungal agents alone or in combination with topical steroids.[1]

Scabies. Scabies, illustrated in Figure 19-6, is very contagious and common to long-term-care and other settings where people live in close proximity with each other. The incidence of scabies has been reported as high as 25% for residents of long-term-care institutions.[17] Scabies is caused by a mite that lays its eggs in burrows on the skin. In 3 to 4 days the larvae hatch, come to the skin, and repeat the process. Several weeks after the initial infection, itching will be reported as a result of the immune response to the mites and their wastes; once the itch is scratched a secondary infection may result. Scabies infections can be recognized by excoriation and papules around the groin, abdomen, axillae, and wrists. Scabies often goes undetected in cognitively impaired older adults because of the inability to report symptoms. Treatment for scabies includes a topical scabicide such as permethrin, and all bed linens should be washed in the hottest possible water (i.e., 140° to 200° F or 60° to 90° C).[1,18,19]

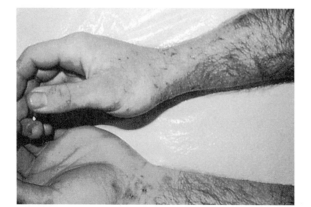

FIGURE 19-6 Scabies. *(From Christsensen BL: Adult health nursing, ed 5, Mosby, St. Louis, 2005.)*

Skin Cancer

The three most common types of skin cancer include basal cell carcinoma, squamous cell carcinoma, and melanoma. Although melanoma is less common than basal or squamous cell carcinoma, it is more deadly. Risk factors for skin cancer include men and women older than age 65 years, patients with atypical moles, patients with more than 50 moles, family history of skin cancer, and a history of severe sunburns. Patients should be educated in the signs of a suspicious lesion, which include asymmetry, border irregularity, diameter greater than 6 mm, or a rapidly changing lesion. Figure 19-7 illustrates a skin cancer. The signs of a suspicious lesion can be remembered with the mnemonic device ABCD: asymmetry, border, color, and diameter. Current recommendations state that any lesion that demonstrates malignant tendencies should be biopsied.[20]

WOUND HEALING PROCESS

Normal Healing

In the healthy older adult, wound healing takes little, if any, more time than it does in younger people. In fact, in older adults, the final scar may be of higher quality under microscopic evaluation compared to younger adults.[21,22]

The inflammatory phase of wound healing commences immediately after the wound is acquired and lasts for the next 2 to 5 days. The body's initial response to trauma is to limit the extent of the injury by achieving homeostasis. Vasoconstriction limits circulation to the area while platelets aggregate and thromboplastin facilitates the formation of a clot. Polymorphonuclear neutrophils release proteolytic enzymes to break down damaged tissue, phagocytize bacteria and tissue debris, and release cytokines along with mast cells and lymphocytes; cytokines act as chemical mediators to progress the wound into the proliferative phase of healing.[23]

The proliferative phase of wound healing begins the transition from injury to closure on or near postinjury day 2 lasting until postinjury week 3. The polymorphonuclear

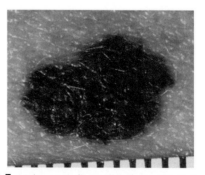

FIGURE 19-7 Melanoma. *(From Goodman CC: Pathology: implications for the physical therapist, ed 3, Saunders, Philadelphia, 2008.)*

neutrophils degrade and are engulfed and replaced by macrophages, which carry on the task of phagocytizing bacteria and debris while also releasing chemical mediators that further guide the wound healing process. During the proliferative phase fibroblasts migrate to the wound bed and lay down an extracellular matrix of mainly type III collagen and elastin; shortly thereafter, angiogenesis leads to the formation of new capillaries in the wound bed. This new tissue, called granulation tissue, has a raspberry-like texture and appearance. While granulation tissue is forming and capillary beds become established, myofibroblasts migrate to the wound edges; myofibroblasts are fibroblast cells that have an actin–myosin complex and are able to contract like a smooth muscle cell. Myofibroblasts contribute to wound healing by contracting the wound edges toward the center of the wound, decreasing the total surface area of the wound base. Once the wound defect has filled in with granulation scar tissue from the bottom up, epithelial cells derived from hair follicles and sweat glands migrate from the edges toward the center to close the wound over. If the wound base is not kept moist, epithelialization takes a significantly longer period of time as the epithelial cells must burrow underneath the desiccated tissue instead of migrating across the moist wound base.[23] In normal aging, the process of epithelialization occurs at about the same rate as that of younger adults and results in a scar that has similar tensile strength.[22]

From week 3 through the 2 years the wound undergoes the process of maturation or remodeling when the thin, friable type III collagen is slowly replaced with stronger type I collagen. Collagen cross-linking increases the tensile strength of the wound, although the final resulting scar is only 80% as strong as the initial tensile strength of the original tissue.[23]

Factors That Delay Wound Healing

Although the basic wound healing process does not change in older adults, the lower physiological reserve of older adults combined with the increased prevalence of comorbid conditions associated with delayed wound healing make the older adult more susceptible to factors that delay wound healing and increase rates of wound infection.[24] Wound healing can be delayed by many factors.[23,25,26] Some of these factors are intrinsic, meaning they emerge from internal physiological abnormalities that impair effective wound healing. Other factors are extrinsic, meaning they arise from external forces deterring normal healing processes. Box 19-1 provides a list of common intrinsic and extrinsic factors associated with delayed wound healing.

If the cascade of events and reactions that lead to wound healing fail to occur in a timely and predictable manner, the wound may become chronic. This is usually an indication of the presence of infection or other foreign matter in the wound. Chronic wounds have been known to have an excess of proteolytic enzymes called matrix metalloproteinases (MMPs) and a paucity of proteinase inhibitors,[21] which leads to an imbalance in the

BOX 19-1 Common Intrinsic and Extrinsic Factors Associated with Impaired Wound Healing

Intrinsic Factors
Immobility
Impaired nutrition
Impaired hydration
Obesity
Cachexia
Infection or colonization
Edema around the wound (inhibits oxygen and nutrient transport)
Decreased circulatory function
Decreased respiratory function
Immunosuppressed state (including use of corticosteroids and NSAIDs)
Radiation therapy
Chronic diseases such as:
 Diabetes
 PAD/PVD
 CAD
 Renal failure
 Anemia
 Cancer
 End of life

Extrinsic Factors
Tobacco use
Pressure that impairs circulation in area
Desiccation, leading to scab or crust
Presence of necrotic tissue (eschar or slough)
Repetitive trauma causing high shear forces
Maceration (typically from incontinence or perspiration)
Lack of participation in wound plan of care

CAD, coronary artery disease; NSAID, nonsteroidal antiinflammatory drug; PAD, peripheral arterial disease; PVD, peripheral vascular disease.

deposition and degradation of collagen in the formation of the extracellular matrix.

Nutrition, Hydration, and Wound Healing

The role of nutrition in the prevention and treatment of wounds in older adults is the source of some controversy with respect to specific measures and supplements. What is clear is that poor nutrition increases risk of impaired integumentary function; and adequate nutrition decreases the risk of integumentary insult and enhances healing of existing wounds. A dietician should be consulted for any older adult who is at risk for, or who has, impaired integumentary status.[27]

Older adults are susceptible to a host of intrinsic and extrinsic factors that may lead to malnutrition, increased risk of developing new wounds, and impaired ability to heal existing wounds. Changes in the digestive system of older adults include decreased production of digestive enzymes and acids, which leads to decreased absorption of nutrients. Impaired dentition may lead to difficulty with chewing, and dry mouth may lead to difficulty swallowing. Chronic illness or impaired mobility can decrease the ability of older adults to shop, cook, or eat independently. Impaired mental function can suppress appetite, as can many medications, including antidepressants, blood pressure medications, and even over-the-counter medications such as aspirin. Older adults may also have a decreased sense of taste and smell, both of which can significantly decrease appetite. Other extrinsic risk factors for malnutrition in older adults include low or fixed income, depression, social isolation, and dietary restrictions necessitated by other comorbidities.[28]

The presence of a wound or infection significantly increases the body's consumption of calories and protein. During the inflammatory response to injury or infection, metabolic activity increases and protein and glycogen stores are released to meet the increased demand for glucose and stress factors such as cytokines and interleukins. Cytokines are cell-mediated proteins that enhance the immune response to injury but also accelerate catabolism, which can rapidly deplete the body's protein stores. As the body's stores of protein are depleted, so too are skeletal muscle strength, immune system function, bowel function, and wound healing.[29]

When nutritional intake is inadequate to support the cascade of inflammatory and immune system responses to injury, lean body mass (LBM) is lost and protein-energy malnutrition (PEM) may result. Patients with PEM are at increased risk of developing new wounds and will experience delays in healing of existing wounds. It is important to note that malnutrition or risk of malnutrition is present in 40% to 60% of hospitalized older adults in the United States. The cardinal signs of PEM are involuntary weight loss with a decrease in functional protein stores. Protein levels are measured with blood tests for serum albumin and prealbumin, discussed later in this chapter. When patients experience a loss of 10% of LBM, wound healing is impaired; with a loss of 20% to 30% of LBM, the risk of developing new wounds increases and healing stops in existing wounds.[29]

Older adults are at greater risk of dehydration than younger people and this can lead to serious health complications including increased time to wound healing, especially with regard to pressure ulcers. It is generally accepted that the increased risk of dehydration among older adults is not a direct consequence of aging but rather the result of age-associated factors such as increased physical dependence and multiple medical comorbidities.[30,31] Clinical assessments of dehydration may include dry mucous membranes, rapid pulse, furrowed tongue, and decreased upper extremity strength. The commonly accepted test of skin turgor at the sternum is not reliable in older adults because of the previously discussed changes in skin elasticity.[30,32,33] Other measures of dehydration are obtained from lab values, including increased levels of serum sodium, increased serum osmolality, and increased ratio of blood urea nitrogen to creatinine.[34]

Nutritional Supplementation to Support Wound Healing

Standard recommendations for nutritional intake include 1.0 to 1.5 g of protein per kg of body weight per day and 35 to 40 kcal per kg of body weight per day. Many powdered and liquid supplements are available to augment oral intake of protein. Many supplements also include arginine and glutamine, both amino acids that increase protein synthesis when the body is under stress.[34,29] Supplemental vitamin C (1 to 2000 mg/day), zinc (50 mg four times a day), and trace mineral supplements should be considered to promote wound healing.[35-38] Vitamin C is a water-soluble vitamin that increases fibroblast proliferation, therefore increasing collagen synthesis. Vitamin C also plays a role in leukocyte phagocytosis of bacteria in the wound bed. Zinc, a trace mineral, is necessary for protein digestion and synthesis. Zinc also plays a role in immune function and collagen synthesis. Zinc levels can be depleted through excess wound drainage. However, zinc supplementation should be provided on a short-term basis only because excess zinc levels can also delay wound healing.[34,29] Anemia commonly requires supplementation to correct the subsequent deficiencies in hemoglobin and hematocrit, which are essential for the transport of oxygen to the wound bed. Different forms of anemia are identified through blood tests and treated with differing supplements. Anemia of chronic disease with iron deficiency is treated by a multivitamin with iron. Folate deficiency anemia is the result of decreased folate absorption and liver disease and is therefore treated with folate supplementation. Pernicious anemia requires vitamin B_{12} supplementation.[34] Nutritional interventions, like all wound interventions, should be evaluated regularly by a qualified professional and modified as needed to facilitate the best possible outcomes.

Enteral nutrition has not been shown to improve outcomes when attempting to improve nutritional status in people with wounds.[27]

ROLE OF PHYSICAL THERAPIST IN THE WOUND CARE TEAM ACROSS SETTINGS

The wound care team typically consists of the patient, any involved family members or caregivers, physicians, nurses, aides, dietician, physical therapists, and occupational therapists. The patient is the most critical member of the wound care team as he or she ultimately determines the extent of the goals for treatment and must participate actively in the plan of care. Family members and other caregivers are integral in providing encouragement and consistency with the necessary interventions. It is of utmost importance that patients and caregivers have a basic understanding of the significance of different interventions in order to ensure full and willing participation in the recommended interventions. For instance, if a caregiver does not possess at least a cursory understanding of the concept of shear, he or she may continue to use less than optimal technique, thus inflicting damage on a pressure wound while assisting the patient in transfers or repositioning.

Physicians provide medical oversight for the plan of care and authorize any interventions that require a physician's order. Nurses typically perform routine risk assessments, skin assessments, and wound and dressing care. Aides serve an important role as the "eyes and ears" of the wound care team. Aides frequently have more direct contact with patients than any other member of the wound care team and may be the first person to notice changes in the patient's integumentary integrity or changes in function, such as mobility, continence, or nutritional intake that put patients at risk for skin breakdown. Dieticians perform nutritional risk assessments and may make recommendations for nutrition and hydration interventions to prevent or facilitate healing of skin impairments. Physical or occupational therapists may be involved in training caregivers in proper transfer

and repositioning techniques, making recommendations for adaptive equipment and the fabrication of splints to assist with wound prevention and healing.

As part of every initial physical therapy evaluation, the physical therapist should perform a screen of the integumentary system with subsequent referral out or management, as appropriate, if an integumentary concern is identified. Physical therapy management may include risk assessment, recommendation for appropriate support surfaces or adaptive equipment, and the prescription of targeted exercise to promote wellness and prevent impairment to the integumentary system. In cases of chronic wounds or those that need more advanced treatment techniques, the physical therapist may use physical agents or other modalities to facilitate wound healing.

SKIN TEARS

Epidemiology

Skin tears, the traumatic separation of the epidermis and dermis, occur with the greatest frequency in adults aged 65 years and older.[1,6] Institutionalized adults suffer 1.5 million skin tears per year.[1,36,39] Older adults may experience skin tears anywhere on the body, though the most common locations are the arms and hands, followed by the lower extremities[1,36] (Table 19-1).

Risk Factors and Injury Prevention Strategies

The risk of skin tears increases with dependence in activities of daily living and with the removal of tapes and adhesives from the skin.[1,38] Any activity that increases the risk of imposing a shear force on the skin, such as assisted transfers in and out of wheelchairs or tub chairs, increases the risk of skin tears. Visual impairment increases the risk of skin tears because of bumping into objects.[1,36,40]

Preventing skin tears means protecting the skin from trauma. Older adults should be encouraged to avoid soaps and lotions containing alcohol, apply lotion twice per day, wear loose, long-sleeved shirts and pants, and

TABLE 19-1	Payne-Martin Skin Tear Classification System[39,40,206]	
Category	**Amount of Tissue Loss**	**Description**
I	Skin tear without tissue loss	Linear type (epidermis and dermis layers separated in an incision-like lesion) Flap type (an epidermal flap that covers the dermis, and wound edges are within 1 mm width) of separation
II	Partial tissue loss	Scant tissue loss: <25% epidermal flap lost Moderate to large tissue loss: >25% epidermal flap lost
III	Skin tears with complete tissue loss	Epidermal flap completely gone

skid-free footwear.[36,38,40-42] The environment can be modified to limit risk of skin tears by eliminating superfluous furniture, providing adequate lighting (including night-lights), and padding edges on furniture, wheelchairs, and bedrails.[36,40,43] Caregivers and institutions should be educated in proper transfer technique to prevent friction, shear, or trauma and should use gauze wrap or stockinette to secure dressings instead of applying tape or other adhesives directly to skin.[36,39,40,42,43]

PRESSURE ULCERS

Epidemiology

Although older adults are not at higher risk for pressure ulcers simply as a consequence of advancing age, the increased prevalence of pressure ulcer risk factors, such as impaired mobility and frailty, are more common in older adults. The prevalence of pressure ulcers among older adults varies widely within and among setting; 3.5% to 29% in acute care/hospital settings; 2.4% to 26% in long-term care settings; and 10% to 12.9% in home health care settings.[36,44,45] The 2009 national prevalence of pressure ulcers for long-stay nursing home residents is 12% for those at high risk for developing pressure ulcers, and 2% for those at low risk. The prevalence of pressure ulcers for short-stay residents is 14% and was not differentiated by high versus low risk.[46] The presence of chronic pressure ulcers is associated with increased 6-month mortality among nursing home residents.[47] The cost of treating a pressure ulcer has been estimated as low as $500 to as high as $50,000 in severe cases.[48] Although prevention of pressure ulcers is a significant concern for facilities that strive to limit patient suffering and cost, it has become a particularly important goal because pressure ulcers have been defined as an avoidable adverse event and Medicare limits reimbursement for costs incurred as a result of hospital-acquired pressure ulcers.[49] Similarly, long-term care facilities can be fined a maximum penalty of $10,000/day for facility-acquired or deteriorating pressure ulcers.[48]

Etiology

Pressure ulcers occur when soft tissue is subjected to pressure and shear forces, particularly over a boney prominence. Once compressed, the soft tissue becomes hypoxic and, eventually, necrotic.[36,50-52] The amount and duration of pressure that soft tissue can tolerate prior to the development of a pressure ulcer varies based on the amount of shear force present and general health status of the person. Shear is a tearing force that causes boney structures to move in the opposite direction of the overlaying tissue.[53] Shear can result from positioning in a chair or bed, particularly when the head of the bed is elevated higher than 45 degrees, causing the patient's deeper tissues to slide down while the skin and superficial tissues

remain in place against the chair or bed. When shear is present, smaller blood vessels are distorted and therefore less pressure is needed to cause occlusion and subsequent tissue hypoxia.[36] Friction, in combination with pressure and shear, is also associated with the development of pressure ulcers.[51] Friction is a mechanical force that occurs when two surfaces move across one another. Friction creates heat and may cause an abrasion. Friction can be caused when a patient transfers but does not fully clear the surface of the bed or chair, causing skin to be dragged along that surface.

Pressure ulcers have traditionally been described as Stage I, II, III, or IV depending on the depth of tissue destruction. In 2007, the National Pressure Ulcer Advisory Panel released an updated staging system[54] with several new descriptions to allow more accurate differentiation between existing stages and to provide more precise descriptions of ulcers that cannot be completely visualized because of the presence of nonviable tissue. This staging system, with definitions of each stage, is displayed in Table 19-2. The four major stages of a pressure ulcer are depicted in Figure 19-8.

As the name suggests, a wound staged at "suspected deep tissue injury" indicates suspicion of damage to deep

TABLE 19-2	National Pressure Ulcer Advisory Panel Pressure Ulcer Stages[54]
Stage	**Description**
Suspected deep tissue injury	Purple or maroon localized area of discolored intact skin or blood-filled blister due to damage of underlying soft tissue from pressure and/or shear. The area may be preceded by tissue that is painful, firm, mushy, boggy, warmer, or cooler as compared to adjacent tissue.
Stage I	Intact skin with nonblanchable redness of a localized area usually over a bony prominence. Darkly pigmented skin may not have visible blanching; its color may differ from the surrounding area.
Stage II	Partial-thickness loss of dermis presenting as a shallow open ulcer with a red-pink wound bed, without slough. May also present as an intact or open/ruptured serum-filled blister.
Stage III	Full-thickness tissue loss. Subcutaneous fat may be visible but bone, tendon, or muscle are not exposed. Slough may be present but does not obscure the depth of tissue loss. May include undermining and tunneling.
Stage IV	Full-thickness tissue loss with exposed bone, tendon, or muscle. Slough or eschar may be present on some parts of the wound bed. Often include undermining and tunneling.
Unstageable	Full-thickness tissue loss in which the base of the ulcer is covered by slough (yellow, tan, gray, green, or brown) and/or eschar (tan, brown, or black) in the wound bed.

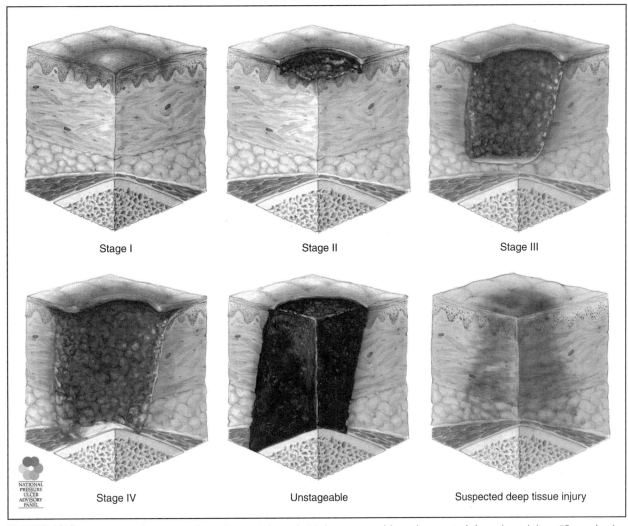

FIGURE 19-8 The stages of pressure ulcers: Stages I through IV plus unstageable and suspected deep tissue injury. "Reproduction of the National Pressure Ulcer Advisory Panel (NPUAP) materials in this document does not imply endorsement by the NPUAP of any products, organizations, companies, or any statements made by any organization or company."

structures. However, the overlying skin is intact, thus only allowing assessment of surface discoloration and not direct observation of a potential underlying wound.[54] As the ulcer evolves, differences in pain, texture, and temperature of the affected area compared to adjacent tissues will become evident. Ultimately, suspected deep tissue injuries may evolve into an open pressure ulcer that can be staged by direct observation. The intact skin overlying both suspected deep tissue injury pressure ulcers and stage I pressure ulcers makes it more difficult to discern wounds in individuals with darker skin tones. In this situation, the clinician should observe for subtle differences in skin tone around the suspected wound in addition to gently palpating for differences in tissue temperature and texture compared to surrounding skin. Complaints of pain or altered sensation over a boney prominence should also trigger suspicion of potential tissue injury.

Stage II pressure ulcers extend through the dermis but not to subcutaneous tissues. If the wound is covered by a blister, it can be more difficult to stage this wound. The general view among experts in the wound care field is that a serum-filled blister represents a stage II pressure ulcer. However, a *blood-filled blister* is indicative of damage that extends beyond the dermis and therefore is classified as a suspected deep tissue injury, not a partial-thickness stage II ulcer.[54]

A stage III pressure ulcer is a full-thickness tissue loss. Although subcutaneous tissue may be visible, bone, tendon, and muscle are not.[54] Many clinicians struggle to differentiate stage II and stage III pressure ulcers because the differences between the two stages can be subtle. There are several tell-tale differences between the two stages that clinicians should keep in mind. Stage II pressure ulcers are shallow because they are, by definition, a partial-thickness wound. Stage II pressure ulcers do not present with slough, necrotic tissue, or undermining/tunneling; if any of these factors are present, the wound is at least a stage III ulcer. A stage IV pressure ulcer has clear evidence of full-thickness tissue loss and may have undermining, tunneling, slough, and/or eschar. Wounds must be described as "unstageable" when the wound base is completely obscured by slough or eschar. Necrotic tissue must be removed before the wound can be accurately staged.

It is important to note that pressure ulcers cannot be "reverse staged" to indicate healing. That is, a stage IV pressure ulcer cannot be called a stage III pressure ulcer once it heals to the extent that bone, tendon, or muscle is no longer exposed. Reverse staging would indicate that the tissues destroyed when the pressure ulcer formed have been replaced. In reality, when a pressure ulcer heals, the void is filled with granulation, or scar tissue. The correct indication of pressure ulcer improvement would be to document a "healing," or "resolving" pressure ulcer of the appropriate stage. Once the pressure ulcer is completely reepithelialized it is still known as a "healed," or "resolved," pressure ulcer because the underlying tissue is composed of scar tissue rather than the original subcutaneous fat, muscle, tendon, etc. Furthermore, should the healed pressure ulcer reopen, it must be documented at its previous stage. For example, if a stage IV pressure ulcer heals (and is then known as a healed stage IV pressure ulcer) but then reopens, it is immediately staged as a stage IV pressure ulcer, regardless of the extent of tissue destruction.[55]

Pressure Ulcer Risk Factors and Wound Prevention Strategies

As the name implies, pressure ulcers are caused by pressure, and therefore, any factor that increases the intensity or duration of pressure on living tissue can be a risk factor for developing a pressure ulcer. Immobility, leading to prolonged pressure, friction, and shear, is the most widely known risk factor for pressure ulcers[56,57] and one that can be most effectively mitigated through physical therapy. Other risk factors for pressure ulcers include impaired sensation,[56] impaired nutrition,[56-58] cognitive impairment,[58,59] and increased exposure to moisture,[1,35,56-60] such as from incontinence of bowel or bladder.

Although urinary incontinence has not been conclusively linked to increased risk of pressure ulcers,[1] it is well documented that exposure to moisture such as urine can cause skin to be more susceptible to friction and other injury.[35,60] Both urinary and fecal incontinence can increase risk of dermatitis and cellulitis,[1] whereas fecal incontinence is a more significant risk for skin breakdown because of the irritation resulting from destructive enzymes in the feces.[60,61]

Urinary and fecal incontinence are not a normal consequence of aging. However, both become more common with increasing age as a result of increasing comorbidities that predispose older adults to being incontinent.[62] Overall prevalence of urinary incontinence in adults age 65 years and older has been reported to be 11.6%; overall prevalence of fecal incontinence in adults age 65 years and older is 3.1%.[63] Prevalence of urinary incontinence increases with increased body mass index (BMI) and cognitive impairment,[63,64] whereas risk of fecal incontinence increases with hospitalization and immobility.[1,65]

There are several pressure ulcer risk assessment tools, and each option uses subscales to measure various aspects of an individual's risk of developing pressure ulcers. No evidence exists to support the use of one tool over another.[66] The most commonly used pressure ulcer risk assessment tools include the Braden,[56] Norton,[59] Gosnell,[58] and Waterlow[57] scales. Subscales vary by tool but generally include factors that increase risk of pressure ulcer. The Gosnell and Waterlow scales include other data such as medications and vital signs that do not contribute to the risk assessment score but are important components of a comprehensive patient examination. According to current literature regarding validity, the Norton scale sacrifices sensitivity for a high degree of specificity. The Braden scale offers a high degree of specificity and sensitivity at a cutoff score of 16.[67]

The most important aspect of completing a risk assessment is to use the information to develop an individual plan of care to prevent the development of pressure ulcers. Although many scales have an overall "cut-off" score at which the individual is considered "at-risk," each subscale can be used as an opportunity to identify an area that might warrant intervention. Table 19-3 summarizes key features of each of these four scales. The National Pressure Ulcer Advisory Panel (NPUAP) recommends that all patients be risk assessed on admission, and that ongoing periodic reassessment differs by setting. In the acute care settings, patients should be reassessed every 24 hours, and more frequently if there is a change in condition. In long-term care settings, periodic reassessment should occur weekly for the first 4 weeks and then quarterly, and with any change in condition. In the home care setting, patients should be reassessed at every nurse visit.[51]

General Approaches to Pressure Ulcer Management

The most fundamental and vital aspect of preventing or treating pressure ulcers is to identify "at risk" patients and mitigate sources of increased pressure. Utilization of risk assessment tools provides insights into primary contributors of risk and the overall amount of risk. From this risk assessment, a comprehensive, individualized plan of care can be developed and carried out by the appropriate members of the multidisciplinary wound care team.[51,60,68] Recommendations for prevention and treatment of pressure ulcers include use of mild cleansing agents when bathing, establishing a bowel and bladder program for incontinent patients, avoiding massage over boney prominences, maximizing nutritional status, and educating caregivers at all levels of care.

TABLE 19-3	A Comparison of Four Scales to Assess a Patient's Risk of Developing a Pressure Ulcer			
	Norton Scale[59] 1962	Gosnell Scale[58] 1973	Waterlow Scale[57] 1985	Braden Scale[56] 1987
Items included in the scale/ subscales	Physical condition, mental state, activity, mobility, and incontinence Subscales rated 1-4	Nutrition subscale rated 1-3; Continence, mobility, and activity subscales rated 1-4. Mental status subscale rated 1-5. Vital signs, skin appearance, diet, 24-h fluid balance, medication, and interventions documented but not scored.	Based on the Norton Scale Subscales include build/weight for height, visual assessment of skin in area at risk, sex and age, continence, mobility, appetite, medication, and special risk factors. Subscale ratings vary by item.	Sensory perception, mobility, activity, moisture, and nutrition subscales rated 1-4. Friction and shear subscale rated 1-3.
Scoring	Scores (sum of subscales) range from 5 to 20; lower score indicates higher risk.	Scores (sum of subscales) range from 5 to 20; lower score indicates higher risk.	Scores (sum of subscales) range from 0 to >20; higher score indicates higher risk.	Scores (sum of subscales) range from 6 to 23; lower score indicates higher risk.
Cut-off scores	Score of 16 is cut-off to indicate risk.	Score of 16 is cut-off to indicate pressure ulcer risk.	Score of 16 is cut-off to indicate risk.	Score of 16 is general cut-off to indicate risk; a score of 18 has been suggested for patients with darker skin tones.[207-209]
Validity	Sensitivity = 0%-80% Specificity = 31%-94% at a cut-off score of 16[67]	Sensitivity = 50%-85%, Specificity = 73%-83%[66]	Sensitivity = 73%-100%, Specificity = 10% at a cutoff score of 15[67]	Sensitivity = 83%-100%, Specificity = 64%-90% at a cutoff score of 16[53,67]

Prevention and treatment interventions in which the physical therapist makes an important contribution include maximizing mobility/activity levels, including transfer training in a manner that eliminates or reduces friction and shear. Chair-bound individuals should be instructed in weight-shifting every 15 minutes. If a patient or caregiver is unable to transfer effectively without creating shear or friction, the use of draw sheets or mechanical transfer devices may be indicated. In addition to implementing mobility interventions, the physical therapist is also called on to make recommendations for appropriate support surfaces.[51,60]

VENOUS INSUFFICIENCY ULCERS

Epidemiology

Frequently and incorrectly called "venous stasis" ulcers, venous insufficiency ulcers account for up to 95% of all lower extremity wounds and can cost up to $40,000 for lifetime treatment of recurrent ulcers.[69] It is estimated that up to 2.5% of the total U.S. national health care budget is spent treating venous insufficiency ulcers.[70] Chronic venous insufficiency is estimated to affect between 10% and 35% of the U.S. population.[69,71,72] Four percent of people older than age 65 years have a venous ulcer.[72]

Etiology

Venous insufficiency ulcers result from venous hypertension in the superficial and deep venous systems of the lower extremities, generally related to one of three conditions: venous obstruction, incompetent valves, or a dysfunctional calf muscle pump.[69,73-77] The calf muscle pump is composed of the calf muscles as well as the superficial and deep veins, which are connected by perforator veins. The calf muscle pump is the main mechanism by which venous blood is returned from the lower extremities to the heart. When the calf muscles contract, blood in the deep venous system is pushed toward the heart; when the calf muscles relax, blood in the superficial venous system is allowed to flow to the deep veins through the perforator veins. Valves within the veins prevent retrograde flow, or reflux, of the venous blood once it has advanced in a cephalic direction.[73-75] With venous insufficiency the valves that typically prevent retrograde flow of blood become incompetent, thus unable to prevent venous reflux.

There are several theories that attempt to explain how venous hypertension resulting from incompetent valves leads to lower extremity ulceration. The fibrin cuff theory hypothesizes that venous hypertension extends to the capillary beds, increasing intravascular hydrostatic pressure and allowing fibrin to escape through the capillary wall, forming a pericapillary fibrin cuff that prevents the usual exchange of oxygen, nutrients, and metabolic wastes to and from tissues.[69,76] The white cell trapping theory states that the decreased capillary flow causes leukocytes to release enzymes, free radicals, and lipids that damage the cell wall, thereby increasing its permeability to larger molecules that leak into the interstitial space.[69,76] A third theory, the trap theory, suggests that large molecules including fibrin leak out of the capillaries and trap substances required for tissue function.[69]

There is no consensus regarding which theory most accurately explains how venous hypertension leads to lower extremity ulceration. Regardless of the specific etiology, once lower extremity tissue is compromised, it is more prone to break down, forming a venous insufficiency ulcer.

Venous insufficiency ulcers commonly occur on the lower leg just proximal to the medial malleolus, in what is known as the "gaiter" region (Figure 19-9). Venous insufficiency ulcers are often chronic, vary in size, have irregular borders, and typically have heavy drainage.[69] The skin surrounding the ulcer may have a ruddy discoloration known as hemosiderin staining, the result of red blood cells leaking into the extravascular tissue. Lower leg tissues may take on a woody texture and an inverted champagne bottle shape, a condition known as lipodermatosclerosis. Lipodermatosclerosis is the result of repeated leakage of fibrin into the lower extremity tissue.

Venous Insufficiency Wound Risk Factors and Wound Prevention Strategies

Risk factors for venous insufficiency ulcers include advanced age; female sex; family history; smoking; obesity; pregnancies; a job requiring long periods of sitting or standing; trauma; arthroscopic surgery of the hip, knee,

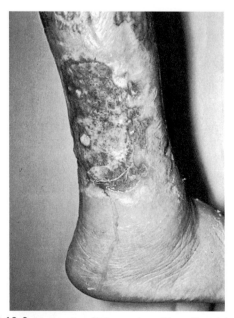

FIGURE 19-9 Venous insufficiency ulcer. *(From Kamal A, Brockelhurst JC: Color atlas of geriatric medicine, ed 2, Mosby Year Book, Europe, 1991.)*

or ankle leading to impairment of the calf muscle pump; deep vein thrombosis (DVT); and congenital abnormalities of the venous system.[77,78] All of these risk factors are associated with dysfunctions of either the calf muscles or the veins of the calf muscle pump.

In addition to compression interventions, ambulation is often an effective treatment for venous insufficiency by increasing venous return from the calf muscle pump. Full ankle plantarflexion and dorsiflexion as well as the attainment of a proper heel-to-toe gait pattern maximize the efficacy of the calf muscle pump.[77-79]

General Approaches to Venous Insufficiency Wound Management

The cornerstone of treatment for venous insufficiency ulcers is compression.[73,80,81] However, compression is contraindicated in the presence of arterial insufficiency.[69,76-80] Therefore, the first step to treating a venous insufficiency ulcer is to rule out underlying arterial disease. Compression is typically achieved through either elasticized or paste-containing bandage systems. Elasticized bandages apply active compression to the extremity whereas paste-containing rigid bandage systems enhance the effects of the calf-muscle pump in facilitating venous return. Occasionally, the limb is treated with an intermittent compression pump. Regardless of ability to ambulate, patients with venous insufficiency ulcers should be educated in elevating the lower extremities to decrease dependent edema.[77]

Current evidence regarding the efficacy of physical agents on venous insufficiency ulcers is mixed. However, several clinical practice guidelines recommend consideration of electrical stimulation,[77,79] negative pressure wound therapy,[79] and pulsed electromagnetic field,[77] particularly for recalcitrant wounds, while recommendations for ultrasound remains the subject of debate.[77,79] Laser and phototherapy are not recommended in the treatment of venous insufficiency ulcers.[79]

In cases of recalcitrant venous stasis ulcers, surgical interventions may be considered. The most common surgical intervention to address chronic venous insufficiency is subfacial endoscopic perforator surgery, which prevents backflow of venous blood from the deep to the superficial venous system.[69,77,79] Other surgical options include superficial venous ablation and free flap transfers with microvascular anastomoses when severe lipodermatosclerosis is present.[79] In addition to these procedures, the use of bilayered artificial skin equivalents in combination with compression therapy has been found to improve venous ulcer healing compared to compression alone.[69,79]

ARTERIAL WOUNDS

Epidemiology

Arterial insufficiency plays a role in as many as 22% of lower extremity ulcers.[81] Arterial disease is defined as an ankle/brachial index (ABI) ≤0.9. Studies estimate that

17% of the population aged 55 to 74 years has some form of arterial circulatory impairment and that approximately 1% of the population older than age 50 years has arterial insufficiency severe enough to threaten the viability of the lower extremity or warrant surgical revascularization.[82] Risk of arterial insufficiency ulceration increases with age: the prevalence of arterial ulceration is 1.5% for people between the ages of 60 and 79 years but increases to 3.5% for people aged 80 to 89 years.[83] Often, arterial insufficiency is not treated early in its progression because symptoms do not commonly present until the disease is in its later stages.[84]

Etiology

Arterial insufficiency ulcers result from ischemia due to lack of arterial blood flow supplying the area of the wound. The most common cause of arterial insufficiency is arteriosclerosis obliterans (ASO), though trauma and thrombosis can also impair arterial blood flow.[85,86] ASO is a progressive disease of the aorta and arteries of the lower extremity. Over time, the lumen of the artery is slowly occluded with plaques, or atheromas, that form between the endothelial layer of the artery, known as the intima, and the smooth muscle layer, known as the media. These plaques are mainly composed of macrophages and cholesterol. In addition to the accumulation of plaque, the involved arteries frequently present with fibrosis and calcification, which cause hardening of the artery, or atherosclerosis.[87] It is uncommon for a lower extremity ulcer to result from pure arterial etiology. However, arterial insufficiency plays a role in the nonhealing status of many wounds with other primary etiologies.[88]

Patients with arterial insufficiency may complain of intermittent claudication, nocturnal leg pain, or leg pain at rest.[80,89] Legs with arterial insufficiency generally lack hair [80,86] and present with thin, cool, shiny skin with minimal or no edema.[86] Arterial insufficiency ulcers tend to occur at the lateral foot but may occur in other locations such as the distal toes. As illustrated in Figure 19-10, arterial insufficiency ulcers typically have well-defined borders with a "punched out" appearance, minimal drainage, and a wound base that may range from red granulation tissue to pale, dry necrosis.[80,86]

Arterial Wound Risk Factors and Wound Prevention Strategies

Risk factors for arterial insufficiency and subsequent ulcers include age greater than 50 years, male gender, diabetes mellitus, smoking, hypertension, hyperlipidemia,[82,86,88] obesity and hypothyroidism,[86,88] elevated low-density lipoprotein (LDL) cholesterol, and increased plasma homocysteine levels.[90] Homocysteine is an amino acid found in the blood.

Controlling risk factors can help prevent wound formation in patients with arterial insufficiency. Diabetes

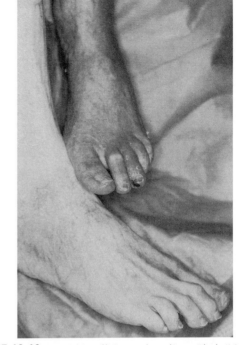

FIGURE 19-10 Arterial insufficiency ulcer. *(From Black JM: Medical-surgical nursing: clinical management for positive outcomes, ed 8, Saunders, Philadelphia, 2008.)*

should be controlled such that the hemoglobin A_{1C} level is less than 7%, indicating acceptable control of diabetes. Hemoglobin A_{1C} is a blood test that demonstrates overall blood glucose control over a period of 2 to 3 months. Smoking cessation should be encouraged,[91-96] and hypertension should be controlled to less than 140/90 mmHg or 130/80 mmHg in people with diabetes mellitus or chronic renal insufficiency. LDL cholesterol should be decreased, possibly with the prescription of statin drugs to less than 70 mg/dL. Hypothyroidism should be treated to prevent the development of arterial insufficiency. However, once arterial insufficiency is present, it will not slow the progression of the disease. Elevated plasma homocysteine levels can be reduced by administering folic acid, vitamin B_6, and vitamin B_{12}.[90]

In patients with intermittent claudication, there is strong evidence supporting the benefit of lower extremity aerobic endurance therapeutic exercise for improving lower limb peripheral blood flow.[88] Therapeutic exercise may also improve other risk factors for ulcer formation including high glucose levels and high cholesterol.

General Approaches to Arterial Wound Management

The treatment that will lead most directly to healing of arterial insufficiency ulcers is revascularization to restore arterial blood flow.[88] Every patient with a lower extremity ulcer should undergo testing for arterial disease.[88] Two noninvasive tests for arterial insufficiency are the ABI and the TBI. Not every patient with an abnormal ABI will require revascularization. However, a referral to the vascular surgeon is always recommended.[88,89] Regardless of the need or plan for surgical revascularization, lifestyle modifications must be encouraged including smoking cessation, and improved control of cholesterol and glucose if necessary.[86,88] Because of the increased risk of infection in ulcers with suboptimal arterial flow and oxygenation, topical antimicrobial dressings should be considered to manage bioburden.[88] Dressing selection for arterial insufficiency ulcers is similar to that of ulcers of any etiology. The selected dressing should maintain a moist wound bed (except in the case of dry eschar in the absence of adequate arterial supply) and should be cost-effective.[88] Selected physical agents may also facilitate improved healing of arterial insufficiency ulcers. Ultrasound has not been well studied in arterial insufficiency ulcers. Despite a lack of high-quality studies, electrostimulation and topical negative pressure wound therapy appear to be promising options worthy of additional research.[88] Intermittent pneumatic leg compression has been shown to improve distal perfusion and may be beneficial before or after revascularization.[88] Hyperbaric oxygen therapy should be considered in patients who are not candidates for surgical revascularization or for those whose ulcers are not healing despite vascularization.[88]

DIABETIC NEUROPATHIC ULCERS

Epidemiology

It is estimated that between 20.9% and 23.1% of adults older than age 60 years have some form of diabetes,[97] and the risk of being diagnosed with diabetes increases with age; moreover, adults older than age 74 years have the highest risk of diabetes.[98] Diabetic foot ulcers are one of the many negative conditions associated with having diabetes. The risk of diabetic foot ulcers increases with length of disease, and the Centers for Disease Control and Prevention (CDC) reports that 9% of people with diabetes older than age 75 years have a history of diabetic ulceration.[99] Other risk factors for development of a diabetic ulcer include white race, Hispanic ethnicity, not being married or cohabiting, obesity, use of insulin, and smoking.[99]

Etiology

Diabetic ulcers of the lower extremity develop as a consequence of neuropathy, arterial insufficiency, or both.[100] Risk factors for the development of an ulcer in people with diabetes include callus formation, trauma, neuropathy, peripheral vascular disease, and history of previous ulcer or amputation.[101] In contrast to the prolonged pressure that causes a typical pressure ulcer, diabetic ulcerations form as a result of repetitive mechanical stress on the weight-bearing structures of the insensate foot. In

a normally functioning foot, weight-bearing forces are distributed across relatively large surface areas, with the majority of the body's weight being borne on the heel and metatarsal bones. Less weight is borne on the midfoot and hallux, and very little weight is borne on the four smaller toes.[102] When biomechanical abnormalities exist, the typical distribution of body weight can become disrupted, with smaller surface areas subjected to larger forces.

Diabetic neuropathy tends to affect the long, fine motor neurons that innervate the lumbrical muscles of the foot. Once intrinsic muscle function is impaired, multiple biomechanical changes can occur, including claw foot, hammer toes, and Charcot arthropathy.[103] Diabetic neuropathy decreases temperature, pain, and vibration sensations, leading to a loss of protective sensation of the foot. The combination of abnormal weight bearing and absence of sensory feedback can lead to the rapid progression of an ulcer before it is even detected. Abnormal weight bearing leads to the development of calluses and ulcers over bony abnormalities, most commonly the first and second metatarsal heads and the hallux.[104] Decreased dorsiflexion and decreased motion at the subtalar joint increase pressure on the forefoot, leading to ulceration[105]; hallux limitus increases pressure under the great toe, which can lead to its ulceration.[106]

Autonomic neuropathy can accompany motor and sensation neuropathy. Autonomic neuropathy causes decreased skin hydration and an inability to inhibit the arteriovenous shunting mechanism, thus increasing overall blood flow in the diabetic foot.[107] However, this blood is shunted away from capillaries of the skin and is therefore unable to contribute to local tissue nutrition.[107,108] Finally, older adults with diabetes are commonly also at risk for atherosclerosis, particularly in tibial and peroneal arteries, which can further contribute to arterial insufficiency.[109]

Several classification systems exist to provide a common language for describing the risk and extent of diabetic ulcers. The Wagner Wound Classification System (WWCS)[110] (Table 19-4) and the University of Texas (UT) Treatment-based Diabetic Foot Classification System[111] (Table 19-5) are the most commonly used. The WWCS,

TABLE 19-4	Wagner Wound Classification System for Diabetic Ulcers[110]
Grade	**Description**
0	No open lesion but may have deformity or cellulitis
1	Superficial ulcer, partial or full-thickness
2	Ulcer extends to ligament, tendon, joint capsule, or deep fascia without abscess/osteomyelitis
3	Deep ulcer with abscess, osteomyelitis, or joint sepsis
4	Gangrene localized to forefoot or heel
5	Extensive gangrene

TABLE 19-5	University of Texas Treatment-Based Diabetic Foot Classification System[111] and Recommended Prevention and Treatment Interventions at Each Category[104]			
Category	Description	Examine/Evaluate	Footwear for Offloading	Surgical Offloading
0	Protective sensation intact	Screen annually	Recommend slippers with firm soles	Elective surgery for bunions/other deformities; nail wedge resection; ensure sufficient blood flow
1	Loss of protective sensation	Screen every 6 months	Wear professionally fitted shoes; extra depth and width footwear with custom total contact orthotic (CTCO)	Elective surgery for hammer toes, bunions, hallux limitus; Achilles tendon release; nail wedge resection; ensure sufficient blood flow
2	Loss of protective sensation with deformity	Screen every 3-6 months	Extra depth modified or custom made; Consider rocker plus CTCO	Elective surgery same as category 1
3	Loss of protective sensation with deformity and history of pathology	Screen every 3 months	Extra depth modified or custom made Rocker plus CTCO	Elective surgery same as category 1 Urgent: if recurrence of ulcer imminent, nonsurgical attempts ineffective
4A	Noninfected, nonischemic wound	See weekly or every other week as needed	Footwear not appropriate: use offloading device (total contact cast, walker, healing sandal, bivalve custom-made walking orthosis)	Urgent and emergent See category 1
4B	Acute Charcot arthropathy			Aggressive debriding of ulcers if needed
5	Diabetic foot infection	See for wound care as needed	See 4A&B	Urgent and Emergent Bypass surgery if required Reduction of ulcer bioburden
6	Critical ischemia	Urgent revascularization indicated		

(Adapted from Orsted H, Searles G, Trowell H, et al. Best practice recommendations for the prevention, diagnosis, and treatment of diabetic foot ulcers: update 2006. Wound Care Canada 4(1):57-71, 2006.)

which has been in existence longer, describes existing ulcerations. In the UT system, the categories are organized to provide explicit recommendations for both the prevention and treatment of diabetic ulcerations. The UT is more descriptive, with both grades and stages, and has been found to be a better predictor of clinical outcome when compared to the WWCS with respect to risk of amputation and prediction of ulcer healing.[112]

Diabetic Ulcer Prevention and Risk Assessment

Preventing diabetic ulcers requires regular screening and assessment of patients with diabetes for lower extremity sensory and circulatory impairments. All patients with diabetes should be periodically examined for decreased protective sensation of the feet using monofilaments. Patients with decreased protective sensation should be educated in daily skin inspections and foot care,[100,103] and examined and evaluated for appropriate footwear.[104] Arterial insufficiency should be assessed using the ABI or TBI.[89,100]

General Approach to Management of Diabetic Ulcers

Although all patients with diabetes should be examined and evaluated for appropriate footwear, those who already have an ulcer require more aggressive offloading. Offloading is defined as "any measure to eliminate abnormal pressure points to promote healing or prevent recurrence of diabetic foot ulcers."[103] Methods of offloading that limit functional mobility and activities of daily living (ADL) generally lead to noncompliance and less successful outcomes. For this reason, offloading should be achieved while maintaining the patient's ability to ambulate, if possible.[103] Options for offloading diabetic feet include total contact cast (TCC),[113] removable walking boots,[113,114] offloading shoes,[113,115] healing sandals,[116] and ankle–foot orthoses (AFOs).[100-104,117,118]

Local wound care to diabetic foot ulcers is similar to that for ulcers of other etiologies. Necrotic or devitalized tissue should be debrided once adequate vascular supply has been confirmed, and a dressing should be selected to facilitate moist wound healing.[100,103,104] Physical agents that should be considered in the treatment of chronic diabetic foot ulcers include hyperbaric oxygen therapy,[100,103] electrical stimulation, and negative pressure wound therapy.[100]

EXAMINATION AND EVALUATION OF SKIN AND WOUNDS IN OLDER ADULTS

Effective skin and wound examination and evaluation rely heavily on observation but also include history taking, review of systems, and the selection of appropriate tests and measures. The examination and evaluation should look beyond the specific skin impairment to the entire patient because of the complex constellation of factors such as medications and comorbid conditions that contribute to skin and wound healing. The frequency of skin and wound examination and evaluation varies by setting: typically wounds are assessed daily or with each dressing change in the acute setting, and weekly in long-term care and home care settings; skin and wound assessment should be completed more frequently if there are any signs of deterioration.[41,119]

History

A concise but accurate history must be collected including medical and social history, diet, and medications. These data provide important insights into the patient's overall health status and risk for integumentary impairments: diseases or comorbid conditions that increase the risk of developing a wound or other skin condition, or that might contribute to delayed healing of a wound or condition that is already present. Medications should be reviewed for any drugs that might delay wound healing, such as steroids or other immunosuppressants. The patient's nutritional status should be assessed with basic questions about appetite and dietary restrictions. Lab tests providing prealbumin and albumin levels should be noted.

Albumin is the most highly concentrated protein in the blood. Lab tests for albumin measure the amount of albumin in the serum (the clear portion of the blood). Normal ranges for serum albumin vary depending on the laboratory completing the test but are generally 3.4 to 5.4 g/dL. Low values of albumin may indicate decreased absorption of protein but can also herald liver or kidney disease and are associated with acute inflammation and shock. High levels of albumin may indicate dehydration. Serum albumin has a half-life of approximately 21 days and therefore may not be a timely indicator of current nutritional status; rather, it is an indicator of nutritional status over the course of several weeks.[120-123]

Prealbumin is another test of serum protein that may indicate protein-calorie malnutrition. The normal range for prealbumin is 17 to 40 mg/dL. Like albumin, prealbumin lab values may appear low in the presence of inflammation. Prealbumin has a half-life of about 2 days and is therefore a better indicator than albumin of a patient's current nutritional status.[120-122]

Review of Systems

The APTA *Guide to Physical Therapist Practice*[137] identifies four areas to be included in the review of systems: the integumentary, cardiopulmonary, neuromuscular, and musculoskeletal systems. Each of these systems can contribute significantly to skin impairments and healing. An initial review of each system helps to focus the specific tests and measures for the physical therapy examination.

The integumentary system is the most obvious component of a systems review when discussing skin and wound care. The physical therapist should be aware that many patients with skin impairments may initially seek physical therapy for other, seemingly unrelated ailments. Intact skin should be observed for any discoloration compared to surrounding skin: areas of darker pigmentation may indicate an area at risk for pressure ulcers, whereas lighter areas may indicate scars where previous wounds have already healed. Palpation of irregular areas or areas where the patient has complained of pain may reveal increased warmth or a difference in texture. An area that is indurated or firmer than the surrounding skin may indicate scar tissue, inflammation, or infection. Areas that are warmer than the surrounding skin may be inflamed or infected. Surgical wounds healing by primary intention can be gently palpated to identify a healing ridge along the incision. A healing ridge is generally palpable by the fifth postoperative day and is a sign of granulation underneath. After 2 to 3 weeks, the healing ridge softens and is no longer palpable.[119,124]

Cardiovascular complaints may range from symptoms of impaired circulation to complaints of impaired endurance that may put a patient at risk for immobility and a subsequent pressure ulcer. Reports of pain may indicate areas that should be examined for signs of tissue damage; complaints of intermittent claudication indicate patients who are at risk for arterial insufficiency wounds. Observe for lower extremity edema or rust-colored hemosiderin staining as this may indicate risk for venous insufficiency wounds.

The musculoskeletal and neuromuscular systems play an integral role in wound prevention and healing. Impaired mobility status puts a patient at risk for many different types of skin conditions and wounds. Muscle weakness may prevent a patient from repositioning. Contractures cause pressure points on splints and make it difficult to adequately clean and dry affected areas of the body. Impaired sensation eliminates one of the body's first warning signs that pressure is building under a bony prominence.

Tests and Measures

If an open area is present, the location should be noted and it should be measured for greatest length, width, and depth.[119,125,126] If any undermining or tunneling is present, this should also be measured and documented relative to its location on the face of a clock.[119,127] Undermining is a pocket of separation between the superficial or deep fascia and the underlying tissues. Tunneling is a linear tract extending beyond the wound opening.[26] Tissue in the base of the wound should be observed, identified, and documented as a percentage of the total wound surface area. Clinicians may observe several types of tissue in the wound base. Granulation tissue is red and bulbous scar tissue that may resemble the surface of raspberries. Clean, nongranulating tissue may have similar color to granulation tissue but with a smoother texture; if striations are present it is likely that muscle is being observed. Slough and eschar are both necrotic tissue and both may range in color from yellow or green to gray or black. Slough tissue is moister than eschar and may appear with a slimy or stringy texture. Eschar is dehydrated and is much firmer than slough; eschar may have the texture of leather or even wood.

The wound edges should be observed and noted as being either open or closed. A closed wound edge is called "epibole" and occurs when the edge of the wound rolls over, prematurely halting the epithelialization process. Open wound edges, identified by a narrow, red, flat border of moist tissue, are necessary to allow epithelialization to occur from the periphery of the wound toward the center.[128]

Wound drainage should be observed for quantity and quality. If there is a thick or purulent texture to the drainage, this may be a sign of infection. Drainage frequently has an odor but the odor of the wound should not be assessed until after the wound has been cleansed. If an odor is still present in the wound after cleansing, this is another sign of possible infection. Other signs of wound infection include increased wound pain, drainage, deterioration of tissue in the wound base, and deterioration in the wound measurements over time.[119,129]

Testing of neuropathy, or lack of protective sensation, can be reliably and easily completed with the use of a 5.07 (or 10 g) Semmes-Weinstein monofilament.[100,103,104] These thin nylon monofilaments are calibrated according to the force required to cause them to buckle when they are briefly pressed against the skin at a right angle to the skin (Figure 19-11). The thinner the filament, the lower the monofilament number and the less force required to induce buckling. The thinner filaments are, therefore, considered more sensitive. Protective sensation in the foot is considered absent if an individual cannot feel the 5.07 monofilament. Monofilament testing should be performed at several sites on the foot emphasizing areas exposed to high weight-bearing pressure.

Ankle and Toe Brachial Index

An ABI should be performed any time a patient has a lower extremity wound in order to rule out arterial involvement in the development of the wound.[88] The ABI is simply a comparison of systolic blood pressure in

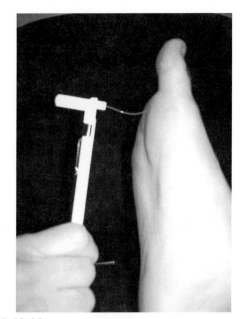

FIGURE 19-11 Semmes-Weinstein monofilament test. *(Courtesy of Erica LaPierre, PT, 2009; VNA of CNY, Syracuse, NY.)*

the brachial artery and the ankle. It is noninvasive and approximates central systolic blood pressure.[80,130] ABI examinations compare favorably in diagnosing lower extremity arteriosclerosis when compared to angiography.[89,131]

In order to take an accurate ABI, the following procedure should be followed.[132] Take brachial blood pressures bilaterally using a Doppler ultrasound to listen for the brachial pulse. Inflate the blood pressure cuff 20 to 30 mmHg beyond the point when the brachial pulse is obliterated. Release the pressure on the blood pressure cuff at a rate of 2 to 3 mmHg per second, noting the pressure when the brachial pulse is once again audible. Document the value for each arm; however, the higher of the two measurements will be used to calculate the ABI. To measure ankle pressure, place the blood pressure cuff around the ankle approximately 2.5 cm proximal to the malleoli. Use the Doppler device to measure the systolic dorsal pedal and posterior tibial blood pressure in both legs using the same procedure as with the brachial pressure. For each leg, use the higher of the two arterial pressures for calculating the ABI. The formula for calculating the ABI is simply the ankle systolic blood pressure divided by the brachial systolic blood pressure. As displayed in Table 19-6, if the ABI results in a value greater than 1.3, the test should be considered invalid because calcification of the arterial walls may be present and preventing complete compression of the artery with the blood pressure cuff. In the event of an ABI result greater than 1.3 a TBI should be performed[133] (Figure 19-12 and Table 19-6).

The toe/brachial index (TBI), like the ABI, is a comparison of blood pressure in the arteries of the great toe

TABLE 19-6	Ankle/Brachial Index Values and Implications for Treatment[89]	
ABI	**Interpretation**	**Recommendation**
1.3 or higher	Abnormal, may suggest calcification of arterial walls which are therefore unable to be compressed by blood pressure cuff. Inaccurate reading.	Assess with toe/ brachial index
1.0-1.2	Normal	Maintenance compression, if needed
0.8-1.0	Mild arterial disease	Compression
0.5-0.8	Mixed venous and arterial disease	Light compression, referral to vascular surgeon
<0.5	Arterial insufficiency	No compression, referral to vascular surgeon

ABI, ankle brachial index

and the brachial artery. TBI is recommended when ABI is greater than 1.3 because the arteries of the toes are not as susceptible to calcification. In cases where the great toe has been amputated or is otherwise not present, the second toe may be used. To measure systolic pressure in the toe arteries, a toe-size blood pressure cuff is applied to the toe just distal to the metatarsophalangeal joint. A Doppler device is used to find the pulse of the toe artery; the blood pressure cuff is then inflated to 20 to 30 mmHg beyond the point when the toe pulse is obliterated. The blood pressure cuff pressure is released at a rate of 2 to 3 mmHg per second until the pulse is once again audible.

The same calculation is used for TBI as ABI with the substitution of toe pressure instead of ankle pressure.

An alternate method of examining the arterial pressure in the toe is to use photoplethysmography (PPG), which uses infrared light instead of ultrasonic waves to measure the pressure in the arteries of the toe.[134] A transducer is placed on the great toe and systolic pressure is measured with a photoplethysmograph (Figure 19-13) instead of a Doppler device. Normal values for toe systolic pressure are greater than 50 mmHg; values less than 30 mmHg indicate ischemia and possible risk of amputation.[134,135] Normal values for TBI are less well documented than for ABI; however, it is thought that TBI of 0.64 or less is associated with arterial disease.[134,136]

Other diagnostic tests for arterial insufficiency include segmental leg pressures, which compare blood pressure at the thigh, calf, and ankle; pulse volume readings, which measure arterial stenosis; transcutaneous oximetry, which tests for microvascular insufficiency; magnetic resonance imaging, which can determine the extent of arterial obstruction; and lower extremity arteriography, which is the gold standard for testing arterial disease although it is the most invasive of these diagnostic tests.[86] When diagnostic tests of circulation such as previously mentioned are required, the role of the physical therapist is to identify the need for further testing and to refer out to the appropriate physician to facilitate the tests.

Physical Therapy Diagnosis

Table 19-7 provides an overview of signs and symptoms that help differentiate arterial, venous, and diabetic ulcers. The major contributing cause of the ulcer helps determine prognosis and treatment recommendations. The APTA Guide *to Physical Therapist Practice*[137] outlines five practice patterns to offer guidance to physical therapists in the management of integumentary impairment. The first pattern describes primary prevention

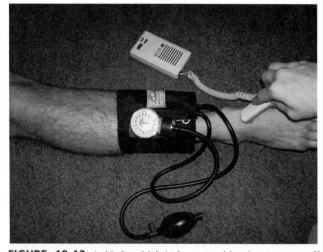

FIGURE 19-12 Ankle/brachial index test: blood pressure cuff placement and Doppler ultrasound placement to measure systolic pressure through dorsal pedal pulse. *(Courtesy of Erica LaPierre, PT, 2009; VNA of CNY, Syracuse, NY.)*

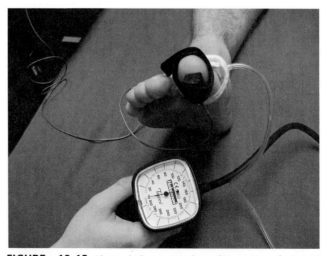

FIGURE 19-13 Photoplethysmography. *(Courtesy of Patrick Remenicky, PT, CWS, 2009; VNA of CNY, Syracuse, NY.)*

TABLE 19-7	Differential Diagnosis of Lower-Extremity Ulcers		
Characteristic	**Venous Ulcers**	**Arterial Ulcers**	**Diabetic Ulcers**
Typical location	"Gaiter" area: medial aspect of lower leg, proximal to malleolus	Lateral foot, distal toes, or at the site of trauma or ill-fitting footwear	First and second metatarsal heads and hallux; may occur any place on diabetic foot subjected to trauma, pressure, or friction
Wound depth and base	Typically shallow; base may be beefy red or covered in thin, yellow fibrin film	May be shallow or deep; typically pale pink or grey, may be necrotic	May be deep, undermining/tunneling may be present; base may be granulation tissue or necrosis
Margins	Irregular margins	Regular, "punched out" appearance	Typically regular and round from pressure, callus may be present
Drainage	Moderate to heavy	Little, if any	Low to moderate; heavy drainage may suggest infection
Surrounding skin	Hemosiderin stained, edematous, may have woody texture with "inverted champagne bottle" shape (lipodermatosclerosis)	Thin, cool, dry, shiny, hairless	May be thin and dry as with arterial ulcers
Pain reports	No consistent pattern: may range from pain-free to severe pain	May report intermittent claudication, night pain, resting pain, pain with elevation, cramping	May be insensate, paresthesia, burning

and risk reduction for integumentary disorders based on conditions or limitations that might put a patient's integumentary integrity in jeopardy. The subsequent four patterns classify impairments based on the depth of tissue destruction, similar to the NPUAP pressure ulcer staging system. The *Guide to Physical Therapist Practice* offers an organizational strategy for physical therapists and assists with selection of appropriate tests and measures, interventions, outcomes, and prognoses.

Physical Therapy Prognosis

Prognosis is defined as "the determination of the predicted optimal level of improvement in function and the amount of time needed to reach that level and may also include a prediction of levels of improvement that may be reached at various intervals during the course of therapy."[137] The length of time anticipated to achieve the skin and wound care goals varies widely and can be as little as 2 weeks for prevention of wounds; 16 weeks to treat a wound extending into fascia, muscle, or bone; and as long as 24 months for scar maturation. Many factors will contribute to the prediction of the optimal level of improvement and function that can be expected for different skin conditions. As clinicians gain more experience, they become more comfortable synthesizing those factors to make a clinical judgment about expected outcomes. Some of the factors that contribute to the formation of a prognosis include the availability of resources, compliance with the treatment plan, caregiver competence, chronicity of the condition, cognitive abilities, comorbidities, degree of impairment, functional abilities, living environment, nutritional status, and psychological and socioeconomic factors.[137]

Outcome Measures

It can be challenging to determine if a plan of care is effective in facilitating wound healing. There are many factors involved in wound examination and evaluation, and not every factor will show significant improvement or deterioration with each examination. It is, therefore, helpful to use one of several outcome measures to quantify the sum of the changes that a wound has undergone. There have been numerous proposed outcome measures to track wound healing. The two most common, the Pressure Ulcer Score for Healing (PUSH) tool and the Pressure Sore Status Tool (PSST) will be discussed below.

The PUSH tool was developed by the NPUAP to provide clinicians an easy-to-use and reliable tool to track the healing of stage II to IV pressure ulcers and as an alternative to reverse staging of pressure ulcers.[138-140] Although developed for use with pressure ulcers, the PUSH tool has also been used to document progress of venous ulcers,[141] but not for other types of wounds. Three subscales including wound length multiplied by width, amount of exudate, and tissue type are graded and added for a total score ranging from 0 to 17, with decreasing scores indicating wound improvement. A PUSH score of 0 indicates that the ulcer has closed. The PUSH tool is not intended to replace a comprehensive examination and evaluation, but rather to provide an additional method to track healing of pressure ulcers.[138,140]

The PSST, also known as the Bates-Jensen Wound Assessment Tool, was also developed to provide a universal method for describing the status of pressure ulcers, although it has also been used in research to measure the progress of diabetic, venous insufficiency, and arterial insufficiency ulcers.[142,143] The PSST consists of two unrated items, wound location and shape, as well as

13 items rated 1 to 5. The 13 rated items on the PSST include wound diameter, depth, edges, undermining, necrotic tissue type, necrotic tissue amount, exudate type, exudate amount, skin color surrounding wound, peripheral tissue edema, peripheral tissue induration, granulation tissue, and epithelialization. Scores on the PSST range from 13 to 65, with lower scores indicating wound improvement.[144]

Interventions for Wound Management

Wound healing, regardless of age and cause, relies on several basic principles. *Wound bed preparation* encompasses all interventions that ready the wound bed to progress through the predictable phases of healing, or to accept more advanced wound care interventions such as physical agents. *Identifying and treating bacterial burden* is the recognition of, and intervention for, managing colonization or infection of the wound. *Filling dead space* requires the thoughtful selection of a wound care product to make total contact with the entire interior space of the wound, including undermining or tunneling. *Maintaining an appropriately moist wound bed* requires the selection of a suitable dressing to absorb excess drainage or to hydrate a dry wound. Maintaining *open wound edges* involves the prevention and treatment of epibole to allow the wound to fill with granulation tissue from the bottom up and to epithelialize from the edges into the center. *Protecting from trauma and bacteria* requires appropriate cleansing techniques and the use of carefully selected dressing products to insulate the wound bed until the subsequent scar can resume the skin's duties of acting as the body's barrier to the outside world.

If there is no improvement in wound status for 2 to 3 weeks, the plan of care should be reevaluated and modifications should be made.[145,146] Modifications in wound treatment may include changes to the topical dressing but should also encompass an evaluation of nutritional status, efficacy of support surfaces and positioning schedules, and consideration of adjunctive therapies, which will be discussed later in this chapter.

Evidence-Based Practice Guidelines in Wound Care

Numerous systematic reviews and clinical practice guidelines have been developed to help wound care practitioners make informed decisions about best practice options for managing wounds. In wound care, we are fortunate to have a number of well-formulated, evidence-grounded clinical practice guidelines presented by experts in the field.[72,82,83,92,98,102] The recommendations of these groups are based on systematic review and integration of the best available literature reviewed and summarized by an advisory panel of content experts. These guidelines represent systems-level resources that translate evidence into practice guidelines.[147]

PRESSURE RELIEF

Mattresses and Cushions

The wide variety of support surfaces available to manage pressure in the wheelchair or bed can make it difficult to choose the most effective surface. Ultimately, it is best to be aware of the benefits and drawbacks of each classification of support surface in order to make individualized choices that will be a good fit for each patient. Support surfaces can be divided into two basic categories: static and dynamic. Static surfaces may include standard hospital bed mattresses, foam overlays, foam mattress replacements, or overlays containing air, gel, or fluid. Static support surfaces tend to be less expensive than dynamic but may not provide the level of pressure management necessary to facilitate pressure ulcer prevention or healing. Dynamic support surfaces include alternating air overlays, low air loss mattress replacements, turning or rotating mattress replacements, and air fluidized systems. Dynamic support surfaces may provide a greater degree of pressure management but are more expensive and may make mobility more difficult for patients, especially those with impaired postural stability because of the increased compliance of the surface.[60] Scientific literature to date offers little evidence that can guide the selection of one support surface over another; however, the Cochrane review on the topic concluded that foam mattress replacements were superior to standard hospital beds.[68,148]

Current clinical practice guidelines recommend that static support surfaces may be considered for patients with pressure ulcers who can assume different positions without bearing weight on the ulcer or "bottoming out"; patients who are unable to change position or who bottom out may benefit more from a dynamic support surface.[68] Bottoming out occurs when less than 1 inch of material exists between the pressure point and the bed when felt with the palm of the hand. In order to check for bottoming out, the therapist should slide his or her gloved hand between the patient's weight bearing area or bony prominence and the surface on which the patient is sitting or lying. For example, to assess wheelchair seating, the physical therapist slides his or her gloved hand between the patient's ischial tuberosity and the wheelchair seat. There should be at least 1 inch of cushioning between the patient's ischial tuberosity and the seat in order to effectively mitigate the force of pressure.[68]

Footwear for Pressure Relief

Specialized footwear is an important intervention in preventing foot ulcerations in people with diabetes. All patients with diabetes should be tested for neuropathy. The presence of neuropathy will help guide footwear choices.

Total contact casts (TCCs) have been identified by many as the treatment of choice for offloading plantar diabetic foot ulcers.[101,104,118] TCCs provide effective pressure redistribution over the plantar aspect of the foot while maximizing patient compliance with offloading as the cast cannot be removed.[103,118] TCC is typically used only in the absence of ischemia[101] and infection,[101,103] although there is some evidence suggesting TCC can be used in the presence of superficial infection or moderate ischemia but not both.[101,149] There are also disadvantages associated with the use of TCC. The disadvantages include high cost, need for specialized staff, inability to visualize the wound, impairment of mobility and ADL, and general discomfort.[101]

One alternative to TCC is a removable walking boot. A walking boot is relatively inexpensive, easily applied without specialized training, and allows for easy removal for wound examination and treatment.[101,103,104,118] Half shoes, wedge shoes, and healing sandals also mitigate pressure on the forefoot[101,118] and provide ease of application and removal similar to walking boots although TCC remains the most effective means of offloading plantar diabetic ulcers. However, wedge shoes are difficult to walk in and may cause pain or decreased postural stability.[118] Compliance is the most important factor in offloading regardless of the method used to achieve the offloading. If the patient is unwilling or unable to participate fully in offloading interventions, ulcer healing will be delayed.[103]

COMPRESSION THERAPY

Compression therapy is the cornerstone of treatment for venous insufficiency ulcers. However, compression is contraindicated in the presence of arterial insufficiency.[69,76-80] Compression therapy requires 30 to 40 mmHg of pressure to counteract the tissue capillary pressure.[69,76,77] A variety of products are available to provide the necessary level of compression. These products include short-stretch bandages and paste-containing bandages as well as three- and four-layer bandage systems. Short-stretch and paste-containing bandage systems tend to lose elasticity and are not effective in nonambulatory or minimally ambulatory patients. In these cases, the increased active compression of multilayered bandage systems is a more effective option.[77] Different bandage systems vary widely in cost and ease of application. However, the current literature states that there is no evidence to support recommending one type of compression bandage over another.[150] What is known is that multilayered systems are more effective than single-layered systems, and high compression is more effective than low compression in healing venous insufficiency ulcers.[150] Continual and long-term management of venous insufficiency is vital to prevent future ulcerations. The most common method of providing long-term control of venous insufficiency is the use of graduated compression stockings. Graduated compression stockings provide the needed 30 to 40 mmHg of compression and should be worn during the day and

removed at night when the lower extremities are elevated. Graduated compression stockings should be replaced every 4 to 6 months as they lose their elasticity.[69,77,78]

An alternative to compression bandages and graduated compression stockings is intermittent pneumatic compression (IPC).[151] This modality consists of an inflatable sleeve placed around the lower extremity and inflated to between 30 and 60 mmHg of pressure intermittently. IPC can be used in conjunction with other forms of compression or as an alternative to compression bandages in patients who are unwilling or unable to tolerate compression bandages well because of the discomfort that may accompany this intervention.[76,77,79] A typical IPC intervention consists of application of 45 mmHg at the foot, graduating to 30 mmHg at the thigh. The device inflates for 0.5 second, maintains peak pressure for 6 seconds, and deflates for 12 seconds. Treatment lasts for 1 hour 5 days per week for up to 6 months.[152]

WOUND DRESSINGS

With thousands of dressing products on the market in ever-increasing classifications, it can be challenging to select an appropriate topical treatment to facilitate wound healing. The choice of wound dressing product should be carefully made to provide a wound environment that maximizes healing potential. There are several key factors that can guide the clinician in selecting the best dressing or combination of dressing products to aid in wound healing: level of exudates, presence or absence of nonviable tissue, presence or absence of infection, amount of dead space to be filled, desired wear time, ease of application, pain with dressing changes, and cost considerations.[68,79,88,100,153,154] These factors, synthesized using clinical judgment, guide the selection of dressings regardless of wound etiology.[68,79,88,100] Table 19-8 provides the basic classifications of dressing products as well as important characteristics to guide in dressing selection.

DEBRIDEMENT

Debridement is the removal of dead or devitalized tissue from the wound bed and is an essential step in preparing the wound to progress through the healing process.[68,77-79,88,100,103,104] Debridement may be accomplished using autolytic, mechanical, and sharp strategies.

Autolytic

Autolytic debridement employs the use of an occlusive dressing to trap wound exudate, thereby hydrating necrotic tissue and keeping in endogenous proteolytic and collagenase enzymes secreted by white blood cells to liquefy nonviable tissue. Autolytic debridement is selective; that is, it will not destroy healthy wound tissue; it will only facilitate autolytic debridement of necrotic

TABLE 19-8	Classes of Advanced Wound Care Dressings[129,153,154,210-216]				
Dressing Classification	Description	Advantages	Disadvantages	Indications	Contraindications
Transparent film	Polyurethane sheet or polymer film, coated on one side with adhesive; available as a sheet	Permeable to water vapor and gas; water proof; allows wound visualization	No absorbency, difficult to apply	IV sites; secondary dressing over other wound products	Highly exudating wounds, infection
Hydrocolloid	Polyurethane foam outer layer, hydrocolloid carboxymethylcellulose/pectin middle layer with adhesive inner layer; available as sheets in various thicknesses and shapes, specific for different body areas (heel, sacrum, etc.)	No secondary dressing required; promotes autolytic debridement	Impermeable to gas and water vapor; may cause periwound maceration with increased drainage; odor may be confused with infection	Minimally exudating wounds; sloughy wounds	Ischemia; infection; vasculitis
Hydrogel	Hydrophilic polymer; available in amorphous sheets or in gel form	Cooling/soothing; facilitates autolytic debridement; absorbs minimal exudate	More frequent changes; may allow proliferation of gram-negative bacteria	Dry, sloughy wounds with minimal exudate	Ischemic ulcers
Collagen/ Biologics	Bovine, avian, or porcine collagen combined with oxidized, regenerated cellulose; available in sheet, gel, or powder form	Encourage deposition of new tissue, bind excess matrix metalloproteases, absorb drainage	May require frequent dressing changes	Chronic wounds	Religious/ethical beliefs may limit use in certain populations
Calcium alginate	Kelp derivative calcium alginate polysaccharide forms gel when in contact with exudates; available in fiber or nonwoven sheets or ropes	Absorbent, gelling action allows autolytic debridement, hemostatic	Requires tape or secondary dressing, odor may be confused with infection, prolonged wear may increase infection	Moderately exudating wounds, after debridement if hemostasis required	Dry wounds, diabetic foot ulcers
Hydrofiber	Carboxymethylcellulose gelling agent; available in sheets or ropes	High absorbency, gelling action allows autolytic debridement, strong fibers are ideal for packing dead space	Requires tape or secondary dressing	Moderate to highly exudating wounds, wounds with dead space	Dry wounds
Foam	Porous polyurethane foam with semipermeable outer layer; available in sheets or rolls	High absorbency, long wear time, thermal insulation, permeable to gas and water	Obscures view of wound	Highly exudating wounds	Dry wounds
Antimicrobials	Silver- or iodine-impregnated dressings; available in most of the above classifications	Ionic silver effective against MRSA, VRE, reduces inflammation, time release for increased wear time	Increased cost	Infected wounds	Choose antimicrobial product classification appropriate to wound characteristics

MRSA, methicillin-resistant *Staphylococcus aureus; VRE,* vancomycin-resistant enterococci.

tissue. However, it may cause maceration to the skin surrounding the wound if the skin is not properly protected. Autolytic debridement is one of the slowest methods of debridement and is not appropriate when fast removal of necrotic tissue is important. Autolytic debridement may not be effective in frail or immunocompromised patients who lack the ability to produce the endogenous enzymes needed to break down necrotic tissue.

Enzymatic

Enzymatic debridement also uses collagenase enzymes to selectively liquefy necrotic tissue. However, in the case of enzymatic debridement, these exogenous enzymes are synthetic and are applied to the wound in the form of prescription ointments. Papain urea was a popular proteolytic enzymatic debriding ointment but lost FDA approval because of lack of high-quality research to verify its efficacy.[155] Collagenase ointments have been shown to remove necrotic wound tissue faster than placebo in a population of older adults.[156]

Mechanical

Mechanical debridement uses deliberate force to nonselectively remove necrotic tissue from the wound bed. One of the oldest and most primitive methods of mechanical debridement is the use of a wet to dry dressing. Wet to dry dressings are painful and nonselective. When the dressing is removed it brings with it both viable and nonviable tissue, causing inflammation and increasing the risk of infection. Other methods of mechanical debridement use the force of water on the wound bed to loosen and remove necrotic tissue. Whirlpool is one of the better known means of mechanical debridement, using propelled water to loosen and remove necrotic tissue, typically from the lower extremity by submerging it into a whirlpool tank with a mechanical agitation component. Unfortunately, if multiple wounds on the same limb are submerged at the same time the risk of cross contamination from one wound to another increases. Whirlpool treatment is time consuming and the tanks are difficult to disinfect in between patients.

In the past few years, pulsed lavage has replaced whirlpool as an effective, sanitary, and convenient means of using the force of water to remove devitalized tissue from the wound bed. Pulsed lavage uses a disposable hand piece to irrigate a wound with saline at pressures between 4 and 15 psi. This range of water pressure has been determined to be forceful enough to remove nonviable tissue and metabolic waste without causing damage to the healthy tissue in the wound bed.[157-165] The saline propelled into the wound base is contained by the tip of the hand piece and is then contained, along with any loosened necrotic tissue, with the use of a suction machine. The evidence to support the specific range of pressures used to irrigate wounds is dated and, in some cases, includes nonhuman trials. However, it does represent the best available evidence to guide the clinician in choosing a wound-cleansing method.

Conservative Sharp Debridement

Conservative sharp debridement refers to the use of scissors, scalpels and forceps to remove necrotic tissue from the wound base to "just above the level of viable tissue margins"[166] and should only be performed by a trained clinician. Sharp debridement can also be combined with enzymatic or autolytic debridement in a technique known as "cross-hatching." Cross-hatching removes eschar by scoring the surface of the eschar in a criss-cross pattern with a scalpel in order to increase its surface area. The eschar is then covered with an occlusive dressing or an enzymatic debridement ointment. Conservative sharp debridement is contraindicated in cases of arterial insufficiency,[68,88,166] malignant wounds, and patients with clotting disorders. Use of anticoagulant therapy is a relative contraindication to conservative sharp debridement.[166] More aggressive sharp debridement "up to and including the viable tissue margins"[166] can be completed by a surgeon under anesthesia.

SURGICAL INTERVENTIONS FOR WOUND CLOSURE

Occasionally surgical intervention is required to close a wound that is recalcitrant to healing such as debrided osteomyelitis or when rapid wound closure is desired.[68] Physical therapists should be aware of the commonly used options described in this section.

Skin grafts typically use the removal of a partial thickness of skin from one area on the body in order to be transplanted to another. This is known as an autograft. The donor skin is often "meshed," or perforated with many small incisions, which allows it to cover a larger surface area on the recipient site. Local wound care is required at both the donor and recipient sites and negative pressure wound therapy and hyperbaric oxygen are common adjuvant therapies after a grafting procedure. Although the physical therapist does not typically treat the graft site itself, physical therapy may be called on to provide wound care, including dressing changes to the donor site from which the graft was obtained.

A second form of grafting is an allograft, where the donor skin is derived from cadaver, live donor, or cultured sources. In the case of allograft, the donor skin acts as a temporary biologic dressing and is eventually removed when the recipient site has improved to the extent that more conventional topical treatments will be effective.

The muscle flap is a less common option in older adults[68] because of the inherent risk-to-benefit ratio of elective surgery. A free flap involves the harvest of a full-thickness section of tissue including muscle and vascular supply that is then placed at the recipient site with microsurgery to connect vascular anastomoses. Free flap transfers are used to treat chronic venous insufficiency ulcers when significant lipodermatosclerosis is present.[79] Pedicle transfers harvest the donor tissue from an adjacent site, keeping the vascular supply intact and rotating the flap onto the recipient site. In cases of muscle flaps, the physical therapist may be most intimately involved in assisting with selection of the appropriate support surface, positioning schedule, and mobility training to facilitate healing of the flap site.

Choosing to Debride

The primary justification for debridement is removal of devitalized tissue to stimulate wound healing. In arterial insufficiency ulcers with dry gangrene or eschar, debridement should only be attempted if arterial blood flow is sufficient to facilitate healing.[88]

Even if wound healing is unlikely, debridement of necrotic tissue may be justified if it has a substantive impact on odor or the patient's perception of body image. This is often the case in the patient in the final stages of a terminal illness in which a wound is present. The individual's specific goals must guide this decision. Debridement can be painful and anxiety producing. If there is little likelihood that wound healing will be achieved or health status improved, then the decision to debride should be consistent with the patient's personal goals and preferences.

PHYSICAL AGENTS

When a wound fails to heal in a predictable timeline the physical therapist should consider the use of a modality to augment wound healing. Evidence favoring the use of selected modalities is mounting while others have failed thus far to demonstrate effectiveness as an adjuvant to the wound plan of care. Table 19-9 provides a summary of the key evidence supporting the use of physical agents for wound care.

Ultrasound

Ultrasound is one of the most commonly used physical agents in physical therapy and typically consists of the application of ultrasonic energy in the 1 to 3 MHz range to produce both thermal and nonthermal effects on tissue. Based on cellular-level studies,[167] researchers have theorized that pulsed (nonthermal) ultrasound applied to the wound bed stimulates mast cell release of histamine, encouraging the migration of monocytes and neutrophils to the wound base. As discussed earlier, neutrophils contribute to the early phagocytosis of tissue debris and bacteria; monocytes become macrophages, which carry out a role similar to neutrophils later in the wound healing process. Others have hypothesized that pulsed ultrasound stimulates increased production of type I collagen by the fibroblasts, which leads to greater tensile strength in the healed wound. The thermal effects of continuous ultrasound applied to the wound base have been theorized to increase local circulation. Although

TABLE 19-9	Summary of Physical Therapy Modalities for Wound Healing						
		Physiological Effect of	Level of Evidence *Based on Oxford Criteria[217]				
Modality	Treatment Goal	Modality	Acute	Arterial	Venous	Pressure	Diabetic
High-frequency ultrasound	Augment wound healing	Accelerates or reactivates normal wound healing	none	none	1a–[168]	none	none
Low-frequency ultrasound	Debride wound bed	Removes bioburden through cavitation and microstreaming	none	1b[174]	4[175]	none	1b[171]
Monochromatic infrared energy	Augment wound healing, increase protective sensation	Increases microcirculation by releasing nitric oxide, a potent vasodilator	none	none	4[204]	4[204]	4[204]
Electrical stimulation	Augment wound healing, decrease infection	Stimulates endogenous bioelectrical activity, bactericidal	none	2a[88]	2a[79]	1b[187-189]	1b[191]
Hyperbaric oxygen	Augment wound healing, decrease infection	Increases tissue oxygenation, bactericidal	none	2a[88]	none	none	1a[200]
Negative-pressure wound therapy	Augment wound healing	Increases wound granulation, decreases bacteria and edema	1b[203]	2a[88]	2a[79]	2a[68]	2a[100]

Note: *1a–*, Based on findings of a systematic review of randomized controlled trials, with worrisome heterogeneity; *1b*, based on findings from individual randomized controlled trials with narrow confidence interval; *2a*, based on conclusions of a systematic review, with homogeneity, of cohort studies; *3b*, based on findings from individual case-control studies; *4*, based on findings from case-series or poor quality cohort and case-control studies.

these physiological changes have been observed in cellular-level research,[167] they have not been clearly replicated in humans with pathology. There is little clinical evidence to support the use of ultrasound in the 1 to 3 Mhz range to promote wound healing, and what evidence does exist is of poor quality.[79,168,169]

In recent studies, ultrasound of different frequencies has been used for its imaging capacity rather than its therapeutic potential. Ultrasound in the 15 MHz range, known as high-frequency ultrasound, has been used to obtain high-resolution images that may aid in the earlier detection of pressure ulcers once a patient has been screened and determined to be at risk.[170] However, high-frequency ultrasound has no known role in the physiological stimulation of tissue healing.

On the opposite end of the frequency spectrum, low-frequency (LF) ultrasound in the range of 40 kHz has been increasingly found to be useful in wound debridement via the theorized mechanisms of cavitation and microstreaming.[171-175] Cavitation refers to the formation and vibration of micron-sized bubbles in the coupling medium and fluids in treated tissues. As these bubbles form and condense, they compress and cause changes at the cellular level in the wound tissue. Microstreaming is the movement of fluids along acoustical boundaries because of the pressure wave created by the ultrasound. Although a recent addition to the world of wound-healing modalities, low-frequency ultrasound is within the scope of the physical therapy practice and units are currently being developed.

LF ultrasound uses an atomized saline solution to deliver ultrasonic energy to the wound base, facilitating wound debridement and promoting increased granulation; this modality has been found to be an effective adjuvant to standard care in chronic ulcers of various etiologies.[171-175] In a randomized controlled trial of patients with chronic diabetic foot wounds, Ennis et al[171] found that patients who received LF ultrasound treatments for 4 minutes three times per week for 4 weeks healed faster than the control group that received sham treatments. In a second study, Ennis et al[172] concluded that patients with lower-extremity wounds of various etiologies healed more quickly, with fewer hospitalizations and surgical interventions when treated with LF ultrasound when compared to historic controls. Kavros et al[174] found that a greater proportion of both chronic lower-extremity ulcers and foot ulcers associated with critical limb ischemia reached at least a 50% reduction in size when treated three times per week for an average of 5 minutes with LF ultrasound compared to a control group that received standard treatment alone. This study was expanded upon in 2008[175] and patients with chronic lower extremity wounds resulting from neuropathy, arterial or venous insufficiency, or multiple factors healed significantly more often when treated three times per week with LF ultrasound compared to matched controls who received standard care.

Monochromatic Infrared Energy

Monochromatic infrared energy (MIRE) uses light-emitting diodes to deliver near-infrared energy at 890 nm to the skin and wound base. MIRE is suggested to heal chronic wounds by increasing the microcirculation under the treatment area through promoting the release of nitrous oxide, which causes vasodilation.[176] In 1994, the Food and Drug Administration approved the use of MIRE for increasing circulation and decreasing pain, paving the way to consider MIRE as a tool to increased circulation in a wound. The suggested treatment protocol is 20 to 30 minutes 1 to 2 times per day 3 to 7 times per week.[177,178] MIRE is contraindicated for use over a malignant lesion, active malignancy, during pregnancy, or with patients who may be pregnant.[178] Very little evidence exists to support the use of MIRE in healing chronic wounds,[179] and though it was initially thought that MIRE could reverse diabetic peripheral neuropathy, the evidence to the contrary is mounting and convincing.[180,181]

Electrical Stimulation

Electrical stimulation is thought to augment wound healing through the use of electrical currents delivered either directly to, or through, the wound base via placement of electrodes in the wound or on the periwound tissue. In theory, electrical stimulation enhances or regenerates the "current of injury" that naturally assists in wound healing. Injured skin relies on a slight electrical current, known as the current of injury, to enhance wound healing.[182-184] The skin is naturally electronegative in relation to its surroundings and deeper tissues because sweat contains NaCl, which accumulates on the skin surface. Sodium pumps on the surface of the skin transport Na^+ ions to the deeper layers of the skin, leaving a greater concentration of Cl^- ions on the skin's surface. The electronegative charge is thought to assist in the skin's natural defense against infection and the elements because pathogens are less likely to proliferate in the presence of a negative charge. A current is naturally formed when the skin is broken due to the electronegative nature of the skin surface and the electropositive deeper tissues; this is known as the "current of injury." The electropositive deeper tissues attract neutrophils, macrophages, fibroblasts and epithelial cells, which all have negative charges. A moist wound base is necessary to perpetuate the current of injury, allowing it to speed the healing process by attracting proliferative cells to the wound base. When the wound is allowed to dry out or desiccate, the current is halted.

Electrical stimulation has been recommended for the treatment of chronic venous,[79] arterial insufficiency ulcers,[88] diabetic ulcers,[100] and stage III and IV pressure ulcers.[68] However, current guidelines are unable to conclude which currents or voltages are most beneficial to different ulcers. Constant low-intensity direct current has been shown to hasten wound healing in pressure, ischemic, and ulcers of unspecified etiologies with a proposed treatment protocol of continuous low-intensity direct current applied to the wound for intensities of between 200 and 800 μA for at least 1 hour per day 5 days per week.[185,186] Many treatment protocols start with the negative electrode in the wound base for 3 days and then the polarity is switched. Other protocols call for switching the polarity every 3 days throughout the course of treatment.

Kloth and Feedar[187] used high-voltage, monophasic pulsed current in the treatment of "stage IV decubitus ulcers" involving a 45-minute treatment 5 days per week at 105 Hz with an interphase interval of 50 μs and a submotor threshold voltage. With this protocol, treatment was initiated with the positive electrode placed in the wound base until a healing plateau was reached; then the negative electrode was used to treat the wound. Once a healing plateau was reached with the negative electrode, the polarity was alternated on a daily basis. In all cases, the dispersive electrode was placed 15 cm cephalad.[187] In a second study of monophasic pulsed current, Feedar et al.[188] proposed a treatment protocol using monophasic pulsed current applied directly to the wound base at a frequency of 128 pps and an amplitude of 35 mA for a 30-minute treatment twice daily starting with the negative electrode in the wound base and alternating to the positive electrode every 3 days. The dispersive electrode was placed 30.5 cm away from the wound. Once the wound was determined to be the depth of a partial thickness wound (this was termed a "stage II" wound in the original paper, which was written prior to the current philosophy to avoid reverse-staging of wounds), the frequency was changed to 64 pps and the polarity was alternated every day. This protocol was found to be effective with stage II through IV pressure ulcers, vascular insufficiency ulcers, and traumatic or surgical wounds.[188]

A recent double-blind randomized controlled trial (RCT)[189] found that direct current treatment of pressure ulcers in a group of older patients and patients with spinal cord injury increased the initial rate of healing but did not result in a statistically significant improvement in overall healing. A second RCT[190] found that high-voltage electrical stimulation led to higher rates of healing on subjects with venous wounds; the subjects themselves were described to have symptoms of chronic venous insufficiency although no specificity was provided about the chronicity of the actual wounds. High-voltage current was also found to produce a higher rate of healing when used to treat diabetic foot ulcers.[191]

A lesser known electrotherapeutic modality is electromagnetic therapy, which uses an electromagnetic field to promote wound healing in contrast to the directly applied current that results from electric stimulation. There is very little evidence to support the use of electromagnetic therapy, and what exists is unable to reach a conclusion on its efficacy or benefit.[192]

Hyperbaric Oxygen Therapy

Hyperbaric oxygen therapy (HBOT) has been recommended in the treatment of diabetic[100,103,193,194] and arterial insufficiency[88] ulcers. Research does not support hyperbaric oxygen for pressure ulcers.[68] Hyperbaric oxygen compared to standard treatment has been shown to facilitate a greater decrease in wound size, greater rate of complete ulcer closure, and reduced rate of amputation of the ulcerated limb.[195] Although it can be provided at home, the typical HBOT treatment takes place at a hospital or outpatient clinic and lasts 90 to 120 minutes on a daily basis; in cases of infection, twice-daily treatment may be ordered. Treatment takes place in a hyperbaric chamber, with the patient breathing 100% oxygen at pressures between 2 and 25 atmospheres. The increased pressure in the chamber drives oxygen into the blood plasma (because hemoglobin in the red blood cells is nearly saturated with oxygen at normal atmospheric pressures), dramatically increasing the partial pressures of oxygen in tissues throughout the body. The increased oxygen levels at the wound site are thought to increase the oxygen gradient between the wound dead space and the periwound.[196] The increased oxygen gradient increases fibroblast division[197] and stimulates wound healing.[103] The increased oxygenation of tissues during HBOT also increases the ability of leukocytes to combat bacteria and increases angiogenesis.[193,198,199] Hyperbaric oxygen therapy has been found to decrease the risk of major amputation when used to treat diabetic ulcers[200] and may increase the 1-year rate of healing.[194] The Underseas and Hyperbaric Medicine Society, which regulates the diagnoses and applications for which HBO is reimbursable, has approved HBOT as a tool to enhance healing in selected problem wounds, including diabetic foot wounds, compromised amputation sites, nonhealing traumatic wounds, and vascular insufficiency ulcers. HBOT is also approved for [refractory] osteomyelitis, skin grafts and flaps, and thermal burns.[201] HBO is not used in every case in which it is indicated because it is not always readily available, requires lengthy treatments, and presents an added cost to the delivery of care. However, it should be considered prior to amputation in chronic nonhealing wounds that lack sufficient tissue oxygenation.

Negative-Pressure Wound Therapy

The use of negative-pressure wound therapy (NPWT) is suggested by the Wound Healing Society for the treatment of stage III and IV chronic pressure ulcers[68] and nonhealing diabetic ulcers[100] as well as before or after flap or graft surgery.[79] However, the most recent Cochrane review of the topic[202] concluded that there is no evidence to suggest that NPWT is more effective in healing chronic ulcers than comparators. Many studies on the effects of NPWT on chronic wounds have been small and not well-randomized and are therefore suscep-tible to bias; other studies did not separate acute and chronic wounds. Only seven studies met the rigorous criteria to be included in the Cochrane meta-analysis and of these, only one demonstrated a statistically significant advantage in the use of NPWT for the treatment of chronic wounds. The main outcome reported in NPWT literature was reduction in wound volume; the Cochrane authors point out that a reduction in time to complete closure would be a more clinically meaningful outcome. Despite the relative lack of evidence to support the use of NPWT in chronic wounds, one study by Armstrong and Levery[203] demonstrated that NPWT led to more patients healing and with a shorter time to closure in a surgical wound after a partial foot amputation related to diabetic complications.

NPWT involves the application of subatmospheric pressure to the wound base, usually in the range of 50 to 175 mmHg 24 hours a day with several dressing changes per week. Negative pressure is applied to the wound by a portable suction device connected to some form of wound dressing via tubing. Different manufacturers suggest different dressings ranging from gauze to polyvi-nyl alcohol foam. NPWT is believed to increase cutane-ous perfusion and the formation of granulation tissue while decreasing bacterial load, wound drainage, and edema. Caution should be taken when using NPWT on a patient with active bleeding or who is on anticoagulant therapy.[179,204,205]

Choosing among the Various Physical Agents

Although many physical agents exist for the treatment of wounds, it can be daunting to determine which is the most appropriate and when to use it. Typically, physical agents are considered after the wound has failed to improve or heal with appropriate dressing, nutrition, or other interventions such as offloading, or compression. NPWT is the one physical agent that is more commonly used in acute surgical wounds, including grafts and flaps. Most facilities have the necessary equipment to provide electrical stimulation, and it has been proven effective in many types of chronic wounds, whereas low-frequency ultrasound equipment might not be as readily available. HBO may be similarly difficult to access, but may repre-sent an alternative to amputation in chronic diabetic ulcers. Physical therapists must consider the resources available and the potential risks and benefits to the wound care patient when deciding which physical agents to use and when to use them.

SUMMARY

The integumentary system undergoes multiple changes with age but is more profoundly affected by the multiple comorbid conditions and systemic medications that occur with increasing frequency in advanced age. Once acquired, wounds undergo the same fundamental cas-cade of reactions and events to progress to closure in older adults but there are more factors that can slow the process of wound healing in the older populations. The physical therapist is an essential member of the wound care team in any setting and can employ his or her knowledge of therapeutic exercise, mobility rehabilita-tion, and environmental adaptations. The management of chronic wounds should often include the thoughtful application of physical agents to augment and speed the healing process. As the demographics of the United States shift toward a greater population of older adults, the absolute number of older adults with impaired in-tegumentary integrity will also likely increase; physical therapists must be prepared to meet the challenge of col-laborating with other health care workers to facilitate wound healing in older adults.

REFERENCES

To enhance this text and add value for the reader, all references are included on the companion Evolve site that accompanies this text book. The reader can view the reference source and access it online whenever possible. There are a total of 217 cited references and other gen-eral references for this chapter.

Management of Urinary Incontinence in Women and Men

Diane Borello-France, PT, PhD

INTRODUCTION

Urinary incontinence (UI), a common health condition among older adults, is defined as the complaint of any involuntary leakage of urine.[1] Although UI affects both genders, women have a greater risk of developing this condition. In a recent epidemiological study of a racially and ethnically diverse cohort of midlife women, prevalence of UI that occurred at least monthly was 46.7%; and the prevalence of more frequent UI (occurring several days per week or more) was 15.3%.[2] Although prevalence of "any UI" does not increase substantially beyond the 5th decade in women, the prevalence of severe UI (daily or a few times/week) does increase from 24.9% (5th decade) to 38.9% (80+ year-olds).[3] In men, UI prevalence estimates are substantially lower, reaching 5% and 34% for younger and older men, respectively.[4-6]

The International Continence Society has defined three types of UI: stress UI, urge UI, and mixed UI.[1] Stress UI is the involuntary leakage of urine that occurs on effort or exertion, or on sneezing or coughing. Involuntary leakage of urine accompanied by or immediately preceded by urgency (a sudden, strong desire to pass urine, which is difficult to defer) defines urge UI. Finally, mixed UI is the involuntary loss of urine associated with urgency and also with exertion, effort, sneezing, and coughing.[1]

Urinary incontinence can seriously affect physical function, psychological well-being, and quality of life. In older adults, UI has been associated with depressive symptoms, poor life satisfaction, social isolation, sleep disturbances, increased risks of falls, and a twofold increased risk of institutionalization.[7-11] Urinary incontinence also poses a significant economic burden to the individual and society. In the United States in 2003, the estimated annual economic cost of UI was $12.0 billion, with 75% of the cost focused on community-dwelling older adults.[12] Individuals themselves incur the burden of routine care, including costs of protective undergarments and laundry. In a study of 528 racially diverse, community-dwelling women with weekly UI, 69% reported incontinence-related costs averaging more than $250 per year (2005 U.S. dollars).[13]

Currently, there are many treatment options for persons with UI, including pharmacotherapy, surgery, pelvic floor muscle (PFM) exercise, and other behavioral interventions. In older adults, mental and physical status, comorbidity, medications, and environment often complicate the etiology of UI.[14] Thus, the physical therapy management of older individuals with UI may not be straightforward. The physical therapist will need to carefully reflect on how these contributing factors affect the patient's prognosis and the efficacy and feasibility of interventions under consideration.

To provide a foundation for clinical decision making, this chapter reviews the (1) anatomy and physiology of normal continence mechanisms; (2) pathophysiology of UI, and risk factors for developing UI; (3) introduces UI-specific tools to determine patient outcomes including UI symptoms, symptom-related distress, quality of life, and sexual function; (4) summarizes the scientific evidence for conservative intervention options for UI (PFM exercise, biofeedback, electrical stimulation, bladder training, and lifestyle modification); and (5) describes pharmacologic and surgical interventions for UI.

CONTINENCE MECHANISM

Continence depends on the neural coordination of activity between the bladder, urethra, and PFMs. As the bladder begins to fill with urine, bladder pressure is low, and the detrusor (bladder) muscle is relaxed.[14] As more urine is stored, bladder outlet resistance must increase to maintain continence. For this to occur, bladder afferents send information regarding bladder fullness to the dorsal horn of the spinal cord. This information is relayed onto spinal interneurons that activate somatic pudendal and sympathetic hypogastric efferents. Somatic pudendal efferent activation causes contraction of the striated urethral sphincter and increased pelvic diaphragm muscle tone. Coincidentally, activation of sympathetic hypogastric efferents inhibits detrusor contractions and promotes urethral smooth muscle contraction.[15,16] Information from bladder stretch receptors is also sent to the pontine continence center, the periaqueductal gray (PAG) matter, and the right anterior cingulate cortex. These areas promote continence by increasing sympathetic efferent activity, bladder compliance, and external urethral sphincter tone; inhibiting parasympathetic activity (activated during voiding); and facilitating pudendal motoneurons.[16]

Once the individual determines an appropriate time and place to void, afferent signals from the bladder are sent to the PAG matter. The PAG matter coordinates voiding by activating the pontine micturition center (PMC). The PMC activates parasympathetic pelvic efferents to the detrusor, causing the bladder to contract. Coincidentally, sympathetic and somatic efferents to the urethra are inhibited allowing urethral relaxation and urine flow.[16]

Continence also depends on the integrity of anatomic structures that support the pelvic organs and affect urethral pressure, including the pelvic ligaments (urethral, cardinal, and uterosacral), endopelvic fascia, urethral smooth muscle and vascular plexus, and PFMs.[14,15,17] Although all of these structures are important to continence, physical therapy interventions for UI are primarily aimed toward improving PFM function.

The PFMs include the perineal membrane and levator ani muscles.[17,18] The perineal membrane is the superficial layer of the PFMs and includes the ischiocavernosus, bulbospongiosus, and superficial transverse perineal muscles. The levator ani is the deep layer of PFM and includes two basic regions (Figure 20-1). The first and most posterior region, the iliococcygeus and coccygeus muscles, originates from a fibrous band on the pelvic wall called the arcus tendineus levator ani. Together, they form a relatively flat, horizontal shelf spanning from the pelvic sidewalls on which the pelvic organs rest.[17,18] The second region of the levator ani muscle includes the pubococcygeus muscle. It originates from the pubic bone on either side and forms a sling around and behind the rectum. It is further delineated into the puborectalis muscle, the portion of the pubococcygeus muscle that passes beside the vagina (in women) and attaches to the lateral vaginal walls.[17,18] It has been suggested that both layers of muscle function as a unit during a PFM contraction.[19]

The levator ani muscles are tonically active, providing constant support to the pelvic organs.[20] In women, they narrow the urogenital hiatus and draw the urethra, vagina, and rectum toward the pubic bone. In this situation, the supporting connective tissues experience minimal tension. If muscular support is lost, connective tissues can stretch or tear, providing a mechanism for pelvic organ prolapse and/or stress UI.[17,20] The levator ani muscles can also be contracted voluntarily during

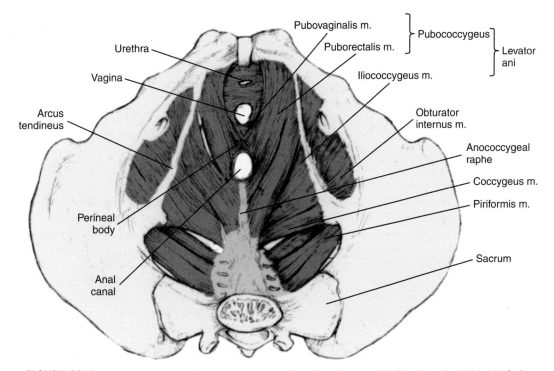

FIGURE 20-1 The pelvic muscles. *(From Mathers LH: Clinical anatomy principles. St Louis, 1996, Mosby.)*

abrupt rises in abdominal pressure (as occurs with a cough or sneeze) to stop urine leakage by compressing the urethra against the symphysis pubis or by preventing urethral descent.[21,22]

In both men and women, the striated urethral sphincter plays an important role in continence. It is composed predominately of slow-twitch (type I) muscle fibers. This muscle is constantly active and assists continence during prolonged periods of bladder filling and urine storage.[17,23]

PATHOPHYSIOLOGY AND RISK FACTORS FOR URINARY INCONTINENCE

Stress Urinary Incontinence

The loss of anatomic support (levator ani muscles, endopelvic fascia, and pelvic ligaments) to the proximal urethra is one mechanism of female stress UI. Without support, the bladder neck and/or urethra descend outside the pelvic cavity during increases in intra-abdominal pressure. Subsequently, the urethra cannot be sufficiently compressed, abdominal pressure exceeds urethral pressure, and UI occurs.[14,24]

Childbirth is one factor that predisposes women to stress UI. Although the exact relationship between pregnancy/childbirth and stress UI is unclear, it is typically attributed to pudendal nerve injury, stretching/tearing of the pelvic ligaments and/or levator ani muscles, or damage to the urethra.[14] As women age to 60 years or older, parity is no longer an independent risk factor for stress UI.[25] Other stress UI risk factors and/or age-related physiological changes in muscle and connective tissue, such as the decline in collagen content and loss of elasticity, may play a greater role than parity in the development of stress UI in older women.[26] Reported risk factors for female stress UI include age, estrogen loss, Caucasian race, family history of stress UI, obesity, smoking, chronic cough/respiratory disease, pelvic surgery, chronic constipation, and neurologic disorders.[26-31] Men with prostate cancer who undergo radical prostatectomy (RP) are at great risk of developing some form of UI. At least 50% of men experience UI immediately following this procedure.[32,33] Although the incidence of UI decreases over time, those who remain incontinent experience a negative impact on their quality of life.[34] Following RP, the proximal urethral sphincter, consisting of the bladder neck, prostate, and prostatic (proximal) urethra, is removed. Consequently, continence depends on the integrity of the rhabdosphincter, the distal urethral sphincter.[35] Stress UI following RP is largely attributed to incompetence of the rhabdosphincter.[36] Surgery-related scar tissue or pudendal nerve injury, reduced sphincter mobility secondary to scar tissues, an underdeveloped/weak distal sphincter, and/or weak PFMs are considered possible causes of rhabdosphincter incompetence following RP.[35-37]

Urge Urinary Incontinence

The exact cause of urge UI in many cases is unknown. However, it is estimated that one third of persons with overactive bladder (OAB) suffer from urge UI.[38] Overactive bladder is defined by the International Continence Society as "urgency, with or without urge UI, usually with frequency and nocturia."[1] Overactive bladder symptoms can be caused by low bladder compliance (a high rise in bladder pressure during bladder filling) and/or detrusor overactivity (the presence of involuntary bladder contractions during the filling phase).[39] Detrusor overactivity can occur due to idiopathic, neurogenic (associated with a neurologic condition, such as stroke, Parkinson's disease, multiple sclerosis, brain injury or tumor, spinal cord injury or tumor, or diabetes mellitus), or nonneurogenic (bladder infection, bladder outlet obstruction, bladder tumors, bladder stones, and aging) causes.[14,39] In women, urethral obstruction secondary to pelvic floor organ prolapse (POP) may lead to detrusor muscle changes and subsequently detrusor overactivity.[14] In men, obstruction caused by benign or malignant prostatic enlargement can result in OAB by altering bladder physiology, neural regulation, restricting bladder emptying, and/or affecting PFM strength.[40] Following surgical removal of the obstruction (as in RP), the bladder may continue to be overactive, potentially causing postsurgical urge UI.[37] Other factors associated with female OAB and/or urge UI include advancing age, hysterectomy, caffeine intake greater than 400 mg/day (about 2.5 cups), weekly consumption of carbonated drinks, obesity, arthritis, and impaired mobility and/or impaired activities of daily living.[3,41-44]

EXAMINATION

History

Given the multifaceted nature of UI, a thorough medical history should be taken from the patient and/or primary caregiver. The history should also review medical conditions that influence bladder function directly, and conditions and/or lifestyle factors that precipitate UI (Box 20-1).[25,39,44] Surgical history, including urethral, bladder, bowel, rectal, and prostate (males only) should be obtained. An obstetric and gynecologic history should be asked of female clients (see Box 20-1). As impaired mobility and activities of daily living are risk factors for UI,[3,44] conditions leading to functional decline, such as arthritis or pain, should be discussed. In such cases, patients should be asked whether they have difficulty getting out of bed, moving from sitting to standing, walking, and removing clothing.

Medications should be reviewed, including those that alter cognition, fluid balance, and bladder and/or sphincter function. Through various mechanisms, medications can directly affect urinary function. Antihypertensives,

---

BOX 20-1 | Medical Conditions That Affect Bladder Function Directly

- Congestive heart failure
- Peripheral venous insufficiency
- Renal disease
- Urinary tract infection
- Bladder tumor
- Bladder stones
- Bladder outlet obstruction (prostatic or bladder neck in men; pelvic organ prolapse, bladder neck, or urethra in women)
- Diabetes
- Neurologic conditions
- Radiation therapy.

Conditions that Can Precipitate Urinary Incontinence (UI) by Increasing Intraabdominal Pressure
- Chronic cough (chronic obstructive lung disease, smoking, asthma, allergies, emphysema)
- Constipation
- Obesity
- Occupation (involving heavy lifting), and/or recreational activities (weightlifting, jogging)

Obstetric History
- Number of pregnancies and deliveries
- Mode of delivery (vaginal versus cesarean delivery; forceps- or vacuum-assisted vaginal delivery)
- Episiotomy and/or anal sphincter laceration during delivery
- Infant birth weight
- UI/FI (fecal incontinence) during or following pregnancy.

Gynecologic History
- Menopausal status (including hormone replacement therapy)
- Surgery (hysterectomy, pelvic organ prolapse, and antiincontinence procedures)

A careful bladder symptom history is important to identify onset, type, frequency, and severity of symptoms, precipitating factors, and need for further medical evaluation. History of other pelvic symptoms should also be obtained. Box 20-2 provides a list of key bladder and bowel symptoms typically asked during a physical therapy examination for UI. For example, pain with urination may be a sign of a urinary tract infection. Straining to urinate and/or incomplete bladder emptying may be a symptom of urethral obstruction. Incomplete bladder emptying may be a sign of poor detrusor muscle contractility, which could lead to urinary retention. Patients should be asked whether or not they experience regular constipation, as it is a known risk factor for stress UI.[26-29] In addition, dual incontinence (defined as monthly UI and fecal incontinence [FI] within previous year) has been reported to occur in about 8% of women and 5% of men with UI.[46] As POP can be associated with urge UI,[14] female patients should be asked if they sense a bulge or pressure in the vagina. Given the high prevalence of UI, particularly in women, several key

BOX 20-2 | Key Bladder Symptom Questions

- When did your bladder problem begin?
- Do you leak urine with laughing, coughing, sneezing, lifting, or exercise?*
- Do you leak urine on the way to the bathroom?*
- Do you have to strain to empty your bladder?*
- Do you feel that your bladder is still not empty after you void?*
- Do you experience pain or burning when you empty your bladder?*
- How often do you empty your bladder during the day?
- How often do you wake up at night to empty your bladder?
- How often do you feel a strong desire or urge to urinate that you can't stop?
- How often do you leak urine during the day?
- How often do you leak urine when you sleep or wake up to empty your bladder?
- Do you use any type of absorbent product (pad, adult undergarment)? If yes, how many do you use in a 24-hour period?
- Do you leak urine during sexual intercourse?
- Are your bladder leaks small (drops), medium (wets underwear), or large (soaks underwear and outer clothing)?

Key Bowel Symptom Questions
- How many bowel movements do you usually have per day?
- Do you experience pain with bowel movements?
- Do you experience frequent constipation? How often?
- Do you experience frequent diarrhea? How often?
- How often do you strain to have a bowel movement?
- How often do you experience loss of liquid or solid stool?
- Do you need a laxative or enema to produce a bowel movement?

*A "yes" response to any of these questions should cause the physical therapist to ask the patient if he or she has sought evaluation or treatment for the symptom(s) from his or her primary care physician or a specialist. If the patient has not been evaluated for the symptom(s) by a physician, the physical therapist should refer them to do so.

neuroleptics, and benzodiazepines can reduce urethral pressure. Diuretics are known to increase the production of urine. Anticholinergics and β-blockers may affect one's ability to empty the bladder completely. Other medications can affect urinary function indirectly via their side effects. Constipation, a risk factor for stress UI, is a side effect associated with narcotic analgesic and iron use. Another risk factor for stress UI, cough, is a side effect of ACE inhibitors.[44,45]

Patients should be asked about their daily fluid intake. Restricting fluids is a coping strategy used by some to reduce urinary frequency, urgency, and incontinence. However, reducing fluids may lead to constipation or urinary tract infection, thus adversely affecting continence. Conversely, a patient may report excessive fluid intake, which may exacerbate bladder symptoms. Time of fluid intake should be discussed, as consumption of fluids during evening hours may contribute to nocturia (waking one or more times at night to void[39]). Caffeine, alcohol, and/or carbonated beverage intake should be reviewed to determine if they are contributing to the patient's UI.

bladder symptom questions in Box 20-2 (identified with an asterisk) should be included in the systems review of any physical therapy client. A "yes" response to any of these questions should lead the clinician to ask the patient if he or she has sought evaluation or treatment for the symptom(s) from his or her primary care physician or a specialist (urologist, gynecologist, or urogynecologist). If the patient has not been evaluated for the symptom(s) by their physician, the physical therapist should refer them to do so.

A bladder diary can be used to capture and quantify bladder function, including voiding frequency, volume of each void, number of UI episodes per day, the size or severity of each UI episode, and daily pad usage.[47] The 7-day bladder diary has been shown to have high test–retest reliability for voiding frequency and number of UI episodes.[48] However, some patients may fail to produce a valid bladder diary. In such cases, the clinician may consider administration of the 3-day bladder diary. Adherence to keeping a 3-day bladder diary has been shown to be superior to 7-day recording. In addition, the mean number of UI episodes recorded during the first 3 of the 7 days has been shown to be representative of the mean number of UI episodes averaged across the entire week.[49]

Physical Examination

Box 20-3 summarizes the components of a basic physical therapy examination for persons with UI. For clients with pelvic pain and/or additional musculoskeletal complaints or conditions, a more detailed and comprehensive examination of the spine, pelvis, and hips may be warranted.

The intent of this chapter is not to instruct the reader on how to perform the procedures outlined in Box 20-3. Therefore, it is recommended that the reader seek continued education and training prior to implementing specific examination procedures into clinical practice. It is also recommended that the practitioner confirm if these examination procedures (particularly the manual pelvic floor examination) falls within their state's physical therapy practice act.

Quantifying Pelvic Floor Muscle Function. The most clinically practical method of examining PFM function is through vaginal, digital examination. Two scales, the Brink[50] and Modified Oxford Grading,[51] have been described for grading digitally (vaginal) examined PFM function. Currently, there is no suggested standard method of assessing PFM trans-anally.

The Brink scale (Pelvic Muscle Rating Scale, Version 2) is based on three muscle contraction variables: intensity of the "squeeze" generated by the muscle contraction, vertical displacement of the examiner's fingers as the muscles lateral to the vagina contract, and muscle contraction duration. Each variable is rated separately on a 4-point categorical scale. The three subscale scores are summed to

---

BOX 20-3 | Components of a Basic Physical Examination for Persons with Urinary Incontinence

General Examination
- Observation for lower extremity edema
- Lower extremity strength and joint mobility
- Lower extremity sensation
- Lower extremity reflexes
- Functional mobility

Specific Examination of Female Clients
Perineal Observation
- Perineal skin for inflammation, excessive vaginal discharge, lesions, scars
- Demonstration of pelvic floor muscle contraction

External Examination
- Sensation around the perineum
- Palpation to identify painful tissues
- Sacral reflexes: anal wink, bulbocavernosal reflex

Internal Examination
- Sensation within the vagina
- Palpation to identify painful tissues
- Pelvic floor muscle bulk
- Pelvic floor muscle contraction
  - Exam rectally if no contraction palpable vaginally
- Presence and quantification of pelvic organ prolapse

Specific Examination of Male Clients
Genital Observation
- Irritation of skin or skin breakdown on penis from urine exposure, genital lesions
- Demonstration of pelvic floor muscle contraction

External Examination
- Perineal and perianal sensation
- Sacral reflexes: anal wink, bulbocavernosal reflex

Rectal Examination (After Medical Clearance Postsurgery)
- Pelvic floor muscle contraction

---

obtain a composite score.[50] Brink et al reported a composite score test–retest reliability coefficient of $r = 0.65$ obtained from a sample (mean age = 55.8 years; 82% with mixed UI) of women attending pretreatment clinic visits.[50] Hundley et al reported good composite score interrater reliability ($r = 0.68$), and correlations between the Brink pressure subscale score and maximal squeeze pressure scores obtained using a perineometer ($r = 0.67$ and 0.71, respectively).[52]

The Modified Oxford scale uses a 6-point numerical scale to grade PFM contraction: 0 = no contraction (nil), 1 = flicker, 2 = weak, 3 = moderate, 4 = good (with lift), and 5 = strong.[51] Testing young, mostly nulliparous females (mean age of 25 years) without symptoms of pelvic floor dysfunction, Bo and Finckenhagen reported the Oxford scale produced only fair intertester agreement. In addition, it lacked the ability to discriminate among women with weak, moderate, good, or strong muscle contractions when measures were compared against vaginal squeeze pressures obtained from a vaginal manometry device.[53] Although the Oxford scale is simpler and perhaps easier to use, the Brink scale's stronger psychometric properties may provide the clinician with a more consistent measurement tool to document the patient's status over time.

Outcome Measures

Symptoms, symptom-related bother or distress, quality of life, and sexual function can be measured with condition-specific standardized assessment tools. If these tools are administered at examination and at discharge from physical therapy, they can be used to determine the outcome or efficacy of the physical therapy interventions for UI.

Shumaker et al developed two widely used, internally consistent, reliable, valid, and responsive clinical outcome measures for women with UI, the Urogenital Distress Inventory (UDI) and Incontinence Impact Questionnaire (IIQ). Both questionnaires were tested psychometrically using a sample of community-dwelling women with stress UI or urge UI.[54] The UDI contains 19 items that measure urinary symptoms (Irritative, Obstructive/Discomfort, and Stress) and their associated bother. The IIQ is a 30-item questionnaire that measures the health-related quality of life (HRQOL) impact of UI across four domains: Physical Activity, Travel, Social Relationships, and Emotional Health.[54] Both questionnaires were shortened to develop the six-item UDI (UDI-6) and seven-item IIQ (IIQ-7). In a sample of community-dwelling women with stress UI, urge UI, or mixed UI, these shorter versions were shown to be reliable and valid against the longer versions.[55]

The reliability of the IIQ-7 has been tested in men after RP. It was found to be internally consistent with good test–retest reliability, and statistically correlated with urine loss measured by pad test and patient responses to a cancer-specific HRQOL measure, the European Organization for the Research and Treatment of Cancer Quality of Life Questionnaire, Version 2.[56] The study investigators, however, highly recommended further validity testing of the IIQ-7 in this particular population.[56]

The Pelvic Floor Distress Inventory (PFDI), developed by Barber et al for women, in many cases, has greater clinical utility compared to other UI-specific QOL tools. The PFDI is similar to the UDI but measures a greater number and scope of pelvic symptoms, including Urinary (identical to the UDI), Colorectal (Bowel), and POP.[57] Its companion measure, the Pelvic Floor Impact Questionnaire (PFIQ),[57] measures the impact of these symptoms on HRQOL and includes three impact subscales: Urinary, Colorectal Anal, and POP. Both the PFDI and PFIQ were found to be internally consistent, reliable, valid, and demonstrated responsiveness in women undergoing surgery for a variety of pelvic floor disorders (UI, FI, POP). As the PFDI and PFIQ are quite lengthy, short forms were developed (the PFDI-20 and PFIQ-7) and also found to have good reliability, validity, and responsiveness. In addition, based on global ratings of improvement defined as at least "a little better" after surgery for pelvic floor disorders, a change of ≥45 points on the PFDI-20 summary score (summary of the three scale scores) and a change of ≥36 points on the PFIQ-7 summary score were found to be clinically important.[58]

The Pelvic Organ Prolapse and Incontinence Sexual Function Questionnaire (PISQ) is an internally consistent, reliable, and valid condition-specific sexual function questionnaire developed for sexually active women with UI and/or POP. It contains 31 items to measure sexual function across three domains: Behavior/Emotive, Physical, and Partner-Related.[59] The PISQ-12 is a reliable and valid shortened version of the 31-item PISQ.[60]

The University of California–Los Angeles Prostate Cancer Index is a questionnaire for men with early-stage prostate cancer. Items measure urine leakage, sexual function and bother, urinary function and bother, and bowel function and bother. It has been shown to have good internal consistency, test–retest reliability, validity, and moderate responsiveness.[61-63]

INTERVENTIONS

The primary physical therapy interventions for urinary incontinence include those aimed toward improving PFM function (PFM exercise, biofeedback, and electrical stimulation), and those aimed toward improving bladder function (bladder training and lifestyle measures). In most cases, patients will require a multicomponent, individualized plan of care. In addition, some patients may have already undergone, or plan to undergo, pharmacologic or surgical interventions to reduce their urinary symptoms. In the following sections, the theoretical rationale and current evidence supporting these interventions will be presented.

Pelvic Floor Muscle Exercise

Pelvic floor muscle exercise is believed to reduce stress UI by improving urethral closure and pelvic organ support. DeLancey suggested that a properly timed PFM contraction can stop stress UI by compressing the urethra against the symphysis pubis.[21] In addition, exercise-induced levator ani muscle hypertrophy may improve urethral pressure and structural support of the pelvic organs, preventing urethral descent during abrupt rises in intra-abdominal pressure.[22]

Several randomized controlled trials and systematic reviews confirmed the efficacy of PFM exercise as an intervention for stress UI and mixed UI.[64-69] However, definitive cure and improvement rates are difficult to conclude, as a variety of continence outcomes were applied across studies. For example, Burns et al found a 16% cure and 44% improvement (50% to 99% reduction in urine loss based on urinary diary) for women who performed PFM exercises compared to 3% cure and 15% improvement rates observed in controls.[64] Using a self-reported cure/improvement scale, Bo et al found that 8% of women were continent, 40% almost continent, and 44% improved as a result of PFM exercise compared to 3%, 87%, and 10% of controls almost continent, unchanged, or worse, respectively.[65] Finally, another randomized controlled trial found 65% of women who performed PFM exercises achieved at least a 50% reduction in pad test weight compared to 0% of controls.[66]

Pelvic floor muscle exercise variables, including the number of PFM contractions performed/day, contraction duration, and duration of care, differ greatly across PFM exercise studies.[67,68,70] Therefore, it is difficult to determine an optimal PFM exercise prescription for women with stress UI. However, several studies that exercised women to improve PFM endurance and power have found favorable results. Burns et al required women to perform up to 200 PFM contractions/day. Quick 3-second, and sustained 10-second contractions were prescribed.[64] Similarly, Wyman et al asked women to perform five repetitions of a 3-second contraction and up to 45 repetitions of a 10-second contraction each day. Wyman et al's protocol resulted in cure for 13% and improvement in 56% (a 50% or higher reduction in UI episodes) of women.[71] Bo et al asked women to perform 8 to 12 contractions three times per day. Each contraction was held for 6 to 8 seconds, and three to four fast contractions were added at the end of each contraction.[65] Finally, Borello-France et al reported an overall 67.9% reduction in UI episodes (41% of women were cured and another 20.5% had at least a 75% reduction in UI symptoms) following a PFM exercise intervention that included a maximum of 60 "fast and strong" (3-second) and 30 endurance (up to 12-second) PFM contractions per day.[72]

Persons with stress UI also need to learn to contract their PFMs during situations that cause urine leakage. The skill of contracting the PFMs prior to and during circumstances of increased abdominal pressure (cough, sneeze, laugh, lifting a heavy object) has been termed the "stress strategy" or "knack."[73,74] Miller et al showed that after 1 week of knack instruction only, women with mild stress UI reduced UI episodes associated with a medium and deep cough by 98% and 73%, respectively.[74] Women with moderate or severe stress UI symptoms may need more time before they gain skill in use of the knack or "stress strategy."

Pelvic floor muscle exercise also plays an important role in the management of OAB and/or urge UI. The rationale for PFM exercise as an intervention for OAB is partly based on the existence of the "guarding reflex."[75]

Earlier in the chapter, the neurourological pathway for the guarding reflex, the increase in external urethral sphincter and PFM activity during bladder filling, was described. Clinical studies have also shown that voluntary contraction of the PFMs can inhibit detrusor contractions, reduce detrusor pressure, and increase urethral pressure.[76,77]

As with stress UI, strong evidence for an optimal PFM prescription for urge UI is unknown.[70] In several studies, a multicomponent behavioral training program that included 45 to 50 PFM contractions/day (working up to a 10-second contraction) was found to reduce UI by a mean 76% to 86% in women with urge UI and mixed UI.[77-79]

In persons with OAB or urge UI, using PFM contractions to suppress urges and prevent incontinence needs to be practiced and learned. The urge-suppression strategy should be applied during situations that trigger urges, such as walking to the bathroom.[78,79] This strategy will be discussed in more detail in the section on bladder training.

The efficacy of PFM exercise to reduce UI in men following RP is less clear. A recent, systematic review that critically examined evidence for postoperative PFM exercise found that only one of seven reviewed studies suggested any benefit.[80] A great deal of heterogeneity was observed across trials for baseline UI status among subjects, subject recruitment methods, PFM exercise interventions, control interventions, study outcomes, and statistical methods. As a result, the authors were unable to determine the value of PFM exercise in men following RP.[80]

Although an "exact PFM exercise prescription" for UI cannot be concluded from the literature, it is nevertheless important to reflect upon the available evidence when determining a patient's plan of care. In addition, it is equally important for the clinician to individualize exercise to the patient's needs and situation. In doing so, basic exercise guidelines should be followed. First, the patient's initial PFM strength and endurance should be considered when prescribing exercise. The total number of contractions per day and the contraction/rest duration for each muscle contraction should be progressed gradually to prevent muscle fatigue and to promote exercise adherence. Second, the goal, and thus the specific parameters of PFM exercise, may differ depending on the patient's circumstance of UI. For example, a patient with stress UI episodes will need an exercise program that focuses on building muscle strength and muscle power. To prevent urge UI episodes, the PFMs may need to function differently. A patient with urge UI will need to have adequate muscle coordination and endurance in order to suppress bladder contractions while walking to the bathroom. Therefore, the focus of exercise may be to promote muscle endurance and coordination. However, many patients will have mixed UI and need an exercise program that to some degree addresses all aspects of muscle function: strength, power, endurance, and coordination. Third, it is important for the patient to be skilled in performing exercises during functional tasks. Initially, most patients are advised to exercise in the supine position. As muscle strength, endurance, and coordination improve, they should be advised to exercise in upright positions, including sitting and standing. Eventually, the exercise program needs to be progressed to include PFM exercises during functional activities (moving from sit to stand; stepping forward, backwards, and sideways; going up a series of steps; or while running in place). General instructions for how to contract PFMs are included in Box 20-4.

Biofeedback

Gaining skill in PFM exercise is a struggle for some clients. It has been reported that after written or verbal instruction, only 30% of women are capable of performing a correct PFM contraction.[81,82] In such situations, biofeedback may be a useful component of the physical therapy plan of care to promote motor learning. Most typically, feedback is obtained using electromyography (EMG) and surface electrodes. Surface EMG can be recorded from special vaginal or rectal sensors that are inserted internally, or from surface electrodes placed externally near the anus. Feedback can also be provided verbally from the therapist based on internal digital palpation of the patient's PFMs.

The efficacy of biofeedback-assisted PFM exercise as an intervention for UI has been shown. Across studies of women with stress UI, biofeedback-assisted PFM exercise resulted in a 61% to 91% average decrease in UI episodes.[64,83,84] A similar 76% to 86% mean reduction of UI has been reported in studies of women and/or men with urge UI.[78,85,86]

Studies comparing the efficacy of biofeedback-assisted PFM to PFM exercise alone have also been done. Numerous systematic reviews and meta-analyses of these studies have consistently concluded that insufficient scientific evidence exists to determine whether PFM exercise augmented with biofeedback is superior to PFM

exercise alone.[42,70,87,88] Therefore, the physical therapist needs to use biofeedback discriminately. It may be most indicated for persons that poorly understand how to contract their PFMs, cannot sense or discriminate a correct PFM contraction, cannot fully relax their muscles following contraction increasing risk of fatigue-induced muscle pain, contract muscles other than the PFMs (gluteal and hip adductor muscles), and strain (Valsalva) while attempting a PFM contraction.

Electrical Stimulation

Electrical stimulation (ES) is an intervention for UI advocated by some clinicians. However, there is little scientific evidence to support its use in the treatment of women with stress UI. Proponents of ES for stress UI believe ES promotes PFM contraction and increases urethral closure pressure.[89] Trials comparing the effectiveness of ES to sham ES in women with stress UI have found conflicting results.[90-93] However, studies that compared ES with PFM exercise have consistently found no difference in stress UI outcomes.[65,94] Goode et al[94] found no benefit of combining ES and PFM exercise compared to PFM exercise alone in the management of women with stress UI and mixed UI. In addition, several unpleasant side effects associated with ES have been observed, including vaginal irritation, pain, bleeding, vaginal infection, and urinary tract infection.[65,90,93,94] As little evidence supports the use of ES in the management of female stress UI, it should be used cautiously. Evidence to support the use of ES in the management of male stress UI has been critically evaluated and also questioned.[95]

Evidence to support the use of ES in women with urge UI is also limited. The rationale behind the use of ES for persons with OAB or urge UI is based on studies that observed bladder muscle inhibition following direct pudendal nerve stimulation.[96,97] One study of women with mixed UI assigned to receive ES or sham ES found no difference between groups across numerous study outcomes, including number of voids, volume of urine loss determined by a pad test, and patient satisfaction.[98] Conversely, a study that included men and women with OAB and compared ES to sham ES found those who received ES had greater improved bladder capacity and self-reported UI improvement.[99] Finally, in a study of men following postprostatectomy, those who received 12 weeks of ES alone versus ES plus PFM exercise did not differ on voiding, incontinence, or HRQOL outcomes. However, both groups in this study rapidly improved, making potential between-intervention differences difficult to detect.[100] Given this controversial evidence, ES should be used sparingly as an intervention for UI. However, persons with stress UI and urge UI need to develop voluntary PFM control. Therefore, ES may be indicated initially for patients who are unable to activate their PFMs. However, as soon as the patient begins to develop consistent active control of their PFMs, the

BOX 20-4	General Instructions for "How to Contract Pelvic Floor Muscles"

- The muscles you need to exercise are those that you would use to prevent the passage of stool or gas from the rectum. You should feel a tightening around the vagina (for females) and anus.
- Never hold your breath when you are doing these exercises.
- Never strain or bear down, like you are trying to produce a bowel movement.
- Always relax these muscles after each contraction.
- Try to relax your buttocks and thigh muscles during exercise. Concentrate on the pelvic floor muscles only.

physical therapist should reevaluate the patient's need for ES.

Vaginal Weights

Vaginal weights are commercially available and may be used for the purpose of progressive resistive PFM exercise. However, there is little scientific evidence to suggest that vaginal weight training is superior to PFM exercise in women with stress UI.[101] In addition, studies that compared vaginal weight training to PFM exercise observed poorer adherence and adverse events (muscle fatigue, abdominal pain, vaginitis, and vaginal bleeding) for those assigned to the vaginal weight training group.[65,102]

Vaginal weights are cone-shaped and sold in sets of progressive increments. They are believed to promote correct PFM contraction (through feedback sensed about cone slippage) and enhance PFM strength (through progressive resistance training). Women begin using the heaviest cone they can hold while standing and walking. They are later progressed to heavier cones as tolerated. Weights are typically used twice daily for 15 minutes.

Behavioral Interventions for Urinary Incontinence

Bladder Training Bladder training is a behavioral intervention most often recommended as an intervention for persons with urge UI. The main goals of bladder training are to improve bladder capacity and restore normal bladder function.[103] Burgio described a model in which the sensation of urgency drives urinary frequency, leading to reduced bladder capacity, OAB, and UI. In this model, the introduction of bladder training (expanding the voiding interval) allows the patient to break the cycle.[103]

Bladder training requires the patient to gradually increase the time interval (usually by 15-minute intervals) between voids until an acceptable voiding schedule is reached. A voiding schedule of every 3 to 4 hours is optimal, but depends on the patient's preintervention voiding schedule. To delay voiding, the patient must be able to suppress the sensation of urgency. Suggested urge suppression strategies include distraction to another (preferably mental) task, taking deep breaths to relax, and contracting the PFMs several times to inhibit bladder contractions. Patients are also taught to avoid rushing to the bathroom, which may increase abdominal pressure and trigger bladder contractions. Instead, they are instructed to walk at a normal pace to the bathroom and pausing, if needed, to contract their PFMs.[104]

Evidence to support the use of bladder training for women with urge UI was demonstrated in a randomized controlled trial of women aged 55 years or older. Women who received 6 weeks of bladder training demonstrated a 57% reduction in UI episodes compared to minor

improvement observed in the control group. In addition, women in the bladder training group demonstrated sustained improvement at a 6-month outcome assessment.[105] The benefit of using bladder training in conjunction with PFM exercise is less certain. A comparative study of three interventions (bladder training alone, PFM exercise alone, PFM exercise combined with bladder training) showed an immediate postintervention advantage to combined therapy on the number of incontinent episodes, HRQOL, and treatment satisfaction in a sample of women with stress UI, urge UI, and mixed UI. However, differences in outcomes between the three interventions did not persist after 3 months.[71]

The efficacy of bladder training as a single intervention for men with RP is unclear. One trial that examined a multicomponent behavioral intervention (PFM exercise, voiding schedules, and behavioral methods to manage urgency and postpone voiding) to reduce urge UI postprostatectomy showed an 80.7% reduction in symptoms. However, the trial included a small number of men, and the combination of interventions made it difficult to draw conclusions regarding the contribution of bladder training to symptom resolution.[85]

Lifestyle Measures

Recommendations to alter factors that increase the risk for UI are often included in the plan of care for persons with UI. Scientific evidence upon which to base specific recommendations is quite limited. For example, despite its potential to impact general health status, the effect of smoking cessation on lower urinary tract symptoms is not known. However, there is growing evidence to support recommendations for weight loss, caffeine reduction, and fluid management.

Aside from recommendations to alter known risk factors, clinicians commonly advise patients with OAB or urge UI to restrict foods believed to irritate the bladder (particularly, artificial sweeteners, citrus fruits, vegetables, and/or juices). However, there is no scientific support to justify these recommendations to persons with OAB or urge UI.[106]

Weight Loss

There is emerging evidence to support weight loss recommendations as an intervention for female UI. In one study, morbidly obese women with stress UI and urge UI experienced significant improvements in UI following a weight loss of 45 to 50 kg after bariatric surgery.[107] Remarkably, another study showed that a weight loss of only 16 kg by women with stress UI, urge UI, or mixed UI enrolled in a conventional weight loss program resulted in a 60% reduction in weekly UI episodes. Observed improvements were sustained 6 months following the weight reduction intervention. In addition, a 50% reduction in weekly UI episodes was found in women who lost as little as 5% to 10% of their baseline weight.[108]

Fluid Management

Many persons with UI restrict fluid intake in an effort to manage their UI. There are very few data to support recommendations for adjusting fluid intake.[106,109] In fact, one study found reducing fluid intake improved UI episodes in women with either stress UI or idiopathic detrusor overactivity, but reduced frequency and urgency in only those with detrusor overactivity.[110] The results of this study should be applied cautiously given the risks associated with restricting fluids, including dehydration, constipation, and urinary tract infection.[111]

Some patients with UI will report excessive water intake and fail to recognize the association between fluid intake and bladder symptoms. Therefore, a recommendation to reduce fluid intake may help improve bladder symptoms, particularly urinary urgency and frequency.

Caffeine Reduction

Evidence to support caffeine reduction recommendations can be gleaned from clinical trials that tested concomitant interventions to reduce female urge UI. In one study, women who consumed more than 100 mg/day of caffeine either underwent bladder training or bladder training combined with recommendations and strategies to reduce caffeine. Those in the combined intervention achieved a 58% (from a mean 238.7 mg/day to a mean 96.5 mg/day) caffeine reduction and reported statistically greater improvements in voiding frequency and urgency episodes compared to women who received bladder training alone.[112] The 96.5 mg/day equates to less than the caffeine content of a 5-ounce cup of brewed coffee (reportedly contains 128 mg caffeine). An 8-oz glass of iced tea and an 8-oz glass of cola soft drink are reported to contain 47 mg and 25 mg of caffeine, respectively.[113] In another multicomponent behavioral intervention study (including caffeine reduction, management of fluid volume, bladder training, and constipation management), 64% of women who reduced caffeine intake were found to have decreased UI episodes.[114]

Some patients are very reluctant to reduce their caffeine intake. Suggesting a trial period of caffeine reduction may be more acceptable. In addition, caffeine reduction should be done gradually to prevent the patient from experiencing severe headaches.

Pharmacologic Interventions for Stress Incontinence

Medications, including estrogens, α-adrenergic agonists, and serotonin-noradrenalin reuptake inhibitors, have been used to treat women with stress UI. However, there is no universally accepted pharmacotherapy for stress UI.[115] The positive effect of estrogen use on the urethral epithelium, subepithelial vascular plexus, and connective tissue promoted its use in women with stress UI.[116] However, randomized clinical trials have found no difference in placebo treatment versus estrogen replacement in reducing stress UI symptoms in postmenopausal women. In addition, it may actually worsen or increase the risk of developing UI in some women.[117-120] Phenylpropanolamine or PPA, an α-adrenergic agonist, acts to decrease stress UI by increasing urethral smooth muscle contraction and thus urethral closure pressure.[121] However, the Food and Drug Administration banned PPA after it was found to increase risk of hemorrhagic strokes in women taking the drug.[122] Finally, studies have examined the effectiveness of duloxetine, a serotonin-noradrenalin reuptake inhibitor, in reducing stress UI. Duloxetine increases the tone of the external urethral sphincter by increasing pudendal nerve output.[115] A recent Cochrane review of clinical trials concluded no difference in stress UI cure rates between duloxetine and placebo treatment.[115]

Pharmacologic Interventions for Urge Urinary Incontinence

Commonly, patients seeking physical therapy for urge UI may have a current or past history that includes a medication for this condition. Therefore, it is important for the physical therapist to be familiar with these medications and their possible side effects. As described earlier in this chapter, activation of parasympathetic efferents to the bladder triggers bladder muscle contractions necessary to promote voiding. Acetylcholine acts on muscarinic receptors in the bladder to produce bladder contractions.[16,116] Anticholinergic drugs are prescribed for urge UI as they block the parasympathetic acetylcholine pathway, resulting in bladder muscle inhibition.[116,123] Anticholinergic drugs are effective in reducing incontinence. A recent review concluded that persons taking anticholinergic medications experienced on average four fewer UI episodes, five fewer trips to the bathroom per day, and moderate improvements in HRQOL.[123]

Oxybutynin and tolterodine are two anticholinergic medications commonly prescribed by physicians to treat OAB and urge UI. Both drugs are available in immediate- and extended-release formulas.[116] Anticholinergic drugs have unpleasant side effects, including dry mouth, dry eyes, blurred vision, constipation, nausea, headache, and dizziness.[123] For some patients, side effects are intolerable causing them to discontinue use of the drug.

The effectiveness of anticholinergic drugs for UI is not age dependent.[42,116,123] However, older persons may be at higher risk for developing drug–drug and drug–disease interactions.[44] Anticholinergic drugs may interact with diseases including dementia, Parkinson's disease, hypertensive renal disease, and diabetes.[44,124] They are contraindicated for persons with acute closed-angle glaucoma and are suspected of inducing cognitive impairment in older adults.[44,124] Persons taking other anticholinergic drugs may experience a load effect, exacerbating certain side effects, such as dry mouth and constipation. This cumulative effect may cause slowed gastrointestinal motility and poor absorption of other important medications.[44] Therefore, the physical therapist needs to be alert to and report to the managing physician any suspected drug-related changes in the patient's status.

Urethral Bulking Agents and Surgical Interventions for Stress Urinary Incontinence

Peri- or transurethral injection of collagen or other synthetic bulking agents into the urethral mucosa creates an artificial urethral seal similar to that provided normally by the submucosal vasculature and urethral smooth muscle.[125] Bulking agents are also recommended for men with stress UI following prostatectomy.[37] These agents can be helpful in reducing stress UI in the short term.[15,68,125,126] However, two to three injections may be needed to see results. In addition, the durability of this intervention beyond 12 months is unknown.[15,37,125,126]

Interventions recommended for postprostatectomy UI are usually conservative, not involving surgery.[80] Therefore, only those surgical options for female stress UI are discussed here. Surgery for female stress UI is typically offered to patients after a trial of more conservative treatment options has failed. The most common surgical procedures for female stress UI include the open retropubic colposuspension, anterior vaginal repair, laparoscopic colposuspension, suburethral sling procedure, and tension-free vaginal tape (a less invasive suburethral sling procedure). These procedures reduce stress UI by correcting urethral closure deficiencies and improving urethrovesical junction support. Recognized complications associated with surgery include new symptoms of urgency and urge incontinence, voiding difficulties, new or recurrent POP, and the need for additional stress UI surgery.[42]

Colposuspension involves lifting the tissues near the bladder neck and proximal urethra in the area of the pelvis behind the anterior pubic bones. It can be performed through a lower abdominal incision (open retropubic colposuspension) or laparoscopically (laparoscopic colposuspension).[126,127] Retropubic colposuspension is considered the gold standard surgery for female stress UI, as it is most effective and results in fewer complications. A recent Cochrane review concluded that this procedure yielded an overall continence rate of 85% to 90%. In addition, approximately 80% of women should expect to be continent up to 5 years following this surgery.[127] The laparoscopic procedure varies from the open procedure with regard to number of sutures applied, the possible use of staples or mesh, and the site of anchor. Given the smaller incision, patients may have less pain and a

quicker recovery compared to the open retropubic colposuspension. However, it appears to be more costly and takes more time to perform.[128] Short-term outcomes are similar between the two procedures. However, long-term success rates appear to be less promising for the laparoscopic procedure.[127,128]

Anterior vaginal repair, or anterior colporrhaphy, uses a vaginal surgical approach. The vaginal mucosa is dissected below the urethra and sutures are placed in the periurethral tissue and pubocervical fascia to lift and support the bladder neck.[42,129] Although this procedure results in lower rates of new or recurrent prolapse, it is less effective compared to open retropubic colposuspension.[42,127]

The traditional suburethral sling operation combines both an abdominal and vaginal approach.[42] The surgeon places strips of material (synthetic or biological) under the urethra and attaches them to the rectus muscle or to the iliopectineal ligaments. Each time the woman strains, the sling tightens, supporting the bladder.[42,130] The tension-free vaginal tape (TVT) procedure is a less invasive sling procedure and is sometimes performed using only local anesthesia. The TVT utilizes a self-fixing polypropylene mesh inserted around the midurethra.[130] A recent Cochrane systematic review concluded that there is a lack of information to judge whether or not suburethral sling procedures are as effective as open retropubic colposuspension, or better or worse than other surgical procedures or conservative management options for UI.[130] However, one large multicenter, randomized surgical trial found that the suburethral sling, using autologous rectus fascia, yielded higher success rates but greater morbidity than the open retropubic colposuspension (specifically, the Burch colposuspension) in women with stress UI.[131]

CASE EXAMPLE

History and Interview

At the time of interview, Mrs. J was a 63-year-old white woman with a diagnosis of mixed UI. She had been referred to physical therapy by her gynecologist. She was living alone and independently in a two-story town house, and working full-time as an administrative assistant to the principal of a nearby high school. Her reported height and weight were 64 inches and 170 lbs, respectively.

When asked about symptoms, Mrs. J indicated that her UI began about 10 years previously, with worsened symptoms over the past 6 months. She indicated a strong sensation of urge associated with UI episodes. Especially, when she stood up and walked to the bathroom.

Mrs. J voided every hour throughout the day and evening. In addition, she woke up three times to void every night. She leaked urine every time she walked to the bathroom, coughed, and sneezed. She classified the leaks as medium to large. To avoid embarrassment, she used three to four maxi pads/day. She denied fecal incontinence but strained and experienced pain while having bowel movements. However, she moved her bowels daily without enemas or laxatives. She reported a diet rich in whole-grain cereals, bread, fruits, and vegetables. She consumed three to four 8-oz cups of coffee and two 12-oz bottles of diet caffeinated soda per day.

Mrs. J was not receiving any other medical treatment for her UI. She indicated that her mixed UI caused her to restrict physical activities and long-distance travel. She previously walked 2 miles per day. She was not in an intimate relationship.

Systems Review

During systems review, Mrs. J denied smoking, allergies, chronic cough, or respiratory disease. She also denied kidney, other bladder (cancer, painful urination, difficulty initiating urine stream, or frequent urinary tract infections), liver, blood, skin, and neurologic disease/disorders. Gastrointestinal problems included straining to have a bowel movement. She denied history of cancer and hearing or vision loss. She indicated arthritis in both knees that caused pain when moving from sitting to standing and walking down stairs. She denied injuries to the back or lower extremities. She reported occasional depression and anxiety but was not seeking medical treatment for either condition. Her medical history was positive for high blood pressure.

Mrs. J's obstetric history included two full-term pregnancies and two operative (episiotomy) vaginal deliveries. She became postmenopausal at age 53 years.

Mrs. J's medical management included β-blocker (Lopressor) for high blood pressure, ibuprofen for knee pain, and estradiol (Estrace) for vaginal dryness. Past surgical history included hysterectomy at age 55 years and cholecystectomy at age 47 years.

Mrs. J's goals for physical therapy were to become "dry" and to reduce the number of trips she made to the bathroom per day. She was anxious to resume her walking program as she gained 15 lbs in the past year.

Examination

Based on Mrs. J's symptoms, functional limitations, and reported disability, the examination included all items listed in Box 20-3 under "General Examination" and "Specific Examination of Female Clients." Significant examination findings included the following. Blood pressure was 130/84 in sitting. Lower extremity knee flexion was limited to 100 degrees bilaterally. Knee extension strength was 4/5 bilaterally. Sensation to light touch was intact throughout all LE dermatomes bilaterally. Lower extremity proprioception was intact, and DTRs were 2+ bilaterally. Mrs. J was independent with bed mobility and sit to stand. She walked independently without an assistive device on level ground. She ascended and descended 10 steps with a handrail independently. She complained of slight knee pain descending the stairs and moving from sit to stand.

The pelvic floor examination was performed after receiving written consent. External examination of the perineum revealed no signs of inflammation or vaginal discharge. Sensation about the perineum was intact to light touch. Episiotomy scar was noted. No pain or tenderness was elicited from palpation of tissues around the perineum. When asked to contract her PFMs, the clinician observed an anal wink.

Internal vaginal examination revealed intact sensation to touch on the lateral, anterior, and posterior vaginal walls. Mrs. J reported 5/10 pain in response to palpation of the left levator ani muscle. Levator ani muscle bulk was symmetrical bilaterally. PFM strength, rated according to the Brink scale, was 7/12 (pressure score = 2, vertical displacement score = 2, and contraction duration score = 3).[50] She demonstrated the ability to contract her PFMs without accessory hip muscle contractions. She required cues to fully relax her PFMs between repeated contractions. Examination of the anterior and posterior vaginal walls during cough assessment revealed no visible POP. A rectal examination was not performed because of Mrs. J's request. When asked to "bear down" as for a bowel movement, Mrs. J demonstrated tightening instead of relaxation of the external anal sphincter.

Evaluation

Mrs. J's symptom profile was consistent with the diagnosis of mixed UI. She reported frequent urination, UI during situations of increased abdominal pressure and associated with a strong sense of urgency, and nocturia. Possible contributing UI risk and lifestyle factors for Mrs. J included age, race, estrogen loss, obesity, and excessive caffeine and carbonated beverage intake. Relevant impairments included PFM weakness, the inability to relax the external anal sphincter during a Valsalva maneuver, and a painful left levator ani muscle. Her knee pain and muscle weakness, although not directly related to her mixed UI, was a relevant factor for intervention planning. Mrs. J's symptoms affected her ability to sleep, exercise, and travel.

Diagnosis and Prognosis

The physical therapy diagnoses for Mrs. J were muscle weakness, mixed urinary incontinence, and urinary frequency. The physical therapy prognosis for Mrs. J was good. She demonstrated a weak but coordinated PFM contraction, was motivated to improve, and willing to make lifestyle changes that could positively affect her outcome. Based on several studies, a 76% to 86% reduction in UI may be expected from a multicomponent intervention program for mixed UI.[77-79]

Goals and Outcome Measures

Mrs. J and the clinician agreed on the following physical therapy goals: (1) 80% reduction in urine leakage episodes, (2) voiding interval of every 2 to 3 hours during day and evening hours, (3) wake to void once per night, (4) use of pads for bedtime only, (5) 0/10 pain with bowel movements, (6) reduction in symptom-related distress, and (7) improved quality of life.

To measure intervention outcomes, the clinician selected a 3-day bladder diary and the PFDI- and PFIQ-short forms (Urinary and Colorectal-Anal subscales only).[49,58] The bladder diary allowed Mrs. J to record the time of each void/24 hours, occurrence of each urine loss episode, and pad usage. The PFDI- and PFIQ-short forms were selected to measure changes in bladder and bowel symptoms, symptom-associated distress, and symptom impact on quality of life following intervention.

Implications for Plan of Care

Based on Mrs. J's symptoms, impairments, and symptom impact on quality of life, the clinician implemented a multicomponent plan of care that included PFM exercise, biofeedback, bladder training, stress and urge strategy training, and education in proper defecation techniques.

Pelvic floor muscle exercises were prescribed to improve Mrs. J's continence mechanisms. They were critical to increase her PFM strength, improve urethral support, and promote skill and success in using the stress strategy to prevent/stop stress UI episodes. Improving PFM function would also enable her to apply the urge strategy to inhibit bladder contractions, prevent urge UI episodes, and promote bladder training. After practicing muscle contractions during the initial session, the clinician educated Mrs. J in a home exercise program. The program consisted of ten contractions, three times per day. The clinician recommended she hold each contraction for 3 seconds followed by 6 seconds of relaxation. The clinician chose this contraction/relaxation ratio based on Mrs. J's weak muscles, incomplete muscle relaxation, and painful left levator ani. Over the course of therapy, the clinician gradually increased the muscle contraction/relaxation ratio to 10 seconds/20 seconds; and the number of contractions to a maximum of 45 per day. This exercise intensity paralleled studies that observed a mean 76% to 86% reduction in UI episodes in women with urge UI and mixed UI.[77-79] By the seventh visit, Mrs. J was able to perform 45 10-second PFM contractions per day without pain. Initially, Mrs. J exercised in the supine position. By the fifth visit, Mrs. J performed exercises in sitting, standing, and while walking. Repeated PFM contractions performed during sit to stand or step-ups were not prescribed because of Mrs. J's knee pain. Instead, Mrs. J was instructed to perform a single PFM contraction each time she stood up throughout the course of her day.

The first three physical therapy visits included a 10-minute session of biofeedback. Given Mrs. J's painful left levator ani muscle, biofeedback was used to ensure full relaxation between PFM contractions. This was essential to prevent exacerbation of pain during exercise and to alleviate straining during defecation.

At Visit 2, the clinician recommended that Mrs. J begin to practice the urge suppression strategy.[73,78] She was advised to initially practice this strategy at home. After gaining success at home, she was told to use the strategy at work. She was also educated in use of the stress strategy.[73,74] She was advised to contract her PFMs quickly and strongly just prior to and during a cough or sneeze.

It was important to initiate bladder training only after Mrs. J reported success using the urge suppression strategy. By Visit 4, Mrs. J began increasing voiding intervals by 10- to 15-minute increments. Her chosen voiding interval goal was 2.5 hours.

Evidence-based lifestyle changes were also recommended. Mrs. J agreed to decrease, but not eliminate, her intake of coffee and diet caffeinated soda. Over the course of 9 weeks, she was able to reduce her caffeine intake by drinking two 8-oz cups of decaffeinated and only one 8-oz cup of caffeinated coffee. She also replaced one serving of carbonated soda with an 8-oz glass of water.

Given that Mrs. J's weight may have contributed to her mixed UI and knee pain, the clinician recommended she investigate a medically supervised weight loss program. Mrs. J expressed the desire to lose weight. However, she desired to pursue weight loss after she completed all of her physical therapy sessions.

Outcomes

After 9 weekly visits, Mrs. J was discharged from physical therapy. She met all of her initial goals. In addition, she exceeded the 80% reduction in UI episodes by 10%. Her PFDI and Colorectal-Anal (decreased from 50 to 28) and Urinary Distress scale (decreased from 79 to 37) scores verified symptom improvement. Similarly, her PFIQ (UDI-7) score (decreased from 67 to 27) indicated improved quality of life.[58] Mrs. J resumed walking 1 mile three times per week.

REFERENCES

To enhance this text and add value for the reader, all references are included on the companion Evolve site that accompanies this text book. The reader can view the reference source and access it online whenever possible. There are a total of 131 cited references and other general references for this chapter.

CHAPTER 21

Conservative Pain Management for the Older Adult

Katherine Beissner, PT, PhD

INTRODUCTION

Pain is a universal experience that has received increasing recognition as a major public health problem and its impact on declining function and prolonging rehabilitation for millions of people.[1] Health professionals often talk about the "pain experience," recognizing that pain has biological, psychological, and social components that result in individualized responses to unpleasant stimuli. Pain is also described as having both a "disease" and an "illness" component. The disease component involves the nociceptive and central nervous system processing of pain; illness reflects the suffering and behaviors associated with pain.

Loeser describes four major types of pain, each requiring a different approach to clinical management: transient, acute, chronic cancer pain, chronic noncancer pain.[2] *Transient pain*, such as stubbing a toe or a needle prick, is an everyday experience that rarely warrants health care intervention. It is a brief activation of nociceptors with negligible tissue damage. *Acute* pain is the unpleasant sensation typically associated with direct tissue injury. Acute pain usually resolves readily through the healing process. Postsurgical pain and pain following a musculoskeletal injury are examples of acute pain. Breakthrough pain, often considered a type of acute pain, is an increase in pain above a tolerable level of ongoing pain.[3,4] *Chronic pain due to cancer* is associated with tissue damage due to the disease process and/or cancer treatment. It is distinguished clinically from other types of pain because the focus of treatment is often on palliative care.[2] *Chronic pain due to nonmalignant diseases* presents a different clinical management problem. Chronic pain and *persistent pain* are terms used interchangeably to reflect an unresolved pain problem that persists after the normal period of tissue healing, continuing because of some factor other than the original injury or illness. Persistent pain is becoming the more commonly used term, and will therefore be used throughout this chapter. Psychological, environmental, and social factors play a large role in the clinical manifestations of persistent pain, and effective treatment addresses these aspects of pain, in addition to symptom relief.[2]

Noting that classification of pain according to its presumed source may help guide treatment, the American Geriatrics Society Panel on Persistent Pain in Older Persons identified four categories of pain based on the presumed source of the pain: nociceptive, neuropathic, mixed or unspecified, and psychiatric.[5] Nociceptive pain arises from stimulation of pain receptors; neuropathic pain from pathology in the peripheral or central nervous system; mixed or unspecified pain from multiple or unknown sources; and in rare cases, pain from a psychiatric disorder, such as a conversion reaction.[5] In the case of psychogenic pain, treatment with analgesic mechanisms is not indicated but psychiatric treatment may be beneficial.

A comprehensive taxonomy of "chronic pain" developed by the International Association for the Study of Pain categorizes a patient's pain according to five attributes: pain location, body system involved (e.g., respiratory, musculoskeletal), pattern of occurrence (e.g., continuous, recurring), intensity, and etiology.[6] Other taxonomies have been developed to classify pain experienced by patients with particular conditions, such as cancer,[7] neuropathies,[8] spinal cord injury,[9] and to incorporate the psychosocial aspects of pain into classification systems.[10,11] Although these classification systems may help to categorize pain types, research into the validity and reliability of the classification systems is mixed, and a valid taxonomy of pain that can be used to guide treatment is not yet available.[12]

SCOPE OF THE PROBLEM: PREVALENCE, CHALLENGES, AND COSTS OF PAIN MANAGEMENT IN OLDER ADULTS

Prevalence

It is estimated that annually more than 76 million people in the United States experience pain, with incidence peaking in middle age (45 to 64 years) and declining in the older population.[13] The 2008 report on health in the United States shows that 48.2% of respondents aged 65 years and older report joint pain (excluding the back or neck) in the 30 days prior to the survey, and almost 32% of older adults reported low back pain lasting 24 hours or more in the prior 3 months.[14]

Because persistent pain lasts extended periods of time, and may never resolve fully, the term *prevalence* rather than *incidence* is used in discussing the extent to which populations are affected with this type of pain. Differences in populations studied and in definitions of persistent pain yield large differences in estimates of its prevalence, from about 20%[15] to 49%,[16] and even higher among residents of nursing homes.[17] On average, older adults have longer pain duration[18] and more pain sites[19] than working-age adults, factors associated with higher levels of functional impairment.[20] Although acute pain is reported more by middle-aged adults, older adults have a higher prevalence of chronic health conditions associated with persistent pain. Epidemiologic studies that categorized prevalence of pain by disease type show that prevalence of rheumatic diseases such as polymyalgia rheumatica, giant cell arteritis, and gout, rise dramatically after age 65.[21] Arthritis, predominantly osteoarthritis, is reported by approximately 50% of adults aged 65 years and older, and activity limitations associated with arthritis are reported by 22.4% of this population.[21] Diagnoses of back and neck pain decrease after a peak in middle age,[22] but severe back pain increases with advanced age.[23]

Pain Management Challenges

Pain management is complex, and it is well recognized that pain is undertreated in the older population (Box 21-1).[24-26] Older adults, concerned with addiction or the potential side effects of drugs, often alter the medication regimen prescribed by their physician.[27,28] Even when taken as prescribed, medication side effects such as fatigue, sedation, dizziness, and confusion can limit a person's ability to participate in therapy, thereby delaying progress and potentially contributing to other serious health concerns.

It is common for older adults to have one or more chronic health conditions that limit the range of analgesic options to manage multiple conditions.[29,30] A study

of older adults seen in a large geriatric pain clinic in Australia between 1991 and 1999 revealed that more than 50% of the subjects had three or more organ systems affected by comorbid conditions,[31] with the most common conditions involving the cardiac (54.4% of subjects) and gastrointestinal systems (35.9%). Those with more medical conditions reported lower levels of physical activity, and higher pain intensity, with approximately 50% of subjects also reporting high levels of depressive and anxiety symptoms.[31] Patients with persistent pain and depressive symptoms report higher levels of disability and diminished physical performance than patients without depressive symptoms.[32] A dose–response relationship exists between the severity of depression and pain-related activity limitations.[33,34] Treatment interactions are seen as well. In a large randomized clinical trial of older adults with pain and depression, treatment directed only at decreasing depression yielded a small but significant treatment effect for pain and pain-related disability.[35]

Pain has a detrimental impact on function. For example, a high level of postoperative pain following surgical stabilization of hip fractures limits early mobility and is associated with longer hospital stays. Morrison et al, in a study of patients post–hip fracture, found that patients with high postoperative pain levels not only had impaired mobility during hospitalization but also that this impaired mobility persisted 6 months after hospital discharge.[36] In a study of older adults (aged 75 to 105 years of age) in southern Sweden, 51% of the oldest old (95+ years) reported pain-related difficulty in functional activities in the prior 3 months, as compared to 36% of the youngest group in the study (aged 75 to 79 years).[37]

The type of functional limitations experienced depends, in part, upon the location of the pain. Limitation in mobility, the most common limitation reported among older adults, is associated with lower extremity pain.[38] Older women with low back pain experienced difficulty with light housework, shopping, and activities of daily living.[39] Those with widespread pain (upper and lower extremities, and trunk) have greater likelihood of having severe difficulties in activities of daily living (ADLs), walking, and lifting.[40]

Although the reported prevalence of pain in older adults with significant cognitive impairment varies widely, there is agreement that the prevalence is high.[41] Accurately assessing pain is particularly challenging in the presence of significant cognitive impairment,[41,42] and accurate pain assessment is key to appropriate pain management.

Another important challenge in understanding pain and pain management is the association of pain with socioeconomic factors. Those with lower education levels and income report higher incidence of pain-related disability,[38,43-46] and cultural aspects of coping also affect patients' pain experience.[47,48] Individuals with lower educational levels tend to use more passive coping

---

BOX 21-1	Challenges of Pain Management in Older Adults

- Underreporting and undertreatment of pain
- Medication adherence and adverse effects
- Impact of pain on function and mobility
- Comorbid conditions—physical and mental health
- Comorbid cognitive impairment
- Association of socioeconomic factors with pain incidence and impact

strategies (e.g., hoping, praying, and catastrophizing) which are less effective than positive, active coping strategies (e.g., positive self-talk, exercise) in terms of impact on disability.[46,47] It is proposed that individuals with higher educational levels have a greater sense of self-efficacy, have more positive interactions with health care providers, and assume greater responsibility for pain management through active coping strategies, thereby reducing pain-related disability despite comparable levels of pain intensity.[46]

The gender differences in pain and pain impact are well documented in the literature. Women experience pain at greater intensity,[49] more locations,[50] and with greater impact on function[21,38] than men. Women have a higher prevalence of persistent back pain,[51] fibromyalgia,[52] and arthritis,[21] including arthritic changes in the lower spine.[53] This pattern is true in patients with primary neurologic diagnoses as well. Among patients with Parkinson's disease[54] and multiple sclerosis,[55] female gender is associated with greater pain and pain-related disability. The mechanisms underlying gender differences in pain intensity and impact are not fully understood, and more research is needed into the potential causes and potential gender-based treatment protocols.[56]

Cost of Pain Management in Older Adults

In addition to the human aspects of pain prevalence and impact, the enormous costs of pain treatment are a universal concern. Costs of chronic or persistent pain management, including lost productivity, increased health care visits, medication use, and diagnostic procedures are burdensome both on the individual patient and the payor system.[57-60] In the United States, it is estimated that more than 50 million people annually seek help for persistent pain problems, at cost greater than $70 billion in terms of medical care and lost productivity.[1]

It is difficult to accurately measure the monetary cost of pain management in the older adult population. However, by examining figures for patients with spinal pain problems, it is clear that the cost of treating patients with pain is growing at an extraordinary rate. Prevalence of persistent back pain and recent attention to the previously widespread undertreatment of the problem has resulted in an astronomical increase in the money spent treating and diagnosing this problem. Although research provides some evidence of advances in effective treatment protocols, these advances are not associated with a proportionate improvement at the population level, and the prevalence of persistent back pain continues to rise.[57] Medicare expenditures for epidural steroid injections and magnetic imaging studies for patients with low back pain have increased disproportionately to the increase in numbers of patients with these conditions.[61] Interestingly, increases in payment for physical therapy services for Pennsylvania Medicare recipients increased a nominal 0.2% between 2000 and 2003, but there was a 59%

increase in payments for steroid injections and almost 42% increase in payments for magnetic resonance imaging (MRI) or computed tomographic (CT) scans. A recent analysis reported a staggering 423% increase in Medicare payments for opiates for patients with low back pain between 1997 and 2004.[62] In 2004 alone almost 20 million prescriptions for these drugs were paid for Medicare beneficiaries with spinal pain conditions.[62] Despite this increased expenditure, there are also increasing numbers of individuals reporting limitations in physical and social function associated with pain.[63]

BIOPSYCHOSOCIAL MODEL OF PERSISTENT PAIN

The biopsychosocial model describes pain as a multidimensional experience that incorporates biological (nociception), psychological (thoughts and emotions), and social (interactions with family or work) mechanisms. Although acute pain certainly has social and psychological impacts that may require a multidisciplinary approach for some patients, the ongoing nature of persistent pain makes these more pronounced, requiring a more uniformly multidimensional approach to care.

Biological mechanisms include the activation of pain receptors, transmission along complex neural pathways, perception of pain, and internal pain suppression mechanisms. A recent summary article highlights neuroscience evidence of genetic factors predisposing individuals to persistent pain and implicates imbalances in neurotransmitters and receptors as contributory toward the development and maintenance of a persistent pain state.[1] It is also clear that pain fluctuates in accordance with the patient's mood state through the impact of hormones on neurotransmitters.[1]

The psychological aspects of persistent pain are thus recognized as being intertwined with the biological components through the impact of thoughts and emotions on the stress regulatory systems, both in terms of heightening sensitivity to noxious stimulation but also in the impact of positive mood states on resilience. Studies examining the management of persistent pain focus on the factors with a negative effect on pain intensity and pain-related disability,[64] including the associations between depression and persistent pain[65] and the impact of maladaptive cognitions on emotions and pain behaviors (e.g., activity avoidance).[66] Although there has been much debate on the direction of causality among depression, anxiety, anger, and persistent pain, it is clear that these factors present concomitantly and all play a role in the patient's pain experience.

Although the "social" aspect of the biopsychosocial model of persistent pain is the least well studied, there is evidence that the relationship between persistent pain and social or intimate relationships is bidirectional. Perceived social support improves persistent pain coping[67] whereas conflict within social networks is associated with higher levels of pain.[68] Small qualitative studies have shown that some patients with persistent pain conditions experience increased tension and conflict in ongoing relationships.[69,70]

AGE-RELATED CHANGES: IS PAIN IN OLDER ADULTS DIFFERENT?

Age differences in the presentation of acute pain and the prevalence of persistent pain conditions have led to research investigating whether there are aging-related anatomic and physiological changes in pain reception, conduction, and perception. Six factors are proposed that may alter the perception of pain in older adults: decreased nociceptor density, changes in the conductivity of nociceptive afferents, changes in central coding of pain, changes in segmental nociceptive reflexes, alterations in descending inhibition of pain, and psychosocial influences that alter the meaning and impact of pain.[71]

Laboratory research with experimentally induced thermal pain confirms that older adults have slower response times than younger adults, but this change in response times is seen only in A-delta fibers. A-delta transmission is associated with "first pain" perception—the initial detection of a noxious stimulation. There is no evidence of slowing of transmission in the unmyelinated C fibers, which yield perception of longer, ongoing pain.[72] Others have found that older adults take longer to report pain than younger adults and that point tenderness takes longer to resolve in older subjects.[73] Aside from these changes in A-delta conduction velocity and slowed pain resolution, studies of changes in sensory perception and pain threshold in older adults using experimentally induced pain models have produced conflicting results but are known to reflect a different pattern of decline than seen in other sensory systems (e.g., hearing, vision).[71] The extent to which these changes in nerve conduction velocity impact the patient's pain experience is not clear. However, in discussing persistent pain in older adults, Karp et al refer to the state of pain homeostenosis—the limitation of an aging person's ability to adjust (physiologically, psychologically, socially) to pain stresses. These authors propose that age-related changes in central and peripheral processing of pain combined with other losses associated with aging (including narrowed social networks, depression, or cognitive decline), exacerbate physiological reserve decline, which, in turn, further decreases the person's capacity to adapt to physical, emotional, and environmental stressors.[74]

It is interesting to note that older adults with persistent pain have more physical limitations in health and function, but for the most part actually show better mental health and better pain coping skills than younger adults with similar pain problems.[75] In this large study (n = 6147, 19.8% aged 60 years and older) drawn from patients at three multidisciplinary pain centers in the United States, older adults reported greater lower body functional limitations than younger adults but lower rates of depression, lower use of passive coping strategies, and higher scores for perceived control and overall mental health.[75] However, in another study of 340 patients between 17 and 93 years of age, 25% of the older subjects were found to have maladaptive coping strategies in which relatively low levels of pain were associated with high levels of depression and disability, a combination not seen in younger age groups.[76]

EXAMINATION AND EVALUATION OF THE PATIENT WITH PAIN

The examination and evaluation of older patients with pain, whether acute or persistent, is similar to the evaluation of younger adults. Although the same components of the evaluation are important, it may be necessary to modify testing procedures for older adults with other health concerns. For example, a patient with chronic obstructive pulmonary disease may be unable to lie flat in either a supine or prone position for muscle testing and range of motion measurement, and will need to have the position modified. This same patient may require frequent rests between testing procedures to avoid fatigue or shortness of breath. Also note that some of the standardized pain assessment instruments that assess pain-related disability may use language biased toward working adults. These may not be relevant for older adults who have retired. Further, it may be difficult to discern whether limitations identified with these instruments are caused by the pain or by other health problems.

Clinically, the experience of nurses and emergency health workers show that some older adults do not complain of pain despite the presence of painful conditions, whereas others complain continuously.[77] Clearly, all older adults are not alike, and in an individualized approach to evaluation and treatment planning a variety of factors must be considered when developing a program geared toward reducing pain and maximizing function.

A full history and physical examination are essential, as the primary purposes of the examination and evaluation process are the identification of physical pathologies that may give rise to pain, and the identification of any associated functional limitations. Comprehensive descriptions of the examination and evaluation process associated with impairments in cardiopulmonary endurance, motor function, joint mobility, motor control, and posture are found elsewhere in this text. The following discussion of the examination focuses on aspects related to the patient's pain.

Patient History

A comprehensive patient history is essential in guiding the physical examination of the patient and should include social history, current work/volunteer status, living environment, general health perceptions, behavioral risk factors, medical/surgical history, current medications, and functional status/activity level. For patients with a chief complaint of pain, particular attention to past medical history is important in identifying conditions that may give rise to pain, affect pain perception, or identify contraindications (e.g., history of cancer) to various interventions. There is consensus that physical therapists should screen for "red flags" (signs and symptoms associated with an increased risk of a serious medical condition that warrants referral out to the appropriate medical practitioner).[78] However, there is concern regarding the lack of empirical evidence on the diagnostic accuracy of many red flags and the potential escalation in costs if every patient with a "red flag" sign or symptom is referred for additional testing.[79]

In 1994 the Agency for Health Care Policy and Research (AHCPR) published guidelines for the management of acute low back pain in adults, identifying red flags for cancer or infection, spinal fracture, and cauda equina syndrome.[80] A more recent set of evidence-based guidelines developed by a European Commission focused on acute low back pain identified 12 red flags: age of onset (less than 20 or greater than 55); history of trauma; thoracic pain; fever; structural deformity; prolonged use of corticosteroids; drug abuse, immunosuppression, HIV; widespread neurologic signs; previous history of malignancy; systemically unwell; unexplained weight loss; and constant progressive, nonmechanical pain (pain that is not altered by movement or changes in position).[81] Although developed for use with patients with spinal pain problems, these red flags may be relevant to patients with extremity problems as well. Boissonnault, in a recent textbook focused on primary care physical therapy, provides a list of red flags for each major body region and recommends that physical therapists screen for applicable red flags as part of every patient assessment.[78] Many of these red flags involve pain symptoms.

Pain History

For all patients for whom pain limits function, it is important to obtain a brief pain history that provides characteristics of pain, past pain history, prior treatment approaches, and the outcome of each approach. When working with older adults with visual or hearing impairments, slight modifications to usual procedures may need to be made. It is important to ensure that the examination area has adequate lighting, that any hearing aid is working properly, and that any written materials are available in large print. Important dimensions of pain to be included in the pain history include the following.

Quality of pain is evaluated in terms of the words the patient uses to describe the pain. Patients can be asked to describe the pain using their own words; or a list of words (e.g., dull, aching, throbbing, stabbing) can be provided, with instructions to circle the words that best describe their pain. Words with dramatic impact (e.g., punishing, cruel, vicious) give cues to the emotional impact of the pain.

Intensity, or the amount of pain perceived, is the most commonly evaluated aspect of pain. When measuring pain, patients' self-report of pain intensity is preferred, because caregivers often underestimate pain intensity. Pain intensity is most commonly measured with the Numerical Rating Scale (NRS), Verbal Numerical Scale (VNS), Verbal Descriptor Scale (VDS), Visual Analog Scale (VAS), and the Faces Pain Scale (FPS).[82] Figure 21-1 illustrates these pain intensity instruments. In a comparison study of these scales using experimentally induced pain, although the VAS had an acceptable interrater reliability, the reliability was the lowest among the five tools (93.5% agreement compared to 100% agreement with the NRS, VDS, VNS, and FPS). The VAS also showed the highest "failure" rate, measured as the frequency of incomplete or incorrect completion (e.g., more than one mark made on a single scale). Each scale was used seven times, and across these testing sessions the VAS had a failure rate of 19.1% for older subjects (age range 65 to 94, $n = 89$) compared to 2.2% for the NRS and lower failures for all other scales.[83] A recently developed pain intensity tool is the Iowa Pain Thermometer (IPT), which uses a shaded thermometer alongside seven verbal pain descriptors ranging from no pain to the most intense pain imaginable (Figure 21-2). Patients use the visual cue of the thermometer to select verbal descriptors of pain intensity. In a study using a sample of 97 subjects with chronic pain (including 36 older adults aged 65 to 87 years), five pain scales (IPT, NRS, VNS, VAS, and FPS) were compared in terms of failure, scale sensitivity, and subject preference. The IPT was judged to be superior to other scales because of its low failure rate and high patient preference rating. However, with the exception of the VAS, the other scales also showed strong performance and provide good options for use in the older population.[82]

Location: identifying the primary pain locations, as well as locations of referred pain is important in determining the potential source(s) of the pain impairment. Pain location is most commonly assessed by having the patient indicate painful areas on a body diagram, or by having the patient point to the painful area(s).

Aggravating and easing factors are the positions and movements that increase or relieve the patient's pain. Relevant questions include determining which positions or movements give rise to pain (or increase pain intensity), and the length of time spent in the position (or movement) before the pain begins. Questions regarding the positions or actions that decrease or alleviate the pain symptoms provide information on appropriate treatment programs and resting positions for patients.

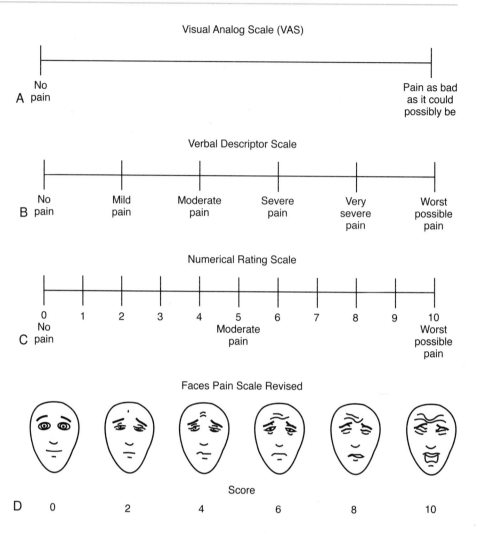

FIGURE 21-1 Pain intensity scales. **A,** Visual Analog Scale (Adapted from Joyce CR, Zutshi DW, Hrubes V, Mason RM. Comparison of fixed interval and visual analogue scales for rating chronic pain. Eur J Clin Pharmacol 1975;8:415-20). **B,** Verbal Descriptor Scale (Data from Melzack R, Torgerson WS. On the language of pain. Anesthesiology 1971;34:50-9). **C,** Numerical Rating Scale (Data from Downie WW, Leatham PA, Rhind VM, Wright V, Branco JA, Anderson JA. Studies with pain rating scales. Ann Rheum Dis 1978;37:378-81). **D,** Face Pain Scale Revised (Hicks CL, von Baeyer CL, Spafford PA, van Korlaar I, Goodenough B. The Faces Pain Scale-Revised: toward a common metric in pediatric pain measurement. Pain 2001;93:173-83.)

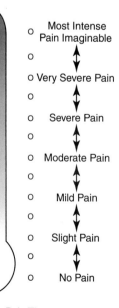

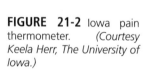

FIGURE 21-2 Iowa pain thermometer. *(Courtesy Keela Herr, The University of Iowa.)*

Standardized Pain Instruments. For patients with chief complaints of pain, or with persistent pain that limits function, therapists should consider using a multidimensional pain inventory as a means for documenting pain symptoms and their impact on function. These instruments are commonly used as outcome measures to quantify the extent to which patients improve over the course of treatment. The Brief Pain Inventory[84-87] and the McGill Pain Questionnaire[88,89] are among the more widely used inventories. The McGill Pain Questionnaire is the most well-known instrument, composed of multiple items assessing the intensity, quality, and behavior of pain, along with the impact of various conditions (e.g., liquor, weather changes, bright lights). Scores on this instrument range from 0 to 78, with higher scores indicating greater pain severity.[88] A short form of this instrument consists of 15 pain descriptors, for which patients rate intensity on a 0 to 3 scale (none to severe), with score range from 0 to 45.[90] Tests of the responsiveness of the Norwegian version of this instrument with patients ranging in age from 23 to 86 indicate that a 5+ change in score represents a clinically important change.[91] A new revision of the short-form McGill Pain Questionnaire has been developed by expanding the number of descriptors to capture aspects of neuropathic pain.[92] The Brief Pain Inventory (BPI) is a 32-item questionnaire that incorporates questions on medical care, location of pain, pain intensity (current, most intense in past week, least intense in past week, average over the past week), pain quality, and the impact of the pain on function, mood, and sleep. The BPI-Short Form is a nine-item questionnaire with subquestions, incorporating items on pain intensity, location, impact, and current treatment.[87] Both versions of the BPI have demonstrated validity and reliability and have been used for patients with a variety of pain diagnoses, including cancer, osteoarthritis,[86,87] and general residential care.[84]

Other standardized instruments used in clinical settings are the Pain Disability Index (PDI) and the Geriatric Pain Measure (GPM). The PDI is a self-report instrument on which patients rate the extent to which their painful condition interferes with seven areas of life function (e.g., recreation, sexual behavior, and family function), using a numerical rating scale from 0 (*no disability*) to 10 (*worst disability*). Summed scores yield a total disability score ranging from 0 to 70. The PDI demonstrates acceptable validity and reliability[93-95] and has been used in outcomes studies for patients with persistent back pain,[96,97] and subacute neck pain[98] as well as other disorders. No research reports were found that used the PDI specifically in the older adult population.

The Geriatric Pain Measure (GPM) was specifically developed for use with older adults in an attempt to measure self-reported pain intensity, and the impact of pain on functional ability, mood, and quality of life.[99,100] The instrument was developed based upon literature review of the existing pain instruments, with items taken from scales shown to have good face validity. Further development was based on expert panel review and pilot testing with a sample of older adults. The instrument consists of 22 items scored dichotomously (yes = 1, no = 0) to measure the impact of pain on social interaction and function, and two items related to pain intensity, scored on a scale of 0 to 10.[100] Item scores are summed to generate scores ranging from 0 to 42, where lower scores indicate less pain. A 12-item version of the GPM includes the pain intensity items and ten items related to pain impact (scored yes = 2, no = 0), with a summed score range from 0 to 40.[101] Both versions of the GPM have demonstrated aspects of validity and reliability[100,101] and a self-administered version has been tested in a sample of 1072 older adults in Europe. However, as a relatively new instrument, use in research studies is limited, and as yet, no standards are set for detecting minimally clinically meaningful changes in GPM scores.

Other options for assessing the impact of a plan of care on patient outcomes include disease-specific instruments such as the WOMAC arthritis disability index,[102] the Roland-Morris Disability Questionnaire for low back pain,[103,104] or the Neck Disability Index.[105] Although not initially developed specifically for use in older populations,

these instruments, and others, have been widely used in clinical research and practice with older adults and are effective in identifying clinically meaningful change. For example, the WOMAC was found to be more responsive to meaningful changes in patient status than the generic health status instrument (SF-36) in comparisons of drug versus placebo treatments of adults (mean age 61.5 years) with osteoarthritis of the hip,[106] and among 697 patients with knee osteoarthritis (mean age = 70 years, range = 38 to 90).[107] A large study (*n* = 1362) determined the minimally clinically important improvement in WOMAC scores for outpatients with hip or knee osteoarthritis (mean age = 64.6 and 67.9 years, respectively) to be −7.9 for hip arthritis and −9.1 for knee arthritis.[108]

The Patient Specific Functional Scale (PSFS) provides individualized assessment of a patient's progress according to functional activities important to the individual.[109] The PSFS has been found to be more responsive to changes in functional status than more standardized assessment tools.[110,111] In the initial examination, the patient is asked to identify three areas in which she or he is having difficulty as a result of their chief complaint. Then each activity is rated on a scale of 0 (*unable to perform activity*) to 10 (*able to perform activity at the same level as prior to the illness or injury*) and scores for the three activities are averaged. At subsequent evaluations, the same items are rated and compared to the initial score. The PSFS has been used in clinical research that included older patients,[109,110,112] though potential age-group differences in instrument sensitivity and specificity have not been studied. Because functional criteria for improvement are individualized, the PSFS is appropriate for use with any population and is considered to be an effective means of documenting clinical changes.[113,114]

Screening Tools. Because of the relationship of thoughts and emotions on pain and pain behaviors, particularly in patients with persistent pain problems, it is important to screen patients with persistent pain for selected psychological attributes, such as depression, fear avoidance behavior, self-efficacy, and coping.

Depression is commonly seen in patients with persistent pain, so screening for depressive symptoms within this patient population is advisable, with referral to an appropriate practitioner if a significant depression is suggested. Recent review articles[115,116] highlight the importance of depression screening for patients with persistent pain and describe several screening tools appropriate for older adults. Chapter 8 provides a detailed discussion of commonly available screening tools for depression.

The Fear Avoidance Beliefs Questionnaire (FABQ) is a useful instrument that can help to identify whether patients have thoughts and beliefs that lead to maladaptive coping strategies such as activity limitation.[117] The instrument assesses the extent to which patients believe that physical activity affects their pain using two subscales, one for the impact of work on pain and the other for general physical activity. Designed for working-age adults with low back pain, FABQ–work scores are associated with self-reported physical disability[118] and are predictive of treatment outcomes for patients receiving workers' compensation.[119] The FABQ–physical activity scale has been shown to be predictive of gait speed[120] and exercise training outcomes in patients not receiving workers' compensation.[121] Little research is available on the use of the FABQ with older populations.

The Tampa Scale for Kinesiophobia[122] also assesses the degree to which fear of movement affects disability, but it has not been examined for use with older adults. Research with younger populations shows this instrument to be useful in assessing the outcomes of rehabilitation programs for patients with a variety of pain problems.[123-127]

Self-efficacy belief, especially as related to an individual's perceived ability to cope with a chronically painful condition, is associated with rehabilitation outcomes. The Arthritis Self-Efficacy Scale (ASES) consists of 20 items related to an individual's beliefs that she or he can manage pain associated with particular tasks.[128] Each item is rated on a scale indicating the certainty with which the person can perform each task, ranging from 0 (*very uncertain*) to 100 (*very certain*). Scores on the ASES are associated with functional performance for patients with a variety of conditions, including knee osteoarthritis,[129,130] fibromyalgia,[131] and rheumatoid arthritis.[132] This instrument may be useful for patients who have persistent pain problems that will require ongoing self-management.

Coping scales are used to measure how patients react to, and cope with, pain. Use of maladaptive coping strategies may interfere with progress in therapy, so identification of coping strategies is indicated when patients appear to have substantial difficulty dealing with their pain. Two self-report instruments are most commonly used: the Coping Strategies Questionnaire (CSQ) and the Chronic Pain Coping Inventory. The CSQ is a 50-item questionnaire assessing the use of five cognitive coping strategies (coping self-statements; catastrophizing; distraction; ignoring pain sensations; and reinterpreting pain sensations) and two behavioral responses (praying/hoping, and increasing activities). For each item, patients rate the frequency of their use of each coping strategy on a 7-point scale, from *never* (0) to *always* (6).[133,134] CSQ scales correlate well with other measures of adjustment and well-being[135,136] and are predictive of disability.[137,138] In particular, the "catastrophizing" scale appears to be particularly helpful in identifying patients with intense pain, depression, and disability.[138]

There are two versions of the Chronic Pain Coping Inventory (CPCI), composed of either 65[139] or 42 items.[140] Both versions are composed of two parts, one focused on illness behaviors (Guarding, Resting, and Asking for Assistance) and the other on positive coping behaviors (Coping Self-Statements, Relaxation, Task Persistence, Exercise/Stretching). The CPCI has been validated for use in patients with chronic[141,142] and subacute[143] pain conditions. The Guarding scale is the strongest predictor of disability among all scales from the CPCI and CSQ,[138,143] and although overall the CPCI is a better predictor of disability than the CSQ, it is less sensitive to the detection of depression.[138,143] Thus, based on research comparing the use of these two instruments, the Catastrophizing scale from the CSQ and the Guarding scale from the CPCI appear to be the most helpful in identifying depressive mood and future disability status.[138,143]

Pain Assessment in Patients with Dementia. There is speculation that difficulty accurately assessing pain leads to a particularly high prevalence of undertreatment of individuals with cognitive impairment. However, pain intensity tools such as the Iowa Pain Thermometer, Visual Analog Scale, Visual Analog Scales with verbal descriptors, Numerical Sequence Scale, and Verbal Rating Scales have all been used with older adults with cognitive impairments with some success. In a study of 160 French-speaking older adults admitted to inpatient dementia units in Geneva, Switzerland, 88% of the sample was able to explain and use at least one pain intensity scale. Highest comprehension was found for visual analog scales with verbal descriptors, and the lowest comprehension was found on the Faces Pain Scale.[144] Similarly, Ware et al found that their U.S. sample of English-speaking subjects with dementia ($n = 28$) were all able to complete at least one intensity scale.[145] Interestingly, all subjects were able to use the Faces Pain Scale, and 90% were able to use the Numerical Rating Scale. Because it appears that many adults with dementia are able to provide valid responses to pain intensity scales, use of self-report instruments is advised. Clinicians should consider having several scale options available to find the one that works best for each patient.

When using self-report measures of pain intensity for adults with severe dementia, there is always some concern over the validity of the ratings. Given that older adults with cognitive impairment have similar facial/behavioral responses to evoked pain as older adults with no cognitive impairment,[146] a number of observation tools have been developed to determine the extent and intensity of pain for those with severe cognitive impairment. Recent review articles[147-149] provide excellent summaries of the instruments that have been used with cognitively impaired older adults. Each review concludes that more research into the psychometric qualities of the instruments is needed, but the Pain Assessment Checklist for Seniors with Limited Ability to Communicate (PACSLAC) and the DOLOPLUS2 have been judged to have the best psychometric qualities.[147] Unfortunately, neither seems appropriate for use within physical therapy treatment sessions. The PACSLAC is a 60-item instrument requiring ratings based upon four dimensions: facial expressions, activity/body movement, social/

personality/mood, and physiological/sleeping/eating. [149a] The DOLOPLUS2 is a ten-item scale requiring observation over an extended period of time rather than current pain level. Physical therapists may work in clinical settings in which these scales are used and may contribute observations/ratings as part of a team evaluating patients with complex pain problems.

Recent studies provide support for the validity and reliability of the Pain Assessment in Advanced Dementia (PAINAD) instrument,[150] a tool designed for use in clinical settings. The PAINAD is based on two more comprehensive pain assessment tools, and includes five items (breathing, negative vocalization, facial expression, body language, and consolability) which are rated on a 0 to 2 scale. Summed scores, assigned by a health care provider, range from 0 to 10, with higher numbers taken to be reflective of more intense pain. Scores on the PAINAD correlated well with numerical response scales for patients with and those without cognitive impairment, and scores were higher during activities anticipated to elicit pain (e.g., during transitional movements). Although easy to use, only three of the six categories of nonverbal pain behaviors recommended to be assessed[5] are included in the instrument, and the limited scope of the assessment leaves questions regarding its sensitivity to changes.[148]

Perhaps a more important weakness of the PAINAD and other instruments that use summation of pain behaviors to yield a pain intensity score is the underlying assumption that more pain behaviors means more intense pain. Pasero and McCaffery caution that instruments that provide checklists are useful in determining whether pain behaviors decrease after an intervention, but are not useful in determining the *amount* of pain the patient experiences.[151] However, at this point summation of pain behavior appears to be the best indicator we have for pain intensity in populations with severe dementia.[152]

Physical Examination

Upon conclusion of the history and assessment of pain, a thorough physical examination should be conducted to identify impairments related to joint mobility, motor function, muscle performance, sensory integrity, integumentary integrity, and cardiopulmonary function. Through tests and measures, the therapist will be able to identify impairments that may contribute to the patient's pain. Throughout the physical examination, it is important to note what positions, motions, and activities give rise to pain as this information will assist in arriving at a diagnosis. Because many patients who have persistent pain problems limit their activity and exercise as a result of concerns with pain, it is likely that impairments in muscle performance, joint mobility, and cardiovascular endurance will be identified in the physical examination. A comprehensive treatment plan will focus on these impairments while using other interventions to help control pain in order to enhance functional recovery.

Information from imaging studies is often available to physical therapists, and this information may be helpful as an adjunct to the physical therapy examination. However, it is important to apply the results of such studies cautiously, as anatomic abnormalities identified on radiographs or scans may not give rise to a patient's signs and symptoms. In a prospective study of asymptomatic adults with no history of low back pain or sciatica, 57% of the MRI lumbar scans on subjects aged 60+ had abnormal results (36% with herniated nucleus pulposus, 21% spinal stenosis).[153] Keeping this in mind, information from any imaging study should be considered alongside the results of the examination in the determination of the physical therapy diagnosis.

PROGNOSIS AND PLAN OF CARE OF THE PATIENT WITH PAIN

The patient's prognosis for recovery is dependent upon many factors, including age, scope and severity of impairments, chronicity of the problem, psychological and socioeconomic factors, and overall health status. In general, younger patients tend to recover more rapidly than older patients, though other factors play a large role in the recovery process. Patients with acute pain that is easily localized and with an identifiable incident of onset have a better prognosis for recovery than those with a widespread persistent pain problem of insidious onset. Subjects with chronic medical conditions that give rise to pain (e.g., osteoarthritis, spinal stenosis) may learn compensation strategies such as strengthening surrounding musculature and minimizing stressors on the affected area. These strategies are likely to decrease pain but unlikely to completely alleviate pain. Note also that other comorbid health conditions affect full participation in rehabilitation. For example, walking programs or other conditioning exercises are recommended for patients with chronic pain. A patient who has chronic back pain and heart disease or chronic obstructive pulmonary disease (COPD) may require a more gradual increase in walking time/distance than would be seen in others without such health problems. Those with a substantial psychosocial component to their pain may require longer interdisciplinary treatment to address their multifaceted pain problem, and patients with significant socioeconomic disadvantages may experience higher levels of challenge to program adherence and progress.

By weighing these and other factors identified through the history and examination with the patient's specified treatment goals, the therapist will make a determination of the patient's expected treatment outcomes. The plan of care is then developed, specifying the long-term and short-term goals, expected treatment outcomes, and interventions.

PHYSICAL THERAPY INTERVENTIONS TO ADDRESS PAIN

Optimally, first-line interventions should directly address the source of pain.[5] A comprehensive examination of the patient to identify impairments associated with the painful condition will direct those interventions. Such interventions may include therapeutic exercise,[154] joint mobilization or manipulation,[155-157] and orthotic or supportive devices.[158-160] These interventions reduce stress and correct malalignments of joint structures, correct muscle imbalances, and enhance the shock absorption capacity of tissue structures. Selection of appropriate treatments must include consideration of contraindications associated with the patient's comorbid conditions (e.g., osteoporosis or osteopenia), and may necessitate adjustment of usual treatment parameters to accommodate comorbid conditions and the patient's current functional status.

Although correction of the cause of pain is always desirable, it is sometimes not possible. Even a thorough assessment may not clearly reveal the source of the patient's pain, or, even if the source is revealed, it may not be possible for physical therapy interventions to directly address the underlying cause of the pain (e.g., osteoarthritis). In these cases, direct treatment of the patient's pain symptoms may increase the patient's ability to tolerate active interventions that address other impairments limiting the patients' function. Passive treatment modalities focused solely on temporarily decreasing pain symptoms (e.g., heat treatments, cryotherapy, transcutaneous electrical nerve stimulation [TENS]) should be used sparingly as part of the physical therapy intervention. These modalities should be a means to an end, the end being decreasing pain to a sufficient extent to allow patients to participate in subsequent active treatments aimed at positively affecting functional abilities.

Thermal Agents

Although thermal agents are frequently used in the physical therapy treatment of patients with pain,[161-163] the literature on the effects of thermal agents on pain in older adults is limited. The Philadelphia Panel, an interdisciplinary group of experts convened to develop evidence-based guidelines for treatment of musculoskeletal disorders, found a lack of evidence to support the use of thermal agents (including ultrasound) for the treatment of low back,[164] knee,[165] and neck pain,[166] but indicated that there is evidence that ultrasound is effective in treatment of calcific tendinitis in the shoulder.[167] Although studies that included older adults were included in the review process, the majority of the literature reviewed focused on younger populations and there was no analysis of potential differential treatment effects according to subject age.

More recent research has shown that when physical agents were applied prior to exercise, older women with knee osteoarthritis generated greater force during isokinetic exercise, suggesting that alleviation of pain enhances muscle performance.[168] Changes in peak torque generated following application of thermal agents were most dramatic in measurements of knee extension, with the advantage of the treatment groups over the control group ranging from 3.35 N-m to 16.05 N-m, depending upon the treatment group and angular velocity tested.[168] These results support the use of thermal agents prior to exercise training to enhance performance during the exercise session, although the long-term effects of this approach to exercise training have not been studied.

Thermal agents are commonly used in the self-management of chronic pain. In a study of 272 community-dwelling adults aged 72 years and older, 28% reported some relief of chronic pain using heating or cooling agents.[169] Among low-income, urban-minority older adults, heating agents were cited as helpful for controlling arthritis pain for 33% of black and 40% of Hispanic subjects.[170] Because heating and cooling agents carry some risk of injury, educating patients about their appropriate use is an important role for physical therapists. General procedures for the application of thermal agents are provided elsewhere.[171-173]

Manual Therapy

We typically think about mobilization and manipulation for their role in the restoration of joint mobility. However, they also have a role in the control of pain. Although there is scant evidence on the use of joint mobilization and manipulation specifically for older adults, research has addressed the use of these treatments for knee and hip osteoarthritis, conditions common in older adults. A recent qualitative systematic review of 39 studies[174] revealed Level B (fair) evidence to support the use of manipulative therapy in combination with exercise for the treatment of knee osteoarthritis, and Level C (limited) evidence in support of the use of the combination of manipulation and exercise for patients with hip osteoarthritis. Limited evidence is also found for the use of these treatments for foot and ankle problems. In one example of a study protocol yielding beneficial effects for patients with hip osteoarthritis, the treatment group receiving a program combining thrust and non-thrust manipulations to the hip joint was almost twice as likely to achieve beneficial outcomes as those in an exercise group. The benefits in terms of pain intensity, function, and range of motion were retained for more than 6 months.[175] In another randomized controlled study of patients with knee osteoarthritis, large-amplitude oscillations of the tibia on the femur improved knee pressure pain threshold about 21% more than a manual contact control treatment. Knee mobilization also decreased the time required to move from sit to stand by more than 5% over pretreatment times, a 13% difference from changes seen in the nontreatment control group that, in contrast, demonstrated an 8% increase in sit to stand time.[176] Because only immediate posttreatment measurements were taken, it is not clear how long these treatment effects are sustained.

A Cochrane review of research on headache treatment concludes that, despite considerable limitations in the design of the studies included in the review, there is evidence to support the use of spinal manipulation for the prophylactic treatment of a variety of headache types. It is important to note that subject ages for studies included in this review extended to age 78 years.[177] The American Pain Society's clinical practice guidelines indicate that there is good evidence that spinal manipulation is effective for the management of persistent spinal pain,[178] and a recent study of younger patients (aged 18 to 45 years) demonstrates benefit of thoracic spine manipulation for management of patients with acute neck pain.[179] A Cochrane systematic review concludes that manual therapy alone is insufficient in the management of persistent neck pain. However, there is strong evidence that either manipulation or mobilization combined with exercise is effective in reducing pain, with up to a 41% improvement in pain ratings over control conditions. This review also concluded that manual therapy with exercise improves function and the patients' global perceived effect of treatment.[180]

TENS

Acute Pain. Recent studies from the international community show increasing support for the use of high-frequency TENS (pulse frequency at or greater than 80 per second) at high sensory intensity for the treatment of postoperative pain. High-frequency sensory level TENS (also known as "conventional TENS") has been shown to be effective in reducing pain intensity and limiting use of pain medications after cardiac surgery[181] and posterolateral thoracotomy[182,183] and was found to decrease pain and increase performance on spirometry after cardiac surgery[184] and abdominal surgery.[185] TENS has also been shown to decrease pain from postoperative wound dressing changes[186] and reduce pain and anxiety among older adults during ambulance transportation following traumatic hip injuries.[187] High-frequency TENS appears to be the most effective TENS application for postsurgical pain and can be used with modulating frequencies to control neurologic accommodation.[188] Table 21-1 summarizes key parameters of the studies examining TENS for management of postoperative pain.

Studies examining the impact of TENS on pain threshold help to highlight the impact of treatment parameters.[191] High-frequency TENS, maintained at a high sensory level but below pain threshold, raises experimentally induced pain threshold, whereas low-intensity TENS (maintained just at the sensory threshold) does not,[191] and high-intensity stimulation at two sites provides greater elevation of pain threshold than stimulation at a single site, especially when stimulation is applied at different frequencies (i.e., high frequency at one site and low frequency at the second site).[192]

In laboratory research with rats, both high-frequency and low-frequency TENS were found to decrease experimentally induced pain. However, the low-frequency effect was not seen when naltrexone (an opiate inhibitor) was administered prior to treatment while the impact of high-frequency TENS was not affected by pretreatment with naltrexone.[193] This indicates that low-frequency and high-frequency TENS achieve pain control through different mechanisms, with low-frequency TENS activating release of endogenous opiates.[193]

Persistent Pain. The evidence for use of TENS in the management of persistent pain is less conclusive. A small study of older adults with persistent pain demonstrated that TENS is tolerated by older adults, and results in a short-term decrease in pain with both high-frequency "conventional" TENS and burst-mode applications.[194] Despite concerns of insufficient evidence to differentiate relative effectiveness among various categories of TENS applications (e.g., "acupuncture-like" vs. high-frequency "conventional" TENS), a Cochrane systematic review concludes that TENS has positive benefits as an adjunctive treatment for patients with hand pain due to rheumatoid arthritis.[195] Subjects achieved a 67% decrease in pain at rest after 3 weeks of acupuncture-like TENS, and a statistically significant but not clinically meaningful reduction in joint tenderness with the application of high-frequency TENS.[195] Further, a meta-analysis of the short-term effects of various treatments for patients with knee osteoarthritis concludes that TENS (including interferential current therapy) is effective in achieving clinically important reductions in pain associated with osteoarthritis of the knee.[196] These authors note that the clinically meaningful changes in pain status were maintained for 1 to 2 months after the treatment period.

Despite these positive conclusions regarding the use of TENS, methodological weaknesses of published studies limit the ability to conclusively support the use of TENS for persistent pain conditions. A recent systematic review of TENS for persistent pain concludes that an insufficient number of high-quality randomized clinical trials exist to evaluate the use of TENS for the management of persistent pain.[197]

Precautions and contraindications important to note when using TENS are consistent with those for the general population. The use of TENS over the thoracic region and its use with patients who have implanted medical devices such as implantable cardioverter defibrillators (ICDs) has been somewhat controversial. There is evidence that TENS interferes with electrocardiac monitoring, and TENS application was comparable to electrocardiographic ventricular fibrillation or ventricular tachycardia. Based upon findings that more than 50% of subjects in a small trial ($n = 30$) had disturbance from TENS, whether applied locally or at the hip, the use of

TABLE 21-1	Summary of Postoperative TENS Studies Including Older Adult Subjects			
First Author, Publication Year	**Condition**	**TENS Type and Comparison Groups**	**Number of Subjects Subject Age**	**Outcomes**
Emmiler, 2008[181]	Postoperative cardiac surgery with medial sternotomy for CABG on valve repair	Frequency: 100 Hz Intensity: Strong, comfortable Duration: 1 hour, repeated once Comparison: TENS Sham TENS Control	N = 60 Mean age: TENS: 59.3 Sham TENS: 63.9 Control: 61.2	TENS group: Decreased pain intensity Decreased analgesics
Erdogan, 2005[182]	Postthoracotomy	TENS frequency: 100 Hz Intensity below motor threshold Comparison: TENS Low-intensity TENS	N = 116 Age range = 20-70	TENS group: Decreased pain intensity (VAS) at rest and with coughing Decreased opioid use Improved pulmonary function (FEV_1) No complications
Solak, 2007[183]	Postthoracotomy	TENS frequency: 3 Hz Intensity to 12 mA 30 minutes Comparison: TENS PCA	N = 40 Mean age: TENS: 47.3 Control: 53.7	TENS group: Decreased postoperative pain Decreased pain intensity on postoperative days 4-60 Decreased analgesics use No side effects
Cipriano, 2008[184]	Cardiac surgery (medial sternotomy)	TENS frequency: 80Hz High intensity (sensory) ×4 hours Comparison: TENS Sham TENS	N = 45 Age range = 41-74	Decreased pain intensity (VAS) Improved vital capacity and tidal volume
Hargreaves, 1989[186]	Postoperative abdominal wound dressing change	Comparison: High-frequency TENS Sham TENS No treatment	N = 75 Mean age: 56.9 years	Decreased pain intensity during dressing changes
Rakel, 2003[188]	Postoperative abdominal surgery	Modulated high frequency (50/100 Hz) Intensity to highest tolerance Comparison groups: TENS No intensity TENS Control	N = 44 Age range = 20-77 Mean: 40	TENS group achieved: Decreased pain during walking Increased vital capacity, increased gait speed Increased gait distance tolerated
Breit, 2004[189]	Unilateral total knee arthroplasty	TENS: Intensity to tolerance × 24 hours No frequency data Comparison groups PCA TENS + PCA Sham TENS + PCA	n = 22 (Mean = 71.5) n = 25 (Mean = 75.4) n = 22 (Mean = 72.2)	No between-group differences in amount of analgesics used
Gilbert, 1986[190]	Postoperative inguinal herniorrhaphy	Frequency: 70 Hz Intensity to maximum tolerable	n = 40 Age range: 24-76	No difference in pain intensity, medication use, or peak expiratory flow rate

PCA, patient-controlled analgesia; *TENS,* transcutaneous electrical nerve stimulation; *VAS,* Visual Analog Scale.

TENS with patients with ICD is not recommended.[198] For patients with pacemakers, electrocardiographic monitoring of the patient during TENS application is recommended prior to independent use by patients.

Low-Level Laser Therapy (LLLT)

Studies regarding the use of low-level laser therapy (LLLT) for the treatment of pain associated with knee osteoarthritis have been generally small. However, a recent systematic review and meta-analysis of five studies with an average subject age of 66.7 years concludes that LLLT, when applied with the assumed optimal parameters, results in a clinically perceptible improvement in pain (24.2% more improvement in pain intensity than placebo controls).[196] The supported parameters are doses of 2 to 12 J for 904-nm laser, and 20 to 48 J for 830-nm laser, applied to two to eight points over the joint capsule.[196]

Other research with a younger sample found LLLT effective in reducing pain associated with temporomandibular joint dysfunction.[199] A Cochrane systematic review found mixed results for the treatment of nonspecific back pain,[200] and a controlled study found LLLT ineffective in reducing shoulder pain in patients with rheumatoid arthritis.[201] Therefore, at this time, LLLT for the management of pain other than that associated with knee osteoarthritis is not supported by the literature.

Protective and Supportive Devices

There is some evidence that protective and supportive devices yield a decrease in pain and increase in function for patients with joint instability or malalignment. Therapeutic taping for patellar realignment is effective in reducing pain and improving function in patients with osteoarthritis of the knee.[158,160] Patients with metatarsalgia associated with rheumatoid arthritis experienced decreased pain using custom-fitted foot orthosis,[202] and patients with sternal surgery or sternal separation experience decreased pain using an external support to stabilize the sternum.[159] However, while the use of supportive devices to prevent glenohumeral subluxation after stroke delays the onset of pain, there is no evidence that such devices are effective in preventing pain or reducing pain intensity.[203] Decisions regarding the use of protective or supportive devices should therefore be individualized to the patient based upon information gained in the examination.

Exercise

Expert consensus statements and review panels consistently indicate that exercise is safe and effective in improving the health of older adults, including decreasing levels of pain.[164-167,204-207] In reviewing the available evidence, the American Geriatrics Society's Panel on Persistent Pain in Older Persons recommends that *all* older adults with persistent pain participate in a physical activity program individualized to the patient's needs and incorporating flexibility, strengthening, and endurance exercises. The panel cites strong evidence (Level I) in concluding that clinicians should always incorporate this recommendation.[5] The decision then rests in the selection of which exercises to incorporate into the treatment program. Clearly, exercises specific to patients' impairments in muscle function and joint mobility are indicated. As recommended earlier, other components should also be incorporated. The following is a brief summary of research regarding the impact on pain of flexibility, aerobic, and strengthening exercises.

Flexibility Exercise. In one study, stretching/flexibility exercise was found to have a more beneficial impact on bodily pain than a program focused on endurance and strength training.[208] However, other research has shown that strength training programs provide a better reduction of pain in older adults with arthritis.[209] Based upon moderate-quality evidence, yoga is among the nonpharmacologic interventions recommended by the American College of Physicians and the American Pain Society for the management of low back pain.[210]

Aerobic Exercise. Although a relatively early study of older adults with a history of arthritis found that joint symptoms were neither exacerbated nor reduced with either cycling, strength training, or a combination of the two,[211] other research shows more favorable outcomes. A small study incorporating a 12-week bicycling program for older adults with persistent back pain yielded improved physical function and decreased back pain symptoms.[212] Individuals with osteoarthritis and comorbid medical conditions had improved pain levels following an 18-month aerobic exercise program, whereas no such improvement was found for participants in a weight training program.[213] Walking programs have been shown to produce health benefits and improved pain scores,[214,215] yet sustaining a walking program is problematic, and cessation of the program results in a loss of the program benefits.[216] Higher levels of program adherence are related to improved outcomes of exercise programs.[215]

Strengthening Exercise. Although physical therapy consisting of light exercise (isometrics, sit to stand, squats, step-ups), massage, taping, and joint mobilization for patients with knee osteoarthritis was no more effective at reducing pain and disability than sham ultrasound,[217] a 4-month home-based progressive strengthening exercise program yielded improved self-reported physical function and decreased pain.[218] This program used squats and step-up exercises and open-chain exercises using ankle cuff weights, with a targeted range of perceived difficulty for the exercises between 6 and 8 on a 0 to 10 scale. Resistance was increased by extending the range of squats/steps, and by increasing the cuff weights in 1-lb increments, up to a maximum of 20 lbs per leg.

Similarly, a center-based (with home exercise follow-up) Fit and Strong program incorporating conditioning, stretching, and strengthening components resulted in improved 6-m walk time and decreased joint stiffness. The strengthening component of Fit and Strong used resistance bands and cuff weights, increased in 0.5-lb increments according to a standardized protocol.[219]

Patient Self-Management Programs. A meta-analysis of the impact of exercise on adults with osteoarthritis revealed that exercise alone does not produce improvements in the psychological well-being of program participants, suggesting the need for other interventions to address the mental burden of persistent joint disease.[220] Given the high impact of pain on psychological and social well-being, incorporating therapies to address these aspects of pain are appropriate for self-management.

The most well-known and well-studied self-management program for patients who have a chronic health condition is the Arthritis Foundation Self-Help program.[221] This group intervention teaches individuals with arthritis or related diseases how to reduce the impact of their disease on their daily functioning. Educational sessions are led by trained laypeople, who teach participants specific coping skills like relaxation, visual imagery, and the use of heating and cooling agents. Sessions also include information on medication management, nutrition, stress reduction, and methods for reducing joint stresses such as using assistive devices and pacing activities. A substantial body of research verifies that this program raises participants' self-efficacy for managing their disease,[222-226] reducing pain,[223,226,227] decreasing disability,[227] improving exercise performance,[224,225] and reducing physician visits.[223,226] Other self-help programs, such as one combining the Arthritis Foundation program with an exercise program,[228-230] a program addressing multiple chronic health conditions,[222,224,231] and an array of other self-help programs[232] provide benefits in terms of pain reduction, improved self-management efficacy, and reduced disability in older adults with persistent pain conditions. The key messages highlighted by these studies are as follows. First, patient education in self-care strategies for managing pain flare-ups, utilizing coping strategies (e.g., use of home-administered heating or cooling agents, relaxation, imagery), and reducing joint stresses through assistive devices is likely to decrease the patient's dependence on health care providers, increase his or her self-efficacy, and improve function. Second, therapists should consider referring patients/clients to local group self-management programs. Group programs allow participants to learn from each other, put their own problems into perspective, and enjoy social support with their peers. Although a meta-analysis of reports on the Arthritis Foundation programs revealed that the effect sizes for reducing pain and disability were small (effect size for pain reduction = 0.12, for disability = .07),[227] the widespread availability of such programs and their low cost may make these interventions worthwhile endeavors for patients with persistent pain conditions.

COGNITIVE–BEHAVIORAL APPROACHES TO PAIN MANAGEMENT

Cognitive–behavioral therapy (CBT) seeks to enhance patients' control over pain using diverse psychological techniques.[233] Underlying this therapy is the notion that a person's beliefs, attitudes, and behaviors play a central role in determining his or her overall experience of pain; that thoughts and emotions influence pain perception and pain behaviors; and that patients can learn adaptive ways of thinking and feeling.[234] Standard CBT pain protocols seek to (1) teach patients specific cognitive and behavioral skills to better manage pain; (2) teach patients to recognize specific thoughts, beliefs, emotions, and behaviors (activity avoidance) that have an effect on pain; and (3) emphasize the primary role that patients can play in controlling their own pain. CBT is provided by psychotherapists and has proven efficacious for reducing pain and disability levels among persons with diverse persistent pain disorders.[235-242] Specific interventions for pain management include instruction in pain theory (e.g., pain does not equal harm, impact of thoughts/emotions on pain perception and behaviors), relaxation training, distraction techniques (e.g., pleasurable activity scheduling, visual imagery), and cognitive restructuring (reinterpreting pain sensations, controlling pain catastrophizing). Although numerous efficacy studies have demonstrated the benefits of this particular therapy, few older adults use cognitive–behavioral techniques for managing pain.[169,243] Although some cognitive–behavioral techniques are incorporated into self-help programs (e.g., relaxation and imagery are taught in Arthritis Foundation self-help courses), more intensive training for these techniques may not be widely available, limiting their use for pain management. Common barriers associated with nonuse of relaxation techniques as a form of CBT-informed self-management among older adults included lack of access to the interventions and internal factors such as time conflicts, and concerns with treatment efficacy.[244]

Although not qualified as cognitive–behavioral therapists, physical therapists are able to adopt a cognitive–behavioral perspective when treating patients[234] by incorporating a cognitive–behavioral approach to instruction and practice on specific coping skills such as diaphragmatic breathing, relaxation techniques, and visual imagery. Other coping strategies associated with both CBT and physical therapy include the concept of pacing activities to avoid pain flare-ups and progressive goal setting. Although the literature from both self-management and psychology validates the effectiveness of these interventions for pain management, currently most physical therapists do not use these techniques as pain management strategies.[161]

It is important to note that some patients with pain problems have substantial psychological distress and may require treatment by a psychologist or counselor skilled in working with patients with pain problems. High levels of anxiety, depression or catastrophizing, and verbalizations of despair are indicators that the patient may need referral to a psychologist and management from an interdisciplinary perspective. Standardized measures such as the Fear Avoidance Beliefs Questionnaire[117] or depression scales may help to identify patients who would benefit from referral to a mental health professional skilled in using CBT in the management of pain.

CASE STUDIES

Case Study 1

Mr. G is a 75-year-old man who fell 2 weeks ago and sustained a left femoral neck fracture. Prior to this injury, the patient lived independently in a one bedroom apartment in a senior housing complex. Mr. G has emphysema and mild depression. His previous medical history is uncomplicated and medications prior to hospitalization included albuterol and a multivitamin. The fracture was stabilized with a compression screw and side-plate fixation.[245] Postoperatively Mr. G reported a high level of pain and was begun on patient-controlled analgesia (PCA) with hydromorphone. The initial physical therapy examination took place on the first postoperative day. Mr. G complained of intense pain during passive range of motion and mobility testing, reporting deep pain in the hip and at the surgical site, which he rated a 6 of 10 on a numerical rating scale. Despite the use of PCA, Mr. G continued to complain of intense pain when his left lower extremity was moved passively, and he was unwilling to initiate active movement because of pain. Mr. G refused further work on transfers or exercise until his pain level was reduced.

Given the known benefits of early physical therapy following hip fracture surgery,[36,246,247] Mr. G's physical therapist was concerned that delayed rehabilitation would adversely affect his prognosis for return to independent living. High-frequency (100 Hz) TENS was applied using a dual-channel stimulator with one set of 2 × 4-in. electrodes at the incision site (one channel) and a second set on the anterior and posterior aspects of the hip joint (second channel). Intensity was adjusted to a strong but tolerable level below the motor threshold. The patient was instructed to increase TENS intensity as needed to maintain the strong sensation. After 20 minutes of TENS application, the patient was able to tolerate active-assisted range of motion of the left lower extremity, and transfer to sitting on the side of the bed. In the afternoon of the first postoperative day Mr. G. transferred to a chair using a rolling walker and assistance of his physical therapist. He was instructed in the use of TENS, and he continued to use it on an as-needed basis until hospital discharge on the third post-operative day. At the time of discharge, Mr. G. was able to independently apply electrodes and adjust machine parameters, was using the TENS unit while ambulating 75+ feet with a rolling walker, and ascending/descending 6-in. curbs; and a 1-month TENS rental was arranged, and home health physical therapy was arranged to ensure continuity of care.

Case Study 2

Mrs. O is a 72-year-old retired school teacher who just moved to a retirement community in the mountains of Vermont. She lives with her husband and enjoys an active retirement, playing tennis twice a week, treadmill walking three times a week, participating in a biweekly weight training class, and taking 2- to 5-mile hikes each weekend. She was evaluated in an outpatient physical therapy clinic with chief complaints of right anterior knee pain that interferes with her ability to "charge the net" in tennis and hike in hilly areas. Pain increases on ascending stairs or hills, and decreases with rest. Mrs. O reports no prior history of knee injuries, and assumes that this problem is due to "old age." Previous medical history includes conservative treatment of shoulder impingement with physical therapy 10 years ago, osteopenia diagnosed 8 years ago, and a recent diagnosis of a mild hearing impairment for which she has sought no treatment. Mrs. O takes alendronate (Fosamax) and a calcium and vitamin D supplement for her osteopenia, a generic multivitamin, and acetaminophen as needed for pain. She reports that the knee pain has caused her to decrease the length of her hikes and to play tennis more cautiously. She wishes to return to a more rigorous exercise schedule primarily due to her concern about her bone strength. She reports that her physician ordered routine radiographs of her knee, with findings of degenerative changes consistent with "mild" DJD.

Pain is described as "stiff" and "achy." Using a numerical rating scale, she rated her pain on initial examination as 3 of 10 and reports a highest-intensity pain of 5 of 10 following long hikes.

Physical Examination. Vital signs: Blood pressure = 125/78 mmHg; respiratory rate = 12 breaths/min; heart rate = 74 beats/min. Palpation reveals mild warmth on the anterior aspect of the right knee as compared to the left. Posture exam shows slight forward head position with the head tilted slightly to the right. Weight is shifted slightly to the left of center. The right patella is noted to be positioned slightly lateral to midline in standing. The patient ambulates independently without an assistive device with slightly decreased stance time on the right. Quick tests show decreased ability to squat, with weight shifted to the left lower extremity during this task. Active range of motion testing reveals limitations in right knee extension. Passive range of motion measurement at the right knee is 0 to 120 degrees of flexion, compared to 0 to 135 degrees on the left. Flexibility testing reveals shortness in the hamstrings bilaterally. Muscle force measurements using a hand-held dynamometer were knee extension L: 50 lbs, R: 35 lbs with pain on testing; knee flexion L: 30 lbs, R: 29 lbs. Strength of gastroc-soleus tested with unilateral heel-ups was L: 10 repetitions; R: 9 repetitions. Mild crepitus was noted bilaterally with testing of knee extensors and on passive range of motion testing. In supine, the right patella is noted to be positioned lateral to midline, but passive mobility allows appropriate patellar alignment.

Evaluation. Mrs. O's signs and symptoms are consistent with the diagnosis of osteoarthritis, but recent increase in pain in the anterior knee aggravated by stairs/hills, pain on testing knee extensor strength, and lateral patella position suggest potential overlying patellofemoral pain syndrome. Given her active lifestyle and motivation, the prognosis for recovery of premorbid function is very good.

Plan of Care. Long-term goals include return to tennis and hiking, with full muscle strength within 1 month. Mrs. O's therapist chose to use patellar taping,[160] hamstring stretching, quadriceps strengthening, and walking on level surfaces[248] as the initial treatment plan. The initial treatment included taping the right patella to provide medial glide, medial tilt, and anteroposterior tilt to the patella followed by exercises including passive stretching of bilateral hamstrings, squats to ~90 degrees of knee flexion, knee extension strengthening including three sets of 10 repetitions of knee extension at 75% of her 1 repetition maximum. Mrs. O was instructed to leave the tape in place for 1 week, continue her exercises at home and at her fitness center, modify her regular exercise regimen to include walking on level surfaces for 30 minutes 3 to 4 days a week instead of the weekend hikes. The planned progression of treatment included teaching the patient self-taping, progression of strengthening exercises as needed, evaluation of balance/stability, and progressing walking to include hills with paved surfaces, gradually returning to walking hills on hiking trails.

Case Study 3

Mrs. D is an 84-year-old woman seen in physical therapy with primary complaints of low back pain present for approximately 3 years but increased in intensity in the past 2 weeks after she experienced a fall in her home. Mrs. D reports she was able to get up from the floor by herself using furniture for support, but indicates that the process was extremely painful and physically draining. She reports that she did not see a physician until 1 week after the fall, when she had a regularly scheduled appointment with her primary care physician. She reports that her physician "insisted" that she come

to physical therapy. Radiography reports indicate no sign of fracture.

The social history reveals that Mrs. D's husband died 4 years ago, and her best friend passed away last year. She lives alone in a small one-level apartment in a senior housing complex. Pertinent medical history includes a diagnosis of osteoarthritis in bilateral knees, degenerative disc disease, and mild central lumbar stenosis. Mrs. D takes acetaminophen for her pain, and vitamin B_{12} and calcium supplements. She reports previous trials of other pain medications but cannot recall which ones. She said she could not tolerate the other medications because they caused drowsiness, dizziness, and constipation. She also reports concerns that she would become dependent upon the drugs, taking them at higher and higher doses. Mrs. D reports spending most of her time in a recliner doing crossword puzzles. She reports difficulty with housecleaning, shopping, cooking, walking, bathing, and dressing due to pain and indicates that she has no assistance with these activities.

Pain Assessment. Mrs. D describes her pain as intense aching sensation throughout bilateral knees and low back, with sharp, shooting, jabbing pain in her back upon moving from supine to sitting and occasionally on sit to stand. Her score on the Geriatric Pain Disability Index is 34 out of 42, indicating severe pain problems. Because Mrs. D describes substantial difficulty with a variety of home activities, and reports limited social interaction, the Geriatric Depression Rating Scale short form was administered. Mrs. D scored 13 of 15 on the GDRS, indicating severe depression, and 27 of 30 on the Fear Avoidance Beliefs Questionnaire–physical activity scale, indicating severe fear avoidance beliefs.

Physical Examination. An abbreviated initial examination was conducted because of Mrs. D's complaints of pain and refusal to attempt formal strength testing. Blood pressure is 140/85 mmHg, heart rate 78 beats/min and regular, and respiratory rate 14 breaths/min and regular. Mrs. D presents as a frail older woman who ambulates with a rolling walker using short step lengths. Observation reveals a flexed posture with forward head, rounded shoulders, flexion throughout the spine, hips, and knees. She refuses to attempt a squat due to stated concerns with pain and falling. Mrs. D moves from standing to sitting independently and cautiously. Sitting to supine is independent but with complaints of pain. Thirty-second repeated chair rise: able to move from sit to stand six times, placing her below the 10th percentile for functional lower body strength. Flexibility testing reveals shortness in bilateral hamstrings, hip flexors, pectoralis major, and the teres major/latissimus dorsi/rhomboid complex. Passive hip extension lacks 15 degrees of neutral on left and 10 degrees on right. Passive hip flexion is 115 degrees on the left, 110 degrees on right. Knee extension lacks 5 degrees of neutral bilaterally.

The Timed Up and Go test took 45 seconds using the rolling walker. She refused the 6 minute walk test.

Evaluation. Mrs. D presents with persistent pain limiting all aspects of her function, and presents at risk for future falls. Scores on the depression and fear avoidance scales indicate the need for interventions to address the psychological aspects of her pain condition. Given the extreme nature of these complaints, a referral to a psychologist with experience working with individuals with pain is indicated. The patient's prognosis for recovery to a more active lifestyle is guarded, given the psychosocial components of her condition. However, given her musculoskeletal impairments, physical therapy interventions addressing muscle function, flexibility, balance, and mobility are also indicated.

Plan of Care. Long-term goals include Timed Up and Go score of less than 30 seconds, 6-minute walk test score of 300 m, and ability to complete 12 repetitions of sit to stand in 30 seconds. Goals addressed with her psychologist included increased participation in active leisure activities, decreased depressive symptomatology, and decreased fear avoidance beliefs. Mrs. D's physical therapist chose to incorporate stretching, mobility training, and strengthening exercises into twice-weekly physical therapy sessions. Mrs. D was also instructed in diaphragmatic breathing and imagery to promote relaxation during exacerbations of pain and the use of home heating agents to control pain. A written home activity plan was developed to encourage the patient to change her position regularly, intersperse activity into her daily routine, and to increase active leisure pursuits outside of her apartment. She was begun on a home exercise program that included practice of relaxation skills, and progressive daily ambulation with her rolling walker in the hallways of her building. Coordination with her psychologist allowed reinforcement of physical and psychological interventions to enhance patient adherence to the program.

REFERENCES

To enhance this text and add value for the reader, all references are included on the companion Evolve site that accompanies this text book. The reader can view the reference source and access it online whenever possible. There are a total of 248 cited references and other general references for this chapter.

CHAPTER 22

Lower-Limb Orthoses
for Older Adults

Joan E. Edelstein, PT, MA, FISPO, CPed

INTRODUCTION

An orthosis is a device worn on the body for a therapeutic purpose. Splint, brace, and support are alternative terms. All orthoses apply forces to the body that can assist or resist motion, or maintain or alter a given posture. The therapeutic goals of applying these forces, highlighted in Box 22-1, are typically to decrease pain, improve gait stability, facilitate mobility, and/or improve endurance. An orthosis can achieve these goals by decreasing or redistributing forces across weight-bearing structures, enhancing joint stability, or improving alignment among body segments.

More commonly, orthoses serve to accommodate, modify, or control permanent deformities or movement dysfunctions. Many older adults have deformities that place abnormal stress on joints. Over time, repetitive stress during weight-bearing activities further damages the joints, resulting in greater pain and instability, thus increasing mobility disability.

Although we do not have clear evidence of the number of older adults using lower-limb orthoses, we do have good estimates of the number of individuals with mobility limitations, which is the group typically considered for orthoses. The Centers for Disease Control and Prevention (CDC) reports that 45% of community-dwelling adults older than age 65 years, and 85% of institution-dwelling older adults older than age 65 years, have difficulty walking.[1] The underlying mobility impairments are usually precipitated by disease or injury, such as arthritis and stroke, which occur with increasing frequency with advancing age.

The CDC's Summary of Health Statistics for United States Adults[2] reports that 40% to 50% of individuals older than age 65 years who responded to a national health interview survey in 2007 indicated they have arthritis or chronic joint symptoms. Osteoarthritis (OA) is predominantly a disease of the weight-bearing joints. About 45% of individuals with osteoarthritis have mobility limitation.[3] The CDC survey also reports that 6.3% of individuals between ages 65 and 74 years and more than 10% of those older than age 75 years have had a stroke, the leading cause of disability among older adults.[2]

For most patients, the benefit of wearing a lower-limb orthosis is improved ability to stand and walk effectively. The person who is limited to household ambulation may feel safe and comfortable enough to venture outdoors with the aid of an orthosis. An older adult who is a community ambulator may increase the distances walked, thereby continuing to enjoy the physiological and psychological benefits of greater physical activity. Evidence suggests that using a lower-limb orthosis allows many individuals with mobility limitations to walk more rapidly, consuming less oxygen.[4-9] These findings may be particularly relevant to the candidate for an orthosis who also has cardiac or pulmonary impairment.

As suggested above, a wide variety of mobility conditions are potentially amenable to orthotic use. This chapter will review the overall principles that can be carried across diagnoses. An orthosis functions by remediating, accommodating, or preventing mobility impairments. An example of the remediation function of an orthosis is a functional electrical stimulator electrically activating dorsiflexors and foot everters during gait of a patient recently poststroke to encourage more normal motor patterns and voluntary control of muscles. Ideally, the amount of electrically delivered motor assistance is gradually decreased as voluntary control returns, at which time the orthosis is discontinued. The patient with an unstable knee from quadriceps paralysis may benefit from an orthosis that provides a counterbalancing force to resist unwanted motion and prevent knee collapse in early stance phase. A knee–ankle–foot orthosis fitted to an older woman with knee OA who has developed genu varum may apply a medially directed force at her knee to control the deformity. Straighter leg alignment provides greater comfort and thus greater ability to increase activity while preventing or slowing progression of malalignment. The septuagenarian with lower-limb arthritis

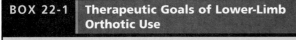

BOX 22-1	Therapeutic Goals of Lower-Limb Orthotic Use

- Decrease pain
- Increase gait stability
- Facilitate mobility
- Improve endurance

or metatarsalgia can walk more comfortably with shoes that provide shock-absorbing soles, or with a foot orthosis that reduces stress on painful foot, knee, hip, or trunk structures.

EXAMINATION OF OLDER CANDIDATES FOR AN ORTHOSIS

History and Systems Review

The history and systems review help guide the examination section of the physical therapist's assessment. In addition to general questions asked of all patients, several additional questions, listed in Box 22-2, should be included for anyone who might be a candidate for an orthosis.

Tests and Measures Relevant to Orthotic Prescription

Observational gait and movement analysis can reveal deficiencies that help guide the choice of specific tests and measures. These tests and measures can provide meaningful data about the potential for an orthosis to improve the patient's movement. For example, an observation of excessive knee flexion in early stance phase leads to a detailed assessment of muscle strength, available range of motion (ROM), and proprioception about the knee. The assessment findings guide decision making about the

BOX 22-2	General Questions to Ask All Patients Being Considered for Orthosis Use

The patient's responses contribute substantially to decision making about orthotic use.

For Those Who Have Worn an Orthosis:
- What type of orthosis and how recently?
- What is your opinion of the positive attributes of each orthosis?
- What is your opinion of the negative attributes of each orthosis?

For all Potential Orthosis Users, Regardless of Their Prior Experience with an Orthosis:
- What are your expectations regarding effect(s) of wearing an orthosis?
- What are your concerns about orthotic appearance?
- What resources are available for purchasing the orthosis?
- What means are available for transportation and obtaining adjustments and other repairs in the future.

benefit of an orthosis to remediate or accommodate the knee instability or prevent deformity.

Data regarding walking speed and distance will provide a baseline against which to discuss likely improvements with the patient and to judge the impact of the orthosis as part of an outcome assessment.

Joint range of motion measurements are essential to formulate an appropriate orthotic prescription. Some orthoses are fabricated to limit available joint motion and thus enhance stability, whereas others provide forces at the very ends of a limited ROM to gradually increase range if worn for a substantial time. Inaccuracy in these measurements would result in an ineffective orthosis.

Muscle strength testing is a basic assessment tool of physical therapists. An orthosis is often used to compensate for weakness in those muscle groups that contribute to normal gait. Prescription of an orthosis to compensate for weakness must consider the extent of the weakness and integrate the data from all other examination findings such as balance, tactile sensitivity, gait analysis, and cardiopulmonary status.

Balance is essential for walking. The ability to maintain balance during static and dynamic upright activities requires the complex interaction of many body systems. Bearing weight on painful joints, or moving joints effectively in the presence of deformities can all contribute to balance deficits. Assessment should determine whether the underlying cause of the balance deficit would likely respond to orthotic use.

Tactile sensitivity should also be checked with Semmes-Weinstein filaments, inasmuch as all orthoses are worn on the body. Even though fabric should be interposed between the skin and the orthosis, it may press excessively, causing discomfort. The patient with proprioceptive deficiency may benefit from stabilizing orthoses. However, weight bearing on insensate feet requires careful choice of shoes and orthoses. Hand function must also be assessed. Manual dexterity is required for donning and doffing the orthosis, unless an attendant is available to assist the patient.

Cardiopulmonary status should be assessed to confirm that the patient has the endurance to participate in and benefit from a gait training program with the orthosis. If visual inspection suggests limb edema, or the patient indicates fluctuations in limb girth, then limb girth measurements should be recorded. Fluctuations in limb girth compromise orthotic comfort and effectiveness. Either the edema must be reduced or the orthosis must be adjustable.

DECISION-MAKING CONSIDERATIONS FOR ORTHOTIC USE (EVALUATION, DIAGNOSIS, PROGNOSIS, AND PLAN OF CARE)

Successful incorporation of an orthosis into the patient's overall plan of care depends on several factors. The practitioner must be knowledgeable about contemporary orthotic designs and the interaction of patient history and physical examination with the appliance. The practitioner must select a design that addresses all factors outlined in Box 22-3. The primary components of orthotic prescription included in a physical therapist's examination and evaluation may focus on (1) making a determination about the need for an orthosis; (2) assessing the fit, benefit, and training needs with a newly fabricated orthosis; or (3) reassessing appropriateness of an existing orthosis. The patient being considered for an orthosis may be categorized within multiple preferred practice patterns of the *Guide to Physical Therapist Practice*.[10] The underlying preferred practice pattern diagnostic category is likely to be within a musculoskeletal or a neuromuscular category.

The first decision point in making a judgment about the appropriateness of an orthosis requires that the practitioner determine whether the primary goal of the orthosis is remediation, accommodation, or prevention of a mobility impairment. Then, the physical therapist must identify the major mechanism through which an orthosis would contribute to the achievement of this goal. The impact of comorbid health conditions and the progressive nature of any disease states must be considered, particularly the effect of an orthosis on the patient's capacity to sustain increased mobility activities.

Orthoses apply force to the body. The basic self-contained force system found in an orthosis is the three-point system, consisting of one force and two counter-forces.[11] For example, the person who has knee instability is likely to benefit from an orthosis that applies a posteriorly directed force at or near the knee and anteriorly directed counterforces above and below the knee.[12]

Evaluation of an older adult's capacity for donning and doffing the orthosis is imperative if the physical therapist is considering long-term use of a device. The individual must be able to don the orthosis accurately, independently, and quickly or have another person readily available and willing to assist. Otherwise, the patient is likely to abandon the device. Selection of fastenings, for example, straps rather than lacing, contributes to donning ease.

Care of the skin and the orthosis is another, and sometimes neglected, prescription issue. Bands and straps should be wide enough to minimize pressure concentration yet not be overly bulky. Excessively wide bands and straps may cause the person to perspire excessively. Streamlined plastic or carbon fiber orthoses are

easier to maintain than those upholstered with leather. Nevertheless, leather remains a useful material for some orthoses as it presents a very comfortable interface between the person's skin, with a thin fabric covering, and the leather interior of the orthosis. Leather is also popular for the upper portion of shoes because it is somewhat porous and conforms very well to the contour of the dorsum of the foot. An orthosis that requires a great deal of care by the patient or caretaker is likely to be abandoned if the amount of care is perceived as outweighing the benefit.

Integrating an orthosis with the patient's other equipment and environment can challenge the rehabilitation team. The patient who relies on a wheelchair for community mobility needs a chair with swinging leg rests to enable transferring to and from the wheelchair while wearing an orthosis. The home environment is another consideration. Many older people live in quarters crowded with a lifetime's accumulation of objects that can occupy the floor area otherwise available for walking with the orthosis. A hot, humid climate can make wearing an orthosis with broad plastic bands uncomfortable. Patients may prefer a metal/leather orthosis with more narrow bands that will still provide adequate structural stability. Mud, snow, and frequent rainstorms influence selection of materials for the orthosis. Carbon fiber and plastic components resist water better than metal ones.

Cost is a practical and necessary consideration with orthotic prescription. Funds must be available, not only to defray the purchase price of the device but also to support physical therapy visits in most instances so that the patient can access the professional expertise that contributes to the maximum advantage of using the device. Although Medicare reimburses most of the cost of orthoses, each older adult's situation is unique. Consequently, the cost of the orthosis and the physical therapy required to enable the patient to achieve maximum benefit may not be fully covered. Although most orthoses are reasonably durable, repairs may be another financial outlay. Generally, the preferred orthosis is the simplest, least expensive design that will address the purposes identified for the patient. For adults with diabetes and related disorders, Medicare covers the cost of appropriate shoes on an annual basis.[13] Coverage generally can be applied to one of three options: a pair of extra-depth shoes plus three pairs of mass-produced or custom-made inserts; a modified pair of extra-depth shoes and two pairs of inserts; or a pair of custom-made shoes.

CHARACTERISTICS OF ORTHOSES

Orthotic Terminology

Orthoses worn on the foot are classified as foot orthoses (FOs), including shoes worn for therapeutic purposes with or without modifications or inserts. A device that

BOX 22-3	Decision about Orthotic Prescription and Design Must Consider the Extent to Which the Orthosis

- Improves the patient's function
- Fits the patient's environment and motivation
- Can be efficiently donned, doffed, and cared for
- Is within the patient's financial resources

extends from the foot to the proximal leg is an ankle–foot orthosis (AFO). The orthosis that extends from the foot to the thigh is a knee–ankle–foot orthosis (KAFO). Addition of a pelvic band and hip joint converts the KAFO to a hip–knee–ankle–foot orthosis (HKAFO). An orthosis that extends from the foot to the trunk is a trunk–hip–knee–ankle–foot orthosis (THKAFO). Identifying the orthosis in a standard manner expedites communication among the patient, family, and clinicians. This generic terminology is preferred, rather than naming orthoses by the person who invented or popularized a given device.

Orthotic Materials

Most contemporary orthoses are made of plastic, which is molded over a model of the patient's limb.[14] Thermoplastics, such as polypropylene, polyethylene, and acrylic, can be heated and shaped; when cool they will retain the shape. Because the process can be repeated indefinitely, thermoplastic orthoses can be adjusted to accommodate changes in the contour of the patient's limb. Orthoses made of thermoplastics are generally white, pink, or amber.

An alternative to thermoplastic are thermosetting plastics, such as polyester laminate. Once the chemical reaction has occurred, the plastic can only be altered by mechanical means, such as adding material, or grinding away material. As a group, thermosetting plastics are more rigid than thermoplastics of comparable dimension and can be tinted to match the patient's skin color. Both thermoplastics and thermosetting plastics are used for the shells and bands of orthoses.

Carbon fiber is a popular material for fabricating orthoses because it is extremely strong and can be used to reinforce weaker materials. Some AFOs are made entirely of carbon fiber. Carbon fiber is usually black. Aluminum, steel, titanium, and magnesium are used in orthoses, particularly for the uprights. Some orthoses also include leather and fabric, especially for straps.[15]

ORTHOTIC COMPONENTS

Components of lower-limb orthoses are described below with emphasis on their distinctive characteristics and relative advantages and disadvantages for specific groups of older adults.

Shoes and Foot Orthoses

Virtually all patients wear shoes, particularly when outdoors. The basic parts of a clinically suitable shoe (upper, sole, heel, and reinforcements) are described below and depicted in Figure 22-1.

The upper designates the part of the shoe that covers the dorsum of the foot. Both leather and canvas are appropriate because they are porous, permitting some

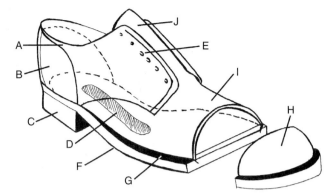

FIGURE 22-1 Basic parts of a shoe. The upper is made up of the quarter (*A*) and its reinforcing counter (*B*), which stabilizes the rearfoot within the shoe; the closure (*E*), the tongue (*J*) across the midfoot; the vamp (*I*) and the toe box (*H*) which encloses the forefoot. The outsole (*F*) is often reinforced with a shank (*D*) and is attached to the upper at the welt (*G*). The standard heel (*C*) is ¾ in. high. (*From Lusardi MM: Orthotics and prosthetics in rehabilitation, ed 2, St Louis, 2007, Saunders.*)

ventilation of the foot. An upper made of thermomolded leather can be heated and adjusted to accommodate bunions and hammer toes. The type of closure influences the ease of donning the shoe. Laces are more adjustable than straps; however, straps, especially if they include hook and pile (Velcro), are easier to manage. The Blucher closure features a distal separation between the two flaps that have eyelets through which laces are drawn, or the flaps that are joined by straps. This closure provides great adjustability in the snugness of shoe fit. The extra-depth upper terminates below the malleoli; because it includes two insoles, the shoe is more spacious than ones with other upper designs. The top insole can be removed to accommodate foot deformities, dressings, or an orthosis.

The sole, composed of an insole and outsole, lies beneath the plantar surface of the foot. The insole is in close contact with the sock-clad foot. The outsole contacts the walking surface. Of particular concern with older adults is an outsole made of material offering sufficient traction to reduce the risk of slipping, and resilient enough to absorb the shock of stance phase.[16] The shoe heel is attached to the sole beneath the anatomic heel. The higher the heel, the greater the load on the forefoot.[17,18]

The shoe is typically reinforced in three places: posteriorly, under the midfoot, and over the toes. The counter reinforces the back of the shoe around the posterior portion of the upper. The counter should fit snugly so that the shoe does not abrade the foot during late stance. The shank reinforces the sole under the midfoot. If the shoe is to be part of an orthosis having a riveted attachment, the shank should be made of corrugated steel. The toe box, located at the distal end of the upper, protects the toes from trauma.

Inserts and internal modifications lie inside the shoe, affecting the forces applied to the plantum.[19] Inserts are removable and can be used in other shoes that have the same heel height. They may be mass produced or custom made, and include heel inserts, three-quarter inserts that do not reduce space for the toes, and full-length inserts that do not slip inside the shoe. Internal modifications, which apply the same forces as inserts, are glued or sewn into the shoe. Although they are not removable, internal modifications ensure that they are used with shoes of appropriate design and proper fit.

Among the most commonly used inserts and internal modifications are resilient full-length inserts. Because they absorb shock and distribute pressure over the entire plantum, they are often used in shoes for people with diabetes or arthritis.[19-23] Trotter and Pierrynowski have demonstrated that although both custom-made and prefabricated inserts typically have an immediate positive effect on gait economy, only custom-molded ones have an effect that lasts at least 4 weeks.[21] An internal heel wedge shifts weight bearing medially or laterally, depending on the wedge shape. A longitudinal arch support applies upward force on the medial border of the foot (Figure 22-2); the apex should be at the sustentaculum tali of the calcaneus. Community-dwelling older adults (mean age = 70 years) using arch supports for 6 weeks were found to have increased comfort in lower-limb joints and improved walking.[24] For older adults, the arch supports should maximize the weight-bearing surface, accommodating any malalignment rather than correcting foot posture.

A metatarsal (MT) pad is a teardrop-shaped pad (Figure 22-3) with its convexity over the metatarsal shafts. It transfers load from the painful metatarsophalangeal joints to the relatively insensate shafts.[25-27] A small change in the location of the MT pad can have a large effect on pressure relief across the MT heads.[25] A toe crest is placed under the plantar surfaces of the toes to increase the bearing area, thereby reducing pressure on the toe tips.

External modifications are additions to the outside of the shoe, particularly the shoe sole. Heel modifications include medial and lateral heel wedges that shift weight bearing to the lateral or medial side of the heel, respectively. A shoe modified with a medial or lateral wedge may redirect forces on the knee.[28-35] Both the beveled and the resilient heel facilitate weight transfer from initial contact to midstance. The resilient heel also absorbs shock in the early stance phase. Rocker bars (Figure 22-4) also enable weight transition through the stance phase.[36,37] The apex of the rocker bar is posterior to the metatarsophalangeal joints. A metatarsal bar on the sole shifts weight posteriorly and, because the bar is rigid, reduces motion at the metatarsophalangeal joints. Heel and sole elevations reduce leg length discrepancy; when used by an individual who has length discrepancy and an immobilized knee, the lift lessens fatigue during walking.[38]

Ankle–Foot Orthoses

Plastic orthoses are lighter, more durable, and easier to clean than metal and leather alternatives.[15]

The foundation of an AFO is usually a plastic insert that conforms to the contour of the plantar surface of the foot. The insert is lightweight, compatible with any shoe having the same heel height as the shoe for which the insert was originally made, and easy to don. An insert foundation, however, requires that the patient wear shoes spacious enough to accommodate the insert. Although the shoe usually terminates below the malleoli, it should fasten relatively high on the dorsum to secure the orthosis to the foot.

The alternate foundation is a stirrup (Figure 22-5) riveted through the shoe sole, the shank piece, and insole. In addition to anchoring the orthosis, the stirrup ensures that, if the orthosis is worn, it will be used with a suitable shoe. The stirrup may be a one-piece solid stirrup for utmost stability or a split stirrup. The split stirrup consists of three portions, with the central part riveted to the shoe shank. The patient can don the shoe, then insert the side portions of the split stirrup in the central section. The split stirrup facilitates donning

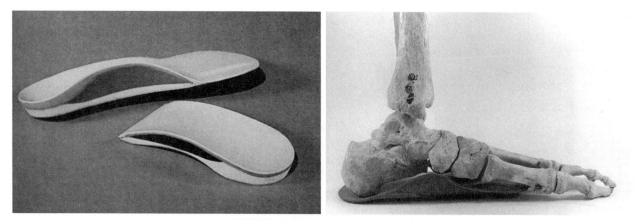

FIGURE 22-2 Longitudinal arch supports.

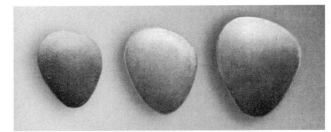

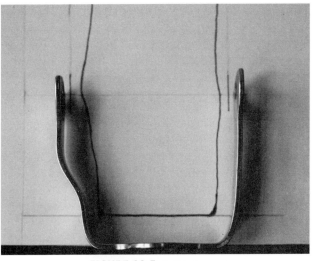

FIGURE 22-5 Solid stirrup.

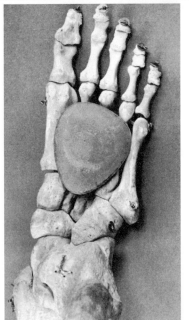

FIGURE 22-3 Metatarsal pads of various sizes.

because the shoe can be separated from the proximal parts of the orthosis; however, the split stirrup is heavier and bulkier than the solid stirrup and, in rare instances, the side portions may separate inadvertently from the central portion.

Ankle control is the primary purpose of most AFOs. The most common indication is inadequate dorsiflexion control during swing phase, which can result in toe drag with the risk of tripping. Dorsiflexion assist can be achieved with a plastic or carbon fiber posterior leaf spring (Figure 22-6). The spring recoils during swing phase, maintaining the ankle in the neutral position, yet allows slight plantar flexion during the early part of

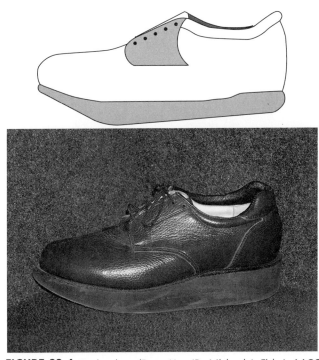

FIGURE 22-4 Rocker bar. *(From Hsu JD, Michael J, Fisk J: AAOS atlas of orthoses and assistive devices, ed 4, St Louis, 2008, Mosby.)*

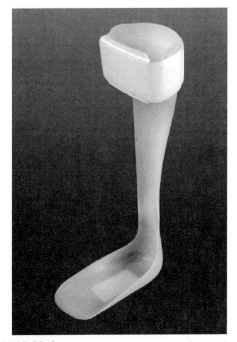

FIGURE 22-6 Posterior leaf spring ankle–foot orthosis.

stance phase, enabling the wearer to obtain a stable position.[39] A steel coil spring has the same biomechanical effect, namely, keeping the foot in neutral position during swing phase and permitting plantar flexion during early stance phase.[40] Tension of the spring can be adjusted with a screw. The drawback of the dorsiflexion spring assist is that it is part of a stirrup foundation.

Rather than spring control, the AFO may have steel or plastic plantar flexion stops that prevent plantar flexion throughout the gait cycle. The stop is simpler than the spring assist; however, it imposes a posterior moment of force on the knee in early stance. The knee, therefore, may flex excessively. Some AFOs have a steel BiCAAL (bichannel adjustable ankle control) joint (Figure 22-7) consisting of anterior and posterior coil springs or rods. The BiCAAL joint enables the clinician to adjust the angle of the orthotic ankle. Tilting the uprights into dorsiflexion aids knee flexion and shifts the wearer's weight forward. Tilting the uprights into plantar flexion has the opposite effect.

Some plastic AFOs have a solid ankle that restricts all foot and ankle motions.[41] Its trim lines are anterior to the malleoli. The solid ankle AFO is streamlined and relatively lightweight. A hinged plastic AFO (Figure 22-8) permits a few degrees of plantar flexion, reducing the tendency of the knee to flex in early stance; hinged orthoses also facilitate stair climbing.[42] Both the solid-ankle AFO and the hinged AFO resist untoward mediolateral and anteroposterior motion. The leather/metal equivalent is an AFO with a limited-motion ankle joint. All these

orthoses should be worn with a shoe with a resilient or beveled heel to facilitate the transition between initial contact and midstance. Propulsion in mid- and late stance is aided by a rocker bar that reduces the distance on the shoe sole through which the individual must pass body weight; stance phase virtually ends when body weight passes the apex of the rocker bar.

Hinged AFOs, however, are bulkier and more fragile than solid-ankle AFOs. A pair of limited-motion stops as part of a stirrup will also limit dorsiflexion and plantar flexion.

Foot control can be obtained with a solid-ankle AFO that restricts mediolateral, as well as sagittal and transverse plane, motions. An older option is a leather valgus or varus correction strap used with a stirrup. Valgus control requires a strap that is attached to the medial part of the shoe sole; the strap buckles around the lateral upright of the AFO, exerting a laterally directed force. If the strap is too tight, it will be uncomfortable and if too loose, will be ineffective.

Superstructure encompasses the portion of the AFO proximal to the foot and ankle controls. Vertical components of the superstructure may be one or two metal uprights, (Figure 22-9, A) whether medial, lateral, or bilateral. A posterior or anterior upright is plastic or carbon fiber. A plastic spiral or hemispiral upright assists dorsiflexion in swing phase and resists inversion during stance phase. A plastic shell covers the posterior half of the leg (Figure 22-9, B). The horizontal part of the superstructure is a band that usually covers the posterior

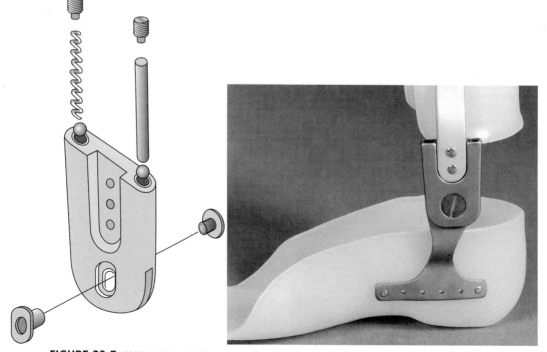

FIGURE 22-7 BiCAAL joint. Either a pair of springs or a pair of rods is located in the channels.

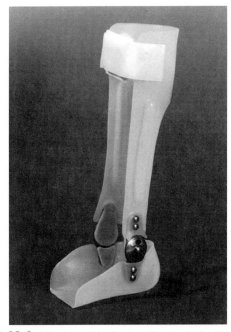

FIGURE 22-8 Hinged ankle–foot orthosis. Orthotic excursion adjusted by screw placement.

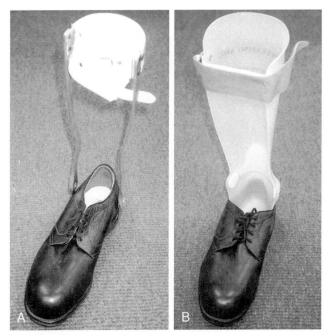

FIGURE 22-9 A, Ankle-foot orthosis with bilateral uprights, stirrup, and calf band is appropriate when limb volume fluctuates significantly. **B**, Thermoplastic hinged ankle-foot orthosis closely follows the contours of the limb minimizing contact pressure.

portion of the leg at the top of the upright(s) (see Figure 22-6). Some AFOs have an anterior band (Figure 22-10).

Knee–Ankle–Foot Orthoses

Choices for shoe foundation, ankle control, and foot control for KAFOs are the same as for AFOs. Most KA-FOs are prescribed to provide knee control in the sagittal plane, to prevent knee collapse, especially during early stance phase. An offset knee joint is a hinge with its axis located behind the anatomic knee axis. Consequently, when the wearer stands, the weight line passes in front of the hinge, stabilizing the individual's knee joint. The offset knee joint does not interfere with swing-phase knee flexion or sitting ease. The drawback is that if the patient walks on a ramp, the orthotic joint may no longer be stable. The most common knee control is a drop ring lock that, when engaged, ensures knee stability regardless of terrain. A steel ring surrounds the distal end of the thigh upright and the proximal end of the leg upright. A spring-loaded retention button prevents the ring from dropping inadvertently; the wearer must push the ring past the button in order to lock the knee hinge. A thigh-level release is a cord attached to the ring; the cord is secured on the lateral upright with a small handle at thigh level so that the wearer can unlock the knee joint without bending.

Individuals with poor balance may prefer a pawl lock with bail release (Figure 22-11). The pawl is a lever projecting from a small wheel in the lock. When the patient rotates the wheel, the pawl catches in the teeth of the lock. The bail is a spring-loaded posterior metal semicircular band connecting the medial and lateral

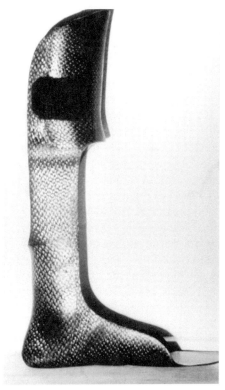

FIGURE 22-10 Ankle-foot orthosis fabricated with carbon graphite and fiberglass to provide maximum stiffness. The combination of a solid-ankle design and an anterior band produces a knee extension force to enhance stance phase stability.

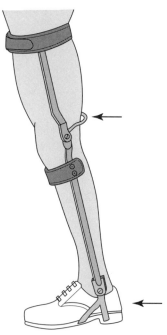

FIGURE 22-11 Knee-ankle-foot orthosis with pawl knee lock with bail release and infrapatellar band. *(From Hsu JD, Michael J, Fisk J: AAOS atlas of orthoses and assistive devices, ed 4, St Louis, 2008, Mosby.)*

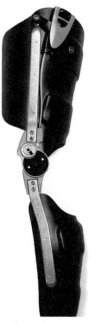

FIGURE 22-12 Swing phase lock system developed by Basko Healthcare in the Netherlands, marketed by Fillauer, Inc. Internal mechanism of the lateral knee joint triggers locking before initial contact then the knee is fully extended and unlocking at the end of stance phase. A medial knee joint that further resists flexion during stance can also be used. *(Courtesy Fillauer, Inc., Chattanooga, TN.)*

uprights at the level of the knee. The patient lifts the bail to release the lock. In its relaxed position, the bail engages the pawl lock. The bail locks the medial and lateral knee joints simultaneously and offers a much larger surface for the patient to grasp, as compared with the small drop ring lock. Both the pawl lock and the drop ring lock can be used only by someone with full passive knee extension.

Individuals with knee flexion contracture require an adjustable orthotic knee joint to accommodate the contracture. Both the fan joint and the serrated lock are readily adjustable. The ratchet lock also accommodates contractures. It also stabilizes the knee hinge in intermediate degrees of flexion, as when the wearer rises from a chair or moves from standing to sitting.

Recently introduced stance control units (Figure 22-12) provide stability during early stance phase, while allowing a more natural movement of the knee into controlled flexion during late stance and swing phase.[43-46] Some units have a cable connecting a foot plate and the knee hinge, whereas others have a locking mechanism within the knee hinge. The patient can select various modes, including stance control, full manual lock, and fully unlocked knee joint.

Regardless of knee hinge and locking mechanism, most patients also require one or two anterior bands or pad to resist knee collapse (Figure 22-13). The suprapatellar band (Figure 22-14) is a rigid plastic band over the distal thigh; the infrapatellar band (see Figure 22-11) lies just below the knee joint. A four-strap leather knee pad

(Figure 22-15) is buckled to the medial and lateral uprights. Although it also provides needed posteriorly directed force when the wearer stands, it may need to be loosened when the individual sits.

A few KAFOs provide frontal plane control either by means of a proximal extension from the medial or lateral side of a rigid plastic calf band, or by a five-strap leather knee pad (see Figure 22-15). The fifth strap is attached to a broad section on the medial side for valgus correction, or on the lateral side for varus correction. The narrow portion of the strap passes behind the knee and may press into the popliteal fossa.

Superstructure of the KAFO includes thigh uprights and one or two thigh bands connecting the uprights posteriorly. A weight-relieving band is a proximal thigh band designed to enable the wearer to support partial weight on the ischial tuberosity.

Hip–Knee–Ankle–Foot and Trunk–Hip–Knee–Ankle–Foot Orthoses

A pair of KAFOs is connected by a pelvic band. The HKAFO restricts hip rotation and abduction and adduction. If the hip joint(s) include a lock, the orthosis also restricts hip flexion and extension. Although these orthoses are occasionally prescribed for patients with low-level paraplegia, the orthoses are difficult to don and cumbersome to wear. The patient usually requires

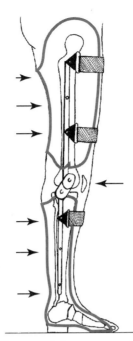

FIGURE 22-13 Diagram of the components and sagittal plane force system acting at the knee in a knee-ankle-foot orthosis.

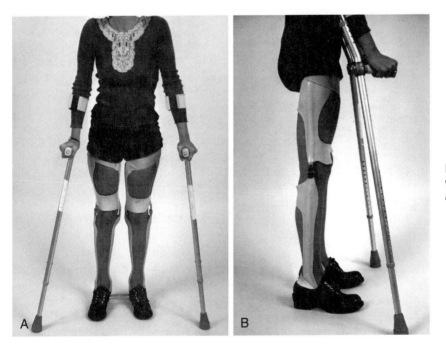

FIGURE 22-14 Knee–ankle–foot orthoses with suprapatellar bands. *A,* Anterior view. *B,* Lateral view.

crutches or other assistive devices when ambulating. HKAFOs are seldom prescribed for older adults.

If a trunk orthosis is added to a pair of KAFOs, the resulting orthosis is a THKAFO. The orthosis controls the paralyzed trunk and lower limbs. The wearer usually ambulates with a swing-to or swing-through crutch gait. Even heavier and more cumbersome than an HKAFO, the THKAFO is rarely used on a regular basis because gait is fatiguing and slow, and transferring from sitting to standing is awkward.

EVALUATING FIT AND EFFECTIVENESS OF AN ORTHOSIS

Before the patient dons the orthosis, the clinician should check its construction, with particular attention to confirming that the interior is smooth. Joints and locks should move easily.

On the sitting and standing patient, one should determine whether the shoe fits properly. The shoe should be slightly longer than the longest toe and as wide as the metatarsophalangeal region. The counter should fit the

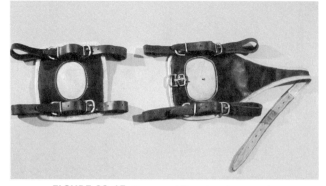

FIGURE 22-15 Four- and five-strap knee pads.

anatomic heel snugly. Any shoe modifications should provide the intended force.

If the AFO has ankle hinges, the medial hinge should be at the level of the distal tip of the medial malleolus and the lateral hinge at the corresponding level, parallel to the floor. This placement minimizes vertical shift of the orthosis when the wearer walks.[47] The calf band should lie below the head of the fibula to avoid pressure on this bony prominence and the adjacent peroneal nerve.

Key features of the KAFO are the placement of the orthotic knee joints. The medial joint should be slightly above the medial tibial plateau so that the orthosis does not interfere with sitting. The lateral joint is at the same height. The medial upright should not impinge on the perineum. The lateral upright should end below the greater trochanter. The top of the calf band and the bottom of the distal thigh band should be equidistant to avoid squeezing the wearer's leg when the individual sits.

When used by the walking patient, ankle restraint, such as that imposed by a solid ankle AFO, posterior stops, or limited motion stops, should contribute to a more secure gait pattern without excessive interference. With a KAFO, the knee control should not interfere unduly with swing phase. Afterward, the orthosis should be removed and the patient's skin checked to make certain that no blemishes attributable to the orthosis are present. Whenever possible, one should assess the patient's gait with and without the orthosis to determine whether the orthosis is beneficial. The ultimate outcome measure of orthotic effectiveness is whether the patient can walk farther and faster with the orthosis as compared with walking without it.

CLINICAL APPLICATIONS

Orthoses are used widely in geriatric physical therapy practice. Typically, the orthosis is part of the physical therapist's integrated management approach. The following section provides examples of typical situations in which a lower-limb orthosis can help older patients achieve their functional mobility goals.

Foot and Ankle Disorders

Changes in the foot and ankle with aging are common and frequently lead to pain and disability.[48-54] Both a 65-year-old plumber with traumatic arthritis due to recurrent ankle injuries and an 87-year-old homemaker with painful feet from age-related atrophy of the plantar fat pads and arthritic metatarsophalangeal changes may achieve increased comfort and stability during ambulation with a lower-limb orthosis.[55]

Foot deformities can negatively affect standing balance.[56-58] Rational selection of shoes contributes to walking stability, decreasing the risk of falling in older adults.[59-63] Individuals with poor balance should wear well-fitting shoes rather than slippers, which tend to shift on the foot during the transition from swing to stance phase. Walking at home with feet clad only in socks invites slipping.[64] Shoe soles should provide adequate traction and shock absorption. Overly thick soles, however, obscure proprioception. High heels also increase falls risk. Menant et al reported that a walking shoe with an elevated 4.5 cm square heel significantly impaired standing balance in older adults.[58] Horgan et al,[57] examining the effect of footwear on balance of 100 typically aging older adults (mean age of 82), concluded that walking in one's typical footwear is better than walking barefoot. No particular type of shoe was found most advantageous. The greatest balance advantage from wearing shoes was in those who had the poorest balance.

Toe deformities, such as hallux valgus, hammer toes, claw toes, and bunionette necessitate shoes with adequate space to accommodate the abnormalities. The upper should be made of soft leather to conform to the dorsal contour of the foot.[65]

Metatarsalgia usually results from persistently wearing high-heeled shoes.[16,18] The heels shift body weight anteriorly onto the forefoot. Atrophy of the plantar fat pad aggravates the discomfort. To the extent that the patient will allow, shoes with lower heels also reduce forefoot pressure. A metatarsal pad within the shoe shifts weight posteriorly, away from the painful metatarsophalangeal joints. A metatarsal bar on the sole combines the weight shift effect with reduction in painful motion.

Pes planus can be addressed with a longitudinal arch support.[19] The degree of orthotic firmness depends on the patient's comfort and body weight. An obese patient requires a more rigid support.

Diabetic peripheral neuropathy, if not conscientiously managed, can be a major catastrophe leading to amputation. Shoes should be well fitting with resilient insoles.[66-71] Hose must also be roomy enough not to constrict the toes. Regular foot inspection by the patient or, if vision is impaired, by a family member or health care professional, is critical to identify superficial abnormalities before they develop into ulcers. Because involvement of the intrinsic musculature is common in diabetes, the shoe upper must accommodate toe deformities, particularly hammer toes. A serious consequence of diabetic neuropathy is Charcot neuropathic joint, often at the ankle. Stabilization with an AFO is important to avoid uncontrolled ankle motion, which can lead to falls.

Osteoarthritis

Shock absorption is a major requirement for arthritic patients. Shoes with resilient insoles with or without supple outsoles absorb impact shock during walking.[72,73] Jannink et al measured plantar pressure and associated pain as 77 patients with degenerative foot disease walked; custom-made orthoses reduced pain in an average of 23% and plantar pressure by at least 9% across all weight-bearing surfaces.[73] Some individuals are more comfortable wearing shoes with heel or sole wedges to offset ankle or knee deformity. For example, the person with genu valgum would probably be more comfortable with medial wedges.

Knee orthoses may be worn by patients with knee OA to reduce load on painful knee joint structures. Brouwer et al,[74] in a systematic review of patients with knee OA, found moderately strong evidence indicating that people using knee orthoses walked for a greater duration than control subjects, and that this difference was maintained at 1-year follow-up. Despite the improved ambulation duration, which has very beneficial functional implications, there was no significant decrease in overall pain or improvement in perceived quality of life in the knee orthosis group. People with grades 1 or 2 OA, mostly medial compartment, did better, as did those younger than age 60 years.

Cerebrovascular Accident

Orthoses can offer patients who have sustained stroke both clearance during swing phase and stance phase control and propulsion. For example, a man with extensor synergy resulting from a stroke may have difficulty initiating stance phase with heel contact. An AFO would usually give him sufficient stability to resume a more stable gait pattern. The same person may also walk more safely when wearing an orthosis that counteracts the tendency of his paretic foot to drag during swing phase.

The shoe closure should be one that the patient can manage with one hand. A shoe on the paretic side with a hook and pile strap that can be cinched medially is often indicated.

The simplest way to enable swing clearance is by adding a ½ in. heel and sole lift to the shoe on the nonparetic foot; the lift also increases weight bearing on the paretic limb.[75] Although the lift is unlikely to disturb pelvic balance, the patient should be monitored for any indication of hip or back pain. A strap connecting the shoe closure to the anterior part of the ankle will also prevent the

paretic foot from dragging during swing phase. As compared with walking barefoot or with only shoes, patients who wore AFOs achieved longer stride lengths.[76] An AFO can either assist dorsiflexion or resist plantar flexion.[77] The posterior leaf spring AFO is a lightweight, relatively inexpensive option.

A more cumbersome AFO is one with a posterior ankle stop or an AFO with dorsiflexion spring assist. These orthoses have a stirrup foundation, adding weight to the orthosis and inconvenience to the wearer. If the patient has marked extensor synergy, the spring may trigger ankle clonus. Orthoses generally enable wearers to increase walking velocity and step length.[78-81] Two of these studies suggest that orthoses are more effective in the earlier phase of stroke rehabilitation rather than later.[79,80] With hinged orthoses, a full-length foot plate improved gait.[82]

Functional electrical stimulation (FES) can be used either as a temporary motor retraining device to enable the patient to learn foot clearance during swing phase,[83-86] or as a permanent means for day-to-day mobility.[85-88] Electrical stimulation is delivered by either a surface or an implanted electrode over the peroneal nerve. Typically, the patient wears around the upper leg a fabric band with an imbedded electrode. Some systems also include an ankle strap holding a floor reaction sensor. The clinician adjusts the stimulation that the patient receives. FES eliminates components within the shoe as well as an orthotic superstructure. When FES is combined with body weight support, preliminary clinical results are positive.[89,90] A systematic review indicates that walking speed increased 38% when a pooled effect was calculated across the eight studies in the review.[86] Other investigators found that subjects who obtained FES at least 5 years after stroke and who used stimulation for a year walked 50% faster than they did with a plastic or metal/leather orthosis.[87]

Peripheral Neuropathies

Some older adults have difficulty during swing phase because of traumatic or diabetic peroneal neuropathy. The same orthotic options that suit individuals with cerebrovascular accident are applicable, namely, contralateral heel and sole elevation if paralysis is unilateral; ankle-shoe strap, and an AFO that assists dorsiflexion or resists plantar flexion, especially the posterior leaf spring AFO. AFO use results in reduced dorsiflexor activity[91] and improved balance possibly associated with additional sources of sensory cues from the orthosis,[92] if shoe soles are not thick. Thick soles deteriorate balance by blunting somatosensory cues.[93]

Spinal stenosis with or without sciatic neuropathy affects swing and stance control because of pain and, occasionally, weakness. If reducing load through the affected lower limb by means of a cane or walker does not suffice, then a solid-ankle AFO or an AFO with a limited-motion ankle joint may improve the ease of walking by restricting painful motion.

Late-Onset Poliomyelitis

People who contracted poliomyelitis in the first half of the 20th century, before the advent of Salk and Sabin vaccines, combine age-related neuromusculoskeletal changes with ongoing deterioration of the anterior horn motor cells in the spinal cord.[94,95]

If the disease occurred in childhood, then the individual is likely to present both leg length and foot size discrepancy. To determine the extent of leg length difference, one should palpate the anterior superior iliac spines, posterior superior iliac spines, and iliac crests of the patient who stands on lift blocks under the shorter leg. When the lift causes the pelvis to reach a level position, the clinician should measure the height of the lift, which indicates the extent of discrepancy. The lift on the shoe should be approximately ½ inch less than the height discrepancy to facilitate swing of the shorter leg. Part of the shoe lift can be concealed inside the shoe. The exterior sole lift should have a rocker shape to aid in stance phase transition.

Foot size discrepancy should be managed so that each foot is well fitted. The patient has three options: (1) two pairs of shoes, discarding the shoes from each pair which do not fit; (2) one pair of mismatched (split size) shoes, which offer a relatively limited range of styles; (3) a custom-made insert for the smaller foot to fit into the larger, contralateral, shoe, which entails a one-time expense but enables the patient to purchase only one pair of shoes whenever new shoes are desired.

A frequent consequence of poliomyelitis is quadriceps paralysis. An AFO with a limited-motion ankle and an anterior band will resist knee flexion.[96] The band provides a posteriorly directed force just below the knee. The alternatives, namely a KAFO with knee locks or a KAFO with stance control joints, also prevent knee collapse. Loads on the orthosis are substantial.[97] These orthoses are more difficult than AFOs for the older person to manage.

An alternate sequel to chronic quadriceps paralysis is genu recurvatum. The older adult is likely to complain of pain in the back of the knee as well as knee instability. An AFO that limits plantar flexion will restrain the leg from shifting posteriorly. The AFO may have a solid ankle or a limited-motion ankle joint. A knee–ankle–foot orthosis (KAFO) with knee locks also protects the knee; however, the orthosis is cumbersome, heavy, and difficult to don.

OUTCOME ASSESSMENT

The effectiveness of orthotic intervention can be measured subjectively by patient satisfaction questionnaires and objectively by clinical parameters of gait efficiency and effectiveness and by laboratory measurement of oxygen consumption with and without the orthosis. Popular clinical tools that assess gait speed and/or distance walked, such as the Timed Up and Go test[98] and the 6-minute walk test[99,100] are appropriate outcome assessment instruments.

Decreased energy expenditure is a major goal of many orthoses. In the area of stroke, studies clearly demonstrate that energy expenditure per distance walked exceeded the oxygen cost of able-bodied adults by 37%.[101] Subsequent research confirms that adults with stroke who wore AFOs walked with greater speed and less energy per distance.[5-9] Changes in the 6-minute walk test are often used as a surrogate score for changes in oxygen consumption. Formal exercise testing of maximal oxygen consumption with and without an orthosis can be performed but may not add sufficient clinically useful information to warrant the increased effort and expense.

WORKING WITH AN ORTHOTIST

Cooperative interaction between physical therapists and orthotists is likely to foster optimum rehabilitation for all patients, particularly older adults. Usually, the patient is examined first by the therapist. A focused report highlighting the patient's musculoskeletal and neuromuscular status facilitates formulation of an optimum orthotic prescription. Ideally, the prescription will reflect consensus among the clinicians and will be acceptable to the patient.

Either the physical therapist or the orthotist should inform the patient regarding what to expect in the orthotic laboratory. The patient will probably select shoes that include features appropriate to the individual's needs. If a plastic or plastic/metal orthosis has been prescribed, the patient's foot and leg will probably be cast in plaster of paris. Multiple length and circumferential measurements of the involved limb will be taken regardless of whether the orthosis is to be plastic, plastic/metal, or leather/metal.

Most likely, while the orthosis is being made, the therapist will engage the patient in a program of therapeutic exercise designed to maintain or increase range of joint motion, muscle strength, standing balance, and cardiopulmonary endurance.

When the orthosis is finished, the therapist, together with the orthotist and other members of the rehabilitation team, will evaluate its fit and construction and the patient's function with it. The team will question the patient regarding comfort and overall satisfaction.

For the remainder of the rehabilitation, the therapist and orthotist should maintain good communication and mutual cooperation, so that any problems in fit or function can be addressed promptly, minimizing the time that the patient does not have the orthosis. A written record of issues relating to the orthosis facilitates communication. Working harmoniously, the members of the clinical team can enable the patient to achieve maximum function.

SUMMARY

Orthotic management can improve acute and chronic mobility limitations, which affect many older adults. FOs and AFOs are the most usual appliances that address foot deformities, spastic or flaccid ankle paralysis, and, occasionally knee disorders. KAFOs and higher orthoses are heavier, more difficult to don, and associated with higher energy cost during ambulation.

Prescription of an orthosis should be based on a thorough examination and evaluation of the patient, taking into account any previous experience the individual may have had with orthoses, as well as the patient's concerns about the utility and practicality of the appliance.

Orthoses, whether made principally of plastic, carbon fiber, or metal, apply forces to the body to limit or assist motion. The shoe is an essential component of all lower-limb orthoses. Many older people benefit from wearing an extra-depth shoe with a Blucher closure. The shoe may be worn with many combinations of inserts and internal and external modifications, depending on the therapeutic goal. AFOs consist of a foundation, ankle control, and superstructure; some patients also require foot control. KAFOs add knee control. Before the patient begins training with the orthosis, the clinician should evaluate its fit, function, and construction.

Clinical application of orthoses encompasses foot and ankle disorders, especially diabetic peripheral neuropathy, osteoarthritis, stroke, peripheral neuropathies, and late-onset poliomyelitis. For older people with disabilities, as compared with walking without an orthosis, the devices are associated with faster gait at lower energy cost. Cooperative interaction among the members of the clinical team, especially the physical therapist and the orthotist, usually affords the patient the best opportunity to improve function.

REFERENCES

To enhance this text and add value for the reader, all references are included on the companion Evolve site that accompanies this text book. The reader can view the reference source and access it online whenever possible. There are a total of 101 cited references and other general references for this chapter.

CHAPTER 23

Prosthetic Management for the Older Adult with Lower Limb Amputation

Carol A. Miller, PT, PhD, GCS

INTRODUCTION

Among the many challenges faced by older adults, the potential loss of ambulatory ability threatens independence as perhaps no other functional limitation can. One can only guess at the magnification of that threat when ambulatory abilities are compromised by lower limb amputation. The continued advancement in general medical care, surgical technique, and the development of more sophisticated prosthetic components provides many options for prosthetic use following amputation that were not available just a few years ago.[1,2] With these advancements, research studies are now better able to elucidate the range of potential functional outcomes for an older person after amputation.[1,3-9]

As a result of improved medical diagnostic testing, surgeons are more frequently able to save the knee by performing transtibial amputations and are also attempting through-ankle (Syme's) amputation, even with older adults with vascular disease.[10,11] The benefit of these distal amputations is decreased energy demand of prosthetic ambulation compared to more proximal or transfemoral levels of amputation.[12,13] Unfortunately, advances in surgical intervention do not always result in decreased morbidity and mortality, particularly in individuals who undergo lower limb amputation as a result of vascular compromise.[14-20]

Although the overall concept of prosthetic design has remained relatively unchanged over the past few decades, the prosthetic components being used to fashion prostheses have been regularly updated to accommodate improved technology and materials. For example, contemporary socket fabrication emphasizes lightweight material (carbon graphite) and endoskeletal design with gel liner suspension systems to improve fit and comfort; advanced knee units including sophisticated microprocessors, and an array of prosthetic feet accommodate different levels of function.[2,21,22] Researchers are only beginning to illustrate the effect of these new prosthetic components on function.[23-28] The impact of these prosthetic improvements on long-term lower limb prosthetic use and functional ability for the older adult with amputation remains unclear.

Each member of the multidisciplinary clinical team shares the responsibility for identifying key factors that affect successful prosthetic management and rehabilitation of older persons. The physical therapist, along with the entire prosthetic team, must incorporate into a prosthetic prescription a thorough understanding of the physiological changes associated with the amputation as well as the impact of comorbid conditions combined with normal aging-related changes to promote maximum patient satisfaction and long-term prosthetic use. In addition, knowledge about psychological readiness, appreciation of socioeconomic factors, and awareness of third-party payer systems for the older adult are essential to determine optimal prosthetic prescription and physical therapy intervention.

The overall goal of this chapter is to establish the scientific basis for clinical decision making by physical therapists regarding prosthetic management and rehabilitation of the older adult. Further, the emphasis of this chapter is on amputation as a sequelae of disease—not trauma or congenital deformity—because loss of limb from disease accounts for the vast majority of amputations among older adults.[10,29] Although there are many similarities between younger and older adults in prosthetic fabrication, fit, alignment, and training to use a prosthesis, critical differences in preoperative and postoperative physical therapy prosthetic management of the older adult are evident and highlighted in the chapter.[21,22,30,31]

AMPUTATION IN THE OLDER ADULT

Incidence

There are approximately 1.6 million persons living with limb loss in the United States, a number projected to increase to 3.6 million by the year 2050.[29] The annual incidence of amputation in an older adult population in the United States is also projected to increase from 28,000 to 58,000 per year by 2030.[3] The major causes for all lower limb amputations include dysvascular disease, trauma, malignancy, and congenital deficiency. Dysvascular disease is the most common cause for lower limb amputation in the older adult.[10]

Currently, the most common levels of surgical amputation secondary to dysvascular disease are transfemoral (25.8%) and transtibial (27.6%), with other lower limb levels such as toe(s) and transmetatarsal accounting for approximately 31% and 10.5%, respectively.[10,32] Other levels of amputation, such as hip disarticulation, knee disarticulation, and hemipelvectomy are much less common for the older adult with vascular disease. Transmetatarsal amputations as a result of ischemia or gangrene of the metatarsals may become a more common surgical approach in the future[11,16]; however, postoperative intervention requires the addition of an orthotic filler inside the shoe but does not require prosthetic intervention.

Amputation due to vascular disease (dysvascular) accounts for 82% of all lower limb loss hospital discharges,[10] which increased from 38.3 per 100,000 in 1988 to 46.92 per 100,000 in 1996.[10,29] This significant increase in dysvascular amputation rate (27%) in the United States is in stark contrast to the decreases (approximately half) in trauma and cancer-related amputations during the same decade of study.[10,29] In addition to the concern over an increasing incidence of lower limb amputation, the absolute number of older adults living with lower limb amputation is expected to continue to increase well into the 21st century, based on the aging of the U.S. population and the increased incidence of diabetes and dysvascular disease.[6,10,15,17,33,34]

Epidemiology

Risk factors associated with lower extremity amputation for the older adult include diabetes and poor glucose control,[17] renal disease,[10] peripheral vascular or peripheral arterial disease, nonhealing wounds with infection, neuroischemic ulcers, older age, male gender, and African American or Hispanic race or ethnicity.[10,14,17-19] Increasing age, especially those older than 55, constitute the largest proportion of individuals with disease-related lower limb amputations.[10,34,35] Men are at a higher risk than women for limb loss, especially for trauma-related causes.[10,34,35] Recent literature concurs that the risk of dysvascular-related lower extremity amputation is greater in African Americans[10,17] and Hispanics when compared to white non-Hispanic persons, even when factors such as age, sex, and presence of diabetes are controlled for in statistical analyses.[18]

An estimated 23 million people in the United States have diagnosed or undiagnosed diabetes, with nearly 52% of these individuals being older than age 60 years.[36] This means that approximately 23% of the U.S. population older than age 60 years has diabetes.[15] King et al predict that the number of people in the United States older than age 65 years with diabetes mellitus (DM) will increase from 13.8 million in 1995 to nearly 22 million in 2025.[37] Peripheral vascular disease (PVD) is the most common cause of lower limb amputation in older adults, particularly vascular disease associated with diabetes. Roughly 70% of all amputations are the result of either diabetes or PVD or a combination of both diseases.[10,14,17,19,38]

Impact and Outcomes (Morbidity, Mortality, Costs)

No one can doubt the serious medical condition of the individual who requires lower limb amputation. All domains of health are negatively impacted, including physical, social, and emotional. Dysvascular disease and diabetes mellitus are both associated with increased impairment and functional limitation among older adults, even those without amputation.[15,17] Leg amputation further affects function and productivity, and reduced quality of life.[39,40] A recent study found that only 25% of transtibial amputees older than age 50 years achieved community mobility,[41] whereas other studies note that transfemoral amputees have an even greater level of mobility disability and increased energy expenditure than transtibial amputees.[42,43]

Alarmingly, in a study on older adults with diabetes, the potential risk for reamputation per person occurred at the rate of 26.7% at 1 year, 48.3% at 3 years, and 60.7% at 5 years, whereas major lower extremity contralateral limb loss occurred at a rate of 11.6%, 44.1%, and 55.3% for 1, 3, and 5 years, respectively.[44] There is also a 20% to 50% risk of losing the contralateral leg due to vascular disease during the 5 years after amputation, which must be taken into careful consideration when considering prosthetic intervention.[17]

Reported survival rates following major lower extremity amputation vary across the literature and depend upon many factors, including the primary cause for amputation. A recent study found that the 1-year mortality rate was as high as 41% in a cohort of older adults with lower limb amputation.[20] When controlling for factors such as age, sex, race, level of amputation, and severity of comorbid conditions, the 1-year survival rate postamputation was greater in those who received inpatient rehabilitation (75%) immediately following acute hospitalization than for those who were discharged to home

(51%) or to a skilled nursing facility (63%). Other studies have reported that a 2-year survival rate after lower extremity amputation averages 50%, with most of the deaths attributable to cardiovascular complications.[14,45] High mortality rates following amputation in persons with diabetes range from 39% to 80% at 5 years.[19] Overall survival rates are significantly worse for individuals with transfemoral amputation (50.6% and 22.5%) than transtibial amputation (74.5% and 37.8%) at 1 and 5 years, respectively.[14]

The costs associated with prosthetic fabrication, fitting, and follow-up can also be substantial. A prosthesis for a person with lower limb amputation can cost thousands of dollars, yet many insurance policies, including Medicare, often only cover 80% of the total amount. In 1997, in an overview report on 15 persons with traumatic below-knee amputation, Lims noted that the mean number of prostheses per patient was 3.4 with a total prosthetic charge of $10,829 (range = $2558 to $15,700) during the first 3 years of wearing a prosthesis.[46] In a medical review of 545 individuals during the first 2 years postamputation, Mackenzie et al estimated the cost of providing a lower limb prosthesis using Consumer Price Index with constant 2002 dollars and found that the average total prosthetic cost was $12,885, ranging from $10,058 for below-knee prostheses to $21,199 for above-knee prostheses.[47] In another study of 935 amputees, it was noted that on average, 24% of all persons with dysvascular amputation reported being fitted with a new prosthesis at least once per year.[24] Today, the costs associated with some of the newer prosthetic designs, such as a transfemoral ischial containment socket with a microprocessor knee unit (C-leg) and dynamic response foot can increase the total cost of the prosthesis to greater than $40,000 (N. Kaselak CPO, personal communication, 2009).

Presently, many of the advances in socket design and components are not fully covered, which can be costly for the patient. Many older adults live on limited income in their later years, especially older women whose income after retirement is generally less than that of their male counterparts. According to Pezzin et al[24] approximately 40% of all persons with dysvascular or trauma-related amputations lived in poverty or near poverty levels when compared to other causes for amputation. The existence of poverty, more prevalent among older persons of racial and ethnic minority groups, may further prevent their ability to pay 20% of the medical bills incurred. Further, those who are underinsured may need other sources of income or support, such as community organizations, to subsidize prosthetic costs. Any of these factors can create financial hardship for the older person after amputation. Thus, the decision about which type of prosthesis, or even whether to provide a prosthesis, may become quite dependent on the older adult's socioeconomic status. In many of these situations, the clinician may choose to take on an advocacy role or make a decision to refer the patient to a skilled case manager for further support.

In summary, many of the medical and sociodemographic risk factors associated with lower limb amputation often mitigate against providing a prosthesis to an older adult. The health care practitioner must recognize, however, that it is critical to understand the interplay between risk factors for diseases, such as diabetes and vascular disease, and health habits that put the individuals at risk for other comorbidities. For example, the older adult at greatest risk for amputation, reamputation, and loss of contralateral limb has a history of diabetes with poor glucose control[17,44] and other modifiable risk factors, such as a history of smoking or poor diet habits that also increase the occurrence of PVD.[35,48] The practitioner must therefore focus on decreasing risk factors, in order to promote successful prosthetic outcomes. It is also essential to remember that the individual's goals, personal motivation, and premorbid status are often the strongest determinants of success with a prosthesis and that numerous studies demonstrate that many older adults with transfemoral or transtibial amputations do achieve functional prosthetic success.[5-9,49]

PROSTHETIC DESIGN

Numerous advances in the design of prosthetic components have occurred over the past few decades. The increased use of modern thermoplastics since the 1980s and more recently carbon graphite has resulted in the fabrication of many different types of prosthetic sockets. There are many changes in suspension liners, knee mechanisms, and ankle/foot designs. Generally, the use of endoskeletal components to reduce the weight of the prosthesis has increased. Many companies produce components targeting older adults. These components are typically made of aluminum, titanium, and other materials that allow for lighter prostheses. In addition, computerized programs such as contoured adducted trochanteric–controlled alignment method (CAT-CAM) and computer aided design–computer aided manufacturing (CAD-CAM) are available to assist the prosthetist in fabrication and follow-up fitting. The daily and long-term effects that these newer prosthetic modifications have on functional abilities yield equivocal results,[23,25,50,51] suggesting that optimal design may vary for different individuals and populations of amputees. A recent study demonstrated that the use and satisfaction with prosthetic limb devices increases among those with shorter timing to first prosthetic fitting and with those who had better communication with the prosthetist and team.[24]

It is well accepted that the prosthetic team must strive to achieve three essential goals in prescription, fabrication, and training: comfort, function, and cosmesis. Comfort must be addressed first and foremost, followed by function and then cosmesis. The prosthesis must provide comfortable containment of the residual limb tissue during the stance phase of gait and provide an effective means of transferring the amputee's weight through the pelvis and residual limb to the floor.[52]

The obvious impact of amputation on function and gait of a person with a lower limb prosthesis is easily attributable to the substitution of prosthetic parts for the normal skeletal segments and joints.[53] Prosthetic factors such as fit and alignment, the type of knee unit, and foot component have been demonstrated to influence gait parameters.[13,52,54-56] The fit, alignment, and adjustment of the prosthesis must provide maximal restoration of function to the amputee with minimal gait deviation, in both the stance and swing phase of a walking cycle.[52-54,57]

During normal gait, lower limb stance and swing phases occur as the result of precisely timed control of joint motion and muscle action. The lower limbs easily adapt to changes in walking terrain and naturally accommodate for obstacles, in which case, energy conservation is optimal. Lower limb amputation causes a loss of limb length; normal joint mobility; muscular control, and local proprioception, especially altering the precise awareness of foot contact on the floor.[58] Even with the many advances made with prosthetic components, the prosthesis at best can only imitate, but certainly cannot replicate, normal gait patterns. Thus, to date, the optimal prosthetic design regardless of the individual's age remains elusive. Because of the complexity of issues that surround the older adult whose health status necessitates an amputation, these seemingly simple primary goals of providing optimal comfort, function, and cosmesis continue to present the medical team with challenging clinical problems.

Components of the Prosthesis

Comprehensive texts[21,22,46,59-61] and recent articles regarding specific prosthetic components and prosthetic training[2,62] for diverse patient populations have been well documented and is beyond the scope of this chapter. To ensure that the patient can properly and safely use the prosthesis, the clinician must understand how the various sockets and components function. Different approaches to functional training are often dictated by the limits or advantages of the components used. Consultation and discussion with a prosthetist is extremely helpful to develop further appreciation of the various types of components most suitable to the older adult patient. Sequences for donning and doffing and the progression of functional training with the prosthesis are quite similar for the older adult and a younger person.

Most prosthetic adaptations are based on collaborative decision making between the patient and the clinic team. The prosthetic prescription should maximize independence in the use and management of the prosthesis, and should be as simple as possible, with components targeted for the potential functional level deemed most appropriate for the individual patient. The prosthesis should be fitted and aligned to maximize stability. A general rule regarding prosthetic prescription for the older adult is that the prosthesis should be lightweight, comfortable, safe, securely suspended, and easy to put on and take off.[63] Table 23-1 summarizes the functional levels that commonly guide prosthetic prescription. Examples of the more commonly prescribed lower limb prosthetic components are shown in Figures 23-1 to 23-3 and are also listed in Table 23-1.[64]

The socket is the most important component of the prosthesis because it requires intimate fit with the residual limb. Thus, socket fabrication and design may be more dependent on the comfort of the patient and the skill of the prosthetist. For example, the transtibial socket is usually patella-bearing, but may require higher walls for stability. Ischial containment sockets with flexible features are becoming more common for the transfemoral amputee rather than the rigid quadrilateral design. Although suction is the preferred method for suspension for achieving intimate fit, this is often difficult for the older adult amputee with conventional donning techniques.[33] Prosthetic donning with atmospheric suction requires the individual to stand and balance primarily on the sound limb, while bending downward to pull the parachute sock through a small suction valve located on the lower end of the socket. Many older adults may not be able to tolerate the amount of forward bend necessary, nor have sufficient hand strength to correctly don this type of suspension. Alternative types of liners and suspension systems, such as the "3-S pin system" (Figure 23-4) or roll-on gel liner (Figure 23-5) may be easier for an older person because the liner and sleeve systems can be initially donned in sitting and then the individual can stand with bilateral upper extremity support to safely secure the prosthesis.

With the transfemoral prosthesis, the knee joint should be reliable, stable, and simple to use. Newer knee joints that combine the features of weight-activated stance as well as polycentric and pneumatic control provide greater stability in stance phase.[2,33] Microprocessor knee units, such as Otto Bock's C-leg (see Figure 23-3), have been reported to decrease the risk of falling and increase confidence of walking.[26,28] The prosthetic foot should also be lightweight for an older adult. Again, all components should be considered durable, stable, simple, and cost-effective.[65]

Insurance Guidelines for Prosthetics

Insurance reimbursement guidelines for prosthetics are usually found with the rules that cover durable medical equipment. Insurance limitations or specific guidelines

---

TABLE 23-1   Potential Functional Levels for Prosthesis Use and Commonly Prescribed Prostheses for the Older Adult

Functional Level K0: Does not have the ability or potential to ambulate or transfer safely with or without assistance, and a prosthesis does not enhance their quality of life or mobility
No prosthesis is prescribed
Amputee Mobility Predictor Score (AMPnoPRO) less than 9.67

Functional Level K1: Has the ability or potential to use a prosthesis for transfers or ambulation on level surfaces at fixed cadence; typical of the limited and unlimited household ambulator
Suspension: Hip control with pelvic belt, Silesian belt, gel locking liner or lanyard for transfemoral; supracondylar or patella tendon bearing with gel locking liner or nonlocking "cushion" gel liner with suspension sleeve for transtibial; suction considered on a case-by-case basis (i.e., an experienced wearer who has always worn suction)
Socket: Ischial containment for transfemoral; patella tendon bearing total contact for transtibial
Socket Inserts/Liner/Sleeve: Locking or cushion gel liners (two per prosthesis)
Knee: Single axis, constant friction, stance phase lock, manual locking or polycentric
Ankle/Foot: SACH or single axis ankle/foot
Amputee Mobility Predictor Score (AMPnoPRO) greater than 9.67 and (AMPPRO) average score of 25.0

Functional Level K2: Has the ability or potential for ambulation with the ability to traverse low-level environmental barriers, such as curbs, stairs, or uneven surfaces; typical of the limited community ambulator
Suspension: Same as for K1, suction considered
Socket[a] and Knee: Same as for K1
Ankle/Foot: Flexible-keel foot or multiaxial foot, axial rotation unit, dynamic prosthetic pylon
Amputee Mobility Predictor Score (AMPnoPRO) greater than 25.28 and (AMPPRO) average score of 34.65

Functional Level K3: Has the ability or potential for ambulation with variable cadence; typical of the community ambulator who has the ability to traverse most environmental barriers and may have vocational, therapeutic, or exercise activity that demands prosthetic utilization beyond simple locomotion
Amputee Mobility Predictor Score (AMPnoPRO) greater than 31.36 and (AMPPRO) average score of 40.5

Functional Level K4: Has the ability or potential for prosthetic ambulation that exceeds basic ambulation skills, exhibiting high impact, stress, or energy levels; typical of the prosthetic demands of the child, active adult, or athlete
Suspension: Same as K1 and K2, suction optional
Socket: Same as for K1 and K2
Knee: Fluid, pneumatic, or computerized knee
Ankle/Foot: Flex foot or flex-walk system, energy-storing foot, multiaxial ankle/foot, dynamic response, shank/foot system with vertical loading pylon
Amputee Mobility Predictor Score (AMPnoPRO) greater than 38.49 and (AMPPRO) average score of 44.67

[a]Suction socket designs, such as the narrow medial lateral, CAT-CAM or CAD-CAM, ischial containment, flexible brim, etc.
Note: The AMPPRO and AMPnoPRO assess functional potential for unilateral amputee subjects with and without the prosthesis; bilateral amputees are tested with AMPPRO only. The total range for AMPPRO scores is 0 to 42 points. Total range for AMPnoPRO is 38 points. If using an assistive device, the subjects' potential total score possibilities increase by 5 points (to 43 and 47 points for the AMPnoPRO and AMPPRO, respectively).
SACH, single axis cushion heel
(*Adapted from the Region C DMERC DMEPOS supplier manual, Spring 2005.*)

for prosthetic socket design are not as restricting as those for component parts. Established insurance guidelines can often affect the patient's, the prosthetist's, and other clinic team members' decisions before a prosthesis is prescribed. As health care changes, with the possibility of increased managed care for all older adults, the clinical team will need to consider the particulars of the individual's health insurance benefits before prescribing the prosthesis. Third-party payers typically require a physician's prescription as a part of the reimbursement process.[30,66]

In the early 1990s, four regional medical directors for prosthetics, orthotics, and supplies collaborated with Medicare to develop criteria and coverage policies for prosthetic prescriptions. The most recent document

was updated in 2005 and is a detailed supplier manual for prosthetics and orthotics, whereby the four durable medical equipment regional carriers (DMERCs) follow the same policies for prosthetic prescription[64]; however, coverage and reimbursement for similar items may vary by region. The Centers for Medicare and Medicaid Services (CMS), which administers the Medicare program, approved these policies as an established set of guidelines that describe the type of lower limb prosthesis that may be covered based on the person's "potential" functional level. Functional level, defined by Medicare, is a measurement of the capacity and potential of the patient to accomplish their expected postrehabilitation daily function.[64] Originally, the guidelines did not include the word *potential*. This term was added to

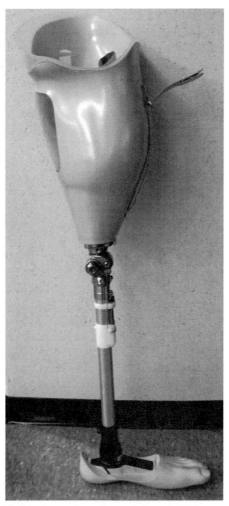

FIGURE 23-1 K2 Level: Ischial containment/flexible socket with gel liner lanyard suspension, weight activated stance control knee, and multiaxial foot.

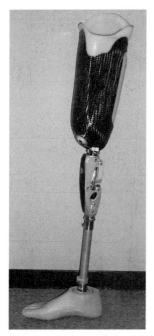

FIGURE 23-2 K3 Level: Ischial containment/flexible socket with lock-in liner, hydraulic knee unit, and dynamic response foot.

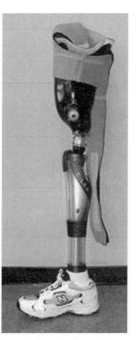

FIGURE 23-3 K3/4 Level: Ischial containment/flexible suction socket with neoprene secondary suspension, microprocessor knee unit (C-leg), and dynamic response foot.

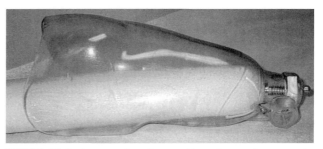

FIGURE 23-4 A suspension sleeve with a pin attachment on its end can be rolled onto the residual limb, requiring less fine motor hand function.

allow the clinical team greater decision-making autonomy in determining the likelihood of prosthetic success. Lower limb amputation potential functional levels from the *Region C DMERC Supplier Manual* for prosthetics is displayed in Table 23-1.[64]

Presently, the guidelines state that the determination of potential functional ability is based on the reasonable expectations of the prosthetist and the ordering physician that consider factors including but not limited to: the patient's past history (including prior prosthetic use if applicable); the patient's current condition, including the status of the residual limb and the nature of other medical problems; and the patient's desire to ambulate.[62,64]

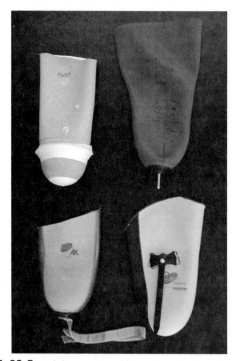

FIGURE 23-5 Gel liners. *Top (L)*, seal or lock-in; *top (R)*, pin system; *bottom (L)*, Velcro lanyard (KISS); *bottom (R)*, "latch-in" lanyard.

PROSTHETIC CLINIC TEAM

Composition, Roles, and Benefits

Typically, for individuals with lower limb amputation, the clinic team will include the patient, a physician (usually a physiatrist), a prosthetist, and a physical therapist. Each one of these members of the prosthetic clinic team contributes an important perspective. Other medical and rehabilitation specialists, such as the case manager, nurse, and psychologist, may be added to the team as needed to assist the older person to achieve optimal recovery after amputation. Unfortunately, the patient's role as a member of the team is often overlooked by the practitioners on the clinical team. Patient and family involvement are extremely important, and these members of the team should be present at each meeting whenever possible.

The physical therapist should provide the team with a thorough examination and evaluation of the patient before the prosthetic prescription. Further, the physical therapist must play a collaborative role with the team in discussing the functional activity level and mobility potential[64] for the patient related to prosthetic prescription. The initial part of the prescription process should involve all team members, including the patient. The prosthetist has particular expertise in the fabrication and alignment of the prosthesis. Further, the prosthetist will bring to the attention of the team knowledge of the most recent advances in components appropriate to the older adult. Continual consultation between the prosthetist

and the physical therapist ultimately creates a very effective means of caring for the patient.

Once the prosthesis is fabricated and fit to the patient, the physical therapist bears substantial responsibility for assisting the patient with adjustment to and acceptance of the device, along with continual assessment of fit and function, during all of the patient's activities of daily living. Finally, the physical therapist must maintain open lines of communication with the prosthetist so that modifications can be made based on the patient's physical performance and the fit and alignment of the prosthesis.

It is unfortunate that clinical teams may not be readily available to every patient with prosthetic requirements; this may especially affect persons residing in long-term care, assisted care facilities, and at home. Quite often for persons with amputation who reside in long-term-care facilities, the therapist initially learns of problems, such as changes in the person's ability to wear and use the prosthesis safely and effectively, from the nursing staff or family members or from an annual screening process. By this time, problems such as improper fit and decreased patient satisfaction may have resulted in a decline in functional abilities.[20] In settings where a clinic team is not readily available, the physical therapist may need to take the initiative to assist the patient and family in locating the originally prescribing prosthetist or consider outreaching for a nearby prosthetist willing to assist in patient consultation.

For the person living in the community, dissatisfaction with fit and function often arises when the patient obtains multiple prostheses from different prosthetists without adequate examination from rehabilitation experts or clinic teams.[20,24] Further, Lims demonstrated a reduction of about 20 days in inpatient hospital stay, a fivefold increase in percentage of patients discharged with prosthesis, and a threefold increase in the effectiveness of long-term rehabilitation over a 5-year period among patients who received team care compared with persons treated in environments without a clinical team approach.[46] Transdisciplinary teams functioning in a coordinated effort offer a sound way to identify and resolve the complex problems that accompany amputations, especially among the very young and very old.[2,21,67]

EXAMINATION CONSIDERATIONS RELEVANT TO PHYSIOLOGICAL CHANGES OF AGING, PROSTHETIC PRESCRIPTION, PROSTHETIC USE, AND REHABILITATION

The physical therapy examination should include a thorough history and systems review and objective tests and measures, with an overall emphasis on the patient's previous functional abilities, social responsibilities, and goals for the future (Box 23-1). The clinician is best able to identify goals and formulate a plan of care for successful

Physical Therapist Examination for Prosthetic Determination

I. Patient History
Medical diagnosis
Past medical/surgical history
Prior functional abilities
Patient's goals

Systems Review
Cardiopulmonary
Musculoskeletal
Neuromuscular
Integumentary
Cognitive/Emotional/Education
Other Systems (i.e., endocrine, gastrointestinal)

Tests and Measures
Pain: (type) residual limb pain, phantom sensation, or phantom pain
Range of motion
Muscle performance
Neuromotor development/Control of movement and coordination:
Integumentary integrity (involved and uninvolved side)
Sensory integrity
Anthropometric characteristics of residuum:
Vascular integrity
Functional mobility, locomotion, and balance

Ambulation   Device   Assistance
Distance   Cognition   Footwear

Evaluation/Physical Therapist Diagnosis
Plan for Prosthetic Prescription

II. Clinic Visits Examination
Device
Patient self-report
Gait deviations
Problem areas (include the prosthetic or patient problem and source)
Fit (document adjustments needed)
Patient/Family instruction (includes wearing time, skin inspection, gait, don/doff of device, exercise, other)
Footwear (includes shoe/sneaker—modifications needed):
Plan for follow-up

prosthetic rehabilitation by completing a comprehensive examination and applying sound knowledge of the influences of the cardiovascular, musculoskeletal, neuromuscular, integumentary, cognitive, and endocrine systems to evaluation of these data. Physiological changes in each of these systems can affect prosthetic fit and function; therefore, the examination information will be presented using a body systems–based approach. In this way, the therapist can organize multiple aspects of examination in relation to the influence that each body system has on prosthetic care for the older adult.

The physical therapist must also be prepared to include in the examination pertinent questions and selected tests to assist the clinician in determining whether prosthetic use is feasible. In 1985, Steinberg[49] recommended careful selection of patients appropriate for

prosthetic use by considering a detailed list of clinical concerns: cognitive dysfunction that interferes with training, advanced neurologic disorders, cardiopulmonary conditions severe enough to impose limitations on effort, ulcers or infections with compromised circulation, and irreducible and pronounced knee flexion contractures in below-knee candidates and hip flexion contractures in above-knee candidates. These factors continue to be identified as essential in the clinical decision-making process for determining an individual's prosthetic potential.[21,22,68]

Age alone does not predict older adults' ability to successfully use a prosthesis. However, age is a risk factor for increased mortality and less-than-optimal functional outcomes.[3,6] Older age has a well-established association with increased likelihood of above-knee amputation, greater incidence of bilateral limb loss, lengthened time necessary for successful rehabilitation, and increased number of comorbid health problems.[3,6,44] Individuals with amputation who have multiple comorbidities, especially diabetes and peripheral vascular disease, are at the highest risk for mortality and have the least success with rehabilitation.[6,14,19,20] Finally, psychosocial factors, such as diminished body image,[69] level of emotional readiness,[70] or the presence of depression and issues related to quality of life[4,71] may hinder prosthetic success in the older adult with lower limb amputation and should be addressed.

History, Systems Review, and Tests and Measures

The initial history and interview should address all essential elements of physical therapy practice,[72] including such items as general demographic information, family and social data, financial concerns, preamputation abilities, and prosthetic goals. The interview also needs to be directed toward the primary cause or causes for the lower limb amputation. For example, questions that specifically address the presence or absence of diseases such as diabetes or dysvascular disease, and lifestyle habits (i.e., smoking) associated with increased risk for lower limb amputation will provide critical information for directing physical therapy care. Further, knowledge of an individual's preamputation functional ability will also assist the physical therapist in guiding the examination and for determining a comprehensive plan of care that addresses patient and family goals.

Cardiovascular and Endocrine Systems

In the older adult with amputation, dysvascular disease is most commonly associated with complications from long-standing diabetes, such as peripheral neuropathy, nephropathy, and vascular conditions, particularly peripheral arterial disease. Therefore, for the purpose of comprehensive examination of the older adult with lower limb amputation, the cardiovascular and endocrine systems will be presented together.

Complications with diabetes, in relation to management of the older adult with amputation, more commonly occur when blood glucose levels are consistently elevated over time.[14,15,17] For the older individual with diabetes, it is important to ask the patient to monitor and report glucose levels at each and every physical therapy session. The need for consultation and referral to the patient's primary medical physician or endocrinologist is not uncommon while a patient is recovering from lower limb loss, as the amount of physiological stress placed on the body following major surgery such as lower limb amputation may make it difficult to initially control blood glucose levels.[73]

Microvascular, or small blood vessel, complications evident in retinopathy, nephropathy, and peripheral neuropathy are discussed under neuromuscular considerations later in this chapter. Macrovascular, or large blood vessel, complications of diabetes include atherosclerotic narrowing of blood vessels, which contributes to coronary artery disease, peripheral arterial disease, myocardial infarction, as well as cerebral vascular disease and stroke.[17,61,74] A significant implication of micro- and macrovascular disease is that the person with lower limb amputation and diabetes will have many more confounding risk factors that could increase demands on the cardiovascular system. Consequently, the medical conditions of these persons require careful monitoring by all members of the medical team to prevent undue stress to the cardiovascular system.

The systems review and initial examination should also include careful monitoring of all vital signs, particularly heart rate (HR) monitoring during all activities in the clinic. One of the best indicators of cardiovascular functional capacity is obtained through the measurement of the maximal oxygen uptake, or $\dot{V}o_2max$. Healthy older individuals in the 6th decade of life use 41% of their maximum aerobic capacity during walking.[43,75] Malatesta et al[76] confirmed these findings and further demonstrated that during all speeds of walking, $\dot{V}o_2 max$ was significantly greater in 80- and 65-year-old adults, when compared to 25-year-olds, at approximately 22% and 13%, respectively. Many studies have indicated that the energy costs of using a prosthesis are substantially increased over normal bipedal locomotion, with estimates ranging from 40% to 60% with unilateral transtibial amputation, 60% to 100% with bilateral transtibial amputation, 90% to 120% with unilateral transfemoral amputation, and more than 200% with bilateral transfemoral amputation.[6,43,55]

Most clinicians do not have access to equipment that measures $\dot{V}o_2max$; however, there is increasing evidence for use of cardiovascular tests, such as the 6-minute or 2-minute walk in individuals with amputation. The 6-minute walk test has been used by physical therapists to assess the quality and integrity of a person's cardiopulmonary response to activity in persons with nonvascular amputation.[12,43,55,77] Clinicians must also take into consideration that many older adults with vascular or diabetes-related amputation, particularly those with transfemoral amputation, cannot walk for a total of 6 minutes until much later in the rehabilitation process, and many others are never able to achieve this goal. For the older person with amputation who is able to complete a walk test, cadence and velocity are likely to be very slow to reduce the significantly increased cardiovascular stress of ambulation with a prosthesis. In light of this, the results of the 6-minute walk test have to be interpreted cautiously. Monitoring vital signs during arm ergometry exercise or with single-lower-limb bicycling[78] may initially offer the clinician an alternative for assessing cardiopulmonary integrity in these patients.

Interestingly, steady-state or resting energy costs for the older persons with amputation compared with a healthy adult of similar age are not significantly different.[12,43,76] As discussed, when compared with normal gait, persons using a lower limb prosthesis will demonstrate much slower walking velocity and cadence, with speed decreasing as level of amputation becomes more proximal. In effect, the person with a lower limb amputation seemingly slows down to reduce the stress on his or her cardiovascular system. Thus, when only the amount of oxygen utilization is compared between a healthy individual and one using a prosthetic limb, and time or distance is ignored, the oxygen utilization per meter can be essentially the same between the two individuals.

Prosthetic factors must also be considered during examination as energy requirements for using a lower limb prosthesis have been a major concern for decades. In earlier years, prostheses were not prescribed for the older adult because of the extensive demands on the cardiovascular system. In the past 2 decades, prosthetics have increasingly moved toward lighter endoskeletal components, especially for the older adult. Newer components, such as hydraulic knee units,[25,28] microprocessor knee units,[55] and dynamic-response prosthetic feet have shown improvements in energy consumption over early design components, even in individuals with dysvascular amputations.[12,13,27] Lighter-weight prostheses, specially fabricated for the older adult ambulator, have been marketed by many different manufacturers; however, the effect of these lighter components on reducing stress to the cardiovascular system remains to be fully studied.

Foremost for the clinician, knowledge of energy cost and oxygen utilization requirements is necessary to formulate an intervention with the appropriate exercise frequency, duration, and intensity. Careful attention should be paid to appropriate intensity of cardiovascular exercise before, as well as during, gait training. Allowing the person with amputation a longer period of time to perform a task and encouragement of slower or more comfortable speeds for gait also may prove helpful.

Musculoskeletal System

With each ensuing decade of life past the middle years comes an increased likelihood of postural changes , even in the absence of disease.[79] Although the precise etiology of these changes is unknown, most often postural change is associated with inactivity and decreased mobility, which has been shown to improve with exercise and adapted physical activity.[79,80] The most common types of postural changes in the lower limb joints of older adults are increased flexion at the hips and knees and loss of dorsiflexion at the ankle. In addition, physiological changes that occur with aging of the musculoskeletal system, such as decreased connective tissue extensibility, decreased muscle strength, and muscle imbalance further promote these postural problems and may limit the effectiveness of the physical therapist's intervention. Depending on the surgical technique employed, removal of the lower limb will create extensive changes in bony alignment and muscle attachment, which in turn will further affect posture and postural control in sitting and in standing.

The musculoskeletal systems review and examination should include pertinent testing of range of motion and lower limb muscle length, strength testing of the trunk and extremities, and posture in both sitting and standing with and without the prosthesis. Extremity and trunk strength, collected through standard manual muscle testing, will be essential for determining the patient's needs for assistive devices in both the pre and prosthetic gait phases of recovery. Postural examination, especially in standing, is important to record and relate to dynamic gait control and function. Range of motion, muscle length and strength for major lower extremity movements should also be assessed.

Girth measures for the residual limb should also be recorded at the distal end and approximately every 2 in. up toward the knee for the transtibial level or greater trochanter for a transfemoral level. These measurements will assist in determining the size for a shrinker (Figure 23-6), an elastic sock-like garment used instead of an ace wrap for control of edema and for shaping the residual limb. A shrinker is generally prescribed once the stitches or staples are removed and will be fitted by the prosthetist. Girth measures should be taken regularly, as limb volume must be relatively stable prior to considering initial prosthetic fitting. Referral to the prosthetist is warranted if the shrinker becomes too loose or too tight as a result of volume change. A properly fit shrinker is essential to effectively control residual limb edema and shape.

Lower limb joint contractures can negatively affect functional outcomes, influence prosthetic fit, alter postural alignment in stance, and contribute to poor gait patterns. Contractures can even prevent ambulation and use of a prosthesis. Most contractures are the result of muscle imbalance, especially after the surgical division

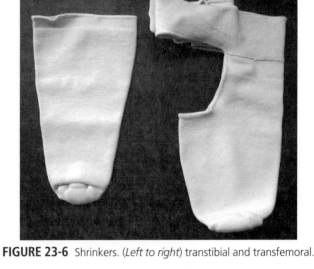

FIGURE 23-6 Shrinkers. (*Left to right*) transtibial and transfemoral.

of muscles, previous impairment, or long-standing poor postural habits. Hip flexion, abduction, and external rotation contractures may occur in a patient after transfemoral amputations, with hip flexion being the most common in this patient group. Hip flexion, abduction, external rotation, and, most commonly, knee flexion contractures may develop as a result of transtibial amputations.

Generally, knee flexion contractures of no more than 10 to 15 degrees for below-knee amputations and hip flexion contractures of no more than 15 to 20 degrees for above-knee amputations can be readily accommodated for in the fabrication and fit of the prosthetic device. Although persons with contractures greater than these can be fitted with prostheses, gait patterns may become more significantly altered with increased deformity. Contractures greater than those identified above may also inhibit safe ambulation and diminish an individual's ability to maintain safe static and dynamic postures.

To promote the ability to transfer and provide acceptable cosmesis, a prosthetist is often able to modify the prosthesis for a person with transtibial amputation and accommodate knee flexion contractures as great as 35 to 40 degrees. In addition, even in the presence of these more significant contractures, some patients have been able to successfully ambulate with a modified prosthesis and an assistive device. Therefore, impaired muscle length or soft tissue extensibility should not necessarily deter the patient or clinician from pursuing a prosthetic fit. Other modifications in prosthetic design, such as the "bent knee" prosthesis, have been used in the presence of extreme knee flexion contractures, sometimes as large as 70 to 90 degrees. However, poor cosmesis is often a problem in these cases and may discourage long-term use of the prosthesis. A walker can also be adapted by adding a weight-bearing surface (seat) that allows the individual with a transtibial amputation and significant knee, and possibly hip, flexion contracture a means to ambulate without the prosthesis.[81]

For the person with transfemoral amputation, it can be quite difficult, if not impossible, for the prosthesis to accommodate a hip flexion contracture greater than 25 degrees and allow for safe ambulation without the use of an assistive device. Stability during the gait cycle can be significantly compromised, resulting in decreased safety and increased risk for falls. With significant contractures at the hip, a prosthesis is not generally provided, even to assist with transfers. If requested by the patient, a prosthesis may be provided to improve cosmesis.

Prevention of these deformities from the outset is the best intervention and should be emphasized throughout the rehabilitation process. Along with patient education, early postoperative management should include stretching and strengthening the remaining lower limb joints and muscles as well as proper positioning to reduce the chances of developing contractures.

Neuromuscular System

In a systematic review of literature, van Velzen et al[81] found that among many physical capacity factors affecting function in amputees, there was especially strong evidence relating balance to walking ability in those persons using lower limb prosthetics. With this in mind, a comprehensive neuromuscular systems review and tests should include the measurement of sensation, motor control, coordination, tone, balance, and locomotion ability, including gait.

Peripheral neuropathies may result from microvascular changes seen with peripheral vascular disease (PVD) but can also be attributed to diabetes alone. Altered sensation in the distal parts of the extremities, especially the hands and feet, is noted in the presence of PVD and in clinical diabetic neuropathy.[74] Any areas on the body with diminished sensation, especially due to diabetes or PVD, can potentially increase a patient's risk of developing bruises, ulcers, and other skin problems. In the long term, this patient may experience additional detrimental consequences, including further loss of limb or loss of the contralateral limb. Prosthetic fit and comfort can be particularly difficult if sensory feedback in the residual limb is affected.

The examination should also include a thorough assessment of pain, to help distinguish the type experienced by the patient and relate the symptoms to the cause of pain.[1,2,6] For example, pain following amputation may be associated with the surgical procedure itself, which is referred to as residual limb pain. Other sensory perceptions of pain or phantom sensation may be expressed as a tingling or numbness in the removed part of the limb. Phantom sensations are often intermittent and respond well to gentle tapping or rubbing as well as limb wrapping (ace wrap or shrinker) and consistent daily use of the prosthesis.

The most difficult type of pain to ameliorate with prosthetic intervention is phantom sensation of pain, a perception of pain in the missing limb that is usually reported as severe, constant burning, cramping, and sharp in nature. The exact mechanism of phantom limb pain remains unclear; however, it is thought to involve disruption in peripheral, spinal, and central nervous system processes.[82] Traditional theory suggests that generated impulses from the affected limb are sent through peripheral and spinal nerves to the thalamus in the somatosensory areas of the brain, causing abnormal sensation.[62,82] Phantom limb pain following amputation is also thought to be the result of abnormal reorganization of the central neuromatrix, which holds past sensory experience in the brain for each body part.[82] Biopsychosocial factors such as depressive symptoms, pain coping mechanisms, cognitive beliefs, and social environmental factors such as social support are also related to long-term adjustment to phantom pain.[83] There are no known prosthetic adaptations that address phantom pain; however, physical therapy interventions, such as transcutaneous electrical stimulation (TENS), ultrasound, ice, and mirror-box therapy have been documented to reduce phantom pain.[1,2,6,21,84]

Peripheral neuropathy, a diabetic complication that ensues over longer periods of time, may also contribute to atrophy of the intrinsic musculature of the hands and feet. Depending on the severity, intrinsic muscle wasting in the hands can affect grasp and may prevent independent donning and doffing of the prosthesis without modification. Hand function, especially grasp, should be tested and documented as a part of the physical therapist's initial examination. Finally, retinopathy, which is often present with microvascular disease, and other aging-associated visual problems such as cataracts and glaucoma, can greatly affect vision and may impede independence in prosthetic donning and doffing without modification.

Prosthetists often are able to make different types of prosthetic modifications to accommodate decreased hand function and impaired vision. Simple modifications can be made to partially accommodate decreased hand dexterity. Today, the most commonly prescribed suspension systems utilize either a roll-on gel liner with pin suspension, or "lock in liner," or a liner with a lanyard system (see Figures 23-4 and 23-5).[59] These newer types of suspension sleeves can be easily rolled onto the residual limb using the heel of the hand, thus requiring less fine-motor hand function. In the pin system, the sleeve is simply inserted into the prosthesis until audible clicks are heard for safe attachment of the prosthesis; a gentle push on the locking mechanism easily releases the sleeve. With the lanyard system, once the sleeve is on, the Velcro strap is pulled through the socket and secured or released to attain adequate suspension. The newer types of suspension systems may also be easier for an older adult with visual impairment. A few factors that may deter the use of the gel liner system include increased difficulty in prosthetic fit, need to still use socks over the sleeve in the event of limb shrinkage during the day, increased fabrication costs, and a potential development of skin allergies from the liner material.

Intrinsic muscle atrophy in the unaffected lower extremity can also influence lower limb alignment and the joint integrity and soft tissue structure of the remaining foot, resulting in greater risk of damage due to trauma. Consultation with an orthotist is recommended in these cases to provide orthoses or other types of accommodative footwear that may reduce trauma and, if possible, delay further excess strain on the muscles of the unaffected lower limb.

The result of limb dysfunction secondary to cerebrovascular accident (CVA), another commonly occurring condition in older adults with macrovascular disease, may affect the person's ability to control the prosthesis if worn on the involved side. Changes in muscle tone, loss of range of motion, weakness, and decreased coordination associated with CVA can also have effects on the contralateral extremities and must be carefully examined. The ability to perform coordinated tasks in a specific sequence is essential for prosthetic donning and doffing as well as functional performance. Few, if any, prosthetic modifications can accommodate for these types of problems. Unfortunately, when the impairments and functional limitations are substantial as a result of a CVA, the patient is typically not considered a strong candidate for safe prosthetic use.

In the past decade, there have been an increasing number of tests implemented to measure motor control, balance, and gait in individuals with amputation, across multiple age groups, levels of amputation, and those with amputation related to nonvascular and vascular disease.[77,85-89] The Timed "Up & Go" (TUG) test,[89] Activities Specific Balance Scale (ABC),[87,88] the L Test of Functional Mobility,[85] and the Amputee Mobility Predictor[86] (AMP with or without prosthesis) have been shown to be reliable and valid instruments for assessing balance and gait function in older adults with amputation. The Amputee Mobility Predictor (AMP)[86] is specifically designed to assess balance, transfer ability, and gait ability in the individual with amputation. The AMP is unique in that the instrument can be implemented with or without the prosthesis and effectively predicts the Medicare guidelines for functional classification level (see Table 23-1), based upon scores achieved on the instrument.[77,86] Therefore, this instrument can be effectively used to assist the clinical team in determining the prosthetic components needed to match the functional ability of the patient.

As already noted with more advanced cardiovascular testing for older adults with amputation, many individuals may not be able to perform these neuromuscular functional tests until much later in the rehabilitation process; furthermore, it must be recognized that many older adults will not be able to complete them at all.

Integumentary System

In essence, the only skin surface on the human body designed to tolerate weight bearing is the plantar surface of the foot. By virtue of the design of lower limb prostheses, one must consider the impact of weight-bearing forces on the skin and soft tissue of the residual limb. Examination of and the promotion of healthy skin integrity is critical because wearing a prosthesis requires an intimate fit between the socket and the person's residual limb. An essential part of clinical examination and management of the patient with lower limb amputation requires careful monitoring of the patient's skin condition before, after, and throughout prosthetic training. Teaching compensatory techniques, such as using a handheld mirror to clearly see the entire residual limb along with careful monitoring of skin condition will reduce the risk of skin damage to all areas affected by sensory loss.

Aging-related skin changes occur and are influenced to varying extents by gender, race, and health conditions. Much more research is needed to accurately delineate the impact of integumentary changes on prosthetic use by older adults. Some aging-related changes in skin that likely affect skin tolerance for prosthetic use include atrophy and fragility of the dermis, decreased solubility and stiffness of collagen, decreased elasticity, reduced viscosity, less eccrine and apocrine sweat, and regression and disorganization of small vessels.[90] The skin's ability to resist shearing forces is especially compromised with aging. Clinically, this is often seen as skin tears, which can easily occur at any interface between the residual limb and the prosthesis.[91] Persons with diabetes or PVD are particularly vulnerable to decreased sweat gland function, decreased tolerance to shear forces, and decreased skin structural stability secondary to a compromised microcirculation.

It is also important to consider the problem of decreased sweat gland function because the gel liners and socks worn within a prosthesis can be extremely warm and often hot. Alteration in perspiration within the socket can result in skin conditions such as folliculitis (inflammation of the hair follicle) that may result in pain and discomfort. If this condition persists, prosthetic use must often be temporarily discontinued, which has significant impact on the person's functional abilities. Patient education regarding personal and prosthetic hygiene and consultation with the prosthetic team are encouraged.

To understand the appropriate timing to schedule prosthetic fitting and initiate safe progression of prosthetic use, the clinician needs to be aware of normal wound healing for the older adult, including wounds that occur through surgical intervention. Wound healing is age dependent[92] but does follow the classical inflammatory, proliferative, and remodeling phases often at a delayed or slowed rate in the older adult.[93,94] PVD and diabetes can delay healing time for surgical wounds. The tensile strength of healing wounds as defined by the force required to disrupt wounds is decreased in persons older than 70 years.[33,95] The distal end of the limb, especially along the scar line, is most vulnerable to damage. Wound dehiscence can occur if fit is improper or if excessive stress is placed on the incision site, particularly when wearing the prosthesis in the early phases of postsurgical rehabilitation. Edema reduction or control of volume of the residual limb may be difficult because of the presence of circulatory disease. Volume changes in the residual limb affect its shape and size, ultimately influencing the type and timing of initial and final prosthetic fit.

Considering the skin changes and longer time for wound healing in older adults, particularly those with vascular disease, the therapist must be certain that the wound is completely healed before initiating training with the prosthesis. Depending on scar healing, prosthetic fitting can possibly occur as early as 3 to 4 weeks post transfemoral amputation, and 5 to 6 weeks post transtibial amputation; however, the average time to prosthesis fitting is generally longer. Lilja and Oberg, using residual laser scanning to assess limb volume changes with 11 older patients with dysvascular amputations, concluded that 3 months postsurgery was a safe approximate of average time for fitting a transtibial prosthesis.[96] In a recent study of 1538 adults, ages 18 to 84 years, Pezzin et al[24] reported that, although the average time from surgery to initial prosthetic fitting varied somewhat by etiology of the lower limb amputation, the average time from surgery to initial fit was between 5 and 6 months. Early or immediate postoperative fitting is sometimes attempted but is not commonly recommended for the older adult because of the nature of amputations.

The most commonly prescribed prosthetic sockets are made of rigid materials that do not readily yield under forces during activities such as gait. Pressure and stability requirements are in opposition within the prosthesis, where a rigid support is required for stabilization during weight bearing, but a soft support is important to reduce pressure on soft tissue and enhance proprioception.[97] The material of the socket and the alignment of the prosthesis have been shown to increase the shear forces and pressure on the residual limb within a socket.[57,98] Flexible sockets are now more commonly prescribed for the older adult. However, although this socket design is more expensive and complex to fit, its increased flexibility reduces shear forces on the skin, making it more comfortable.[21,51,59]

In the past, residual limb socks or liners, made of materials such as cotton and wool, were worn directly over the skin to create a more intimate fit within the nonsuction socket. Today, synthetic gel liners made of silicone are much more commonly prescribed, and if necessary, socks can be worn over the liner to achieve a snug fit within the socket if there are changes in limb volume secondary to edema.[21,51,59] The gel liners, such as alpha liners, Silipos sleeves, among many others provide cushioning to the residual limb within the socket, may be helpful in reducing shear on the residual limb and providing more uniform pressure. In turn, hopefully, improved comfort is achieved, especially for the older person with fragile skin.

One concern is that the materials used in the newer liners or socket fabrication materials may cause allergic reactions in the form of a rash or dry irritated skin[25]; therefore, skin condition must be monitored carefully. As with other prosthetic modifications, research regarding the effectiveness for preventing skin breakdown and improving comfort and function in the older amputee is clearly needed.

Finally, it is important to examine the skin integrity of the contralateral limb as we are reminded that the risk for loss of the contralateral limb or need for higher levels of amputation is great in older adults with dysvascular disease. Changes in the quality of lower limb pulses (weak, normal, strong/bounding) when compared to the same vessel on the sound limb; presence of edema; and any alterations in the amount of hair, color, and degree of warmth should be documented. Padding areas of the prosthesis, such as over any rivets used for suspension mechanisms or over prominent areas of the socket wall or ankle/foot components, may be needed to reduce the risk of tearing skin on the uninvolved limb.

Cognitive System

Although intellectual ability is normally maintained well into the mid-70s or later, other aspects of cognitive function, including the speed of memory processes and abstract thinking, decline with age.[99,100] Cognitive changes, if present, can have significant implications for an older individual's ability to incorporate new skills in motor behaviors to replace lost abilities.[33,100] Chapter 8 provides a detailed summary of mental and affective tools to assess cognitive function in older adults. Memory, attention, concentration, and organizational skills are necessary for effective use and maintenance of a prosthetic limb.[101,102]

If cognitive changes are present, all members of the health care team, and especially the physical therapist, must actively become involved in consistent, ongoing education. Repetition of tasks may prove helpful for the patient and family to learn new tasks such as donning and doffing of the prosthesis. Even patients with minimal to moderate cognitive impairments have learned to use a prosthesis with consistent repetition in a structured environment.

ESTABLISHING A PHYSICAL THERAPY DIAGNOSIS, PROGNOSIS, AND PLAN OF CARE TO GUIDE PHYSICAL THERAPY REHABILITATION

Lower limb amputation as the result of disease is associated with multisystem failure that will require comprehensive multidisciplinary intervention. Further, for older adults, lower limb amputation may be just one of many losses across many aspects of their life. The individual may be experiencing role loss due to a loss of work or ability to participate in other meaningful activity, financial stresses as a result of retirement, increasing dependence from the physical challenges of the amputation combined with aging and comorbid health conditions. The inability to deal with all of the biological, social, and functional losses due to amputation may potentially lead the individual toward despair, depression, and withdrawal from society.[71]

In regard to diagnosis, the very nature of a major surgical amputation will significantly affect most, if not all, of the primary body systems considered in the physical therapy examination, but will most directly affect the musculoskeletal, integumentary, and neuromuscular systems. Considering the primary cause for amputation in the older adult, dysvascular disease, the therapist will often need to consider secondary diagnoses related to cardiovascular disease and endocrine system compromise, specifically diabetes-associated impairments. Using the *Guide to Physical Therapist Practice*,[72] most individuals with a primary diagnosis of lower extremity amputation will fall under "Pattern 4J: Impaired Motor Function, Muscle Performance, Range of Motion, Gait Locomotion, and Balance Associated With Amputation." If the patient also has significant dysvascular disease, then a second pattern may be used, such as "Pattern 6D: Impaired Aerobic Capacity/Endurance Associated With Cardiovascular Pump Dysfunction or Failure." Considering the significant intimacy of prosthetic wearing on the integumentary system, a third pattern may also be required: "Pattern 7A: Primary Prevention/Risk Reduction for Integumentary Disorders."

Factors Relevant to Prognosis

In order to effectively implement a plan of care, the physical therapist will need to comprehensively consider all essential findings from the examination as it relates to the potential for recovery. These findings should collectively reveal a patient's sense of health and well-being across multiple domains, including physical, psychological, and social health. Awareness of epidemiologic data regarding morbidity and mortality along with sound knowledge of prosthetic requirements for function must also be taken into account in order to successfully predict functional potential and recovery for the older adult with lower limb amputation.

Psychosocial Implications and Rehabilitation

Psychosocial issues relevant to successful prosthetic management warrant careful consideration of an individual's readiness, cognitive status, and extent of depression, if present.[71] In some cases, the influence of the involvement of significant others or family is a key determinant of successful prosthetic use. The cost of obtaining and learning to use the prosthesis may pose a significant financial burden to the patient and family and therefore must be considered.

Most importantly, the patient must have a desire to use the prosthesis. The loss of a limb is almost always considered initially devastating by the individual, and this perception exists regardless of age. A person's evaluation of his or her body image can both positively and negatively influence self-esteem, anxiety, and depression.[69,71,103] Specific education about the advantages and disadvantages of using a prosthesis for cosmesis, functional activities, and ambulation may assist the patient and others involved to understand the scope and limitations of the rehabilitation outcomes expected for that individual. Support groups, peer visitors, or volunteers who can demonstrate different prosthetic components and their level of success are sometimes psychologically beneficial to the patient who is preparing to use a prosthesis. Because psychological readiness is so extremely important to outcome, the patient may require psychological intervention before or concomitant with the physical therapist's intervention.

Rehabilitation professionals need to be aware of their own biases against older adults, particularly older adults with disabilities and chronic conditions who may be noncompliant or depressed. Rybarczyk et al,[104] in a well-devised study of nearly 1000 rehabilitation professionals, found that perceptions of the "ideal" younger patient and "ideal" older patient with an amputation were quite similar. However, if the same generic patients were identified as depressed or noncompliant, then the rehabilitation professional had a more negative reaction to the older patient and deemed the older patient less "worthy" of rehabilitation than the identically described younger patient.

Prosthetic Factors Influencing Prognosis and Rehabilitation

It is important to remember that many studies show that a high percentage of older adults discard their prosthesis within months or the first year of training.[6,40] Rehabilitation after the loss of the second limb is more likely to be successful if rehabilitative efforts were successfully undertaken after the loss of the first limb.[23] Intensive rehabilitation efforts by an interdisciplinary team have shown positive outcomes for use of a prosthesis and functional success,[31,46] particularly intensive inpatient rehabilitation.[6,31,40,46] Inpatient rehabilitation has been demonstrated more effective than care at home alone.[20] Finally, based on what has been reported in the literature, the physical therapist must remember that successful use of a prosthesis is multifactorial, with complex and imprecise predictors of success.[40,105]

With increasing frequency, persons postamputation are being discharged to home directly from acute care. Home health services provide follow-up care, with or without physical therapy involvement, until wound healing is complete and the patient is ready for prosthetic fitting. For the person with lower limb amputation, this may mean discharge from home health rehabilitation services before prosthetic limb fitting. Under optimal circumstances, the person has achieved independence in wheelchair management and mobility and independence in basic activities of daily living at a wheelchair level before this discharge.[33] In addition, with home care or inpatient services, the added time during wound healing phase allows time for the patient and the rehabilitation team to focus on the preprosthetic program, which can afford the best opportunity to formulate realistic treatment goals.[60] The overall costs of rehabilitation for the older adult, however, may also be increased if the patient needs an extended period of home care or outpatient services to function successfully after amputation. As stated earlier, older adults with amputation who receive inpatient rehabilitation immediately following acute hospitalization have better outcomes than patients who go home or are discharged to a nursing care facility, even after controlling for all likely confounding factors influencing outcomes.[20]

Delay in prosthetic fitting may make prosthetic training at a later date more difficult. Less frequent physical therapy sessions lead to more gait deviations and may ultimately require both an increased frequency of treatment and longer episodes of physical therapy care. Psychological readiness and motivation can also be adversely affected by delay in fitting.[70] Some patients become so proficient in functioning with a wheelchair that they become less enthusiastic about the effort needed to learn to be proficient in ambulating with the prosthesis and express a higher fear of falling with use of a prosthesis.[6,31,40,46] Regardless of the setting for early intervention, once the wound is healed, successful prosthetic use will be enhanced by coordinated rehabilitation team efforts.

Finally, there is no doubt that in the initial phases of prosthetic use, more frequent prosthetic revisions and patient and family training are necessary to ensure safe use and prevent complications of skin breakdown. Systematic methods of examining the person with amputation and his or her prosthesis not only determine whether the goals of comfort, function, and cosmesis have been met but also serve as a basis to correct problems.[21,59,68] In the home arena, the members of the team may simply need to communicate more frequently by telephone or other means to allow constant dialogue between physician, prosthetist, and therapists. Further, each member of the team and those members of the patient's immediate family affected by the limb loss need to independently examine and evaluate the patient to better determine appropriate management so that the patient achieves an optimal functional level, which attends to his or her quality-of-life needs.[66]

Plan of Care

Physical therapy intervention for the older adult with lower extremity amputation is very well described in textbooks, videos, and related literature.[12,21,22,60,68,86,106,107] Comprehensive physical therapy rehabilitation generally includes planning progressive interventions that address the postsurgical or preprosthetic and the prosthetic phase for recovery. The preprosthetic phase intervention should focus on promoting increased strength, preventing loss of range of motion while emphasizing hip and knee extension to avoid contracture. Cardiovascular training, with appropriate vital sign monitoring, is essential during all stages of recovery and can initially be easily performed using arm ergometry. Although there are few studies investigating the effect of aerobic training on function in older adults with lower limb amputation,[108] single-limb bicycling has been shown to improve endurance and anaerobic threshold in individuals with lower limb amputation.[78] Trunk or core strengthening, as well as balance activities performed in sitting and in single-limb stance are critical in preparation for prosthetic gait, especially for the patient with transfemoral amputation.

The prosthetic phase of gait training for the older adult is also well described.[21,22,68,109] Initial sessions should focus on education regarding prosthetic management, donning and doffing techniques, and skin inspection. Gait training will begin most often in parallel bars and emphasize standing balance activities and progression of the prosthetic limb. Balance activities in standing should progress from static tasks to dynamic reaching.

Patient education is an essential tool for prosthetic training. One effective tool that a physical therapist may use is an educational questionnaire that addresses all aspects of residual limb care and prosthetic management (Box 23-2). The educational program is tailored to the cognitive, visual, and auditory level of the patient. The questions can be asked frequently, to ensure safety with limb care once the patient is independent of therapy. Home programs on videotape or with pictures can be helpful for those who have difficulty with written items.

If possible, the physical therapist will also want to promote cardiovascular endurance through gait training with the use of a rolling walker or any other mobility device so that the patient can achieve an exercise intensity greater than 50% $\dot{V}O_2$ max.[108] This type of activity and level of intensity has been shown to optimize prosthetic use and success in the older adult.[108] Progressive

BOX 23-2	Educational Questionnaire for Independent Prosthetic Use

Prosthetic Socket and Liner Management
Where should your leg feel the pressure in the socket?
What does the gel liner do?
What is the difference between the liner and the socks?
How often should you clean the socket? How often and how do you care for the gel liner/socks?

Sock Management
Name the different types of socks (thickness: number of plies) and how many you should wear?
What is the proper way to put on your socks?
How should you wash and dry the socks?
What do you do when your leg feels loose in the socket?
What do you do when your leg feels tight in the socket?
Why is it important to always carry extra socks with you when wearing your artificial leg?

Skin Care
What is the importance of checking your skin regularly?
How long should areas of redness last on your skin?
What do you do when you have an area of skin breakdown?

gait training that addresses all aspects of household ambulation and community ambulation on curbs, ramps, and uneven surfaces is appropriate for older adults with amputation.

In certain cases, a patient may be referred to physical therapy because the individual is having difficulty with an existing prosthesis and might report a decline in functional ability. The physical therapist should examine the patient to first determine whether or not prosthetic factors are contributing to the patient's concerns, and if so refer to the prosthetist. Once all prosthetic adjustments are made, functional prosthetic training will generally follow the same sequence of activities outlined earlier, progressing from easy to advanced prosthetic activity as tolerated. In addition, all education, exercise, and gait activities must specifically address the impairments and functional limitations noted during the physical therapy examination.

OUTCOME MEASURES AND ASSESSMENT

Tools Used to Assess Overall Outcome of Prosthetic Rehabilitation

In the past and even today, measuring morbidity and mortality rates is considered most influential in evaluating health outcomes for the older adult with amputation, especially when the amputation is the result of disease.[7,10,14,15,19,39,44,45] Many of the outcome measures being used in rehabilitation today for individuals with amputation such as The Timed "Up & Go" (TUG) test,[89] Activities Specific Balance Scale (ABC),[87,88] the L Test of Functional Mobility,[85] and the Amputee Mobility

Predictor[86] (AMP with or without prosthesis) were previously described throughout this chapter. In addition, there are a few excellent review articles summarizing the use of multiple outcome-based tools for patients with amputation, which includes assessment of the psychometric properties of the various instruments.[77,110]

Although there is an increasing number of performance-based rehabilitation measures being used to assess functional outcomes in the older adult population,[77,85,86,88,89,110] the ability to predict long-term outcomes for older adults with amputation remains limited.[8,77] To date, only one instrument, the Amputee Mobility Predictor, provides sufficient prediction to be used to assess functional prosthetic potential under the Medicare guidelines.[86] Yet, prosthetic use following amputation is not the only sound measure of functional ability following lower limb loss; therefore, wheelchair mobility and function related to quality of life in older adults with lower limb amputation also warrant investigation.

What has been gleaned, to date, from the results of outcome-based studies is that older adults with amputation have marked physical limitations,[7,81] psychosocial difficulties,[71,103] and diminished quality of life when compared to healthy adults of similar age.[39] Using the Sickness Impact Profile, Peters et al[9] further found that older individuals with amputation and diabetes compared with age-matched individuals with diabetes alone had lower physical dimension scores but scored similarly in the psychosocial dimensions. From a positive perspective, other studies reveal that at least 50% of older adult with amputation are able to return to community mobility, including driving.[5] Fear of falling is increased and balance confidence among older adults with amputation is also reduced when compared to age-matched adults.[85,87,88] Psychosocial adjustment and motivation, which is often measured by assessing extent of depression or examining satisfaction with life with and without the prosthesis, is also significantly affected by amputation.[70,71] Finally, reported outcomes from studies using the Medical Outcomes Survey: SF-36 further reveal that older adults with amputation, especially as the result of disease, have markedly reduced perceptions regarding quality of life.[110,111]

Although amputation often occurs in the late stages of serious illnesses that preclude return to work and former community activities, there are many older adults who do return to these activities following extensive rehabilitation.[5,24] Clearly, the significant impact that lower limb amputation has on all aspects of health in the older adult makes any one measurement insufficient for determining outcomes. Perhaps the greater challenge in understanding health outcomes for the older adult with amputation is in trying to determine which factors should be measured. In an extensive systematic review of literature of 25 different prosthetic outcome measures from 1995 to 2005, Condie et al[110] explored generic outcome measures such as the Timed Up & Go, Timed Walk Tests, Barthel Index, and Functional Independence Measure, and the amputee-specific tests included review of tests such as the Amputee Mobility Predictor, Functional Measure for Amputees, and Houghton Scale. The authors note that there was no single measure that emerged as being universally appropriate for measuring lower limb prosthetic success.

SUMMARY

Many factors influence the successful prosthetic use for the older person who has experienced a lower limb amputation. Careful examination of the person's psychosocial, socioeconomic, and physiological status assists the clinician and entire prosthetic clinical team in formulating a prognosis and designing appropriate interventions that lead to successful prosthetic functional outcomes. Physical therapists may more often encounter older adults in the home setting who require prosthetic prescription and application, given the present trends in health care service delivery. The complexity and high illness burden of the typical older adult with amputation is apparent, and recent evidence suggests that there is a potential benefit of providing more intensive inpatient rehabilitation. In every rehabilitation setting, advocacy and consultation with other members of the prosthetic team are essential to assist older adults to achieve their maximum functional potential using a prosthesis.

Improvements in surgical techniques for amputation and advancements in prosthetic design occur each year. The effect that these scientific advances have on the quality of life and functional mobility of the older adult who uses a lower limb prosthesis is only beginning to be elucidated and requires greater investigation. Moreover, outside of the traditional standard physical therapy care being provided today, such as general strengthening, balance tasks, and progressive prosthetic gait training, there appears to be limited, if any, evidence-based physical therapy studies examining treatment strategies that promote optimal prosthetic function for the older adult with amputation.

CASE STUDY

History and Interview

Mr. J was a 62-year-old man who sought outpatient physical therapy 3 months following a left transfemoral amputation, secondary to vascular insufficiency and gangrene. He had a failed femoral popliteal bypass graft on the left (autograft was from the right lower limb), which resulted in poor restoration of blood flow and necessitated amputation. Although not commonly used in older adults, the surgical technique for the above-knee amputation included myoplasty, muscle-to-muscle attachment of his abductors/adductors. The patient reported to outpatient physical therapy using a wheelchair and was already walking with his prosthesis and a rolling walker; he had received his initial prosthesis 1 week earlier and was able to ambulate in parallel bars at the prosthetic facility.

Mr. J's past medical history revealed multiple significant medical conditions as follows: hypertension, peripheral artery disease, coronary artery disease, status post coronary artery bypass graft × 4, and type II diabetes mellitus. Medications included: metoprolol (Toprol XL), valsartan (Diovan), and insulin (Novolin 70/30). The patient denied symptoms of recent episodes of chest pain or signs of claudication in the right lower extremity at the time of this initial outpatient evaluation. His history also included use of alcohol (one to two drinks per day) and moderate tobacco smoking (one pack per day). The patient lived in a ranch-style home with a significant other; he worked as a welder in a machine shop and enjoyed fishing (dock and boat). The patient and family goals for rehabilitation were for him to receive training with his prosthesis, learn to walk, get back to fishing, and if possible return to work. The discharge plan was for the patient to achieve independent community ambulation with his prosthesis, with the potential to return to work.

Systems Review

Based upon this patient's extensive history and interview, a brief review of all body systems was indicated. Impairments were grossly noted in the musculoskeletal, neuromuscular, cardiovascular, integumentary, and endocrine systems. The patient did not present with any cognitive impairment; however, he was somewhat tearful during the interview as he was deeply concerned about his ability to return to work and was worried about disability. He was not overweight; however, his reported diet was not optimal for diabetic control or his cardiac condition. He reported having difficulty controlling his blood pressure and blood glucose levels since the amputation; however, he was being carefully monitored by his cardiologist and medical physician, with changes to his medications ongoing.

Examination

The physical therapy examination focused on addressing all impairments and functional limitations related to Mr. J's goals to return to community ambulation and work. Functional ability with and without the prosthesis, lower extremity and core trunk strength, gait and balance, and education about correctly managing the prosthesis were emphasized.

- Cognitive status/emotional behavior/education: Intact cognition. Although tearful at times, it appeared that his emotional status was consistent with significance of illness; he felt that he was coping effectively at that time. Education regarding prosthetic use was indicated—patient required verbal cues for prosthetic management and limb care.

- Pain: He reported 2/10 pain ("soreness") in the residual limb, which occurred during attempts to increase walking distance or with decreased use of an assistive device; he had symptoms of tingling sensation in his missing foot consistent with phantom sensation and did not report any symptoms of phantom pain.
- Range of motion: Remarkable for hip flexion contractures of −10 degrees left (residual side), −5 degrees right using the Thomas test.
- Motor performance: Grossly 3+/5 left lower extremity, 4−/5 right lower extremity; bilateral upper extremities 5/5; trunk extensors/abdominals 4−/5.
- Integument integrity: The left residuum healed effectively; the scar was pliable and not adhered, there was no evidence of any skin lesions. Observation of the skin of the right lower leg was noted to have a shiny appearance, "patchy" hair growth, and evidence of healed graft wounds.
- Bed mobility/transfers (without and with prosthesis): Independent.
- Cardiovascular response to ambulation (initial):
  - Resting vitals (sitting): heart rate = 82 bpm; blood pressure = 154/92 mmHg
  - Peak vitals postambulation with rolling walker 500 feet (not timed): heart rate = 98 bpm; blood pressure = 188/98 mmHg; O_2 saturation = 97%; he did not show any signs of shortness of breath during activity.
- Function/balance/gait: Mr. J was independent in bed mobility and transfers with and without the prosthetic and in all aspects of wheelchair mobility and ADL abilities at home. The patient required contact guard to maintain standing balance with the prosthesis and without upper extremity support but had difficulty reaching outside of his base of support—indicating fair dynamic standing balance. He ambulated with the prosthesis independently more than 200 feet with a rolling walker with minor gait deviations in the home and community; contact guard to minimum assistance was required to ascend/descend four steps with railing, and to safely ambulate on ramps or curbs.

Prosthetic Clinic Assessment

Mr. J. was evaluated in the prosthetic clinic 10 weeks after amputation and was measured for his initial prosthesis. Even though the patient had multiple medical issues, he was progressing well at home with functional tasks and was very motivated to walk. At approximately 12 weeks, the patient received his prosthesis with a left flexible brim ischial containment socket, gel liner with pin suspension, a multiaxial safety knee, and dynamic response foot.

- Prosthetic checkout: At the first outpatient physical therapy visit, a well-fitted prosthesis was noted with no areas of excessive pressure, proper alignment, and patient report of comfort in sitting and standing; the patient required verbal cues for management of prosthesis and correct donning and doffing techniques.

Evaluation, Diagnosis, and Prognosis

Mr. J came to outpatient physical therapy highly motivated to begin physical therapy. Of primary concern to him was his inability to ambulate safely with or without a device and difficulty performing instrumental activities of daily living, such as grocery shopping or doing housework. His two children did not live within the state, and although he discussed a significant other he did not seem to indicate she helped him with everyday activities in his home. He was also unable to work, which created tremendous financial hardship to him, as he was often unable to make copayments for therapy. He was given guidance on ways to apply for "indigent care" through the outpatient hospital system and received indigent care services within 1 month into physical therapy treatment. The patient's tearfulness and expressed sadness were also of concern when he was asked how he was coping. The physical therapist discussed options to address these issues by asking if he would like to seek counseling, receive peer visits (amputee volunteer), or attend an amputee support group. Mr. J really liked the idea of having a peer visit, so this activity was set up in consultation with his prosthetist.

Based upon examination findings and the *Guide to Physical Therapist Practice*,[72] this patient's primary diagnosis fell under Pattern 4J: Impaired Motor Function, Muscle Performance, Range of Motion, Gait Locomotion, and Balance Associated With Amputation. Because of the severity of his cardiac condition, a second pattern was used: Pattern 6D: Impaired Aerobic Capacity/Endurance Associated with Cardiovascular Pump Dysfunction or Failure.

Mr. J's prognosis was considered good to excellent for his goal for independent community ambulation, but it was not clear if he could return to work because of the high physical intensity of his job. There were some concerns regarding his cardiovascular signs at rest and with ambulation; therefore, referral to his cardiologist and consistent vital sign monitoring during all physical therapy activities were warranted. His vital signs may be indicative of more significant disease and could delay progress. Although he had a complex medical history, the examination findings illustrated that this patient had the potential to achieve his goals and the functional demands of a transfemoral community ambulator.[62] Mr. J's ability to return to work, however, would depend upon modifications to his job, as standing long hours and heavy lifting are difficult tasks for a person with transfemoral amputation.

Plan of Care

Mr. J's postsurgical inpatient rehabilitation and home physical therapy program involved mat activities that emphasized lower extremity stretching and strengthening exercises. He also reported working on dynamic sitting balance activities with a balloon or ball toss and performed cardiovascular training on an arm ergometer, with vital signs monitored as appropriate. The patient was instructed in skin monitoring and the use of a shrinker garment for edema management and shaping of the residual limb. All aspects of functional mobility were addressed, including performance of ADLs, wheelchair mobility, and hopping with a walker.

Once his prosthesis was received, Mr. J was referred for outpatient prosthetic phase physical therapy training. Education regarding skin care, management of limb shaping, gentle massage, tapping continued—he was now also able to use the roll-on gel liner as a means of shaping throughout the day, which is what he preferred. Mr. J was able to learn to ambulate with a rolling walker independently during the week from referral to his first physical therapy session; he had little fear of falling and was actually quite safe. Physical therapy began prosthetic gait training in parallel bars with emphasis on weight acceptance on the prosthesis, dynamic weight shifting and limb advancement, and immediately progressed the assistive device to a rolling walker. Progression of therapeutic exercise, core training, balance and gait training was conducted using a treatment approach that is well described by others and beyond the scope of this case report.[21,106,109,112] Patient education for prosthetic management was also addressed throughout treatments.

Cardiovascular endurance training was also performed using single-limb bicycling and arm ergometry. Using the Karvonen formula, the patient's target heart rate for exercise was calculated at 113 bpm {[(220 − 62) − 68] × 0.5 + 68}, which was based on literature suggesting that training effects can be achieved at 50% Vo_2 max.[108] Within 2 months of attendance at outpatient physical therapy two to three times per week for endurance training, the patient's ambulation on a treadmill progressed to 1.0, 1.2, and 1.4 mph with bilateral upper extremity support for 2- to 3-minute bouts, as tolerated. The physical therapist remained in close contact with the medical team to ensure safe progression of exercise and activity, considering his complex cardiac status and diabetes.

Goals and Outcome Measures

Mr. J had multiple medical problems with a significant history of diabetes and cardiovascular disease, which could have prevented his progress at any stage of his recovery. The patient also had a history of smoking and did not have optimal eating habits, placing him at risk for worsening of his arterial disease. Yet, the patient continued to make steady progress in all aspects of physical therapy as he was highly motivated and willing to work with the entire rehabilitation team to achieve his goals and the highest level of success.

After 3 and 6 months of physical therapy on average of two times per week, the patient required prosthetic socket changes and adjustments, secondary to residual limb shrinkage/shaping and advancements in all aspects of function with the prosthesis. At 9 months, in consultation with the prosthetist, we recommended that he receive a new prosthesis that included components required for a K3 level so that he could achieve his community-level goals. To better determine his Medicare functional "potential" level, the Amputee Mobility Predictor[86] was completed. Mr. J scored a 38/47, which was indicative of the patient's ability to meet the criteria of a K3 level, so we began discussing use of the C-leg. In view of the significance of his problems, some would argue that he also had relative contraindications for an advanced prosthetic fit, especially at the K3 level. However, providing him with a permanent transfemoral prosthesis would allow for more intimate fit and control through suction suspension and for greater ease of ambulation with reduced fall risk by using the C-leg microprocessor knee.[26,28]

Although it was clear that Mr. J would achieve his goal for prosthetic ambulation, he was unable to return to work because of the high demand of his welding job, which required standing for long hours and heavy lifting. His cardiac condition also would not allow for this type of work, and at the cardiologist's recommendation he applied for disability. This patient also had issues related to limited insurance coverage from his work (would not cover the K3 recommended components) and difficulties in filing for disability after amputation, which resulted in a delay in prosthetic fitting with the C-leg. In addition, his "inability to work" greatly compromised his financial status and further delayed healing recovery, emotionally and socially. Written letters of request to receive disability were submitted by the physical therapist and cardiologist. After two attempts, his request for disability benefits was finally approved 1 year following his surgical amputation. While awaiting his disability status and benefits, many physical therapy visits were provided pro bono so that he could continue with therapy and attain his optimal potential for functional recovery. Once he was granted Medicare disability, he received an ischial containment, flexible-brim suction socket with a C-leg microprocessor knee and dynamic response foot as recommended.

At the time of discharge from outpatient rehabilitation, approximately 18 months after the initial outpatient clinic visit, the patient achieved independent community ambulation on all surfaces without an assistive device; he felt safe and comfortable doing instrumental activities of living, such as grocery shopping, and was also able to return to fishing on the dock and by boating with friends (he did carry a cane when he went boating "just in case").

Mr. J's case continued to be followed by the prosthetic clinic, as needed, for monitoring fit, alignment, and wear. If prosthetic adjustments were made he was referred, by the prosthetist, for a physical therapy assessment. Early rehabilitation and coordinated efforts of the entire prosthetic clinic team played a significant role in promoting this patient's maximum functional potential. The coordinated efforts of the outpatient physical therapist and the prosthetic clinic team included support and encouragement, which allowed him to achieve his goals as quickly as possible.

REFERENCES

To enhance this text and add value for the reader, all references are included on the companion Evolve site that accompanies this text book. The reader can view the reference source and access it online whenever possible. There are a total of 112 cited references and other general references for this chapter.

PART V

Special Populations and the Continuum of Care

Wellness for the Aging Adult

Marybeth Brown PT, PhD, FAPTA,
Dale Avers, PT, DPT, PhD, Rita A. Wong, EdD, PT

The World Health Organization defines health as "a state of complete physical, mental, and social well-being and not merely the absence of disease or infirmity."[1] Wellness is often described in terms of these three interconnected domains of physical, psychological (mental), and social well-being. Wellness is viewed by some as a process,[2,3] and by others as an outcome achieved through health promotion and disease prevention processes.[4] Regardless of whether wellness is viewed as a process or an outcome, wellness programs give participants tools to approach life and activities in ways that promote optimal health and maximize personal potential.

Health promotion and disease prevention programs typically focus on enhancing wellness within one or more of these three health domains.[5] Wellness becomes a philosophy of life that utilizes health promotion and disease prevention strategies to achieve the goal of optimal aging. Optimal aging implies maximizing one's ability to function across physical, psychological, and social domains to one's satisfaction and despite one's medical conditions. The three overarching domains of physical, psychological, and social health are often further divided into dimensions (Table 24-1). Hettler, the founder of the Wellness Institute, is frequently quoted for his view of wellness as a process with six interconnected wellness dimensions: physical, emotional, spiritual, social, occupational/vocational, and intellectual (Figure 24-1).[3] Although these dimensions are frequently described in the wellness literature, there is little scientific evidence to confirm or reject these dimensions as the primary underlying factors making up the broad construct "wellness." Despite the lack of a clear understanding of the various components of the construct of wellness, wellness is generally accepted as a multidimensional entity, with inclusion of factors associated with physical, psychological, and social health making intuitive sense.

PHYSICAL HEALTH DOMAIN

The physical dimension of wellness is primarily influenced by such factors as exercise, nutrition, sleep, avoidance of disease-causing agents, early detection and treatment of diseases and medical conditions, and avoidance of iatrogenic complications.[2,4,6] Exercise and nutrition are discussed later in this chapter.

Sleeping well is important for physical health and emotional well-being, especially if there is a history of prior depression.[7] A good night's sleep is especially important with age because it improves concentration and memory formation, allows the body to repair any cell damage that occurred during the day, and refreshes the immune system, which helps to prevent disease.[8] Conversely, a lack of sleep is linked with the risk of depression.[9] Older adults' sleep habits change with aging, with having increased periods of wakefulness and less REM sleep.[10] Chronic diseases are associated with poor sleep habits, complaints of poor sleep quality, and interruptions in sleep patterns.[11] Specific sleep habits such as engagement in physical exercise, one nap in the middle of the day, avoidance of caffeine and snacks in the evening, relaxation techniques, and a consistent sleep schedule can promote healthful sleep.

Cigarette smoking is a major public health concern. Conservative estimates are that 30% of deaths from lung cancer, and 80% of deaths from chronic obstructive pulmonary disease are linked to cigarette smoking.[12] Smoking is also a factor in cardiovascular disease. It is never too late to quit smoking, with benefits occurring in as little as 1 year in those with cardiovascular disease.[13]

Few studies have been conducted regarding the value of participating in preventive medicine services after the age of 75 years. However, common sense might dictate that getting regular checkups to identify problems before they impact wellness, maintaining a healthy weight, engaging in physical activity, and getting enough physical exercise promotes physical wellness. These habits may make it less likely for hospitalization and medications that often have associated iatrogenic complications.[6]

Physical therapists can promote the goal of optimal aging through the accommodation of the primary, secondary, or tertiary prevention needs for those whose health conditions span the range of minor physical impairments and sedentary lifestyle to major disability. Similarly, physical therapists possess the requisite knowledge of the

TABLE 24-1	Wellness Domains	
Health Domain	**Wellness Dimension**	**Description**
Physical	Physical	Physical functioning to the degree that allows one to perform roles in family and society
Mental	Emotional	Sense of well-being and the ability to cope effectively with life's "ups and downs"
	Spiritual	Aspect of life that provides meaning and direction that connects to something greater than one's self
	Intellectual	Ability to learn and use information effectively; to reason and use self-efficacy in wellness endeavors
Social	Social	Meaningful relationships and presence of a social support structure
	Occupational/ Vocational	Purpose in life, a reason to get up in the morning

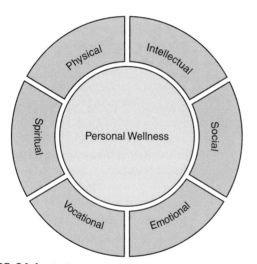

FIGURE 24-1 Six dimensions of wellness. *(Courtesy of Lifetime Wellness, Ltd., Longview, Tex.)*

consequences of poor health behaviors and strategies to promote more positive behaviors through patient education.[14] Wellness is a way of life that often requires behavioral and lifestyle changes to accomplish, changes only accomplished when individuals are educated in behaviors and conditions that limit or enhance wellness.[5]

Nutrition

Poor nutrition and excessive weight loss in older adults,[15] as well as excessive weight gain (obesity),[16] are associated with excess mortality, frailty, and lower quality of life. Maintaining a healthy body weight promotes optimal aging. Effect size for the relationship between optimal aging and having a normal body weight ranges from 1.58 to 3.05.[16] Weight loss in obese individuals is associated with improved functional status and amelioration of frailty in older adults.[17] Dietary interventions may decrease the risk or progression of macular degeneration, stroke, heart attacks, and lipid abnormalities, osteoarthritis and osteoporosis, and a number of cancers.[18-20] There is growing evidence that older adults can benefit from regular use of a daily multivitamin containing age-appropriate recommended amounts of folic acid and vitamins B_6, B_{12}, D, and E, as older adults are often deficient through dietary intake.[21-23] Subopitmal vitamin D levels have been associated with poor balance, weakness, and increased risk of hip fracture.[24-26] Table 24-2 provides a summary of the key nutritional considerations outlined in the USDA-approved modified nutritional guidelines for older adults, advocated by many gerontologists.[6] Physical therapists should be ready to advise older adults on basic nutrition principles to manage weight or accommodate high levels of physical activity.[27] The physical therapist will also work with nutrition specialists who can provide individualized assessment of nutritional needs and recommendations for nutritional modifications in managing special diets (e.g., control of diabetes or morbid obesity).

Exercise

Exercise is the single most important health-promoting activity for older adults.[28] Current recommendations for physical activity to achieve health benefits are a minimum of 150 minutes per week of *moderate to intense* aerobic activity and strengthening of the major muscle groups 2 or more days per week (Table 24-3). However, the Centers for Disease Control and Prevention reports

TABLE 24-2	Recommendations from the Modified USDA Food Pyramid for Older Adults
1. Whole, enriched, and fortified grains and cereals such as brown rice and 100% whole wheat bread
2. Bright-colored vegetables such as carrots and broccoli
3. Deep-colored fruit such as berries and melon
4. Low- and nonfat dairy products such as yogurt and low-lactose milk
5. Dry beans and nuts, fish, poultry, lean meat, and eggs
6. Liquid vegetable oils and soft spreads low in saturated and trans fat
7. Fluid intake (water is best)
8. Physical activity such as walking, housework and yard work

(Adapted from Lichtenstein AH, Rasmussen H, Yu WW, et al: Modified MyPyramid for older adults. J Nutr 138(1):5-11, 2008.)

TABLE 24-3	2008 Physical Activity Guidelines for Older Adults
	2 h and 30 min (150 min) of moderate–intense aerobic activity (i.e., brisk walking) every week AND muscle strengthening exercise on 2 or more days a week that work all major muscle groups (legs, hips, back, abdomen, chest, shoulders, and arms)
OR	1 h and 15 min (75 min) of vigorous–intense aerobic activity (i.e., jogging or running) every week AND muscle strengthening exercise on 2 or more days a week that work all major muscle groups (legs, hips, back, abdomen, chest, shoulders, and arms)
OR	An equivalent mix of moderate- and vigorous-intensity aerobic activity AND muscle strengthening exercise on 2 or more days a week that work all major muscle groups (legs, hips, back, abdomen, chest, shoulders, and arms)

For generally fit older adults the guidelines listed in Table 24-3 apply. Otherwise, obtaining a health clearance from the individual's physical therapist or physician is advisable to set appropriate physical activity goals. (*Data from Centers for Disease Control, Division of Nutrition, Physical Activity and Obesity, National Center for Chronic Disease Prevention and Health Promotion. Physical activity for everyone: guidelines: older adults. http://www.cdc.gov/physicalactivity/everyone/guidelines/olderadults.html. Accessed April 4, 2010.*)

that only 34% of individuals between ages 65 and 74 years, and 17% of individuals aged 75 years and older, exercise regularly.[29] This is consistent with Fiatarone Singh's findings that only 30% of older adults are physically active.[30] Physical therapists are uniquely qualified to guide older adults to improve physical wellness through individualized fitness and physical activity programs. Physical therapists, as movement specialists, can provide information, guidance, and help that is particularly relevant to older adults striving to optimize their aging—by maintaining and enhancing function and adapting physical activity and exercise programs to accommodate pain or other disability that challenges movement ability. Communicating and marketing the value of physical therapist–designed and –led wellness programs are key to promoting the functional abilities and wellness of aging adults.

PSYCHOLOGICAL WELLNESS

Psychological wellness includes the emotional, cognitive, and spiritual dimensions of wellness. Emotional wellness emphasizes control of stress and effective coping with life situations. High stress levels with poor coping can lead to negative physiological (e.g., cardiovascular, musculoskeletal), emotional (e.g., depression, anxiety, anger), and behavioral (e.g., inability to work, inefficiency) responses. Cognitive wellness emphasizes the skills, self-efficacy (a person's confidence in his or her ability to accomplish a task or achieve a goal), and interest in engaging intellectually in the world. Strategies to promote cognitive health are contained in Chapter 8 on cognition.

Spiritual health includes the values, morals, and ethics that guide an individual's search for a state of harmony and inner balance. Spirituality is about a person's existence and relationships with self, others, and the universe. Spirituality does not necessarily connote religiosity.[31] The spirituality dimension may increase with age, perhaps

because of increased time to reflect about their role in the universe and the meaning of life.[32]

Ryff and Keyes[33] in a confirmatory factor analysis of a large group of adults across a wide age range compiled six distinct dimensions associated with psychological wellness that integrate elements from several theorists such as Erikson, Maslow, and Rogers. Taken together, these six dimensions encompass a breadth of wellness that includes positive evaluations of one's self and one's life, a sense of continued growth and development as a person, the belief that life is purposeful and meaningful, the possession of good relationships with other people, the capacity to manage one's life and the surrounding world effectively, and a sense of self-determination. A healthy psychological outlook can reduce the intensity and duration of illnesses, creating the so-called mind–body interaction. Although the absence of mental distress or illness does not equate to psychological well-being, attention to these six domains can promote a sense of well-being and hope that encompasses psychological health.[34]

SOCIAL WELLNESS

Social wellness includes the social and occupational dimensions of wellness. In general, social well-being involves the ability to develop and maintain healthy relationships with others, to feel connected to a community or group, to interact well with other people, and to have a support structure to call on during difficult times. Social supports significantly influence the ability to cope with life's stressors. Social networks also help to protect older people against harm and promote emotional and physical well-being. For older adults, social connectedness is often a priority need and helps people find a balance between quality of life and compromised health. People considered socially well are usually involved with others, rather than isolated, and they report satisfactory levels of perceived social support.

Five major factors make up the construct of social wellness.[35] These five factors are:

1. Social integration ("I feel close to other people in my community")
2. Social contribution ("My daily activities are worthwhile to my community")
3. Social coherence ("I can make sense of what's going on in the world")
4. Social actualization ("Society is improving for people like me")
5. Social acceptance ("People care about the social issues that are important to me")

In a large-scale set of two studies that included adult subjects between 18 and 74 years of age, Keyes found that social well-being increased with age (although more slowly with increasing age) in all categories except for social coherence, which decreased with increasing age.

Social supports and caregiving can be both formal and informal. Formal caregiving involves paid services, usually from agencies and organizations that address basic needs of individuals such as personal care, meals, and transportation. Informal (unpaid) caregiving, typically provided by family, friends, and significant others, often is the main source of emotional and psychosocial support for the older adult. A healthy social network provides a safety net for older adults. Older adults who lack adequate social supports are more vulnerable to safety risks such as older person abuse and substance misuse and are at risk for depression, impaired decision making, isolation, loneliness, poor health, and decreased life expectancy.[36]

Occupational/vocational wellness is closely linked to social wellness. A basic tenet of occupational/vocational wellness is a balance between work, home, and leisure activities, with the opportunity to engage in meaningful activity.[37] Occupational wellness refers to one's attitude about one's work and to having an occupational or vocational interest in life. An occupationally well person is one who is involved in paid and nonpaid activities that are personally rewarding and make a contribution to the well-being of the community at large. As older individuals leave paid work, purposeful employment (occupation) can be replaced with purposeful and meaningful activity such as volunteer activities (vocation). Vocational wellness occurs through matching core values with interests, hobbies, employment, and volunteer work. Retirement can bring opportunities for vocational wellness. Employment or vocational endeavors can provide a sense of purpose, enrichment enhanced mental health indices, and overall wellness in older adults.[38]

The dimensions of wellness described earlier demonstrate the capacity of aging adults to live optimally throughout their days. Wellness is a concept to strive for regardless of health conditions. Although physical therapists deal primarily with the domain of physical wellness, familiarity with the other domains of wellness will enhance the physical therapist's ability to promote optimal aging.

PHYSICAL ACTIVITY AND EXERCISE–FOCUSED WELLNESS PROGRAMS

In the past decade, there has been an explosion in the literature to support the efficacy of purposeful activity for the older adult, whether community, clinic, or home based. The essence of this work demonstrates that fundamental and meaningful change in strength, balance, flexibility, function, and community participation is possible with exercise regardless of age.[30,39,40] Therefore, the inclusion of activity promotion, purposeful physical engagement, and/or exercise should be a goal of any wellness program for individuals between the ages of 50 and 100+ years.

PHYSICAL THERAPISTS' SCOPE OF PRACTICE

Providing health promotion and wellness services in the area of physical fitness and patient education in healthy lifestyle principles is identified in both the *Guide to Physical Therapist Professional Practice* and in the *Normative Model of Physical Therapist Professional Education*[41,42] as practice expectations of physical therapists. However, wellness is not generally viewed as a health care service within the traditional medical model oriented around illness. Most insurance companies do not reimburse health care providers for delivery of wellness interventions. As such, there are few regulations on who can deliver wellness services. Thus, many wellness practitioners are not licensed within any health profession. In seeking wellness services, older adults should carefully scrutinize the background of the provider to determine their comfort level with the practitioners educational background.

However, when licensed health professionals such as physical therapists deliver wellness services they must function within the scope of practice allowed by their state licensing laws. Each state has its own laws regarding the practice of physical therapists. Some states allow full and direct access to patients; other states require a physician referral for any access to a patient. Most states allow physical therapists to evaluate and screen individuals without physician referral but then have varying provisions regulating the implementation of an intervention. For several states, the language of the state physical therapy practice act makes a clear statement allowing physical therapists to provide wellness and fitness programs without physician referral when the purpose is for prevention of illness or improved functional ability (in the absence of an acute illness or injury). However, other state practice acts do not provide this option. Thus, physical therapists must be familiar with the licensing regulations in their state and organize wellness services to comply with these regulations.

The ability to legally evaluate and provide wellness services to older adults is a separate consideration from the ability to be reimbursed by health care insurers. Frequently, patients' rehabilitative needs far exceed their Medicare benefits. For example, older individuals with fractured hips or stroke frequently show the greatest trajectory of improvement between 2 and 6 months; after that time, most patients have completed their reimbursable rehabilitation.[43,44] Other clients with chronic conditions may be ineligible for traditional physical therapy because they require "maintenance," an area Medicare benefits do not currently cover. General deconditioning (e.g., following treatment for cancer or even severe flu), neurologic disease such as Parkinson's disease and dizziness are examples of chronic conditions that fall into the cracks of our health care system. These patient groups are given as examples of older adult clients who may benefit substantively from follow-up care or wellness for which the expertise of a physical therapist could be particularly useful.

Screening for Physical Activity and Wellness Programs

Screening is an essential part of a physical activity/ exercise-focused wellness program to determine the appropriateness of individuals to participate and may help to stratify individuals to the appropriate program or level within a program. Screening is a precursor to baseline and outcomes assessment, which will be discussed in the next section.

Although validated screening tools for adults older than age 70 years do not exist, several tools are widely used in the general population. The Physical Activity Readiness Questionnaire (Par-Q) is a popular screening form to identify contraindications to exercise. However, the Par-Q has several limitations, such as unnecessary elimination of individuals.[45] The Par-Q is accompanied by a MED PAR-X form that can be used to communicate with the client's medical team. The Par-Q consists of seven questions that address possible contraindications to exercise and is freely available.[46] A positive answer on any of these seven items indicates a need to further investigate the individual's readiness for more intense physical activity. For example, the Par-Q question "Is your doctor currently prescribing drugs (for example, water pills) for your blood pressure or heart condition?" can help identify medications such as β-blockers that can blunt the physiological exercise response. The Par-Q question of "Do you have a bone or joint problem (for example, back, knee or hip) that could be made worse by a change in your physical activity?" is often answered yes because clients have experienced increased pain and/or discomfort with physical activity as a result of

a total joint replacement or arthritis. Asking a few questions about their pain can often determine if a physical activity modification is needed, thus promoting confidence that exercise may improve the clients' symptoms.

In response to the limitations of the Par-Q, the Exercise Assessment and Screening for You (EASY) tool was developed.[47] This six-question online screening tool[48] (Table 24-4) identifies potential health problems that require health care provider clearance before exercising, provides education about each problem and the value of exercise, and helps older adults choose appropriate exercises that may not first require a physician's approval. The EASY tool emphasizes the benefits of exercise and physical activity for all individuals while educating the older adult about how to exercise within the individuals' limitations. The EASY tool provides instant recommendations regarding the safety of exercise or the need for the client to see a physician before exercising.

Regardless of which screening tool is used, additional questions about the presence of osteoporosis and falls history are helpful in an older clientele. Certain movements such as excessive thoracic flexion, common in the presence of osteoporosis, have been linked to thoracic fractures,[49] and fractures result more easily with falls.[50] In addition, fear of falling may be more acute in individuals who know they have a heightened risk of fracture.[51] The physical therapist can provide valuable information and exercise cueing to avoid potential problems if awareness of osteoporosis is present. Table 24-5 describes screening questions for osteoporosis. Although no tool exists as a criterion standard of fall risk,[52] the American Geriatrics Society recommends asking about a history of falls in the previous 12 months and conducting the Timed Up and Go (TUG) test when screening for fall risk.[53] Others would suggest a positive history of falls is sufficient to determine fall risk.[53]

TABLE 24-4	Exercise and Screening for You (EASY)
1. Do you have pains, tightness, or pressure in your chest during physical activity (walking, climbing stairs, household chores, similar activities)?	
2. Do you currently experience dizziness or lightheadedness?	
3. Have you ever been told you have high blood pressure?	
4. Do you have pain, stiffness, or swelling that limits or prevents you from doing what you want or need to do?	
5. Do you fall, feel unsteady, or use assistive device while standing or walking?	
6. Is there a health reason not mentioned why you would be concerned about starting an exercise program?	

(Adapted from Exercise and Screening for You. http://www.easyforyou.info/ index.asp. Accessed July 3, 2010.)

TABLE 24-5	Screening for Osteoporosis
The physical therapist can ask for:	
The results of previous dual-energy x-ray (DEXA), heel scan indicating (T-Score of −2.5 or more)	
Family history of osteoporosis (mother, sisters, grandmother)	
Low body mass index	
History of vertebral or wrist fractures[135]	
Observe presence of kyphosis[135]	
Loss of height of >4 cm[135]	

Baseline and Outcomes Assessment

Baseline measures for physical activity/exercise-focused wellness programs can help establish program goals and identify specific areas to target, such as flexibility, strength, and aerobic fitness. Baseline measures can also be used to stratify clients to an appropriate exertional and skill level. Ideally, baseline information should be gathered that determines health issues, prior exercise history, functional deficits, impairments such as poor cardiovascular endurance, strength deficits, and balance issues. In addition, clients' adherence and self-efficacy can improve when regular feedback is given about their progress.[54-56]

Many objective and responsive tools are available to measure different aspects of physical ability, and many of these tools have age-based normative data. The specific measurements or assessments used depend on the amount of time available, the condition of the client, and the focus of the program. For example, if a walking program is the focus of the wellness activity, then the assessment may be heart rate response to walking in a 6-minute walk test, gait speed, 1-mile walk, or a 24-hour pedometer reading. If the intended outcome is improved balance, then baseline measures of balance capacity should be used. Several tests that range from well-validated and reliable tests with normative data to timed tests such as stair climb,[57] time to put on a jacket,[58,59] and floor rise[60] are listed in Table 24-6.

Knowledge of the clients' physical activity history can provide valuable baseline information if a goal is to improve physical activity. Knowledge of clients' physical activity history can help determine a starting point for the physical activity/exercise class. A detailed history of prior training is likely important if preparing older adults for an intense exercise activity such as a competitive senior Olympic sport. If working with a group of frail seniors in an assisted living facility, the only question that may be needed is, "Have you ever been active?" Then follow up with an inquiry about frequency and intensity of the activity. Several valid, self-report physical activity tools exist.[61] Several of the more reliable and valid measures of routine activity are listed in Table 24-7.

Outcome measures for program evaluation can be used to provide individual feedback on progress, to evaluate and determine whether the class has met its purpose, and to provide data on the program's effectiveness. Individual client feedback focused on the clients' wellness goals can be provided at the end of the program. Consideration should be made for the time it takes to realize a change in the desired outcome. For example, 12 months or more may be needed to achieve weight loss goals, to increase physical activity to recommended wellness levels, or realize quality-of-life changes.[62-64] However, specific strength and endurance gains may occur in as little as 12 to 15 weeks.[65-67] Recognizing that several months may be required to achieve functionally important physical changes, it is important to provide feedback that highlights the short-term successes the patient is achieving along the longer-term path to more functionally visible outcomes, for example, sticking with a commitment for regular attendance and participation in physical activity, lower perceived exertion with the same workload, and additional repetitions of exercises or distance walked without a rest. Early success in physical activity endeavors positively reinforces commitment to pursuit of long-term physical activity goals. Individual results can be provided in terms of age-based norms for additional value to the client.

Program evaluation can also be determined by factors such as class attendance, clients' adherence, and satisfaction with the various components of the program, such as self-perception of health and lifestyle changes. Summary scores of performance-based outcome tools can provide an indication of general strength gains, weight loss, and balance improvement in the group. Program evaluation outcomes should relate to the purpose and focus of the program.

Types of Physical Activity and Exercise Programs

There are literally hundreds of opportunities for physical therapists to promote wellness for the older adult client. Fortunately, there are resources available, some in book or monograph form, many on the Internet, and numerous video-based protocols that may be used to assist in the design of an activity program. Several types of programs are presented here. Utilizing preexisting resources is encouraged when a specialty wellness activity program is chosen. Physical activity/exercise–focused wellness programs can be developed in any venue such as health clubs, outpatient offices, older adult residences, senior centers, health-related clinics, nursing homes, rehab hospital gyms, religious facilities, or individually. Wellness programs can also take the form of consultant-type services.

Balance and Fall Prevention Programs. Many older adults are justifiably afraid of falling as their balance is beginning to fail and reaction times are slower than they

TABLE 24-6	Baseline Measures for Physical Activity/Exercise–Focused Wellness Programs	
Measure	**Description**	**Normative Values**
Short Physical Performance Battery (SPPB)	Quick, easy to perform test consisting of timed 5× chair stands, usual gait speed, and balance tests. Scored on an ordinal scale with a total possible score of 12. Test is free and instructions are available at www.grc.nia.nih.gov/branches/ledb/sppb/download_sppb.doc	Individuals scoring 9 or less reflects mobility disability.[136]

Gait speed[137]	Can use any distance of 4 m or more. Usual (customary) and fast gait speeds can be recorded.	1.2 m/s is approximate time it takes to cross the street.
		Norms for community-based older adults[138]:
		  60-69 y: males 1.59 m/s (usual); 2.05 m/s (fast)
		  60-69 y: females 1.44 m/s (usual); 1.87 m/s (fast)
		  70-79 y: males 1.39 m/s (usual); 1.83 m/s (fast)
		  70-79 y: females 1.33 m/s (usual); 1.71 m/s (fast)
		  80-89 y: males 1.21 m/s (usual), 1.65 m/s (fast)
		  80-89 y: females 1.15 m/s (usual); 1.59 m/s (fast)

Single limb stance test.[35] This test is self-explanatory although a few rules do apply such as not being able to put the free limb against the stance limb or wiggling in place. It is up to the therapist (dictated by safety) whether or not to assist the client into the test position and then let go when they are ready or have them do the entire activity unassisted. Make note of the choice.	Ability to stand on one leg is associated with balance and normal gait and is known to decrease with age.[139] Time of stance should be measured with arms folded across chest and one leg lifted from floor, not touching the other leg.	10 s eyes open is the recommended minimal standard for adults older than age 60 y[139]
		Age-based means[140]:
		  60-69 y: mean 26.9 s (eyes open); 2.8 s (eyes closed)
		  70-79 y: mean 15.0 s (eyes open); 2.0 s (eyes closed)
		  80-99 y: mean 6.2 s (eyes open); 1.3 s (eyes closed)

Tandem and semitandem stance	Can be used in addition to single leg stance and is included in the SPPB.	

Timed Up and Go test	Demonstrates ability to get up from a chair, walk, and turn and sit down again.
	May be too low level for higher-functioning older adults.
		TUG times can be considered worse than average if they exceed[141]:
		  60-69 y: 9.0 s
		  70-79 y: 10.2 s
		  80-99 y: 12.7 s

Activities-Specific Balance Confidence Scale, or ABC[142]	Measures balance confidence during common community-based tasks and is known to be responsive to improved balance.[142] Is a self-report, paper-based test.	None available

Chair stand test	30-s chair stand test or timed 5-repetition chair stand test have been used as proxies for leg strength and power. Arms cannot be used.	8 or fewer repetitions indicate risk for mobility disability.[143]
		Norms for 30-s chair rise[143]:
		  60-69 y: women 11-17; men 12-19
		  70-79 y: women 10-15; men 11-17
		  80-89 y: women 8-14; men 8-15
		  ≥90 y: women 4-11; men 7-12

Distance walk test	Time taken to walk 400 m (approximately ¼ mile) or distance walked in 6 min can be used as proxies for endurance tests. The rate of perceived exertion can be used as a measure of effort.[88]	Taking more than 5 min 30 s to complete 400-m test is indicative of risk of developing functional limitations.[144]
		Mean time of 5 min 11 s was recorded in healthy older adults.[145]
		6-min walk test norms[138]:
		  60-69 y: men 572 m; women 538 m
		  70-79 y: men 527 m; women 471 m
		  80-89 y: men 417 m; women 392 m

Continued

TABLE 24-6	Baseline Measures for Physical Activity/Exercise–Focused Wellness Programs—cont'd	
Measure	Description	Normative Values
Flexibility: 　Back Scratch	Back Scratch (Apley's) tests shoulder mobility while the Modified Sit and Reach tests hamstring and lumbar mobility.	Norms for Back Scratch test[146]: 　60-69 y: women −3.5 to +1.5 in.; men −7.5 to 0.0 in. 　70-79 y: women −5.0 to +1.0 in.; men −9.0 to 1.0 in. 　80-89 y: women −7.0 to −1.0 in.; men −9.5 to −3.0 in. 　≥90+ y: women −8.0 to −1.0 in.; men −10.5 to −4.0 in.
Modified Sit and Reach		Modified Sit and Reach norms[146,147]: 　60-69 y: women −0.5 to +5 in.; men −3 to +4 in. 　70-79 y: women −1.5 to +4 in.; men −4 to +2.5 in. 　80-89 y: women −2.5 to +3.0 in.; men −5.5 to +1.5 in. 　≥90+ y: women −4.5 to +1.0 in.; men −6.5 to −0.5 in.

TABLE 24-7	Measurements of Physical Activity	
Physical Activity Scale	Description	Comments
Physical Activity Scale for the Elderly (PASE)[148]	PASE comprises self-reported occupational, household, and leisure activities during a 1-wk period providing prompts with examples of specific activities. Can be administered by phone, mail, or personal interview. Focus on activities commonly performed by older adults by giving more weight to these activities instead of sports.	Correlates with 6-min walk and other physical performance measures.[61] May not be responsive to change following physical activity/exercise interventions.[149] Requires a license and purchase[150]
Pedometer	Simple, inexpensive tool to record steps and/or minutes of activity. Generally, 10,000 steps per day is considered to afford a health benefit.[133]	In people walking slower than 0.8 m/s, may not be accurate or register steps.[151] Individuals who used a pedometer were more likely to achieve the recommended amount of activity as compared with those without a pedometer.[132]
Accelerometer	Computerized measures of step count and movement that may be more applicable for research.[152]	Can be attached at the ankle. Requires a computer to interpret number of steps.

were in younger years. Balance programs are quite valued, particularly if they capitalize on popular programs such as Tai Chi. Tai Chi is known to be effective in improving balance and reducing fall risk, and its movements and principles can be incorporated into any balance activity.[68-70] Tai Chi was also shown to reduce symptoms of knee osteoarthritis[71] and reduce blood pressure.[72]

Tai Chi is not the only approach to enhancing balance in older adults. Literature has demonstrated that balance will improve if multimodal programs are used.[73,74] The programs should include challenge to static and dynamic balance provided two to three times a week for at least 8 weeks, environmental assessment and remediation, visual assessment and remediation (if needed), vestibular assessment, and promotion of strength, particularly of the muscles controlling the ankle.[73,75,76]

Missouri has the dubious distinction as the state with the highest falls-related death rate in the country. It also ranks in the top three states for recorded falls in the older adult population. Consequently, the state government has grown alarmed and a coalition of practitioners was formed to create Falls Free Missouri, which is an

excellent Web-based resource.[77] The Falls Free Missouri Web site provides information such as risk factors and statistics on falling but more importantly, includes action steps that may be taken to reduce falls. Falls prevention programs are relatively easy to provide with minimal allocation of financial and human resources. In addition, this approach is an excellent way to enhance public awareness and foster community loyalty to the facility.

Strength Training. The efficacy of strength training for older adults has been demonstrated by numerous investigators. From the seminal article by Fiatarone et al.[78] in 1990 to more contemporary issues of power versus velocity versus traditional weights, a multitude of evidence overwhelmingly supports the inclusion of strength training for all older adults, including those who are frail, have multiple comorbidities, and have never done any type of resistance activity.[75,79-87] Indeed, resistance training is endorsed, even encouraged by the American Association for Retired Persons (AARP) and the American College of Sports Medicine.[88,89]

Strength training can be done in a myriad of ways, including traditional free weights, isotonic-type machines, elastic bands, functional activities (e.g., weighted chair stands, stair climbing), incorporating high-velocity training and emphasizing power-based training into class-type activity or individual exercises. Because resistance training is so strongly recommended for older adults, it should be incorporated into most activity programs.[28,40,90] Strength training in dose-specific recommendations known to increase strength should be followed as described in Chapter 5 on exercise.[40,91]

Exercise for Frail Older Adults. Eighty-plus-year-old individuals are the fastest growing group in the United States and are at greatest risk for loss of independence.[92] A large proportion of this population is highly deconditioned, with poor muscular and cardiovascular endurance as well as muscle weakness, associated with sedentary lifestyle and periodic bouts of bed rest from illnesses and hospitalizations. More than 50% of individuals older than age 80 years are physically inactive; at least 60% have difficulty with functional activities such as stooping, crouching, kneeling, lifting or carrying 10 pounds, and standing from an armless chair; and 30% have difficulty with very basic activities of daily living such as dressing and bathing.[93] Individuals who have low physical activity levels, need help with daily activities, fatigue easily, are weak, have slow motor performance and balance abnormalities are likely to be classified as frail.[94] Many frail older women test poorly on measures of function and balance.[95]

Wellness classes are greatly needed for frail and near-frail older adults. However, this is the most challenging group to tackle given preexisting medical conditions, the lack of endurance, low physical activity levels, and generalized weakness.[96] Nonetheless, developing and implementing programs for the frail is interesting, gratifying, and wonderfully challenging. Exercise focused on remediating frailty and improving function in frail older adults can be task specific, as research has shown that task-specific exercise is equivalent to resistance training.[97-103] Task-specific exercise has the advantage of being relevant to the frail older adult, which may promote participation.

General conditioning exercises are extremely effective for prefrail older adults and can be done in groups.[72,104-107] These classes should focus on strengthening activities, particularly the lower extremities, dynamic balance (in standing position), and functional activities such as getting up and down from the floor, stair climbing, and walking distances of 0.25 to 1 mile. An advantage of group classes is the socialization they provide that may promote exercise adherence.[108,109]

Exercise to Enhance Bone Quality/Quantity. One of every two women older than age 50 years is on a trajectory to develop osteoporosis if she does not have it already.[110] Consequently, wellness programs that emphasize bone loading are important and highly pertinent. Key components to all of the approaches to enhance bone health are core strengthening exercises for abdominals and back extensors, possible use of a weighted vest (if there is no kyphosis), strengthening exercises for the scapular retractors and upward rotators, and lower-extremity loading.[111,112] A summary of activity- and exercise-based strategies to improve the quantity and quality of bone include the following:

1. Exercises must include weight-bearing activity; weight-bearing that is over and above what is done in a typical day.[113-115]
2. Resistance exercise will increase bone mineral density if exercise adherence is maintained for 6 months or longer.[115,116]
3. Weighted vests do work, but evidence suggests a minimum of a 2-year commitment to wearing the vest.[113] For gains to be maintained, vest use must be continued.[114]
4. Back extensor and core strengthening to reduce the risk for vertebral fractures.[112,117]

Aerobic Training. The vast majority of older adults have cardiovascular deconditioning, most of which is the consequence of sedentary lifestyle.[118,119] The presence of cardiovascular disease does not preclude aerobic training; to the contrary, the presence of disease makes aerobic training even more important.[120-122] There is no evidence indicating a worsening of cardiovascular disease with exercise[123,124]; in fact, exercise actually improves the disease state (e.g., congestive heart failure, post–myocardial infarction) and raises the level of conditioning.[125] The only time exercise is contraindicated for heart disease is if a client is in the midst of an acute crisis.[88] One thing that should be borne in mind is that because so many older adults are so very deconditioned, nearly all exercise constitutes an aerobic challenge. It is not necessary to consider aerobic exercise within the narrow framework of running, cycling, Nordic track, elliptical trainer, or stair stepper. Musical chairs, dance, Tai Chi, brisk walking, and resistive strengthening functional activities are often of sufficient intensity to achieve an aerobic training effect.

Enhancing Physical Activity and Mobility. Mobility challenged older adults are everywhere but most visibly within assisted care facilities. These men and women are often one fall or illness away from admission to the nursing home. Many of the so-called mobility programs for sedentary older adults and frail individuals are chair-based, which is counterintuitive to mobility. Wellness activities for this population should heavily emphasize functional activities, including handling pots and pans, carrying items, sweeping and vacuuming, putting clothes away, and stooping to pick up items from the floor. Gait activities are also important and should include changing direction suddenly, walking slowly and very quickly in response to a command, walking the equivalent width of a street in time to cross with the light, and stepping up and down from a curb. Obstacle courses and circuit training kinds of activities can be fun, meaningful, and effective for individuals struggling to stay independent.[126-129]

Walking Programs. Walking programs are very easy to set up, require little supervision, and can provide numerous benefits such as socialization, sense of well-being, self-efficacy, and health benefits such as decreased pain (in the presence of knee osteoarthritis)[130] and improved glycemic control.[131] Pedometers are effective in tracking steps and can promote physical activity more so than encouragement alone to be more physically active.[132] Pedometers with the sponsor's name on them can also be an effective marketing strategy. Recommendations of 10,000 steps/day (5 miles) are associated with health benefits.[133,134]

One of the most successful walking programs in this country came out of Waukesha, Wisconsin, over a decade ago. The basic idea was to start a program with a nucleus of interested people and "grow" that program over the first and second summers by having each member recruit another walker. There are walking trails throughout Waukesha that are clearly labeled to provide distances, information about where to go from that particular way-point, and suggestions for an exercise that can be done at each station. Participants have t-shirts and there is a strong sense of belonging. Hundreds of older adults have joined the walking club over the years with their "train the trainer" concept.

CONCLUSION

Given the burgeoning older adult population, an increasing life span, and the fact that nearly 50% of all those older than age 80 years have already lost their independence, it has become critical to stave off frailty and extend productive and capable years for older adults. Because increased physical activity and exercise is most important for health and physical and cognitive well-being, every physical therapist should be involved in promoting physical activity and exercise programs. Physical therapists have the skills required to prevent the spiraling decline in independence among the aging and aged population. The efficacy of physical activity and exercise programs has been demonstrated. Elements of endurance as in walking, strengthening, and balance should be incorporated. All that is required is willingness to begin and an appropriate assessment of resources.

REFERENCES

To enhance this text and add value for the reader, all references are included on the companion Evolve site that accompanies this text book. The reader can view the reference source and access it online whenever possible. There are a total of 152 cited references and other general references for this chapter.

CHAPTER 25

Home Health Physical Therapy

Christine E. Fordyce, PT, DPT,
Claire Gold, MSPT, MBA, COS-C, CPHQ

INTRODUCTION

Providing care in the home is a unique way to deliver geriatric rehabilitation to older adults who are homebound. On any given day, the home care clinician may be the only health care professional to see the patient. Although home care offers a great deal of autonomy, the home care clinician must be able to coordinate the patient's care with other members of the team, work in collaboration with other health care providers, and teach available caregivers. Home care has several advantages. The clinician spends one-on-one time with the patient in average durations of 45 to 60 minutes, with a relatively low full-time caseload of about 5 to 6 patients a day. Most home health agencies and patients allow the therapist to set the time of the visit, often accommodating the therapist schedule. The therapist can work with the family and/or caregiver within the patient's actual setting to provide care that is relevant to the patient's environment and needs. Home care also presents unique challenges for the physical therapist. Although the home care setting has inherent autonomy, it also presents situational isolation from other health professionals, documentation requirements, variability, and unanticipated circumstances and requires efficient time management.

Clinicians caring for older adults in their homes need to be prepared to make the best practice decisions. Whether or not the home is one of cramped living conditions, overflowing with saved items, or a well-maintained residence with lots of space, the therapist is literally a guest in someone's home and must be able to project a sincere attitude of caring while conveying a respect for the desire of the older adult to remain at home. This chapter will discuss these unique features as well as federally mandated characteristics of the home care provision benefit under Medicare Part A and the sequence and scope of an episode of care.

DEFINITION OF HOMEBOUND

To receive coverage under the Medicare benefit, patients must be "homebound" or "confined to the home."[1] An individual is considered confined to home if the individual has a condition, as a result of an illness or injury, that restricts the individual's ability to leave the home except with the assistance of another individual or with the aid of a supportive device (such as crutches, a cane, a wheelchair, or a walker), or if the individual has a condition such that leaving home is medically contraindicated.[1] Although an individual does not have to be bedridden to be considered confined to home, the condition of the individual should be such that there exists a normal inability to leave home, and leaving home requires a considerable and taxing effort.[1] However, "considerable and taxing effort" is not defined and therefore is left to the interpretation of the therapist, agency, and intermediary. Thus, as part of the initial home health visit and on all subsequent visits, the clinician must identify the functional criteria that support the patient's homebound status. Examples of homebound conditions are described in the Medicare Home Health Benefit Policy Manual listed in Box 25-1.[1] Therapy services can also be provided to patients in their homes under the Medicare Outpatient Part B benefit. For this benefit, patients do not need to be considered homebound but the travel time to the patient's home is not reimbursable.

"Fixing to Stay"

Typically, older adults want to remain in their homes as long as possible, even to die at home. This preference is fundamental to understanding the needs of the older adult home health patient. It cannot be overemphasized: older adults are "fixing to stay," a term used by the American Association of Retired Persons (AARP) in a national telephone survey of 45-year-and-older Americans about their housing preferences, difficulty getting around the house, and concerns about being able to remain in their homes.[2] The researchers concluded that an overwhelming number of their 2000 respondents intended to remain in their current residence for as long as possible and 63% of survey participants believe that their current residence is where they will always live. Furthermore, only 9% expressed a preference for moving to a facility where care is provided, and only 4% of the respondents expressed a preference

In order for a patient to be eligible to receive covered home health services under both Part A and Part B, the law requires that a physician certify in all cases that the patient is confined to his/her home. An individual does not have to be bedridden to be considered confined to the home. However, the condition of these patients should be such that there exists a normal inability to leave home and, consequently, leaving home would require a considerable and taxing effort. If the patient does in fact leave the home, the patient may nevertheless be considered homebound if the absences from the home are infrequent or for periods of relatively short duration, or are attributable to the need to receive health care treatment.

Any other absence of an individual from the home shall not so disqualify an individual if the absence is of an infrequent or of relatively short duration. For purposes of the preceding sentence, any absence for the purpose of attending a religious service shall be deemed to be an absence of infrequent or short duration.

It is expected that in most instances, absences from the home that occur will be for the purpose of receiving health care treatment. However, occasional absences from the home for nonmedical purposes, e.g., an occasional trip to the barber, a walk around the block or a drive, attendance at a family reunion, funeral, graduation, or other infrequent or unique event would not necessitate a finding that the patient is not homebound if the absences are undertaken on an infrequent basis or are of relatively short duration and do not indicate that the patient has the capacity to obtain the health care provided outside rather than in the home.

Generally speaking, a patient will be considered to be homebound if they have a condition due to an illness or injury that restricts their ability to leave their place of residence except with the aid of: supportive devices, such as crutches, canes, wheelchairs, and walkers; the use of special transportation; or the assistance of another person; or if leaving home is medically contraindicated.

Some examples of homebound patients that illustrate the factors used to determine whether a homebound condition exists would be:

- A patient paralyzed from a stroke who is confined to a wheelchair or requires the aid of crutches in order to walk;
- A patient who is blind or senile and requires the assistance of another person in leaving their place of residence;
- A patient who has lost the use of their upper extremities and, therefore, is unable to open doors, use handrails on stairways, etc., and requires the assistance of another individual to leave their place of residence;
- A patient in the late stages of ALS or neurodegenerative disabilities.

In determining whether the patient has the general inability to leave the home and leaves the home only infrequently or for periods of short duration, it is necessary (as is the case in determining whether skilled nursing services are intermittent) to look at the patient's condition over a period of time rather than for short periods within the home health stay. For example, a patient may leave the home (under the conditions described above, e.g., with severe and taxing effort, with the assistance of others) more frequently during a short period when, for example, the presence of visiting relatives provides a unique opportunity for such absences, than is normally the case. So long as the patient's overall condition and experience is such that he or she meets these qualifications, he or she should be considered confined to the home.

- A patient who has just returned from a hospital stay involving surgery who may be suffering from resultant weakness and pain and, therefore, their actions may be restricted by their physician to certain specified and limited activities such as getting out of bed only for a specified period of time, walking stairs only once a day, etc.;
- A patient with arteriosclerotic heart disease of such severity that they must avoid all stress and physical activity; and
- A patient with a psychiatric illness that is manifested in part by a refusal to leave home or is of such a nature that it would not be considered safe for the patient to leave home unattended, even if they have no physical limitations.

The aged person who does not often travel from home because of feebleness and insecurity brought on by advanced age would not be considered confined to the home for purposes of receiving home health services unless they meet one of the above conditions.

(From Medicare benefit policy manual, Chapter 7, Home health services. http://www.cms.hhs.gov/manuals/Downloads/bp102c07.pdf Updated 2005. Accessed April 29, 2010.)

for moving to a relative's home if unable to care for self.[2] Therapists treating older adults in their homes need to be cognizant and accepting of this preference as it provides an ultimate therapeutic goal.

ROLE OF THE PHYSICAL THERAPIST IN HOME HEALTH

The fundamental roles of the older adult–oriented home care physical therapist are to promote independence in essential activities of daily living (ADLs), promote reintegration of the patient into the community, and to minimize the risk for either recurrent acute care hospitalizations and/or nursing home admission. According to a 2009 study of 1480 participants conducted by the National Alliance for Caregiving, 60% of family caregivers report

assisting a relative with at least one activity of daily living. As such, home care therapists play a key role in teaching caregivers a variety of safety techniques, including proper patient positioning for transfers and fall prevention.[3] The patient's home environment provides a rich context for the therapist to gain insight into the patient's functional abilities, in particular, the performance of essential ADLs such as bathing, dressing, walking inside the house, and transferring from a chair. Frequently, hospitalization or inactivity leads to the development of or restriction of essential ADLs.[4] Furthermore, individuals who lose their ability to perform valued functional and social activities are more likely to become dissatisfied with their quality of life and are likely to experience depression, increasing the likelihood of being homebound.[5] The effect of decreased physical activity and functioning promotes further decline on the slippery slope of aging[6] and increases the risk for physical frailty, recurrent disability, multiple hospitalizations, and eventual nursing home admission.[4] The home care physical therapist has a critical role to play in this transitional setting between a higher level of function and institutionalization.

Rehospitalization

The process by which patients move from hospitals to other care settings is increasingly problematic as hospitals shorten lengths of stay and care becomes more fragmented. Within 30 days of discharge, there was a 17.6% rate of hospital readmissions in 2008,[7] with home health patients the most vulnerable.[8] A study on Medicare Fee for Service home health beneficiaries in 2004 revealed that almost one of every five discharges (19.6%) are readmitted within 30 days and 34% of discharges were readmitted within 90 days. The study also estimated Medicare's cost for these unplanned readmissions was $17.4 billion.[9] The most frequent reasons for unplanned readmissions were acute myocardial infarction, heart failure, pneumonia, sepsis, dehydration, postoperative infection, and gastrointestinal bleeding.[9] Unplanned rehospitalizations are almost always urgent or medical emergencies and often signal failure of the transition from the hospital to another source of care.

In 2007 and 2008, more than 5500 home health agencies joined the first Home Health Quality Improvement National Campaign[10] funded by the Centers for Medicare and Medicaid Services (CMS), an agency of the U.S. Department of Health and Human Services. As a follow-up to this initial project, the CMS funded a second campaign that was launched in January 2010. The contractors for the 2010 campaign, West Virginia Medical Institute and Quality Insights, the Medicare quality improvement organization (QIO) for West Virginia, provided campaign participants with best-practice tools or "intervention packages" designed to avoid potentially preventable hospitalizations. CMS looks to QIOs, nonprofit organizations under contract with CMS, to implement projects that affect process improvements to address issues in medication management, postdischarge follow-up, and plans of care for patients who move across health care settings. As such, QIOs conducted interviews in 2007 with providers in community forums to identify gaps across the transition from hospital to home.[10] The three main drivers of unplanned rehospitalizations that emerged were that (1) the patient and family was not engaged in the health care process, (2) there were gaps in processes within a provider or provider group (e.g., not having a focused plan of care for CHF patients, or not having a uniform discharge transfer tool), and (3) there was not an existing process to communicate information between providers at discharge including the next care provider and the primary care physician (PCP). The overriding goal of this two-phased campaign that started in 2007 is to unite the home health stakeholders and providers across multiple health care settings in a shared vision of reducing avoidable hospitalizations and improving medication management. The evidence of national and individual home health agency's success is demonstrated with publicly reported comparative measures (Box 25-2).

Rosati et al[11] identified several risk factors for medical adverse events among home health care recipients listed in Box 25-3 and found that home health agencies that focused on these risk factors were more likely to improve

---

BOX 25-2 | Publically Reported Comparative Measures for Home Health Agencies

The quality measures available include:
1. Three measures related to improvement in getting around:
   a. Percentage of patients who get better at walking or moving around
   b. Percentage of patients who get better at getting in and out of bed
   c. Percentage of patients who have less pain when moving around
2. Four measures related to meeting the patient's activities of daily living:
   a. Percentage of patients whose bladder control improves
   b. Percentage of patients who get better at bathing
   c. Percentage of patients who get better at taking their medicines correctly (by mouth)
   d. Percentage of patients who are short of breath less often
3. Two measures about how home health care ends:
   a. Percentage of patients who stay at home after an episode of home health care ends
   b. Percentage of patients whose wounds improved or healed after an operation
4. Three measures related to patient medical emergencies:
   a. Percentage of patients who had to be admitted to the hospital
   b. Percentage of patients who need urgent, unplanned medical care
   c. Percentage of patients who need unplanned medical care related to a wound that is new, is worse, or has become infected

(From Medicare—the official U.S. Government site for people with Medicare. Home health compare. http://www.medicare.gov/HHCompare/Home. asp?dest=NAV|Home|DataDetails#TabTop. Accessed April 29, 2010.)

BOX 25-3 | Risk Factors for Medical Adverse Events

- Pattern of one or more hospitalizations or emergency room visits in the past 12 months
- History of falls
- Chronic conditions such as congestive heart failure, skin ulcers, or congestive obstructive pulmonary disease
- Social and cognitive factors such as inadequate support network, low literacy level, dementia, needing help with managing medications, and low socioeconomic status

(Modified from Rosati RJ, Huang L, Navaie-Waliser M, Feldman PH: Risk factors for repeated hospitalizations among home healthcare recipients. J Healthc Qual 25(2):4-10; 2003.)

the effectiveness and efficiency of their efforts to prevent rehospitalization of their patients.[11] Home health physical therapists who address a patient's fall risk and decline in physical functioning can play a key role in the prevention of unplanned hospital readmissions. A continued focus on reducing the factors contributing to rehospitalization to promote cost containment will continue in the foreseeable future, with physical therapists continuing to play a significant role.

Variability of the Home Environment

In addition to the medical management of the patient, providing physical therapy care in the patient's home presents unique personal challenges. The clinician has to be sensitive to and respectful of any boundaries the patient sets with respect to their home environment and aspects of care provided. The home health clinician may encounter a wide variety of socioeconomic, ethnic, and cultural situations. Sensitivity to patient beliefs and background is needed to help gain trust and establish rapport with the home health patient. Clinicians in the home setting are likely to encounter a variety of cultural dynamics. Depending upon the patient's culture, self-care may not be an important personal goal and therefore it may be inappropriate to insist that an older adult patient provide self-care, especially when family members are available and willing to provide care.[12]

In some cultures, older adults are considered to be "entitled" to rest and to be cared for by loved ones. In fact, the majority of cultures do not consider self-care to be an important goal of aging, including Asian, Hispanic, and almost all other cultures other than Anglo-American. These cultures value family interdependence over independence and therefore may feel it is inappropriate for an older adult to insist upon self-care when family members are available to provide care. Moreover, younger caregivers may be quite willing to attend to older loved ones as a natural and normal family dynamic. However, although there is great diversity in American culture, American culture typically promotes continued self-reliance and the maintenance of independence with age for the most part. Independence in traditional American culture is not only the expectation but a source of self-esteem, whereas dependence can be a source of significant emotional and psychological distress. See Box 25-4 for a cultural assessment checklist.[13]

Some clients/patients may prefer to have family members present during physical therapy sessions and, depending upon the degree of family involvement, there may be the need for additional teaching and explanations. By contrast, the physical therapist may be able to work more effectively with the patient when there are no family "observers" as the patient may be reluctant to demonstrate functional independence in front of family caregivers. Sensitivity to cultural differences, such as acceptability of being touched, in particular by someone of the opposite gender, verbal and nonverbal expressions of pain, and patient-specific goal setting allows clinicians to adapt care in a manner that is congruent with their patients' cultural expectations.[14]

Lastly, providing care in the home involves having to adapt to a variety of structural barriers, sensitivity to the homeowner who may not be the patient, as well as lifestyle preferences of the patient and/or caregivers. Patients typically have daily routines, routines that when disrupted can be sources of stress and conflict. Home health therapists have to take these concerns into account when scheduling treatment times. In addition, homes can range widely from being very tidy to being cluttered, presenting fall risk hazards. All of these variables can make it challenging to prescribe an effective exercise program, and a substantial degree of creativity is needed to make the best of a particular situation.

REIMBURSEMENT AND DOCUMENTATION

The Medicare Payment Advisory Commission (MedPAC) classifies Home Health as a postacute setting,[15] and payment is administered under the Medicare Part A program. MedPAC advises the Center for Medicare and Medicaid Services (CMS) on setting payment rates for all Medicare providers. Similar to other settings, Medicare sets payment rates based on the patient's medical complexity and expected resource use. In 2006, Medicare spent $12.9 billion on home health services for 2.8 million beneficiaries, representing a growth of about 44% since 2002. The number of home health agencies (HHAs) also increased, from 6553 in 2002 to 8463 in 2006, with more than half of the increase occurring in just two states—Florida and Texas.[16] Medicare home health spending is expected to grow by an average of 6.2% annually between 2007 and 2016.[15]

Medicare pays HHAs a predetermined base payment under what is called the prospective payment system (PPS).[17] The base payment is adjusted for the health condition and care needs of the Medicare beneficiary. The payment is also adjusted for the geographic differences in wages for HHAs across the country. The adjustment for the health condition, or clinical characteristics, and service needs of the beneficiary is referred to as the case-mix adjustment. The home health PPS will provide HHAs with payments for each 60-day episode of care for each beneficiary. If a beneficiary is still eligible for care after the end of the first episode, a second episode can begin; there are no limits to the number of episodes a beneficiary who remains eligible for the home health benefit can receive. Although payment for each episode is adjusted to reflect the beneficiary's health condition and needs, a special outlier provision exists to ensure appropriate payment for those beneficiaries that have the most expensive care needs. Adjusting payment to

BOX 25-4 Cultural Assessment Checklist

Health/Illness Issues
- Are there health problems that carry a stigma in the culture?
- Are there culture-bound illnesses (i.e., illnesses that are only identified within the culture)?
- Are there tests/procedures/treatments that violate cultural norms?
- In past experiences with the health care system, what has the patient found helpful? Offensive? Confusing?

Life Span Rituals/Practices
- What beliefs, values, and practices surround life events (birth, childcare, aging, death)? Ask as appropriate to patient's situation.
- When the patient has a terminal disease, should one "tell the truth" or "maintain hope"?

Biophysical/Risk Factor Variation
- Are there genetic variations or endemic diseases frequently encountered within the patient's group?
- Do members of the culture commonly engage in practices that are harmful?

Pain Assessment
- Does the patient tend to be stoic or expressive when in pain?
- What does pain mean to the patient?
- Is pain generally described in quantitative or qualitative terms?
- Is the numerical scale confusing?
- What is the patient's attitude about taking pain medications?
- Ask the patient: What is the worst pain you have ever had? How did you cope with it? How did you treat it? How well did the treatment work?

Nutrition Assessment
- What is eaten and when is it eaten? Perform a 2-day diet recall.
- Are there dietary patterns that may be in conflict with the plan of care (e.g., fasting)?
- Is there potential for food–drug interactions with traditional foods?
- What foods are thought to promote health? What foods are considered good for sick people?
- Does the patient ascribe to the cold–hot theory of disease and treatment?
- Are there religious food prescriptions and restrictions?

Medication Assessment
- What is the patient's attitude toward Western medications? Are they valued or distrusted?
- Could there be genetic variations in the way the patient responds to medications?
- Are there traditional remedies, such as herbs, teas, or ointments that the patient uses?

Daily (Health) Practices and Routines
- Are there special rituals/practices associated with bathing, toileting, hair/nail care?
- Are there gender/age/social class restrictions on who can help a person with ADLs?
- How important is modesty? How is modesty shown?
- Are there special morning/evening rituals or practices that are important to the patient?

Psychosocial Assessment
- Who is considered "family"? What impact does the illness have on the family?
- Who is the head of the family? Who makes decisions for the patient?
- With whom should we discuss your care? Is there someone who helps you make decisions?
- How will family members be involved in the patient's care?
- Who helps when you are sick? How do they help you? How would you like them to help you?
- What health/support services are available through the patient's cultural community?

Degree of Acculturation
- How strictly does the patient/family adhere to the belief/values/practices of their culture of origin?
- Is the patient/family traditional (maintains ways of culture of origin)? Acculturated (understands and is able to move in/out of old/new culture)? Assimilated (has internalized the new culture's norms)?

Religion/Spiritual Needs
- Are there spiritual practices that providers and caregivers can help the patient to keep (e.g., special prayer times)?
- Are there religious articles that the patient likes to use, wear, or keep close?
- Are their special rites/blessings for the sick? Spiritual leaders/healers the patient finds helpful?
- Are there dietary prescriptions or restrictions that should be kept?

Language and Communication
- What language is the patient most comfortable speaking?
- The patient has a right to a medical interpreter. Would the patient like one?
- Is the patient able to read in English or in preferred language?

Continued

BOX 25-4 | **Cultural Assessment Checklist—cont'd**

Patient's Explanation of Health Problem
- What do you call the problem you are having? (Use the patient's term instead of "the problem" when asking the rest of the questions.
- When and how did your problem begin? Why do you think the problem started when it did?
- What do you think caused this problem? Why do you think you developed this problem and not someone else? What might others in your family/community think is wrong with you?
- Do you know someone who has had this problem? What happened to that person? Do you think this will happen to you?
- What are the chief problems this condition has caused you?
- What problems has it brought into your life? What do you think will happen?
- What do you fear most about the problem? How serious is this problem? Do you think it is curable?
- How have you treated the problem so far? What have you done to feel better? Have you tried remedies like herbs or remedies from your homeland?
- How do you/your family/your community members think the problem should be treated? Who in your family/community/religious group can help you? Are you consulting other healers?

Nonverbal Communication Patterns
- Is eye contact considered polite or rude?
- Is personal space wider/narrower than American norms?
- When, where, and by whom can the patient be touched?
- What is the meaning behind certain facial expressions and hand/body gestures?
- Is special meaning attached to loud or whispered conversations?

Etiquette and Social Customs
- How would you like to be greeted and addressed by our staff?
- What behaviors are expected of guests? Taking shoes off?
- Accepting food/drink?
- Is punctuality important?
- Is it polite to engage in "small talk" before getting "down to business"?
- Should discussions be direct and forthright or subtle and indirect?
- What topics are not acceptable? Is it appropriate to share emotions and feelings? Discuss reproduction, sexual, or elimination issues? Discuss the possibility of negative outcomes?

At Times Like This, Many People Draw on their Religious/Spiritual Beliefs to Help Them.
- Is there anything the nurses can do to help you find the spiritual strength you need at this time?
- Are there spiritual practices that we can facilitate for you?
- Is there a religious leader/healer whom you might find helpful?

Your Nurses and Therapists Want to Be Polite and Respectful to You and your Family.
- How would you like to be addressed by our staff?
- Are there certain cultural courtesies we should practice when we come to visit you?
- Are there things we might do that you would find offensive?
- Could you please let us know if anything we do seems rude or offensive so we can fix it?

Everyone Has Cultural Beliefs and Customs that They Find Help Them to Heal.
- Are there special beliefs or customs you would like to keep related to this health problem?
- Are there special herbs/foods/treatments that you have found helpful?
- Are there healers from your community who might also be able to help you?
- How does your family think this illness should be treated?
- What do you think about that treatment?
- What are the characteristics of a good doctor? Of a good nurse?

(Modified from Narayan MC: Cultural assessment and care planning. Home Healthc Nurse 21:611-618, 2003.)

---

reflect the HHA's cost in caring for each beneficiary, including the sickest, should ensure that all beneficiaries have access to home health services for which they are eligible.

Payment for each home health 60-day certification period, or episode rate, is based on a complex formula of factors. Factors include the impact of specific diagnoses within certain groups called case-mix weight diagnoses, the patient's clinical needs, functional status,

and service utilization (i.e., amount of medically necessary therapy visits). The computation of the episode rate is derived from responses to specific data elements extracted from a unique home health assessment instrument called the Outcome and Assessment Information Set (OASIS).[18] The OASIS allows for the computation and reporting of measures that are calculated from standardized data elements. In addition to quality measurement, a subset of OASIS items is used to calculate payment algorithms under the prospective payment system.[18]

The OASIS instrument, in use since July 1999, is used by the HHA nurse or therapist to assess the patient's condition. The OASIS instrument has been revised several times with the latest version, implemented January 1, 2010, called the OASIC-C. Physical therapy is one of the three qualifying disciplines authorized to collect the

initial OASIS data as part of the patient's comprehensive assessment at the start of care. Skilled nursing and speech–language pathology are the other two qualifying disciplines authorized to collect OASIS data at the start of care. However, the Medicare Conditions of Participation for Home Health[19] require a registered nurse to make the initial visit and collect the OASIS data if skilled nursing is ordered at the time of referral[20] (Box 25-5).

BOX 25-5 | **Conditions of Participation: Home Health Agencies, Subpart C—Furnishing of Services**

PART 484—Conditions of Participation: Home Health Agencies
Subpart C—Furnishing of Services
Sec. 484.55 Condition of participation: Comprehensive assessment of patients.
Each patient must receive, and an HHA must provide, a patient-specific, comprehensive assessment that accurately reflects the patient's current health status and includes information that may be used to demonstrate the patient's progress toward achievement of desired outcomes. The comprehensive assessment must identify the patient's continuing need for home care and meet the patient's medical, nursing, rehabilitative, social, and discharge planning needs. For Medicare beneficiaries, the HHA must verify the patient's eligibility for the Medicare home health benefit including homebound status, both at the time of the initial assessment visit and at the time of the comprehensive assessment. The comprehensive assessment must also incorporate the use of the current version of the Outcome and Assessment Information Set (OASIS) items, using the language and groupings of the OASIS items, as specified by the Secretary.

(a) Standard: Initial Assessment Visit.
(1) **A registered nurse must** conduct an initial assessment visit to determine the immediate care and support needs of the patient; and, for Medicare patients, to determine eligibility for the Medicare home health benefit, including homebound status. The initial assessment visit must be held either within 48 hours of referral, or within 48 hours of the patient's return home, or on the physician-ordered start of care date.
(2) **When rehabilitation therapy service (speech–language pathology, physical therapy, or occupational therapy) is the only service ordered by the physician, and if the need for that service establishes program eligibility, the initial assessment visit may be made by the appropriate rehabilitation skilled professional.**

(b) Standard: Completion of the Comprehensive Assessment.
(1) The comprehensive assessment must be completed in a timely manner, consistent with the patient's immediate needs, but no later than 5 calendar days after the start of care.
(2) Except as provided in paragraph (b)(3) of this section, a registered nurse must complete the comprehensive assessment and for Medicare patients, determine eligibility for the Medicare home health benefit, including homebound status.
(3) When physical therapy, speech–language pathology, or occupational therapy is the only service ordered by the physician, a physical therapist, speech–language pathologist or occupational therapist may complete the comprehensive assessment, and for Medicare patients, determine eligibility for the Medicare home health benefit, including homebound status. The occupational therapist may complete the comprehensive assessment if the need for occupational therapy establishes program eligibility.

(c) Standard: Drug Regimen Review.
The comprehensive assessment must include a review of all medications the patient is currently using in order to identify any potential adverse effects and drug reactions, including ineffective drug therapy, significant side effects, significant drug interactions, duplicate drug therapy, and noncompliance with drug therapy.

(d) Standard: Update of the Comprehensive Assessment.
The comprehensive assessment must be updated and revised (including the administration of the OASIS) as frequently as the patient's condition warrants due to a major decline or improvement in the patient's health status, but not less frequently than—
(1) Every second calendar month beginning with the start of care date;
(2) Within 48 hours of the patient's return to the home from a hospital admission of 24 hours or more for any reason other than diagnostic tests;
(3) At discharge.

(e) Standard: Incorporation of OASIS Data Items.
The OASIS data items determined by the Secretary must be incorporated into the HHA's own assessment and must include: clinical record items, demographics and patient history, living arrangements, supportive assistance, sensory status, integumentary status, respiratory status, elimination status, neuro/emotional/behavioral status, activities of daily living, medications, equipment management, emergent care, and data items collected at inpatient facility admission or discharge only.

(From U.S. Department of Health and Human Services. Part 484: Conditions of participation: Home health agencies, Subpart C—Furnishing of services. http://frwebgate.access.gpo.gov/cgi-bin/get-cfr.cgi?TITLE=42&PART=484&SECTION=55&YEAR=1999&TYPE=TEXT. Accessed April 6, 2010.)

This initial visit serves to assess if the patient meets home health coverage criteria, the patient's condition and likely needs for skilled nursing care, therapy, medical social services, and home health aide services. OASIS items describing the patient's condition, as well as the expected therapy needs (physical, speech–language pathology, or occupational) are used to determine a case-mix factor that reflects the relative costliness of patients in a particular case-mix category. This payment adjustment is the case-mix adjustment. There are 153 case-mix groups, or Home Health Resource Groups (HHRG), available for patient classification.

The 60-day-episode payment for a home health patient is calculated from the day the OASIS is completed. OASIS regulations require that the expected number of therapy visits needed be projected at the beginning of each episode by the clinician conducting the home health OASIS assessment. This projection is adjusted up or down from the initial projection based on the needs of the patient that emerge during the 60-day episode. As a disincentive for home health agencies to provide more care than is appropriate, incremental increases in therapy result in a declining rather than constant amount of payment per additional therapy visit.[21]

At the end of each 60-day episode, the actual number of therapy visits provided to a patient is reconciled against the projected number of therapy visits planned. Depending upon the difference (more than projected visits were provided vs. less than projected provided), the home health agency may be subject to an adjustment in their final Medicare episode payment.[21]

Home Health Documentation Requirements

The Medicare Conditions of Participation for Home Health mandate an initial comprehensive, individual, and specific assessment of each patient. Whether the therapist is documenting on paper-based forms or electronically, the initial home health visit can average 90 minutes to complete the initial comprehensive assessment. In addition to the OASIS instrument, therapists may also have to document the patient's medication profile that includes all of the prescription and over-the-counter medication, including herbs and supplements. When a home health case is "therapy only," the physical therapist may find that a great deal of time is spent on the initial home health visit resolving medication discrepancies between the hospital discharge medication list and the patient's actual medications in the home. Follow-up with the primary care physicians and specialists to resolve discrepancies or to obtain a referral for a nurse is often necessary. Until the therapist becomes familiar with the OASIS instrument and more practiced in

completing medication profiles, the initial home health visit with an OASIS assessment can take as much as 2 hours. Most importantly, the primary focus for a physical therapist conducting a home health admission is to ensure that the patient is safe at home and to refer to other disciplines/services when appropriate. An explanation of the services covered by Medicare for Home Health is presented in Box 25-6.

OASIS rules and conventions are described in detail in the OASIS Implementation Manual and are periodically updated with information available at the CMS website.[1] Competence in assessment of all areas of the OASIS may require additional education in differential diagnosis, pharmacology, skin assessment, depression screening, and home safety assessment. Given the uniqueness of the home health admission, the therapist new to the home care setting can benefit greatly from a guided practical orientation with a peer mentor. The mentor can role-model how to efficiently conduct the sequence of interview questions that correspond with OASIS data items. Some OASIS assessment "quick tips" are described in Table 25-1.[22]

Specific observations of the patient's functional abilities such as transfers, dressing, and walking are also necessary for accurate responses to OASIS items and serve as the basis for planning the teaching that a therapist would provide the patient. The length of time a patient or family or caregiver may require education interventions should be determined by assessing each patient's individual condition and other pertinent factors such as the skill required to teach the activity and the unique abilities of the patient. It is important to know that teaching activities must be related to the patient's functional loss, illness, or injury. When a patient or caregiver is incapable of learning, more visits to provide patient/caregiver education are subject to Medicare payment denials. Medicare's home health benefit is not intended to provide training and education to patients, families, or caregivers for an infinite period of time.

THE INITIAL VISIT

This section will describe the features of best practices for the first visit for a home care patient under Medicare Part A. The authors suggest contacting the patient prior to the initial visit to arrange a time that is convenient and to request the patient have a Medicare card and all medications (including over-the-counter) available and ready for review. Also, the patient may prefer to have a family member or friend present. Calling ahead is useful because Medicare does not require a patient to be home 24/7 to be considered homebound. Asking the patient or family member to have the Medicare card and medications ready will help to make the

BOX 25-6   Skilled Services for Home Health Covered by Medicare Part A

Skilled Nursing (SN)
- Observation and assessment of the patient's condition
- Medication management/assessment and teaching
- Tube feedings
- Nasopharyngeal and tracheotomy aspiration
- Catheters, wound care, heat treatments, medical gases, rehabilitation nursing, venipuncture, psychiatric evaluation, therapy and teaching

Speech–Language Pathology (SLP)
- A change in functional speech or motivation
- Clearing of confusion
- The remission of some other medical condition that previously contraindicated speech–language pathology services

Occupational Therapy (OT)
- Selecting and teaching task oriented therapeutic activities designed to restore physical function
- Planning, implementing and supervising therapeutic tasks and activities designed to restore sensory-integrative function (vision and cognition)
- Planning, implementing and supervising individualized therapeutic activity programs as part of an overall "active treatment" program with a patient diagnosed with psychiatric illness
- Teaching compensatory techniques to improve the level of independence in the activities of daily living
- Designing, fabricating and fitting of orthotic and self-help devices
- Vocational and prevocational assessment and training
- Patient must have a continued need for OT when: the services meet the definition of OT and the patient's eligibility has been established by virtue of a prior need for skilled nursing care, SLP or PT in the current or prior certification period

Medical Social Services (MSW)
- Assessment of the social and emotional factors related to the patient's illness, need for care, response to treatment and adjustment to care
- Assessment of the relationship of the patient's medical and nursing requirements to the patient's home situation, financial resources and availability of community resources
- Appropriate action to obtain available community resources to assist in resolving the patient's problem
- Medicare does not cover the services of MSW to complete application for Medicaid
- Counseling services that are required by the patient
- Services of MSW are covered if they are necessary to resolve social or emotional problems that are or expected to be an impediment to the effective treatment of the patient's medical condition AND the plan of care indicates how the services necessitate the skills of a qualified MSW to be performed safely and effectively
- Covered on a short term basis and agency must demonstrate that a brief MSW intervention is necessary to remove, clear and direct impediment to the effective treatment of the patient's medical condition or to the patient's rate of recovery

Home Health Aide (HHA)
- Patient care
- Simple dressing changes that do not require skills of a licensed nurse
- Assistance with medications which are ordinarily self-administered and do not require the skills of a licensed nurse to be provided safely and effectively
- Assistance with activities which are directly supportive of skilled therapy services but do not require the skills of a licensed nurse to be provided safely and effectively
- Assistance with activities which are directly supportive of skilled therapy services but do not require the skills of a therapist to be safely and effectively performed such as routine maintenance exercises and repetitive practice of functional communication skills to support SLP services
- Provision of services incidental to personal care services: however the purpose of HHA visit may not be only to provide incidental services (light cleaning, preparation of a meal, taking out the trash, shopping, etc.)
- Must be intermittent and patient is being case managed by SN, PT, OT or SLP

(From Centers for Medicare & Medicaid Services: Medicare benefit policy manual. http://www.cms.hhs.gov/manuals/Downloads/bp102c07.pdf. Accessed April 29, 2010.)

time spent in the patient's home more efficient. Items recommended to have available on the first and subsequent visits are listed in Box 25-7. It is valuable to carry everything in a clinical travel bag. In addition to the bag, home health therapists should always carry a cell phone and keep car keys on their person at all times in case of an emergency.

THE PHYSICAL THERAPY ASSESSMENT

The Comprehensive Start of Care OASIS and Consent (Full Disclosure)

Opening a Case. Arguably the primary focus of opening a case is to complete the OASIS, assure the patient is safe to be in his or her home, and refer to other skilled

TABLE 25-1	OASIS Quick Tips
Action	**Assess (Components of the OASIS)**
Greet your patient at the door. Review and sign agency admission paperwork. Ask about vision problems (e.g., cataracts, glaucoma, diabetic retinopathy) or use of corrective devices. Ask the patient to count fingers at arms length.	*Assess:* Ambulation/locomotion, dyspnea, cognitive functioning, urinary/bowel incontinence, grooming, confusion, anxiety, hearing and ability to understand language, speech and oral expression of language
Ask if there is anything the patient cannot do or has trouble doing because of pain or discomfort. Ask the patient if he or she is more irritable or less tolerant of frustrations?	*Assess:* Ambulation/locomotion, pain, anxiety, confusion, dyspnea, grooming, ability to dress upper and lower body, transferring
Have the patient go to the bedroom. Observe the patient sitting and rising from the bed (or his or her ability to turn if bedfast). Ask the patient to get a shirt out of the closet or dresser and put it on, or ask the patient to obtain a coat or jacket he or she would wear to a doctor appointment. Ask the patient if anyone lays clothes out for him or her. Perform skin scan. Minimally, ask the patient to remove shirt, remove shoes and socks, and lift pant legs.	*Assess:* Ambulation/locomotion, pain, skin lesion or open wound, pressure ulcer, stasis ulcers, respirator treatment (look for CPAP), anxiety, confusion, dyspnea, behaviors demonstrated at least once a week, grooming, ability to dress upper and lower body, transferring
Ask the patient what he or she ate at his or her last meal. Ask what he or she would do in the event of a fire.	*Assess:* Memory deficit, impaired decision making, behaviors demonstrated, cognitive functioning, confusion
Have the patient walk to the bathroom and sit and rise from the commode. Ask the patient to step into the tub or shower. Ask if the patient ever has help in the tub or needs reminders. Ask the patient what type of assistance he or she needs to wash his or her entire body in the tub or shower. Ask the patient if he or she ever has "little accidents," dribbling, stress incontinence, or trouble holding stools. Normalize this occurrence based on age or disease status.	*Assess:* Management of oral medications, management of inhalant medications, management of injectable medications, patient management of equipment, O$_2$, IV, cognitive functioning, confusion, anxiety, behaviors demonstrated, reported or observed, hearing and ability to understand language, speech and oral expression of language
Have the patient walk you to where he or she keeps his or her medications. Have the patient ambulate 20 feet and negotiate stairs (if indicated). If the patient is chairfast or bedbound, observe dyspnea while performing ADLs.	*Assess:* Pain, vision, dyspnea, hearing and ability to understand language, cognitive functioning, confusion, anxiety, ambulation
Have the patient open a medication bottle, pour out a pill, tell you the color, read the dosage instructions, and tell you the correct times to take the medication.	*Assess:* Management of oral medications, management of inhalant medications, management of injectable medications, patient management of equipment, O$_2$, IV, cognitive functioning, confusion, anxiety, behaviors demonstrated, reported or observed, hearing and ability to understand language, speech and oral expression of language

CPAP, continuous positive airway pressure; *IV,* intravenous *OASIS,* Outcome and Assessment Information Set.

(*Adapted from Colorado Foundation for Medical Care. Home health: toolkits and resources. http://www.cfmc.org/hh/hh_toolkits.htm.*)

services when appropriate. As mentioned previously, opening a case for an experienced clinician typically takes 1 to 2 hours depending on the complexity of the patient and home situation. The OASIS document serves as a guideline for the clinician to ensure a comprehensive assessment.

TIP: ASSESSMENT OF URINARY AND BOWEL INCONTINENCE

The OASIS assessment requires the physical therapist to assess for urinary and bowel incontinence. When interviewing the patient, he or she may deny this condition especially in the presence of family members and/or friends. The clinician may need to do some "detective work" (or sense of smell) to answer this question correctly. During the assessment of ADL/IADLs section of the OASIS when the patient is up and moving around the house, look for adult diapers in the bathroom and/or next to the patient's bed.

The results of the OASIS will help the clinician determine if there are issues in an area beyond the scope of physical therapy. The clinician is ethically obligated to refer to the appropriate service for additional assessment and intervention. For example, if the patient is having difficulty in the OASIS area of Living Arrangements, Supportive Assistance, and Emotional/Behavioral status, the physical therapist may consider a referral to social work services. If the patient is having difficulties in the areas of sensation, cognition, vision, ADLs or instrumental activities of daily living (IADLs), the clinician may consider a referral for speech–language pathology or occupational therapy. An occupational therapist can also assist the patient with equipment needs/management. If the patient is having difficulties in the areas of integumentary, respiratory, cardiovascular, urinary, gastrointestinal, or medication management, the clinician may consider a referral to a skilled nurse. The need for a home health aide should

BOX 25-7 | Items for the Clinical Bag

The Clinical Bag—Essential Items to Pack for the Trip
Blood pressure cuff
Cardiopulmonary resuscitation mask
Disinfectant wipes for equipment
Gait belt
Girth measurement tape
Goniometer
Hand soap
Paper towels
Personal protective equipment (gloves, mask, gowns)
Reflex hammer
Sterile wound care supplies
Stethoscope
Stopwatch
Tape measure
Thermometer

Additional Useful Items
1000 feet or more measuring wheel
Balance pad
Elastic tube/bands
Masking tape
Pedal ergometer
Pulse oximeter
Weighted vest

also be assessed at the start of care. The patient who is receiving home health services under the Medicare part A benefit is entitled to receive all the services needed. Medicare has defined guidelines for what is considered skilled services in home health.[23] See Box 25-6 for a detailed explanation of skilled services covered by Medicare Part A in Home Health. Once the systems review has been completed using the OASIS as a guide, a medication reconciliation is required.

The Medication Reconciliation

Pharmacology competencies for the physical therapist are defined by the American Physical Therapy Association (APTA).[24] These competencies state that the physical therapist should, at a minimum, list all medications (over-the-counter and prescribed) on the medication profile for the patient's clinical record. Importantly, it is not within a physical therapist's scope of practice to provide instructions about how to take drugs or assess for possible drug interactions. However, the physical therapist should be aware of adverse drug reactions for the patient's safety, and recognize when it is necessary to contact the patient's physician to obtain an order for a skilled nursing assessment. Tips for assessing the patient's ability to manage medications are described in Table 25-1 (OASIS assessment quick tips).

Physical therapists should then perform a reconciliation of the medication list. This reconciliation includes assessment of whether the medications correlate with past medical history or current diagnosis. For this skill, the physical therapist needs to have knowledge of medications and their appropriate usage. The therapist should also reconcile the patient's symptoms with possible adverse drug reactions. For example, if a patient complains of dizziness and is taking multiple medications to lower blood pressure, the patient may be experiencing an adverse drug event. Finally, the therapist should assess whether there are medication implications for the therapy plan of care. In the previous example, if the patient is experiencing dizziness from hypotension, a clinical hypothesis regarding decreased exercise tolerance should be explored.

When reviewing medications with the patient, the home care physical therapist should consider if a skilled nursing assessment may be warranted. It should be noted that there are different regulations by state on medication reviews and providing patient education about high-risk medications by physical therapists. For example, as a result of the implementation of OASIS-C, in January 2010 the New York State Department of Health ruled that a physical therapist may complete the comprehensive assessment *only* if the home health agency has implemented a policy and procedure that requires collaboration between the physical therapist and other agency staff.[25] It is important for home health therapists to be aware of their state regulations regarding medication review.

Older adults aged 65 years or older are at a higher risk for adverse drug reactions (ADR) than younger individuals.[26,27] The increased risk occurs for several reasons. Older adults are prescribed more medications and have more chronic conditions than younger individuals.[28] In addition, the older adult may metabolize the drug less efficiently, especially in the presence of disease. Medication errors, either patient-initiated or prescribing errors, can cause an ADR. Physical therapists need to be aware that errors that lead to adverse events most often occur after the medication regimen is prescribed—while the patient is administering the drug and fails to adhere to medical advice about medication use.[28] If the patient or family member is unable to tell the clinician what medications the patient is taking or the usage and purpose of the medication, it is likely that the patient is at risk for an adverse drug event.

Several red flags pertinent to the physical therapist may become apparent during the medication reconciliation. For example, older adults taking more than four medications are at increased risk for falls because of the accumulated and/or enhanced side effects of the medications.[29] The Beers criteria for potentially inappropriate medication can be used to screen the medication profile for inappropriate or problematic drugs. Although the list was approved by expert consensus panels of geriatricians and was widely published, a percentage of older adults continue to use these medications.[26] Adverse drug events occur most often because of prescribed medications[30];

however, it has been suggested that community-dwelling older adults who take medications identified on the Beers list are at a greater risk for an adverse drug event.[31] The Beer's list of potentially dangerous drugs for older adults is shown in Box 25-8. The Screening Tool of Older Persons' Potentially Inappropriate Prescriptions (STOPP) published in 2008 is another valuable reference for the home care physical therapist.[32] The STOPP criteria focus on avoiding use of medications potentially inappropriate in older adults, similar to the Beers list. The criteria are organized by organ system. Examples of the STOPP criteria include theophylline as monotherapy for chronic obstructive pulmonary disease, nonsteroidal anti-inflammatory drugs (NSAIDs) with heart failure, NSAIDs together with warfarin, vasodilator with postural hypotension, and bladder antimuscarinic drugs with dementia. The authors recommend that the home health therapist have a copy of the Beer's list and STOPP when in the home to utilize as a quick reference tool during medication reconciliation.

Apart from a medication review, the therapist could determine if the patient or caregiver has difficulty with managing the medication regimen such as being able to visually recognize each drug, describe the purpose, verbalize when to take each medication, and determine if the patient uses any type of medication-organizing system. The therapist should be aware of the strain on caregivers when the burden of managing and

---

BOX 25-8 | Beers List of Potentially Dangerous Drugs for Older Adults

alprazolam (Xanax)	guanethidine (Ismelin)
amiodarone (Cordarone)	halazepam (Paxipam)
amitriptyline (Elavil)	hydroxyzine (Vistaril, Atarax)
amphetamines	indomethacin (Indocin, Indocin SR)
anorexic agents	isoxsuprine (Vasodilan)
barbiturates	ketorolac (Toradol)
belladonna alkaloids (Donnatal)	lorazepam (Ativan)
bisacodyl (Dulcolax)	meperidine (Demerol)
carisoprodol (Soma)	meprobamate (Miltown, Equanil)
cascara sagrada	mesoridazine (Serentil)
chlordiazepoxide (Librium, Mitran)	metaxalone (Skelaxin)
chlordiazepoxide-amitriptyline (Limbitrol)	methocarbamol (Robaxin)
chlorpheniramine (Chlor-Trimeton)	methyldopa (Aldomet)
chlorpropamide (Diabinese)	methyldopa-hydrochlorothiazide (Aldoril)
chlorzoxazone (Paraflex)	methyltestosterone (Android, Virilon, Testred)
cimetidine (Tagamet)	mineral oil
clidinium-chlordiazepoxide (Librax)	naproxen (Naprosyn, Avaprox, Aleve)
clonidine (Catapres)	Neoloid
clorazepate (Tranxene)	nifedipine (Procardia, Adalat)
cyclandelate (Cyclospasmol)	nitrofurantoin (Macrodantin)
cyclobenzaprine (Flexeril)	orphenadrine (Norflex)
cyproheptadine (Periactin)	oxaprozin (Daypro)
desiccated thyroid	oxazepam (Serax)
dexchlorpheniramine (Polaramine)	oxybutynin (Ditropan)
diazepam (Valium)	pentazocine (Talwin)
dicyclomine (Bentyl)	perphenazine-amitriptyline (Triavil)
digoxin (Lanoxin)	piroxicam (Feldene)
diphenhydramine (Benadryl)	promethazine (Phenergan)
dipyridamole (Persantine)	propantheline (Pro-Banthine)
disopyramide (Norpace, Norpace CR)	propoxyphene (Darvon) and combination products
doxazosin (Cardura)	quazepam (Doral)
doxepin (Sinequan)	reserpine (Serpalan, Serpasil)
ergot mesyloids (Hydergine)	temazepam (Restoril)
estrogens	thioridazine (Mellaril)
ethacrynic acid (Edecrin)	ticlopidine (Ticlid)
ferrous sulfate (iron)	triazolam (Halcion)
fluoxetine (Prozac)	trimethobenzamide (Tigan)
flurazepam (Dalmane)	tripelennamine guanadrel (Hylorel)

(Data from Fick DM, Cooper JW, Wade WE, Waller JL, MacLean JR, Beers MH: Updating the Beers criteria for potentially inappropriate medication use in older adults: results of a US consensus panel of experts. Arch Intern Med 163(22):2716-2724, 2003.)

administering the patient's medication regimen falls to the caregiver.[33] This strain is more pronounced in caregivers of patients with moderate cognitive impairment as opposed to those patients with normal or very low cognitive functioning.[33] When a home health therapist recognizes caregiver strain, it may be appropriate to refer to skilled nursing or a medical social worker to help the patient and caregivers cope with these types of issues. Thus, physical therapists, as frontline professionals, have an important role to play in the home health setting by evaluating the extent to which the patient or caregiver are competent in the management of the patient's medication regimen. Some elements of an interdisciplinary medication assessment are listed in Box 25-9.

The home health physical therapist may consider adding a small medication resource book to his or her tool bag for immediate reference. The Internet is also another useful source of information. Potentially serious drug interactions can be quickly identified using "Drug Interaction Checkers" available on most Internet-based resources. Box 25-10 provides examples of websites that these authors have found valuable.

Fall-Risk Screening

An important area to assess at the first visit is fall risk. Reducing fall risk and fall-related injuries can prevent significant declines in function and independence and allow older persons to remain in their home.[34] Risk factors for falling are diverse and many of them, such as balance impairment, muscle weakness, polypharmacy, and environmental hazards, are common but potentially modifiable in the homebound patient. Approximately 20% to 55% of all unintentional falls and fall-related

injuries in older adults occur inside the home.[35] In addition, patients are more vulnerable to sustaining a fall within 1 month of hospital discharge.[7] The evidence is strong for multifactor falls risk assessments and individually tailored follow-up interventions that include appropriate exercise intensity and specificity.[36] The home health therapist is in an ideal position to address all the fall-related factors within a functional and relevant environment.

The home health assessment of potential fall risk begins with a history of a prior fall or a fear of falling. A prior fall predicts a decline in function, hospitalization, and adverse events among older adults and remains independently predictive of a likelihood of future hospitalization as well as a future fall.[37] In addition, falls occurring indoors and an inability to get up after a fall are positive predictors of falls in older adults.[38] Therefore, the physical therapist should routinely assess the homebound older adult's ability to rise from the floor, both as a potential predictor of fall risk and as a safety issue should the person fall. If the person cannot safely rise unassisted, a Lifeline or similar device may be recommended.

Fear of falling is also a predictor of fall risk. Many older individuals limit their mobility and become increasingly sedentary and homebound because of their awareness of declining balance, near falls, and/or a fear of falling. Interviewing a patient about his or her fear of falling including the completion of a fear of falling index such as the Falls Efficacy Scale or the Activities Balance Confidence Scale (ABC) may provide useful information that will inform goals and intervention strategies.

Home health therapists need to be aware of the possible underreporting of falls and near falls. Older adults may feel that reporting a fall might result in nursing home placement and/or notification of the fall incident to other family members who might arrange for relocation. Therefore it is likely an older adult may deny or minimize a fall history and/or a fall injury. Because only 20% of older adults who fall seek medical attention, the health care provider may not know about a fall.[35] Our recommendation is to assume fall risk and create a safe environment for the homebound patient to report a fear of falling and/or near and actual falls.

Home Safety Assessment

Home assessment should be carried out at the first visit. Safety and mobility barriers are the prime focus for the physical therapist. Because approximately 20% to 55% of all unintentional falls and fall-related injuries in older adults occur inside the home,[35] it is imperative that the therapist address any potential hazards.

Homes are a common setting for nonfatal unintentional injuries.[2] Although most falls occur on level surfaces, 16% occur on the stairs or from a height, and 4% occur in the

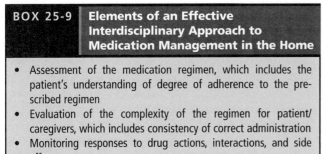

BOX 25-9 | **Elements of an Effective Interdisciplinary Approach to Medication Management in the Home**

- Assessment of the medication regimen, which includes the patient's understanding of degree of adherence to the prescribed regimen
- Evaluation of the complexity of the regimen for patient/caregivers, which includes consistency of correct administration
- Monitoring responses to drug actions, interactions, and side effects
- Provide education

BOX 25-10 | **Useful Websites for Drug Interactions and Information**

www.drugs.com
www.rxlist.com
www.drugdigest.com
www.epocrates.com
www.webmd.com/drugs

bathroom. Approximately 75% of these falls happen during the performance of routine daily activities, and 44% occur in the presence of one or more environmental hazards.[39] Environmental hazards have been found to be common in the homes of community-dwelling older adults and pose a fourfold risk of falling in those without a previous fall. Interestingly, environmental hazards are not associated with a cause of a fall in older adults *with* a history of falls; perhaps because older adults who have fallen may be more cautious of their surroundings, more aware of fall hazards, and more sedentary.[40]

The home health therapist may be familiar with the resistance of many older adults to changing their home environment on the recommendation of the therapist. Resistance to recommendations may be because the patient does not believe the hazard will cause a fall, the patient may be resistant to change and the associated costs of the change, or the patient may resist the perceived lack of control in incorporating a change to his or her home. Strategies that may be effective in overcoming resistance include sensitive communication with the patient and family member or friend about why the changes are necessary and the implications associated with falls and health status in older adults and providing the patient with a list of community resources. These types of resources may be found from senior centers, rehabilitation centers or physician offices, and on the Internet. Some states may provide financial assistance for home modifications. In addition, any recommendations should be presented in a way that allows the older adult to remain in control of his or her home environment. Presenting recommendations in terms of choices, such as grab handles or a slip-proof stair covering, may allow the older adult to feel more in control.

The fundamental goals of home safety assessments and interventions are to improve and maintain the older adult's ability to function safely at home in all seasons. For example, an antislip shoe device reduced the rate of falls in icy conditions.[41] A home safety assessment is especially effective in people with severe visual impairment and in those at higher risk of falling. However, home safety interventions do not necessarily reduce falls, perhaps because of the low rate of compliance.[41] Despite this evidence, it seems prudent to advise the patient and family about potential risks in the home.

Home safety checklists should address three basic areas: the presence of environmental hazards, problem areas, and lack of supportive or safety features (Box 25-11).[40] Checklists are commonly available to help organize the home safety assessment. For example, the Centers for Disease Control and Injury Prevention publishes a "Home Fall Prevention Checklist for Older Adults" that is available in English and several other languages.[42]

In addition to the home safety assessment, the home health therapist also has a role in recommending modifications to improve mobility. These recommendations may be to remove or modify potential hazards

---

BOX 25-11 | Home Safety Checklist

All Living Spaces

____ Remove throw rugs.
____ Secure carpet edges.
____ Remove low furniture and objects on the floor.
____ Reduce clutter.
____ Remove cords and wires on the floor.
____ Check lighting for adequate illumination at night (especially in the pathway to the bathroom).
____ Secure carpet or treads on stairs.
____ Install handrails on staircases.
____ Eliminate chairs that are too low to sit in and get out of easily.
____ Avoid floor wax (or use nonskid wax).
____ Ensure that the telephone can be reached from the floor.

Bathrooms

____ Install grab bars in the bathtub or shower and by the toilet.
____ Use rubber mats in the bathtub or shower.
____ Take up floor mats when the bathtub or shower is not in use.
____ Install a raised toilet seat.

Outdoors

____ Repair cracked sidewalks.
____ Install handrails on stairs and steps.
____ Trim shrubbery along the pathway to the home.
____ Install adequate lighting by doorways and along walkways leading to doors.

(*Adapted with permission from Rubenstein LZ: Falls. In: Yoshikawa TT, Cobbs EL, Brummel-Smith K, editors: Ambulatory geriatric care. St Louis, 1993, Mosby.*)

---

to mobility, such as adapting stairs with a ramp, or recommend an assistive device. Examples of adaptive or structural changes are listed in Table 25-2.

Emergency Situations

Being prepared for emergency situations in the home is considered best practice in home health. Because of the autonomous nature of the home care practice, the therapist is often alone with the patient and needs to be adaptable to creating a safe and clear space for treatment as well as remain cognizant of the patient's and therapist's personal safety. The authors recommend that the home health therapist always utilize a gait belt when working with patients in the home and to keep a cell phone on one's person at all times in case of an emergency when the patient cannot be left.

It is assumed that the home health therapists are aware of their limitations and know when to call for help. Options include 911, the patient's physician, or a clinical manager of the home health agency. Basic clinical assessment skills such as taking baseline vital signs and assessing the patient's perceived rate of exertion during exercise are standard requirements for most home health agencies. Moreover, current certification in Basic Life Support for Healthcare Providers is the minimum requirement for

TABLE 25-2	Home Safety Interventions	
Environmental Risk Factors	**Home Modifications**	
Throw rugs and mats	Replace nonsecure mats with nonslip bathmats and rugs	
Poor lighting	Use night lights	
Electrical cords	Remove electrical cords	
Stairways without rails	Addition of stair rails	
Adaptive Equipment		
Tub transfer bench/shower chair		
Cane/walker		
Bedside commode		
Elevated toilet seat		
Grab bars		
Hospital bed		
Wheelchair		

(Data from Cumming RG, Thomas M, Szonyi G, et al: Home visits by an occupational therapist for assessment and modification of environmental hazards: a randomized trial of falls prevention. J Am Geriatr Soc 47(12):1397-1402, 1999.)

patient safety. A cardiopulmonary resuscitation mask should be included in the therapist's tool bag.

The potential for a situation that requires activation of emergency medical services (EMS) always exists. A DNR (Do Not Resuscitate) Form, called "Emergency Medical Services Prehospital Do Not Resuscitate (DNR) Form" in some states, is an official document. When completed correctly, this form allows a patient with a life-threatening illness or injury to forgo specific resuscitative measures that may keep the individual alive. Home health providers are trained to inquire at the start of care if the patient has a Prehospital DNR form and to identify where the document is kept. The Prehospital DNR form is designed to express the patient's wishes when the patient cannot speak for himself or herself. The patient should be instructed to keep the DNR notice easily visible—mounted by a magnet on the refrigerator door is recommended by state medical associations. However, EMS personnel are taught to proceed with cardiopulmonary resuscitation when needed, unless they are absolutely certain that a qualified DNR advance directive exists for that patient. If, the DNR form or a medallion such as medical emergency bracelet is not found, after spending a reasonable (short) amount of time, EMS personel will proceed with life-saving measures. It is important to keep in mind that in a situation when every second has potentially life-or-death consequences, decisions need to be made quickly. EMS personnel are taught to provide life support if they are in doubt. Home health clinicians are usually advised by their clinical managers to do the same until EMS personel arrives on the scene.

TIP: STORING MEDICAL INFORMATION

Medical information can be stored in the refrigerator in an empty vial or pill bottle designated with a sticker that would alert emergency responders such as paramedics or firefighters to its contents.

Personal Safety

The authors strongly believe that employee safety is fundamental to being able to provide patient care, and policies that promote a culture of safety for employees as an organizational priority are essential. Although incidents of violence in the home health environment are rare, situations do occur. Incidental personal safety factors such as unrestrained pets, clutter, and poor lighting in homes were found to be commonplace in a 2006 survey of 833 home health nurses.[43] Another study found that 63% ($n = 465$) of home health nurses surveyed reported one or more exposures to violence, with the most prevalent exposure being verbal abuse.[44] Exposure to violence or other threats to personal safety was associated with the presence of illicit drugs, firearms, or violent family members. For these reasons, cell phones and other mobile communication devices are considered essential for home health care workers.[45]

When risk factors for violence are suspected, prescreening of the patient's home, using a security escort and/or supervisory visits by a home health agency clinical manager may be necessary. Patients can be required to sign a contract that they understand that the home health agency may terminate their care if a home health employee is exposed to violence or any threatening activity in the home, including an unrestrained animal.

Functional Assessment Testing

Functional assessment testing can provide valuable information in any setting but is particularly relevant in the home health setting because of its specificity to home care activities. Functional assessment is an effective way to objectively document a patient's functional status, progress through the episode of care, and justify homebound status. Functional assessment testing can also justify discharge from physical therapy services. The functional tests described in Table 25-3 are particularly relevant for the homebound patient transitioning to the community. We have included scores we feel indicate safe mobility at home and in the community that may help with goal setting. Scores on these tests can help justify skilled services. For example, a patient who scores greater than 13.5 seconds on the Timed Up and Go test may be at risk for falls,[67] thus justifying homebound status because of the increased risk for falls and supervision needed.

Gait speed has been shown to be the single best predictor of functional decline and disability and therefore should always be assessed in the home setting.[68] Slower gait speeds of 0.56 m/second or less can also indicate increased fall risk.[69] The scores of usual and fast gait speed can indicate the patient's homebound status and when an individual has progressed to community

TABLE 25-3	Functional Assessment for the Home Setting
Functional Assessment Testing in the Home	**Scores**
4-Square Step Test[46,47]	<15 s
5-Repetition Sit to Stand Test[48]	<10 s
6-Minute Walk Test[49-51]	1200 feet in 6 minutes
Activities-specific Balance Confidence Scale[52,53,56]	>85%
Berg Balance Scale[54-57]	>50
Borg RPE[58]	<12 for normal activities
30-s Timed Chair Stand Test[59]	>12 in 30 s
Dynamic Gait Index[60]	>19
Gait Speed[61,73]	>0.8 m/s (usual); 0.33 m/s difference between usual and fast
Performance Oriented Mobility Assessment/Tinetti Assessment Tool[62,63]	>12 on balance portion[64]
Physical Performance Test[65]	26/28 (without stairs); 34/36 with stairs
Timed Floor Rise	<20 s[66]
Timed Up and Go[67]	<12 s

ambulation (Table 25-4). Gait speed is easy to measure with distances of as little as 8 feet.[73] An assistive device can be used. Normative values for gait speed in older adults exist that can aid in goal setting (Table 25-5). For these reasons, the authors strongly recommend usual and fast gait speed be recorded for each home health patient. In addition, we recommend having the functional tests and scores listed in Table 25-3 handy at each visit to aid efficiency.

GOAL SETTING

There is some evidence that when the therapist and patient work together to establish meaningful goals for the patient, the patient has improved enthusiasm, buy-in, and outcomes.[74] Many home health patients will have the potential and desire to become community-dwelling ambulators, returning to their prior or higher level of function. Others may be more limited or not desire to be integrated into the community. Therefore, it may be advisable and necessary to involve the patient's family members in the goal-setting process. Family members can help with information on prior level of function that is useful in setting realistic goals. For example, the patient may indicate a desire to return to full community integration, including driving. However, when discussing this goal with the family, the therapist find may out the patient has had several near-accidents and is oftentimes confused about the actual location when out in the community. Some warning signs that it is unsafe for the individual to drive are listed in Box 25-12. This information may require a refocusing of the patient on shorter-term goals with the expectations that the individual may come to a realization of limitations. The Ozer–Payton–Nelson (OPN) model,[75] described elsewhere in this text, may be useful in establishing meaningful and realistic goals.

In setting goals to reintegrate a patient into the community, it may be useful to refer to Shumway-Cook et al's required tasks of community-dwelling older adults.[76] The authors observed older adults for a 1-week period to identify required tasks in community-dwelling

TABLE 25-4	Functional Gait Speeds for Older Adults	
Functional Level	**Gait Speed**
Household ambulator at risk for fall	0.5 m/s (1.64 ft/s)[70]
Community ambulator	0.8 m/s[71]
Usual adult walking speed	1.2 m/s-1.3 m/s
Well-functioning older people at high risk of health-related outcomes	<1.0 m/s[71]

TABLE 25-5	Normative Values for Gait Speed in Older Adults		
Gender	**Age Range (years)**	**Gait speed [ft/sec (m/s)] over 8 ft**	**Gait speed [ft/sec (m/s)] over 20 ft**
Female	50-59	3.61 (1.10 m/s)	3.64 (1.11 m/s)
	60-69	3.28 (0.99 m/s)	3.30 (1.01 m/s)
	70-79	3.01 (0.92 m/s)	3.05 (0.93 m/s)
	80+	2.50 (0.76 m/s)	2.57 (0.78 m/s)
Male	50-59	3.66 (1.12 m/s)	3.68 (1.12 m/s)
	60-69	3.38 (1.03 m/s)	3.39 (1.03 m/s)
	70-79	3.13 (0.95 m/s)	3.14 (0.96 m/s)
	80+	2.77 (0.84 m/s)	2.73 (0.83 m/s)

(Modified from Bohannon RW: Population representative gait speed and its determants. J Geriatr Phys Ther 31(2): 49-52, 2008.)

<table>
<tr><td>

BOX 25-12 Warning Signs That Indicate Someone Should Begin to Limit Driving or to Stop Altogether

1. Almost crashing, with frequent "close calls"
2. Finding dents and scrapes on the car, on fences, mailboxes, garage doors, curbs, or the like
3. Getting lost
4. Having trouble seeing or following traffic signals, road signs, and pavement markings
5. Responding more slowly to unexpected situations, or having trouble moving foot from the gas to the brake pedal; confusing the two pedals
6. Misjudging gaps in traffic at intersections and on highway entrance and exit ramps
7. Experiencing road rage or having other drivers frequently honk at driver
8. Easily becoming distracted or having difficulty concentrating while driving
9. Having a hard time turning around to check over shoulder while backing up or changing lanes
10. Receiving traffic tickets or "warnings" from traffic or law enforcement officers in the last year or two

</td><td>

BOX 25-13 Examples of Evidence-Based Goals for Home Health Patients Who Have Potential to Become Community Ambulators upon Discharge

- The patient will score <13.5 s on the Timed Up and Go without an assistive device.
- The patient will score ≥ 50/56 on the Berg Balance Test.
- The patient will score <12 s on the 4 Square Step Test.
- The patient will reach >10 in. on the Functional Reach Test.
- The patient will score >85% on the Activity-specific Balance Confidence Scale.
- The patient will ambulate >1000 ft without an assistive device with a gait speed of greater than 0.8 m/s with a reported Borg RPE of 10 or less.
- The patient will score ≥25/28 on the Performance Oriented Mobility Assessment/ Tinetti Assessment Tool.
- The patient will score >19/24 on the Dynamic Gait Index Test.
- The patient will score <14.2 s on the 5 Repetition Sit to Stand.
- The patient will score X reps (insert # of reps based on the norms for the patient's age and sex in 50th percentile or greater) on the Chair Stand Test.
- The patient will ambulate X feet (insert # of feet based on the norms for the patient's age and sex) on the 6-Minute Walk Test with a reported Borg RPE of 10 or less.

</td></tr>
</table>

(Data from AARP. Driver safety program. http://www.aarp.org/home-garden/transportation/info-05-2010/Warning_Signs_Stopping.html. Accessed April 5, 2010.)

older adults for the purpose of helping home health therapists set goals. They found that older adults routinely:

- walked a minimum of 1000 feet per errand (often making 2 to 3 separate trips at a time),
- carried packages averaging 6.7 pounds while walking,
- frequently encountered stairs, curbs, and slopes, and
- engaged in frequent postural transitions (changes in direction, reaching up, looking up, moving backward, etc.).[76]

Ideally, the goals set for patients who desire to return to the community should reflect these community standards. Box 25-13 lists some examples of evidence-based goals useful for a home health physical therapist.

The therapist and patient need to work closely to determine what goals are realistic and measurable to achieve the understanding that the episode of care is limited to achieving specific goals. For example, if the patient does not desire to return to the community but expresses a desire to be able to get out of a chair, walk to the bathroom, transfer on and off the toilet, and return to the chair with the use of a walker without becoming short of breath, a long-term goal stating "Patient will transfer independently on/off a chair, ambulate 45 feet with a walker from the chair to toilet and back with a reported Borg RPE of 10 or less" is appropriate. At the time of the goal negotiation, the expected duration of care is determined. In collaboration with the patient, the number and frequency of visits are

agreed upon and a treatment consent form is signed with this information in writing. This consent form clearly articulates the therapist's and the patient's expectations for the episode of care and could be considered a contract.

There may also be cases where a patient may well intend to be a community ambulator and home health care is used as part of the continuum of care to transition the patient to outpatient care. An example might be a patient who is discharged to home from the hospital a few days after total hip arthroplasty (THA). That patient may have a goal of getting to outpatient therapy as soon as possible, so goal setting would include increasing ambulation distance, endurance, and car transfers.

It is the opinion of the authors that often patients are discharged far too early from home health services. Criteria for community mobility have been clearly established by Shumway-Cook et al and should be used as goals for the patient desiring to be reintegrated into the community.[76] In addition, objective fall risk should be considered when preparing for discharge. When a person demonstrates substantial fall risk per the Berg Balance Scale as an example, the person may benefit from further therapy to decrease fall risk. Unfortunately, the authors have seen arbitrary standards for justification of discharge that have no basis in Medicare guidelines. For example, one therapist may discharge a patient from home health services simply because the patient went out to get a haircut. Another therapist may discharge a patient because the patient can ambulate 200 feet or can drive. However, under Medicare guidelines, a homebound patient is allowed to leave the home to get a haircut, attend physician appointments, and participate in religious services. They are also permitted to leave their home for special occasions such as holidays or visiting relatives as long as the trip away from home is physically taxing (see Box 25-1). It is important to note that no Medicare guideline establishes a prescribed ambulation distance to determine homebound status. Box 25-14 lists some examples of statements that may justify continued homebound care.

Home health physical therapists have a professional obligation to provide the needed patient services while complying with CMS guidelines and regulations. Objective documentation and thorough examination of the patient will help drive an appropriate plan of care. Each subsequent visit note must stand alone to justify medical necessity. The purpose of this section was to assist the home health therapist to think critically about patient-centered goals and justify the provision of in-home therapy services under Medicare guidelines.

EPISODE OF CARE

Projecting Number of Physical Therapy Visits and Episode Timing

A 60-day certification period applies to home health patients admitted for home health services under the Medicare Part A benefit. A detailed description of what Medicare considers skilled physical therapy services is available on the CMS website.[23] Briefly, the skilled services should be appropriate, reasonable, necessary, and safe for the patient. Skilled physical therapy will be covered throughout the 60-day certification period under the condition that supporting documentation justifies the need for skilled services. The documentation needs to include homebound status at the time of start of care and on every subsequent visit note.

The frail individual's predicted episode of care is particularly challenging with respect to predicting the frequency and duration of services because frailty is linked with a poor prognosis.[77] Frailty is a biological condition characterized by three or more of the following characteristics: unexplained weight loss of 10 lbs or more in the past year, self-reported exhaustion, weakness (as measured by grip strength), slow walking speed, and low physical activity.[78] A patient who is frail will require more visits on average, spread out throughout the certification period to move them to a higher functional level. However, if the person is so frail that the individual is almost bedbound (Figure 25-1), fewer therapy visits will be needed to educate the patient and family on safe mobility and a home exercise program.

Application of clinical decision making is imperative when determining frequency and duration of physical therapy services. Appropriate exercise for the older adult—including intensity, overload, and specificity—is needed to effect change. Use of these principles will help the home health physical therapist determine frequency and duration for the home health episode of care and avoid a premature discharge. In all cases, the home health therapist is responsible for ordering the number of therapy visits that are medically necessary. The patient's needs must remain the therapist's foremost concern when determining the number of therapy visits,

BOX 25-14	Examples of Statements That Can Justify Home Care

- After returning home from an outing, the patient requires 2 hours of rest as a result of exhaustion from the trip.
- The patient scored >14 s on the Timed Up and Go and therefore requires the assistance of one person to safely exit the home as a result of fall risk.
- The patient reports a Borg score of >12 while ambulating inside the home and is therefore homebound as a result of the taxing effort ambulation requires.
- Decreased cognition as evidenced by the Mini Mental Status score indicates the patient requires the assistance of one person to exit the home safely.
- The patient lives in an apartment building and is unable to safely negotiate stairs as a result of partial weight-bearing status after total hip arthroplasty to exit home.
- The patient reports a Borg RPE of >12 after descending and ascending 14 stairs required to enter his or her home and is therefore homebound as a result of the taxing effort required to leave the home.
- The patient is unable to ambulate >1000 feet with a gait speed of >0.8 m/s and reported Borg RPE of ≥11 and is therefore homebound because the patient is unable to safely ambulate community distances at a gait speed required for community ambulators.

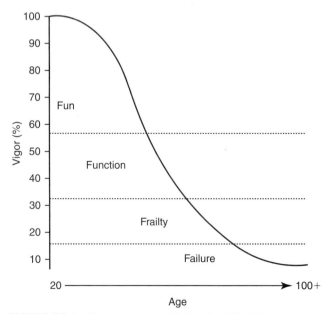

FIGURE 25-1 Slippery slope and frailty. *(Modified from Schwartz RS: Sarcopenia and physical performance in old age: introduction. Muscle Nerve Suppl: 5:S10-S12, 1997.)*

regardless of reimbursement models. Considering that all therapy visits must be medically necessary, each visit note must justify the visit.

Initial Patient Education Interventions

Skilled home health therapy includes patient education interventions *and* the patient's as well as caregivers' response to education. Patient education at the start of care may include information about the patient bill of rights, the agency's complaint process, the agency's disaster plan, home safety interventions, pain management interventions, home exercise program, orthopedic precautions, fall prevention strategies, and the plan of care. Any patient education provided must be documented at the initial and subsequent visits. Suggestions for documentation of patient education are explained further in the subsequent visit section of this chapter.

The volume of information to be shared and taught may necessitate several educational sessions. Effective patient education is considered a skilled intervention as teaching must be tailored to meet the older adult's physical, cognitive, and psychosocial functioning level. Clinicians who take the time to assess their patients' individual abilities, learning preferences, and motivational differences will find teaching to be more rewarding and meaningful for the patient. Chapter 10 on motivation and patient education provides many useful tips on how to be an effective patient educator.

Start of Care Case Conference and Physician Communication

Communication with Physician Regarding Plan of Care. A verbal order from the physician (or an agent of the physician) for an initial physical therapy evaluation must be obtained prior to the first visit. If further visits are required, the physical therapist must verbally contact the physician (or the physician's agent) to negotiate the specific plan of care, including frequency and duration of anticipated services. The physician must sign a paper copy of the verbal referral; however, the clinician does not need to wait to get the signed referral from the physician before service is rendered as long as verbal communication regarding the proposed plan of care has occurred.[23] The verbal referral prior to the start of care and subsequent signatures on paper copies are typically managed by the home health agency.

Discharge Planning at the Start of Care. As in all settings, discharge planning in home health begins at the start of care. The patient is required to sign a consent form at the first visit that includes the agreed upon frequency and duration of home physical therapy. Rarely can an older adult afford the luxury of being sedentary; thus some plan for continued physical activity and exercise should be discussed with the patient within the first

few visits. The patient may be discharged to outpatient services, self-care, or a home program with assistance from a family or friend. The home health physical therapist is expected to coordinate the discharge plan with the physician, the patient, and anyone else who may be involved in the patient's care. In many cases, a patient who is expected to reintegrate into the community could benefit from additional outpatient physical therapy services to help move the person to as high a level of function as possible. This will help prevent future functional decline by building up functional reserve and protecting the person against future hospitalizations.[79,80] Discharge planning will be discussed later in this chapter.

Subsequent Visits

Documentation. Documentation for each home health visit may differ from other clinical settings. Issues need to be documented each visit as appropriate, such as complete vital sign assessment, objective pain assessment, documentation of subjective/objective assessment, and the reassessment of the physical therapy plan. The therapist may also document the observance of universal precautions or the use of "clean bag" technique to reduce the risk of using contaminated equipment between patients. Documentation of discharge planning and homebound status should be noted throughout the episode of care.

Documentation of skilled teaching and progress toward goal should also be included on every visit. For example, the home health therapist may document the provision of patient education regarding THA precautions knowing that the patient will require further teaching. The teaching intervention may be documented in the following way: "The patient was provided with education on THA precautions; further teaching is required because the patient was only able to verbalize two of three hip precautions." This example includes what the patient was taught *and* the patient's response to teaching. This example requires follow-up documentation on subsequent visit notes because "further teaching is required" was documented. When full understanding of THA precautions is demonstrated by the patient, the home health therapist may document the following: "The patient verbalized understanding of THA precautions." If understanding the THA precautions was a goal for the patient, the therapist would also document that goal was met on that date in the progress toward goals section on the note.

The home care setting is rich with opportunities for patient and family education. These opportunities can be used as justification for ongoing physical therapy services. The Home Health Section of the American Physical Therapy Association (APTA) provides guidelines for documentation of plan of care and subsequent visits (Box 25-15).[81]

BOX 25-15 | **Documentation Requirements for Home Health Care**

Guideline: The physical therapist or physical therapist assistant will:
1. Prepare appropriate documentation for the patient's/client's clinical record, including any OASIS-related documents, if applicable;
2. Complete documentation in a timely manner in compliance with the agency's policies and procedures; and
3. Utilize documentation principles consistent with APTA's Guidelines: Physical Therapy Documentation of Patient/Client Management [BOD G03-05-16-41].

Criteria:
1. Each visit/client encounter requires that documentation be completed the day of the visit and included in the patient's/client's clinical record.
2. The patient's/client's health record includes, but is not limited to:
   a. Documentation of examination, evaluation, diagnosis, prognosis (including plan of care), intervention, and outcomes;
   b. Progress notes/visit records;
   c. Written exercise and activity programs
   d. Summations of care;
   e. Physician's order, if required;
   f. A plan of care reflecting the patient's/client's current status; and
   g. Outcome measurement tools and scales (e.g., OASIS, Tinetti, Pain Visual Analog Scale).
3. Specific documentation should include, but is not limited to:
   a. The treatment provided;
   b. The patient's/client's/caregiver's response to treatment;
   c. The progress/lack of progress toward the attainment of the anticipated outcomes;
   d. Physical therapy outcomes updated as appropriate;
   e. Visit frequency; and
   f. Visit date and time:
      i. Time the visit started,
      ii. Time the visit was completed, and
      iii. Total time spent with the patient/client.
4. Communication about the patient/client among the physical therapist, physical therapist assistant, and other care providers are to be documented and include, but are not limited to:
   a. Current problems;
   b. Current goal status;
   c. Interventions provided;
   d. Physical therapy visit frequency and duration; and
   e. Supervisory activities.
5. Communication/conferences with the patient/client/family members/other care providers involved in or supervising patient/client care are to be documented, including date and time.

(From American Physical Therapy Association. Home Health Section—Guidelines for the provision of physical therapy in the home. http://www.homehealthsection.org. Accessed April 29, 2010.)

Coordination of Patient Care

Although the home health visit may occur in isolation from other health care team members, communication about the case occurs frequently between clinicians and clinical managers in the office. This communication is so important it is termed *care coordination* and is required for each patient under CMS Conditions of Participation. Care coordination is characterized by communication between all members of the interdisciplinary team. Specific documentation of patient notification of care provided, the disciplines involved, frequency of proposed visits, notification 48 hours prior to planned discharge, and any changes to the plan of care is required. The Conditions of Participation also require the agency to notify the physician of changes in the patient's condition that may necessitate a change in the treatment plan that was established on the first visit. For example, if the physical therapist determines 2 weeks after the start of care that the patient is exhibiting a change in cognition or having signs of skin breakdown, a referral for a skilled nursing assessment is warranted because of the change in the patient's medical condition. An interim order from the physician is required for the newly required skilled nursing assessment. Also, if a patient is not progressing as anticipated and/or not participating with therapy, the physician must be notified that services may no longer be skilled and thus need to end prior to what was originally planned. In such an example the home health therapist may work with the physician and possibly the agency's social worker to coordinate options for a different level of care for those individuals who are not safe in the home and yet not progressing sufficiently with rehabilitative efforts.

Coordination of care also requires communication between disciplines and typically with the agency's clinical manager; however, these requirements are agency specific. Care coordination needs to take place at the start of care, resumption of care, recertification of care, and at discharge. There are other cases where documentation of communication between the interdisciplinary team and the clinical case manager are warranted, such as when reporting patient complaints/infections and incidents, lack of progress toward goals, and when providing supervision of other associates (home health aide, physical therapist assistant, and licensed practical nurse).

In the home health setting the case manager is responsible for overseeing the care plan and coordination of that care with all disciplines. The physical therapist, registered nurse, speech–language pathologist, or occupational therapist is allowed under Medicare guidelines to be the patient's case manager. If nursing is involved in a patient's care, the nurse is considered the patient's case manager by default. When physical therapy but not nursing is involved, the physical therapist is the case manager regardless of what other disciplines are involved on the case.

The interdisciplinary team is expected to work together to set goals with the patient to ensure a cohesive plan of care. Physical and occupational therapists work particularly closely with each other when both are involved in the same episode of care because of the similarity in goals and focus. Both professionals collaborate on the duration and frequency of the plan of care and specific intervention focus. Care coordination is also important when scheduling visits with patients to ensure that the services are not overlapping. If two individuals are needed to provide a service, two visits may be covered by CMS.[1] An example given by CMS is an occupational therapist is at a patient's home supervising the certified occupational therapist assistant. In this instance, only one visit is billable to Medicare. CMS reimburses for joint visits (e.g., physical therapy and occupational therapy) only in special circumstances.[1]

Resumption of Care. If a patient is hospitalized or placed in a facility for any reason during an episode of care, the case manager is responsible for completing an OASIS transfer assessment. If the patient is then subsequently discharged home within the same 60-day episode, the clinician completes an OASIS resumption of care assessment. The guidelines for completion of the various OASIS assessments are available from CMS.[82]

Recertification. At the end of the 60-day certification period, the patient may still require skilled services. There are no limitations as to the number of times a patient can be recertified as long as the criteria for skilled services is met as defined by CMS.[23] The case manager completes the recertification OASIS assessment.[82] If physical therapy is still appropriate to the needs of the patient, additional physician orders[23] are required for the subsequent 60-day recertification period and the new plan of care. Physical therapy goals should be reevaluated and updated for each new 60-day certification period to justify the medical necessity for continuing skilled services.

Discharge. The appropriateness of physical therapy discharge should be assessed prior to the last day of services to determine if the patient's goals were met. Discharge should be based on functional assessment testing that indicates the individual has met stated goals and community requirements, as appropriate. Referring to the Shumway-Cook recommendations for community ambulation may be helpful.[76]

Care coordination with all disciplines at the time of discharge is necessary. Skilled services of various disciplines of the interdisciplinary team may be discharged at different times during the episode of care. The last discipline on the case will be responsible for completion of the OASIS discharge assessment, with the exception of home health aides. Disciplines that discharge prior to the OASIS discharge are responsible for completing less labor-intensive documentation in accordance with CMS, state, and agency guidelines.

A home health physical therapist may help facilitate the patient's discharge from home health and any transition to outpatient physical therapy by communication with the physician and outpatient clinic of the patient's choice. If the patient does not go to outpatient physical therapy at the time of discharge, it is recommended that the physical therapist ensure that the patient and

the family/caregivers understand the home exercise program instructions. The Home Health Section of the APTA provides additional information on discharge planning and documentation requirements for home health (see Box 25-15).[81]

CMS uses the Start of Care OASIS and Discharge OASIS scores as a way to determine the effectiveness of the services provided by the home health agency. The results for all agencies are available for public reviewing at "Home Health Compare" on Medicare's website.[83] Box 25-2 lists the quality measures for home health agencies. Written notification and signature of the patient is required 48 hours *prior to* discharge from Home Health Services. The purpose of this is to make sure that the patient is aware that the discharge planned by the home health agency may be disputed by contacting Medicare. A copy of the information is left with the patient and kept in the clinician record. The patient has a right to appeal the agency discharge by contacting Medicare.

PHYSICAL THERAPY INTERVENTION IN THE HOME

Exercise is one of the most often utilized interventions in the home health setting as it has been shown to be effective in improving functional abilities given appropriate intensity and specificity. The lack of formal exercise equipment can make the provision of evidence-based exercise challenging, requiring creativity to achieve the necessary parameters of an effective exercise program. Box 25-16 provides some suggestions for exercises and activities easily done in the home. Box 25-7 lists a few items that are useful and feasible to carry with the therapist when prescribing exercise in the home. The drive spent between patients can often be used to develop creative exercises that are functional and of interest to the patient.

Home Exercise Programs

The literature shows that it is best practice to give a patient only two to three exercises for the home exercise program to ensure correct form and perhaps compliance.[84] Home health patients are typically seen two to three times a week initially during the episode of care; therefore exercise performance between sessions may be necessary depending on the goals of treatment. If strengthening is a goal and the patient is seen three times a week, it would be best to space out the physical therapy visits and prescribe endurance and/or flexibility exercises between sessions. An exercise program of sufficient intensity does not require additional exercises for the patient on days they do not have therapy as rest for that specific muscle is necessary. Rather, a home program could consist of a physical activity prescription such as a daily walking program with alternating days working on speed or strength. The home health therapist may also

BOX 25-16	Examples of Exercises for Home Health

Examples of Practical Exercises in and outside the Home
Car transfers
Dynamic balance activities
Floor transfer training
Heel raises, progress to unilateral heel raises
Quick toe tapping
Repeated sit to stand, progress to one leg sit to stand
Stair climbing
Step ups
Walking on uneven surfaces outside

Examples of Task-Specific Activities
Repeatedly getting in/out of bed
Repeatedly performing dressing tasks
Reaching up into cupboards lifting cans of food, dishes, or weights
Carrying items (dishes and/or pots) across room from kitchen to dining area
Putting in/removing items from refrigerator and/or stove
Repeatedly opening and closing refrigerator and/or exterior door of home
Transferring up and down from commode repeatedly
Bending over to pick up pet's food/water dishes from floor
Stand at bedside and put shirts onto hanger and then hang shirts in closet
Vacuuming and/or sweeping
Transferring clothes from washer to dryer

choose to have the patient work on task-specific activities on the nontherapy days (see Box 25-16). The home exercise program should be updated as the treatment progresses. Written exercise prescriptions with pictures may be useful for patients. The exercises should be reviewed regularly with the patient to ensure that technique is safe and correct. In some cases, the most effective way to prescribe a home exercise program is to involve family members, especially in cases where the patient has an existing cognitive or visual deficit.

Physical Therapist Assistant Utilization

Under CMS guidelines, the physical therapist assistant (PTA) can provide therapy without onsite supervision of the physical therapist, another unique aspect of the home care setting. However, physical therapist supervision and utilization must be in accordance with CMS and state regulations. The Home Health Section of the APTA provides information on the role of the physical therapist assistant in the home as well as the necessary qualifications (Box 25-17).[85]

Individual states can also regulate how the PTA is utilized in the home care setting. For example, in New York State, the physical therapist and the PTA must make the initial joint visit together, with the physical therapist performing a follow-up visit every sixth occa-

sion or 30 days (whichever comes first). In the states of New York and California, the physical therapist cannot supervise more than two PTAs at any given time.[86] In California, the physical therapist is required to make a supervisory visit of the patient at least every 30 days after the initial evaluation by the physical therapist, and the PTA does not need to be present for this visit.[87] However, within 7 days of the care being provided by the PTA, the supervising physical therapist is required to either review, cosign, and date all documentation by the PTA or conduct a weekly case conference and document it in the patient record. These examples demonstrate how each physical therapist should be aware of his or her state's requirements regarding supervision of PTAs in the home care setting.

TECHNOLOGY

Technology, composed of four categories, has a growing presence in the home health environment. These categories include (1) point of care; (2) office automation; (3) telehealth and telephony; and (4) technology such as laptops, tablets, personal digital assistants, or other Web-based portals.[88] There is wide disparity in the current use of technology among home health agencies and providers centered around the point of care and office automation types. However, the need for increased technology in all of its capacity is evident. An increased use of home-based technology will help to ensure that older adults have the health care they need in the future. Unlike prior generations, baby boomers will be very comfortable and familiar with technology as an integral part of their daily lives.

Technology adoption in home health becomes imperative as paper-based systems are increasingly overwhelmed by the burden of multiple regulatory agencies and the complexity and number of aging adults. Home health agencies are embracing point-of-care technology as electronic systems become more affordable and intuitive.

Telehealth is the use of electronic information and telecommunications technologies to support long-distance clinical health care, patient and professional health-related education, public health, and health administration. Technologies used in telehealth typically include videoconferencing, the Internet, store-and-forward imaging (the use of transferring medical data), streaming media, and terrestrial and wireless communications. Although new applications are increasing, significant barriers currently exist such as affordability and having reliable safeguards to secure and protect patient identifiable information. Many older adults and their families would welcome a low-cost desktop video system that provides 24/7 monitoring, to facilitate earlier identification of functional decline, medication administration problems, and/or acute exacerbations of chronic diseases. Telephone-based systems are already available,

BOX 25-17	Guidelines for the Use of the Physical Therapist Assistant in Home Health

Guideline: The physical therapist assistant will provide patient/client care as directed by a physical therapist:

1. In accordance with APTA's Standards of Practice for Physical Therapy [HOD S06-03-09-10] and the Criteria [BOD S03-06-16-38];
2. In accordance with APTA's Code of Ethics [HOD S06-00-12-23] and Guide for Professional Conduct, and the Standards of Ethical Conduct for the Physical Therapist Assistant [HOD S06-00-13-24] and Guide for Conduct of the Physical Therapist Assistant;
3. In accordance with APTA's policy on Direction and Supervision of the Physical Therapist Assistant [HOD P06-05-18-26];
4. In accordance with APTA's policy on Access to, Admission to, and Patient/Client Rights Within Physical Therapy [HOD P06-03-16-13];
5. In accordance with applicable municipal, state, and federal laws and rules and regulations;
6. In coordination with the supervising physical therapist; and
7. In coordination with the patient's/client's other care providers.

Criteria:

1. The Physical Therapist Assistant (PTA) will perform skilled interventions and related tasks that have been selected and assigned by the supervising physical therapist, consistent with the plan of care.
2. The PTA will provide instruction to the patient/client/caregiver:
   a. Verbal; and
   b. Visual (e.g., demonstration, written, pictures, video, etc.).
3. The PTA will provide documentation to the agency for inclusion in the patient's/client's clinical record.
   a. Documentation to be completed in a timely manner in compliance with applicable state and federal home-health-related rules and regulations, agency requirements, and/or third-party payer requirements.
4. The PTA will monitor and communicate to the supervising physical therapist any changes in the patient's/client's condition.

Guidelines for the Provision of Physical Therapy in the Home

1. The PTA will monitor and document the patient's/client's response to therapeutic physical therapy intervention:
   a. Communicating to the supervising physical therapist where appropriate the patient's/client's response to physical therapy intervention; and
   b. Referring to the following algorithm as a problem-solving process utilized by PTAs in provision of selected interventions: Clinical Problem-Solving Algorithm Utilized by PTAs in the Delivery of Physical Therapy Interventions.
2. The PTA will participate in care management processes, such as:
   a. Individual and multidisciplinary care conferences;
   b. In-services/continuing education;
   c. Chart audit activities;
   d. Quality improvement activities; and
   e. Other agency initiatives that affect multidisciplinary care.
3. The PTA will maintain confidentiality of information relating to the physical therapist assistant–client relationship in accordance with:
   a. The agency's confidentiality policies and procedures;
   b. APTA's Standards of Ethical Conduct for the Physical Therapist Assistant [HOD S06-00-13-24]; and
   c. The Health Insurance Portability and Accountability Act (HIPAA).
4. The PTA will demonstrate knowledge of available community resources/services.

(From American Physical Therapy Association: Home Health Section—Guidelines for the provision of physical therapy in the home. http://www.homehealth section.org Accessed April 29, 2010.)

such as personal emergency response systems (e.g., pendants or bracelets that a patient wears at home to activate an alarm that goes to a call center). However, large, regional providers of either a subscription-based commercial service or a publicly funded "telehome care utility" service that offers equipment rental and a menu of patient monitoring options would need to be developed before these types of monitoring systems are readily available.

The future trend of postacute rehabilitation is "virtual home-based rehabilitation." In this model, the therapist would first conduct an initial in-person assessment and then use two-way interactive real-time video-conferencing to conduct subsequent visits. By staying "connected," the rehabilitation model could be extended beyond the current face-to-face model. A telehealth approach might provide a more affordable means of tracking the progress and outcomes of large populations of older adults over an extended period of time. However, private and government insurers will have to develop new reimbursement policies that include a fee structure and standards for "virtual care" or rehabilitation beyond the in-person encounter. The benefits of telehealth technologies and being able to monitor patients remotely are described in Box 25-18, Point of Care Technologies.

CARE TRANSITIONS AND PATIENT SELF-MANAGEMENT: A VISION FOR HOME HEALTH

According to the American Geriatrics Society (AGS) position statement "Improving the Quality of Transitional Care for Persons with Complex Care Needs," practitioners across health care settings often operate independently, which interferes with the ability to have seamless

BOX 25-18	Point-of-Care Technologies

Point of Care Technologies: Laptops, tablets, personal digital assistants (PDAs) or other Web-based portals used while a clinician is seeing a patient

Benefits

- Improves efficiency of clinical processes by making it easier to access and communicate vital information
- Provides real-time information and centralizes medical record entries contemporaneously with care
- Facilitates use of protocols for assessments and medications management
- Improves the accuracy of the information required for electronic validation of OASIS assessments and eliminates data reentry to correct manual errors
- Reduces the cycle time for billing
- Improves coordination of care and communication between all
- Enhances consistency and compliance with orders by providing easy access to plan of care, follow-up notes, and visit schedules

Office Automation: Software for home care agencies to track and manage information beginning with the client intake process to workforce management and back office accounting

Benefits

- Improves efficiency of scheduling of staff and clients by using intelligent scheduling support
- Matches staff with clients based on client preferences, staff availability, geographic location, skills required, previous schedule history, and profitability
- Improves human resources management by automating time and attendance records, e.g., verifies schedules
- Improves general and administrative management through better reporting, financial management, and immediate claim calculation
- Automates the documentation of OASIS data and provides validation prior to submission
- Manages clinical information quickly and easily
- Streamlines physician order tracking process by confirming orders are signed and received by the agency prior to billing and allows physicians to electronically sign their orders
- Enables agencies to designate trained case managers to oversee care for certain diagnoses
- Tracks patient care so that adverse events are quickly communicated to the entire care team

Telehealth: Technologies that include two-way video conferencing, remote vital sign collection and transmission, and education in the home

Benefits

- Documenting vital signs and symptoms from the home without the intervention of a clinician empowers patients to better control contributing factors that can exacerbate their health conditions, such as diet, exercise, alcohol, insulin and medication use, and stress levels, translating into higher patient satisfaction
- Using two-way interactive video improves communications between patients and caregivers, giving the caregivers and patients data in real time, thus enhancing the overall diagnosis
- Monitoring patients remotely improves patient care by collecting vital patient information on a daily basis from the patient's home without the need for a clinician or caregiver to be present, thus eliminating gaps in patient monitoring

Telephony: Telephony is communications via a voice messaging system through specialized dissemination to a category of caregivers or broadcast to the entire workforce

Benefits

- Collects activity codes, supplies, and mileage helping to ensure that information is accurately and immediately captured
- Improves scheduling and manages missed visits, no-shows, and reassignments in real time

transitions of the patient among care settings.[89] During transitions, patients are at risk for medical errors, service failures, and ultimately poor clinical outcomes. Intervention strategies to improve care transitions involve a timely transfer of health care information from the acute care setting to post–acute care health care providers and vice versa. Organizational tools such as care transition coaches who support patients and teach self-management skills will enhance health information exchange across care settings. When patients and their caregivers are able to easily track key medical information, health care concerns, medications from all prescribers, and their history of provider contacts, patients' competence in self-management and likelihood to remain independent at home increase. Thus, the authors feel that should tools become widely used to promote seamless transitions, home health becomes the only truly scalable infrastructure to deliver transitional, postacute, and primary care/chronic care management for older adults.

SUMMARY

Although Medicare may limit the definition of home health to short-term, intermittent, treatment-focused medical care for homebound patients, these restrictions historically came from when home care was initially designed to be *incident* to acute care. Moreover, rehabilitation programs for older adults were considered possible only if delivered in facilities with therapy gyms and an array of therapeutic equipment. Home health is now recognized as a transition in the continuum of care that provides a window of opportunity to affect the functional abilities of older adults. There are many functional assessment tests and interventions that are extraordinarily adaptable to being performed in the patient's home. The provision of evidence-based exercise in the home allows for comparisons of outcomes across settings and overall sound clinical decisions about the patient's readiness to progress to self-management. All physical therapists should advocate for their patients to reintegrate into the community and progress to outpatient care or community-based exercise programs. The challenges in the home health setting present opportunities for physical therapists to demonstrate their expert clinical decision making while practicing in the most functional environment for their patients.

REFERENCES

To enhance this text and add value for the reader, all references are included on the companion Evolve site that accompanies this text book. The reader can view the reference source and access it online whenever possible. There are a total of 89 cited references and other general references for this chapter.

CHAPTER 26

Patient Management
in Postacute Inpatient Settings

Greg W. Hartley, PT, DPT, GCS, Sabrina Camilo, PT, MSPT, GCS

INTRODUCTION

Postacute care of the geriatric patient has undergone massive change since the Balanced Budget Act of 1997 (BBA).[1] According to the United States Department of Health and Human Services, Agency for Healthcare Research and Quality, there was a 30% increase (from 4 million to 5 million) in the rate of patients discharged to nursing homes or rehabilitation facilities between 1997 and 2006.[2] New payment methodologies like prospective payment systems (PPSs) have significantly altered patterns of patient placement upon discharge from acute care settings.[3] These changes have forced physical therapists working in these postacute environments to broaden the rehabilitation services offered and to expand upon traditional roles, most especially skilled nursing facilities (SNFs). This chapter will focus on several, but not all, *inpatient* postacute care settings. Rehabilitation hospitals will be discussed briefly since regulatory changes in this environment have subsequently impacted the patient population of other postacute care environments.[4] The bulk of the chapter will focus on the nursing home environment, both short-term skilled (subacute) care and long-term care (LTC). Specifically, this chapter will address how physical therapy practice has evolved to keep pace with the changing population in these settings. In the United States, Medicare is the predominant payor in all of these settings, and since Medicare is the predominant payor for geriatric patients, a discussion of Centers for Medicare and Medicaid Services (CMS) regulations that impact the provision of physical therapy services in these settings will be provided where applicable.

INPATIENT REHABILITATION FACILITIES

Profile of an Inpatient Rehabilitation Facility and Its Patients

Rehabilitation hospitals, or inpatient rehabilitation facilities (IRFs), are either free-standing hospitals or units within an acute care hospital whose purpose it is to provide multidisciplinary, team-oriented services to patients with intense rehabilitation needs. For the purposes of Medicare (and most other payors) in order for a patient to be admitted to an IRF, patients must meet specific criteria, including reasonable and necessary care and a significant rehabilitation potential. Patients must also require the coordinated care of at least two therapy disciplines, which includes physical therapy, occupational therapy, and speech–language pathology. One of the two disciplines must be either physical therapy or occupational therapy. Patients are also required to participate in a minimum of 3 hours of therapy per day, at least 5 days a week at the time of admission. Therefore, IRFs must be reasonably assured that patients require these services and can fully participate at the time of admission. Trial admissions are not permitted. Care must be coordinated and team oriented, with an emphasis on discharging patients to the community.[5] These criteria were revised in 2009 and made effective January 1, 2010.[5]

For geriatric patients in a rehabilitation hospital, Medicare is most often the payor. Since 2002, CMS has reimbursed IRFs prospectively, a system referred to as the Prospective Payment System (PPS).[6] Because of the level of care that is required in IRFs, CMS's payments are typically higher than other settings.[7] Because payment is at a higher tier, CMS requires IRFs to meet specific criteria in order to be paid under the PPS. Chief among these criteria is a requirement that at least 60% of all patients have a diagnosis that qualifies for the setting.[5] There are currently 13 diagnoses, or diagnostic categories, that qualify. These diagnostic categories are collectively called the CMS-13. The qualifying diagnoses in the CMS-13 are listed in Box 26-1. The remaining 40% of patients admitted to IRFs may have any diagnosis; however, the patients must still meet all of the requirements, including admission requirements, a need for multidisciplinary rehabilitation, and intensity of service (3 hours/day).[5,6]

CMS regulations for IRFs have undergone significant change since PPS became the means of reimbursement

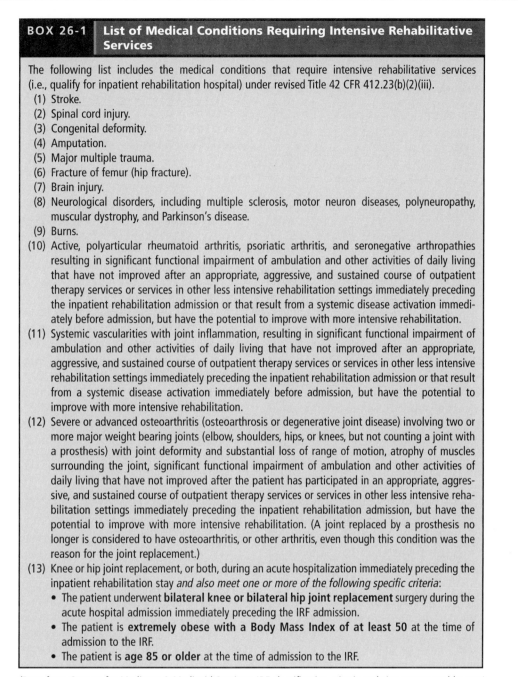

BOX 26-1   **List of Medical Conditions Requiring Intensive Rehabilitative Services**

The following list includes the medical conditions that require intensive rehabilitative services (i.e., qualify for inpatient rehabilitation hospital) under revised Title 42 CFR 412.23(b)(2)(iii).

(1) Stroke.

(2) Spinal cord injury.

(3) Congenital deformity.

(4) Amputation.

(5) Major multiple trauma.

(6) Fracture of femur (hip fracture).

(7) Brain injury.

(8) Neurological disorders, including multiple sclerosis, motor neuron diseases, polyneuropathy, muscular dystrophy, and Parkinson's disease.

(9) Burns.

(10) Active, polyarticular rheumatoid arthritis, psoriatic arthritis, and seronegative arthropathies resulting in significant functional impairment of ambulation and other activities of daily living that have not improved after an appropriate, aggressive, and sustained course of outpatient therapy services or services in other less intensive rehabilitation settings immediately preceding the inpatient rehabilitation admission or that result from a systemic disease activation immediately before admission, but have the potential to improve with more intensive rehabilitation.

(11) Systemic vascularities with joint inflammation, resulting in significant functional impairment of ambulation and other activities of daily living that have not improved after an appropriate, aggressive, and sustained course of outpatient therapy services or services in other less intensive rehabilitation settings immediately preceding the inpatient rehabilitation admission or that result from a systemic disease activation immediately before admission, but have the potential to improve with more intensive rehabilitation.

(12) Severe or advanced osteoarthritis (osteoarthrosis or degenerative joint disease) involving two or more major weight bearing joints (elbow, shoulders, hips, or knees, but not counting a joint with a prosthesis) with joint deformity and substantial loss of range of motion, atrophy of muscles surrounding the joint, significant functional impairment of ambulation and other activities of daily living that have not improved after the patient has participated in an appropriate, aggressive, and sustained course of outpatient therapy services or services in other less intensive rehabilitation settings immediately preceding the inpatient rehabilitation admission, but have the potential to improve with more intensive rehabilitation. (A joint replaced by a prosthesis no longer is considered to have osteoarthritis, or other arthritis, even though this condition was the reason for the joint replacement.)

(13) Knee or hip joint replacement, or both, during an acute hospitalization immediately preceding the inpatient rehabilitation stay *and also meet one or more of the following specific criteria*:

- The patient underwent **bilateral knee or bilateral hip joint replacement** surgery during the acute hospital admission immediately preceding the IRF admission.
- The patient is **extremely obese with a Body Mass Index of at least 50** at the time of admission to the IRF.
- The patient is **age 85 or older** at the time of admission to the IRF.

(Data from Centers for Medicare & Medicaid Services: IRF classification criteria website: www.cms.hhs.gov/ InpatientRehabFacPPS/03_Criteria.asp#TopOfPage. Accessed July 15, 2010.)

for IRFs in 2002. One of the most significant changes occurred in 2004 with the elimination of unilateral total joint replacements from the CMS-13 list of qualifying diagnoses.[8] After analysis by CMS, it was determined that these patients could achieve similar outcomes in a less expensive setting (SNF, home health, outpatient).[8] Some patients may continue to qualify for the rehabilitation hospital setting (in the other 40%) if they meet requirements for IRF admission, including requiring more than one discipline (e.g., physical therapy and occupational therapy as well as a coordinated team approach

that cannot be provided in a less "intense" environment. But in general, patients with uncomplicated unilateral total joint replacements no longer qualify for an inpatient rehabilitation hospital level of care. When possible, these patients when able go directly home from acute care, where they typically receive home health care or outpatient therapy. However, in many cases, patients are not able to go directly home after acute care.[9] Patients in this category are frequently discharged from acute care to SNFs, whereas they might have been sent to a rehabilitation hospital several years ago. The effects of the changes in CMS policy have contributed to a change in SNF patient populations over the past several years, particularly in urban areas, where IRFs are more abundant.[10] As a result, the total population of patients with major joint replacement in IRFs has decreased more than 10% between 2004 (when the elimination of this diagnostic group became effective) and 2008 as the numbers of these patients in SNFs has been increasing.[11,12] The payment system in SNF was reconfigured in 2006, adding new payment groups to accommodate the patients who require some medical monitoring but do not require the intense level of services provided in IRFs.[13] Subsequently, CMS findings indicate that many SNFs have reconfigured themselves to better care for this type of patient (i.e., subacute rehabilitation).[12]

Inpatient rehabilitation facilities are paid under the PPS when Medicare is the primary payor. The prospective payment system in IRFs is based on data gathered via a tool called the Inpatient Rehabilitation Facility–Patient Assessment Instrument (IRF-PAI).[14] Diagnoses, comorbidities, and demographic data are combined with information gathered from the Functional Independence Measure (FIM) tool.[15] Initial FIM scores, along with the other demographic and diagnostic data combine to determine which case-mix group (CMG) the patient will be assigned to. Each CMG is associated with a payment amount. This payment, set upon admission, is the payment the facility will receive for the care of the patient for that entire admission. Payment is based on an expected or average length of stay for that particular CMG. If the patient is discharged to the community (e.g., home, assisted living facility), the IRF receives the entire payment regardless of the patient's length of stay. However, if the patient is discharged to another health care delivery site (e.g., SNF, acute care), the IRF receives a prorated payment based on the anticipated length of stay. For example, if the anticipated length of stay was 16 days, and the patient is discharged to an SNF on day 7, the IRF receives 7/16 of the total projected payment.[16,17] Knowledge of the payment system is important for physical therapists. Clearly, it is in the best financial interest of the rehabilitation hospital to discharge patients to the community and not to another health care facility. Therapists must be cognizant of this incentive when developing goals and making discharge recommendations. In addition, physical therapists must understand the importance of accurately capturing FIM scores. These data are used to determine payment and to generate outcome reports that are shared with external agencies like CMS and the Joint Commission.[16]

Although rehabilitation hospitals play a large role in postacute rehabilitation, the vast majority of Americans needing postacute rehabilitation receive this care in an SNF. Although this is partly related to the IRF criteria described earlier, it is more likely related to accessibility issues.[18-23] Many communities simply do not have access

to an IRF.[11,12] Accordingly, the remainder of this chapter will focus on patients/residents in short-term (skilled/subacute) and LTC facilities.

SKILLED NURSING AND LTC FACILITIES

Profile of a Skilled Nursing Facility and Its Patients (Residents)

A SNF is a nursing home that has been certified by CMS to provide Medicare-reimbursable short-term skilled nursing/therapy services. Among SNF residents, the most common diagnoses are hip fracture, stroke, pneumonia, and heart failure.[24] Because the participation and payment rules for SNFs were created as a "subset" of nursing home rules and regulations, clients in an SNF are referred to (by CMS) as "residents" (a product of LTC language).[25] Historically, patients treated in SNFs were those with lower functional levels and required longer courses of treatment (nursing or rehabilitation) in order to return to the community. If a return to the community was not possible, patients could potentially stay as an LTC resident. Historically, SNFs also had a greater variety of diagnoses than rehabilitation facilities (there is no "60% Rule" in SNFs), with more individuals having lower functional levels.[20] Although SNFs have continued to care for the complex, lower functional-level patients who may (at least initially) require less intense rehabilitation services and longer lengths of stay, SNFs also care for a myriad of patients with advanced rehabilitation needs who require relatively short stays, have the potential to return home or to the community quickly, and who tolerate intense levels of rehabilitation services. In fact, in the calendar year 2006, the average length of stay for patients with Medicare in SNFs nationwide was 26.4 days.[26] The regulatory changes in other settings have meant more patients in SNFs have elective joint replacements, "acute" rehabilitation needs, and the potential to make rapid, substantial progress with an expected discharge to the community.[12] The growth in this group of patients has led to greater use of the term *subacute* to describe this cohort more effectively. In addition, the growth of Medicare Advantage (MA) programs has also affected rehabilitation utilization in SNFs. More and more, patients enrolled in MA programs are referred to SNFs instead of other, higher-cost settings such as IRFs.[27]

The availability of SNFs and IRFs makes a difference in where patients ultimately receive postacute care.[18-23] One study confirmed that utilization of services (and therefore total health care costs) is frequently determined by what services are available in the community.[28] For example, the study found that where more intensive care beds are available, more intensive care is provided. Likewise, where there are more specialists, more referrals to specialists are provided. Similar studies have confirmed that the same practice holds true for postacute care placement.[22,23] However, in the authors' experiences, it is observed that many MA programs will not authorize treatment in IRFs even when the patient has a qualifying complex diagnosis and IRF beds are available. This is an internal administrative decision made by each participating MA program.

Overview of SNF Prospective Pay System (PPS)

The Medicare payment structure for SNFs is a PPS but is entirely different from the IRF system discussed earlier.[13] The SNF benefit under the Medicare system can potentially last up to 100 days per qualifying episode. Residents must have had a 3-day stay in an acute care facility at least 30 days prior to admission to a SNF in order to meet criteria for *skilled* services. There are no specific diagnostic criteria for admission; however, residents must require *skilled* services of a nurse, therapist, or both. If Medicare is the primary payor, payment to the SNF is based on a calculated per diem which is, in large part, determined by the amount of rehabilitation services provided.[29] To determine the exact amount of this per diem payment, residents are assessed using the minimum data set (MDS).[30] The MDS is an instrument that analyzes clinical information as well as utilization of resources and categorizes the resident into a "resource utilization group" or RUG for payment purposes. The MDS and RUG levels are periodically refined, and the MDS 3.0 was implemented in 2010.[31]

With the MDS 3.0 and the fourth generation of RUGs (RUGs IV), there are 66 different RUG levels. Of those, 23 are directly associated with the amount of rehabilitation provided.[13] The RUG level is associated with a per diem payment that lasts for a specified period of time. MDS assessments are required on admission (day 1), day 14, day 30, day 60, and day 90 (and also when there is a significant change in status or a readmission).[30] There are "grace days" that can be used for each assessment due date, allowing some flexibility for when the reports are actually generated and which dates are actually used; however, when a RUG level is assigned, the SNF is paid the associated rate for that RUG for the specified assessment window (day 1 through day 14, day 14 through day 30, and so on). A RUG level is assigned for each time interval, so payment can and does vary for each interval.

As mentioned, the amount of rehabilitation physical therapy, occupational therapy, and/or speech-language pathology plays a significant role in determining the RUG, that is, payment level. Therapists determine the frequency and duration of services (utilization) on admission. The amount of therapy, inclusive of physical therapy, occupational therapy, and Speech, provided in a week (measured in minutes/week) determines which one of several rehabilitation RUGs best classifies the resident. Please refer to Box 26-2 for a detailed explanation of the Rehab RUGs.[29]

BOX 26-2 | **Major RUG-IV Classification Category Requirements**

Ultra High Rehabilitation
Residents receiving physical or occupational therapy, or speech–language pathology services
Rehabilitation Rx 720 minutes/week minimum
AND
At least one rehabilitation discipline 5 days/week
AND
A second rehabilitation discipline at least 3 days/week

Very High Rehabilitation
Residents receiving physical or occupational therapy, or speech–language pathology services
Rehabilitation Rx 500 minutes/week minimum
AND
At least one rehabilitation discipline 5 days/week

High Rehabilitation
Residents receiving physical or occupational therapy, or speech–language pathology services
Rehabilitation Rx 325 minutes/week minimum
AND
At least one rehabilitation discipline 5 days/week

Medium Rehabilitation
Residents receiving physical or occupational therapy, or speech–language pathology services
Rehabilitation Rx 150 minutes/week minimum
AND
5 days any combination of three rehabilitation disciplines

Low Rehabilitation
Residents receiving physical or occupational therapy, or speech–language pathology services
Rehabilitation Rx 45 minutes/week minimum
AND
3 days any combination of three rehabilitation disciplines
AND
Restorative nursing, two or more services, 6 or more days/week

Rx, treatment.

Logically, per diem payments are higher for RUGs with higher rehabilitation utilization because of the increased cost of providing rehabilitation. It is important to note that physical therapists determine the RUG level when they set frequency and duration of treatment. Clearly, this puts decision making, reimbursement, resource utilization, and staffing levels in the hands of the therapist; such authority is a clear example of autonomous practice in the SNF setting.

A third factor is added to the amount of therapy services provided to determine the final RUG level. This factor includes how much assistance the resident requires with several activities of daily living (ADLs) and how much medical care and oversight the resident requires. Specifically, if in addition to rehabilitation services, the resident requires tracheostomy care, a ventilator or respirator, or isolation for active infectious disease while a resident, the resident will qualify for a higher payment. Varying degrees of ADL assistance without the medical complexity are associated with slightly lower per diem rates.[30]

As mentioned, if residents require a skilled service, they may stay in an SNF for up to 100 days.[29] After that point, the "skilled" benefit is exhausted under Medicare guidelines, and the resident must be discharged or convert to LTC. As one can infer, the SNF benefit was *originally* intended for individuals with conditions that required daily skilled care over a longer period of time when rapid recovery or discharge was not necessarily anticipated. This provision would include those who are not able to tolerate the intensity of services provided in a rehabilitation hospital, who do not meet the other requirements for rehabilitation hospitals, when the expected length of recovery is relatively long, or in cases where the individual may not be discharged to the community. However, this "typical" resident has changed in recent years. Although SNFs have always been providers of postacute rehabilitation, the emphasis on rehabilitation has grown. This is in large part due to the transition of patients who in the recent past would have gone to an IRF or other postacute settings.[12,27] Now, because of regulatory changes, payor mix changes, accessibility, and some outcome data, these individuals are increasingly going to SNFs.[18-23] Recent CMS data indicate that the so-called "rehabilitation RUGs" are the most frequently used RUGs, representing 86% of RUG scores for the fourth quarter of 2009, nationwide.[32] As recently as 2005, the use of rehabilitation RUGs was 11% lower.[32]

Clearly, rehabilitation services are a large part of the services provided by SNFs. Of the *rehabilitation* RUGs used during the same quarter, more than half (54.4%) were in the ultra high, very high, and high categories (Figure 26-1).[32]

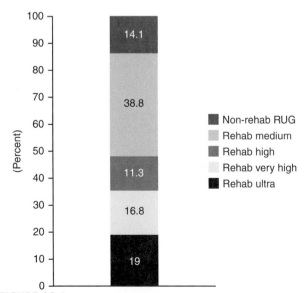

FIGURE 26-1 National RUG III Medicare frequencies: fourth quarter 2009 (5-day assessment). *(From CMS MDS 2.0 Public Quality Indicator and Resident Reports 32.)*

An exception to the PPS reimbursement system in an SNF occurs when a resident has a Medicare Advantage (MA) Plan (formerly known as "Medicare Plus Choice"). In those cases, Medicare beneficiaries sign up with private managed care organizations that contract with and are paid by CMS to manage the beneficiary's care.[33] As of December 2008, 10.1 million (23%) of the nearly 45 million Medicare beneficiaries have enrolled in MA plans.[34] Enrollment has steadily grown each year. MA plans offer a different approach to health care delivery than beneficiaries experience under fee-for-service Medicare. Instead of focusing almost exclusively on treating beneficiaries when they are sick, these plans also place an emphasis on preventive health care services that help to keep beneficiaries healthy, detect diseases at an early stage, and avoid preventable illnesses. In addition, many MA plans help reduce beneficiaries' out-of-pocket costs by providing additional benefits not covered in the Medicare program and reducing cost sharing for Medicare-covered benefits.[35] Facilities that accept patients/residents with MA must contract directly with each MA plan. Payment is typically a flat fee per day. It is not uncommon for MA case managers to determine the level of care, including the amount of therapy that will be covered, based primarily on the individual's admitting diagnosis.

All of these factors combined (i.e., payment and regulatory changes, growth of the Medicare Advantage program, and a lack of accessibility) have led to more acutely ill patients with high rehabilitation needs filling the beds in America's SNFs. These individuals are treated with aggressive rehabilitation, and most are discharged home in a short time.[36] So, although the SNF benefit *allows* for slower recovery for individuals who require longer lengths of stay, there is a large and growing cohort of residents who have a relatively short stay in an SNF.[37] Although SNFs are legally classified as nursing homes, the skilled patient (as opposed to the nonskilled, long-term resident) is clearly different today than 20 years ago.

Profile of the LTC Resident

In some cases, residents do stay in a nursing home as an LTC resident once the SNF benefit is exhausted or when they no longer require skilled services. The leading reasons for LTC admission are decrease cognition, incontinence, decreased falls leading to a decrease in functional status.[38] About 1.46 million residents of all ages lived in 16,435 nursing facilities in 2006. Of those, 90% were age 65 years or older.[38] In 2006, only 3.5% of people older than age 65 years lived in nursing facilities, a decline from 7.5% in 1982.[39] It is unknown exactly why the percentage decreased so much during this time. It could be due to economic reasons as the cost of care has risen drastically. Alternatively, it might be related to improved social support systems, accessibility, or a greater focus on health promotion and wellness over the past several years. However, the percentage is likely to increase again in future years as the numbers of individuals surviving into their 8th, 9th, and 10th decades of life will represent the fastest-growing segment of the population.[40] Disability rates are strongly related to age; about 50% of the population ages 85 years and older has a disability, compared with only 10% of the population ages 65 to 74 years. Among the population aged 65 years and older, 69% will develop disabilities before they die, and 35% will eventually enter a nursing home.[41]

By definition, long-term *institutional* care is custodial. Of course, LTC can be interpreted to include much more than institutional care. The broader definition of LTC would include assisted living (where less supervision is provided, but typically some supervised services are offered), adult day care (per day/daytime supervised care), home care or sitter services (nonskilled home care under the Medicare Part A benefit), and many other local or community-based services, whether paid or unpaid. As the population of aging adults who require these services increases, the availability and variety of these alternative LTC settings and services will also expand. However, for the purposes of this chapter, the focus will remain on institutional LTC.

In the LTC setting, no *regular, skilled* intervention is provided. The staff administer medications and provide ongoing restorative, recreational, and social activities for residents. Because LTC is, in fact, nonskilled, Medicare does not cover this cost. LTC is paid out of pocket, by private insurance, or by Medicaid for residents who qualify based on their income.[42] Medicaid is the primary payor for most nursing facility residents. Almost two thirds (65%) of LTC residents had Medicaid as the primary payor in 2009. The remaining nursing facility residents had other sources of payment such as private LTC insurance or paid out of pocket.[43] *Institutionalization* is a term that unfortunately conjures up images of an older person being abandoned forever at the door of some dark building. However, admission to LTC institutions is not permanent in many cases. In fact, in a report to Congress, the Centers for Disease Control and Prevention, National Center for Health Statistics, indicated that 29.2% of all LTC residents are discharged to the community because they have either stabilized or recovered.[44] The average length of stay for all nursing home residents (which includes the skilled residents as well as the long-term residents) is 341 days, which includes those who are discharged to the community, those who are discharged to acute facilities, and those who die in the facility. Of those who die while a resident, the average length of stay is 729 days.[44] Table 26-1 describes the most common diagnoses for residents in LTC settings *at the time of admission*.[45]

If permanent residence is required, a wide variety of services are available to residents to ensure quality of life for the remainder of life. In long-term settings, staff

TABLE 26-1	Percent Distribution of Long-Term Care Residents by Primary Diagnosis at Admission, United States, 2004	
Diagnosis		**Percentage Distribution**
Diseases of the circulatory system		23.7
Mental disorders		16.4
Other mental disorders		14.2
Diseases of the nervous system and sense organs		14.0
Supplementary classification		9.6
Posthospital aftercare (including fractures)		8.8
Alzheimer's disease		8.5
Heart disease		8.3
Diseases of the respiratory system		6.7
Acute, but ill-defined, cerebrovascular disease		5.8

(Data from Centers for Disease Control, National Center for Health Statistics, National Nursing Home Survey, 2004. www.cdc.gov/nchs/data/nnhsd/Estimates/nnhs/Estimates_Diagnoses_Tables.pdf#Table33.)

performs periodic screens for the need for rehabilitation services. When the need for skilled therapy is identified, residents are treated under the Medicare Part B (outpatient) benefit, assuming Medicare is their payor, or a similar benefit if the individual has a Medicare Advantage product or private insurance. The same rules that apply to regular outpatient (Part B) also apply in the LTC setting. For example, documentation requirements, billing, and coding rules are the same. A study commissioned by CMS indicates that in 2006, 29.2% of all Part B therapy claims were billed from a SNF, more than private practice settings (26.6%) or hospitals (20.0%).[46] From these data, one can hypothesize that many of the residents who reside in LTC have the potential to benefit from physical therapy.

PHYSICAL THERAPY PATIENT MANAGEMENT IN THE LTC SETTING

The clinical management of the LTC resident who is not receiving the "skilled" benefit (i.e., not in SNF) will be the focus of the remainder of the chapter. Long-term residents are different from those patients who are in a nursing home for short stays receiving skilled services. As discussed previously, in today's health care environment, SNF residents present clinically as "subacute" patients, and the clinical management of those types of patients and diagnoses is dealt with in various other chapters of this text. Long-term residents are those patients who, for whatever reason, reside in the nursing home for extended periods of time, often for the reminder of their lives. There are a wide variety of functional abilities among these patients. Although many individuals are frail, not all fit that description. Of the settings discussed in this chapter, long-term residents show the most variability in functional abilities, ranging from being an independent ambulator to being totally bed-bound.

In the LTC setting, the goal is often to return the resident to a prior level of function or higher. The prior level of function, though, may be lower than that of a patient in a rehabilitation hospital or even SNF. For example, the prior level of function may be ambulation of short distances with a rolling walker, or perhaps it is simply the ability to sit independently. However, therapists should not underestimate the residents' ability to make significant improvements, sometimes beyond the prior level of function. Residents whose status commonly declined by virtue of disuse and with physical activity along with physical therapy, can reasonably expect the achievement of a higher functional level. This variability of patient function coupled with altered mental status (in some cases) and complex regulations can make for challenges as well as opportunities in the LTC setting. These opportunities create a perfect environment for autonomy in decision making and teamwork with other health professionals, especially nurses and physicians. In the LTC setting, the therapist must function as a team member who will delegate tasks and follow through with other team members. Collaboration between team members is vital to the success of any LTC therapeutic program and can be one of the greatest challenges of this setting. Next we will highlight important differences and nuances in the physical therapy assessment and management of residents in the LTC setting.

Frailty in LTC

Frailty is highly prevalent with increasing age and thus it is imperative for the good management and treatment of older adults, especially those in LTC settings, for physical therapists to understand it.[47] When one thinks of frailty, the picture that commonly comes to mind is one of a bed-bound contracted resident in a nursing home or an extremely kyphotic, osteoporotic older woman sitting in a wheelchair. But the frail older adult extends beyond those stereotypes, and it is important to realize that frailty is not a disease but rather a combination of a variety of medical problems. The term *frail* should be considered a cluster of medical conditions and not a characterization—differentiated from disability or advanced old age.

Geriatricians define frailty as a biological syndrome of decreased reserve and resistance to stressors resulting from cumulative declines across multiple physiological systems and causing vulnerability to adverse outcomes.[47] Fried et al provide a standardized definition for frailty that is widely accepted.[47] These authors suggest that someone should be considered frail if that person has three or more of the following five characteristics:

1. Unintentional weight loss (10 lbs or more in a year)
2. General feeling of exhaustion (self-report)
3. Weakness

4. Slow walking speed
5. Low levels of physical activity[47]

In a study of 5317 older individuals who were living in the community, Fried et al found that 6.9% of these individuals were frail.[47] They also found that frailty was a reliable predictor of a general decline in health. Frailty was highly associated with cardiovascular disease, low education and poverty, hospitalization, and death. The frail older adult faced increased risk for falls, deteriorating mobility, and disability. As frailty is not a disease per se, other diseases and medical problems are related. Rothman et al suggest that the frailty phenotype might be strengthened by the inclusion of cognitive impairment. In their study to determine the independent prognostic effect of seven potential frailty criteria, including five from the Fried phenotype, it was found that cognitive impairment was associated with chronic disability, long-term nursing home stay, and death and the magnitude of these associations was comparable to that of the weight loss criteria.[48]

The problems or conditions that cause frailty are multifactorial and interrelated in a cycle of cause and effect represented in Figure 26-2.[49] Sarcopenia, or loss of muscle mass, can lead to weakness, difficulty walking, falls, and eventually immobility. Less oxygen (Vo_2) reaches the tissues and organs of someone with atherosclerosis, which can lead to cognitive impairment. Vascular disease caused by atherosclerosis can result in nutrient deprivation of the muscles, slow walking speeds, and ultimately sarcopenia. Decreased balance can initiate the vicious cycle in which a fall can lead to fear of falling and decreased mobility. Depression can cause failure to thrive, weight loss, and decreased mobility. Cognitive impairment can lead to a decline in mental processing time and reaction speed, resulting in falls. The relationship of multiple physical factors that are associated with frailty was examined by Brown et al.[50] They combined chair rise and Romberg test to the original seven functional items of the Physical Performance Test (PPT)[51] to examine the relationship of factors believed to be associated with frailty, including isometric and dynamic strength, range of motion (ROM), sensation, coordination, balance, and reaction time. Their findings strongly indicate that frailty is multidimensional, and evaluation of only one domain does not provide complete insight into this phenomenon. It is important to highlight that they also found that balance items were the most strongly associated with frailty.[50]

The Modified Physical Performance Test used by Brown et al and presented in Box 26-3 can be used to determine the severity of an older adult's frailty. Each of the nine items on the PPT is worth a maximum of 4 points, for a perfect score of 36. For purposes of their study, the group with PPT scores ranging from 32 to 36 was considered "not frail," the group with scores ranging from 25 to 32 points was

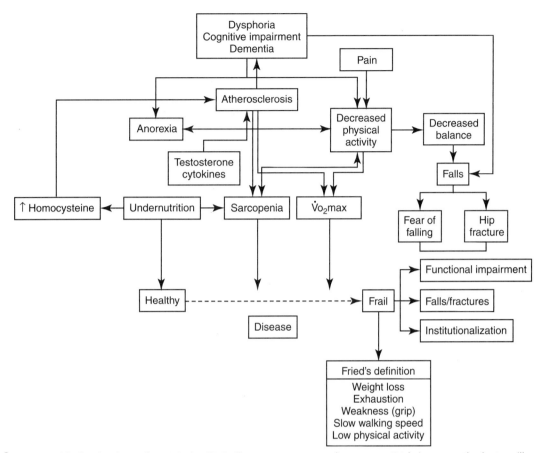

FIGURE 26-2 Causes of frailty. *(Redrawn from Morley JE: Frailty: management and treatment. Website: www.thedoctorwillseeyounow.com/content/art2070.html?getPage=2.)*

considered to have "mild frailty," and the group with PPT scores between 17 and 24 points was considered to have "moderate frailty." It has been their experience that those scoring below 17 points no longer function independently within the community.[50]

Understanding the relationship of multiple impairments to frailty will better enable the clinician to develop appropriate treatment strategies for the remediation of frailty. Residents who are frail and in LTC may take longer to achieve goals than patients in other settings. However, the frail older adult should not be excluded from any therapeutic interventions as this patient population can benefit from strength training just as the healthy older adult. Physical activity and exercise are of extreme importance to break the frailty cycle. Boltz suggests that the starting point of the cycle is muscular weakness. He defines frailty as "a state of muscular weakness and other secondary widely distributed losses in function and structure that are usually initiated by decreased levels of physical activity."[52] Older persons may be less active as a result of habit or limitations caused by certain conditions. The decline in physical activity initiates sets of negative outcomes, as seen in Figure 26-2, that accelerate the deterioration process. Acknowledging that the state of frailty is keyed by

muscle weakness leads directly to the simple preventive and remedial strategy of physical exercise.[52] The type of exercise program that will be most beneficial remains to be determined but is likely to include balance activities, resistance training, and endurance types of exercise.[50]

Screening in LTC

The continuous-care nature of LTC requires ongoing and regular screening of the functional status of each resident. Although there is no regulation that designates a specific discipline to conduct screens, physical therapists are aptly qualified to perform them. Screenings are not meant to replace an evaluation and should be used to determine a change in status, for better or worse. Important information on residents' status can be obtained from the MDS, but the therapist should obtain information beyond the MDS. A more comprehensive picture of any change is usually obtained from nursing staff, nutritionists, and residents themselves. The therapist performing the screening should then visually inspect and/or observe the resident. Changes in ability to transfer, to ambulate, any new onset of pain, worsening or development of contractures, new difficulty in eating, swallowing or speaking, and difficulty propelling the wheelchair

BOX 26-3	Modified Physical Performance Test Items

1. Book lift.
   A 7-lb book is lifted from waist height to a shelf 12 in. above shoulder level. Scores are based on the time required to complete the task.
2. Put on and take off a coat.
   Subjects put on and take off a standard lab coat of appropriate size as quickly as able. Scores are based on the time required to complete this item.
3. Pick up penny.
   Subjects pick up as quickly as possible a penny that is located 12 in. in front of the foot. Scores are based on the time required to complete the task.
4. Chair rise.
   Subjects sit in a chair that has a seat height of 16 in. They then stand fully and sit back down, without using the hands, five times, as quickly as possible.
5. Turn 360
   Participants turn both clockwise and counterclockwise quickly but safely. They are subjectively graded on steadiness and ability to produce continuous turning movement.
6. 50-ft. walk.
   Subjects walk 25 ft in a straight line, turn, and return to the initial starting place as quickly as possible, safely.
7. One flight of stairs.
   The time required to ascend 10 steps.
8. Four flights of stairs.
   Participants climb four flights of stairs. One point is given for each flight of stairs completed.
9. Progressive Romberg test.
   Subjects are scored according to their ability to maintain a reduced base of support: feet together, semitandem, and full tandem, for a maximum of 10 seconds.[50]

BOX 26-4	Medicare Coverage for Skilled Therapy in LTC (Part B)

- Service must be of a level of complexity and sophistication, or the condition of the patient must be of a nature that requires the judgment, knowledge and skill of a qualified therapist. This means that the services can only be performed by a qualified therapist. If a CNA, family member or other caregiver can perform the treatment, then it probably does not meet this criterion. Document tests and measures, functional assessments, special techniques and specialized teaching that only you can provide as part of your scope of practice.
- Positive Expectation for Improvement: The condition of the patient is expected to improve materially in a reasonable and generally predictable period of time or services must be necessary for the establishment of a safe and effective maintenance program. Ask yourself what do you see in the patient's environment and behavior that suggests intervention would be beneficial (i.e., social support, prior level of function, motivation and attention, ability to follow directions).
- The services must be considered under accepted standards of medical practice to be a specific and effective treatment for the patient's condition. This requires knowledge of the research. Know the tests and techniques that have been found to be effective within our scope of practice.
- The service must be reasonable and necessary for the treatment of the patient's condition including amount, frequency and duration of services. Documentation of a change of condition, ongoing problems and risk factors can add support to the necessity of your treatment. Documentation of the patient's complications and safety issues related to his or her impairments and functional deficits is important to meet this criterion.

(From Medicare benefit policy manual, Chapter 15: Covered medical and other health services. http://www.cms.hhs.gov/manuals/Downloads/bp102c15.pdf. Accessed July 15, 2010.)

should be noted. Inspection of the prosthesis, braces, or splints can identify problems that may impair mobility and/or comfort and safety. Periodic assessment of the fit of the prosthesis or orthosis is necessary as the resident may experience muscle atrophy and weight loss over time. When function is measured over time, a snapshot of the resident's ability to maintain basic self-care activities is obtained and indicates if there has been a decline, improvement, or stabilization of a condition.[53] After recognizing resident's change in functional status, physical therapists working in an LTC setting may determine that skilled intervention is required or they may refer the resident to a restorative nursing program. Therapists should attempt to make this decision process as objective as possible. Therefore, it is of paramount importance for the physical therapist to understand payor definitions of skilled therapy.

Medicare sets forth its definition of skilled physical therapy services in § 220 and § 230 of Chapter 15 of the *Medicare Benefit Policy Manual*.[54] The CMS definition of skilled therapy is presented in Box 26-4. It is incumbent upon the physical therapist to understand the requirements of each specific payor; however, many payors will follow CMS's lead.

Gait training and ambulation are clear differentiators of a skilled service and a nonskilled service. Gait training provided by a physical therapist or physical therapist assistant is considered skilled care under CMS criteria under three conditions: (1) when a therapist needs to give specific instructions, verbally or manually, to a resident in order to improve the gait pattern; (2) a gait assessment needs to be made to determine the impairments causing any abnormalities; or (3) recommendations need to be made for assistive devices. When a therapist determines that no improvement can be made in the gait pattern, but a resident should continue walking to maintain the functional status or simply improve distance ambulation for endurance, it can be performed in a restorative nursing program and does not require the skill of a therapist. It is also important to differentiate between manual cues and physical assistance. A resident can be in a restorative nursing program even when physical assistance is required to ambulate as long as the referring therapist believes it is safe, and the person assisting is providing support to the resident where no significant functional improvement is expected.

Active ROM or passive ROM provided in order to maintain the range does not require the skills of a physical therapist and can be performed in a restorative nursing program. However, exercise to improve ROM or to maintain range in a complex circumstance, such as in a joint near an unstable fracture, should be performed by a physical therapist or physical therapist assistant. It is important to understand that goal setting and plans of care in an LTC setting will be different when compared to goals and plans of care provided in a rehabilitation hospital where patients tend to quickly improve in function. LTC residents may not require treatment for mobility deficits at all. The potential for skin breakdown alone may warrant admission to skilled services for positioning, education, devices, contracture management, and prevention. As with all patients, a thorough history and chart review are the first two steps to determine the need for skilled therapy.

EXAMINATION AND EVALUATION

History

Although information provided in the chart, such as history of condition, MDS scores on ADLs, nutritional status, and laboratory values, is important when determining the plan of care and setting goals, history taking should not be limited to the medical chart. Interviewing the resident and staff most involved with the resident is key. Certified nursing assistants, restorative nursing staff, nutritionists, and any other staff that have regular interaction with the resident can provide information, such as how much assistance the resident needs and whether the resident's ability to perform ADLs has changed recently. The individuals in regular contact with the resident may be the first ones to realize a resident's change in functional status and behavior.

Any history of falls and mitigating circumstances for the falls should be noted. Some facilities may have fall assessment teams, often directed by a physical therapist, where the team analyzes the reasons for a particular fall or looks for patterns that may be contributing to falls and then discusses and plans ways to intervene.

The incidence of falls in LTC institutions is about three times the rate for community-dwelling older adult persons.[55] This increase is caused both by the nature of persons living in institutions and by more accurate reporting of falls in institutions. Falls are a major determinant of functional decline, nursing home placement, and restricted activity.[55] LTC residents are generally more frail than older adults living in the community. They also may have difficulty with concentration or memory and may need help getting around or taking care of themselves.[55,56] All of these factors are linked to falling, and determining the cause of the fall through an extensive

BOX 26-5	Comparison of Causes of Falls in Nursing Home and Community-Living Populations Ranked by Prevalence
Nursing Home	**Community-Living**
Gait or balance disorder or weakness	Environmental related
Dizziness or vertigo	Other causes
Environmental related	Gait or balance disorder or weakness
Other causes	Drop attack
Confusion	Dizziness or vertigo
Visual disorder	Unknown
Drop attack	Confusion
Unknown	Postural hypotension
Syncope	Visual disorder

(*Data from Rubenstein LZ, Josephson KR, Robbins AS: Diagnosis and treatment: falls in the nursing home. Ann Intern Med 121(6): 442-451, 1994. http://www.annals.org/content/121/6/442.full#T2*)

history can be fundamental in establishing an appropriate intervention and prevention. Box 26-5 compares the causes of falls in nursing-home and community-dwelling individuals.[57]

Physical therapists are often the ones identifying residents at risk for falls resulting from medications, including their adverse effects and polypharmacy concerns, and this information should be shared with the nursing and medical staff. Sometimes falls may be reduced by just decreasing or reducing a medication. In a trial conducted by Tinetti et al in a community-based population, medication review was specifically identified as part of a multifaceted intervention.[58] In this study, sedatives were withdrawn and the number of medications was decreased. The intervention group demonstrated a relative fall-risk reduction of 31%. Other studies targeting the reduced use of psychotropic, cardiovascular, and analgesic drugs have also reported success in decreasing the risk of falls in older people.[59-63] The role of the physical therapist in identifying these risk factors by taking a thorough history cannot be underestimated. For example, adverse drug reactions such as orthostatic hypotension and dizziness are common, and medications should be reviewed carefully for their contribution to the cause of falls. Ooi et al reported that more than half of 900 nursing home residents studied had at least one episode of orthostatic hypotension during the trial period.[59] Their operational definition for orthostasis was a 20 mmHg or greater decline in systolic blood pressure (BP) 1 or 3 minutes after changing from a supine to a standing position. Orthostatic hypotension was most frequent before breakfast. Those patients with persistent orthostasis tended to complain of dizziness or lightheadedness, be independent in ambulation, have hypertension (systolic greater than 160 mmHg or diastolic greater than 95 mmHg) or mood disorders, be taking psychotropic medications, and have multiple comorbid conditions.[59] These characteristics can help the therapist consider the contribution of orthostasis to falls and fall risk.

Systems Review

The senses of hearing and vision are expected to decline as a normal part of aging, and losses are common findings in most nursing home residents. Hearing loss is the most prevalent of all sensory losses, affecting an estimated 30% to 46% of individuals over age 65 and 90% of individuals over age 80.[64] Vision losses from cataract, glaucoma, diabetic retinopathy, and macular degeneration have all been shown to decrease quality of life.[65] Population-based studies have reported the prevalence of functional visual impairment to be 16% among individuals age 80 years and older and 39% for those older than age 90 years.[65,66] In a sample of 198 nursing home residents, researchers asked residents whether they had difficulty hearing in a group, while watching television, or while talking on the telephone. This three-question method was significantly more effective than the use of a single hearing loss question in predicting which residents had hearing loss as measured by audiometric assessment.[67]

Residents often wear corrective lenses. However, approximately 25% of residents in LTC settings who wear corrective lenses still have moderate vision impairment, that is, vision less than 20/70.[68] Information about residents' hearing and vision is important when the therapist is determining the best way to teach and cue a patient and should be noted in the initial evaluation and the plan of care. Specific visual pathologies such as cataracts, macular degeneration, or glaucoma have different presentations and visual effects that can impede physical therapy interventions. Awareness of visual pathology presentations will help the therapist provide the most effective education and cueing. Therapists need to be cautious to differentiate poor cognition from poor hearing, and lack of interest from poor vision.

Control of bowel and bladder functioning also should be noted. Approximately 49% of residents in LTC are incontinent of urine.[69] Incontinence is reported to be highly associated with impairment in ADL, the presence of dementia, restraint use, the use of bedrails, and the use of antianxiety/hypnotic medications.[69] For many residents, incontinence or bowel/bladder accidents may likely be due to impairments in ADL.

Residents may have chronic conditions affecting the heart and lungs, and many have mobility constraints, which may affect skin condition. Therefore, cardiac, pulmonary, and integumentary systems require special attention. Aerobic capacity and endurance tests include vital signs at rest and after activity, autonomic responses to positional change, and functional tests of endurance.

Tests and Measures

Strength. Muscle strength is a predictor of function in the older adult, and because most LTC residents have difficulty with ADLs, it can be safely presumed that most LTC residents have severe strength deficits.[70] For example, to stand from a normal chair without the use of arms requires leg strength of nearly half of the body weight.[71] If a resident cannot walk without weight bearing on his or her arms secondary to leg weakness, it can be presumed the resident has lost 75% of his or her reserve strength.[72] Therefore strength assessment is vital to the physical therapy examination. However, the traditional manual muscle testing (MMT) has inherent limitations, especially in the LTC setting. MMT is not a quantitative assessment method for strength and has been shown to lack accuracy when used as a screening test.[73] Bohannon et al have shown that MMT has severe ceiling effects for grades higher than 5/5 with a range from 85.4 to 650.0 Newtons.[74] MMT may not be easily performed in some patients with cognitive impairments, ROM, or mobility limitations. Therefore, MMT will not correlate with functional tasks on certain patients. Therapists may over- or underrate strength by observing function. For example, Bohannon found that if a patient is able to stand up from a chair without the use of his or her arms, it is safe to assume that strength on the quadriceps is at least 4+/5.[75] The therapist may determine the resident has "normal" strength and not incorporate appropriate strength training. Besides strength deficits, the resident may also exhibit poor balance or be afraid of falling, affecting task performance. The resident may have difficulty understanding instructions or simply not want to perform the task, issues insensitive to MMT. For these reasons, we advocate a functional testing perspective.

Functional Assessment. Functional assessment plays a vital role in demonstrating and documenting the outcomes of rehabilitation and should be an assumed standard of practice for all geriatric practitioners.[75,76] Many assessment tools that measure and analyze gait and balance require some level of resident comprehension and willingness to participate. Considering the great number of residents suffering from dementia and depression in LTC settings, the use of some of the standard tests may be challenging for the therapist.[77-79] We have listed some functional tools we find most valuable for residents of LTC settings, including functional markers for different abilities (Table 26-2).[80]

The data obtained from the tests and measures are used to make a clinical judgment (evaluation) and to establish a diagnosis and prognosis. The physical therapist has great autonomy in the LTC setting and will determine the dosage of interventions and when to

TABLE 26-2	Functional Markers for Older Adults		
Functional Marker	Physically Independent	Frail	Physically Dependent
Timed Up and Go	10 to 20 s	>20 s	>30 s
Gait speed	0.8 to 1.5 m/s	0.35 to 0.8 m/s (walker)	<0.35 m/s (walker)
6-Minute Walk	1800 to 1500 feet	1500 to 800 feet	<800 feet
Walk 1 mile	18 to 33 min	Unable	Unable
Floor transfer	10 to 30 s (with or without assistance)	>30 s with assistance	Unable
Berg Balance Scale (56 total)	>48	30 to 48	<30
10 stairs (up or down)	5 to 15 s	15 to 30s	>30 s
30-s chair rise	>15	<8	0
Timed 5-repetition chair rise	10 to 15 s	>15 s	Unable
Reach to toe while sitting (sit and reach test)*	+2″ to 0″	0″ to − 4″	<4″
Back scratch test*	+0″ to − 4″	− 4″ to − 8″	<8″
Tandem stance	5 to 10 s	<5 s	Unable
Single-leg stance	10 to 30 s	<10 s	Unable

*Flexibility norms differ for females and males, with females having higher flexibility norms than males.
(Avers and VanBeveren, Course notes, SUNY Upstate Medical University, October 2009.)

discharge from skilled therapy. It is imperative to constantly reassess the individual to determine when to refer them to a maintenance (restorative nursing) program.

INTERVENTIONS

Exercise

Probably the most crucial type of training in LTC is active participation in meaningful activities. Residents may not understand why they are asked to perform certain exercises and may not see the potential benefit of exercise performance.[81] Older adults must see the connection between their resistance training improvements and the performance of ADLs.

One of the strongest motivators affecting exercise adherence in older adults is self-efficacy, the confidence in one's ability to carry out a planned behavior.[82,83] When an exercise directly improves ADLs, it may then generate exercise adherence. A second motivator is outcome expectation, which is the belief that specific consequences will result from specific personal actions.[82,84] Older adults who adhered to exercise are characterized by an inner motivation to exercise, a belief that they were able to exercise safely (self-efficacy), a recognition of the benefits of exercise (outcome expectation), and the ability to set specific activity-related goals.[82] Self-efficacy has been shown to be a predictor of stair-climbing ability, balance, and general functional decline in older adults.[85] In addition, it is also a strong predictor of exercise participation, especially in women.[86] Efficacy scores increase as older

individuals become more confident of their abilities.[83] Martin Ginis et al compared a weight training alone treatment (WT) to an innovative WT plus educational treatment (WT+ED) to investigate strength gains, ADL self-efficacy, and performance.[81] The WT+ED participants increased self-efficacy for performing ADLs beyond the effects attributable to strength training alone. The findings suggest that ADL performance–related strength education can help older adults understand the relationship between exercise program strength gains and the application of those gains to ADL performance.

Exercises that are meaningful to the older adult not only improve exercise adherence but also provide gains in functional capacities. It has been documented that older adults can adapt physiologically to exercise training similarly to younger adults, if specificity is incorporated.[87] de Vreede et al performed a randomized controlled trial to determine whether a functional-task exercise program and a resistance exercise program have different effects on the ability to perform daily tasks.[86] It was found that functional task–specific exercises are more effective than resistance exercises at improving functional task performance in healthy older adult women and may have an important role in helping them maintain an independent lifestyle. Manini et al had similar results in a study to determine the efficacy of 10 weeks of resistance (RT), functional (FT), or functional plus resistance (FRT) training in 32 older adults (75.8 ± 6.7 years).[87] Participants completed 20 training sessions within approximately 10 weeks. The authors found that those who performed only FT improved in both components of functional ability (task modification and timed performance), but did not have consistent adaptations in muscle strength. Those individuals who performed only RT increased muscle strength, but only reduced task modification and not timed performance. Individuals who performed 1 day of each training type had less dramatic changes in muscle strength and functional ability than the other two groups but had consistent improvements in both components of functional ability and muscle strength.[87] These data suggest an important role of task specificity when designing exercise programs to improve physical function in lower-functioning older adults.

Age is not an appropriate characteristic to determine application of specific interventions. Too often, in the authors' opinion, physical therapy practice in LTC reflects low expectations by the therapist and often by the resident. Frequently, LTC residents are viewed as too frail or too cognitively impaired to benefit from best practices such as high-intensity strengthening, motor learning principles, electromodalities, and task-specific training. Unfortunately, there is a tendency to be too conservative when prescribing exercises to older patients even though studies have long shown that older adults can gain as much benefit from intense strength training as younger individuals.[88] Prescribing exercise that is intense enough to provoke a strength-training effect of at least 60% of a 1 repetition maximum (RM; or 15 RM) for 1 set will achieve functional gains and can be motivating as well.[89]

Older adults themselves may have misconceptions and lack of knowledge about strength training and therefore be resistant to an intense exercise regimen. In another study by Manini et al, 129 older adults (77.5 ± 8.6 years) responded to questions about their opinions, experiences, and knowledge of strength training recommendations.[90] Forty-eight percent of older adults believed that strength training would not increase muscle mass, 45% said that increasing weight is not more important than number of repetitions for building strength, and 37% responded that walking is more effective than lifting weights at building strength. Clearly, physical therapists have an important role educating older adults on the benefits and appropriateness of strength training.

It is well known that the frail older adult can achieve improvements in strength, balance, and endurance with training at any age.[91,92] A large controlled trial of a strengthening regimen for frail older adults was conducted by Fiatarone et al.[93] In this study, 100 nursing home residents (mean age = 87 years) were randomly assigned to one of four groups: high-intensity strengthening, nutritional supplementation, strengthening and nutritional supplements, or a placebo exercise/nutrition control group. Strengthening was targeted to the hip and knee extensors, at an intensity of 80% of the subjects' 1 RM. The residents performed three sets of eight repetitions three times per week for 10 weeks. The outcome measures included strength (1 RM), gait speed, stair-climbing power, nutritional intake, body composition, and physical activity. The strengthening intervention significantly improved muscle strength and increased quadriceps cross-sectional area, habitual gait speed, stair-climbing power, and overall level of physical activity. The nutritional supplement did not provide additional benefit to the changes seen with exercise alone. The design and number of subjects in this study provide the most convincing evidence that high-intensity strengthening exercises in frail, institutionalized older adults is safe and effective in improving both impairments and functional limitations.

Evans studied a population of 100 frail, institutionalized older adults (age range 87 to 96 years) randomly assigned to high-intensity strength training for the quadriceps muscle.[94] Initial strength levels were extremely low in these subjects, with a mean 1 RM of 8 kg for the quadriceps. The absolute amount of weight lifted by the subjects during the training increased from 8 to 21 kg. The average increase in strength after 8 weeks of resistance training was 174% ± 31%. The substantial increases in muscle size and strength were accompanied by clinically significant improvements in tandem gait speed and index of functional mobility. Repeat 1 RM testing in seven of the subjects after 4 weeks of no training showed that quadriceps strength had declined 32%. Additional research has shown that strength training, when done at appropriate levels of intensity based on the 1 RM, may minimize or even reverse the syndrome of physical frailty prevalent among very old individuals.[94] Based on evidence, we advocate and strongly encourage the prescription of moderate to vigorous exercises centered on a program established according to the patient's 1 RM. However, the frail older adult can still make gains that may be more related to improved motor learning and movement efficiency than actual strength gains with a low- to moderate-intensity program.

The intensity principle should be applied to aerobic conditioning as well, using a percentage of heart rate reserve. Foster et al compared the effects of moderate- and low-intensity exercise in women with a mean age of 78.4 years residing in retirement homes.[95] The women were randomly assigned to either an intervention group that walked 3 times a week at a heart rate that corresponded to 60% of their heart rate reserve or an intervention group that walked 3 times a week at a heart rate that corresponded to 40% of their heart rate reserve. After 10 weeks of training, both groups showed improvements in maximal oxygen consumption, but there was no difference between groups. Similarly, MacRae et al performed a randomized controlled trial investigating the effects of a walking program on walk endurance capacity, physical activity level, mobility, and quality of life in nursing home residents.[96] The 22-week intervention required that the residents in the intervention group walk at their habitual pace for a maximum of 30 minutes per day. The results showed that the daily walking routine improved residents' walking endurance but did not improve the other outcome measures.[96] The results of these studies suggest that low-intensity exercise (of sufficient duration) may be enough of a stimulus to produce some cardiovascular changes in these individuals, but functional change appears to require directed, intense, preferably task-specific training of sufficient intensity.

Gait Training

Older adults often recognize changes in their gait patterns and speed and feel that they cannot walk "the way they used to." Gait speed has been shown to be a predictor of functional decline, nursing home placement, and mortality.[97-100] Oberg et al and also Bohannon reported that habitual gait speed may decrease by 9% to 11% and fast gait speed may decrease by 8% to 18% between the fourth and eighth decades.[101,102] When gait speed slows below 1.0 to 1.2 m/s, older adults are reported to have more difficulty crossing the street safely before the traffic light changes.[103,104] Potter et al reported that older adults with a gait speed of <0.25 m/s were more likely to be dependent in one or more ADLs.[105] Gait speeds of 0.5 m/s or less are not uncommon in an LTC setting and indicate the severe loss of strength associated with frailty and sedentary behavior. Lower-extremity therapeutic exercise has been reported to improve muscle force-generating capacity and flexibility, which are needed for gait.[106] Thus, improving lower-extremity muscle force and flexibility, along with aerobic fitness and upright balance training, are expected to result in an improvement in gait speed. We advocate the measurement of gait speed over a 4-m walkway for every resident. Usual and fast gait speed should be measured with an expectation of 0.33 m/s difference between usual and fast gait speed, which may indicate a measurement of reserve. Many clinicians may find that residents only have one walking speed and thus an intervention could be to walk for short distances as fast but as safely as possible.

Gait training in the institutionalized older adult should be no different than in other settings where the therapist analyzes stance and swing phases, observes step length and symmetry, notes compensations, and generates hypotheses as to the causes of the limitations (impairments). Therapists should realize that causes of gait dysfunction in the institutionalized older adult may be of a chronic nature and that some of the impairments may not be reversible. However, any impairment noted should not be assumed to be attributable to "geriatric gait" but rather an indication of an underlying gait impairment that may be corrected or modified. Although the impairment may not be reversible, the functional limitations may improve if treatment is directed at balance, speed, and compensatory strategies. Improving gait to decrease the risk of falls is of extreme importance in most LTC settings. Slowed gait speed in the older

adult population has been related to an increased risk for falls, which, in turn, often leads to a loss of independent living and to institutionalization.[107,108]

UNIQUE CHALLENGES IN THE LTC SETTING

Fall Risk Reduction

Falls prevention is an important component of caring for the aging adult. Although what constitutes successful fall intervention in LTC has not been determined, some program characteristics are promising. For example, Shimada studied a group of 32 LTC facility residents and outpatients aged 66 to 98 years who were randomly assigned to a usual exercise group or to a treadmill exercise group.[109] Perturbed gait exercise on a treadmill continued for 6 months. The number of falls and the time to first fall during a 6-month period, balance and gait functions, and reaction time were evaluated before and after intervention. The number of falls on the treadmill exercise group was 21% lower than that in the usual exercise group. Gait training with unexpected perturbation seems to have a beneficial impact on physical function in disabled older individuals. Ray et al evaluated a falls prevention intervention in nursing home residents who were at a high risk of falling.[110] The 267 control subjects resided in different nursing homes than the 232 residents who received the intervention. An interdisciplinary falls consultation team conducted the intervention and attempted to decrease unsafe practices in the following four domains: environmental and personal safety, wheelchairs, psychotropic drugs, and transferring and ambulation. Residents' rooms were assessed for environmental hazards, wheelchairs were assessed and modified as needed, psychotropic drug use was evaluated in ambulatory residents, safety in transfers and gait was evaluated, and inservices were given to all nursing home staff regarding causes and consequences of falls and for recognizing environmental hazards. The outcome measures were the number of recurrent fallers and the number of injurious falls. An average of 15 recommendations were made per patient. The intervention group showed 19% fewer recurrent fallers and 31% fewer injurious falls. The program was more effective among the residents who had three or more falls the prior year and when compliance with the recommendations was achieved. These results suggest that high rates of falls can be lowered through interdisciplinary approaches in LTC settings. Physical therapists should be active members of the falls reduction teams, present in most facilities.

Restraint Reduction

The Omnibus Reconciliation Act of 1987 specified that residents have the right to be free from restraints, and therefore, restraints are used only when all other alternatives to prevent injuries have failed.[111] Most institutions have programs in place to reduce the use of restraints. In the LTC setting, physical therapists are often consultants, and assume leadership roles in finding alternatives for the use of restraints. Some of the alternatives for the use of restraints include engaging residents in physical activities, increasing participation in leisure activities, and increased supervision from staff, which can be difficult and sometimes overwhelming. Commonly used alternatives to restraints are low beds, mattresses on the floor to prevent injury in case of a fall out of bed, wheelchair or bed alarms, and beds with no railings. Some facilities have adopted the use of hip protectors to reduce the likelihood of fracture if a fall were to occur; however, the evidence on hip protectors is equivocal.[112]

There are many reasons why residents prefer having a bed rail, including the sense of security it seems to offer and the bed rail's ability to enable rolling. Bed rails are common in LTC but are considered a restraint if the resident is unable to lower the rail independently. And while the rail may seem to prevent injury and falls, the opposite is actually the case. Between January 1, 1985, and January 1, 2009, the Food and Drug Administration (FDA) received notice of 803 incidents of patients caught, trapped, entangled, or strangled in hospital beds.[113] The reports included 480 deaths, 138 nonfatal injuries, and 185 cases where staff needed to intervene to prevent injuries. Physical therapists should consider these facts when assessing functional independence in the LTC setting.

Contracture Management and Risk Reduction

Contractures are a common consequence of prolonged physical immobility among nursing home residents and further reduce mobility and increase the risk of other ill effects of decreased mobility, such as pressure ulcers.[114] Almost two thirds of the LTC residents in a study performed by Wagner et al had at least one contracture, with the most common locations being the shoulder and knee.[115] ROM is often limited in nursing home residents and needs to be assessed carefully, especially in the bed-bound residents.[69,114,115] Accurate measurement is the best way to detect contractures and provides the therapist objective numbers to refer back to in case there is a reported decline and a new evaluation needs to be performed. There have been only a few studies that have evaluated interventions for contractures. Fox et al studied the effectiveness of a bed positioning program for the treatment of patients with knee flexion contractures.[114] The bed positioning program consisted of stretching a patient's knee into extension and then securing and maintaining the position for a period of 40 minutes four times per week. There was no improvement in participant's ROM. The result of the study does not support the use of bed positioning programs for treating patients with knee flexion contractures. Light et al investigated

an intervention for decreasing knee flexion contractures in institutionalized older adults by comparing high-load brief stretch to low-load prolonged stretch.[116] The protocol suggested by Light et al consisted of a 1-hour duration stretch, twice a day for 4 weeks. The intensity of the stretch was such that the slack was taken up in the muscle. The stretch was maintained by a traction unit that hung off a plinth. High-load brief stretch consisted of a proprioceptive neuromuscular facilitation technique to hold the muscle at its end range for 1 minute, followed by a 15-second rest, and then the process was repeated three times. Low-load prolonged stretch techniques were found to be more effective than high-load brief stretch in reducing knee flexion contractures.

Mollinger and Steffen measured knee flexion contractures in nursing home residents for 10 months.[117] They reported that 75% of their sample of 112 residents had unilateral knee flexion contractures of greater than 5 degrees. The presence of knee flexion contractures was associated with resistance to passive motion, cognitive impairment, impaired ambulation, and complaints of knee pain. Their results suggested that residents whose knee flexion contractures approached 20 degrees may also develop subsequent ambulation impairment; therefore, skilled intervention may be indicated in these patients.

When contracture is already present, the therapist should not only take the accurate ROM measurement but also assess the nature of the contracture by differentiating fixed contractures (with no give in ROM by passive stretch) from a nonfixed restriction (with a gain in ROM with stretch) and rigidity from spasticity (neurologic) in order to establish the best intervention.

Pressure Ulcer Management and Risk Reduction

Physical therapists are often the first ones to observe redness or tender points in nursing home residents, frequently in bed-bound, nonverbal patients. Careful skin inspection should be part of the physical therapist's assessment. Sharing the findings with nursing staff, and providing alternatives for position is a primary task of the physical therapist in this scenario.

The prevalence of pressure ulcers varies from 2% to 24% among long-term patients.[118] The incidence and prevalence is more than 60% in high-risk patients, including older individuals with femoral fractures.[118] Risk factors for pressure ulcers include immobility or restricted mobility, loss of bowel and bladder control, poor nutrition, and impaired mental awareness.[119,120] Preventive interventions, such as frequent repositioning, tissue load management, and ensuring adequate nutrition, has been shown to help prevent pressure ulcer formation among patients at risk.[121]

The most practical method for reducing pressure is to turn and position the patient frequently. In a study demonstrating the effectiveness of repositioning, higher nursing staff ratios may have resulted in demonstrating increased effectiveness of pressure sore prevention.[122] Because of the limitations and cost of turning the patient frequently, a number of devices have been developed for preventing pressure injury. The only devices that consistently relieve pressure on the trochanter, ischium, and sacrum are low-air-loss and air-fluidized beds, and their long-term effectiveness is controversial.[123] Malnutrition has been linked to an increase in the risk of skin ulcers and to delayed healing.[124] During periodic screenings, therapists should speak with dieticians and certified nursing assistants involved in feeding to identify residents who are malnourished or at high risk for malnourishment, thereby attempting to indirectly reduce the risk of pressure sores. Some useful questions that can be asked are the following:

- Has there been any weight loss?
- If the resident wears dentures, do they fit appropriately and are they being used?
- Does the resident eat independently or with assistance?
- If the resident requires assistance eating, has there been a recent change in the level of assistance required?

In summary, the list below highlights the role of the physical therapist in managing and preventing pressure sores in the institutionalized older adult:

- Educate nursing staff whenever needed on proper transfers and lifting techniques to avoid skin injury from friction/shear.
- Recommend a turning and repositioning schedule for residents that are at risk.
- Leave residents with pillows or other devices to keep bony prominences from direct contact with each other.
- Teach residents to perform small and regular weight shifts.
- Recommend proper pressure-reducing devices for the wheelchair and bed and be familiar with current products available.
- Keep residents as active as possible; promote mobilization by referring to restorative programs and encouraging participation in social events.

RESTORATIVE PROGRAMS

When it is determined by the therapist's evaluation that a resident is not appropriate for skilled services, physical therapists also have an active role in teaching nursing staff the most appropriate transfer techniques, aids for proper positioning, donning and doffing braces and splints, guarding techniques during ambulation, and development of a restorative nursing program to maintain current status and prevent risk of functional decline. Physical therapists often

refer patients to these restorative nursing programs upon discharge from skilled physical therapy as a type of "step-down" program for the residents or if the therapist determined that the resident does not require the skills of a physical therapist. Restorative programs may include turning and positioning programs, wheelchair mobility and endurance programs, ambulation, ADL programs, active ROM programs, and restorative dining programs, among others. Programs that encourage walking as part of the resident's daily routine (e.g., walking to the dining room) have been reported to increase overall ambulatory endurance, decrease fall rates, decrease incidences of incontinence, and inhibit functional decline.[96,125-128]

Trained restorative aides generally carry out restorative nursing programs. These programs can be quite effective if both nursing and rehabilitation staff are committed to their success. Programmatic features that should be present in a restorative nursing program include:

- method of screening to assess functional abilities or to classify patients according to program requirements or guidelines,
- means of reassessment to determine whether residents continue to need the services,
- documentation/communication system to convey information about patients to all staff involved in the program on an ongoing basis and to ensure accountability, and
- method of objectively evaluating the effectiveness of the program and determining whether program goals have been met.[127]

Communication between the therapist referring the resident to a restorative program and the clinician running it is fundamental. Some facilities keep a log with descriptors of their residents' participation and restorative goals that have or have not been achieved. This may be a quick and effective way to supervise a resident's performance. A good time to interview the staff member responsible for the restorative program is during a periodic screen. The physical therapist should ask about residents' participation in the program and whether they are achieving the desired results. It is not uncommon for residents to improve slowly, over time, while on a restorative program. Do not confuse this with skilled therapy, where significant functional gains are expected in a reasonable time frame.[54] Any major changes in performance, for better or worse, should warrant a complete physical therapy evaluation.

DEALING WITH DEMENTIA AND DEPRESSION

Dementia is the most common reason for placement of the older adult in nursing facilities.[76] Depression affects up to 25% of patients in a nursing home setting and is associated with significant morbidity, mortality, disability, and suffering for patients and their families.[74,128,129] The presence of dementia or depression may pose challenges for the physical therapist that require creativity in engaging the resident. The resident who is depressed may be more likely to participate in activities that were enjoyed prior to the onset of depression. For example, if the resident enjoyed dancing, it could be incorporated into treatment by having the resident move according to the music to improve balance, or move according to the beat during gait training. Balls and competitions could be used for residents who enjoy sports. Consideration of how to build self-efficacy as described earlier can be included. Residents who are cognitively impaired may not understand exercising for the sake of exercising, or in severe cases, not even understand the instructions given. Therapists often struggle with this challenge, and unfortunately may exclude the resident from skilled therapy claiming that the resident is unable to participate. However, therapists should attempt to include the confused resident in activities that are meaningful, or make sense. For example, a resident who was a housewife for her whole life may be able to fold towels and sheets. The therapist can use that activity to work on balance, standing tolerance, or upper extremity motion. A resident who refuses to stand up from a chair when asked to may automatically stand up to answer the phone or the door and may agree to "go for a walk" to look for something or someone.

Often, persons with Mini Mental State Examination (MMSE) scores lower than 25 are excluded from physical rehabilitation programs.[79] However, evidence suggests that cognitively impaired older adults who participate in exercise rehabilitation programs have similar strength and endurance training outcomes as age- and gender-matched cognitively intact older participants.[74] These findings are consistent with those of Littbrand et al.[130] The result of Littbrand et al's study suggests that a high-intensity functional weight-bearing exercise program is applicable for use, regardless of cognitive function, among older people who are dependent in ADLs, living in residential care facilities, and have an MMSE score of 10 or higher. Goldstein et al studied 58 patients with hip fracture, 35 with and 23 without cognitive impairment to compare outcomes (physical function and discharge destination) and to identify cognitive skills related to functional gains.[131] They found that patients with hip fractures and cognitive impairments can achieve positive outcomes as defined by functional gain (as determined by the FIM) and discharge destination. Clearly, cognitively impaired individuals should not be excluded from rehabilitation programs.

Blumenthal et al assessed whether patients receiving aerobic training achieved reduction in depression compared to standard antidepressant medication (sertraline HCl) and a greater reduction in depression compared to placebo controls.[129] Their findings indicate that the efficacy of exercise in patients seems generally comparable with patients receiving antidepressant medication and both tend to be better than the placebo. Clearly, given these results, physical therapists need to be engaged in the discussion and treatment of patients with depression in LTC and other settings.

Physical therapists are introducing LTC residents to virtual technology applications such as the Nintendo Wii. Anecdotally, there appear to be increases in the treatment program adherence, some preliminarily positive outcomes, and increased patient engagement in the clinic.[132] The Nintendo Wii is a computer gaming console that offers simulated sports games, fitness, and other activities. The uniqueness of the console is that the controller is wireless and can detect acceleration and orientation in three dimensions. Although more definitive research is needed, improvements in balance have been demonstrated in nursing home residents.[132] A number of the sports games can be played in a sitting position, and opens many possibilities for the wheelchair-bound population. Cognitively impaired patients may also participate.[132] The key challenge is for the therapist to choose the appropriate program. Boxing, for example, is considered a good starting place as all that a participant needs to do is to swing alternate arms forward repetitively. There are also potential social benefits from such games. Residents may gather around to see other residents in action. For residents, simulation technology can stimulate the fun of attending or participating in a sport event. Although beneficial to patients with dementia or depression, these types of simulators have a much broader applicability in the modern clinic.

FUTURE TRENDS IN POSTACUTE CARE

Health care delivery and systems in the United States are changing rapidly. The CMS is interested in developing a new assessment tool.[133] The tool is intended to replace similar items on the existing Medicare assessment forms, including the Outcome and Assessment Information Set, MDS, and IRF-PAI tools.

Any initiatives from states and the federal government to ensure the solvency of Medicare and Medicaid programs are likely to affect postacute care settings in great measure. In coming years, there may be massive changes in health care payment methodology, systems of delivery, and continuity of care. Postacute care settings, including LTC, will see widespread implementation of electronic documentation and medical record keeping. The American Recovery and Reinvestment Act of 2009 alone dedicated some $19 billion toward assisting health care entities and providers with implementation of electronic medical records.[134]

It is clear that our current system will need to change to keep up with the large numbers of aging baby boomers who will create the biggest demand on the Medicare system the program has experienced since its inception. Physical therapists will continue to have an important role in the delivery of care in postacute care settings. Knowledge of evidence-based interventions, which are both clinically effective and fiscally efficient, will be especially important. Health promotion and wellness efforts should become standard practice for geriatric physical therapists as our society shifts toward a more preventive model of health care delivery. The postacute care environments, especially LTC, offer many opportunities for physical therapists to make substantive contributions to changes in how the aging adult regains function and is able to have a meaningful, productive quality of life.

REFERENCES

To enhance this text and add value for the reader, all references are included on the companion Evolve site that accompanies this text book. The reader can view the reference source and access it online whenever possible. There are a total of 134 cited references and other general references for this chapter.

CHAPTER 27

Hospice and End of Life

Richard Briggs, MA, PT, Karen Mueller, PT, PhD

THE CONCEPT OF A "GOOD DEATH"

Health care outcomes, regardless of one's discipline, are generally focused on the enhancement of patient quality of life. For each person, quality of life is a subjective, broad, and multifaceted construct, which includes all elements that provide life satisfaction. Physical therapists have a critical role in optimizing quality of life through the application of skills related to the evaluation and treatment of conditions affecting movement and function from the moment of birth until the moment of death.

Nevertheless, because the typical expectation of physical therapy intervention is related to the attainment of improved function, the benefits of our services to those facing end of life are often not considered. To that end, patients in a hospice setting may be told that "nothing more can be done" by health professionals who are unaware of the value of physical therapy in maintaining safe and comfortable function in the presence of physical decline. Unfortunately, such lack of awareness may prevent the optimization of quality of life in persons for whom death may be imminent yet still potent with opportunities for rich interactions.

It does not have to be this way. The indignities of a lonely, painful, and helpless death are among the greatest fears of Americans.[1] Fortunately, in the past few decades, these fears have forced a reexamination of end-of-life care, resulting in the development of the compassionate, patient-centered approach that defines hospice and palliative care.

Central to the hospice approach is the construct of a "good death," the inevitable outcome to which all effective end-of-life care is directed. This construct is the obvious antithesis of our worst fears. Simply put, a good death is one where the dying person is free of discomfort, in the presence of those they love and in the environment of their choosing.

This patient-centered approach is certainly not a foreign concept in other areas of health care. For example, just as expectant mothers can orchestrate the manner in which their labor and delivery proceed, dying patients can be given similar options for the ways in which they affect their end of life. One of the most important contributions of hospice and palliative care is to assist patients in making and carrying out these choices.

Physical therapists have an important role in supporting a good death through a host of interventions to reduce pain, optimize the patient's remaining function, and enhance the quality of life for whatever time is left. In end-of-life care, physical therapy outcomes may not be solely functional but can include improved sleep quality, decreased physiological and psychological stress, improved respiratory function, and a decreased need for analgesic medication. More importantly, skilled physical therapy intervention can help the patient and family to maintain safe, energy-efficient mobility in the presence of declining systemic function, a process that can best be described as "rehabilitation in reverse."

A primary goal of this chapter is to examine the current structure and process of hospice and palliative care, a growing health setting for all Americans, particularly those in their later years. In addition, the roles, benefits, and outcomes of physical therapy intervention in the realms of hospice and end-of-life care will be explored. Most importantly, the information presented here should enable the reader to advocate for the ongoing involvement of physical therapists in this important area of care. Accordingly, because hospice and palliative care is a newer area of physical therapist practice, rich opportunities exist for engagement in outcome studies to support the value of these services. Finally, we should remember that participation in hospice and palliative care is an elegant reflection of the American Physical Therapy Association's 2020 Vision Statement, which directs us to "maintain active responsibility for the growth of the physical therapy profession and the health of the people it serves."[2] Given that the overall outcome of interventions in hospice and palliative care relates to a death with dignity, it is important to first understand the physiological elements of the dying process. This knowledge is critical in providing compassionate support to patients and families as they navigate the poignant experience of this natural process.

THE PHYSIOLOGICAL PROCESS OF DYING

It has been stated that "we die of old age because we have been worn and torn and programmed to cave in. The very old do not succumb to disease, they implode their way to eternity."[3] As this quote suggests, advances in medicine have prolonged our lives so that the typical American death is most likely to occur in the old and very old from a chronic condition involving a period of physiological decline. Accordingly, the Centers for Disease Control and Prevention reported that of the 2,448,017 U.S. deaths that occurred in 2005, the four leading causes were heart disease (27%), cancer (23%), stroke (6%), and chronic lower respiratory tract disease (5%).[4] In fact, 90% of all American deaths occur from these or other chronic conditions. Although a slow and progressive deterioration can be disheartening for the patient to experience and challenging for the family to observe, a centered presence in the face of impending death optimizes opportunities for meaningful closure. Accordingly, patients can rally when least expected, often to fulfill one last important goal. For example, in the days before his death, Bill, a 70-year-old man with end-stage brain cancer, decided that he would leave his bed in order to have one last meal at the table with his family. Physical therapy services were requested and provided to help Bill carry out this goal. In other cases, patients may also linger in an unresponsive state for a period of time, dying shortly after a long awaited loved one finally arrives. Joseph, a 72-year-old man with liver cancer, died the day after his six adult children finally arrived from their locations around the country.

The end-of-life process is unique for every individual. There are many different ways in which the journey to the end of life begins so that each person dies in his or her own unique way, and in his or her own time.[5] Supporting this individual process is the purpose and focus of hospice care.

In the context of hospice care, approaching death is viewed as a physical, psychological, and spiritual event. Patients and their families require information and compassionate support to assure that their collective needs are honored during this critical time. The interdisciplinary hospice approach involves considerable involvement of the patient's nurse, who will administer medications for comfort. The hospice chaplain may be involved for spiritual support at the request of the individual or family, especially when impending death provokes questions by the dying person or family members related to the presence of or the prospect of life after death. Trained hospice volunteers may provide caregiver respite or provide a reassuring presence at the bedside. The hospice social worker may assist the family in a number of practical ways, such as addressing financial concerns. Physical therapy interventions such as edema reduction, breathing exercises for relaxation, positioning, and gentle massage or stretching may be performed in the days

or even hours before death. In one Swiss study of 56 older adult patients dying from cancer and other conditions, 44 (79%) received respiratory interventions from physical therapists (including side-to-side positioning for lateral chest excursion, chest mobilization, and guided breathing) up until their last 24 hours.[6] The following section includes a description of common physiological changes that accompany the death process, but it is important to note these will vary among persons.

The Dying Process

Physiological Changes Associated with Death. The dying process involves the decline and ultimate failure of all major organ systems. Depending on the nature of the contributory disease, this process may take anywhere from several months to several hours. Box 27-1 depicts the broader progressive changes that occur in the final months of life.

As a patient declines in function, physical therapy intervention can be helpful in providing education, adaptive devices, or alternative movement strategies to optimize safe function. These interventions are fully described in the section on models of physical therapy practice in hospice and palliative care further in this chapter.

Of equal importance to providing appropriate interventions is working closely with the hospice team to ensure that all forms of pain and discomfort are minimized. This is important not only for the patient but also for family members who, whenever possible, must be freed of the burden inherent in watching a loved one suffer. In the weeks or days before death, multisystem

BOX 27-1	Progressive Changes in the Terminal Phase
Month 6	Generally, patient is ambulatory, coherent, some adverse effects from curative measures/medications, initial stages of grief, anger, denial.
Month 5	Some weight loss, weakness, symptoms manifested, showing signs of stress, growing acceptance of terminal state, fear, depression.
Month 4	Continuing weight loss, decreasing appetite, physical manifestations, symptoms more pronounced. Grief work, planning, resolving.
Month 3	Physical deterioration apparent, symptomatology and pain increase, beginning of withdrawal, acceptance of terminal disease.
Month 2	Progressive physical deterioration, symptoms increase, pain management primary, may be bedridden, increasing withdrawal, resolution and closure.
Final month	End stage: pronounced withdrawal, requires total care, intensive management of symptoms and pain, no appetite.

(Adapted from National Hospice and Palliative Care Organization (NHPCO): Time line phases of terminal care, 1996. Reprinted with permission.)

decline results in a host of signs, which are illustrated in Table 27-1 and further described in this chapter.

It is very common for patients to sleep most of the time in the days before death. They may no longer be interested in food or fluid, and family members must be assured that for the dying person, the process of digestion can be uncomfortable or even painful. Furthermore, as death approaches, patients may have increased difficulty swallowing. Even in the absence of discomfort, dying patients do not need, nor can their bodies assimilate, the energy provided from food. When patients refuse food and fluids, or in cases where they are withdrawn in accordance with an advance directive, family members need assurance that the patient will not experience hunger or any sense of deprivation. In such instances, the hospice nurse will work with the patient and family to provide medications and other interventions to ensure optimal comfort. The ethical and legal aspects of intentional food and fluid withdrawal will be further discussed later in this chapter.

"Terminal restlessness" is a specific form of delirium and agitation that occurs in the final weeks, days, or hours of life. It is very common, although the degree may vary greatly, affecting up to 85% of terminally ill patients, and includes signs such as restlessness, agitation, confusion, hallucinations, or nightmares.[7] The experience of terminal restlessness can be highly upsetting for families and patients alike. One patient of the authors described his terminal restlessness as a feeling of "just wanting to crawl out of my skin." Terminal restlessness is thought to be the result of failing metabolic processes occurring as death approaches. In addition, terminal restlessness may be exacerbated by physical distress from severe constipation, decreased oxygen exchange, or changes in body temperature. Thus, terminal restlessness could be described as a condition involving considerable physiological and psychological pain, occuring at all levels of consciousness. Unresponsive patients may demonstrate terminal restlessness by pulling at their bed clothes, making random movements, or attempting to remove their medical appliances. Patients who are more wakeful may repeatedly ask to get up or attempt to do so without help. They may talk about seeing and speaking with deceased friends or family members (for example, a patient may sit up in bed and tell family members, "They're coming!"). Understandably, the behaviors of terminal restlessness can be disconcerting for patients and families. Reassurance, support, and skilled pharmacologic intervention, often involving the use of sedating medications, are important measures that can reduce the duration and severity of these symptoms.

"Active death" typically occurs in the final days or hours and involves observable signs of systemic failure.[8] Terminal restlessness may increase. Respirations may become extremely irregular and include periods of very rapid breathing, followed by several seconds of apnea (Cheyne–Stokes breathing). Other types of irregular breathing patterns may occur as well, along with "death rattles" from congested and fluid-congested lungs. Urine output decreases significantly, and the urine may be dark. Blood pressure will often drop 20 to 30 points below the patient's normal blood pressure range, with systolic pressure as low as 70 mmHg and diastolic readings as low as 50 mmHg. This lack of perfusion may result in extremities that are very cold, blue or purple. Patients may also complain of numbness in their distal extremities.

The patient may be unresponsive, or even comatose. Family members need to be assured that the patient hears them as hearing is one of the last senses to fail[8]

TABLE 27-1	Multisystem Physiologic Signs of Approaching Death	
System	**Sign or Symptom**	**Contributing Factors**
Central nervous system	Confusion, delirium Disorientation Increased time spent sleeping (from a few hours a day to most of the day) Decreased levels of responsiveness, eventual coma Anxiety and restlessness, hallucinations or reports of seeing things, hearing voices	Hypoxemia from disease process or decreased function, metabolic imbalances such as acidosis, toxicity from renal or liver failure, pain, adverse effects of opioid medication (this may be reversible)
Musculoskeletal	Weakness, loss of function, fatigue	Progression of disease process, prolonged inactivity
Cardiopulmonary	Drop in blood pressure Heart rate variability and irregularity Breathing rate may be very rapid, alternating with periods of apnea, or very slow gurgling in chest	Disease process, organ failure, adverse effect from chemotherapy (not reversible) Respiratory failure may result in fluid accumulation in lungs
Integumentary	Cool and clammy skin, distal extremities may be bluish Edema	Loss of cardiovascular perfusion Pump failure Loss of muscle tone
Gastrointestinal	Loss of interest in food and fluid Constipation or diarrhea Incontinence, decreasing urine output as death approaches	Adverse effects of medications (opioid medications are constipating)

and thus should be encouraged to talk to their loved one even if they do not receive a response. In contrast, other patients may be relatively wakeful and able to converse with family members almost to the moment of death.

As stated previously, dying is not only a physical event. Many patients experience significant psychological and social signs as well. Table 27-2 illustrates the spectrum of these, along with their possible causes and helpful interventions.

TABLE 27-2	Psychosocial and Spiritual Signs, Symptoms, and Interventions of the Actively Dying	
Signs and Symptoms	**Cause/Etiology**	**Interventions**
Fear of the dying process. Fear of the dying process may be greater than the fear of death.	Cause of fear will be specific to the individual. Fear of the unknown: how they will die, what will happen during the dying process. Fear of painful death and suffering such as breathlessness, physical pain, loss of mental competence and decision-making ability, loss of control, loss of ability to maintain spiritual belief systems and faith. Fear of judgment, punishment related to guilt, and subsequent pain and suffering during the dying process.	Explore fears and cause/etiology of fears, including physical, psychosocial, and spiritual. Educate patient and family on physical, psychosocial, and spiritual signs and symptoms of dying process. Ask patient/family how they would like the dying process to happen. Normalize feelings. Provide reassurance that patient will be kept as comfortable as possible. Provide presence and increase as needed.
Fear of abandonment. Most patients do not want to die alone. May present as patient anxiety, pressing call button frequently, or calling out for help at home. Family members may continuously stay at bedside to honor patient wish to not be left alone.	Fear of being alone. Fear of who will care for them when they are unable to care for themselves.	Provide reassurance that everything will be done to have someone with the patient. Provide presence. Explore options for increasing presence around the clock, including health care professionals (nurse, social worker, nurse's aide) and family, friends, volunteers, church members, etc. For family member doing bedside vigil, encourage frequent breaks, offer respite. Family members may also be anxious and need permission from nurse to care for themselves.
Fear of the unknown.	Fear of what will happen after they die: afterlife or cultural/faith system beliefs in relation to death. Fear that belief systems regarding afterlife will be different than perceived and/or lived.	Exploration of fear. Companionship, presence. Pastoral care or patient's clergy for exploration of life, afterlife, faith system beliefs. Support cultural and faith system beliefs.
Nearing death awareness. Patients state they have spoken to those who have already died or have seen places not presently accessible or visible to family and/or nurse. May describe spiritual beings, bright lights, "another world." Statements may seem out of character, gesture or request. Patients may tell family members, significant others when they will die.	Attempt by the dying to describe what they are experiencing, the dying process and death. Transition from this life. Attempting to describe something they need to do/accomplish before they die, such as permission to die from family, reconciliation, see someone, reassurance that survivor will be okay without them.	Do not contradict, explain away, belittle, humor, or argue with the patient about these experiences. Attentively and sensitively listen to the patient, affirm the experience, and attempt to determine if there is any unfinished business, patient needs. Encourage family/significant others to say goodbye, give permission for patient to die as appropriate. Support to family and other caregivers. Educate about the difference between nearing death awareness and confusion, education to family, and other caregivers.
Withdrawal from family, friends, the nurse, and other health care professionals: decreased interest in environment and relationships and family may feel they have upset or offended patient.	Transition from this life, patient "letting go" of this life.	Normalize withdrawal by educating family about transition. Presence, gentle touch. Family members may need to be educated, encouraged to give permission to patient to die. Family may need to be encouraged to say goodbyes.

(From The Hospice of the Florida Suncoast, 1999. Reprinted with permission.)

One of the many benefits of hospice involvement is the preparation of the patient and their family about the signs and symptoms related to the death process. Such preparation dispels inaccuracies (i.e., death is painful), reducing fear, regret, and guilt over not doing enough for their loved one. Most of all, skillful management of death-related discomfort allows the patient and family to be comfortably and lovingly present to each other throughout the process. Finally, when a loved one dies peacefully in the manner of a "good death," family members can focus their grief on mourning their loss and finding comfort in their memories.

Nearing Death Awareness. A variety of altered mental states may be experienced as the end of life approaches. The "out of body" experience has been reported after brushes with death, such as an accident.[9] Others have reported incidents of knowledge of things that they attribute to awareness of another dimension.[10] All of this work recognizes the mystery that surrounds the dying process, which exceeds the physical indicators that medical professionals can use to quantify the ceasing of life in the body.

Callahan and Kelley[11] recommend from their years of working with individuals during end-of-life experiences that clinical caregivers as well as family members learn from close listening and observation of the person in their care. Caregivers who do not have an understanding of this communication may experience more anxiety.

The dying person may speak in metaphoric language. For example, imagine this dialogue between a mother and daughter.

"I need to go home," states the older patient. "Mom, you are home. This is your house. See the family photos on the mantle above the fireplace, and there is your favorite chair," replies her daughter in frustration after several repetitions. Could there be another sense of *home* to which she is referring, perhaps even a spiritual resting place consistent with her life-long beliefs?

Another example of misinterpreting metaphorical speech would be this hypothetical conversation between a father and son. "The door is locked," declares Mr. Thompson emphatically as he arouses from a lethargic state. His family is glad to hear him communicate. Son Robert steps from the bedside to the sliding glass door across the room. "No, Dad. Look, the door is open," he responds as he demonstrates the sliding door out to the patio moving freely. Perhaps there is some unfinished business Mr. Thompson needs to address, or his way of indicating that he does not believe he is ready to die.

Patients will commonly report seeing things that are not visible to others. Insects, reptiles, or other animals may be reported as hallucinations related to the introduction or dosing changes of opioid medications but the visualization of people is worth exploring. Often these may be recognizable to the dying individual as previously deceased friends or family members, who are perceived as calling and communicating in some way with the dying person. Understanding this as a relatively common but often unacknowledged experience, perhaps because of a societal reluctance to grapple with complex metaphysical issues, may provide recognition that this is a normal end-of-life process occurring, and afford some individuals comfort that the dying loved one will not be alone after passing away as may be consistent with their personal beliefs.

Other patients may voice their beliefs about the timing of their deaths in ways that may not seem to coincide with apparent physical parameters. The insights offered by those in our care offer us an opportunity to support their caregivers and loved ones in helping meet the desire to have a peaceful death. By listening carefully, then recognizing such communication, physical therapists can educate family members, allowing them to become more intimately involved in this experience of accompanying their dying loved one and preparing for their own time of bereavement.

AN OVERVIEW OF HOSPICE AND PALLIATIVE CARE

Hospice vs. Palliative Care

In the realm of end-of-life care, two related terms, hospice and palliative care, are often used. Both terms pertain to the optimization of comfort and quality of life of patients with life-threatening conditions. Although hospice programs have delivered palliative care for more than 30 years, it is also used in many other settings that focus on the treatment of the chronically, but not terminally, ill. As discussed later in this chapter, hospice is a specific set of services that is covered by the Medicare Hospice Benefit. Patients admitted to hospice must meet certain requirements, including a physician-determined prognosis of less than 6 months and the acknowledgement that they are no longer seeking curative measures.

The World Health Organization (WHO) defines palliative care as an approach that improves the quality of life for patients and families facing life-threatening illness.[12] Thus, palliative care is broader in scope, including patients at any stage of their disease process, who may also be seeking curative treatment. Unlike that for hospice, Medicare does not have a specific "palliative care benefit." However, Part B may cover services such as poststroke rehabilitation that have palliative components (i.e., quality of life, comfort).[13]

In reality, the philosophy of palliative care is nothing new to physical therapists as it relates to preserving human dignity and maintaining an optimal quality of life whatever the circumstances. The professions' long history of compassionately enhancing the quality of life for all patients is only one of the ways in which we are well positioned for important contributions in palliative care.

In many communities, hospice and palliative care services are offered through the same facility. Reimbursement for palliative care services is administered through the patient's primary medical insurance, enabling patients in palliative care to receive coverage for monthly visits from the hospice/palliative care nursing staff. Patients may remain on palliative services for months or years while seeking curative or supportive measures for their condition. For example, Edwin, an 84-year-old gentleman with a stroke, remained on palliative service for 3 years, receiving monthly nursing visits from the palliative care nurse. In addition, Edwin's wife requested a physical therapy mobility consult. Thus, Edwin received three visits from the hospice/palliative care physical therapist for patient and family education in transfer safety. One day, Edwin suffered a myocardial infarction at home, whereupon his wife summoned an ambulance. He died at the hospital the next day. In contrast to Edwin, patients with a progressive disease may transfer to hospice when their condition becomes terminal. At this point, their care is reimbursed through hospice benefits.

Clinical Scenario. Elaine was a 54-year-old woman with a 2-year history of cervical cancer. During this time, Elaine had received three courses of chemotherapy, with good results. Elaine sought palliative care services through her local hospice for the purpose of expert pain management. She received monthly visits from the palliative care nurse, who assisted Elaine in determining appropriate pharmacologic measures for pain control. Elaine's medications were covered by her primary insurance. In the meantime, Elaine underwent an additional course of chemotherapy, and this episode left her considerably weaker than prior courses. As a result, Elaine was unable to engage in her aerobics classes at her local gym. A physical therapy consult was requested to assist Elaine in modifying a fitness routine. The physical therapist worked with Elaine to develop a slowly progressive walking program, using a pedometer to measure her progress. Elaine remained on palliative services for an additional 8 months, whereupon her physician determined that further curative measures were unlikely to be successful. Elaine transferred to hospice and received services for another 2 months before her death.

The Medicare Hospice Benefit

The Medicare hospice benefit was enacted by Congress in 1982 and since that time has been the major source of payment for U.S. hospice services. In 2007, Medicare provided services for 84% of all patients served.[14] In order to qualify for hospice, a physician must provide certification of a terminal condition with a prognosis of less than 6 months. In addition, patients must certify that they are no longer seeking curative measures for their condition. Finally, patients must be entitled to Medicare Part A services (inpatient). Patients who elect the Medicare hospice benefit begin with two initial 90-day periods, which can then be followed by unlimited

60-day periods as long as documentation shows the continued need and appropriateness for services. A patient may revoke their hospice benefit if they decide to pursue curative measures.[15] Medicare requires that all covered services (nursing, physician, psychological, and spiritual support) be available on a 24-hour basis to ensure support and comfort whenever needed. The levels of service and types of care covered under the Medicare hospice benefit are illustrated in Box 27-2 and Box 27-3.

The Interdisciplinary Model of Care

Today, hospice care involves an interdisciplinary medical, psychological, and spiritual approach to the promotion of comfort and quality of life in patients with a terminal illness and a life expectancy of 6 months or

---

BOX 27-2 | Specific Services Covered by Medicare Hospice Benefit

- Nursing services*
- Physician services to provide palliation and management of the terminal illness and related conditions*
- Medical social services provided by a social worker under the direction of a physician*
- Counseling services (chaplain, psychosocial, bereavement)*
- Home health aide services
- Homemaker services
- Medical supplies
- Drugs related to the care of the terminal illness
- Durable medical equipment
- Any other medical supplies
- Physical therapy, occupational therapy, and speech therapy if indicated
- Laboratory testing and other diagnostic studies related to the care of the terminal illness

*Denotes core service required for Medicare reimbursement.

BOX 27-3 | Levels of Care Provided by Hospice Benefit

Home-Based Care

1. Routine Home Care: Patient receives hospice care at the place he or she resides.
2. Continuous Home Care: Patient receives hospice care consisting predominantly of nursing care on a continuous basis at home. Continuous home care is only furnished during brief periods of crisis and only as necessary to maintain the terminally ill patient at home.

Inpatient Care

3. General Inpatient Care: Patient receives general inpatient care in an inpatient facility for pain control or acute or chronic symptom management that cannot be managed in other settings.
4. Inpatient Respite Care: Patient receives care in an approved facility on a short-term basis in order to provide respite for the caregiver.

less. Medicare-certified hospice facilities require the involvement of several distinct health professionals who comprise the interdisciplinary team (IDT). These professionals represent four domains of care that include (1) *physical* (physician and nurse), (2) *functional* (consulting therapists, nurses, and nurse's aides), (3) *interpersonal* (social workers, psychologists, and counselors), and (4) *spiritual* (chaplain, psychologists, and social workers).[16] Coverage for core services, medications, and equipment is provided to Medicare-certified hospices through a specified daily, or per-diem, rate. As of April 2009, Medicare reimbursed hospices at a daily rate of $140.15 for each patient receiving routine home care, $817.26 for continuous home care, and $622.66 for inpatient hospice care.[17] Volunteers, who complete a comprehensive training course on the philosophy of hospice, are an important element of each domain of hospice care. Accordingly, volunteers assist with light housework or meal preparation. They can also provide supportive companionship for patients and family members.

Physical therapists are not a required "core service" on the hospice IDT, meaning that Medicare does not require their services to be provided for all patients. Rather, physical therapists are part of a group of professionals (including occupational therapists and speech–language pathologists) who must be made available to any patient on an "as needed" or "consultative basis." Thus, the Medicare hospice benefit includes coverage for physical therapy provided in a hospice setting on a consultative basis. This policy is supported by the 2008 Medicare Conditions of Participation for hospice (section 418.92), which was revised to include the following language: "Physical therapy, occupational therapy, and speech–language pathology must be—

1. *Available, and when provided, offered in a manner consistent with accepted standards of practice; and*
2. *Furnished by personnel who meet the qualifications specified in part 484 of this chapter (individuals who are licensed in the relevant disciplines)."*[17]

Although this mandate suggests that physical therapy is an important component of the IDT, individual hospice programs must develop their own guidelines for our inclusion. Research is currently underway to help determine these guidelines as well as to support the cost-effectiveness of physical therapist inclusion as a core service on the IDT. Figure 27-1 illustrates the disciplines that comprise the IDT. **Interdisciplinary Team Meetings.** The Medicare Conditions of Participation[17] mandates that each patient in a Medicare-certified hospice receive an interdisciplinary plan of care at the time of admission, which must be updated by the team at least every 2 weeks. Thus, most hospices hold weekly IDT meetings, which facilitate the coordination of care for both new and existing patients. The reports of each core discipline provide a comprehensive picture of

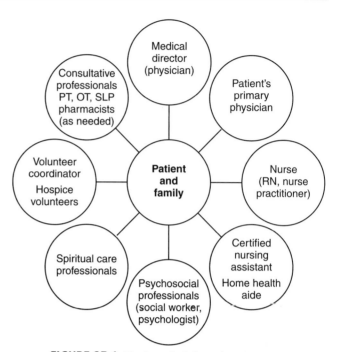

FIGURE 27-1 The interdisciplinary hospice team.

the status of each patient and his or her support system. The patient and his or her family members may also request the option to attend the IDT.

The IDT model of hospice care prevents many of the communication pitfalls that can impede quality of care and create patient dissatisfaction. By the thoughtful coordination of every aspect of care, patients and their families can have every element of their quality of life addressed at a time when it is most needed. Because physical therapists are not considered a core member of the IDT, they may not feel that their presence at the weekly meetings is appropriate or necessary. However, it has been the experience of these authors that a consistent presence at weekly IDT meetings is invaluable for educating team members about the value of our services. In addition, we can identify patients who could benefit from a physical therapist examination and intervention.

Case Scenario. Alicia was an 86-year-old woman who was admitted to hospice after a series of several strokes that resulted in failure to thrive. Alicia had a long prior history of back pain that had recently exacerbated. At the IDT meeting, a long discussion ensued about appropriate options for pain control, as Alicia wanted to avoid sedation as much as possible. At that point, the physical therapist suggested a trial of transcutaneous electrical nerve stimulation (TENS), describing the use and benefits of this modality in the treatment of back pain. The team agreed that a trial of TENS might provide Alicia with a nonsedating approach to pain control. A physical therapy consult was initiated and TENS turned out to be a successful pain control option for Alicia.

History of Hospice Care

The term *hospice* derives from the Latin term *hospitum*, which originally described a place of shelter for sick and weary travelers. Nirmal Hriday (Pure Heart), one of the first known homes for the dying, was established in 1952 by Mother Teresa in Calcutta, India.[18] Working in the most destitute slums of Calcutta, she and her sister nuns took indigents who were dying off the streets to nurse them at this home, enabling "persons who lived like animals to die like angels, loved and wanted."[18] This noble work continues today in more than 500 worldwide centers.

Dame Cicely Saunders, MD (1918-2005), is recognized as the founder of the modern hospice movement. As a nurse working at an English cancer hospital after World War II, she was disturbed by the pain and isolation she witnessed among dying patients. These observations compelled her to enter St. Thomas's Medical School in 1951 at the age of 33, qualifying as a physician in 1957.

Following the completion of her medical studies, Saunders sought additional training in pharmacology, when she explored the effective use of analgesic medications for the treatment of pain at end of life. In an environment where medication underutilization was common because of fears of addiction, she challenged rationales that were grounded mainly in conjecture. Accordingly, instead of requiring patients to wait until their pain medications wore off before requesting another dose, Saunders advocated medicating at a level to produce continual analgesia and wrote several papers that described and provided support for her approach. Furthermore, instead of the sterile and lonely hospital rooms where she had worked as a young nurse, Saunders proposed treating dying patients in a warm and comfortable setting with a home-like atmosphere. In 1967, Saunders opened St. Christopher's Hospice in London where she put her vision into action.[19] Saunders served as the medical director of St. Christopher's until 1985, and was awarded England's Order of Merit in 1989. By the time she died in 2005, at the same hospice she established, there were more than 8000 hospices worldwide.

The U.S. hospice movement began in 1974 upon the opening of the Connecticut Hospice in Branford. Many of Cicely Saunders' original ideals have been successfully integrated into current hospice practice, contributing to the hospice movement's significant growth and making it the preferred approach to end-of-life care.

Growth of Programs and Services. Since the inception of hospice in 1974, the number of American hospices has steadily grown, numbering 4700 in 2008.[14] Hospice services are delivered through a variety of facilities that include freestanding facilities (58%), programs in home health agencies (20%), or units attached to hospitals (21%) and nursing homes (1%).[20] In 2008, the National Hospice and Palliative Care Organization's annual *Facts and Figures on Hospice Care*[20] reported that of the 2.4 million U.S. deaths occurring that year, 930,000 (38.8%) occurred in a hospice setting. Furthermore, 1.4 million Americans received hospice services during that time. Interestingly, 220,000 patients (15.7%) were discharged from hospice, either because of an extended prognosis or a desire to pursue curative measures. This is a noteworthy statistic, which dispels the misperception that hospice is an irrevocable or predictably ominous choice for patients with terminal illness.

The ability for patients to choose where they die is a major tenet of hospice. For 70% of Americans, their own home is the setting of choice.[21] In 2002, only 25% of patients achieved their preference. The concept of hospice care as the setting of choice for the support of advance directives has also begun to emerge. Accordingly, the number of clients served by hospice each year has grown by approximately 10% each year between 2005 and 2009.[20] Furthermore, 70% of the 930,000 patients who died under hospice care in 2008 were able to do so in their primary place of residence. Of this 70% who died in their primary residence, 42% of deaths occurred in private residences, and 22% in nursing homes. These statistics are one important outcome measure that supports the value of hospice care in meeting the needs of dying patients.[20]

Profile of Hospice Patients

According to 2008 outcome data from the National Hospice and Palliative Care Organization, 54% of all hospice patients were female. The vast majority (83%) of these hospice patients were age 65 years or older.[20] Thus, hospice is and will continue to be primarily a geriatrics treatment setting, with numbers increasing significantly with the aging of the baby boomer generation.

Currently, hospice patients are overwhelmingly Caucasian (83%). The existence of racial and ethnic disparities in end-of-life care has been confirmed in several studies.[22,23] A systematic review of 13 retrospective cohort studies found statistically significantly lower hospice utilization rates among African Americans compared to Caucasians.[22] Another retrospective study examined Medicare hospice database records of 40,960 Caucasian, Hispanic, African American, and Asian beneficiaries who received services for end-stage cancer between 1992 and 2001.[23] The results of the study showed that Caucasians had the highest hospice utilization rate (42%) followed by African Americans (37%), Hispanics (38%), and Asians (32%). The study also found that nonwhite groups had higher numbers of hospitalizations for longer periods of time as well as a higher likelihood of an ICU admission in their last month of life. Finally, members of these nonwhite racial groups were also more likely to die in the hospital.[22] The reasons for these ethnic and racial disparities are not yet clear, and further research is needed to explore the impact of cultural differences, belief systems, and patient preference on selections related to end-of-life care. As the American population becomes increasingly diverse, health care professionals may need to explore culturally sensitive approaches for educating patients of different racial and ethnic backgrounds about the value of hospice care.

Diagnoses. The major diagnostic categories of the patients seen in U.S. hospices during the years 2006 and 2007 are shown in Table 27-3. An interesting trend with respect to these diagnostic categories is the increasing number of patients with Alzheimer dementia and debilitation. Currently it is estimated that 5 million Americans are living with Alzheimer's disease, and projections are as high as 16 million by 2050.[24] Patients with this disease may survive and deteriorate for a period of years while their family members struggle to provide care.

As patients with Alzheimer's disease become more debilitated, they may ultimately develop a host of conditions that are considered indications of the end stage of the disease. In order to be considered for hospice coverage, Medicare guidelines require patients with Alzheimer's disease to exhibit at least one of the following signs in the previous 12 months: muscle wasting and malnutrition (inanition) with a 10% decrease in body weight, septicemia, decubitus ulcer, aspiration pneumonia, recurrent fever, or urinary tract infection.[25] Unfortunately, by the time they qualify for hospice care under the current guidelines, many patients with end-stage Alzheimer's disease are completely dependent in all care and show significant cognitive impairments. The extent of these impairments can challenge caregivers, especially in the realm of determining patient needs for pain medications and other

comfort measures. As patients with end-stage dementia enter the hospice system in increasing numbers, further guidelines may need to be established to determine appropriate indications for pain control and comfort as they approach end of life. Because the burden of caregiving can be considerable in such cases, hospice staff can also provide assistance to family members so that patients can remain in their homes during this process.

Length of Stay. The average length of stay for patients in hospice in 2008 was 67 days.[20] However, 30% of patients died or were discharged in 7 days or less, and 13% died or were discharged in 180 days or more. This statistic indicates that overall, patient survival is well within the Medicare requirement of an expected prognosis of 6 months or less. Furthermore, it indicates that a majority of patients and families receive services long enough to benefit from hospice's compassionate and expert approach to comfort measures.

It can be emotionally difficult for family members when admission to hospice is delayed in light of a compelling need. This can occur when lack of health care provider awareness precludes a timely referral, or when the disease process becomes so acute that the patient dies in the hospital. In an illustrative case, Cheryl, an 83-year-old woman with ovarian cancer was admitted to the hospital with severe pain. Her attending physician, perhaps fearing the possibility of an overdose, refused to prescribe opioid medications at the level needed for analgesia. When Cheryl's son arrived from another state 2 days later, he arranged for Cheryl's immediate transfer to a hospice residence where she died only hours later, still without adequate pain control. Cheryl's case raises troubling questions. How can health care providers be better educated about the value of hospice services? How can candidates for hospice services be identified in a timelier manner? What are sources of barriers to effective pain control at end of life, and how can they be mitigated? As the consequences of the economic downturn of the late 2000s unfold, it will be important to identify any additional barriers to timely hospice admission.

Hospice Outcomes

Data on hospice outcomes are slowly emerging and showing promising results. One of the most encouraging outcomes, from a study of 4493 patients, indicates that admission to hospice prolongs life by a mean of 29 days.[26] The authors of this study suggested that the reason for this finding was the administration of adequate pain control and its favorable impact on enhancing comfort and quality of life.

Another promising trend is that hospice care is a cost-efficient approach to reducing Medicare expenditures, 25% of which have been reported to occur in the last year of life.[27] A recent study from Duke University reported that the use of hospice services reduced Medicare expenditures by $2309 during this same time period.[28]

TABLE 27-3	Diagnostic Categories of Patients Admitted to U.S. Hospice Programs, 2006-2007	
Primary Diagnosis	**2007 (%)**	**2006 (%)**
Cancer (malignancies)	41.3	44.1
Noncancer diagnoses	58.7	55.9
Heart disease	11.8	12.2
Debility unspecified	11.2	11.8
Dementia, including Alzheimer's disease	10.1	10.0
Lung disease, including chronic obstructive pulmonary disease	7.9	7.7
Stroke or coma	3.8	3.4
Kidney disease, including end-stage renal disease	2.6	2.9
Motor neuron diseases, including amyotrophic lateral sclerosis	2.3	2.0
Liver disease	2.0	1.8
HIV/AIDS	0.6	0.5
Other diagnoses	6.5	3.7

(Courtesy of National Hospice and Palliative Care Organization.)

As a further testimonial to the benefits of hospice care, recent outcome data from the National Hospice and Palliative Care Organization indicates that in 2008, orders for do not resuscitate (DNR) were respected 100% of the time, patient wishes to avoid hospitalization were honored 98% of the time, and in 73% of cases, pain was brought to a tolerable level within 48 hours of hospice admission.[29] At the current time, there are few studies examining the interdisciplinary role and outcomes related to physical therapy intervention in hospice. This may be partially explained by a general lack of awareness among consumers, health care providers, and even hospice personnel about the value of our services. It is encouraging that the Hospice Patients Alliance (www.hospicepatients.org), a national resource center for hospice patients, families, and caregivers, describes (and promotes) physical therapy interventions for the improvement of safe mobility, reduction in pain, and determination of appropriate equipment needs on their website. Materials such as these can help improve awareness of the role physical therapy has in optimal end-of-life care. Fortunately, an increasing number of hospice websites are now posting information on physical therapy services.

Areas of physical therapy intervention in hospice have been described in a few studies and considerable agreement among them suggests that pain control, relaxation, respiratory care, and mobility are the major areas of focus.[6,30-35] These interventions are discussed next.

MODELS OF PHYSICAL THERAPY PRACTICE IN HOSPICE AND PALLIATIVE CARE

Advanced and progressive disease requires a different orientation to goal setting and treatment than care for those who are likely to regain a premorbid level of function. Dietz identified palliative care strategies in patients with cancer, recognizing the need to address ongoing problems and minimizing complications.[36] Briggs[37] further defined models of care in the palliative spectrum by integrating the framework from the *Guide to Physical Therapist Practice*[38] in response to a variety of reimbursement structures. Briggs' models include rehabilitation light, rehabilitation in reverse, case management, skilled maintenance, and supportive care. As the models are described, keep in mind that they are not necessarily exclusive of one another and may be used together or in succession as a framework to support important interventions of end-of-life physical therapy practice.[39]

Rehabilitation Light

Some patients are admitted to hospice care after a long course of disease and uncontrolled symptoms, or when experiencing the adverse effects of treatment interventions such as chemotherapy, surgery, or radiation treatment.

Likely their pain management has been poor. Initial nursing care may improve symptom control so that for the first time in many weeks or months, the person may feel like he or she might be able to make some headway toward a stronger and more functional state. Physical therapy at a traditional frequency of two to three times each week might be more than the person can tolerate, and is often considered cost-prohibitive in the per diem reimbursement model of a hospice benefit program. An alternative model is a slowly progressive modified "rehabilitation light" program that provides exercise and functional training during each weekly or biweekly visit. Activities can include targeted strengthening exercises that minimize the number of exercises and functional activities such as a timed sitting program or other ambulation activity that provides both increased strength and endurance as well as improved quality of life. Home exercise program follow-through is an essential part of this approach. Progress toward goals may be extremely slow, though measurable, over a few weeks or even several months. The rehabilitation light approach uses the skilled care of the therapist in providing timely and appropriate exercise instruction and functional training, and it works within the hospice framework emphasizing quality of life despite a terminal diagnosis. Close contact and communication with the interdisciplinary team is vital to ensure all team members recognize and concur with this approach to care, as it may initially appear to conflict with the hospice goal of acceptance of a natural death. The following case scenario illustrates the use of the rehabilitation light approach.

Case Scenario. Thelma, age 78 years, was discharged from the hospital with end-stage renal disease, and begrudgingly chose hospice, as the only alternative offered was to begin dialysis three times a week. She faced multiple other conditions, including chronic obstructive pulmonary disease, diabetes, obesity, an indwelling catheter, osteoporosis, and a fractured metatarsal, but maintained a lifelong outlook that she would overcome these conditions. She accepted hospice care, but did not plan on dying. Initially bed-bound, and on a pressure-relieving mattress because of her inability to reposition herself, she tolerated minimal exercise, but wanted to know what she could do to work toward the goal of getting out of bed to the commode. Beginning with a sitting program in the semielectric bed, within a month she was able to sit at bedside. Each day she worked on her own on a few basic exercises with the support of her granddaughters. At each weekly visit she was able to do more, like come to stand and then transfer with less assistance as her foot pain subsided to allow more weight bearing. By the end of the second month, transfers with family assist to the commode or wheelchair were happening almost daily, though actual sitting tolerance was less than an hour. After continued work in standing for strength, balance, and self-support with weight shifting, Thelma took several steps with a front-wheeled walker by month 3 and declared, "I want to be able to walk out to the kitchen so I can enjoy a cigarette." Slowly, progressive gait training ensued, followed by instruction of caregivers to assist with limited ambulation, with a wheelchair following. By 6 months, she had achieved her goal as well as transfers with a tub transfer bench and wheelchair negotiation of a ramp to the yard. Physical therapy goals had been met with Thelma reaching her maximum potential, and she was shortly discharged from hospice, to live another 2 years. This case demonstrates how physical therapy intervention can help achieve a person's desired outcome by using restorative therapy principles within the palliative care model of the hospice care environment.

Rehabilitation in Reverse

Traditional rehabilitation progresses a person from a lower to higher level of functional ability. Rehabilitation in reverse is the utilization of skilled patient training and instruction to caregivers as a person moves through the transitions from an independently mobile level to a more dependent one as the disease progresses and as strength and balance wane. Transfers may also become increasingly difficult, necessitating the use of equipment (wheelchair, bedside commode, shower bench) and the assistance of another person. Eventually, bed mobility may require assistance for positioning and comfort, and determination of the proper bed surface for skin pressure management. Throughout this course, the physical therapist can use his or her skill and knowledge of optimal ways to move and assist, allowing the patient and family to negotiate this transition toward the end of life. By being able to problem-solve function dilemmas and anticipate the loss of activities, the physical therapist can enhance the family's ability to adjust along an unpredictable course of decline and prevent unsafe conditions resulting in falls or caregiver injuries. At each new functional level, the therapist might consider what are the short-term goals for the visit, in light of the long-term hospice goal of a safe and comfortable patient-directed death at home. Frequency for such care may be quite variable, and the use of PRN (as needed) visits can be appropriate. Regular communication with the patient, family, and other hospice IDT staff may help identify when visits are needed. The following case scenario illustrates rehabilitation in reverse.

Case Scenario. Frank, age 84 years, developed back and abdominal pain while traveling in a recreational vehicle one summer and eventually was diagnosed with advanced adenocarcinoma. Frank and his family decided not to pursue treatment but rather to try to enjoy the remaining time they had together, at home. When Frank was admitted to hospice, nursing was able to manage his pain while social work fostered family support, with daughters traveling for respite and help when needed. Frank had been losing weight but had been active doing household and garden chores. Some unsteadiness in the yard one day made the IDT and family concerned about the possibility of falling and a physical therapy referral was made. Frank's lower extremity strength was decreased, with significant muscle atrophy visible although his gait appeared symmetrical. However, any challenge or advanced balance activity revealed unsteadiness. He was willing to accept a standard cane, after a trial and instruction in several alternative assistive devices. A therapy visit frequency of two to four times a month was established to follow his adaptations. Within a week he requested a quad cane, which was properly fitted. He was instructed in the quad cane's use within his home, on the steps to the driveway, and about his shop. Frank declined any exercises, stating his preference was to spend his time and energy doing what he loved most. By the end of a month, it was evident that bilateral support was needed as he walked about with the cane in one hand while constantly reaching for support on the nearest wall or furniture. A trial of a front-wheeled walker was offered, providing new freedom, despite some difficulty in navigating about his favorite spots.

His wife and daughters watched over him with concern as they could see his continued weight loss and declining energy level. Within the second month, a second near-fall occurred, making it apparent that the options of having a family member provide contact assist, or use of a wheelchair would become necessary. This transition required more instruction, and significant discussion of his physical course. Soon Frank was spending almost all of his time sitting, and the wheelchair became his more ready companion. Moving from sitting to standing was becoming more difficult, so instruction was provided to Frank and his family on his wheelchair setup and body positioning for a transfer, as well as assistance techniques. His reluctance to use a bedside commode required an increasing number of transfers throughout the day and night, a strain on all involved. Frank was preparing to let go, as his sense of meaningful participation in life was ebbing. A sudden change in level of awareness and physical status required family training on bed positioning and turning for pressure relief. After 3 days of intermittent consciousness, Frank died in his own bed, with his wife and two daughters nearby.

This case illustrates the type of effective care a physical therapist can provide in the face of a terminal diagnosis and declining mobility, rather than the traditional care of expecting participation in progressive-resistive exercise to achieve goals of enhanced mobility. Interestingly, the patient and family's acceptance of Frank's impending death made this approach feasible and appropriate.

Case Management

Case management is a frequently used model of care for nursing and physical therapy in many specialty clinics to provide long-term, ongoing care for challenging and changing conditions such as amyotrophic lateral sclerosis, spinal cord injury, amputation, and diabetes. In home health, case management is used to provide similar follow-up, care, and instruction for people with complicated care, multiple comorbidities, and unskilled or multiple caregivers.[40] This model is useful in palliative and hospice care as well. With a person who is relatively stable though gradually declining over weeks or months, periodic reevaluation can identify physical and functional changes that need to be addressed to prevent complications. Interventions can include instructing the caregivers in providing optimal assistance, updating the home exercise program, and outlining problems that might be anticipated. Monthly or bimonthly visits with appropriate instruction and follow-up intervention can accomplish this end. The case of Evelyn illustrates case management.

Case Scenario. At 94 years, Evelyn retained a regal demeanor, sitting in her chair holding court with four generations of offspring attending to her, although she did not allow much to be done for her. With end-stage heart disease as an admitting diagnosis, along with osteoarthritis, cataracts, and hearing loss, life had become a challenge. She insisted on doing almost everything herself, despite exerting high levels of energy expenditure. An initial physical therapy visit offered recommendations to make the environment safer and easier to move around, and adjust her equipment for improved comfort and efficiency. Monthly visits were scheduled to reassess her safety and mobility, and to instruct various caregivers in different ways to assist as Evelyn's condition became more fragile. Begrudgingly she allowed more help with bathing, dressing, and other tasks.

Because sitting was her primary position of comfort both day and night, skin integrity and pressure relief concerns were addressed. Adapting her chair to an optimal height with the fabrication of a platform underneath the entire chair elevated the seat height while maintaining the other comfort features and eliminated the instability of multiple cushions. She enjoyed doing some exercises while she sat, if someone did them along with her, and the family was more than willing to comply. Her family's concerns about potential falls were discussed repeatedly and at length in the context of physical limitations, quite variable patient willingness to have assistance or use devices, and Evelyn's right to self-determination. Evelyn was under hospice care for 8 months, long enough to celebrate her 95th birthday. Just a week later, her daughter found her in her chair one morning, having expired peacefully during the night.

Traditional physical therapy might have been offered on a very short-term basis to achieve a specific short-term goal and then the patient would have been discharged as she did not have rehabilitation potential. However, under hospice, supportive, palliative care can be provided, easing the transition to dependency and facilitating a safe and comfortable patient-directed death.

Skilled Maintenance

When a patient must perform an activity that is medically necessary, skilled maintenance has been identified for use under Medicare home health guidelines.[40,41] In traditional home health situations, care that might, under usual circumstances, be taught to a caregiver may require skilled physical therapist intervention because of specific complexity. An example might be the performance of range of motion to a joint proximate to an unstable fracture. In hospice, skilled maintenance is used to perform an important functional activity, which the patient is no longer able to perform alone or with a family caregiver, yet can complete with the assistance of the physical therapist. For example, because of extensive weakness, tone or balance deficits, or caregiver limitations, a therapist may be needed to provide help with ambulation or bed transfers. Under hospice rules, when these activities provide for significant quality of life, they are considered skilled care. Consultation with the IDT is important to establish a care plan that provides for the frequency needed, as well as patient and family support through the process of letting go of activities during the course of care.

Case Scenario. Roger, age 74 years, was a retired rancher and businessman. His life was changed with the diagnosis of an astrocytoma, and the resultant physical trauma of brain surgery to resect the tumor, radiation treatments, and the array of medications to control seizures, swelling, and other adverse effects. He was eventually admitted to hospice, and a physical therapy consult was initiated because the patient's wife was having difficulty helping him transfer because of the dense left-sided paresis and spasticity he experienced. The primary focus of physical therapy was problem-solving environmental challenges and transfer techniques to allow his petite spouse to assist with the patient's transfers to every surface.

In conversation, it became clear that Roger's sense of self had been dramatically affected by confinement to a chair. What he missed more than anything was being able to walk about his home and gaze through the windows at "his spread." A trial of gait with a hemicane, a plastic ankle–foot orthosis, and gait belt on the next visit revealed Roger's ability to walk up to 50 feet with help to maintain balance, weight shift, and control the advance of his left leg during swing phase. He was elated at this recovered ability, and his physical therapist decided with the patient that it could become a part of a weekly physical therapy visit. Other issues arose, including travel plans to a national rodeo and training other family caregivers.

As the disease progressed, Roger lost the ability to walk, even with assistance, but was able to stand at the counter with support to look out over land he loved. The opportunity to continue being mobile until it was no longer possible, even with assistance, gave meaning to his existence.

Supportive Care

Supportive care is often provided throughout the course of care, and is comprised of the psychosocial support associated with end-of-life process, as well as physical measures. The frequency of supportive care measures is variable. Physical measures may include range of motion and massage. Physical therapy pain management techniques should coincide with the frequent use of a medication regimen by nursing. Some mechanical pain that is not treatable with even high levels of opiates can be diminished using a physical therapist's knowledge of biomechanics and positioning.

Pressure relief becomes an issue with progressive weakness, decreased mobility, insufficient nutrition, and fragile skin. Both seating and bed surfaces should be considered in order to manage a failing body's integumentary system. A more complete discussion of these clinical supportive care measures follows in Clinical Issues.

CLINICAL ISSUES—CONSIDERATIONS FOR CARE

As with the models for practice in hospice and palliative care, the circumstances of declining function and often very limited performance status demand the attention of the physical therapist to reexamine elements of clinical practice in this light. Subtle changes in the way knowledge is used and clinical skills are applied can result in substantially improved short-term outcomes for those individuals in the last stage of life.

The Role of Exercise

Exercise plays a critical role in maintaining strength to allow adequate functional mobility for quality of life. When determining the appropriateness of exercise for a body that is failing at the end of life, the cause of the weakness should be considered to determine if increased strength is possible and/or realistic. Weakness that can be reversed may be caused from chemotherapy or radiation therapy,[42] prolonged hospitalization,[43] or a period of immobility or forced bed rest.[44]

The client's prior exercise and fitness history is also significant.[45] A person with substantial prior participation in some strength and endurance activities will respond in a different way than someone who has never participated in exercise as a lifestyle behavior. Ability to differentiate effort, fatigue, and workload from soreness or pain will play a role in performance and success as well. Some patients will decline an exercise program as

part of their end-of-life care, choosing only to participate in activities that provide quality of life—a decision that must be respected by the therapist.

The limited physical capacity that may be present in a chronically debilitated person can guide us toward the use of "rehabilitation light" as previously discussed. Focusing the exercise program on maximum strength outcomes with a limited number of exercises can enhance success. Recent evidence indicates that a home exercise program for people older than age 65 years with two exercises results in a better performance outcome than with eight exercises.[45]

All exercise should address functional goals[46] and thus be directly seen by the patient as a means to an end, rather than something to keep them occupied. Positively reinforcing experiences gives feedback that will provide the best outcome. If the patient feels overwhelmed or experiences significant delayed-onset soreness following activity, it is likely that the decreased quality of life satisfaction will inhibit further participation.[47]

Even patients with severe chronic obstructive pulmonary disease have been found to benefit from a biweekly supervised home exercise program over a 4-month period, with a 3% gain as opposed to 28% deterioration in the nonexercising control. These results are not overwhelming evidence of the effectiveness of exercise training, but the patients in this study belong to a severely disabled population with a progressive disease and a grim outlook.[48]

Measuring resting heart rate (RHR) and activity-related heart rate is useful in determining physical performance status, when related to the predicted maximum heart rate (age-adjusted maximum HR) (using 220 – age, or less, or 220 – RHR × exercise level). With a failing body, resting heart rate may be much higher than 100 beats per minute. A 75-year-old man with a predicted maximum heart rate (PMHR) of 145 and a RHR of 120 is already performing at more than 80% of maximum (82%). After walking 30 feet to the bathroom using a wheeled walker, he nearly collapses with a HR of 144, more than 99% of PMHR. This adverse event represents not only a significant fall risk from collapse but also an effort comparable to that of a sprint performance on a running track. An explanation of this relative maximum aerobic effort is often affirming to the patient and reassuring to the family. Similarly, patients with progressive weakness and muscle atrophy will experience difficulty moving from sitting to standing, especially from their favorite chair. Physical therapists have a critical opportunity to educate patients, their families, and their caregivers regarding maximal physical capacity for anaerobic muscle contraction and the work that is done just to move from one position to another. Sharing these examples with both patient and family can lead to an affirmation that perceived exertion is extremely high while in the process of decline and also some recognition of the effort it takes to accomplish even the smallest of tasks.

In conclusion, it is important that the physical therapist offer the option of specific exercises and activities that are both accomplishable and meaningful to the patient's life condition, along with education that puts exercise and physical performance in the perspective of physical changes toward the end of life. If such a program is well integrated into a daily routine, the optimal understanding and outcomes will be achieved.

Equipment and the Environment

The ability to move from sitting to standing may require greater effort or assistance with increased weakness. Adapting a favorite recliner chair to an optimal height can be achieved by instruction to the family in fabrication of a platform underneath the entire chair, often of 4 to 6 inches. This elevates the seat height, maintains the other comfort features, and eliminates the instability of multiple cushions. Some families may choose to purchase an electric lift recliner as another option. Other equipment in the home such as a bedside commode or shower bench might need to be elevated accordingly.

Energy conservation can be of great significance, as patients are often performing at near maximal energy output levels and fatigue rapidly as noted earlier. Standard measurement for walker heights allows for significant elbow flexion. In younger populations and people with adequate strength, the energy costs of this upper extremity use may be easily within their ability. In tests of upper extremity forces with variable walker heights while maintaining a stressful lower extremity non–weight-bearing status, evidence shows that more complete elbow extension can reduce elbow force moments.[49] With the older adult in terminal decline, adjusting a walker height to allow almost complete elbow extension can provide energy savings that will allow safer and easier ambulation for an extended time during their illness.

Comfort Care Measures

Comfort care of the terminally ill has risen to the forefront with increased awareness of the physical and psychosocial variables that affect and accompany the process.[50] One of the primary goals of end-of-life care through hospice is pain relief and comfort. Physical therapy has much to offer through appropriate direct interventions and the education and training of family caregivers.

Edema is a frequent symptom as the body fails, whether from adverse effects of treatment (surgery and radiation), decreased mobility and stasis of position,[51] or failure of body systems as disease progresses. Swollen limbs can become extremely uncomfortable from the internal pressure on sensory receptors. Manual lymphatic drainage and other massage techniques can provide temporary and longer-term relief in many such situations. Positioning and wrapping with short stretch bandages also may be helpful to reduce limb size, and make it easier to allow easier functional mobility with unweighted limbs.[51] By demonstrating these techniques effectively and teaching the caregivers to follow a modified program that is not overly taxing of the family, caregivers can be taught by a physical therapist to provide a successfully satisfying activity with their loved one. It is understood and should be explained that in some cases the efforts to control edema may fail because of the body's system failure, and this is not a failure of the caregivers. Despite this eventual outcome, comfort from the touch of massage may still be enjoyed.

As is discussed in the earlier section on Nearing Death Awareness, end-of-life experiences may include a sense of "needing to go," as the person undergoes transitional changes and separation. Younger and more able-bodied patients can become very restless, and walk or pace endlessly. This phenomenon becomes a more challenging management problem if the terminal restlessness occurs in someone unable to get up from bed safely.[52] Therapeutic techniques such as holding and rocking (in bed or at the bedside) may be used, and also taught to caregivers as a way to provide the physical and vestibular sensation of movement and the "going" that is so keenly desired.[53] This is an excellent adjunct to the medications frequently offered by the hospice team to control this symptom.

Range of motion is another intervention that must be considered from a different perspective. Range of motion may be provided to maintain enough range to allow for personal care or limiting finger flexion to prevent palm injury. If movement is painful, range of motion should be limited to this practical standard. Some people may very much enjoy the stimulus of having their otherwise immobile and understimulated limbs moved for comfort. With proper instruction, caregivers or other volunteers may be able to do passive or assistive range of motion regularly. Another application of range of motion in end-of-life care is to provide the gentle stimulus of passive, assistive, or active movements of the lower extremities, along with the verbally guided visualization images of a favorite walk that the person might have enjoyed (e.g., to a park, the ocean, or community locations). This "walking together" can provide the patient and caregivers with a sense of doing something purposeful and pleasurable as they reflect on their memories and life closure issues together.

Understanding the nature of falls, as discussed elsewhere in this text, is important during the decline at end of life. Many of the changing physical parameters will increase fall risks. These risks can be magnified by the person's ego and desire to maintain independence. Engaging the patient and family in discussions of this disparity of physical ability and desire can lead to informed decision making to solve this dilemma and make for a safer environment of care. People who perceive that they are being "called by others" or "going to the light" may try to get up even though no longer physically able.[11]

PAIN AND SYMPTOM MANAGEMENT

Defining Pain at End of Life

A painful death is among the greatest fears surrounding the end-of-life process; accordingly, one of the most important goals in the management of terminally ill persons is timely and effective pain management.[16] The hospice approach to pain supports this goal, specifically in terms of reducing the level of related distress to a tolerable level within 48 hours of admission.

Although pain can be academically defined as "an unpleasant sensory experience associated with actual or potential tissue damage,"[54] the definition used in hospice is "whatever the patient says it is."[55] Thus, any patient report of pain is acknowledged and addressed in a compassionate and efficacious manner.

In the hospice setting, pain assessment is considered the "fifth vital sign,"[1] an important indication of the patient's physiological homeostasis and well-being. In addition, pain is viewed as an impediment to the patient's spiritual, psychological, and emotional processes of life review and meaningful closure with loved ones. Hospice nurses are experts in the area of pharmacologic approaches to pain management. Working with the patient and family, they can quickly identify strategies to reduce, and in many cases eliminate, discomfort. Physical therapists can also provide the nonpharmacologic interventions described in the previous section on comfort measures, which may enhance the effectiveness of medications. In many cases, physical therapy interventions such as massage, guided breathing for relaxation, TENS, and gentle movement can even reduce the need for pharmacologic agents.

In cases where the patient is unresponsive, delirious, or aphasic, potential causes of pain are identified and addressed. For example, an unresponsive patient with a severe urinary tract infection would most likely be treated for pain. In addition, if a patient has previously reported a consistent pattern of pain during periods of consciousness, it will probably be assumed that this discomfort remains even when they are no longer able to verify this.

Prevalence of Pain at End of Life

Although the prevalence of pain at end of life will vary depending on the nature of the terminal disease process, research indicates two thirds of patients with advanced cancer experience pain. Pain and discomfort are multidimensional constructs. One assessment known as the Memorial Symptom Assessment Scale-Short Form (MSAS-SF)[56] is a patient self-report of the spectrum of cancer-related sources of physical and psychological

distress (Figure 27-2). The MSAS-SF also enables patients to rate the extent to which particular symptoms affect them, using a 5-point continuum between *not at all* (0) and *very much* (4).

The two most common forms of discomfort in 299 patients with advanced cancer completing the MSAS-SF included pain (72%) and lack of energy (70%).[56] Furthermore, more than 50% of these patients rated these symptoms as affecting them "quite a bit" or "very much." Finally, between 35% and 39% of these patients reported occasional psychological distress such as worrying, feeling irritable, and feeling sad. Clearly, the physical and psychological effects of advanced cancer frequently affect most patients.

The multidimensional element of pain, particularly at end of life, was first recognized by Cicely Saunders, who defined pain as "not just an event, or a series of events, but rather a situation in which the patient is held captive."[57] Saunders defined the collective impact of these discomforting "events" as "Total Pain," which is illustrated in Figure 27-3.

In developing the interdisciplinary model of hospice care, Saunders considered that each professional member had a role in helping ease the various contributions to a patient's total pain. For example, a hospice chaplain could address spiritual pain, whereas a social worker might mitigate the issues of bureaucratic pain (i.e., the frustration of filling out the endless and tedious forms required for insurance claims). By addressing the many contributions to distress, patients' energy resources can then be marshaled for meaningful and comforting activities, thus enhancing their quality of life. In the context of total pain, Saunders' approach to management was to employ both pharmacologic and nonpharmacologic measures proactively rather than reactively.

Without a doubt, effective pain management is one of the most important of Saunders' many contributions to the development of a standardized approach to compassionate end-of-life care. She was among the first to demonstrate that inadequate pain management at the end of life hastens death by increasing physiologic stress, myocardial oxygen demand, and the work of breathing."[57] Furthermore, inadequate pain relief increases the burden of total pain, causing significant anguish for both the patient and family. Accordingly, given the prevalence and intensity of physical pain among terminally ill patients, Saunders advocated the use of opioid medications in sufficient doses to maintain a consistent level of relief. Her well-known maxim in this regard was "constant pain needs constant control."[57] Nevertheless, despite considerable evidence for their use, barriers exist within society and the medical system that can prevent adequate dosing of the highly effective opioid medications. Because of their potential for abuse and addiction as well as opioids' popularity as street drugs, many states have restrictive laws that can limit their availability in both rural and inner-city pharmacies.[1] Accordingly, it is

Patient's Name _____ Date ___/___/___ ID # _____

MEMORIAL SYMPTOM ASSESSMENT SCALE – SHORT FORM [MSAS-SF]

I. INSTRUCTIONS: Below is a list of symptoms. If you had the symptom **DURING THE PAST WEEK,** please check YES. If you did have the symptom, please check the box that tells us how much the symptom DISTRESSED or BOTHERED you.

Check *all* the symptoms you have had during the PAST WEEK.	IF YES: How much did it DISTRESS or BOTHER you?					
	Yes (√)	Not at all (0)	A little bit (1)	Some-what (2)	Quite a bit (3)	Very much (4)
Difficulty concentrating						
Pain						
Lack of energy						
Cough						
Changes in skin						
Dry mouth						
Nausea						
Feeling drowsy						
Numbness/tingling in hands and feet						
Difficulty sleeping						
Feeling bloated						
Problems with urination						
Vomiting						
Shortness of breath						
Diarrhea						
Sweats						
Mouth sores						
Problems with sexual interest or activity						
Itching						
Lack of appetite						
Dizziness						
Difficulty swallowing						
Change in the way food tastes						
Weight loss						
Hair loss						
Constipation						
Swelling of arms or legs						
"I don't look like myself"						
If you had any other symptoms during the PAST WEEK, please list them below, and indicate how much the symptom DISTRESSED or BOTHERED you.						
1						
2						

II. Below are other commonly listed symptoms. Please indicate if you have had the symptom **DURING THE PAST WEEK,** and if so, how **OFTEN** it occurred.

Check *all* the symptoms you have had during the PAST WEEK.	IF YES: How **OFTEN** did it occur?				
	Yes (√)	Rarely (1)	Occasionally (2)	Frequently (3)	Almost constantly (4)
Feeling sad					
Worrying					
Feeling irritable					
Feeling nervous					

FIGURE 27-2 The Memorial Symptom Assessment Scale-Short Form. *(Chang VT, Hwang SS, Feuerman M, et al. The memorial sypmptom assessment scale-short form (MSAS-SF). Cancer 89: 1162-71, 2000. Copyright 2000, American Cancer Society. Reproduced with permission of Wiley-Liss, Inc., subsidiary of John Wiley and Sons, Inc.)*

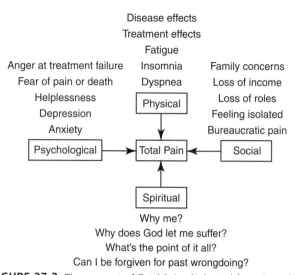

FIGURE 27-3 The concept of Total Pain. *(Adapted from Saunders C. Nature and management of terminal pain. In Shotter EF, editor: Matters of life and death. London, 1970, Dartman, Longman and Todd.)*

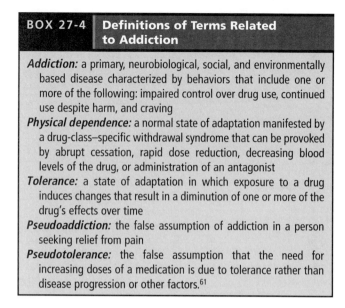

critical for health professionals working in pain management to understand the true nature of addiction as well as physical dependence, tolerance, pseudotolerance, and pseudoaddiction, in order to avoid perpetuating existing barriers to appropriate pain management at end of life. In reality, both past and recent studies have found addiction rates of anywhere between 0% and 7% in patients receiving opioids for end-stage cancer pain.[58,59] In end-of-life care, concern for patient comfort is first and foremost. Moreover, nurses and other health professionals working in a hospice setting may need to educate and advocate for their patients in order to ensure their access to appropriate medications and need for optimal comfort.

In order to educate health professionals, the American Academy of Pain Medicine generated a consensus document in 2001 defining the terms *addiction, physical dependency,* and *tolerance.*[60] These definitions are defined in Box 27-4.

Types of Physical Pain

In order to achieve the outcome of consistent analgesia, it is important to understand the physiological sources that contribute to pain. For example, physical pain can derive from organs, neural tissue, or musculoskeletal components, each of which produces a distinct type of discomfort and requires a specific class of pharmacologic agents. An understanding of pain's sources and behavior promotes the physical therapist's effective advocacy and pain management. In general, *nociceptive* and *neuropathic pain* are the two major types of pain common at the end of life.

Breakthrough Pain. In the presence of advanced disease (particularly with cancer), it is not uncommon for patients to experience brief intermittent episodes of severe pain lasting from several seconds to several minutes. In most cases, this "breakthrough pain" occurs in the presence of overall effective baseline analgesia. Although these episodes can occur without apparent provocation, they may also correlate with changes in activity. Use of a pain diary such as the one illustrated in Figure 27-4 can be helpful in identifying triggers (and premedicating accordingly, if needed). Breakthrough pain can be effectively managed, usually by providing a fast-acting medication in a specific percentage of the patient's overall daily dose.

Pain Assessment

Decisions related to appropriate medications for pain control are based on patient or caregiver reports. It is important for health professionals to recognize that patients, especially older ones, may be reluctant to report the true nature, extent, and severity of their pain. Barriers to accurate reports are numerous, including cultural differences, fear of being seen as complaining, lack of knowledge about pain control, and fears of medication adverse effects, tolerance, or addiction.[1]

It can be helpful for patients to maintain a pain diary, which allows them to record the impact of activities and other factors on their pain levels. Figure 27-4 illustrates an example of the American Cancer Society's pain diary, which is also available on their website (www.cancer.org/docroot/MON/content/MON_1x_Pain_Control_Record.asp). The pain diary includes useful questions that can help physical therapists in the

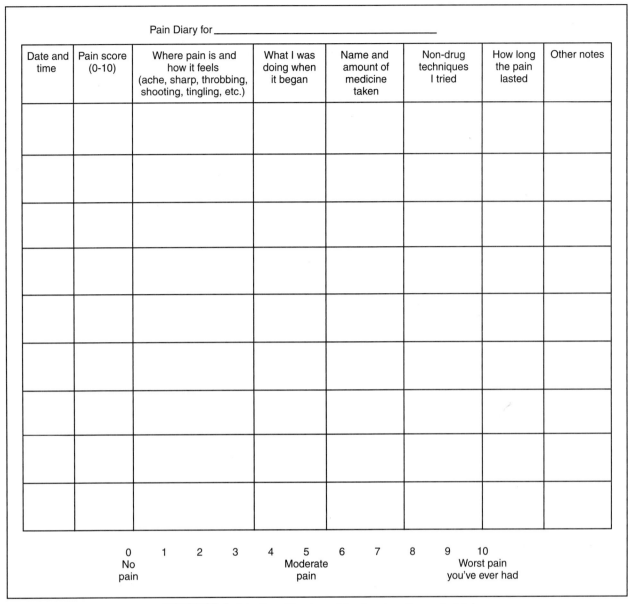

FIGURE 27-4 Pain diary. *(Courtesy of the American Cancer Society.)*

assessment of pain such as location, nature (e.g., stabbing, throbbing, shooting), pain rating, and provoking factors.

Pharmacologic Measures for Pain Control

There are several effective medications that can be used for pain control in patients facing the end of life. This section will provide a brief overview of the three major classes of medications commonly used in a hospice setting. These include nonopioid analgesics, opioid analgesics, and adjuvant analgesics.

The selection of the appropriate class of medications is determined by the source of the pain as well as its severity. The WHO has developed a pain ladder that

can also be used to determine the appropriate medications in end-stage cancer (Figure 27-5).

Nonopioid Analgesics. This class of medications includes acetaminophen and nonsteroidal anti-inflammatory drugs (NSAIDs). The WHO pain ladder recommends nonopioid analgesics for mild pain, which is less than 3 on a 1 to 10 numerical scale where 0 is *no pain* and 10 is the *worst imaginable* pain.[16(p100)]

Acetaminophen (Tylenol) is considered one of the safest medications for long-term use in the management of mild pain and the reduction of fever.[61] Its main mechanism of action is the inhibition of cyclooxygenase (COX), an enzyme responsible for the production of prostaglandins. Acetaminophen is particularly effective for use in nociceptive somatic pain of musculoskeletal origin. This

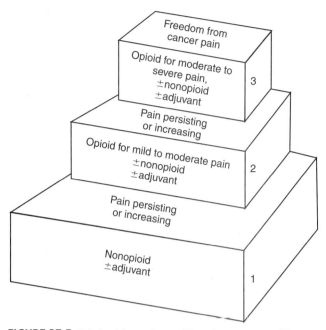

FIGURE 27-5 Pain level for patients with end-stage cancer. *(Courtesy of the World Health Organization's pain level for patients with end-stage cancer. http://www.who.int/cancer/palliative/painladder/en/)*

drug can be used in isolation for mild pain and also has a potential coanalgesic effect when used with opioid medications.

NSAIDs produce analgesia by reducing the biosynthesis of prostaglandins and thus preventing inflammation and reducing fever. Examples of common NSAIDs include aspirin, ibuprofen, and naproxen. Like acetaminophen, these NSAIDs also inhibit the cyclooxygenase pathway. NSAIDs are also useful for mild nociceptive pain of musculoskeletal origin. Because prostaglandins are found in high concentrations in the periosteum, NSAIDs can be useful for mild bone pain. The typical dosing of this medication is 500 to 1000 mg every 4 to 6 hours for aspirin and 200 to 400 mg at the same intervals for ibuprofen. The maximum daily recommended dose for aspirin is 4000 mg, and that for ibuprofen is 2400 mg. These medications have a ceiling effect so that doses beyond the recommended maximum do not improve the analgesic effect, but instead increase the risk of adverse effects.[61] NSAIDs can produce gastric irritation through its inhibition of prostaglandins, which in turn decrease the mucosal coating in the stomach. This reduction in mucosal coating can render the gut lining more vulnerable to injury from acids, pepsin, and bile salts, thus increasing the risk of gastrointestinal bleeding. Kidney dysfunction can also occur as a result of inhibition of renal vasoactive prostaglandins which decrease blood flow to organ arterioles and reduce the glomerular filtration rate. This complication is more likely to occur in the presence of dehydration.[1]

A newer type of NSAID selectively blocks the cyclooxygenase 2 (COX-2) enzymatic pathway and appears to decrease the risk of gastrointestinal bleeding, renal dysfunction, and generalized bleeding that can occur with the COX-type NSAIDs.

Opioid Analgesics. Opioid analgesics are considered the most effective medications for the management of moderate to severe pain. Accordingly, the WHO pain ladder recommends these as the preferred medication in such instances.[61]

Moderate pain is defined as between 4 and 6 on a 0 to 10 numerical scale, where 0 is *no pain* and 10 is the *worst imaginable pain.* Severe pain is defined as between 7 and 10 on the same numerical scale.[16(p 100)] These medications bind to opioid receptors in the brain, blocking the release of neurotransmitters involved in processing pain perception. Thus, opioid medications are effective for all types of pain, and are also useful in treatment of dyspnea.

Opioid medications can be derived from the resin of the opium poppy (codeine, morphine) or manufactured synthetically (fentanyl, methadone). Thus, there are numerous types of opioid medications available, such as MS Contin, Oramorph, oxycodone, OxyContin, hydromorphone, Vicodin, and Lortab.

Morphine is considered the "gold standard" of the opioid analgesics and is used as a measure of dose equivalence. Dosing of opioid medications thus depends on the type of medication given as well as the route of administration.

In end-of-life care, optimal pain control is the ultimate goal of pharmacologic treatment; thus, dosing is determined by the level required to attain this outcome. Fortunately, many of the opioid medications can be delivered in either extended- or immediate-release formulations, allowing for a more consistent level of control. Often, both types of medications are used.

Opioid Adverse Effects. Fortunately, allergic reactions to opioid medications are extremely rare, and the only contraindication to their use at end of life is a history of a hypersensitivity reaction such as rash or wheezing. One of the more common opioid adverse effects is constipation, and it is thus recommended that a prophylactic bowel regimen be started immediately upon the initiation of these medications. In addition to stimulant laxatives and the encouragement of adequate fluid intake when possible, interventions such as abdominal massage, range of motion, and upright mobility training can also assist bowel evacuation.

Sedation is another common adverse effect of opioid use, particularly with the initial doses. This effect will often wear off after the first 24 to 48 hours. If improvement does not occur, stimulant medications may be added (the use of such medications is described in the following section on adjuvant medications). It is also important to recognize that although many patients may view sedation as a barrier to quality waking time with family and loved ones, others may consider it a welcome opportunity for rest, particularly if insomnia has been problematic.

One of the most feared (yet relatively rare) complications of opioid use is respiratory suppression. Fortunately, this adverse event is usually preceded by sedation, which provides an opportunity for symptom reversal through the use of an opioid antagonist such as naloxone. Indications for reversal generally include lack of arousability and a drop in oxygen saturation. The highest risk for respiratory depression occurs with the first doses of opioids in patients without a prior history of their use (opioid naïve). Opioid-tolerant patients who have achieved good pain control generally do not develop this complication.

Nausea and vomiting can occur, particularly during the initial dosing of opioid medications. This adverse effect is thought to result from the combined effects of delayed gastric emptying and vestibular sensitivity, which can also occur from these medications. Fortunately, most patients habituate to this adverse effect in the first few days. Should this not occur, antinausea medications can be added.

Myoclonus can occur, particularly with high-dose morphine therapy. This is thought to result from the accumulation of metabolites, especially in the presence of renal dysfunction. This adverse effect can thus often be eliminated with a morphine alternative. In addition, diazepam may also be used.

Pruritus (itching) is most commonly seen with the use of morphine, although it is sometimes seen with the use of other opioids. Antihistamines can be used to counteract this adverse effect and are generally effective.

Adjuvant Analgesics. This class of medications includes an array of agents that produce analgesic effects. These include antidepressants, anticonvulsants, corticosteroids, local anesthetics, and calcium channel blockers. Although these medications can be effective for milder pain when used in isolation, they are most typically used in conjunction with opioids. They can be particularly effective in the presence of severe neuropathic or bone pain.

Routes of Administration. Analgesic medications can be administered through a variety of methods. Although many patients with advanced disease are able to take medications orally (either in pill or liquid form), others may require alternative forms of delivery. Thus, medications can be administered through a variety of routes, including mucosal, transdermal, rectal, or topical approaches. One of the most common routes for patients without oral function is through rectal or vaginal suppositories. Medications can be also delivered through intravenous or intrathecal methods; however, whenever possible, the least invasive approach is used.

Intramuscular injections are generally not used in end-of-life care as they are painful in themselves, and because rates of vascular drug absorption are highly variable when using this approach. In selecting the preferred route of delivery for pain medications, the hospice nurse will work closely with the patient and family to determine the most effective, consistent, and efficient approach.

PALLIATIVE SEDATION

For some individuals, the end-of-life process may involve levels of pain that are intractable even with aggressive pain management efforts. In such cases, the only remaining approach is to induce sedation in order to alleviate conscious awareness of pain. Palliative sedation (PS) is defined as "the monitored use of medications (sedatives, barbiturates, neuroleptics, hypnotics, benzodiazepines or anesthetic medication) to relieve refractory and unendurable physical, spiritual, and/or psychosocial distress for patients with a terminal diagnosis, by inducing varied degrees of unconsciousness."[62]

The American Academy of Hospice and Palliative Medicine describes mild and deep levels of PS, which vary in terms of the level of consciousness preserved.[63] With mild sedation, smaller doses of short-acting medications such as midazolam at an infusion rate of 0.5 mg/hour are used, promoting enough alertness to allow the patient to engage in conversation. Should mild sedation not be sufficient, a deeper level may be required and in this case, higher doses of midazolam may be used in addition to longer-acting medications such as benzodiazepines and morphine sulfate.[64] In having two progressive levels of PS available, patients and their families can maintain a level of choice, which enables them to fully direct their care with the assistance of the hospice team.

Ethical Framework for Palliative Sedation

The intent of palliative sedation is to provide comfort when all appropriate methods of pain control are inadequate. Patients and families must clearly understand that the overall intent of PS is to provide relief from unendurable suffering, but not to hasten death. Nevertheless, the end result for many patients undergoing PS will be the eventual cessation of respiration followed by death. Although death is an expected outcome from the disease process itself, the addition of PS cannot be definitively excluded as a contributory factor. Thus, the ethical framework in which PS is grounded is that of "double effect," which suggests that the beneficent intention of reducing suffering may produce the unintentional effect of death. In addition, the principle of proportionality suggests that the selection of PS should be proportionate to the extent of patient suffering, treatment alternatives, expected benefits, and possible harm.[65] A 1997 ruling of the United States Supreme Court stated, "There is no constitutional right to physician-assisted suicide. Terminal sedation is intended for symptom relief and is appropriate in the aggressive practice of palliative care."[64]

Initiating Palliative Sedation

The decision to initiate PS is based upon the assessment of patient symptoms and often, the patient's stated desire to be free of his or her discomfort. Once it is clear that

PS is the only remaining treatment option, the patient or health care surrogate (the individual appointed to make medical decisions on the patient's behalf) must be clearly instructed in the goals and expected outcomes of treatment. Informed consent is typically required. Members of the hospice team are also available to provide any support that may be needed by the patient or family.

In most cases, PS is initiated at the onset of terminal restlessness, an indication that death is imminent within days or hours. Although the most common indication for PS is agitated delirium, others include pain, seizures, and dyspnea and severe anxiety. Many patients have more than one symptom, which greatly compounds their distress. One patient of the authors described the feelings of terminal restlessness as "a horrible sense of doom and fear, like a weight crushing down on me."

There are many different medications that can be used for PS. They include central nervous system depressants such as midazolam, benzodiazepines, lorazepam, and pentobarbital. Most of these medications are administered intravenously. Another common formulation known as a hospice suppository contains metoclopramide to prevent gastrointestinal distress, diphenhydramine to dry up secretions, morphine sulfate (for pain), lorazepam for anxiety, and haloperidol for delirium. These suppositories are inserted rectally every 3 to 8 hours as needed and are often a preferred method for home use.

The frequency with which PS is used at end of life in the hospice setting is estimated to between 20% and 52%.[66] A recent prospective cohort study performed on a consecutive sample of 77 dying patients showed that 42 (54.5%) received PS. Interestingly, the patients who received PS had a significantly longer survival period than patients who were not sedated, a finding that has been demonstrated in other studies as well.[67] Patients in this study had a mean time to death of 22 hours, with a range of 2 to 160 hours, with family members actively involved in the decision to initiate PS. These families perceived that it promoted a peaceful and comfortable death. Similar time frames have also been reported in other studies.[68,69]

When a patient is undergoing PS, family members should be encouraged to talk to them and touch them. Gentle massage can be helpful in assisting the letting go process, and patients may respond with a change in breathing that suggests relaxation. Sometimes, patients may respond in other poignant and life-changing ways.

ADVANCE DIRECTIVES: PLANNING AHEAD FOR DEATH WITH DIGNITY

As this chapter has suggested, a person facing end of life has many options for care and comfort. A major source of family stress often revolves around attempts to determine what a family member would want when the patient has not identified or disclosed his or her choices.

An advance directive is a legal document that provides a clear statement of the patient's desires for care in the event of imminent death (a living will) and the appointment of a person to make decisions on their behalf should they become incapacitated (medical power of attorney). A third element of an advance directive includes an optional DNR document, which is usually printed on bright orange paper and displayed in a prominent place in the patient's home and medical chart. Patients who elect hospice services do not need to have a signed DNR in place. State-specific advance directives can be downloaded through the National Hospice and Palliative Care Organization website (www.caringinfo.org/PlanningAhead/AdvanceDirectives/Stateaddownload.htm). Many patients who are in other settings such as skilled nursing or acute care will have advance directives and a signed DNR in place. Physical therapists working with patients in these settings should know whether or not they have a DNR in place. This information can be found in the medical chart. In most cases, a bright orange sign reading "DNR" will be placed on the outside of the chart, where it can be easily noted.

Confronting the Reality of Death

Being comfortable with dying is a challenge for many therapists and individuals because of the limited exposure during our training and clinical practice and the nature of modern culture. The process of understanding the meaning and nature of death, then being able to speak of living and dying with comfort and ease, takes time and practice through repeated exposure and experience. This development can occur through reading, conversations with professional peers, and eventually during work with people approaching the end of life. This section will introduce conversation topics that arise in clinical settings and promote adjustment to the dying process.

Decline, if not reversible, will lead to death. Fully understanding the universality of death as more than an abstract concept can make us open to the possibility of improvement, maintaining a functional level, or further decline and death during the course of clinical care. Death is not failure by the patient or the therapist, but the natural course of life. The ability to give voice to this natural event as it occurs during the process of care can provide a sense of understanding that will support the coping of patients and family members.

Death is an experience fraught with an array of emotion. Patients often have limited experiences with death during their lifetimes and may find themselves struggling with unfamiliar circumstances and feelings as their conditions progress. How health professionals address the events that occur at the end of life can offer support and understanding to allow the completion of this process with less distress and better understanding. Patients and family members have identified geriatric and oncologic medical care that includes physical and intentional presence, developing an understanding of their individualized experience, and maintaining the patient's humanity and dignity as essential to their spiritual well-being.[70]

Reframing Physical Loss and Dying

Loss and suffering are a natural, albeit unpleasant, part of the dying process. Often there is a component of significant physical loss such as the inability to walk, stand, or even get out of bed during this experience. The physical therapist can use clinical observations made during initial examination or ongoing assessments to affirm the person's maximal efforts at mobility and function in light of a progressive or deteriorating condition. Understanding these losses can change the aspects of suffering that are then experienced and one can discover a meaning to life by the attitude taken toward this unavoidable suffering.[71]

Spiritual Awareness

In the past century, perhaps because of the advances of medicine, emphasis has been on the physical changes that occur as the body deteriorates in the process of dying rather than on the spiritual changes with dying, as in past centuries. Previously, societies have examined death as a spiritual event and created treatises such as the Christian *Ars Moriendi* or "Art of Dying"[72] and the Buddhist *Tibetan Book of the Dead*.[73] Evidence of spiritual well-being is found to improve coping with terminal illness.[74] It is important that members of the IDT meet the spiritual needs of patients and families receiving hospice care, even if their spiritual/religious tradition or beliefs differ from one's own.[75]

Dealing with Death and Dying

In physical therapy practice of aging adults, it is common to provide care to individuals who are facing death either imminently or in the not so distant future. Many physical therapists' first experience of death is with an older patient with whom they have grown close through the therapeutic relationship. When confronted with the inevitability of the patient's death, a physical therapist may feel anxiety or feel incapable of coping with such a situation.[76] A common and natural emotional reaction is fear that can be perceived by the patient from the therapist's body language and facial expression as pity.[77] The therapist's recognition that death is inevitable and naturally occurring can bring about a freedom from the fear and a recognition that everyone has choices in how one's days can be lived. Listening to the patient with empathy and unconditional positive regard is a way of communicating compassion[77,78] without using nonsensical statements such as "I know how you feel" (you don't) or "It will be alright" (it may not) or worse, "You shouldn't

feel that way" (why not?). In order to provide compassionate care by being present to the dying individual, health professionals must face their own fears of loss, suffering, and death. To be effective, physical therapists need to recognize their own as well as the aging adult's feelings, have a sense of their strengths and weaknesses, and be aware of their thoughts and feelings about death and dying, as these may all have an impact on how care is provided. Awareness that any discomfort the therapist feels is a personal reaction and may not be shared by the older adult who is at the end of life can help the therapist with appreciating the continuity of life.

Unfinished Business

Often, the older patient may be comfortable with death, even anticipating it as a means of meeting a spouse or other loved one who predeceased him or her. However, the patient's family may still be resisting the finality of death and may express discomfort as wanting more therapy, pushing the patient to do more, to not give up, etc. This lack of acceptance of the loved one's death may be a result of unfinished business. Clinically this can be addressed through using the various practice patterns identified earlier in this chapter to sustain a sense of hope rather than the abandonment that may be felt from a discharge from having "failed" therapy. The personal issues of unfinished business can be addressed as well.

Unfinished business has been identified by Elizabeth Kubler Ross[79] and others[80] as tasks and relationships that need completion or resolution before the end of life, or to get through any difficult situation. Byock[81] has outlined four communication tasks of the dying and their families: "Please forgive me," "I forgive you," "Thank you," and "I love you." Offering these words of goodbye may help families find closure. Being in the presence of those close to the end of life and struggling with their own issues of pending loss will in many cases bring to the level of awareness of the family and/or practitioner feelings and emotions related to their own past or anticipated life losses.

Being able to process and resolve one's own personal issues of unfinished business is a healthy and life-affirming process that is recognized as anticipatory grief for patients and families. Patients can be teachers to therapists as well. Those at the end of life may report increased comfort and peace as this occurs. They may report a clarity and meaning in life that was not evident previously. For the health and well-being of physical therapists as end-of-life caregivers, reflection around such issues can promote more effective listening ability and long-term work satisfaction. Most hospice workers have a spiritual belief system, which may not be connected to an organized religion or be well defined, but consist of some belief in something beyond the self, some way of making meaning of the world and life.[82] Patients and families can be guided to access their own religious or spiritual support system, or that of the hospice program, to cope with the realities and unknown of death.

SUMMARY

End-of-life care is a challenge for both the new and experienced physical therapist. Clinical expertise is developed through an ongoing practice of reflection and mindfulness.[83] Knowledge of aging and disease processes, pain and symptom management, and the different patterns of care used to support a palliative care approach is essential. Understanding the physical therapy role within the hospice interdisciplinary team approach is important for successful practice integration. Personal exploration of one's own feelings and issues with loss, grief, and death is necessary to maintain personal health while providing the best intervention and support to individuals as they die.

REFERENCES

To enhance this text and add value for the reader, all references are included on the companion Evolve site that accompanies this text book. The reader can view the reference source and access it online whenever possible. There are a total of 83 cited references and other general references for this chapter.

CHAPTER 28

The Senior Athlete

Barbara J. Hoogenboom, PT, EdD, SCS, ATC,
Michael Voight, PT, SCS, OCS, ATC, CSCS

INTRODUCTION

As the population of the United States ages, more individuals are living longer and staying physically active into old age. As the baby boom generation enters the over-65 age category during the years 2010 to 2030, the increase in the population of healthy older-age individuals will be dramatic, and the number of older-aged athletes is expected to increase concurrently.[1] This athletic subgroup of aging adults represents a truly unique example of those who are aging exceptionally well (Figure 28-1). Athletic endeavors in this unique aging population range from weekend or fitness activities to competitive athletics and the Senior Olympics. Although many senior athletes are examples of successful aging and continue to be active, vigorous, and competitive, the reality is that the senior athlete is slower and weaker than in his or her youth. The reasons for the inevitable declines in athletic performance are important to understand. Some senior athletes have been active for a lifetime; others began their fitness and competition during the fitness craze of the 1970s and 1980s, coming to athletics later in life. Masters and age-group distance running, cycling, and swimming records are broken at a staggering rate. The Masters' marathon record was shattered at the Boston Marathon in 1990 when John Campbell (as a newly minted 40-year-old) finished among the top five runners of all age groups, in 2:11:04. The fastest senior marathon time is held by then 80-year-old Helen Klein, who in 2002 ran the California International Marathon in 4:31.32. She has run an amazing 59 marathons and 136 ultramarathons! In 1991, at age 83, Johnny Kelley ran his 60th Boston Marathon. Jenny Wood Allen of Scotland completed the 2002 London Marathon at age 89 years, making her the oldest woman ever to finish a marathon.[2] Although there is inevitable decline in performance levels with age, the physical limits of the human body are constantly being challenged by senior athletes of all sports and walks of life.

This chapter will focus on those individuals who physically challenge themselves by participating at high levels in competitive or recreational sports throughout their adulthood. These individuals have been referred to as the physically elite elderly[2] and are "a testament to the remarkable resilience of the human body when it is kept properly maintained."[2(p288)] They combine good inheritance (genetics)[3,4] and luck while maximizing their potential and longevity by successful training and good health habits. Those who participate in athletics into older age offer an amazing view of successful aging and provide a model for how adults can defy the physical effects of aging and maintain outstanding physical abilities and a high quality of life well into the eighth and ninth decades of life (Figure 28-2). Certainly, the demand for sports rehabilitation services for these aging athletes will increase as they age and continue their unique activity levels.

The physical therapist who expects to treat the older athlete must have experience and a good working knowledge of aging and the mechanisms of athletic injuries. The ideal individual would have firsthand experience with caring for athletes before, during, and after athletic participation and know both the physical and psychological demands sports place on the participant. This clinician should be versed in a diversity of areas, including anatomy, cardiovascular and muscle physiology, nutrition, biomechanics and kinesiology, physical training, flexibility and conditioning programs, protective/preventive taping and/or bracing, and rehabilitation. Understanding age-related physiological changes and their ramifications relating to physical exercise and rehabilitation is vital to the patient's safe and successful functional return to participation and, in some cases, competition. Knowledge of pathologic changes, comorbidities, and their effects on the ability to participate in athletic activities is critical in the design and implementation of a rehabilitation program for the older athlete.

This chapter defines the senior athlete and describes typical systems changes and characteristics found in these individuals. Musculoskeletal problems and injuries common to the senior athlete are discussed and presented. The role of comorbidity also is considered. A unique assessment is presented with pertinent examples for use with the senior athlete. Practical considerations for rehabilitation, equipment recommendations, and return to

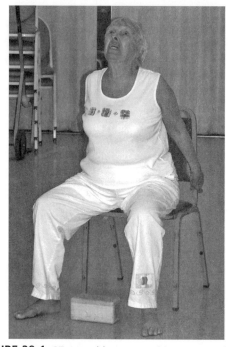

FIGURE 28-1 87-year-old yoga practitioner, group leader.

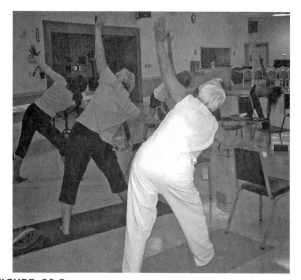

FIGURE 28-2 Yoga group at senior retirement center, led by 87-year-old leader.

athletics are considered. Finally, case studies are used to illustrate the interrelationship among the variables that affect treatment of the senior athlete.

DEFINING THE POPULATION: WHO IS THE SENIOR ATHLETE?

The physically elite older adult represents a small percentage of the young-old (65-74 years), old (75-84 years) and old-old (85-99 years),[2] many of whom are able to outperform individuals years younger. There is often confusion about the definition of a senior athlete. The terms "masters athlete," "geriatric athlete," "aging athlete," and "senior athlete" are not synonymous. Masters athletes may not be senior athletes. Masters athletes are competitors in a given sport who exceed a minimum age criteria, which are often in the 20s, 30s, and 40s. For example, in competitive swimming in the United States and Canada, the minimum master's age is 18 years (Table 28-1).[5] The average nonathletic but well older adult is not discussed in this chapter, nor is the care of former athletes reviewed unless those athletes are still actively engaged in regular physical activity. For the purpose of this chapter, there are three groups that comprise the population described as the senior athlete. Although there may be an overlap, these groups have some apparent differences that influence their need for rehabilitation services. Each group is dealt with in turn. Table 28-2 provides both a Centers for Disease Control and Prevention (CDC)–related definition[6] and a description of the level of activity for the wide variety of athletes that may be considered "senior athletes."

The first group consists of former competitive athletes who have continued to exercise recreationally, for example, the football or field hockey team player who is now conditioning on a more individual basis, using an activity such as running, swimming, or cycling. Many of these individuals may have sustained a significant injury during their earlier competitive play and therefore may not currently participate in competitions or tournaments; rather, they have adopted independent or group fitness as a part of their way of life. The older recreational athlete encompasses lifelong athletes who trained intensively for a period in their lives and currently may or may not be training at a relative intensity that is comparable with their earlier training levels. The physical performances of these noncompetitive athletes are hard to describe and quantify. This group utilizes a wide variety of sports and training intensities; however, these athletes share the dedication to fitness, healthy living, and regular activity that support this categorization. Virtually all the athletes who played team sports as competitive performers and who are still exercising are training at some other sport or activity, often at the recreational level.

The second group is composed of lifelong athletes. Again, these athletes are involved in a spectrum of activities and training intensities, making their participation rates and physical performances hard to describe and quantify. Most are lifetime "sports people," some of whom are recreationally active and others who compete (Figure 28-3). They play tennis or golf; they run, cycle, or compete in triathlons. They may even participate in several different activities, but their involvement has been primarily in one sport or group of sports, some at the local level and others at the national or elite level. The definition of a competitive senior athlete for the purposes of this chapter is "one who participates in an organized team or individual sport that requires regular competition against others, places a high premium on

TABLE 28-1	Masters/Seniors Sport Organizations and Competitions		
Sport Organization	Ages	Age Divisions	Events
World and National Masters Athletics	35-100+	5-y increments	All stadia (in stadium) and nonstadia track and field events
Masters Running	Age 35+	5-y increments	Road races
Senior Golf (USGA)	50+	No age divisions	Designated Senior Golf tournaments
Masters Swimming (USMS)	18-100+	5-y increments	Designated Masters swimming events
Worldwide Senior Tennis Circuit (USTA)	30 and up	5-y increments	Designated Senior Tennis events

(*Data from www.world-masters-athletics.org, www.seniorjournal.com, www.usga.com, www.usms.org, and www.itftennis.com.*)

TABLE 28-2	Descriptions of Types of Senior Athletes, Using CDC Guidelines			
Descriptors	Sedentary	Recreational	Competitive	Elite
Level and intensity of exercise	< CDC recommendation for substantial health benefits	CDC recommendation for substantial health benefits: 150 min/wk of moderate-intensity* aerobic activity or 75 min/wk of vigorous-intensity* aerobic activity PLUS muscle strengthening 2 or more days/week	CDC recommendation for greater health benefits: 300 min/wk of moderate-intensity* aerobic activity or 150 min/wk of vigorous-intensity* aerobic activity, PLUS muscle strengthening 2 or more days/wk	> CDC recommendation for greater health benefits, PLUS specific and varied intensities of training for high-level competitions in select sports
Typical activities	ADLs and low-level functional tasks only	Home or health club, individual or group exercisers, without competitive participation	Runners, cyclists, tennis players, and golfers who compete in small, local events	Registered "senior" or "masters" athletes who train and compete nationally and internationally

*Moderate intensity is equivalent to brisk walking; vigorous intensity is equivalent to jogging or running (www.cdc.gov).

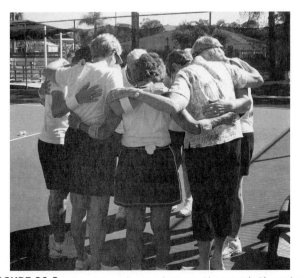

FIGURE 28-3 Women's senior tennis team, Riverwoods Plantation, Estero, FL.

excellence and achievement, and requires systematic training."[7] A significant subgroup of athletes in this recreational group are the aging athletes who are considered physically elite. They train and compete at high levels, regionally, nationally, and internationally in events such as the National Senior Games or the Worldwide Senior Tennis Circuit. This population may have a disproportionate amount of the overuse type of injury. For these individuals, athletic activity is as much a part of their routine as dressing or eating meals. They are reluctant to stop participating in their chosen activity, even in the face of significant pain or dysfunction.

The final group is made up of the nonathlete who began to exercise late in life (arbitrarily, after age 40 years). This is a small but significant group who may be recreationally or competitively active. These individuals present a unique set of problems related directly to beginning physical activity at an older age and indirectly to their reasons for beginning to exercise. In many instances, exercise has been initiated by a health crisis. Common examples of this type of individual may include the patient who has experienced coronary symptoms (or may be a prime candidate for them) that is the direct result of a number of controllable risk factors including improper diet (obesity) and lack of exercise. In many cases, the physician has prescribed a progressive walking program as a beginning or introduction to exercise and positive health behaviors. The fact that a person's walking program was begun as a result of a heart attack does not protect him or her from musculoskeletal injury, but an injury or previous dysfunction may interfere with motivation for recovery from the cardiac event.

Opportunities and Organizations for Senior Athletes

The three groups of senior athletes may differ in the quality, frequency, and intensity of their exercise. Many older athletes are involved in racquet sports, running, triathlon, walking, and low-impact sports such as golf and bowling. Each of these sports can be played in a highly competitive manner against an opponent, a score, or time.[8] Competitive senior athletes can be found in any of the three categories of athlete previously described. Competitive amateur Masters Events have been established for years and are sponsored by more than 50 countries, for example, swimming,[5] weight lifting, running,[9] and cycling.[9] Each of these sporting events encourages participation of the aging athlete by offering a wide variety of age categories. As an example, the United States Masters Swimming Organization boasts more than 50,000 members in more than 450 local clubs located throughout the United States.[5] Professionally, the "senior" golf tour[10] and Masters Races for runners are the most high-profile events. The increase in the number of aging active adults implies that the number of events and competitors will continue to grow.

The National Senior Olympics formed in 1987, and now known as the National Senior Games (after its name change in 1990), provides multisport competitions every odd year for adults aged 50 and older.[2,9] The events include archery, badminton, basketball, bowling, cycling, golf, hockey, horseshoes, race walking, racquetball, road races, shuffleboard, softball, swimming, table tennis, tennis, track and field, triathlon, and volleyball. There are both summer and winter National Senior Games, with the summer games being the most popular, drawing more than 12,000 participant athletes from more than 90,000 seniors who attempted to qualify in 2007.[9] The winter games are much smaller, drawing less than 500 participants for five winter sports. These competing senior athletes "raise both physical and psychological ceilings and shatter the barriers of expectations that society has for the aged."[2(p290)]

AGING AND PHYSICAL CHANGES SPECIFIC TO THE SENIOR ATHLETE

All senior athletes, regardless of the category in which they fall or the activities they perform, experience some predictable age-related changes. Senior athletes are generally less flexible[8,11,12] and have lower muscle masses,[4] lower aerobic capacities,[1,4] and less well tuned thermoregulatory mechanisms[13] than they did at a younger age. They are likely to have osteoarthritis of the weight-bearing joints, although not necessarily brought on by their previous level of physical activity or exercise.[14,15] In fact, it has been demonstrated that older, recreational athletes do not sustain joint changes related to their activity or intensity.[16] Age-related changes affect training, injury, treatment, and recovery of the older athlete and must be considered when designing their rehabilitation program. It is well known that vigorous exercise throughout middle and older ages is associated with reduced disability and increased longevity.[17] For example, runners who were running 60 minutes/week with a mean age of 78 years had strikingly lower disability rates, especially women, and had prolonged survival in a 21-year longitudinal study. Clearly, lifelong athleticism has the potential to slow the functional consequences of aging (Figure 28-4).[1,17-21]

Musculoskeletal

It is well accepted that continued or progressive exercise and training affect an aging musculoskeletal system in many ways.[22-24] Similar to the younger athlete, the older athlete incurs acute or traumatic injury (macrotrauma) as well as overuse injury (microtrauma).[8] Unlike the younger athlete, however, these injuries are superimposed on an aging musculoskeletal system and recovery may take longer. Therefore, prevention takes on a more important role in this population. Proper equipment selection and use, for example, shoes, racquet, and stretching and training techniques must be encouraged to prevent problems and will be discussed in a subsequent section.

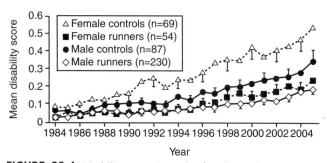

FIGURE 28-4 Disability rates in male, female, and nonrunners. *(Data from Chakravarty EF, Hubert HB, Lingala VB, Fires JF: Reduced disability and mortality among aging runners: a 21-year longitudinal study. Arch Intern Med 168(15):1638-1646, 2008.)*

Changes common to the aging joint include deterioration of joint surfaces, breakdown of collagen fibers, and a decrease in the viscosity of synovial fluid, which can result in loss of flexibility and an increase in joint stiffness. Osteoarthritis is a common manifestation of these changes and will be discussed in a later section of this chapter. Although a decrease in bone mineral density (BMD) is common with advancing age, the senior athlete performing higher levels of vigorous *weight bearing* exercise and resistance training (as promoted by the CDC[6]) may experience less bone density loss. In fact, the results of a 5-year longitudinal study of male master runners aged 40 to 80 years demonstrated maintenance of BMD despite moderate decreases in training volumes as the runners aged. These runners demonstrated a slower decline from peak bone mass, indicative of bone maintenance, not loss.[25] However, master cyclists and swimmers who performed little weight-bearing activity showed less bone density than age-matched controls.[26]

Changes affecting the muscular system include a decrease in the size, number, and type of muscle fibers. The loss of muscle occurs at a rate of 1% to 3% annually and fat increases at about the same rate, 1% per year. Muscles experience a decrease in respiratory capacity and an increase in fat and connective tissues. These changes affect the gross appearance of an older athlete. Individual motor units lose fibers, which result in a decrease in the force-generating ability of that muscle. There is an effective loss of type II fibers, which results in a higher percentage of type I fibers.[2,27] Although this change in percentage may increase the muscle's ability to sustain performance during endurance activities, it may limit the muscle's ability to generate strength and power. Thus, as muscle fibers are replaced with fat and connective tissue, muscle fibers are lost, especially type II fibers, the muscle's ability to forcefully contract is diminished, accounting for the general loss of force production seen with aging. Women are more vulnerable to loss of function secondary to type IIa muscular atrophy,[27] and women appear to experience greater declines in muscular strength and power (particularly in the upper extremities) than men.[21] Muscular strength as defined by Olympic weight lifting capacity declines linearly at the rate of 1% to 3% annually until the seventh decade, and then accelerates significantly.[28] The rate of strength decline is directly related to the specific activity of the individual. For example, weight lifters experience less strength decline (0.5%/annually), whereas runners experience a slower decline of endurance (Figure 28-5).[29]

The positive changes that occur in muscle as a result of resistance training in the older athlete of both genders should encourage strength training as an important countermeasure against the sarcopenia of aging.[4,11,18,23,27] Progressive resistance training (PRT) is an important part of an overall fitness program for senior athletes. PRT has been successfully implemented in the aging population in order to increase strength, muscle size,

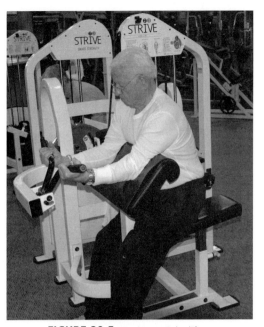

FIGURE 28-5 Senior weight lifter.

diminish age-related atrophy, and prevent specific injuries.[27] Most senior athletes incorporate a component of PRT in their workouts in order to slow the loss of lean body mass.

Cardiopulmonary

Longitudinal studies of the wide variety of markers of cardiovascular fitness show a predictable decline with increasing age. Physiological functional capacity (PFC) has been studied extensively in runners and swimmers by Tanaka and Seals,[19,21] who found only modest declines until age 60 to 70 years, with an exponential decrease thereafter. Age-associated declines in physiological determinants of performance may occur at different rates in men and women, especially in short-distance events as compared to long-distance events. Physically active individuals, however, demonstrate less of a decline than sedentary individuals (Figure 28-6).[2,3,30] In fact, if body composition and physical activity are kept constant, declines in $\dot{V}O_2$ max can be decreased from 10% per decade to 5% per decade.[4,31] Although the PFC declines with advancing age are somewhat predictable, the rate of decrease in maximal aerobic capacity is determined largely by the corresponding reduction in exercise stimulus. Simply stated, those who undergo the largest decrease in exercise volume or intensity will also demonstrate the largest decrease in PFC.[21]

The maximum percentage of $\dot{V}O_2$ max that can be used during exercise increases up to 90% in elite endurance athletes as compared to sedentary controls. Results of a study of elite mountain runners demonstrated the maintenance of a 3.5-fold greater endurance capacity as measured by oxygen uptake at the anaerobic threshold

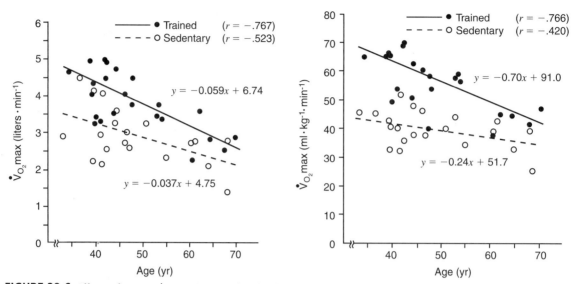

FIGURE 28-6 Effects of age on V̇o₂max in trained and sedentary men. Note that even though both trained and sedentary subjects show predictiable age related declines, trained subjects generally performed better than sedentary subjects at all ages. *(Adapted from Suominen HE, et al: Effects of "lifelong" physical training on functional aging in men. Scand J Soc Med 14(suppl):225-240, 1977.)*

(V̇o₂ AT) up to the age of 70+ years when compared with untrained peers. Maintaining a higher endurance capacity into the seventh decade of life is a sign of extremely successful aging, which positively affects quality of life, functional ability, and longevity (Figure 28-7).[3]

The loss of heart rate variability (HRV), frequently seen in sedentary aging adults, is associated with increased mortality and prevalence of cardiac events. When runners older than age 60 years with a 40-year history of endurance training were studied and compared with sedentary matched controls, researchers found that the age-related decline in HRV was mediated by lifestyle. For example, long-term participation in endurance training produced an increase in HRV and exercise work capacity, which are established predictors of enhanced cardiovascular function and positively affect longevity.[32] Conventional wisdom about aerobic fitness, performance limits, and age-related decline is challenged by the performances of senior athletes. In

fact, the limits of functional performance in the older athlete are largely unknown. Maintaining excellent cardiopulmonary endurance capacity at the age of 70 years is a sign of extremely successful aging, and senior athletes who do so have achieved superior fitness by lifelong participation in physical activity. Such participation, when combined with favorable genetics produces a high quality of life and enhanced longevity.[3]

Injuries and Physical Changes

Currently, there is a lack of consensus on whether older athletes experience different rates or types of injury, when compared with younger athletes.[11] Matheson et al[8] studied the distribution of injuries between older and younger individuals and found a greater incidence of meniscal injury, degenerative joint disease, and various inflammatory conditions along with a lower incidence of patellofemoral pain and stress fracture in older athletes.[8] In a study of

FIGURE 28-7 Multisystem effects of the typical response to aging through training, endurance is maintained, partially decreasing negative effects of age. *(From Tanaka H, Seals DR. Endurance exercise performance in Masters athletes: age-associated changes and underlying physiologic mechanisms. J Physiol 586:55-63, 2008.)*

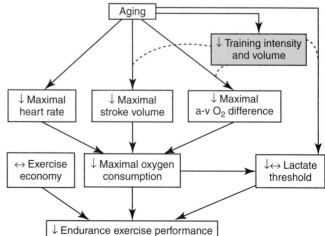

masters athletes involved in track and field, Kettanen et al[33] reported that about half were injured in the course of a year, and a third of those who were injured had to be out of training for a month or longer. Another study of 70- to 81-year-old athletes who participated in a variety of sports found that 81% sustained at least one sport-related injury, 38% of which were related to overuse.[34] Injuries sustained by the older athlete can be described as macro- and microtrauma by the mechanism of injury. Although the injuries may be similar to younger athletes, unique features exist, which will be discussed next.

Acute, Traumatic Injury (Macrotrauma). Acute musculoskeletal trauma is different in the older athlete than in the younger athlete. Because many older athletes participate less in collision sports, major contusions, fractures, and multiple ligament trauma occur less frequently. The exception to this is in sports such as cycling, hiking, climbing, and skiing, where falls and accidents do occur as a potential consequence of participation. Because of the loss of density in aging bone and the increased stiffness of ligamentous tissues, the senior athlete is more likely to sustain a fracture than to rupture a ligament in a macrotraumatic event. Likewise, because of increased collagenous stiffness, senior athletes are more likely to tear or avulse a muscle than sustain a muscular strain during athletic participation. For the purposes of this chapter, *traumatic injuries* will be operationally defined as those injuries resulting from a single traumatic event, which often involves uncontrolled force or momentum. When macrotraumatic injuries such as fractures, dislocations, ligamentous sprains, and muscle strains or tears occur, they can be devastating to the senior athlete because of the length of time it takes to recover.

Detraining or deconditioning occurs as a result of lack of exercise and occurs more rapidly than the time it takes to achieve conditioning for persons of all ages. The rate of detraining may occur faster with aging as a result of the insidious decline that occurs in all systems.[3,33,35] The aging muscle, with less mass and fewer sarcomeres, may show rapid atrophy and further loss of muscle mass after injury and the requisite immobilization or healing time frame. The period of rest required after joint or muscle injury can mean the end of athletic activity for an older athlete because of this detraining effect.

Overuse Injury (Microtrauma). Most competitive athletes suffer from injuries that fall into the overuse category and older athletes are no exception. For the purposes of this chapter, *overuse injuries or microtraumatic injuries* will be operationally defined as those injuries resulting from training but not attributable to a single traumatic event. Many microtraumatic injuries related to sport participation or training for sport occur in or around the musculotendinous unit. These injuries include muscle strains, bursitis, and a wide variety of tendinopathy. In-depth discussion of varied presentations and differentiation of tendon pathology is beyond the scope of this chapter, but many senior athletes present

with these types of injuries. For many reasons, older athletes may actually be more prone to overuse injuries than younger athletes (Figure 28-8).[36,37] First, older athletes have stiffer collagenous tissues and are less flexible than younger athletes.[30,36,38] Second, most have at least some arthritic changes in weight-bearing joints that can lead to altered movement strategies secondary to pain.[18] Third, muscle mass is reduced, offering less shock absorption and protection against external forces.[4,23,39]

Muscle soreness, a common symptom experienced by many active older adults, is attributed to microscopic injury to muscle and connective tissue. Generalized muscle soreness is often noted by senior athletes at the beginning of an exercise program or when new types of exercise are added to an existing program, and is considered normal or a necessary prerequisite to strengthening. Delayed-onset muscle soreness (DOMS) is similar in the aging population as in younger populations and typically occurs 24 to 48 hours after exercise. Eccentric exercise appears to pose the biggest risk for development of DOMS.[23,40] Prolonged muscle soreness (significant pain that lasts longer than 48 hours after exercise) should be evaluated as it could indicate muscle or tendon injury that may be the result of overtraining either by frequency, duration, or intensity. In fact, cross-training may be more effective to avoid orthopedic stress than low-intensity training between heavier training sessions.

Joint pain and associated effusion are common in the active aging population. Pain with specific movements or pain that occurs after certain activities that is not "joint pain" or DOMS can occur and are more like the "overuse" injuries that occur in younger athletes. Joint-related

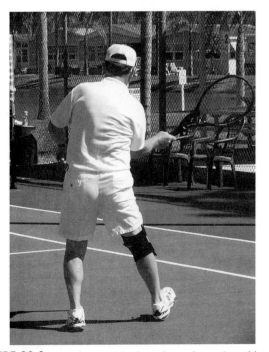

FIGURE 28-8 Use of supportive knee brace by senior athlete for tennis.

pain usually can be attributed to a specific set of circumstances, change in routine or volume of activity, or to structural abnormalities. For example, the older athlete with medial knee pain may in fact have tendinitis of the pes anserine region. Other examples may include pain in the subacromial region as a result of impingement of the suprahumeral space, or plantar fasciitis, which may indicate a need for orthotic fabrication. Structural abnormalities may be a consequence of age, such as in the osteophyte found in aging shoulders; postural changes or muscular weaknesses; or structural abnormalities, which may be chronic such as in the individual who has always had knee varus. It is important to note that anatomic pathology is not always correlated with dysfunction and impairments of activities of daily living (ADLs). Several authors have found that rotator cuff tears (RCTs), acromioclavicular osteoarthritis, and subacromial spurring occur independent of normal function, and in fact 54% of individuals older than age 60 years had magnetic resonance imaging (MRI)–confirmed RCTs, 75% had acromioclavicular (AC) arthritis, and 33% had subacromial spurring but were clinically and functionally asymptomatic.[41,42] Pain near a joint in the aging athlete should not be automatically interpreted as osteoarthritis or another microtraumatic source but rather should be carefully and systematically evaluated using both a clinical exam and movement-based exam, with the goal of identifying anatomic abnormalities and their effect on function.

Osteoarthritis and Joint Arthroplasty. Articular degeneration, commonly known as osteoarthritis (OA), is the most common joint pathology of aging and occurs over time. Characterized by joint space narrowing, osteophytes, swelling, morning pain and stiffness, and eventually joint deformity, articular degeneration can be accompanied by muscle weakness. Weight-bearing joints are most prone to OA.[16,43] The prevalence of osteoarthritis in the hip and knee is high, even in older athletes.[44-46] However, primary osteoarthritis of the hip was found in only 4% of former runners as compared to 8.7% of nonrunning controls,[47] indicating that running alone is not a risk factor for development of osteoarthritis. Running will be discussed in greater detail in a subsequent section.

Exercise programs to maintain strength and range of motion in senior athletes are strongly supported in the literature.[1,2,4,31,33,39,48] Exercise designed to maintain or improve muscular strength is especially important for the senior athlete because of not only the general maintenance of lean body mass but also the shock-absorbing capacity of muscle that can support arthritic joints. Exercise programs can decrease joint pain with functional activities, but the long-term effectiveness in prevention of progression of OA is somewhat unclear.[2,22,43,48] Specifically, muscle training exercises that are performed in closed kinetic chain positions increase joint stability and functionally train muscles as shock absorbers. Muscle, when strong and flexible, serves as a shock-absorbing

system to protect and offload the aging, potentially arthritic weight-bearing joints of the senior athlete.[35] Treatment of the senior athlete with osteoarthritis of the lower extremities should focus on progressive resistive exercise and patient education regarding functional activities, with emphasis on activities that minimize compression and shear (so-called joint-sparing techniques) to avoid a progression of impairments. Exercise modifications, when necessary, should focus on those activities that minimize weight bearing and joint compressive loading, for example, stationary cycling, rowing, swimming, and walking instead of running[2,15,16,36,48] or the athlete should be counseled to vary types of training between those that offer greater and lesser joint forces.

Degenerative arthritis of the hip is quite common in the aging athlete because it is one of the most commonly affected weight-bearing joints. Groin pain, hip muscle weakness, and subtle losses of range of motion are the primary symptoms of hip dysfunction and may be indicative of progressive hip degeneration, including labral lesions[49] and other mechanical pathologies. Athletes with symptomatic degenerative arthritis of the hip must limit or avoid weight-bearing athletic activities in order to avoid progression of the articular breakdown.[15,36,47] Continued progression of the degenerative joint disease, however, often results in the need for hip arthroplasty. Baby boomers will drive an increase in demand for total joint arthroplasty, while concurrently expecting return to athletic activity as an outcome of the joint arthroplasty.[50] Many senior athletes, of all levels of participation, undergo total joint arthroplasty in order to continue participation in their sport. As a result, total hip arthroplasty is being performed in younger (younger than age 50 years), more active individuals, and the longevity of the prosthesis itself is increasing.[50]

Like OA of the hip, OA of the knee may progress to such an extent that the senior athlete chooses a total knee arthroplasty (TKA) as a strategy for pain relief and improvement of function. As the outcomes of total knee replacement have improved, both in terms of range of motion and functional stability, younger athletes (younger than age 50 years) have opted for TKA in an attempt to stay active, return to certain sports, and remain competitive.[50] Box 28-1 illustrates current recommendations after knee arthroplasty for a wide variety of sports. Total joint arthroplasty is associated with improved function, improved quality of life, and longer life. In the past few years, technological advancement in this area of orthopedic surgery has allowed for more sports to be considered "safe" after total joint replacement and adequate rehabilitation. Athlete expectations for return to athletic activity are high, and the limits of safe return to sport are constantly being challenged. However, people who participate in athletic activity after joint replacement subject the prosthesis to increased force, increased joint-bearing-surface wear, increased stress at the prosthetic–bone interface, and

BOX 28-1	Recommended Activities after Knee Arthroplasty		
Allowed	**Allowed with Experience**	**No Consensus**	**Not Recommended**
Bowling	Horseback riding	Baseball	Basketball
Canoeing	Rowing	Fencing	Football
Cycling (stationary)	Skating (ice)	Gymnastics	Jogging
Cycling (road)	Skiing (cross-country)	Handball	Soccer
Dancing (ballroom)	Skiing (downhill)	Hockey	Volleyball
Dancing (square)	Stationary skiing	Rock climbing	
Golf	Tennis (doubles)	Roller skating	
Hiking		Singles tennis	
Shuffleboard		Squash/racquetball	
Swimming		Weight lifting	
Walking (normal)		Weight machines	
Walking (speed)			

Data from Healy WL, Sharma S, Schwartz B, et al. Athletic activity after total joint arthroplasty. J Bone Joint Surg Am 2008;90:2245-2252, based upon a survey of expert members of the Knee Society, conducted in 2005. The survey was based on expert opinion, not evidence. The trend for increasing athletic activity after total knee arthroplasty is based on improved outcomes, improvements in surgical technique, and innovations in joint implants.

BOX 28-2	Sport Participation Recommendations after Hip Arthroplasty		
Allowed	**Allowed with Experience**	**No Consensus**	**Not Recommended**
Bowling	Cross-country skiing	Fencing	Basketball
Canoeing	Downhill skiing	Baseball	Football
Cycling (stationary)	Horseback riding	Gymnastics	Jogging
Cycling (road)	Ice skating	Handball	Soccer
Dancing (ballroom)	Rowing	Hockey	
Dancing (square)	Stationary skiing	Rock climbing	
Golf	Tennis (doubles)	Squash/racquetball	
Hiking	Weight lifting	Singles tennis	
Shuffleboard	Weight machines	Volleyball	
Swimming			
Walking (normal)			
Walking (speed)			

Data from Healy WL, Sharma S, Schwartz B, et al. Athletic activity after total joint arthroplasty. J Bone Joint Surg Am 2008;90:2245-2252, based upon a survey of expert members of the Hip Society, conducted in 2005. The survey was based on expert opinion, not evidence. The trend for increasing athletic activity after total hip arthroplasty is based on improved outcomes, improvements in surgical technique, and innovations in joint implants.

higher potential for traumatic injury than those with lower levels of activity.[50] The return to sport after total joint arthroplasty typically takes about 6 months[50] and remains controversial based on the sport and the athlete. Return to sport is guided by the surgical procedure (minimally invasive vs. traditional approaches), surgeon recommendations, and previous participation in athletic activity. Box 28-2 illustrates current recommendations, based on expert opinion, for return to sport after total joint arthroplasty for a wide variety of sports.[50] Surgeons and therapists have a responsibility to recommend activities that promote long-term durability and health of the prosthesis, and unfortunately there is little hard evidence on which to base recommendations.[2,50] The astute therapist will provide an individualized plan for return to activity based on all factors surrounding the surgery and any postoperative movement dysfunction.

MOVEMENT DYSFUNCTION AND ASSESSMENT IN THE SENIOR ATHLETE

The examination of the active older adult should begin with awareness of aging changes and high expectations for performance. For example, an awareness of fitness norms for specific tasks will help the therapist determine an individual's fitness level. Currently, there are several norm-referenced tests for older adults. These include the Senior Fitness Test, YMCA fitness test, and ACSM fitness tests. The use of norm-referenced, functional skill–based tests is advocated because of the limitations of testing impairments that may or may not relate to the functional skill needed. Generally speaking, the aging athlete is examined in the same method as his or her younger athletic peer. A sport- or movement-specific examination is imperative to understanding the contributions of athletic activity to functional limitations or pain. Motion, related to and produced by all the neuromusculoskeletal contributions of the human body, although variable by age remains the prerequisite for function.

Traditional rehabilitation approaches used with athletes are often based on identification of inflamed tissues (and subsequent symptomatic treatment of those tissues) rather than on the correction of the mechanical cause of the tissue irritation. The symptom-based approach makes the assumption that the painful tissue is the source of the pain and subsequent dysfunction. Although clinicians are trained to examine both the local area of complaint and the whole patient, typically the sequence of assessment is specific to general, with the examination focused on reproducing the athlete's pain. For example, if a senior athlete complained of knee pain, the clinician typically would first observe and evaluate the knee, attempting to provoke the senior athlete's complaint. Following this, the clinician might ask the patient to perform some general movements of function. By looking at the knee first, an opportunity was missed to watch the body move as a whole and lost is the overall perspective of what the athlete can functionally achieve. All too often clinicians become too focused on the special tests that serve to confirm a pathologic diagnosis that they fail to refine, qualify, and quantify the functional parameters of the problem at hand. Reversing the sequence of assessment by examining gross movements before looking at component impairments, the therapist may determine where to focus specific assessment. By taking this approach, gross movements may provoke or reveal symptoms in the problem area as well as in other areas. Observing functional movements that the patient is able or unable to perform and those that produce pain may provide a clearer picture of the cause of the problem. One exception to initiating the examination using functional movements is the presence of chemical pain, that is, acute postsurgical or postinjury inflammation. Pain or inflammation of chemical origin is capable of influencing and producing movement dysfunction. Initial treatment emphasis would be directed locally in order to mediate the problem prior to a complete functional examination.

THE SELECTIVE FUNCTIONAL MOVEMENT ASSESSMENT

Mobility and stability coexist to create efficient movement in the human body. Mobility and stability are the fundamental building blocks of strength, endurance,

speed, power, and agility and therefore of all athletic activities. When these building blocks are decreased, the older athlete may compensate quality and therefore develop altered biomechanical habits to allow continued performance of an activity. When required movements are changed to accommodate less than optimal musculoskeletal integrity, negative changes and compensations such as altered joint arthrokinematics can occur.[51] Accommodations to altered mobility and stability can produce inefficiency and thus require more energy, resulting in an increased chance of poor performance, pain and likelihood of injury, especially with years of accumulation of these accommodations combined with the aging changes of the musculoskeletal system.

The Selective Functional Movement Assessment (SFMA) is one way of quantifying the qualitative assessment of functional movement and is not a substitute for the traditional examination process. Rather, the SFMA is the first step in the functional orthopedic examination process, which serves to focus and direct choices made during the remaining portions of the exam, which are pertinent to the functional needs of the older athlete. The SFMA uses functional movement patterns to identify impairments that potentially alter specific functional movements. The approach taken with the SFMA places less emphasis on identifying the source of the symptoms and more on identifying the cause. An example of this assessment scheme is illustrated with a runner who presents with low back pain. Frequently, the symptoms associated with the low back pain are not examined in light of other secondary causes such as hip mobility. Lack of mobility at the hip is compensated for by increased mobility or instability of the spine. The global approach taken by the SFMA would identify the cause of the low back dysfunction.

The authors believe that it is important to start with a whole-body, functional approach such as the SFMA prior to specific impairment assessments to direct the evaluation in a systematic and constructive manner. Traditional muscle length and strength as well as special tests are used subsequently to help the clinician identify the impairments associated with the dysfunctional movement. In the case of a senior athlete, functional ability involves participation in sport at their desired level: fitness, recreational, or competitive.

The functional assessment process emphasizes the analysis of function to restore proper movement of specific physical tasks.[51] Use of movement patterns with the application of specific stresses and overpressure serve to determine if dysfunction and/or pain are elicited. The movement patterns will also reaffirm or redirect the focus of the musculoskeletal problem. Maintaining or restoring proper movement of specific segments is a key to preventing or correcting musculoskeletal pain.[51] The SFMA also identifies where functional exercise may be beneficial and also provides feedback regarding the effectiveness of such exercise. A functional approach to exercise utilizes key specific movements that are common to the senior athlete regardless of the specific sport they participate in.[52] Exercise that uses repeated movement patterns required for desired function is not only realistic but practical and time efficient.[52]

The Scoring System for the SFMA

The SFMA uses seven basic movement patterns to rate and rank the two variables of pain and function. Function comprises mobility and stability (Box 28-3). The term *functional* describes any unlimited or unrestricted movement. The term *dysfunctional* describes movements that are limited or restricted in some way, demonstrating a lack of mobility, stability, or symmetry within a given movement pattern. *Painful* denotes a situation where the selective functional movement reproduces symptoms, increases symptoms, or brings about secondary symptoms that need to be noted. Therefore, each pattern of the SFMA must be scored with one of four possible outcomes.

The seven basic movements or motions that comprise the basic SFMA screen look simple but require good flexibility and control. An older athlete who is (1) unable to perform a movement correctly, (2) shows a major limitation with one or more of the movement patterns, or (3) demonstrates an obvious difference between the left and right side of the body has exposed a significant

finding that may be the key to correcting the problem.[51] The seven basic movements of the SFMA are listed in and further explained in Table 28-3. Each movement is performed first in the loaded position and then in the unloaded position if dysfunction is observed in the loaded position (Figures 28-9 to 28-16).

The first five movements examine a combination of upper quarter, lower quarter, and trunk movements. The shoulder and cervical assessments examine upper quarter movement quality. Each movement is graded with a notation of FN, FP, DP, or DN (see Box 28-3). All responses other than FN are then assessed in greater detail to help refine the movement information and direct the clinical testing. Detailed algorithmic SFMA breakouts are available for each of the movement patterns, but it is beyond the scope of this chapter to describe. Once dysfunction and/or symptoms have been provoked in a functional manner, it is necessary to work backward to more specific assessments of the component parts of the functional movement by using special tests or range-of-motion comparisons. As the gross functional movement is broken down into component parts, the therapist should examine for consistencies and inconsistencies as well as level of dysfunction for each test as compared to the optimal movement pattern. Provocation of symptoms as well as limitations in movement or the inability to maintain stability during movements should be noted. Biomechanical adaptations producing dysfunctional patterns are common in aging persons but should be considered having rehabilitation potential.

Loaded and Unloaded Implications. By performing parts of the test movements in both loaded and unloaded conditions, the clinician can draw conclusions about the interplay between the older adult's available mobility and stability. If any of the first five movements are restricted when performed in the loaded position (e.g., limited, and/or in some way painful prior to the end of the range of motion [ROM]) a clue is provided regarding functional movement. For example, if a movement is performed easily (does not provoke symptoms or have any limitation) in an unloaded situation it would seem logical that the appropriate joint ROM and muscle flexibility exist and therefore a stability problem may be the cause of why the patient cannot perform the movement in a loaded position. In this case, a patient has the requisite available biomechanical ability to go through the necessary ROM to perform the task, but the neurophysiological response needed for stabilization that creates dynamic alignment and postural support is not available when the functional movement is performed.

If the patient is observed to have a limitation, restriction, and pain when unloaded, the patient displays consistent abnormal biomechanical behavior of one or more joints and therefore would require specific clinical assessment of each relevant joint and muscle complex to

BOX 28-3	Scoring System for the SFMA, Based upon Function and Pain Reproduction
Label of Outcome of Pattern Performance	**Description of Outcome**
Functional nonpainful (FN)	Unlimited, unrestricted movement that is performed without pain or increased symptoms
Functional painful (FP)	Unlimited, unrestricted movement that reproduces or increases symptoms or brings on secondary symptoms
Dysfunctional painful (DP)	Movement that is limited or restricted in some way, demonstrating lack of mobility, stability, or symmetry, that reproduces or increases symptoms, or brings on secondary symptoms
Dysfunctional nonpainful (DN)	Movement that is limited or restricted in some way, demonstrating lack of mobility, stability, or symmetry that is performed without pain or increased symptoms

SFMA, Selective Functional Movement Assessment.

TABLE 28-3	The Seven SFMA Tests		
The Top-Tier Tests	**Test Description**	**Reason for Test**	**Scoring Criteria**
1. Multisegmental flexion (Figure 28-9)	Toe touch maneuver: • Stand with feet together and toes pointing forward. • Bend forward from the hips and try to touch the ends of the fingers to the tips of the toes, without bending the knees.	Tests for normal flexion of the hips, spine, and length of the muscles of the lower back and legs.	Touches toes without bending knees Posterior weight shift of pelvis Uniform spinal curve No lateral spinal bend
2. Multisegmental extension (Figure 28-10)	Overhead UE reach with concurrent spine and hip extension: • Stand with feet together and toes pointing forward. • Raise the arms directly overhead with arms extended, trying to get the elbows in line with the ears. • Bend backward as far as possible making sure the hips go forward and the arms go backward at the same time.	Tests for normal extension in the UEs, hips, and spine.	Arms extend to clear the ears. Anterior superior iliac spine moves anterior over the toes. Spine of the scapula moves posterior and clears the heels. Symmetrical spinal curves.
3. Multisegmental rotation (R & L) (Figure 28-11)	Total body rotation: • Stand with the feet together, toes pointing forward, and the arms abducted away from the sides. • Rotate the entire body as far as possible to the right, using LE, trunk and cervical rotation, remaining upright (no extension). • Return to the starting position and repeat to the left.	This maneuver tests for normal rotational mobility in the neck, trunk, pelvis, hips, knees, and feet.	Pelvis rotates >50 degrees. Trunk rotates >50 degrees. No loss of body height or extension of trunk. Symmetrical motion to the right and left.
4. Single-limb stance (R & L) (Figure 28-12)	Single-limb balance test: • Stabilize on one leg with the contralateral LE flexed to 90 degrees, attempt to hold for 10 s, eyes open • Repeat on opposite limb • Repeat with the eyes closed, attempt to hold for 10 s	This is used to evaluate the patient's ability to effectively stabilize on each leg independently for 10 s.	Eyes open >10 s Eyes closed >10 s Level pelvis (no Trendelenburg) No loss of height
5. Overhead deep squat (Figure 28-13)	Stand to squat activity: • Stand with feet shoulder width apart and toes facing straight ahead • Raise the UEs above the head and hold slightly wider than the feet • Instruct patient to squat all the way down while keeping the hands above the head. • Patient should be cued to perform a full deep squat with the heels remaining on the ground and the hands above their head without pain or discomfort.	This maneuver is used to assess bilateral mobility of the hips, knees, and ankles. When combined with the hands held overhead, this test also assesses bilateral mobility of the shoulders as well as extension of the thoracic spine.	Thighs break parallel, >90 degrees flexion. Hands stay over the feet (do not progress anterior). Feet point forward. Weight is evenly distributed between the two LEs.
6. UE movement patterns A. Medial rotation with extension (Figure 28-14, A) B. Lateral rotation with flexion (Figure 28-15)	A. Back scratch B. Back patting	A. Assesses medial rotation, extension, and adduction of the shoulder. B. Assesses lateral rotation, flexion, and abduction of the shoulder.	Compare both sides and look for gross imbalances from right to left.

TABLE 28-3	The Seven SFMA Tests—cont'd		
The Top-Tier Tests	**Test Description**	**Reason for Test**	**Scoring Criteria**
Clearing tests: A. Impingement sign (Figure 28-14B) B. Horizontal adduction	Provocation tests to look for glenohumeral impingement, instability, capsular tightness, and AC joint pathology.	Impingement test: This pattern looks for impingement and a functional instability problem of the glenohumeral joint. Horizontal adduction: This pattern looks for AC joint problems, anterior impingement, and posterior capsule tightness.	Is pain reproduced?
7. Cervical movement patterns (Figure 28-16)	Flexion and extension motions alone, plus a combined motion of flexion, side bending, and rotation (performed bilaterally).	Cervical spine clearing for ranges of motion and muscular extensibility, bilaterally.	*A—Chin to chest:* Limited movement can indicate a reduced capacity of the short neck flexors and may also indicate reduced mobility. Chin should touch sternum without pain. *B—Face to ceiling:* This move evaluates the amount of cervical spine extension available. Face should extend to within 10 degrees of parallel without pain. *C—Chin to shoulders:* This move is a combination pattern that incorporates side-bending and rotation. Normal range is midclavicle bilaterally without pain. (Mouth should stay closed).

AC, acromioclavicular; *LE,* lower extremity; *SFMA,* selective functional movement assessment; UE, upper extremity.

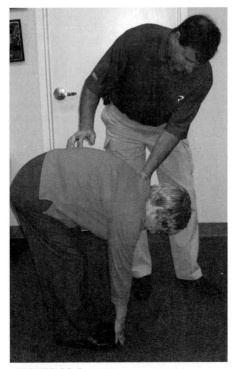

FIGURE 28-9 Multisegmental flexion test.

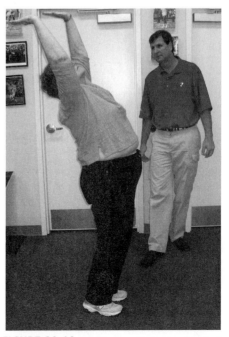

FIGURE 28-10 Multisegmental extension test.

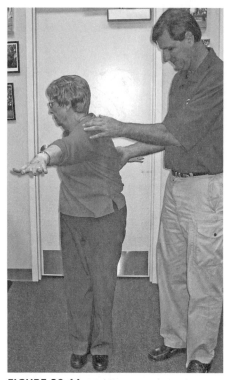

FIGURE 28-11 Multisegmental rotation test.

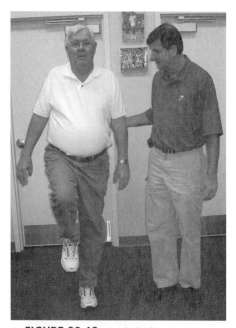

FIGURE 28-12 Single-limb stance test.

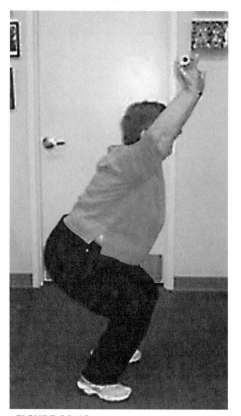

FIGURE 28-13 Overhead deep squat test.

How to Interpret the SFMA

As mentioned earlier, each movement pattern should be ranked and rated according to Box 28-3. The criteria listed in Box 28-4 help to give qualitative analysis to the four possible descriptors (FN, FP, DP, DN).

Once the SFMA has been completed, the therapist should be able to do the following: (1) Identify the major sources of dysfunction and movements that are affected. (2) Identify patterns of movement that cause pain where reproduction of pain indicates either mechanical deformation or an inflammatory process affecting the nociceptors in the symptomatic structures. The key follow-up question must be "Which of the functional movements caused the tissue to become painful?" (3) Once the pattern of dysfunction has been identified, the problem is classified as either a mobility or stability dysfunction, determine where intervention should commence.

With the SFMA, the choice of treatment is not about alleviating mechanical pain; rather the SFMA guides the therapist in choosing interventions designed to improve the dysfunctional nonpainful patterns first. This philosophy of intervention does not ignore the source of pain; rather, it takes the approach of removing the mechanical dysfunction that causes the tissues to become symptomatic in the first place.

Pain-free functional movement is the goal of healthy aging. Pain-free functional movement necessary to

identify the barriers that restrict movement and that may be responsible for the provocation of pain. Consistent limitation and provocation of symptoms in both the loaded and unloaded conditions may be indicative of a mobility problem.[51] True mobility restrictions often require appropriate manual therapy in conjunction with corrective exercise.

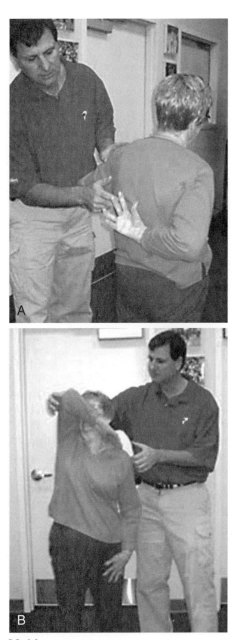

FIGURE 28-14 **A,** Medial rotation test. **B,** Impingement pain reproduction test.

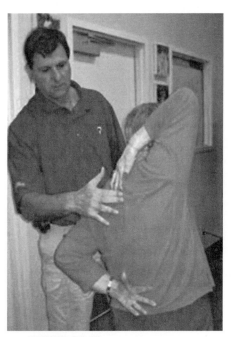

FIGURE 28-15 Lateral rotation test.

allow participation in sports is composed of many components: posture, ROM, muscle performance, and motor control. Impairments in any of these components can potentially alter required functional movement. The therapeutic plan of care needs to be focused on the athletes' functional impairments that are a result and/or cause of pathology. The clinician can then use the traditional parts of the clinical examination to refine and deduce the specific pathoanatomic structures responsible for the functional limitation. The authors believe the SFMA, though untested in research literature, incorporates the essential elements of many sports activities and provides a schema for addressing movement-related dysfunction. More information can be obtained at www.functionalmovement.com.

GENERAL REHABILITATION CONSIDERATIONS FOR THE SENIOR ATHLETE

The rehabilitation of injuries sustained by older athletes is approached in a similar manner to comparable problems in younger athletes. In our experience, older athletes respond well to treatment, but recovery takes longer as rate of tissue repair slows with age[4,18,36] and which may result in more residual dysfunction. For example, when compared to a 20-year-old, a 60-year-old athlete may require double the time and an athlete older than age 75 years may require three times as long to return to sport.[4,18] This does not, however, diminish the motivation to return to sport, and the rehabilitation provider must remember to treat the injury, not the "age." Many aspects of intervention common to the younger athlete can be generalized to the older athlete, but several unique differences inherent to the aging athlete must be addressed and are described next.

Pathologies related to normal consequences of aging as well as residual injuries affect older athletes' response to training and rehabilitation.[18] Systemic disease, degenerative disease, and previous injury can have a significant impact on athletic performance in the older adult and will likely influence the choice of athletic activity. Systemic diseases whose incidence increases with age include cardiovascular disease and diabetes. Exercise has been shown to have a generally positive effect on these diseases.[7,17,32,45,53] The therapist needs to be aware of the kinds of screening necessitated by the presence of systemic disease. For example, aging athletes with diabetes should be carefully examined for signs of foot problems related to diminished peripheral sensation secondary to degeneration of myelin and a compromised vascular

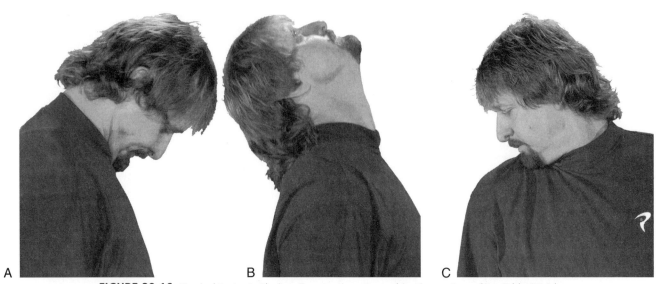

A   B   C

FIGURE 28-16 Cervical tests: **A,** Flexion; **B,** extension; **C,** combination pattern. (See Table 28-3.)

BOX 28-4	Qualitative Questions for Assessing Performance during the SFMA Tests

1. Did performance of the test produce pain? If yes, you must score DP or FP, depending on whether the pattern was performed functionally or dysfunctionally.
2. Is the pattern asymmetrical or symmetrical? If asymmetrical, you must score it a DP or DN, depending on whether pain is present.
3. For unilateral active movements, if the motion is symmetrical and equal, is the effort the athlete uses to perform the movement perceived as equal? If not, score DP or DN depending on whether pain is present.
4. Does the performance of the movement fall under the "norms" of performance, based on your clinical experience or published data? If yes, score FP or FN depending on whether pain is present.

---

system resulting from arteriosclerosis. Other factors associated with diabetes mellitus include coronary complications, kidney failure, blindness, cataracts, and muscle weakness. Blood glucose should be carefully monitored in the senior athlete with awareness of the effects of intense performance on blood glucose levels.[53]

Degenerative disease states, as previously mentioned, occur in most older individuals.[4,44,48,50] Although senior athletes may have radiographic evidence of osteoarthritis, careful physical examination is essential before the osteoarthritis can be incriminated as the cause of exercise-related symptoms. Frequently, the presence of osteoarthritis is sufficient for a physician or rehabilitation professional to attribute activity-related pain to arthritis, when in fact it may be mere coincidence that the patient's complaint is in the general area of a joint with osteoarthritis. Careful attention to the onset and mechanism of injury and the subsequent presentation of

symptoms and functional limitations will guide the rehabilitation professional in designing an appropriate plan of care, in spite of the presence of osteoarthritis. Degenerative disc disease also can be a problem in the older athlete, but again, radiographic evidence is not sufficient to ascribe symptoms to its presence. Care should be taken to carefully evaluate other possible causes of pain, such as hypomobility, inflammation, and overuse.

Impairments

Movement patterns utilized by an individual are developed by their activities, habits, hand dominance, and previous injuries. A temporary lack of activity may be the impetus for deterioration of movement patterns. A lack of variety of movements, sedentary lifestyle, prolonged static postural stress, or poor body mechanics can all lead to muscular imbalances. Overuse activities frequently lead to adaptive shortening/tightening of muscles. Disuse may lead to weakening or inhibition of muscles. A common example of inhibition is the tightening of the iliopsoas, perhaps from prolonged sitting or ineffective recruitment of the gluteus maximus leading to the neurologic inhibition of its antagonist, the gluteus maximus. Frequently, senior athletes will present with mobility dysfunction secondary to their aging musculoskeletal system. True mobility restrictions often require appropriate manual therapy in conjunction with corrective exercise. For example, evidence exists for the effectiveness for joint mobilizations addressing capsular restrictions in aging joints.[54,55] Soft tissue restrictions may be treated with manual therapy and/or stretching. The patient may be taught to perform their own soft tissue mobilizations, static or dynamic stretches, or self-mobilizations to reinforce the manual work done in the clinic (Figure 28-17). Once the patient has the mobility

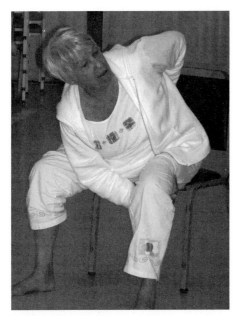

FIGURE 28-17 Seated yoga stretch for trunk rotation, performed by 87-year-old yoga practitioner, group leader.

to perform the movement, they may progress to corrective exercises.

If the problem is determined to be a stability dysfunction, frequently the clinician will need to use external stabilization techniques or teach the patient to recruit certain key stabilizing muscles before an exercise program can begin. This may include the use of taping procedures, supports or braces, PNF patterns, abdominal stabilization techniques, as well as functional corrective exercises. Senior athletes may have compromised stability because of a long history of incorrect or repetitive movements throughout their lifetime. It is never too late to teach proper movement within the confines of correct movement patterns and optimal stability. It is important to remember that mobility problems take precedence over stability problems: the clinician MUST *correct mobility deficiencies before stability*. In accordance with the SFMA guidelines, corrective exercises are initiated for those movements that are dysfunctional and nonpainful (DN) first. The chosen corrective exercise should challenge the patient, yet they should be able to perform it correctly. Incorrect performance will only further reinforce the faulty motor pattern, resulting in suboptimal outcomes.

Big Picture: Core and Balance

A brief discussion of core stability is important to excellent treatment of the senior athlete. The authors believe that many therapists overlook the importance of the trunk and its impact on efficiency of movement, yet trunk function, also known as core stability, plays a key role in returning the senior athlete to preinjury level of training and competition. When appropriate, improving the mobility, stability, and neuromuscular performance of the core prevents injury and enhances sport performance in both upper- and lower-extremity–dominant sports. Although not new, the concept of proximal stability to facilitate distal mobility is frequently overlooked in orthopedic and sports rehabilitation.

The spinal column, essentially a stack of blocks that sit atop one another, acts as the anchor for the remaining skeletal parts (the extremities). The position of the base of the spinal column along with the position of the pelvis determines to a great extent the functional position of the extremities during movement. Anterior–posterior trunk muscular balance determines pelvic position, and along with efficient neuromuscular programs of the transversus abdominis and the multifidi serve to provide a stable base on which the lower extremities can function. Trunk and pelvic muscle length, strength, and motor control should be evaluated in all athletes, and imbalances or poor performance should be addressed, attempting to see and rectify "big picture" problems relating to core imbalances or instability. This principle is especially important in the senior athlete because of the typical postural changes often exhibited in the aging population that affects balance and efficiency of movement. The authors believe that addressing core function and control in all senior athletes is important, regardless of the primary site of injury. This is especially true in the case of overuse injuries where improper biomechanical stresses may lead to dysfunction over a prolonged period of time. Balancing the musculature and "re-educating" motor programs involves a combination of many interventions, including exercises for the transverse abdominals and multifidi, teaching diaphragmatic breathing, as well as enhancing the function of the gluteals (Figures 28-18 and 28-19). Exhalation during a forceful sporting technique, such as the backhand stroke in tennis

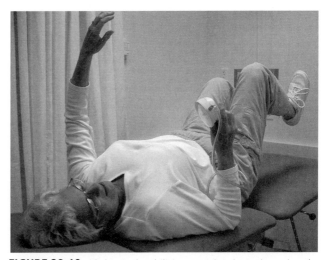

FIGURE 28-18 Abdominal stabilizing exercises in supine using the Stabilizer for biofeedback. Focus is on transversus abdominis and multifidus to stabilize against limb movement.

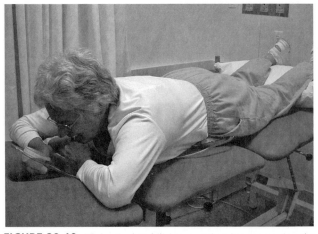

FIGURE 28-19 Abdominal stabilizing exercises in prone using the Stabilizer for biofeedback. Focus is on transversus abdominis and multifidus against limb movement.

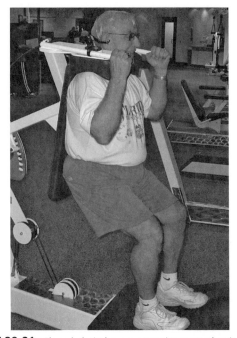

FIGURE 28-21 Closed-chain lower extremity strengthening (squat) performed by a senior athlete.

may assist the senior athlete in achieving a rigid trunk that provides a stable base on which to move.

Strength. Atrophy of skeletal muscle is a well-known consequence of aging. Muscular hypertrophy and strength is much easier to lose than to gain, and positive adaptations in skeletal muscle that occur as a result of resistance training can begin to reverse in as little as 48 hours.[56] As skeletal muscle mass decreases, an associated reduction in muscle strength and general function often occurs. Muscular resistive training programs have been a cornerstone of fitness and wellness regimens used by athletes regardless of age, and may be especially important as they have been shown to prevent or partially reverse age-related muscular atrophy (Figures 28-20 and 28-21).[18,22,23,27,29,57,58] Such programs serve as an important method to maintain lean body mass and combat the typical decrease in lean–fat body mass ratios that occur during aging. Strength and lean body mass typically peak in the third decade of life, and subsequently decline thereafter as a normal consequence of aging.

How much of this muscular strength decline is related to inactivity and can be prevented by consistent, well-targeted progressive resistive training? Collectively, the available literature supports that muscular hypertrophy and strength increases between 7% and 174% with resistance training depending on training dose (intensity and sets), and improved neural or functional adaptations occur similarly in young and older individuals.[58-61] The exact method by which strength training influences sarcopenia remains controversial, and could be related to whole muscle factors (mass, hypertrophy) or myocellular level qualities.[27] Skeletal muscle plasticity and subsequent response to training markedly diminishes after the age of 80 years, and therefore Raue et al suggested that all older individuals should engage in resistance training in the sixth and seventh decades in order to maintain and gain muscular mass to remain functional into the eighth and ninth decades.[27] Senior athletes are best served by being directed to maintain a muscular resistance training program as an integral part of their training.

Stretching. Injury prevention has always been an integral part of sports physical therapy. Flexibility decreases with age, and this may affect tissue tolerance of the many demands of a wide variety of sporting activities. Because even a minor injury can lead to a dramatic decrease in the senior athlete's sports participation, prevention is extraordinarily important for the senior athlete. There is moderate to strong evidence that the routine application of static stretching does not reduce overall injury rates, and preliminary evidence that it may positively affect the rates of musculotendinous injury.[62,63] Improper or inconsistent stretching techniques, for

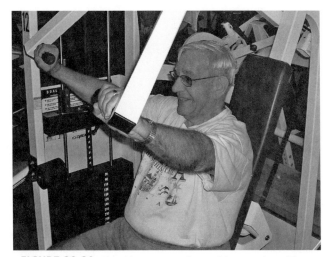

FIGURE 28-20 Shoulder press performed by a senior athlete.

example, ballistic techniques, can cause muscle strains and soreness, especially in the aging athlete whose flexibility is decreasing. Although it may not be harmful, statically stretching a cold muscle is not as efficient as stretching a warm muscle. There is some evidence for the necessity of holding a static stretch for 60 seconds in older persons as compared with 30 seconds in younger persons (Figure 28-22).[64]

Warm-Up. In the opinion of the authors, there is no substitute for an adequate warm-up by senior athletes before exercise. Athletes who have always avoided this aspect of training find it increasingly essential as they age. The best warm-up for a specific activity is 10 to 15 minutes of low-intensity engagement in that activity in order to increase intramuscular temperature of the requisite muscles.[62,65] For example, if tennis is the activity, then the players should begin by total body movements for warm-up, progress to hitting balls across the net, slowly at first and then with increased velocity and movement. If running is the activity, the runner should begin the few minutes walking and progressing to an easy jog, gradually picking up speed. This rule is easily generalized to other sports.

Warm-up is often confused with stretching. Although stretching may be a component of the warm-up for some athletes, stretching can be as much of a problem as it can help, and outcomes of the research exploring the effects of preparticipation stretching are mixed. Muscle can be adequately warmed by the previously mentioned warm-up techniques, and the authors suggest that older athletes engage in more global activities to warm the muscles before stretching or, even better, to incorporate stretching into their cool-down routine. As a rule of thumb, athletes who have always stretched before exercise should not be discouraged from doing so. In general,

low-velocity, nonballistic stretching is best for the muscles and soft tissues of the aging athlete. Stretching in functional patterns and with low-velocity sport-specific movements may be helpful to prepare for athletic activity. It seems logical to suggest stretching as a remedy for the flexibility changes that occur with aging. However, it should be noted that the reason for the loss of flexibility or range of motion with aging may be less a result of soft tissue tightness and more a result of joint changes. Some changes include joint surface deterioration, breakdown of the collagen fibers, and a decrease in the viscosity of synovial fluid. In these cases, stretching may not be particularly helpful.

Sport-Specific Training and the SAID Principle

Two important and closely related concepts are sport-specific training (SST) and the specific adaptations to imposed demands (SAID) principle.[66] SST is defined as training that consists of stretching, strengthening, and aerobic or anaerobic conditioning that is targeted to optimally prepare an athlete for his or her chosen sport.[67] SAID principle uses similar thinking and applies specificity of training by imposing demands on the athlete that simulate or reinforce his or her sport. "Demands" that can be incorporated include speed of motions, sport patterns, or specific exercise movements in the context of the athlete's chosen sport. Both principles require the therapist to understand and "impose" correct demands on athletes, no matter their age, in order to return them to sport. Therefore, careful selection of the proper interventions will allow the therapist to best prepare an athlete for return. The SFMA relates well to both the SAID principle and the SST principles. By using the fundamental movements inherent to the SFMA to identify impaired movement patterns, the therapist will be led directly to specific interventions that promote improved functional abilities. Each of these fundamental movements provides a glimpse into foundational movement patterns on which ADLs and athletic ability are constructed. An excellent example of this is the deep squat maneuver. Many ADLs and athletic movements incorporate squatting motions (unilateral or bilateral) in their performance. If the deep squat test is impaired, at a low level, sit-to-stand function is impaired, and at a higher level, jumping or propulsion would be impaired.

The Drive to Compete and Remain Active

"Muscle mass declines, but determination doesn't"[2] depicts the senior athletes' amazing desire to continue training and competing in their chosen sport. The physical therapist must understand and acknowledge this fact and realize that although senior athletes may take longer to rehabilitate, their eagerness to return to sport is no

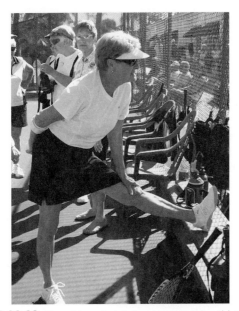

FIGURE 28-22 Hamstring stretch in senior tennis athlete. Note: This athlete has had bilateral total knee replacements.

different from their younger counterparts. This philosophical approach is vital for those who work with senior athletes and attempt to return them to their chosen levels of function. Senior athletes use training and competition for maintenance of fitness, "enjoyment of the competition,"[52] and to achieve their age-related peak performance.[17] The best outcomes and most satisfied athletes will occur when physical therapists honor the senior athlete's motivation and drive to compete.

SPORT-SPECIFIC REHABILITATION APPROACHES FOR COMMON SENIOR SPORTS

As previously described in this chapter, senior athletes are often injured in the course of training and performing their chosen endeavors. Where there are injuries there is a need for rehabilitation! Rehabilitation of the senior athlete follows the same basic guidelines as rehabilitation of a younger athlete; in fact, interventions used for younger athletes are almost always appropriate for use with older athletes, including manual therapy, therapeutic exercise, select modalities, functional retraining, and sport-specific training. Although specific treatments for every injury encountered by the senior athlete fall beyond the scope of this chapter, this section will highlight basic ideas and differences the rehabilitation provider may encounter.

Aerobic fitness is one important consideration of total fitness in all senior athletes. Walking is possibly the single most popular form of physical activity for the older individual.[35] Accessible in all geographic areas, walking provides one of the highest compliance rates, greatest benefits, and lowest risk of injury in older persons. Walking for general aerobic fitness should be a potential suggestion for exercise prescription for the older adult who is beginning or returning to exercise. It is recommended that 10,000 steps be achieved each day to achieve health benefits.[68] Several activities have been described as popular for seniors, including walking, swimming, cycling, rowing, dancing, and less commonly running.[8,35,52] In their assessment of older athletes, Matheson et al[8] described a decreased frequency of running coupled with an increase in participation in racquet sports, walking, and other low-intensity sports with age. Also, running in the older age group showed the greatest differences in gender ratios of participants, with males outnumbering females.[8] Several sports with high participation by senior athletes (running, swimming, golf, and tennis) will be specifically addressed.

Running

For those healthy, anatomically stable adults, running serves as an excellent choice for aerobic exercise, fitness, and training. Some individuals run for exercise and fitness, whereas others compete throughout a lifetime.

Natural selection related to adverse anthropometric dimensions that influence biomechanical efficiency (such as height, physique, percentage body fat, and leg alignment) and economy of movement tend to eliminate athletes from running throughout a lifetime. More specifically, taller, heavier individuals with anatomic variations such as varus or valgus angulation of the lower extremities are less likely to be able to sustain a lifetime of running.[3,8,15,47]

Running places repetitive, dramatic stresses on joints and supporting structures of the lower extremity. However, available evidence indicates that moderate running in individuals without anatomic variances poses no increased risk for development or acceleration of OA.[15,16,36,43,47,69-71] Forces transmitted through the lower extremity during the midstance phase of running gait may equal 250% to 300% of total body weight,[47] and thus the frequency of OA may be increased in joints previously injured or which have anatomic flaws.[8] Despite the debate over the traditional concept that vigorous exercise causes OA, currently no research data support the concern that athletic participation makes OA more likely.[72] In fact, strengthening exercise for the core, pelvis, hips, and thighs is widely recognized as a treatment for OA.[35,73,74]

In an 8-year longitudinal study of more than 900 subjects, Fries et al concluded that older persons who engage in vigorous running and other aerobic activities have lower mortality and slower development of disability than members of the general population. The authors also concluded that these positive benefits probably related to increased aerobic activity, increased strength, and better fitness of organ systems rather than postponed development of OA.[14] Researchers have also concluded that vigorous running activity over many years is not associated with increased musculoskeletal problems in older age and that age-related musculoskeletal disability appeared to develop at a lower rate in runners.[14,15]

Much like the previously described body systems, running performance declines with age primarily because of a decline in $\dot{V}o_2$max. Performance in a 10-km run modestly decreases in elite runners older than age 35 years, with progressively greater declines occurring after the age of 50 to 60 years.[21] Gender differences are somewhat more pronounced after the age of 45 to 49 years, with women showing greater declines in performance. This may be due to greater decline in $\dot{V}o_2$max in females, or may be an apparent difference due to selection bias represented by smaller numbers of female runners in older age groups.[32]

Runners of all ages must use proper footwear. The shoe, a powerful tool for controlling human movement and affecting the function of the lower quarter, can also prevent or contribute to injury.[14] Relative decreases in strength and flexibility that occur throughout a lifetime may contribute to decreased shock absorption by the foot in closed kinetic chain activities. When shock absorption of the foot diminishes, as is the case in many senior athletes, it is essential to have a well-designed shoe to compensate. Consequently, shoes remain the single most important piece of equipment for the runner or walker.[47]

Swimming and Aquatic Exercise

Swimming and aquatic exercise are popular modes of exercise for many aging athletes. Traditionally, the "old" swimmer is someone older than age 25 years, and as previously mentioned, masters swimming competitions are available for those older than age 19 years.[5] The advent of organized aquatic exercise programs contributes to increasing numbers of participants in water-based exercise. The discussion in this chapter focuses on the swimmer or aquatic exerciser older than age 50 years.

Aquatic-based exercise programs offer an excellent medium in which to exercise, especially in the presence of osteoarthritis. Seniors who are returning to exercise after not exercising for a time may be attracted to the water-based exercise classes common in fitness clubs. These classes offer an excellent method for the achievement and maintenance of general fitness. The buoyancy of the water allows for aerobic training with decreased weight bearing and overuse to the joints of the lower extremities and spine. Nevertheless, injuries occur in this type of exercise. Exercising in a pool with a subtle transition from shallow to deeper levels may produce a functional leg length discrepancy in the senior athlete. The leg closer to the deeper end of the pool functions at a slight disadvantage, and the ankle must plantarflex to a greater degree than the leg closer to the shallow end, thereby increasing the plantarflexion stresses. Prevention and treatment of this injury requires proper warm-up and cool-down, with emphasis on stretching of the gastrocnemius and soleus. Use of specialized aquatic footwear and exercising on a level pool surface are recommended.

When an athlete uses lap swimming for exercise or ongoing training for swimming or triathlon competitions, it is likely that sometime in their career they have experienced shoulder pain or dysfunction. Many young and older swimmers alike experience conditions of overuse of the shoulder complex. Sixty percent of elite swimmers and probably a greater percentage of subelite swimmers experience the condition referred to as "swimmer's shoulder."[30,75] Swimmer's shoulder, a nonspecific diagnosis, refers to several pathologies including but not limited to pain in the anterior aspect of the shoulder, likely because of inflammation of the subacromial bursa, the tendons of the rotator cuff, and the long head of the biceps.[30,75] Rarely is bursitis a primary condition; rather, it is frequently related to tendinitis.[75] In younger swimmers, rotator cuff tendinitis and impingement is often

secondary to glenohumeral instability,[76] whereas in older swimmers, the same pathologies are more likely due to hypomobility and stiffness of the glenohumeral joint or thoracic spine or insufficient steering provided by dynamic stabilizing musculature of the scapulothoracic joint.

Glenohumeral pain and impingement/tendinitis symptoms often plague swimmers, secondary to the greater force per stroke placed on the shoulder complex in sprinters and secondary to fatigue in distance swimmers. Because sprint swimming is used less frequently for training in most senior swimmers, injury often presents when training volume increases. As volume increases, fatigue is likely to take its toll, and technique often suffers. Common technique errors include decreased body roll and improper arm position during the recovery phase of the "freestyle" (both forward and backward) stroke. Both of these training errors frequently contribute to shoulder complex dysfunction. The freestyle stroke requires adequate glenohumeral flexion/extension motion, concurrent with adequate spinal rotation and extension.

The freestyle stroke, most commonly used for distance and recreational training, is broken down into four phases of movement (Figure 28-23): (1) hand entry into the water and early pull-through, (2) late pull-through, (3) early recovery, and (4) late recovery. The latissimus dorsi and the pectoralis major muscles serve to propel the body over the arm, the pectoralis working primarily during early pull-through and the latissimus working during late pull-through. The primary muscles used during recovery are the middle deltoid, supraspinatus, and infraspinatus. The arm abducts and externally rotates as the swimmer draws it out of the water. The serratus anterior is also very active during the recovery phase. The scapula must go from full protraction at hand entry to full retraction at the transition between late pull-through and early recovery phase. The subscapularis and serratus anterior remain active throughout all phases of the freestyle stroke, and prevention of anterior shoulder impingement is directly related to proper scapular mobility and dynamic positioning.[77]

Body roll during the freestyle stroke is described as transverse plane movement of the body in relation to the horizon. Normal body roll during the freestyle stroke is between 70 and 100 degrees.[77] Body roll allows for easier recovery of the arm as it draws out of the water as well as offering improved mechanical advantage to the opposite shoulder during pull-through in the water. The less the body roll, the greater the abduction required of the glenohumeral joint during recovery. Diminished body roll due to fatigue during training or insufficient glenohumeral range of motion may affect the swimmer by placing greater stresses on the shoulder complex. In short, the better the maintenance of shoulder complex range of motion and flexibility, the less the body roll is needed. Therefore, stretching of the glenohumeral joint and

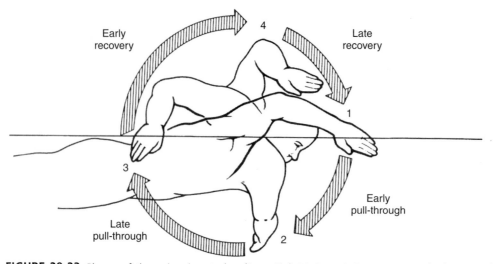

FIGURE 28-23 Phases of the swimming stroke. *(From Pink M, Perry J, Browne A, et al: The normal shoulder during freestyle swimming. Am J Sports Med 19:569-576, 1991.)*

scapulothoracic articulations are important in training as well as injury prevention. Of critical importance are the muscles that tend to become tight due to postural shortening, the latissimus dorsi and internal rotators.[30,75]

The major movement of shoulder adduction and internal rotation provides powerful propulsion during the pull-through phase. These two movements, if occurring in excess, place the anterior shoulder in a closed down position, thus making the subacromial space smaller, causing the potential for increased impingement. Coaching the technique modification of "high elbow position" can minimize this impingement force. As the arm draws down from an overhead position during recovery, the proximal arm adducts in a plane nearly parallel to an imaginary line connecting both shoulders, allowing for maximal force generation without excessive impingement on the anterior shoulder. The high elbow position is also important during the mid–recovery phase because it limits excessive abduction at the glenohumeral joint, thereby shortening the lever arm and decreasing torque at the joint.[30,77]

The side predominantly used for breathing is most often affected with rotator cuff dysfunction. The decrease in spinal and glenohumeral range of motion and flexibility noted in the aging swimmer are frequent contributing factors. As the senior athlete loses rotational flexibility of the cervical, thoracic, and lumbar spines, they actually have to increase the reliance on body roll to maintain the ability to breathe, thereby stressing the shoulder on the side toward which the breath is taken. In the senior swimmer with cervical osteoarthritis, range-of-motion limitations, or pain, the use of a mask and snorkel may allow the athlete to continue swimming and decrease the stresses on the neck and shoulder. The use of the snorkel allows the swimmer to maintain a neutral,

facedown position, avoiding the cervical rotation necessary for breathing.

Rehabilitation of the senior swimmer's shoulder complex must go beyond the traditional shoulder girdle stretching, strengthening, and use of modalities for pain control and reduction of the inflammatory response. Rehabilitation must focus on the biomechanical faults and improper training techniques commonly used by the senior swimmer. Range-of-motion and stretching exercises specific to any tight muscle group of diminished motion is important. Strengthening of the appropriate muscles should be performed in the position that mimics the swimming stroke. For example, strengthening of the supraspinatus should be performed in a position that replicates the recovery phase, as compared to a standing, arm at the side position. Strength and endurance exercises should focus on dynamic positioning of the scapula and thoracic spine for the different stroke phases. Cervical, thoracic, and lumbar trunk rotation coordinates with arm and leg movements necessary for proper body roll. Stabilization and power generation from the pelvic and trunk regions is also important, requiring adequate spinal positioning and control. Senior swimmers often position themselves in the position of anterior pelvic tilt, thus increasing thoracic kyphosis and closing down the anterior shoulder during all stroke phases. The physical therapist must be astute at instructing the athlete in how to position the pelvis in neutral, stabilize it there by using small local musculature, and activate the global muscles to achieve propulsion and body roll. The therapist must be ready to evaluate the stroke technique of the senior swimmer with regard to elbow position during recovery, arm position during other phases of the stroke, as well as breathing technique.

Some common training errors include the improper use of fins, hand paddles, and kick boards. Many senior swimmers bring training techniques and equipment from their younger years that may be too much stress for the aging body.[38] The use of fins may be encouraged, as they allow the senior swimmer to improve their upper extremity technique due to the increased swimming speed offered by the fins. Fins are also helpful in building strength in the lower extremities due to the longer lever arm and increased resistance they provide. The use of fins by the senior athlete is contraindicated in the presence of remarkable weakness or knee pain. The long lever arm may cause increased transmission of forces to the knee, overpowering weak musculature or exacerbate an already painful condition by overloading a biomechanically stressed joint (osteoarthritis or meniscal injury). The use of upper extremity training devices such as hand paddles or webbed gloves should be discouraged because of the increased resistance they offer while pulling the arm/hand through the water. This may contribute to the development of impingement. Finally, if a senior athlete is using a kickboard for a lower extremity workout, or to rest the upper extremities, it should be placed under the chest or near the face in order to avoid the outstretched upper extremity position, which occurs when the board is placed above the head. Positioning the kickboard above the head with outstretched arms and palms flat on the board places the shoulders in a fully flexed and internally rotated position, thereby increasing the pressure on the anterior shoulder.

Golf

The rapid growth of the game of golf, especially in the over-50 age group, attests to the need for knowledge in treating the older golfer. The senior golfer has the time and often the disposable income necessary to play golf and enjoys golf as a form of recreation and exercise; thus, he or she will be a principal player in using the golf courses and purchasing equipment (Figure 28-24).[78]

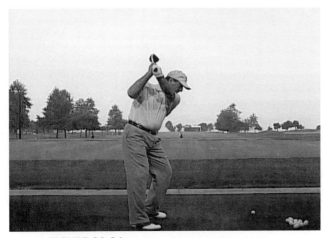

FIGURE 28-24 Senior golfer, top of backswing.

In male amateur golfers, the lower back is the most commonly injured area, followed by the lateral elbow, hand and wrist, shoulder, and knee. Women most commonly injure the lateral elbow, followed by the back, shoulder, hand and wrist, and knee.[37] These injuries are generally of the repetitive kind. Repetitive practice, related to volume, ranks as the most common cause of injury in the amateur golfer, followed by poor swing mechanics. Both professional and amateur golfers believe that their injuries (as mentioned earlier in frequency) were caused by stresses occurring near the impact phase of the golf swing as compared to microtraumatic causes.[78]

Understanding the dynamics of potential injury helps locate areas of preventive maintenance. The golf swing, probably the most researched sporting technique in the literature and equipment manufacturing industry, is described in five stages: (1) setup, (2) backswing, (3) transition, (4) downswing, and (5) follow-through. All phases of the golf swing impact the production of a successful, accurate shot strategically placed to set up the next shot to the hole.

Although swing styles vary (Jim Furyk vs. Ernie Els), and swing philosophies and teaching methods differ (Natural Golf vs. Stack-N-Tilt), ball flight is based on several physical variables: club face angle, club path, club angle of attack, solidness of ball impact, and club head speed. No two golfers on the PGA tour have the same swing style, yet they are all successful. Different golfers have different swing capabilities based on their physical structure and physical capabilities. Therefore, instead of focusing on swing style, it is more important to determine the efficiency of the particular swing. This is especially important for the senior golfer. The question is not how similar a swing is to a professional on video analysis; rather the question should be "How efficient is the swing compared to a known standard (derived from analysis of the best golfers in the world)?" Data collected from three-dimensional motion analysis systems have determined how golfers generate speed and transfer this speed or energy throughout their bodies, using a certain sequence in order to transmit this speed to the club head. This is called the "kinematic sequence." The amazing thing is that all great ball strikers have the same kinematic sequence or the same signature motion by which they generate speed and transfer that speed throughout their body. During the downswing in golf all body segments must accelerate and decelerate in the correct sequence with precise and specific timing so that the club arrives at impact accurately and with maximal speed. The correct sequence of motion for the major segments is pelvis, trunk, arms, and finally club. This motion must occur sequentially, with each peak speed being faster but later than the previous one. This sequence reflects an efficient transfer of energy across each joint and facilitates an increase in energy from the proximal segment to the distal one. The muscles of each joint produce this increase in energy. On the other hand, if the timing of energy transfer is wrong, energy can be dissipated instead of added and as a result, speed will be lost. Also if one body part has to compensate because another is not doing its job, then injury may result.

There are three things that have been shown to create efficiency or kinematic sequence breakdowns: (1) improper swing mechanics, (2) physical limitations, and (3) improperly fit equipment. Determination of the senior golfer's physical capabilities and limitations is therefore critical in establishing a swing that is efficient and prevents injury. The SFMA, mentioned earlier in this chapter, is an integral part of the physical therapist's exam to determine these physical limitations. It is also important to work closely with a respected golf professional for correction of swing mechanics and equipment.

Critical zones of stress during the golf swing exist in the trunk and impact the extremities during the different phases of the swing (Figure 28-25). The critical zones of restriction of mobility include the cervical region, upper quarter, trunk (especially the thoracic spine and ribs), and the proximal lower quarter. These zones undergo shear, lateral bending, compression, and torsional forces and must have the ability to change directions quickly and smoothly. Golfers who use proper warm-up and maintain fitness during their golf participation are less likely to have injury to these critical zones. Those who do not are more likely to sustain an overuse injury, especially as their connective tissues become stiffer with age.

Although many senior golfers undergo a total hip or knee replacement, return to golf is often a primary goal. A survey of orthopedic surgeons in the Hip Society and Knee Society revealed that no respondent to the survey in the Hip Society felt that a total hip replacement prevented patients from playing golf. Of those responding to the survey in the Knee Society, 93% felt that a total knee replacement did not hinder playing golf.[24] Most seniors resume full golf at 3 to 4 months after surgery, but medical professionals advise them to start slowly with chipping and short shots and progress to hitting the longer shots. Some recommendations, listed in Box 28-5, provide guidelines for individuals with total hip or knee replacements who wish to return to golf. These recommendations are for right-handed golfers; therefore, the terms "right/left" need to be reversed for the left-handed golfers.[78]

Club head speed primarily creates distance when hitting the golf ball. The senior golfer, like the younger golfer, ranks distance as important, and both age groups constantly look for ways to gain length in the drive. Declines in performance in various facets of golf are described with advancing age, although the rate per year depends on the skill. For example, greens in regulation (0.36%/year) and driving distance (0.23%/year) had the greatest rate of decline, whereas scoring average (0.14%/year) and putts per round (0.11%/year) decline more slowly. This makes sense as muscular power declines more rapidly with age than other motor properties.[79]

Improved club technology, refined golf swing mechanics, and physical conditioning, including strengthening and flexibility interventions, all contribute to increasing club head speed at impact of hitting the golf ball. The physical therapist plays an important role in helping the senior athlete gain mobility in the critical zones

BOX 28-5	Recommendations for Return to Golf after Total Joint Replacement

- Avoid playing in wet weather to decrease chance of slips/falls.
- The golfer may be able to play better without golf spikes, which puts less stress on the replaced hip/knee.
- The golfer must learn to play "more on the toes" to avoid torsional loading on the replaced joint.
  - During backswing: the left heel should be elevated.*
  - During downswing: the right heel should come up off the ground.*
- The patient with a total hip replacement should learn to play with a greater hip turn, i.e., rotate the trunk more. To create more full body turn, have the golfer narrow their stance or to create more internal rotation of the hip, fan the feet outward.
- Right-handed golfers with a right total knee replacement may benefit from "stepping through" the swing with the right leg. This assists in weight-shifting to unload the replaced joint.
- Right-handed golfers with a left total knee replacement may benefit from an "open stance" to decrease stress and torque on the replaced joint.
- Consider using a pull cart or caddy to decrease the stress on the replaced joint during carrying. Walking is encouraged.

*Right handed golfer.
(Data from Stover CN, McCarroll JR, Mallon WJ, editors: Feeling up to par: medicine from tee to green. Philadelphia, 1994, F.A. Davis Company.)

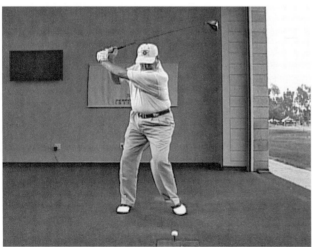

FIGURE 28-25 Senior golfer, beginning downswing phase of swing.

mentioned previously and educating the athlete in strengthening and dynamic stability exercises specific to the golf swing.

Like other athletes, golfers must select equipment carefully with knowledge that proper-fitting golf clubs contribute to safe and successful golfing. The understanding of golf equipment and fitting of this equipment is usually beyond the scope of knowledge and expertise of most physical therapists. Therefore, respected golf professionals in your geographic area can work with you to provide expert equipment modifications for any senior golfer.

Tennis

The United States Tennis Association (USTA) defines the senior tennis player as someone aged 45 and older. The senior divisions encompass ages 45 to 85. The last age category of 80- to 85-year-olds, established in the early 1980s, came as a response to the growing numbers of competitive players at these ages.[80] Although both male and female age divisions exist, more males than females currently compete in the senior age categories. Most senior players who play at a competitive level attribute their well-being to the playing of tennis itself. Senior athletes who play two or more times a week seem to fare better than those who play intermittently.[81]

Tennis involves physical demands of quickness, agility, muscular strength and power, flexibility, eye–hand coordination, and reaction time (Figure 28-26). All of these factors decrease with age. How do senior athletes continue to play at a competitive level? Although senior tennis players cannot play at the same level as when they were younger, they can maintain a high level of performance well into their seventies, although rarely do they play singles tennis. If you "don't use it, you lose it" may be exemplified in tennis more than other sports such as running or swimming. Examples include the demands for foot speed to move the body around the court and quickness and precision of upper extremity movement to contact the ball in all strokes. These demands require trunk, upper and lower extremity muscular strength, power, and endurance.

Lifelong tennis participation can cause both macro- and microtraumatic injuries to several regions of the body,[82] with a higher incidence of injury occurring in the overuse or microtrauma category. Some of the common macrotraumatic injuries include medial meniscus tear in the knee, tear of the medial head of the gastrocnemius, rupture of the Achilles tendon, and rotator cuff injury. Controversy still exists over the decision whether to attempt surgical intervention for some of these acute tears in 80-year-old athletes, depending largely on their decision regarding return to competitive athletics. Many competitive senior athletes elect for surgical repair and work hard during rehabilitation, over the course of several months, in order to return to competitive tennis

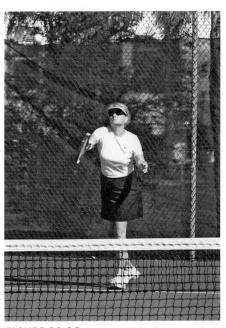

FIGURE 28-26 Senior tennis player, serving.

and other sports. They do not settle for anything less and do not expect the physical therapist to treat them differently than younger athletic counterparts.

For the senior tennis athlete, the potential for chronic injuries increases with age, playing time, and with use of ill-fitted equipment.[82] The four areas most often involved are the knee, elbow, shoulder, and back. The degeneration of the meniscus or articular cartilage surfaces causes degenerative changes in the knee, creating increased forces at the knee. Chronic lateral epicondylitis, known as "tennis elbow," commonly plagues the senior athlete and may result from the loss of strength and flexibility in the arm, accentuated by a poorly fit tennis racquet (Figure 28-27). Rotator cuff tendinitis may also result from strength loss seen with aging. However, we believe that the lack of spinal and upper quarter mobility, evident with the overhead volley and serve, put the senior athlete's shoulder more at risk than loss of strength. Back pain, also a common injury for the senior tennis athlete, can lead to significant limitations in playing level.[81]

A thorough examination of senior athletes performing tennis strokes will lead the physical therapist directly to the critical areas of dysfunction due to lack of range of motion, loss of strength, poor technique, or poorly fit equipment. Looking at the big picture and having that picture in mind as you prepare the athlete for return after a significant hiatus from the game, such as after surgery, is necessary to get the athlete back to preinjury competition level.

The authors of this chapter also believe the pelvis, lower extremity, trunk balance concept, as previously discussed, plays a predominant role in the success of a tennis player. The core serves as an important link

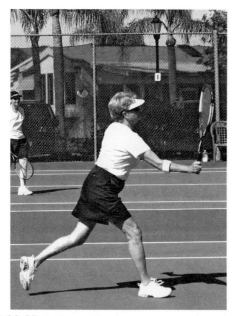

FIGURE 28-27 Senior tennis player, note stretch/reach position, and use of elbow brace for overuse of the forearm.

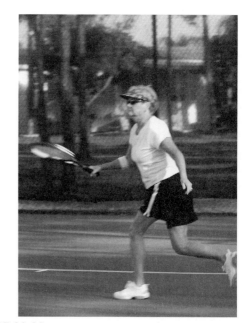

FIGURE 28-28 Training the senior tennis player in stroke-specific position.

between the lower and upper extremities, both regions important for different facets of the movements involved in tennis. For example, if the tennis athlete fails the SFMA deep squat test because of trunk or core instability (the trunk is not maintained in an upright, stable position), this area must be targeted with stability interventions. Most players perform tennis strokes in the semiflexed position or go from an extended trunk position to trunk flexion rapidly and with significant rotational force. The pelvic girdle and anterior and posterior trunk muscles provide significant stabilization and power for tennis strokes. If aging or disuse has decreased the efficiency or synchrony of these muscles, the extremities must do more of the task and thus be at risk for overstrain. Once senior athletes develop baseline trunk strength, they must strengthen the trunk muscles in stroke-specific positions and in quick movement patterns to develop the power needed for strong, accurate shots. The large muscles in the lower extremity such as the quadriceps, hamstrings, hip adductors, and gastrocnemius provide additional power that is transmitted to the trunk and proximal musculature during stroke execution. Rehabilitation should therefore address strength and power of these muscles in addition to the stabilizers of the core (Figure 28-28).

Once strength and power of key muscles are addressed, mobility and flexibility become key principles. Mobility and flexibility of the body segments must be used in combination to get to the ball and hit an accurate shot, which are essential skills of tennis. Performing the overhead volley and serve requires a significant amount of trunk extension. If that trunk mobility is not present, the shoulder must abduct and externally rotate more to compensate, thus putting increased stress on the aging

rotator cuff. The decrease in glenohumeral external rotation and abduction present with aging causes the senior tennis player to use more elbow and wrist movement to hit the ball with power. This alteration in stroke mechanics places the senior tennis athlete at risk for overuse injury to the distal upper extremity.

The ground strokes of tennis require a significant amount of trunk rotation, and the arms and legs must be able to cross midline with ease while maintaining balance over the base of support (Figure 28-29). When performing the backhand, if trunk rotation is limited or the lower extremities do not cross midline, the shoulder girdle must horizontally adduct excessively to reach the ball. This alteration may cause shoulder impingement, rotator cuff tears, or other upper quarter and cervical injuries. Again players have shortening of collagen tissues and concurrent declines in neuromotor control of balance. Flexibility and balance losses need intervention before the athlete can expect to be able to play tennis without recurring chronic injuries.

Strategies exist that help to keep the senior tennis athlete competitive and injury free. Many senior tennis athletes play doubles instead of singles tennis to compensate for their loss in quickness and agility (Figure 28-30). They also play on clay courts when possible as this creates a softer surface. The tennis racquet must be adjusted specifically to fit the senior athlete. Most senior tennis players still like to play the power game rather than the finesse game and feel the bigger the racquet head, the longer the racquet body length, and the tighter the strings, the better. However, the decreased strength and flexibility that comes with age, make it difficult to handle the powerful racquets used by young professionals and may be increasing the risk of injury. Therapists, there-

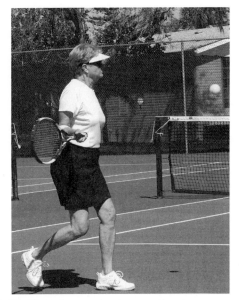

FIGURE 28-29 Senior tennis player performing a ground stroke (forehand).

fore, must address the issue of racquet dimensions with senior athletes. A tennis professional can assist with proper fit, according to the athlete's physiological status and type of game.

Length of racquet body, size of racquet head, tension of strings, grip size (which often changes as a person ages because of the arthritic hand), racquet weight and distribution from handle to head, and the texture of the strings must all be considered. Tennis racquet length varies between 27 inches, most often used by junior tennis players, and 29 inches, the newer "long body." Older tennis players often purchase a longer racquet to compensate for losses in quickness and agility. The selection of a longer racquet is not without consequence, however,

as it creates a longer lever arm to transmit forces to the entire upper extremity. Increased forces to the upper quarter place the athlete at risk for overuse injury.

Racquets weigh between 8.8 to 13 ounces and should have an equal weight distribution between the handle and head of the racquet. Many seniors also use large-head tennis racquets. Larger racquet heads have approximately 135 square inches of contact space and have a larger "sweet spot" with which to contact the ball. Larger racquet heads require adequate strength to control not only the racquet but also the force of the ball hitting the racquet. A larger racquet head does not always enhance the power and accuracy of the player.

String tension is another feature of a properly fit racquet. Correct string tension ranges from 45 to 70 pounds of pressure. Average tension is 60 pounds. The higher the string tension, the more force is absorbed by the soft tissues of the upper extremity. Encourage the senior player to use a tension that his body can handle and rely more on finesse to outscore the opponent. Texture and gauge of racquet string vary. The finesse game requires the ball to be in contact with the racquet head longer, so a larger string gauge and more textured string enhances spin and speed of the ball.

Lastly, grip size, determined by measuring the distance between the first palmar crease and the distal end of the third digit of the hand, varies. Grip size ranges from 4 to 4¼ inches, and correct sizing is essential for protecting the hand. It is important to reevaluate grip size as a player ages because of arthritic changes that can occur in the hand. These changes may cause alterations in gripping ability and also in grip size. There are special grip adapters for the arthritic hand. A properly fitting tennis racquet will enhance the player's ability to make those difficult shots and continue playing at a competitive level, no matter what the age.

CASE STUDIES

Case 1

Mr. E. is a 74-year-old retired lawyer who presented postoperatively after having his rotator cuff repaired 1 week ago. He is right hand dominant, and in his retirement enjoys singles tennis on a three- to four-time-per-week basis. He noted a gradual onset of right shoulder pain and weakness during all overhead and outstretched upper extremity (UE) activities over the previous year, and reports that his tennis game had "gone down the tubes" because he was unable to serve or perform overhead shots secondary to pain. Additionally, his forehand and backhand had become painful (6/10 on a 0-10 Visual Analogue Scale, 10 being the worst score). He also reported difficulty sleeping secondary to pain (5-6/10). Preoperatively, his physician had performed standard radiographs that demonstrated a type III acromion with spurring throughout the acromioclavicular (AC) joint,

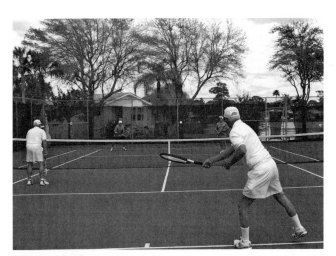

FIGURE 28-30 Doubles tennis play in senior athletes reduces the need for running and court coverage.

and an MRI that demonstrated a medium-sized (3-cm), full-thickness rotator cuff tear.

Surgery included a mini-open double row rotator cuff repair of the supra- and infraspinatus using three bone anchors and an acromioplasty. Cuff quality at the time of the repair was described as "fair to good," with a good repair achieved. He had been performing Codman's pendulum exercises and cervical/elbow/forearm/wrist/hand active range of motion (AROM) three times daily, while wearing a sling the rest of his day. Patient's goals at initial evaluation were to decrease his postoperative pain (8/10), return to ADLs using his right (R) hand, and return to competitive tennis. His physician has stated that he may not perform AROM for 8 weeks postoperation, no overhead activities for 6 months, and no tennis for 12 months. Upon initial examination the patient had passive range of motion (PROM) of 88-degrees flexion, 65-degrees abduction, 10-degrees external rotation (in adducted position), and 45-degrees internal rotation. All PROMs were limited by pain, and no AROM was allowed. Posture was consistent with sling usage: neck in slight R lateral flexion, R shoulder slightly elevated, and in the position of adduction and internal rotation. R upper extremity arm swing during gait restricted secondary to sling use. Patient demonstrated mild forward head, increased thoracic kyphosis, and decreased lumbar lordosis, generally. Significant spasm noted in the pectoralis major and minor, and accessory movements of the glenohumeral joint are restricted and painful in the inferior and anterior directions. Strength was not tested acutely postoperatively, but strength deficits were demonstrated in all scapular muscles and humeral internal rotators (3+/5), external rotators (3/5), and deltoid (2+/5) when they were able to be tested at 8 weeks postoperation. Prognosis for return to ADLs and sport over a 6-month time frame was considered good secondary to quality of tissue and quality of repair achieved.

Problems/Treatment

1. Loss of postural symmetry, abnormal UE movement with gait. Initially this was addressed with active postural correction via instruction and cervical and appropriate upper quarter AROM. He was also taught diaphragmatic breathing to improve thoracic and cervical positioning and also to assist with pain management. When removed from the sling, arm swing during gait was addressed. Further postural assessment in conjunction with return to sport phases of rehabilitation was necessary.

2. Pain throughout the upper quarter. Initially cryotherapy was used for both glenohumeral joint pain (postoperative, chemical pain) and also for spasm of trunk musculature. In this case, as is typical, postoperative pain was manageable within a few weeks postsurgery.

3. Diminished PROM and AROM, and decreased strength of the upper quarter musculature. Initially

this was accomplished using accessory mobilizations (grades 1 and 2 for pain reduction) and PROM. When soft tissue healing and resolution of chemical pain was appropriate, the SFMA was used for movement pattern assessment. The patient failed the total body extension, the overhead deep squat, and the shoulder screening tests. The central themes to be noted as to why these gross movement screens were failed are encompassed by insufficient scapular stability and diminished rotator cuff stability/glenohumeral joint mobility. Scapular mobility was also carefully assessed and addressed, including timing of movement, PNF diagonals, and eventually stability and mobility exercises consistent with the demands of tennis. When AROM was allowed, gentle, gradual demands were placed on the rotator cuff in steering, stabilizing, and rotating functions. This was accomplished by gradually adding rhythmic stabilization in open and closed chain exercises for stability, open chain rotational strengthening against gravity and then light weights and Theraband (Blackburn exercises), and eventually more complex motor tasks unique to tennis. It is essential that all tasks be performed with correct scapulohumeral biomechanics to encourage proper scapulothoracic and rotator cuff synergy. The patient was only allowed to progress to more difficult exercises with progressive resistance if scapulohumeral rhythm was correct.

4. Return to tennis. Preparation for return to tennis was initiated at 14 months postoperatively, with physician approval. The patient was eventually able to pass all SFMA screening tests, and it was deemed appropriate to begin SST with regard to tennis-specific activities. To address this functional goal, it is important to look at the base of strength the patient possesses. Criteria for Mr. E to move to this phase were: equal AROM to left, MMT of 4+/5 or greater in all UE musculature, isokinetic internal–external rotator torques greater than 90%, and total work greater than 80% of the uninvolved arm. (Note that it may take several tests over the months to achieve these isokinetic scores.) Return to sport activities included dynamic trunk/core strengthening using resisted stroke movements, elastic resistance, and dynamic lumbar stabilization in tennis-based tasks; sport-specific movements with pulleys, tubing, the Intertial trainer, and the Bodyblade (forehands, backhands, overhead/serving); and LE footwork, balance, and drills for lateral movements and cross-over stepping necessary for tennis. When allowed to return, we suggested that Mr. E. begin with ground stroke practice, and avoid serving and game situations. He gradually returned to full tennis activities with the progression from doubles (minimal sets), no serves doubles, increased sets with serves doubles, whole game singles, diminished play singles, regular play. Because this rehabilitation progression takes many months, it

should be noted that this patient was only seen once or twice a month in the final stages.

Case 2

Mr. S is a 65-year-old male and avid golfer who presented with complaints of chronic low back pain without a specific mechanism of injury. Chief complaints consisted of generalized stiffness of the thoracic and lumbar spines after prolonged sitting, standing, or walking. He denied radicular symptoms and was able to sleep undisturbed by pain. He reported some difficulty getting to sleep as a result of back stiffness especially after golfing. He golfs both recreationally and in a seniors, competitive league, an average of three times per week. He walks the 18-hole course pulling his clubs. He also reported having purchased a new large-headed driver and attempting to "retool" his swing to increase his distance from the tee. The patient's primary goal was to be able to golf a minimum of three times per week without spinal pain.

Mr. S was unable to complete the SFMA tests of forward bending, multisegmental extension, multisegmental rotation (bilaterally), single limb stance (bilaterally), the deep squat test, and the cervical rotation test (bilaterally). Based on these gross patterns of movement dysfunction, specific clinical testing revealed that Mr. S exhibited pes planus feet bilaterally, an exaggerated anterior pelvic tilt, exaggerated thoracic kyphosis, protracted scapulae (bilaterally), and mild forward head with hyperextension of the upper cervical region. He is minimally overweight in the abdominal region. Dramatic soft tissue tightness is noted in the lumbar spinal extensors, thoracolumbar fascia, bilateral iliotibial bands, anterior chest wall (pectoralis major and minor), and cervical suboccipital muscles. No specific trigger points or tenderness was noted. Gross trunk motion diminished by 50% in all planes with complaint of soft tissue tightness and pulling. Cervical rotation limited to 50 degrees bilaterally. Hip rotations (both IR and ER) limited 50% bilaterally. Segmental assessment revealed remarkable decreases in anterior/posterior and rotational joint play from C6-T4, as well as decreased upper cervical (OA and AA) rotation to the left. Remarkably decreased flexibility was noted in the gastroc/soleus complex, rectus femoris, iliotibial band, psoas, piriformis, pectoralis minor, and scalenes, bilaterally. He was unable to actively recruit his transversus abdominis, and tested very poorly for upper and lower abdominals (2/5). UE and LE strength was generally 4+/5 to 5/5, with exception of lower trapezius, middle trapezius, hip external rotators, and hip abductors (3+/5).

Problems/Treatment. The above-noted soft tissue tightness and joint restrictions all place great compression and torsional forces on the spinal segments during ADLs, which are magnified during golf. Initial treatment consisted of joint mobilizations to address the restrictions, followed by postural corrections to support optimal functional alignment. Mobilizations with movement were used to mobilize the spine in rotational movements similar to the golf swing. Mr. S. was instructed in soft tissue and spinal positional self-mobilizations using towel rolls, foam rollers and wedges. His home program also consisted of passive and dynamic stretching for the low back, anterior chest wall, and lower extremities. Patient was instructed to perform self-mobilizations once daily, and flexibility once daily in addition to before and after his aerobic exercise or round of golf. As previously mentioned, mobility problems must be managed prior to adding interventions for stability. Mobility deficits in the hip and thoracic spine were providing abnormal stresses on the lumbar spine.

Mr. S also needed to address his trunk strength and dynamic core control in addition to initiating an overall fitness program. Core exercises were targeted to address the core stabilizers (transversus abdominis, multifidi), the proximal hip musculature (gluteus minimus, gluteus medius, hip external rotators), and posterior scapular muscles. Strengthening was initiated in straight planar movements, with progression to complex diagonal and rotational movements necessary for golf. Chops and lifts and total body rolling motions were used to "balance" out the rotational stability and dynamic motor performance of the trunk. Emphasis was placed on engaging the core muscles throughout reproduction of the golf swing, as well as maintaining a neutral pelvic posture. Using the dynamic stability of the core was beneficial in increasing club head speed, without excessive spinal pressure. An aerobic fitness program was formulated for Mr. S, which consisted of proper warm-up and cooldown phases combined with exercising in his target heart rate zone. Initial target heart rate was calculated using 60% of his maximal heart rate using the Karvonen formula. The target heart rate zone was increased to 70% to 75% in the fifth week of exercise. Aerobic exercise (in his case bicycling or walking) was performed a minimum of three times per week.

Body mechanics instructions for lifting and carrying the golf bag, picking up golf balls, and other ADLs were provided. Dynamic core activation during motions of the golf swing against resistance along with developmental postures and closed chain neuromuscular training (core, hip rotators) served to ready Mr. S for return to playing golf.

Finally, Mr. S was referred to a local golf professional where analysis of Mr. S's golf swing was conducted because he had reported trying to "tune up" his swing in order to gain more distance on his drives. During this analysis, his functional range-of-motion restrictions helped confirm the importance of the manual stretching and mobility interventions. He was instructed to return to a less demanding golf swing with more upright posture on follow-through to decrease the stresses on his thoracic and lumbar spinal segments. Excessive trunk lateral bending was also observed, and this should be avoided by keeping the shoulder over the hips throughout the swing. While setting up to strike the ball, he was cued to use the 30-degree rule: knees flexed to 30 degrees, with 30-degree forward flexion at the hips, and 30-degree external rotation of the lower extremities (to compensate for lack of hip internal rotation, which helps decrease stress on the lumbar spine), which facilitates pelvic and trunk muscular activation to provide dynamic stability to the body during the golf swing. In addition, Mr. S was coached regarding a club change and thorough warm-up procedure for return to golf, which were critical in his success. Communication between the golf professional and the physical therapist helped to facilitate positive outcomes for this patient. The patient was eventually able to pass all SFMA screening tests, except the multisegmental rotation test secondary to OA at the hips and, therefore, after communication with the golf pro, it was determined that Mr. S should continue to modify his technique to work around the limitations present at his hips.

CONCLUSIONS

How do they do it? When studying seniors who run into their eighth decades, perform yoga, climb mountains, hit tennis and golf balls, and play team sports into their sixth and seventh decades, health professionals of much younger ages are in awe (Figure 28-31). The fact that many individuals older than age 60 years participate in noncompetitive, physically demanding activities bears repeating. Frequently, these individuals remain unnoticed unless they become injured and seek rehabilitation. When the question "What do we know about athletic injuries in the older population?" is asked, the answer is "Not much." Much of the literature is anecdotal. Few epidemiologic studies have been conducted on this group of elite older adults; however, descriptions of the performances of the senior athlete are important and have value in understanding the physical and physiological changes that occur with successful aging.

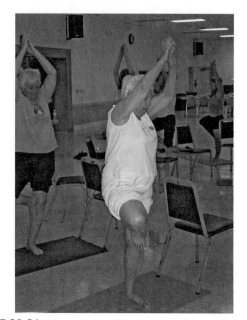

FIGURE 28-31 Balance in an 87-year-old yoga practitioner/leader, demonstrated in "tree pose."

Older athletes who are injured present a unique set of circumstances to the rehabilitation professional. These seniors may regard themselves as athletes, and high levels of participation are an important part of their lives. Physical therapists need to respect this value while suggesting ways to adapt to the sport. Addressing the concerns and rehabilitation of the aging athlete requires knowledge, patience, diplomacy, and a healthy respect for the patients' desires to return to activity.

REFERENCES

To enhance this text and add value for the reader, all references are included on the companion Evolve site that accompanies this text book. The reader can view the reference source and access it online whenever possible. There are a total of 82 cited references and other general references for this chapter.

Older Adults with Developmental Disabilities

Toby M. Long, PT, PhD, FAPTA, Kathleen Toscano, MHS, PT, PCS

INTRODUCTION

The population of individuals older than age 65 years is close to 13%.[1] Included in this group are individuals with a developmental disability who up to a few years ago would not be expected to live to the age of 65 years, much less beyond that.[2] Physical therapists are integral members of the team that serves individuals with developmental disabilities and will be expected to contribute to their care as they get older. A *developmental disability* is defined as a condition that occurs before age 22 years, continues indefinitely, is a substantial obstacle to the ability to function, and results in a functional limitation in three or more of the following: self-care, receptive or expressive language, learning, mobility, self-direction (or motivation), capacity for independent living, or economic self-sufficiency.[3] This definition includes individuals with intellectual disabilities, cerebral palsy, Down syndrome, autism, and a host of other conditions that encompass a wide range of physical and mental changes that alter the functional abilities throughout the life span. The purpose of this chapter is to discuss the role of the physical therapist in providing intervention services to an older adult with a developmental disability. Covered specifically are the legislative mandates and philosophical underpinnings of providing services to this population, the unique aspects of aging in selected disability categories, the services rendered by the physical therapist, and the facilities where services may be provided.

The *U.S. Healthy People 2010*[4] initiative targets the top American health care concerns. The two main goals of the U.S. Healthy People 2010 initiative are to increase the quality and numbers of years of healthy living and eliminate health disparities. People with disabilities are represented in the objectives used to track progress for these goals. Two other national initiatives, *Closing the Gap: A National Blueprint to Improve the Health of Persons with Mental Retardation*[5] and the *Surgeon General's Call to Action to Improve the Health and*

Wellness of Persons with Disabilities,[6] focus on promoting a healthy lifestyle, healthy aging, and preventing further impairment, disability, and disease. *Closing the Gap* is a national campaign designed to help improve the health of people with intellectual disability. The goals of the Surgeon General's initiative, *Call to Action on Disability*, are to:

- Increase understanding nationwide that people with disabilities can lead long, healthy, and productive lives.
- Increase knowledge among health care professionals and provide them with tools to screen, diagnose, and treat the whole person with a disability with dignity.
- Increase awareness among people with disabilities of the steps they can take to develop and maintain a healthy lifestyle.
- Increase accessible health care and support services to promote independence for people with disabilities.

Globally, the World Health Organization's (WHO) program *Healthy Aging—Adults with Intellectual Disabilities*[7] and four other WHO documents[8-11] outline the key issues facing aging adults with developmental disabilities globally and offer specific recommendations to support healthy aging, including an emphasis on rehabilitation.

Consistent with these prevention- and wellness-focused initiatives, there has been a paradigm shift in how disability is viewed. The medical model, an impairment-based model that regards disability as a biological abnormality requiring treatment, is being replaced with a social model. The social model conceptualizes disability as a condition that occurs primarily within the context of psychological, social, and environmental constraints that may interfere with functioning.[12] This change in perception supports community-based programming that takes into consideration the needs, wants, and preferences of the individual.

Four major events occurred during the 1970s enabling the growth of community-based services and supports:

- Passage of the Intermediate Care Facilities/Mental Retardation Program of Title XIX (Medicaid) of the Social Security Act (1971)[13];
- Landmark ruling on the right to treatment in the Wyatt v. Stickney case (1971)[14];
- Passage of Section 504 of the Rehabilitation Act (1973)[15];
- Passage of the Education for All Handicapped Children's Act (now called IDEA) (1975).[16]

Building on these initiatives, several major legislative efforts were passed mandating that older persons with developmental disabilities be afforded services to meet their unique needs (Box 29-1). In addition, the Americans with Disabilities Act of 1990[19] ensures access to and participation in senior citizen centers, day care sites, and social service centers for individuals with developmental disabilities. Most recently, the Supreme Court[22] ruled that the states are required to provide community-based services for those with intellectual disabilities if appropriate and if the individuals with disabilities agree to treatment in the community. Thus, legislation is in place which ensures that individuals with developmental disabilities are becoming members of the community at increasing rates.

DEMOGRAPHICS

It is estimated that there are between 3.2 and 4.5 million individuals with sensory, mental, physical, or other developmental disabilities that impair their ability to effectively care for themselves.[2] Of these, 641,000 are older than age 60 years, and this number is projected to double by 2030.[2] According to Cooper et al,[23] individuals with developmental disabilities represent about 1% of the population. Of these, 12% are older than age 65 years. As the number of individuals with developmental disabilities has grown, so has life expectancy. Life expectancy has increased by approximately 250% since the 1930s from 19 years of age to 70 years.[24] Unless the individual has a significant disability such as Down syndrome, cerebral palsy, multiple disabilities, or a severe level of cognitive impairment, the life expectancy and age-related medical conditions of older adults with developmental disabilities are similar to that of the general population.

In the population of older adults with developmental disabilities, women tend to outlive men by about 3 to 1.[24] Surviving cohorts of women who have an intellectual disability are more often mildly or moderately impaired, whereas men tend to be severely impaired. The ratio of older men to women with cerebral palsy, however, tends to be higher than that found in the general population of individuals with developmental disabilities. Also, there exists an interaction between gender, age, degree of retardation, and longevity.[24] Women with milder disabilities, such as mild intellectual disability, tend to live longer. Women with developmental disabilities present with unique considerations, placing them at greater risk for developing health-related problems than women without developmental disabilities. They receive significantly less preventive care than other women and lead very sedentary lives, which often results in greater risk for cardiovascular diseases. For example, participation in breast cancer screening is much less likely if the woman is older and has a disability or functional limitations.[25]

Whereas the majority of the general geriatric population live alone or with a spouse, the majority of older adults with a developmental disability live in varied types of community residences.[26] Community-based residential facilities are designed as home-like living environments that combine supervision and care with support of a family or group setting. There are four basic types of community-based residential facilities:

1. *Intermediate care facilities (ICFs):* These provide the most intensive group home setting for individuals with health problems, multiple disabilities, or very

---

BOX 29-1	Legislation Affecting Services to Older Adults with Developmental Disabilities

Older American Act Amendments (OAA) 1987[17]
- Mandated that older persons with developmental disabilities be served under the Act's provisions
- Mandated that the Administration on Aging (AOA) collaborate with the developmental disability service system to design and implement appropriate services
- OAA programs were opened to older adults with developmental disabilities
- Developmental Disabilities Bill of Rights and Assistance Act (1987)[18]
- Extended the provisions of the Developmental Disabilities Services and Facilities Construction Act of 1970
- Identified service delivery models to accommodate growth in population and need for trained professionals
- Promoted community-based residential services

Americans with Disabilities Act (ADA) (1990)[19]
- Provisions include access to and participation in senior citizen centers, day care sites, and social service centers for individuals with developmental disabilities

The Domestic Volunteer Service Act (1975)[20]
- Authorized senior companions to assist adults with developmental disabilities
- Omnibus Budget Reconciliation Act (1981)[21]
- Before admission to a nursing home, a screening must be performed for every person with a developmental disability
- Annual review of every person with a developmental disability who resides in a nursing facility
- Persons with developmental disabilities who are found to be inappropriately placed in a nursing home must be discharged

limited daily living skills. No more than eight individuals reside together in this type of setting.

2. *Community residencies (CRs):* These are group home settings for individuals with moderate abilities to care for themselves. Individuals whose primary disability is moderate mental retardation or autism often reside in these facilities. Up to 12 adults may live together in a CR.

3. *Supportive residencies:* These are for individuals with a significant level of independence. These facilities are often apartments and usually consist of two to three "roommates." Monitoring by a supervisor is done weekly or as needed.

4. *Family care homes:* These are for individuals of all degrees of disability. An individual resides with a family who has been trained and licensed to care for individuals with a developmental disability.

In addition to these community-based residencies, older individuals with a developmental disability may reside in skilled nursing facilities, nursing homes, or private residential facilities for persons with developmental disabilities.

THE DEVELOPMENTAL DISABILITIES SERVICE SYSTEM

Federal legislation passed since the 1970s supports the community-based model of care and provides systems to increase the likelihood that adults and older persons with a developmental disability will become integral members of the community. The system of services for the general population of older Americans, funded primarily through federal monies, is defined as an age-based service system, that is, the age of the individual determines eligibility for service. The services are designed focusing on the needs of the group of older citizens. In contrast, the service system for older adults with a developmental disability is considered to be needs-based and provides individualized, specialized services. Provisions for age-specialized models of service exist within this system, which is primarily state funded. The current focus of service provision is to bridge these two service delivery systems to encourage collaboration and joint planning between the systems to ensure that an individual's needs are best met in the most efficient community-based manner as possible. This contemporary model of service provision has evolved from the "normalization" movement of the 1960s.[27] This movement was grounded in the belief that individuals would develop optimally if they were integrated into society and afforded the same experiences as those without disabilities.

The community-based model of care operationalized the normalization philosophy. By the mid-1970s states began to develop community-based residential and treatment programs. Individuals who had the opportunity to take advantage of these programs were more functional and independent than their counterparts in institutions and on some parameters than those living with their parents.[28] Thus, the movement toward deinstitutionalization took hold, and by 1991 a nationwide movement took place to close all state-supported residential facilities and develop community-integrated living and vocational and leisure programming. As noted previously, legislation has been passed that supports the community-based model of care and provides systems to increase the likelihood that adults and older persons with a developmental disability will become integral members of the community. Thus individuals with developmental disabilities now live and receive the services and supports they need in their local communities. They are no longer relegated to institutional settings away from family, friends, and their community. Clients are now able to access a variety of appropriate service providers, such as physical therapists, through direct access or upon physician referral.

AGE-RELATED HEALTH CARE ISSUES SPECIFIC TO ADULTS WITH DEVELOPMENTAL DISABILITIES

Obesity and Cardiovascular Disease

Obesity affects individuals with all types of developmental disabilities. Research, however, has focused on individuals with an intellectual disability who have been found to have a higher incidence of obesity than adults without an intellectual disability. Yamaki[29] estimated that the obesity rate for adults with intellectual disabilities was significantly higher than that of the general population at each of the four 4-year observation periods of the National Health Interview Survey. For instance, in the time period between 1997 and 2000, 36.4% of adults with intellectual disabilities were considered obese as compared to 20.6% of adults without intellectual disabilities.[29] More recently, Rimmer and Wang[30] found that the rate of obesity in people with intellectual disabilities was twice as high compared to that of the general population. Seventy percent of adults with Down syndrome and 60.6% of adults with intellectual disabilities were found to be obese. What is especially alarming is that extreme obesity was 4 times greater in adult individuals with Down syndrome (19%) and 2.5 times greater for adults with other forms of intellectual disabilities (12.1%) as compared to the general population. In addition to various health conditions such as hypertension, diabetes, heart disease, stroke, and stress, obesity also results in significant societal and personal limitations such as employment and leisure activities.[31] As seen in the general population, obesity in older adults with intellectual disabilities results in higher medical costs for obesity-related chronic health conditions.[32,33] Furthermore, it requires a greater effort on the part of caregivers to assist obese individuals with intellectual disabilities, thus placing caregivers at greater risk for health problems such as low back pain.[31] Lack of physical activity, poor diets, and environmental factors have been linked to obesity in persons with intellectual disabilities.[31]

Cardiovascular disease (CVD) has also been found to affect those with developmental disabilities. As in the general population, CVD is the leading cause of death in those with an intellectual disability, except for those with Down syndrome.[34] Factors that would indicate a higher CVD incidence in this population include longer life expectancy, physical inactivity, and higher dietary fat intake.[34]

The three most common types of developmental disabilities seen by physical therapists are intellectual disabilities, cerebral palsy, and Down syndrome. Until recently, little research had been conducted documenting the changes seen in individuals with these disabilities as they age. It was not until the mid-1980s that the medical community felt the need to conduct such research because up until that time, few individuals with disabilities lived beyond middle age. Longevity for individuals with Down syndrome and those with cerebral palsy is increasing. With increasing longevity, there has been a concomitant interest in the aging process for these individuals.

Down Syndrome

Age-related changes in the behavior of individuals with Down syndrome have been documented.[35-37] The age of onset of the decline and underlying reasons for this premature decline have yet to be determined. However, there is a growing body of literature that discusses two possibilities for this decline: Alzheimer's disease[36,37] and depression.[38]

Alzheimer's Disease. Although the exact incidence of Alzheimer's disease in individuals with Down syndrome is unknown, an estimated 40% to 45% of these individuals between 50 and 70 years of age will develop Alzheimer's disease. This incidence is three to five times greater than in the general population.[36] Furthermore, the age of onset is much earlier in those with Down syndrome (age 35 to 45 years) than seen in the general population.[36] Current research suggests a causative link between the excess material in chromosome 21 and apolipoprotein production and deposition—the neuropathologic finding seen in individuals with Alzheimer's who are not developmentally disabled.[36]

Early symptoms of Alzheimer's disease in older adults with Down syndrome are similar to those in the general population: loss of memory and logical thinking, diminished abilities to perform activities of daily living (ADLs), changes in gait and coordination, and loss of bowel and bladder control. Individuals with Down syndrome also develop seizure activity, a symptom not common in the general population. It is recommended that individuals with Down syndrome receive psychological testing annually starting at age 30 years to determine and monitor loss of skills. Because of the known cognitive impairments of individuals with Down syndrome, declines in ADL skills may be a better indicator of Alzheimer's disease than memory and cognitive loss.[36] A checklist has been developed that can be used reliably to identify early signs of Alzheimer dementia in adults with Down syndrome.[39] Other tools, such as the Adaptive Behavior Scale,[40] the Client Development Evaluation Report,[41] and the Vineland Adaptive Behavior Scales, Second Edition,[42] also have been used to identify functional decline in individuals with Down syndrome. These tools have been found to be valid with this population.

Depression. There is indication that some individuals with Down syndrome are erroneously diagnosed as having Alzheimer's disease when, in fact, they are depressed.[38] Because depression is a treatable condition and Alzheimer's disease is only manageable at this time, distinguishing between the two is important for caregiving purposes. The prevalence of depression in individuals with Down syndrome is between 6% and 12%.[38] In addition to Alzheimer's symptoms associated with other conditions such as hypothyroidism and hearing loss mask the identification of depression in individuals with Down syndrome. Although severely depressed individuals also show a loss of adaptive skills, the pattern of loss tends to be up and down rather than a continuous decline as seen in dementia. Also, individuals with depression respond positively to intervention and will regain skills that were once thought to have been lost. In addition to changes noted in adaptive skills, it is important to document changes in affective behaviors, such as sadness; crying; increases in self-injurious, assaultive, or aggressive behaviors; and somatic complaints.[38,43] A framework that distinguishes among depression without dementia, depression with dementia, and dementia without depression is needed to guide rehabilitative interventions.[38]

Cerebral Palsy

Little information exists on how the aging process affects persons with cerebral palsy, and there is no reason to suspect that cerebral palsy alters the genetically driven process of aging. Life expectancy for individuals with cerebral palsy has not been studied extensively. Of the studies conducted in the 1990s, data indicate that individuals with cerebral palsy who lack mobility, are severely or profoundly intellectually disabled, and cannot feed themselves have a decreased life expectancy.[43] However, the chronic physical impairments and conditions associated with cerebral palsy may affect the onset or severity of age-related changes.

Older adults with cerebral palsy are at high risk for secondary conditions that cause a loss of function and deterioration of their quality of life. Complications related to musculoskeletal changes including increasing scoliosis, contractures, hip subluxation or dislocation, pathological fractures, and pain contribute to a loss of independent living skills as individuals with cerebral palsy age. Lower extremity contractures are prevalent in individuals with cerebral palsy who do not walk (up to 91%) and can be problematic for transfers, positioning, hygiene, and skin protection.[44] In addition, scoliosis appears to show a significant progression over time, which can lead to difficulty sitting and positioning, and has further effects on mobility, comfort, pelvic positioning, independence, skin integrity, and respiration.[45]

Pain, related to musculoskeletal dysfunction, overuse syndromes, and degenerative arthritis, is often reported in adults with cerebral palsy[44] Sixty-seven percent of women within one community complained of pain greater than 3 months' duration, 62% had daily pain, and 53% reported their pain to be moderate to severe in intensity.[46] The most common areas of musculoskeletal pain are the hips, knees, ankles, and lumbar and cervical spine.[46] In 2004, Jahnsen et al[47] found that 33% of adults (aged 18 to 72 years, mean is 34 years) with cerebral palsy report chronic pain; this compares to 15% in the general population. They also found that pain was associated with low life satisfaction, deteriorating function, and chronic fatigue.[48] Even though pain is reduced with intervention, most adults with cerebral palsy experiencing pain do not seek help from health care providers about their discomfort.[49] In addition, it may be difficult for caregivers to fully appreciate and interpret nonverbal pain behavior from persons with severe cognitive and communication impairments.[49] Thus, it is important to monitor individuals for behavioral changes that can be linked to pain, especially in older adults.

The Pain Assessment Instrument for Cerebral Palsy (PAICP)[50] was developed to assist practitioners in measuring the extent of pain experienced by nonverbal clients with severe cerebral palsy and a cognitive age of at least 4 years. The PAICP demonstrates adequate test–retest reproducibility and construct validity for use in measuring pain in this population.[50] The instrument consists of six drawings of typically nonpainful daily situations and six drawings of activities that are typically painful. Respondents are asked to rate each activity as painful, not painful, or possibly painful. Use of this instrument may give physical therapists and caregivers a better understanding of those activities that provoke pain in these individuals.

A consequence of chronic, unmanaged pain is a higher level of psychological distress.[51] Individuals who experience chronic pain are often forced to change their lifestyle (i.e., reduce work hours, begin to use a wheelchair or other assistive device, or look for additional home services).[52] Chronic pain is a significant and potentially life-altering problem for adults with cerebral palsy, negatively affecting work and daily life as well as functional skills and quality of life. This is a population that

therapists who specialize in the area of pain management will want to reach out to ensure they receive appropriate service.

Fatigue is another problem that is often reported by adults with cerebral palsy and is associated with diminishing functional independence.[48] Adults with cerebral palsy report a higher rate of physical, but not mental, fatigue than the general population, and the number reporting fatigue increases with age. The greatest predictors that were associated with fatigue were low life satisfaction, bodily pain, limitations in emotional and physical role function, and deterioration of functional skills.[48] Fatigue was not strongly associated with type of cerebral palsy; however, it was most prevalent in those reporting a moderate degree of motor impairment. These results reveal that physical fatigue is an issue in adults with cerebral palsy, it increases with age, and it has an impact on preserving functional skills and life satisfaction.

Pain, fatigue, and musculoskeletal changes can ultimately lead to loss of function and independence. Very little information is available on diminishing independence in this population as they age. Work done in Sweden in 2000[52] indicates that 43% of the 221 adults with cerebral palsy who responded to a survey (61% return rate) had either decreased their walking ability or stopped walking by the age of 35. During the same time period, Buttos et al[53] also found a significant decrease in walking ability in their sample of adults with cerebral palsy. Most lost their ability to walk between 20 and 40 years of age.[53]

In addition to the resultant problems directly related to the musculoskeletal impairments of cerebral palsy, women with cerebral palsy are more likely to be diagnosed with late-stage breast cancer than the general population.[25] Women with cerebral palsy underuse mammography, often leading to delayed diagnosis of breast cancer and less favorable outcomes.[25] Barriers to obtaining this service include lack of information about the benefits,[54] transportation challenges, inability to be positioned appropriately[55] in the mammography machine, communication challenges,[56] and negative attitudes from staff.[57] Appropriate services and knowledgeable service providers must be available to provide intervention that meets both the unique challenges presented by the population as well as the age-related health care challenges. Physical therapists are in an ideal position to consult with mammography technicians and instrument manufacturers in making mammography more accessible for adult women with cerebral palsy.

Intellectual Disabilities

Intellectual disability is characterized by significant limitations in both intellectual functioning and adaptive behavior (conceptual, social, and practical skills).[3] According to Krahn et al,[58] the health status of many individuals with intellectual disabilities is adversely affected by a range of disparities, which if addressed, can improve health outcomes. Persons with intellectual disabilities have relatively high rates of epilepsy, behavioral/mental health problems, fractures, skin conditions, respiratory disorders, and poor oral health. Older adults with severe to profound levels of intellectual disability are at increased risk to die from intestinal obstruction, cardiovascular diseases, pneumonia, trauma, and other physical disabilities.[59] There are also reported cases of unrecognized problems with vision and hearing and an unnecessary increase in the use of medications for psychiatric concerns.

EXAMINATION AND EVALUATION

A key role of the physical therapist working with individuals with developmental disabilities is to comprehensively examine the patient/client because a comprehensive examination forms the basis for clinical decision making. The components of a comprehensive examination are described in the following text and listed in Box 29-2.

History

Documenting pertinent history of the patient/client's health and behavioral changes can help the therapist make decisions on the appropriateness of specific therapeutic strategies. In addition to the patient/client's developmental disability, confounding problems such as congestive heart disease, hypertension, or diabetes also may be present. These comorbidities could influence recommendations or treatment strategies. It is likely that

BOX 29-2	Components of a Comprehensive Physical Therapy Examination for an Individual with Developmental Disability

History
Medical
Surgical
Therapeutic
Intervention
Medications
Cognition
Behavioral Response
Neuromuscular Status
Flexibility
Strength
Muscle tone
Posture
Endurance
Functional Skills
Balance
Gait
Activities of daily living
Use of assistive technology

individuals with developmental disabilities, especially cerebral palsy, will have a history of surgical intervention. As multiple surgical procedures may lead to scarring and deformity, it is essential to document the time frame of when the surgery occurred and how it has affected the person over time. Medications for treatment of conditions directly related to the developmental disability and those related to additional conditions should be thoroughly documented. Long-term use of anticonvulsive medications may lead to physical findings such as ataxia and tardive dyskinesia[60] or behavioral changes. Most individuals with a developmental disability will have had many years of various therapeutic interventions, and summarizing those interventions and their effects will prove invaluable for treatment planning. Documenting the use and effects of additional interventions, such as occupational therapy, special instruction, and therapeutic recreation that the client participates in, will assist in designing comprehensive programming that is collaborative—not redundant—with other disciplines.

Behavioral Response

Individuals with a developmental disability, especially those with severe or profound intellectual disability, autism, or emotional disturbance, may demonstrate behavioral characteristics that can interfere with functional use of motor skills. Documentation of the person's response to interactions and performance demands during the examination will assist with designing appropriate treatment plans. Documenting behavior also will help differentiate between behavioral characteristics that are consistent with the individual's developmental diagnosis and with those that are consistent with aging or other disabilities or medical conditions, such as depression. Documentation of antecedents to a behavioral outburst or change in behavior will assist the team in designing appropriate interaction plans and behavioral support strategies. Also, the therapist should document the method used by the individual, for example, verbal, gestures, or sign language, to communicate needs.

Neuromusculoskeletal Status

Traditional tests of neuromusculoskeletal status, such as manual muscle tests and goniometry, may not provide the information needed to make functionally oriented habilitation plans. The physical therapist should judge through observation the patient/client's degree of *flexibility*, *strength*, and *balance* within activities that are functional for the individual. It is likely that the patient/client may have long-term limitations in range of motion and decreased strength that he or she has learned to compensate for and do not contribute to his or her functional limitations. In addition, the therapist must be aware of the individual's interests and activity level to determine whether an impairment results in functional limitation. For example, a person with an intellectual disability who swims on a regular basis may consider a decrease in shoulder range of motion a significant limitation over a person who does not swim. This same approach should be taken when examining endurance and muscle strength. Assessment of strength and endurance should be performed within the context of functional activities that are meaningful to the individual, are age-appropriate, and are consistent with the patient/client's desired outcomes. Table 29-1 outlines a variety of tools that are used to evaluate functional status of an individual with a disability and are discussed in depth

subsequently. One of these tools, the Functional Outcome Assessment Grid (FOAG),[61] also incorporates the assessment of neuromuscular components in the performance of specific functional activities.

Motor Function and Functional Activities

Motor function skills are those that underlie activities that the individual does or would like to do on a regular basis and are meaningful to both the patient/client and caregivers. These skills are evident in examining mobility within the home and community and ADLs. Gait

TABLE 29-1	Tools Commonly Used to Evaluate Functional Status and Assist with Program Planning in Individuals with a Severe Level of Disability	
Tool	**Purpose**	**Components**
Functional Outcome Assessment Grid (FOAG)[61]	To determine performance factors that limit or support the accomplishment of specific functional tasks	*Performance areas:* 1. Posture and alignment against gravity 2. Movement patterns 3. Movement of body in space 4. Secondary physical disabilities *Administration:* Direct observation of attempts to accomplish task. Components of each performance area are rated as to how intensely they influence the accomplishment of a functional task
Functional Skill Scale of the Pediatric Evaluation of Disability Inventory (PEDI)[66]	To determine functional capabilities and performance, monitor progress, and evaluate therapeutic or rehabilitative program outcome	*Functional Skill Scale subtests:* 1. Self-care: eating, grooming, dressing, bathing, toileting 2. Mobility: transfers, indoors and outdoors mobility 3. Social function: communication, social interaction, household and community tasks *Administration:* Caregiver report, structured interview, or through observation. Environmental modification and amount of caregiver assistance is also systematically recorded.
Scales of Independent Behavior (SIB)–Revised[67]	To measure functional independence and adaptive functioning across settings Norm referenced and standardized for older adults	*Adaptive behavior clusters:* 1. Motor skills 2. Personal living skills 3. Social interaction & communication skills 4. Community living skills *Problem behaviors:* Support score predicts level of support required based on the impact of maladaptive behaviors on adaptive functioning. Functional limitations in adaptive behavior can be identified. *Administration:* Structured interview or checklist procedure.

Supports Intensity Scale (SIS)[66]	To measure the practical supports needed by adults with intellectual disabilities in functional living areas by ranking activities according to frequency, amount, and type of support required	*Identifies supports needed in:*
		 1. Medical
		 2. Behavioral
		 3. Life activity
		     Home living
		     Community living
		     Lifelong learning
		     Employment
		     Health and safety
		     Social
		 Administration: Comprehensive interview of patient/client and those who know him or her well.

patterns and balance are components of motor function that influence mobility.

Historically, older adults with developmental disabilities were administered developmental motor assessments that determined the developmental age level of their skill performance. It is inappropriate to test an adult with measures used to determine developmental skill level in children. It is, however, important to document skills that have been linked to functional activities and ADL (basic and instrumental), mobility, and recreation. In addition to the functional assessment tools widely used across a broad scope of health status (Katz Index of Independence in Activities of Daily Living,[64] Functional Independence Measure,[65] Older American Resources and Services,[66] the Philadelphia Geriatric Center Multilevel Assessment Instrument[67]), older adults with developmental disabilities can be assessed more specifically using dimensions contained on the Pediatric Evaluation of Disability Inventory,[62] the Scales of Independent Behavior–Revised,[63] the Supports Intensity Scales,[68] and the FOAG.[61]

Pediatric Evaluation of Disability Inventory. The Pediatric Evaluation of Disability Inventory (PEDI)[62] is a standardized, norm-referenced inventory that can be administered by caregiver report, structured interview with a caregiver, or through professional observation of a client's behavior. The PEDI is divided into two scales. The Functional Skill Scale has three subtests: self-care, mobility, and social function. Environmental modification and amount of caregiver assistance is systematically recorded in the Modification Scale and Caregiver Assistance Scale. Although standardized on children from ages 6 months to 7 years 6 months, the items on the PEDI can be administered to older individuals to describe patterns of strengths and needs to assist with program planning. The Modification Scale and the Caregiver Assistance Scale also provide valuable information for program planning and documenting benefits from intervention aimed at decreasing the burden of care for an individual.

Scales of Independent Behavior–Revised. The Scales of Independent Behavior–Revised (SIB-R) measures functional independence and adaptive functioning in the school, home, and employment and community settings.[63] It has been specifically designed to be used with children, adults, and the older adult population. The SIB-R is a norm-referenced test[63] that has been standardized on individuals aged 3 months to 90 years and older. The full scale is divided into 14 subscales, which are organized into four clusters: motor skills, social interaction and communication, personal living skills, and community living skills. Of particular interest to the geriatric population are items related to domestic skills, such as homemaking and community orientation. The design of the SIB-R also allows comparison of an individual's functional independence with cognitive status. A Screening Form and a Problem Behavior Scale are also part of the SIB-R package.

Supports Intensity Scale. The Supports Intensity Scale (SIS) is unique in that rather than measuring ability or inability the SIS measures the support needed by an adult with a developmental disability in 57 life activities and 28 behavioral and medical areas.[68] The assessment is completed through an interview with the patient/client and those who know him or her well. The SIS measures support needs in the areas of home living, community living, lifelong learning, employment, health and safety, social activities, and protection and advocacy. The scale ranks each activity according to frequency, amount, and type of support. Finally, a Supports Intensity Level is determined based on the Total Support Needs Index, which is a standard score generated from scores on all the items tested by the scale. The SIS is an excellent program planning tool, especially for those individuals who are known to have significant impairments and activity limitations. According to the manual, content validity, criterion-related validity, and construct validity were calculated using a variety of methodologies. All scores were intercorrelated, and coefficients exceeded the minimum level needed to demonstrate criterion-related reliability.[68] Results indicate that the SIS is suitable for measuring unique characteristics of support needed by an individual and not abilities as measured by adaptive behavior scales or achievement tests and that the scores correlate with level of intelligence (the lower the intelligence quotient, the higher the level of support needed).[68]

Functional Outcome Assessment Grid. The FOAG[61] is based on the top-down model of assessing the influence of impairments on patient/client-specified functional outcomes. Using the desired outcome as the starting point, the therapist determines barriers to the accomplishment of the task and strengths that will assist the patient/client in accomplishing the task. Using this model, the purpose of the FOAG is to assist the team in implementing functional outcomes. The FOAG is individualized, based on team consensus of desired outcomes for the patient/client. Although there are six functional outcome areas that can be assessed, each area can be assessed independently. The six areas—caring for self, communication, learning and problem solving, mobility, play, and leisure—are associated with four disability categories: physical, sensory, special health care needs, and other. The patient/client is observed attempting the desired outcome, and the therapist rates component skills, such as muscle tone, strength, and flexibility, on a 5-point scale from no problem to significant problem that affects or prevents skill performance. Program plans are then designed that bypass obstacles, promote strengths, and/or improve deficits. This tool is an informal program-planning strategy, providing therapists with a systematic approach to link impairments and functional limitations to client-desired outcomes.

Gait, Fall Risk, and Locomotion. In addition to using specific assessment tools, documenting the *gait* pattern of the patient/client is important. Individuals with developmental disabilities, especially those with cerebral palsy, have well-documented gait deviations and neuromuscular impairments. Gait assessment should document those impairments but, more importantly, determine the functional limitation imposed by the gait deviations. It is preferred that a gait assessment be performed in various natural settings and over a variety of terrains to determine the impact of the gait characteristics on the ability of a person to maneuver functionally. As noted in the older adult population without developmental disabilities, the patient/client may show a decrease in speed of ambulation and an increase in energy expenditure as he or she ages. Increased energy expenditure may be more pronounced in individuals with postural deviations.[69]

Fall risk and balance also should be assessed. Again, traditional balance tools used with younger individuals with developmental disabilities, such as the ability to walk a balance beam or stand on one foot, may not be the most appropriate methods to determine balance in the context of function. Maintenance of balance within functional activities, such as individuals maneuvering in their own environments during routine activities, may be more helpful for program planning.

Many balance tools have been found reliable and valid in detecting risk for falls in the general older adult population, but further research is needed to determine if these tests are valid in detecting fall risk in individuals with developmental disabilities.[70-72] Bruckner and Herge[73] found that modifying the Timed Up and Go test[74] is a reliable method of determining fall risk in ambulatory older people with developmental disabilities. However, there was no correlation found between fall history and performance on the modified test. Using the Tinetti Performance-Oriented Mobility Assessment Tool,[75] Adams et al[76] found that the tool was a reliable way to assess mobility in individuals with intellectual disabilities. The use of observation to assess mobility was found to be the most useful aspect of the tool for those individuals with intellectual disabilities or behavior problems.

There are also cognitive and injury risk assessment tools that could be helpful for falls risk assessment. These tools do not directly assess balance and gait, but because changes in cognition or mental status can be a risk factor for falls, use of tools that assess mental status may be helpful.[77] A change of scores in the Mini-Mental State Examination (MMSE)[78] was shown to predict falls for the general population as well as individuals with a cognitive impairment (odds ratio is 0.88 to 1.06).[79] As seen in the general population of older adults, those with developmental disabilities who are at risk for falling have more than one factor contributing to that risk.[73,80,81]

Assistive Technology. Many individuals with developmental disabilities use *assistive technology*. Assistive technology consists of simple adaptive equipment devices, such as adaptive spoons, to very complex computer-driven communication systems. The use of assistive technology

may increase for adults with developmental disabilities as they become older. As seen in older adults without developmental disabilities, the use of mobility devices will increase. This is especially true for the use of wheelchairs for individuals with cerebral palsy. A thorough assessment of the fit and appropriateness of a wheelchair or ambulatory device should be part of a comprehensive examination. The assessment of the use of assistive technology should be performed within the environment that it is to be used. Assessing the devices also will require assessment of the environment to determine whether it is conducive for the size, shape, and weight of the device. Before a person is placed in a community residential facility, the physical therapist may be asked, as part of the team, to assess the environment to ensure appropriateness for an individual's needs.

The evaluation of an older adult with a developmental disability must be comprehensive and meaningful to the person's activity level and living situation and must be individualized to meet specific needs. The therapist must consider the patient/client's impairments, functional limitations, skill acquisition, environment, and desired functional outcomes in planning the evaluation strategies and procedures. Functionally based examinations are clinically useful.

PROGRAM PLANNING AND IMPLEMENTATION

Individuals with developmental disabilities living in a community need access to supportive care providers and skilled health care clinicians who are knowledgeable about the person, the condition of the individual, and the system of services and supports available to them. Accessing appropriate services is challenging because of an array of disparities seen in the health, rehabilitation, and social service arenas. Older adults with developmental disabilities experience lower rates of preventive care and health promotion than that of the general population.

A greater awareness of such disparities has resulted in numerous intervention programs and practices aimed at promoting successful aging in those with developmental disabilities. *Person-based practices* promote the health of persons with developmental disabilities by educating and supporting the individual in such areas as nutrition, physical activity, preventive care, rest, and the management of stress. The *Healthy Lifestyles Curriculum*,[82] the *Exercise and Nutrition Health Education Curriculum for Adults with Developmental Disabilities*,[83] and *Women Be Healthy: A Curriculum for Women with Mental Retardation and Other Developmental Disabilities*,[84] although not developed specifically for the older adult, are structured, center-based health promotion intervention programs that have been shown to effectively change health behaviors in adults with developmental disabilities. The *M.E.E. Calendar*,[85] a less structured approach, provides a variety of activities that can be done with older adults to promote fitness and activity, maintain language skills, and facilitate problem solving. *Provider-based practices* call for the standard and systematic inclusion of information on developmental disabilities within curricula for service providers.[86,87] Professional organizations, such as the American Physical Therapy Association[88] are including a variety of programs to increase knowledge and skill among their members. *Policy-based practices* have focused on creating a system of care to improve coordination among agencies providing services to those with developmental disabilities. Service coordination, interdisciplinary care, and interagency collaboration are receiving a great deal of attention. The Special Olympics Healthy Athlete[89] program is one attempt to provide hearing, vision, and musculoskeletal screenings during the Special Olympics Games. In the United States, there has been a desire to increase communication between interagency and interdisciplinary groups for addressing mental health needs in people with intellectual disabilities.[90] These practices recognize that adults with developmental disabilities are aging and with increasing life expectancies there will be a need for a greater array of comprehensive, integrated services.

Habilitation vs. Rehabilitation

Older adults with developmental disabilities generally necessitate habilitation programs. *Habilitation*, as distinguished from rehabilitation, refers to services that assist an individual in gaining skills and abilities.[91] Rehabilitation attempts to restore skills that have been lost as a result of injury or medical condition.[91] Habilitation is required by law, under Medicaid regulations, and financed by Title 19 of the Social Security Act. Habilitation services for the older adult are generally provided by an interdisciplinary team. The *Individualized Service Plan* (ISP) is the document that records the outcomes, goals, and programmatic strategies decided by the team to be necessary for the client to attain or maintain an optimal level of independence.

The interdisciplinary team is the team approach that is most commonly used with older persons with developmental disabilities.[92] The team consists of various professionals, in addition to physical therapists—for example, occupational therapists, physicians, speech-language pathologists, nurses, psychologists, nutritionists, special education teachers, and social workers—who independently evaluate the individual and then meet together and share their findings with each other and the individual. Based on this information and the desired outcomes of the patient/client and caregivers, the team formulates a comprehensive plan that will best meet the needs of that individual.

The role of the physical therapist on the team is determined by the needs of the client and the priority outcomes established on the ISP. The therapist may be a direct provider of service, a consultant to other team members, or a monitor of programs carried out by direct care providers. Although individuals have long-term disabilities, the role of *direct provider* of physical therapy may be intermittent. The level of intensity will be related to the prioritized outcomes of the ISP or the need for services after an acute illness or injury. More often, the therapist may be an indirect provider of service. As a *monitor* of services, the physical therapist establishes functional goals that are consistent with the outcomes prioritized on the ISP and trains other individuals (usually direct care providers) in a specific program aimed at achieving goals. The physical therapist creates a data collection system for the person implementing the program and monitors the client's progress at an appropriate frequency. Figures 29-1 and 29-2 are examples of simple data collection systems designed for individuals living in an intermediate-care facility. The data collection system must be very simple to increase the likelihood that it will be completed by the staff. Also, the staff carrying out the program implementation must be trained and supervised. Monitoring of the program data collection and intermittent retraining must be performed on a regular basis with adaptations to the program as necessary.

The role of *consultant* requires the physical therapist to respond to specific requests of the patient/client, caregivers, or program staff. Unlike monitoring services, the physical therapist providing consultation is not directly responsible for the outcomes of the individual client.

Goal: Tom will walk with his walker from the living room to his bedroom in 5 minutes.

Date	4/1	4/2	4/3	4/4	4/5	4/6	4/7	4/8	4/9	4/10
Record time in minutes	10	10	9	10	8	9	8	8	7	8
Initial										

FIGURE 29-1 Example of a simple data collection system identifying a mobility goal and displaying the scores achieved over a 10-day period by Tom Charles, a 77-year-old man with mild-moderate level of intellectual disability and decreased endurance due to acute emphysema.

Goal: Chris will transfer from a chair into his walker independently.

Date	4/1	4/2	4/3	4/4	4/5	4/6	4/7	4/8	4/9	4/10
Assistance needed to steady the chair (Y/N)	Y	Y	Y	Y	Y	N	N	Y	N	N
Assistance needed at arms to pull up to stand (Y/N)	Y	Y	N	Y	Y	N	Y	Y	N	N
Initial										

FIGURE 29-2 Example of a simple data collection system identifying a mobility goal and displaying the scores achieved over a 10-day time period for Chris Allen, a 59-year-old with moderate spastic diplegia.

The physical therapist is responsible for providing to the consultee information that is helpful to assist the patient/client in meeting the outcomes. *Case consultation* focuses on the needs of an individual patient/client. The physical therapist, for example, may provide suggestions to a caregiver about how to involve a patient/client with cerebral palsy in leisure activities. *Colleague consultation* targets the needs of other service providers. Discussing with direct caregivers proper body mechanics to prevent back injury when transferring a patient/client would be an example of colleague consultation. The purpose of *system consultation* is to effect system change, with the focus being on the service delivery system rather than a specific client. In-service training, program development, or evaluation are examples of system consultation.

Regardless of the role the physical therapist takes in implementing the therapeutic program, an appropriate documentation system must be established. Documentation is important and should meet the needs of those involved in the program, third-party payers, and the service system (developmental disabilities or aging). If the therapist is acting as a direct service provider, progress and the response to intervention should be documented at each visit. The plan for future intervention also should be included. If service is being provided on an indirect basis, a system for documentation must be created for those implementing the program. Figures 29-1 and 29-2 provide examples of simple documentation systems. As indicated previously, this documentation should provide an objective measurement of the individual's progress, and the system must be clear and concise so that it is not burdensome to caregivers. Therapists also must follow the regulations of the Medicaid and Medicare systems (see Chapter 30). Unfortunately, this may require duplication of documentation in various formats to meet the requirements of the various regulatory systems.

Resources

Because the challenge of providing services to this population is an emerging area of service delivery, it may be helpful to consult current journals in geriatrics and developmental disabilities. Periodicals such as *Intellectual and Developmental Disabilities*, *American Journal on Intellectual and Developmental Disabilities*, and *Journal of the Association for Persons with Severe Handicaps* may be helpful. *Topics in Geriatric Rehabilitation* has recently published a special issue, *Aging with a Developmental Disability*. Also, the Administration on Developmental Disabilities has funded selected University Centers for Excellence in Developmental Disabilities to develop training and service programs specifically for older persons with developmental disabilities. These programs offer multimedia information and are available to train service providers in providing appropriate care to older

adults with developmental disabilities (Box 29-3). The National Institute on Disability and Rehabilitation Research also funds a Rehabilitation Research and Training Center on Aging with a Developmental Disability at the University of Illinois at Chicago.

CASE STUDIES

Case 1

Zachary is a 67-year-old man with mild-moderate intellectual disability and cerebral palsy of the spastic diplegic type, Gross Motor Function Classification System[93] level 3-4. He is able to communicate verbally. He lives in an intermediate-care facility and attends a day treatment program. As a child, he walked with crutches and long leg braces. He had hamstring lengthenings and heelcord lengthenings at age 10 years and again when he was 14 years old. As he got older, he continued to walk with crutches but without the braces. By the time Zachary reached age 60 years, his gait had slowed considerably

> **BOX 29-3 University Centers for Excellence in Developmental Disabilities with Specific Programs for Older Persons with Developmental Disabilities**
>
> - Center for Child and Human Development, Georgetown University, Box 571485, Washington DC 20057-1485, 202-687-2071. http://gucchd.georgetown.edu
> - Eunice Shriver Center, 200 Trapelo Road, Waltham, MA 02115, (617) 734-7509. http://www.umassmed.edu/shriver
> - Institute for Study of Developmental Disabilities, Indiana University, 2853 E. 10th St., Bloomington, IN 47408-2601, 812-855-6508. http://www.iidc.indiana.edu
> - Institute for Human Development, University of Missouri-Kansas City, 22200 Holmes St., Third Floor, Kansas City, MO 64108, 816-235-1770. http://www.ihd.umkc.edu
> - Mailman Center for Child Development, University of Miami, School of Medicine, P.O. Box 016820, D-820, Miami, FL 33101, 305-547-6635. http://www.ihd.umkc.edu
> - North Dakota Center for Developmental Disabilities, Minot State University, 500 University Ave. W, Minot, ND 58071, 701-857-3580. http://www.ndcpd.org/
> - Partners for Inclusive Communities, University of Arkansas for Medical Sciences, 2001 Pershing Circle, Ste 300, North Little Rock, AR 73114, 501-682-9900, http://www.uams.edu/partners
> - Rehabilitation Research Training Center on Aging with Intellectual and Developmental Disabilities (RRTCADD, Department of Disability and Human Development (DHD); College of Applied Health Sciences, University of Illinois at Chicago (UIC) 1640 West Roosevelt Road, M/C 626, Chicago, IL 60608-6904, Phone: 312-413-1520. http://www.rrtcadd.org/About_Us/Home.html
> - Strong Center for Developmental Disabilities, University of Rochester Medical Center, 601 Elmwood Ave., Rochester, NY 14642, 716-275-2986. http://www.urmc.rochester.edu/pediatrics/divisions/developmental_disabilities/index.cfm

and he was encouraged to use a wheelchair by the staff at his day treatment program. A manual wheelchair was purchased for Zachary when he was 62 years old. By 67, Zachary had gained 17 pounds and his wheelchair needed to be replaced. The range of motion in Zachary's legs had become more limited, making even stand-pivot transfers difficult.

Planning and implementing a program appropriate for Zachary involved a comprehensive examination as previously described. Through an interview with Zachary and his caregivers, it was found that Zachary was somewhat depressed regarding his inability to walk. He also was found to have an interest in improving his ability to manage transfers to and from the toilet independently. The caregivers stated that Zachary enjoyed swimming and was independent in the shallow water at the pool.

The information gained from the person-centered planning interview[94,95] (Box 29-4) was enhanced by the structured interview of the SIS and the SIB-R. These data coupled with the information gained from the neuromuscular assessment allowed the therapist to create appropriate goals and a realistic plan that was driven by the outcomes identified through the person-centered planning process according to the desires of Zachary and his caregivers. The team decided that one outcome would be a return to independence in the bathroom.

In order to regain independence in the bathroom, independence in stand-pivot transfers was one goal. To achieve that goal, the therapist instructed Zachary's caregivers on performing transfers with the client and encouraging greater assistance from Zachary. The plan involved having Zachary practice this transfer each time he needed to use the bathroom. To create a program that was more likely to help Zachary reach his goals, the staff at the day treatment program also received training and agreed to follow the plan as designed. The therapist monitored progress weekly for 1 month and then monthly for another 2 months to ensure progression toward the goal. In addition, building on Zachary's

interest in swimming, the physical therapist in collaboration with the recreational therapist designed a swimming program that would (1) promote cardiovascular fitness and weight loss and (2) improve lower extremity strength. Both of these goals would assist him in reaching his stand-pivot goal as well. Activities included swimming laps and practicing standing and walking in the water. The recreation therapist monitored the program monthly with an agreement to contact the physical therapist with any questions or concerns.

In collaboration with the team that included Zachary, his caregivers, the social worker, and physician, a new, appropriate wheelchair was prescribed and obtained for Zachary. The therapist assessed the wheelchair on a quarterly basis for safety, fit, and function. The therapist taught the staff appropriate wheelchair care and maintenance.

Zachary and his caregivers were pleased with the program because it took into consideration everyone's needs and Zachary's desired outcome. Zachary was pleased because he was able to practice "walking" in the water, which he enjoyed. He was motivated to practice the stand-pivot transfer because he wanted to regain the ability to transfer independently. This intervention program proved to be quite successful. At the end of 3 months, Zachary had lost weight; was able to complete a standing-pivot transfer with only stand-by assistance; and his new wheelchair was modern and streamlined, allowing him to maneuver in his home more efficiently. The success of this program was due to the collaboration among all team members including Zachary and the fact that it was based on Zachary's desired outcomes. The physical therapist, in collaboration with her team members, successfully monitored his program and consulted with daily caregivers and Zachary.

Case 2

Lisa is 71 years old and has a diagnosis of mild intellectual disability. She lives in a supervised apartment with two other older women and attends an integrated adult day care program at a local nursing home. Lisa ambulates independently on all surfaces including stairs. She is independent in ADLs. She is able to take a bus to a destination, after she has been shown three to four times. Lisa has always enjoyed riding a stationary bike, but her knees and hips have begun to bother her. She has been diagnosed as having osteoarthritis, and her physician suggested that she find an alternate activity to replace the stationary bike riding.

The community in which Lisa lives funds her residential program as well as her day program through the state Medicaid program. Medicaid programs for adults with developmental disabilities in her state (as in many) require that a physical therapist be a member of the team and available to consult with the client, any caregivers, or administrative staff as appropriate. Being a

---

BOX 29-4	**Key Elements of a Person-Centered Planning Interview**

- Respect the individual as a key informant
- Address questions to the client directly
- Maintain a conversational tone throughout the interview
- Clarify information with follow-up questions to the client first and then to other team members as needed
- Begin the conversation by eliciting information on the dreams and aspirations of the client
- Identify natural supports prior to determining professional services
- Focus on desired outcomes and capacities, not deficits or impairments
- Maintain a reflective, creative, positive environment where all members of the team contribute equally to problem solving

direct-access state, the physical therapist received a referral from Lisa's home supervisor to consult with the team regarding Lisa and the suggestion that she find an alternative to stationary bike riding. Upon interviewing Lisa and the supervisors, it was discovered that Lisa once enjoyed swimming, but since she had moved to this apartment 7 years ago, there had been no opportunity for this activity. Following a chart review, a systems review, and a screening for strength, balance, and ambulation ability, the physical therapist determined that Lisa was not in need of his direct services but he felt that she could benefit from a non–weight-bearing exercise program to avoid knee pain. The physical therapist collaborated with the apartment supervisor, recreational therapist, and social worker to involve Lisa in a regular swimming program at the local indoor pool at the community fitness center. The social worker found a companion to accompany Lisa on the bus to the pool. The recreation therapist arranged with the staff at the pool to have Lisa participate in a water aerobics class. The adult day care staff were made aware that Lisa would be coming in late on Wednesdays and Fridays—the days she would participate in the aerobics program. The physical therapist was available to consult with the home care providers, recreation therapist, and pool staff, if necessary.

Lisa and the staff were pleased with the progress. Lisa experienced a problem often seen in the aging population, but her developmental disability made it difficult for her to access appropriate care and activities. The therapist in consultation with other members of the interdisciplinary team found an activity that Lisa enjoyed and created an effective program for her. Through a collaborative effort, a program was implemented that met the patient/client's needs.

SUMMARY

Information regarding aging individuals with developmental disabilities has recently begun to receive attention in the literature.[94,95] Older persons with developmental disabilities have begun to be recognized by service providers and policy makers as a large heterogeneous group who require specialized services integrated into the service system of the general population of older adults.

This chapter reviewed the legal mandates and social policy impetus guiding service to this group. The role of the physical therapist in examining individuals and assisting team members with designing appropriate, holistic habilitation plans was presented. Although little information is available on specific aspects of the aging process in adults with developmental disabilities, aspects of aging in persons with Down syndrome and cerebral palsy were discussed.

Physical therapists are in a unique position to assume leadership roles in the care of older adults with developmental disabilities and develop integrated programs of habilitation. In addition, a critical role for physical therapists will be to design and foster leisure skill programming for these persons that will promote and maintain functional skills. Physical therapists also are in a position to effect system change, specifically recognizing the importance of leisure skill programming and creating reimbursement strategies that will take leisure skill programming into consideration.

REFERENCES

To enhance this text and add value for the reader, all references are included on the companion Evolve site that accompanies this text book. The reader can view the reference source and access it online whenever possible. There are a total of 95 cited references and other general references for this chapter.

PART VI

Societal Issues

Reimbursement and Payment Policy

Jean Oulund Peteet, PT, MPH, PhD, Rhea Cohn, PT, DPT

INTRODUCTION

It is virtually impossible to understand reimbursement for physical therapy services provided to older adults without understanding federal programs and payment policies. These programs and policies must also be considered within the context of the American health care system and its complex blend of public and private financing. Although the United States offers technologically advanced health care, it has been the only developed nation that did not provide universal health insurance,[1] leaving some 47 million Americans without access to care.[2] In 2006, 74% of Americans thought that the health system had serious failings or was in crisis.[3] Universal health insurance programs rely on social insurance and expect that a large number of people will each contribute small amounts of money to fund the program. The reluctance of the United States to embrace universal coverage is the result of fundamentally different political philosophies and attitudes concerning the role of government and the private sector in formulating health care policies and underwriting health care policies.[4,5] Thus, presidents and legislators had attempted more than five times in the past 50 years to pass legislation for universal access to health care and previously only partially achieved it for older adults through the Medicare law enacted in 1965 and for a portion of low-income people through Medicaid legislation enacted along with the Medicare law.[6]

Employment-based private insurance remains the primary source of insurance coverage used by some 51% of the population in the United States.[2] This fact describes the current context of health care policy formulation for individuals of any age and the backdrop to all health care reform proposals affecting older adults. For example, many ideas about how to control rising costs flow bidirectionally between the governmental and private sectors. Federally funded benefits and payment schedules are scrutinized and often utilized by the private sector

payers for their insurance products and supporting payment policies. Employees are dependent on the health insurance options that are offered by their employer; however, participation is voluntary and requires employee cost sharing to some degree or other. Analogous features are found in Medicare programs and insurance products. Large group employers usually offer more than one health insurance option to their employees. Small group employers usually offer only one health insurance option. Large group employers can often negotiate better premium rates because their risk pool is larger. Small group employers and individuals purchasing their own insurance have access to smaller risk pools, thereby decreasing their ability to negotiate more affordable premiums. Also, one very sick employee in a small business will have serious consequences for future premium rates for the other employees. Therefore, health insurance premiums are generally more expensive for small business owners.

In contrast to the private sector, Medicare has standard benefits and premiums for all individuals who qualify. As more people older than age 65 years remain employed, a greater number of older adults will likely have primary health insurance coverage through their employer and Medicare will become their secondary payer. In summary, the interplay between the public and private sector regarding health care dynamically influences similarities and differences in beneficiary qualifications, policy options, coverage, and premiums as well as reimbursement for services.

Although the Medicare program is available for people age 65 years and older, access to all desirable health care services is still a problem for older adults because the Medicare program lacks coverage for many aspects of preventive care, has limits for hospital and skilled nursing facility (SNF) care, and lacks coverage for long-term care provided at home or in nursing homes. Medicare enrollees may choose to obtain supplemental or secondary coverage that will help offset their financial obligations for services provided under the Medicare program or for services that are not covered.

Comprehensive health reform legislation, the Patient Protection and Affordable Care Act (PL 111-148), was signed into law by President Obama in March 2010 and addressed many of the limitations described previously. The law impacts both federally funded programs as well as the private insurance market. This complex law includes provisions to expand insurance coverage to meet the requirement that all Americans have health insurance, to control health care costs, and to improve quality of care. Implementation of this law will be phased in through the year 2014; however, the effects will be felt for many years.[5a]

This chapter will help readers understand the health insurance programs for older adults and the complexities of reimbursement methods and reforms to control costs and improve quality. Application of this knowledge will enable readers to effectively advocate for patients, for older adults as a population, and for policy changes that benefit society as a whole. Health care is a rapidly changing industry, and readers are encouraged to refer to the Centers for Medicare & Medicaid Services (CMS) and the American Physical Therapy Association (APTA) websites to read up-to-date information on legislation, regulatory interpretation, and opportunities for professional legislative advocacy.

ACCESS TO HEALTH CARE

The Title 18 Amendment of the Social Security Act in 1965 was landmark legislation that established Medicare, a federal health insurance program for older adults for hospital care (Medicare A) and voluntary insurance for physician services (Medicare Part B). Medicaid, a federal and state funding program providing public assistance for low-income people was established at the same time. These two programs facilitated access to health care for individuals age 65 years and older as well as many younger people with disabilities by providing insurance to help pay for their health care expenses.[6]

These programs are two among other programs that provide health insurance to Americans. The mix of private and public financed health care coverage makes the health care system in the United States complex and costly. In 2008, the United States spent more than 16% of its gross domestic product (GDP) on health care—more than any other industrialized nation in the world.[7] In contrast, Canada spent only 10%.[8] Factors contributing to lower costs in Canada were (1) administrative costs 300% lower than in the United States, (2) lower costs per patient day in hospitals, and (3) lower physician fees and pharmaceutical prices.[9] The United States is spending an increasing percentage of its GDP on health care, and cost escalation is compelling the federal government to reconsider how to fund and regulate these public programs.

Funding for Health Care Coverage

The health care system in the United States can be segmented by funding source as well as the categories of services covered by the funding (Figure 30-1). Although government funding (i.e., Medicare or Medicaid) is the primary payment vehicle for older adults of all income levels, those adults who continue to work full-time past age 65 years usually have employment-based or private

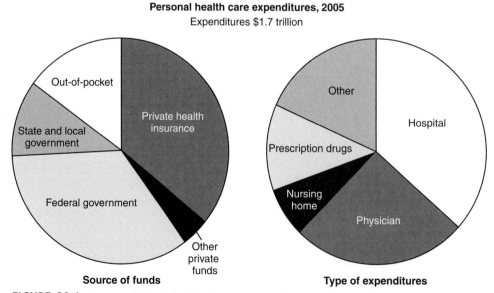

Personal health care expenditures, 2005
Expenditures $1.7 trillion

Source of funds
Out-of-pocket
Private health insurance
State and local government
Federal government
Other private funds

Type of expenditures
Other
Hospital
Prescription drugs
Nursing home
Physician

FIGURE 30-1 Sources of funds for health care expenditures and types of expenditures. *(Sources: Centers for Disease Control and Prevention, National Center for Health Statistics, Health, United States, 2007, Figure 6. Data from the Centers for Medicare & Medicaid Services.)*

insurance that will have specific coverage and limitations. For these people, Medicare may be a secondary payer.[6] Figure 30-1 illustrates that hospital and physician services account for more than half of the health care expenditures in the United States, making these services important for examining the potential for improved efficiency and cost savings.

Historically, health care services were paid based on the number and type of services provided in both the public and private sectors. Therefore, as the number of services provided increased, so did the potential for revenue growth for those providing care. This method promoted an escalation in health care expenditures across all settings, regardless of who might be responsible for reimbursement of the services. In 1983, well ahead of cost control in the private sector, the federal government changed this paradigm and established prospective payment systems for hospitals, and in 1997 extended these systems to SNFs and home care services. Under prospective payment, Medicare reimburses acute care hospitals based on the patient's specific diagnosis grouping, known as diagnosis-related groups (DRGs) rather than paying for each individual service provided in the hospital. SNFs are paid a per diem rate based on a classification gleaned from an evaluation tool known as the Minimum Data Set. Home health agencies use yet another tool, Outcome and Assessment Information Set, that assists with the classification of payment.[6]

Although each of these prospective payment systems are configured differently, they all provide a common incentive—provide care in a cost-effective manner because the payment for the admission will essentially be the same, regardless of the number or type of services provided. Prospective payment has not yet been developed for outpatient services. It should be noted, however, that current outpatient payment methodologies are broadly perceived as unsustainable and the federal government continues to explore alternatives. Medicare and Medicaid, not unlike private insurers, want to become more active purchasers of health care and, at the same time, influence how their beneficiaries access services.

Cost Control Methods across All Settings

Health care insurers, purchasers of health care coverage, and providers alike are concerned about costs and several methods have been, and are being, used to control health care costs.[5] First, payments to providers are controlled by different reimbursement methodologies. Fee for service, per diem, episode of illness, and capitation are the primary methods. Table 30-1 provides a definition of these methods and illustrates that each method carries a different level of risk for providers. Fee for service is the least aggregated method of payment whereby a provider or hospital is paid a fee for each procedure or service provided. The most

TABLE 30-1	Examples of Provider Payment Methods for All Insurance Types	
Type	**Definition**	**Provider Risk**
Fee for service	An amount assigned to a specific procedure or service	Lowest
Per diem	An amount associated with all services provided in each day of care	
Episode of illness	An amount for all procedures and services associated with an episode of hospitalization	
Capitation	A fixed payment given to providers at specified intervals for all care provided to patients in a managed care plan	Highest

aggregated method is capitation, where providers receive a fixed payment based on the number of enrollees in a defined geographic area for a patient's care during a month or year, regardless of the type or number of services provided. Capitation is less common than it was 10 years ago and has primarily been used for primary care physicians. Payers can control costs by selecting a payment method, such as fee schedules or contracted payment rates with preferred providers.[5] Because hospitals and providers were historically paid on a fee-for-service basis contributing to escalated costs, there was a rise in managed care plans in the private market in the 1990s.[5] These plans utilized payment mechanisms that favored more aggregated payment methodologies. The evolution of payment methodologies continues as payers search for the most effective way to control costs and ensure the provision of appropriate services.

A number of broader strategies are also used to control costs. Regulations and competition are two commonly used strategies to limit the amount of money that providers receive. The traditional fee-for-service Medicare program is an example of a program that uses regulatory strategies and an adjustable fee schedule conversion factor to control costs. The Balanced Budget Act of 1997 is the most dramatic example of legislation that reduced reimbursement for services.[10] The reduction in payments along with stricter and comprehensive regulations are intended to control utilization of services and expense to the program.

Competitive strategies focus on making purchasers (employers and employees) more price-sensitive. Employers negotiate with insurers to maintain or lower premium rates, revise employee deductibles and copayments, and determine a reasonable benefit package for their employees. A few large group employers have begun to design their employee health insurance benefit to promote use of prevention services that will ultimately save costs associated with inappropriate use of hospitalizations, imaging, and emergency department visits.[11] Employees and individuals purchasing their own insurance coverage usually select a plan based on price; however, educated consumers may also consider the details of the benefit package.

There are economists who oppose the traditional insurers' response to competitive market forces, that is, raising rates or diminishing the benefit package. It can be argued that a more beneficial long-term approach would be to encourage utilization of services that will provide higher quality outcomes at lower costs. Another payer strategy to decrease financial exposure is to select enrollees based on the likelihood of enrollees having or developing a particular health condition, hoping to assume as little risk as possible for future expenditures.

Insurers can also control their expenses by reducing the payments to providers and hospitals. A response by providers to such reductions can be increased utilization of services or procedures, or contracting with insurers who offer better reimbursement for the delivery of the service. Medicare and other third-party payers carefully monitor utilization of services by all providers. If an unexpected and unwarranted increase in utilization is detected, the usual response is yet another type of payment control mechanism. Private payers usually monitor use of services either concurrently (while the services are being provided) or retrospectively (after the care is complete). This review of services, known as "utilization management," is a third type of cost control mechanism highly utilized by managed care plans.[4,5]

Most payers have defined benefits for coverage of physical therapy services. This fourth method of controlling costs helps the payers predetermine their liability for physical therapy services. A benefit for physical therapy could be defined by a specified number of visits per year (e.g., 20 visits per year) or a specific number of visits per condition. Medicare has intermittently had a financial cap on services provided under a physical therapy plan of care.[12] Medicare and many other payers specify that physical therapy must be for restorative care rather than maintenance care. Although many providers, including physical therapists, realize the potential benefits from prevention services, this is usually not a covered benefit. All of these controls help the payers know the extent of their financial liability for physical therapy services, thereby reducing their risk and, ultimately, their costs.

Patient cost-sharing is yet another type of cost control mechanism and is very typical throughout the industry. When instituted, patients may pay a portion of the premium and also assume responsibility for the deductible and copayments. Medicare uses this method as does the private sector. Medicare beneficiaries typically have a copayment of 20% for some services, an annual deductible, and/or a per diem fee associated with hospital or

BOX 30-1	Common Cost Control Mechanisms

1. Choice of payment methodology for providers
2. Utilization management
3. Benefit restrictions
4. Increased patient cost-sharing
5. Limitations on covered services
6. Financial caps on services

facility-based services.[13] One concern with this mechanism is that cost sharing creates inequity for lower income patients as they pay a higher percentage of their total income toward health care.

Employers, providers, patients, and payers all assume some level of risk. Varying payment methodologies shift risk among these groups and influence consumer behaviors related to accessing services and choosing providers. Each of these cost controls is in some way "painful" to one or more of these entities and understanding the impact a cost control has on any entity, whether patient, provider or payer, is important to understanding that entity's response to the control.[5] No matter who is affected or in what ways, physical therapists must always bear in mind that payment methodologies and cost control strategies will always either support or restrict access to care. Moreover, it is highly unlikely that any particular combination is "all good" or "all bad." On the contrary, the best system will optimize the "pros" for all entities and simultaneously minimize the "cons" of various mechanisms for each entity as well. Box 30-1 details common cost control mechanisms.

HEALTH INSURANCE PROGRAMS: MEDICARE

The Department of Health and Human Services, part of the executive branch of the federal government, administers the Medicare program and funds it through contributions from employees who have paid into the Social Security system. This entitlement program has no premium for Part A (hospital services) but does have a premium ($96.40 to $110.50/month in 2010) for the voluntary component, Part B (medical services and durable medical equipment). People can also purchase supplemental private insurance known as Medigap to help pay for Part A and B uncovered services. Box 30-2 provides examples of services provided under Medicare A and B. Box 30-3 details coverage of Parts A, B, C, and D of the Medicare program. Both Medicare A and B require the patient to make out-of-pocket payments for deductibles and coinsurance costs. The deductible and copayments only apply to covered services. If a particular service is not covered, the patient must be notified in advance and would have to assume full financial responsibility for that service.[13]

BOX 30-2 | Medicare Part A and Part B: Examples of Covered Services

Medicare Part A (Hospital Insurance)
- Hospital stay
- Skilled nursing facility stay
- Inpatient rehabilitation facility
- Home health care
- Hospice care

Medicare Part B (Medical Insurance)
Helps to cover:
- Doctor's services, outpatient care
- Outpatient mental health therapy services
- Occupational, physical, and speech–language pathology services
- Outpatient diagnostic tests

Examples of Medicare Part B Covered Preventive Services
- Abdominal aortic aneurysm screening
- Bone density measurement every 2 years
- Cardiovascular screening every 5 years
- Colorectal cancer screenings
- Diabetes screenings for people with high-risk factors
- Flu shots
- Glaucoma tests
- Mammograms
- One-time "Welcome to Medicare" physical exam
- Pap tests
- Prostate cancer screenings
- Smoking cessation counseling

Examples of Part A and Part B Non-Covered Services
- Acupuncture
- Chiropractic services
- Custodial care
- Deductibles, coinsurance or copayments
- Dental care and dentures
- Eye exams
- Foot care
- Hearing aids and exams

BOX 30-3 | Medicare Choices

Original Medicare Part A and Part B
- Run by federal government
- Provides Part A (Hospital Insurance)—no premium for adults who are eligible for Social Security or Railroad Retirement Benefits
- Provides Part B (Medical Insurance)—requires a monthly premium
- Beneficiary pays deductibles and coinsurance
- Beneficiary can add drug coverage (Part D) and purchase a Medigap policy from a private insurer to cover some out-of-pocket expenses

Medicare Advantage Plans–Part C (similar to Health Maintenance Organizations and Preferred Provider Organizations)
- Run by Medicare-approved private companies
- Provide Parts A, B, and D
- A Medigap policy is not needed
- Costs vary by plan

Other
- Medicare Cost Plans, Demonstration and Pilot programs, Programs of All-Inclusive Care for the Elderly (PACE)

Medicare Part D Drug Coverage
- Run by Medicare-approved insurance companies
- Beneficiary pays a monthly premium
- Beneficiary can change plans once per year

Medicare Part C offers an alternative to the traditional Medicare fee-for-service coverage, which allows a beneficiary to choose to join a Medicare-approved health plan that is operated by a private insurance payer. Costs vary by plans and the plans provide coverage for Parts A, B, and D (Prescription Drug Coverage). These plans are more comprehensive than traditional Medicare coverage, and patients do not need a Medigap policy if they choose this plan.[13] This type of coverage is attractive to beneficiaries because they will have lower out-of-pocket costs; however, they are limited to a restricted provider network. A newer alternative is the Medicare Part C fee-for-service health plan. These plans are most often offered to retirees of large companies that need to devise ways to cover lives dispersed across many areas of the country. This permits the employer to standardize a retiree's coverage, regardless of residence, within the framework of a Medicare Part C model.[14]

Medicare Part D, implemented in 2006, provides optional prescription drug coverage to all Medicare enrollees. Plans vary in cost and in drugs that are covered. To obtain Medicare drug coverage, patients must join a plan run by an insurance company that is in their state.[6] Medicare Part D provides coverage of medications up to a certain dollar amount ($2840 in 2011); there is no additional coverage until they have reached the ceiling of the "donut hole" ($4550 in 2011)[13] (Table 30-2). Therapists need to be sensitive to the possibility that their patients may be without drug coverage for a portion of the year and this could seriously affect the levels of participation in therapy as well as the outcome of care.

Medicare Coverage in Different Settings

The Medicare program offers varying coverage in different practice settings for services and durable medical equipment (DME). Benefits in the acute care hospital, inpatient rehabilitation, SNFs, outpatient settings, home health, hospice, the community, and DME coverage can be accessed through Chapter 15 of the Medicare Benefit Policy Manual.[16] It is important for providers to access this manual and its updates on a regular basis to minimize the risk for claims denials.

TABLE 30-2	Example of Medicare Drug Costs			
Ms. Smith joins the ABC Prescription Drug Plan. Her coverage begins on January 1, 2010. She doesn't get "extra help" and uses her Medicare drug plan membership card when she buys prescriptions.				
Yearly Deductible	**Copayment or Coinsurance**	**Coverage Gap**	**Catastrophic Coverage**	
Ms. Smith pays the first $310 of her drug costs before her plan starts to pay its share.	Ms. Smith pays a copayment, and her plan pays its share for each covered drug until what they pay (plus the deductible) reaches $2840.	Once Ms. Smith and her plan have spent $2840 for covered drugs, she is in the coverage gap. She will have to pay all of her drug costs beyond the $2700, until she reaches $4550. Some drugs will be discounted through 2020 when she will have full coverage in the gap.	Once Ms. Smith has spent $4550 out of pocket for the year, her coverage gap ends. Now she only pays a small copayment for each drug until the end of the year.	

Source: Medicare and You 2010.[13]

Acute Care Hospital. Medicare Part A covers acute care inpatient hospital stays for 90 days of care per episode of illness with 60 lifetime reserve days. The "episode" begins when a person is admitted, and ends when the person has been out of the hospital or SNF for 60 consecutive days. Box 30-4 provides an example of the out-of-pocket costs a person would pay in 2011 for a hospitalization.[13]

Medicare groups patients with similar clinical problems into DRGs and reimburses hospitals based on the DRG and the Inpatient Prospective Payment Rate (IPPS) per discharge that includes a complex method of accounting for the patient's condition, treatment, and the market conditions of the hospital's location. The hospital receives the same payment whether the patient stays in the hospital 3 days or 3 weeks (although outlier payments are added for excessively complex patients). In 2009, Medicare implemented a transition to a system that is known as Medicare severity (MS) DRGs that increase the number of DRGs and recognizes comorbidities and major complications. Rates are annually updated and Medicare has created an incentive for hospitals that provide specific-quality data to the U.S. Department of Health and Human Services to receive the full rate increase.[17]

Inpatient Rehabilitation. Inpatient rehabilitation facilities (IRFs) provide intensive services such as physical, occupational, or speech therapy for patients after surgery, an injury, or illness. To qualify for Medicare coverage, patients must be able to benefit from and tolerate 3 hours of therapy for 5 of 7 days each week or participate in 15 hours of therapy in 7 days. When patients are transferred from an acute care hospital to an IRF, they have no additional deductible. However, they will have a deductible to meet if admitted from the community. Acute hospital days and IRF days all count toward the Medicare Part A inpatient hospital limits.[18]

Reimbursement to IRFs has been under a prospective payment system (PPS) since 2002. IRFs receive a predetermined per-discharge rate based on the patient's diagnosis, cognitive status, functional status, market area wages, and a system of case-mix categories that reflects the expected resources needed to provide care. The rate covers all capital and operating costs associated with providing intensive rehabilitation. Medicare increases payment rates for rural areas (because of fewer cases in those areas, longer length of stays, and higher costs per case), makes adjustments for teaching institutions, and for patient stays that are outliers providing a lower rate for short stays and a higher rate for high-cost stays.[18]

An important rule applied to IRF admissions is the 60% rule (formerly known as the 75% rule) whereby in order for an IRF to receive payment, 60% of their admissions must have one or more of 13 qualifying medical conditions. Box 30-5 lists those conditions as of 2009.[18] The 60% rule intends to promote proper placement of postacute care patients into the most cost-effective setting. If a patient covered by Medicare cannot tolerate 3 hours of therapy each day or if the patient's condition does not warrant comprehensive rehabilitation combined with 24-hour skilled nursing and medical supervision, Medicare will not cover the

BOX 30-4	Example of Out-of-Pocket Costs for Medicare Services[13]

Sonia is 68 years old and has Medicare parts A and B. She experiences a cerebral vascular accident with multiple medical complications. She spends 65 days in the hospital, followed by 25 days in a skilled nursing facility (SNF), and then receives home health services (nursing, physical therapy, occupational therapy, speech–language pathology) for 21 days. Her out-of-pocket costs in 2011 for these settings would be:

Hospital deductible		= $1132.00
Hospital daily cost		
after 60 days	$283 × 5 days	= $1415.00
SNF daily cost after		
20 days	$141.50 × 5 days	= $707.50
Home health care		= 0.00
TOTAL		**$3254.50**

See Table 30-2 for out-of-pocket costs she would incur for drugs once she is home.

BOX 30-5	Inpatient Rehabilitation Facility Conditions That Qualify for Medicare Under the 60% Rule[16]

Stroke
Spinal cord injury
Congenital deformity
Amputation
Major multiple trauma
Hip fracture
Brain injury
Neurologic disorders (such as multiple sclerosis, Parkinson's disease
Burns
Three arthritis conditions for which appropriate, aggressive, and sustained outpatient therapy has failed
Joint replacement for both knees or hips when the surgery immediately precedes admission when body mass index is greater than or equal to 50 or age is >85 years.

admission to an IRF. Instead, that patient may be a more appropriate candidate for an SNF, which is considered a less intense level and lower cost level of care.

Like acute care facilities, prospective payment provides an incentive for IRFs to control costs, either by managing the number and type of services being provided or minimizing the length of stay. The outcome of care could potentially be negatively affected if an IRF were to provide insufficient or inadequate care because of reducing the delivery of necessary services with the goal of increasing profit from the prospective payment.

Skilled Nursing Facilities. Skilled nursing facilities may provide 24-hour skilled care and/or custodial (also known as maintenance) care, either for short-term skilled nursing and/or rehabilitation or for long-term care. Medicare and most private insurance will cover care provided in an SNF for a limited time if the patient had been hospitalized for 3 days, enters the SNF within 30 days of an acute care hospitalization discharge, and requires skilled care from a registered nurse and rehabilitation therapies. The patient must be making functional gains to qualify. In an SNF stay covered by Medicare Part A, the patient has no financial obligation for the first 20 days. Starting on day 21, the patient is responsible for a daily copayment, and there is a 100-day maximum stay.[13,15]

In a SNF, Medicare covers physical therapy evaluation and treatment programs, as long as the patient meets the requirement of being able to make functional progress. Progress needs to be demonstrated in the documentation. Therapists may provide the treatment or supervise a physical therapist assistant to administer the treatment program. When the patient is no longer making functional gains that support the continued use of skilled providers, Medicare will cover the instruction of a maintenance program to ancillary personnel. Again, documentation needs to support this instruction. Therapy

services are included in the prospective bundled payment made by Medicare to the SNF.[13]

Outpatient Therapy Services. Outpatient therapy services include physical therapy, occupational therapy, and speech-language pathology, and can be provided in different settings. Figure 30-2 illustrates how therapy tends to be distributed by setting. More than half of outpatient services are provided in nursing homes and private practices under the Part B benefit. In order for Medicare to cover these services, they must be provided by qualified provider (i.e., not an aide), be appropriate and effective for a patient's condition, and be reasonable in terms of frequency, intensity, and duration.[19] Technically, a referral to therapy from a physician is not required under the Medicare program; however, a physician must sign the therapy plan of care within 30 days of the initial therapy treatment. Therefore, if state law permits, a therapist can evaluate a patient covered by Medicare without a referral, and subsequently ask the physician to sign the plan of care. The physician must recertify the plan of care every 90 days, but may request to recertify the plan of care sooner. The patient must have impairments that have the potential to improve with therapy interventions. Medicare will not cover any treatment intended to maintain the same level of function or that is a general exercise program. Medicare will, however, cover the instruction of a home exercise program to the patient or

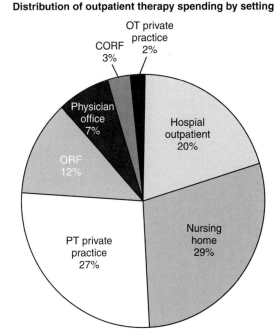

Distribution of outpatient therapy spending by setting

FIGURE 30-2 Medicare outpatient therapy services by setting. *CORF,* comprehensive rehabilitation facility; *ORF,* outpatient rehabilitation facility; *OT,* occupational therapist; *PT,* physical therapist. *(From Medpac: Outpatient Therapy Services Payment System. http://www.medpac.gov/documents/MedPAC_Payment_Basics_08_OPT.pdf.)*

caregiver.[19] Medicare covers some services when provided by a physical or occupational therapist assistant only if a qualified therapist is supervising the assistant as regulated by Medicare. If state law regarding supervision is more stringent than the Medicare regulations, Medicare will follow state laws. Medicare does not permit physicians to directly supervise physical or occupational therapy assistants when services are provided "incident to" the physician's services. States may allow physician assistants, nurse practitioners, and clinical nurse specialists to provide therapy services. Medicare does not recognize aides, chiropractors, athletic trainers, and nurses as qualified providers of therapy services and these providers cannot bill Medicare for such services.[19]

Congress has been involved since 1972 in setting forth laws that both enable physical therapists to provide outpatient services and also restrict those services through spending caps.[21] Therapists are paid under Medicare's physician fee schedule (PFS). Public Law 92-03 of 1972 allowed qualified physical therapists in independent practice to provide services in a patient's home or the therapist's office, thereby increasing patients' access to care. However, since 1979, Medicare has imposed various reimbursement caps on Part B services provided by physical therapists, occupational therapists, and speech–language pathologists.[20] These caps do not affect outpatient rehabilitation services provided in inpatient hospitals, inpatient skilled nursing facilities, and most home health settings that are covered under Medicare Part A.

Home Health Services. Home health services may include medically necessary intermittent skilled nursing, physical therapy, occupational therapy, speech-language pathology, medical social work, home health aide services, and DME for homebound patients. Medicare Part A covers these services and includes 100 days of service after a hospitalization. The patient has no copayments for these services. Since 2000, the CMS has utilized a prospective payment system for home health services and pays home health agencies a preestablished rate for each 60-day episode of illness. Patients who require five or more visits are categorized in 1 of 153 home health resource groups based on the measurement tool, the Outcome and Assessment Information Set (OASIS). Clinical and functional status, expected resource use in the different groups, and geographic factors are considered in developing the payment rates.[22] Private practice physical therapists may see patients in the patient's home under the Part B benefit and the reimbursement is based on the Physician Fee Schedule used for Part B services. The claim form must note that the service was provided in the home.

Historically, home health agencies provided services that assisted people with their functional limitations including activities of daily living and instrumental activities of daily living. However, the demands and incentives placed on hospitals that promote shorter length of stays have caused home health services to provide more specialized services such as nutritional feeding via feeding tubes, intravenous antibiotic infusions, home renal dialysis antibiotic, morphine pumps, and chemotherapy. This decrease in length of stay has concomitantly increased the level of complexity of the patient conditions in the home health setting, requiring therapists in the home care setting to use knowledge and skills generally associated with therapists in acute care settings.[5]

Hospice Care. Hospice care gives patients the choice to maintain quality of life, remain alert and pain-free, and to receive end-of-life care at home, in a hospital or nursing facility. End-of-life care is costly; some 27% of Medicare dollars are spent in patients' last year of life.[23] Hospice care is a lower-cost alternative. Public or private hospice organizations provide supportive services and pain relief to terminally ill patients who are expected to live 6 months or less as determined by their physician. Care is provided in the patient's home or in hospice care based in a hospital or nursing facility. Medicare Part A helps to pay for these services when the following conditions are met: (1) a doctor certifies that a patient is terminally ill; (2) a patient chooses to receive care from a hospice instead of curative treatment for the terminal illness; and (3) care is provided by a Medicare-participating hospice program. Box 30-6 details the services that hospices can provide. Physical, occupational, and speech therapy are covered under Medicare, as are all other services, when treatment is for pain relief and symptom management.[13]

Hospice services are growing and Medicare estimates that spending for hospice by 2018 will double, representing the largest growth rate of all Part A services.[24] Medicare pays for these services through a daily rate schedule that includes four base payment amounts based on the type of hospice care provided: routine care, continuous home care, inpatient respite care, and general inpatient care. Most care (95% of days paid for under hospice) is provided at the routine home care level. Patients pay no copayment for these services and only $5/day for inpatient respite care.[25]

Community Services, Prevention, and Wellness. The United States health care system in 2006 spent less than 3% of the $2.1 trillion health care dollars on services to

---

BOX 30-6 | **Medicare Hospice Benefits**[23]

Skilled nursing service
Drugs for pain control symptom management
Physical, occupational, and speech therapy
Dietary, spiritual, family bereavement and other counseling services
Home health aide and homemaker services
Short-term inpatient respite care and symptom and pain management
Other services needed for palliation and management of the terminal illness

prevent illness,[5] despite research showing that the risks of the top causes of death in the United States, including cardiovascular heart disease, cancer, and cerebrovascular disease, are in large part reducible[26] if people adopt behaviors such as eating a low-fat diet, not smoking, and increasing their physical activity.

Historically, Medicare has been a health insurance program focusing on treating health problems within health care settings. Medicare covers some preventive screenings and services as detailed in Box 30-2. However, these services have little if any impact on primary prevention of the major causes of death when initiated at the time of Medicare enrollment, age 65 and older. Because Medicare is primarily a program for older adults, it cannot address the need for risk reduction in health plans or programs that cover children and young adults.

Recognizing that a large number of Medicare beneficiaries have one or more chronic conditions that are costly and require the expertise of multiple specialists, Medicare is testing a new model termed "medical home." In a "medical home," the high-need older adult will be part of a physician-directed medical practice that coordinates access to care, utilizes an electronic medical record, and monitors use of pharmaceuticals and specialty services. Medical homes will be paid an additional amount per patient to cover their added value for managing the patients' multiple needs.[27] The medical home initiative is meant to promote coordination of services for beneficiaries who are using multiple providers and resources. The intent is not only to provide cost savings for the program but also to coordinate and improve the care provided to the beneficiaries.

Another targeted program for high-need older adults is the Programs of All Inclusive Care for the Elderly (PACE). In this program, medical, social, and long-term-care services as well as drug coverage are provided through community-based care to seniors who otherwise would need nursing home level of care.[6] Medicare and Medicaid fund PACE jointly and although the program has demonstrated cost savings through lower hospitalization rates, it only serves a very small portion of older adults who are high need.[28] As Medicare works to control costs, it will necessarily continue to focus on helping older adults stay well and avoid use of unnecessary medical services.

Durable Medical Equipment. Medicare covers equipment a patient needs at home to treat his or her health problem under its DME benefit through Part A benefits. DME is also available under Part B benefits. DME is equipment that is reusable, such as wheelchairs and walkers.[29] Thus, all patients have access to this benefit and Box 30-7 shows the conditions and categories of coverage. The categories are additionally sorted into some 2000 product groups and within these groups, the payment rate is the same using a fee schedule that Medicare sets.[29] Medicare has seen widespread abuse in the area of DME and closely monitors acquisition and payment for DME. In response to the abuse, the new Competitive Bidding Program is being implemented in an attempt to rein in costs of the DME benefit and ensure that beneficiaries are receiving appropriate equipment.[29a]

REGULATIONS AND PRACTICE IMPLICATIONS

Medicare Contracting Reform

The Medicare program is vast and administrative duties are contracted to certain entities known as contractors. In the past, carriers and fiscal intermediaries (FIs) were the entities that managed claims for Part A and Part B services. The Medicare Prescription Drug, Improvement, and Modernization Act (MMA) passed by Congress in 2003 required the CMS to replace the existing FI and carrier contracts for Part A and Part B services with competitively procured contracts. The provisions contained under section 911 of the MMA are collectively referred to as Medicare Contracting Reform.[30] The CMS was given 6 years, between 2005 and 2011, to complete the transition of Medicare Fee-for-Service claims processing activities for Part A and Part B services from the FIs and carriers to 15 Medicare Administrative Contractors. These contractors will be a single point of contact for providers and beneficiaries and also become a modern administrative information technology platform. Also, each Medicare Administrative Contractor will interact with one Program Safeguard Contractor regarding investigations of fraud and abuse.

The Medicare program has two layers of coverage. First, Medicare will cover specific services, procedures,

BOX 30-7	Durable Medical Equipment (DME) Covered Under Medicare[27]
Conditions of Coverage	**Categories of Covered Equipment**
• Withstand repeated use • Primarily service a medical purpose • Generally not be useful to a person without an illness or injury	• Inexpensive or routinely purchased equipment • Items that require frequent and substantial servicing • Prosthetic and orthotic devices • Capped rental items • Oxygen and oxygen equipment

or technologies on a national basis as outlined in national coverage decisions (NCDs). The CMS publication 100-03, National Coverage Determinations Manual, is the source document for the NCDs.[31]

Contractors must follow the guidance issued in NCDs. If an NCD does not specifically exclude or limit an item or service, or if the item or service is not mentioned in an NCD, a Medicare contractor may choose to write a local coverage determination (LCD). An LCD contains "reasonable and necessary" information about coverage.[32] Each contractor has a website that includes its LCDs. The contractors are required to publish articles that provide guidance for providers regarding any pertinent coverage decisions.

The practical application of this information is critical to understanding and obtaining payment under the Medicare program and decreasing provider risk for denial of payment. Providers should not assume that all services are covered under the program and if they are in doubt, should access the NCDs and LCDs prior to developing a plan of care with the patient. If a service is not covered as defined by an NCD or LCD, then the provider should discuss this with a patient in advance of providing the treatment and inquire if the patient would assume the financial responsibility if the service or item is provided. This conversation must be documented using the Advance Beneficiary Notification form and included in the medical record.[33] If the patient does not want an additional financial obligation above and beyond his or her deductible and copay, then the provider needs to consider alternative treatment options and document the alternative plan in the medical record. If the service is not covered under the LCD as being "reasonable and necessary," the patient cannot be charged for the service or item, even if it is rendered. Knowledge and implementation of information contained in NCDs and LCDs will decrease the provider's risk pertaining to fraud, abuse, and claims denials.

Medicare Cost Control Mechanisms

Under Medicare, payment to facilities and home health agencies is made under a prospective payment methodology. Currently, payment for Medicare's Part B services is made under a fee schedule called the "Physician Fee Schedule."[34] Medicare has multiple mechanisms to control costs for services covered under Part B. Despite the current controls, the program is actively considering alternative payment mechanisms that will not only control costs but also align provider incentives with the goals of the program. At the time of this writing, the most visible controls that are currently in place and the most important to understand include the fee schedule conversion factor, the benefit definition, coverage guidelines as previously discussed, the therapy cap, the Correct Coding Initiative program, and the Recovery Audit Contractor program.

The calculation for payment of services under the Part B Physician Fee Schedule changes each year, and changes are usually effective January 1 of each year. The payment changes because of revisions in the valuing of the Current Procedural Terminology (CPT) codes, the geographic practice cost index, or the conversion factor.[35] The annually assigned conversion factor, a dollar amount that is included in a formula with the value of the code and the geographic practice cost index, changes the payment rate year to year. So although the relative value of each billing code may not change, the actual payment for services will change because of the updated conversion factor.

The Medicare Benefit Policy Manual (Publication 100-02, Chapter 15, Sections 220-230) details the benefit available to beneficiaries related to Part B therapy services.[36] The manual includes information regarding conditions of coverage, reasonable and necessary therapy services, use of qualified personnel, supervision, documentation requirements, and the plan of care. Correct implementation of this information is critical or the provider may be at risk of denial during claims processing or payback after an audit.

For many years, Medicare has utilized an annual payment cap on Part B therapy services as a means to control costs.[37] The cap on physical therapy services is combined with services provided by speech–language pathologists. The cap for occupational therapy services stands alone. The cap in 1997 was raised to $1500 under the Balanced Budget Act and continues to exist in 2010, at $1860 per beneficiary for physical therapy and speech-language pathology, and a separate $1860 limit for occupational therapy.[21] This method of controlling costs has been politically controversial and has been applied with and without an exceptions process. Therapy providers affected by the cap, along with their professional organizations, have aggressively advocated for removal of the cap. The APTA has been a steadfast voice on behalf of its members to have the caps removed, as have the American Occupational Therapy Association and the American Speech Language Hearing Association. These associations stressed that the caps are an arbitrary restriction placed on therapy providers and negatively affected patients who either require multiple episodes of therapy within a calendar year or have a serious condition requiring extensive therapy (e.g., stroke). Although an exceptions process, which excluded patients with some diagnoses from the cap, was enacted in 2005 under the Deficit Reduction Act, it places additional administrative burden during the claims submission process.[20] Although these spending restrictions may result in cost savings to the Medicare program, patients and providers alike continue to challenge these laws.[12] Medicare's interest in an alternative payment methodology is partly a result of the recognition that the cap is arbitrary and negatively affects their beneficiaries who have complex and long-term rehabilitation needs.

The National Correct Coding Initiative (NCCI) was developed as a means to control improper and duplicative billing under the Medicare program for Part B services.[38] NCCI is an extensive list of claims edits that are applied when claims are processed. The contractors use the edits to reduce their liability for inappropriate claims. At the time of claims submission, there is the option for some code pairs identified as duplicative services to be modified on the claim form. The use of a modifier will alert the contractor that the services were provided in different time intervals and, consequently, should not be considered duplicative. Use of the modifier on the claim form requires complete and thorough documentation to support the claim. Anyone submitting claims to the program should familiarize themselves with the NCCI edits prior to submitting claims or they will assume an unnecessary level of risk for claims denials.

The Medicare program has a variety of mechanisms to investigate overpayments made by contractors. Not only do the contractors themselves have an audit mechanism but they will also rely on the four new Recovery Audit Contractors (RACs).[39] The RAC program is being phased in and medical necessity reviews will begin in earnest in 2010. The RACs have a financial incentive to identify over- and underpayments made by the program. Initially, the RACs will look at hospital and facility claims, but services provided under Part B as well as providers of DME will also be audited. Any provider that submits claims to a Medicare contractor should track the implementation of this program and be prepared for an audit. The four RACs are required to offer educational sessions to providers in their region. It is highly recommended that any provider participating in the Medicare program be knowledgeable about this initiative.

Documentation

The medical record serves many purposes, including being a formal record of the patient's status and the services that were provided to the patient. Even more critical and challenging for physical therapists is that the medical record must reflect the decision making of the provider and substantiate the need for skilled care, regardless of the site of the provision of care. Some third-party payers, including Medicare, have detailed documentation requirements, and the payment for services is often dependent on the information contained in the medical record. The documentation must substantiate the services that are reported on claim forms. Otherwise, the services are at risk for nonpayment should the documentation be audited.

For Part B services, Medicare's detailed guidance for documentation is located in the Medicare Benefit Manual, Publication 100-02, Chapter 15, Sections 220-230.[40] The Medicare Benefit Manual states that the guidance reflects the *minimum* requirements for documentation and that any state laws that are stricter will supersede Medicare's requirements. The documentation needs to defend the patient's need for skilled services or *medically reasonable and necessary* care. The Benefit Manual states:

> Services are medically necessary if the documentation indicates they meet the requirements for medical necessity including that they are skilled, rehabilitative services, provided by clinicians (or qualified professionals when appropriate) with the approval of a physician/NPP, safe, and effective (i.e., progress indicates that the care is effective in rehabilitation of function).[41]

Not all payers have such detailed documentation guidance. However, all therapists should familiarize themselves with the Medicare Benefit Manual language as some private payers have adopted Medicare's guidance. If a provider is able to comply with Medicare's documentation requirements, it will most likely meet the requirements of other payers. The Benefit Manual has detailed information pertaining to evaluations and reevaluations, progress notes, treatment notes, and discharge notes. It should also be noted that each contractor's LCDs may have guidance pertaining to documentation. Providers should access those documents and carefully follow the instructions.

A payer expects that the documentation will reflect the need for skilled services and include information pertaining to the patient's progress. So rather than just noting a specific impairment measurement, it is recommended that the provider translate that measurement into a functional finding that reflects the need for skilled services. For example, instead of noting only that the patient has "Fair plus" strength of the quadriceps, it would be far more informative for a reviewer to also see how that impairment affects the patient's function. Box 30-8 provides an example of documentation that includes the translation of the impairment into activity limitation.

The APTA has a Web-based tool for members called "Defensible Documentation." This interactive tool provides therapists with a wealth of information pertaining to documentation and its importance relative to reimbursement for services.[42]

BOX 30-8	An Example of Documentation That Includes the Translation of an Impairment into Activity Limitation Language
Strength	**Functional Deficit**
F+ right quadriceps	Patient requires a standard cane on all surfaces; unable to climb stairs without a railing or minimal guarding of one person.

In summary, the Medicare program provides access to health care for all older adults. There are restrictions in benefits, and cost-sharing with beneficiaries is required for some services. Although the historical focus of the program has been coverage for illness and injury, the program is beginning to focus attention on prevention services as a means to both improve beneficiary health and lower costs. The program has transitioned to prospective payment in hospitals, SNFs, and home health. Services covered under Part B continue to be paid under a fee schedule. Medicare has signaled its intent to become a "value-based" purchaser and resources are increasingly being devoted to promote better use of the limited resources. Therapists and other providers need to closely monitor Medicare's activities in this area. The changing population demographics will continue to be a driving force for Medicare to be fiscally prudent in its spending.

Fraud and Abuse

All third-party payers are concerned with overutilization of services and cost controls. However, it is a priority of payers, particularly Medicare and Medicaid, to identify activities that improperly utilize limited public monies needed for their beneficiaries' health care. The Office of Inspector General (OIG) is responsible to protect the programs covered by the Department of Health and Human Services such as Medicare and Medicaid. Through a coordinated program of audits, investigations, and inspections and the publication of advisory opinions and compliance guidance, the OIG manages activities related to fraud and abuse.

The Anti-Kickback statute and the Physician Self-Referral laws are very important for all providers to understand. The rationale behind these two statutes is that the government does not want to encourage incentives that would increase inappropriate utilization of services and distort medical decision making. The Anti-Kickback Statute of the Social Security Act makes it a criminal offense to knowingly and willfully "offer, pay, solicit, or receive any remuneration to induce or reward services covered by a Federal health care program."[43] Remuneration is anything of value including cash or in-kind services. The criminal penalties are significant for violation of the Anti-Kickback statute. Besides monetary penalties, a provider can be prohibited from participating in the Medicare program and may be sent to prison. Examples of violations include leasing space to a referral source that is below market value, discounting or waiving patient copays or deductibles, and giving physicians elaborate gifts such as season tickets to sporting events. Exceptions are in place, but providers need to be aware of these regulations. For example, if a provider fails to collect copays and deductibles after multiple attempts, then an exception might be made. However, the provider should not have a pattern of waiving fees or providing discounts that could be construed as inducement. Providers should have written policies and procedures for these exceptions, and there should be no identifiable pattern of discounting or waiving fees.

Submitting claims that misrepresent the services that were provided is another form of fraud. Unbundling CPT codes (billing separately for each component of an all-inclusive procedure code), reporting more services than what were actually provided, or misrepresenting who provided the services are all examples of intentional erroneous billing. Guidance for compliance activities is available on the OIG website.[44] and professional associations such as the APTA offer considerable information and education pertaining to fraud and abuse.[45]

The Physician Self-Referral Prohibition statute, sometimes called the "Stark Law," prohibits physicians from referring to designated health services or entities in which the physician or a family member has a financial interest, unless an exception is permitted. Physical therapy is considered a designated health service. However, exceptions have been identified. For example, if the service is being provided by someone who is supervised by that physician, the exception is permissible under the "in office ancillary services" provision. This law applies only to physicians and intent does not have to be apparent. Civil penalties are applied for Stark law violations and these are less onerous than the criminal penalties under the Anti-Kickback statute.[43]

Providers in all settings should be aware of the legal ramifications of the provision and billing of services they provide. They should not assume that the billing office or billing service is appropriately reporting their services. Rather, they should regularly ask to see bills that are generated and compare them to internal fee slips and documentation. The treating therapist whose name is on the claim form is responsible for the bills that are generated and will have to defend any claims that are audited.

Value-Based Purchasing

There has been a significantly increased interest since the late 1990s in value-based purchasing. Value-based purchasing models attempt to link payment to quality and efficiency of care as a means to control excessive health care costs and promote appropriate utilization of services. This increased interest comes from the recognition that traditional models of health care delivery, including managed care, have had limited impact on the rising costs and utilization of services in the United States. Decision making by the patient as well as the employer, who is the usual purchaser of health care, must be influenced in order to realize cost savings. Value-based purchasing is based on the premise that allowing consumers access to information regarding quality of health care services as well as cost, coupled with financial incentives to the best-performing providers, will have a meaningful impact on the utilization of services.[46]

Key elements of value-based purchasing include the availability of information to support the decision making of employers or individuals purchasing health insurance, a quality reporting and management system that promotes continuous improvement, incentives for providers and consumers that promote and reward certain behaviors and practices, and educational initiatives directed at consumers that reinforce the desired decision-making and health behaviors.[46] The Institute of Medicine's study "Rewarding Provider Performance: Aligning Incentives in Medicare" notes that a system is needed that rewards both higher value and better outcomes.[47] The Institute of Medicine recommended that Medicare should focus on the three conditions that affect 32% of patients covered under the Medicare program and account for 61% of the payments: chronic heart failure, coronary artery disease, and diabetes.

Consumer education can take many forms, including enrollment counselors, public service announcements, brochures, computer decision-making tools, as well as health plan and provider report cards. It is thought that an educated consumer will make wise and desirable health care choices. Research has indicated, however, that consumer decision making regarding choice of provider is often based on location of the provider, word-of-mouth recommendations, and out-of-pocket financial obligation.[47]

The CMS is a leading driver of the promotion and interest in value-based purchasing. In a 2007 testimony to the House of Representatives Subcommittee on Health, a CMS official noted that "it is a top priority at CMS to transform Medicare from a passive payer to an active purchaser of high quality, efficient health care."[48] The goal is that Medicare intends to pursue an active and thoughtful purchasing strategy that promotes efficient utilization of services and public reporting of comparative data pertaining to facilities and providers that will be used by consumers to make decisions pertaining to accessing medical care.

To this end, the CMS has begun to develop value-based purchasing programs. For example, the Tax Relief and Health Care Act of 2006 provided the CMS instructions to institute the 2007 Physician Quality Reporting Initiative that included a bonus payment for successful reporting of specific measures pertaining to care delivery by physicians and nonphysicians. Funding for this program was expanded for 2009 and 2010.[49] During the development of this initiative, the CMS has continued to collaborate with various external stakeholder groups such as the American Medical Association, the National Committee on Quality Assurance, National Quality Forum, and the Ambulatory Care Quality Alliance to facilitate measure development that can be utilized by health plans, physicians and nonphysician providers, and facilities.

The CMS is also aware that it must try to influence the utilization of services over an episode of care rather than only considering resource use at the individual provider level. Historically, the CMS has drawn conclusions of utilization based on retrospective reviews of claims. It monitors trends in utilization by provider groups and individual providers. It would be more meaningful, however, to analyze the full use of services for a specific condition when assessing resource use and outcomes of care. For example, evaluating utilization of all services over an episode for patients with low-back pain (e.g., physician services, imaging services, medications, and physical therapy) may be more meaningful than evaluating services provided by individual providers. The development of this analysis capability is in progress and could have a major impact on the development of future payment models and incentives for providers.

The CMS has shown its intention to develop value-based purchasing at all levels of care. In 2003, the CMS began its hospital value-based purchasing initiatives with the Premier Hospital Quality Incentive Demonstration project. Payments to the participating hospitals are contingent upon their performance on specific quality measurements. Measures being utilized by the broad spectrum of participating hospitals include process of care and patient outcomes measures.[50] The demonstration has been so successful that extended funding was made available to continue through 2009.

As of October 1, 2008, the CMS limits payment to certain hospitals for ten categories of specific conditions caused by medical error. Payments to those hospitals will not be increased for the hospital-acquired complications. Categories on the list that are pertinent to physical therapists include fall or trauma resulting in serious injury and stage III and IV pressure ulcers.[51] This is yet another example of value-based purchasing by the CMS.

In 2005, the CMS announced its intention to fund a Nursing Home Value-Based Purchasing demonstration project. Quality performance in four domains would be assessed for nursing homes: staffing, appropriate hospitalizations, Minimum Data Set outcomes, and survey deficiencies.[52] The CMS currently offers information on nursing home quality to the public through the Nursing Home Quality Initiative that was started in 2002. "Nursing Home Compare" is easily accessible on the Internet and provides information on Medicare and Medicaid certified nursing homes.[53] This kind of public reporting is expected to ultimately be available at the individual provider level based on information obtained from the Physician Quality Reporting Initiative program.

The significance of value-based purchasing should not be underestimated. Physician and nonphysician providers treating older adults will be affected by these programs, regardless of site of practice. It is expected that quality measure reporting will continue, and public reporting of facility and individual providers will become more pervasive and increasingly transparent to the consumer. Incentives had been built into inpatient facility payments to affect costs over an episode of care but now outcomes and medical errors are being monitored and reported publicly. Similar incentives are being developed for outpatient providers, and Medicare is developing the analytic tools to analyze costs, quality measurements, and outcomes over an episode.

In summary, the Medicare program provides vital health care benefits for older adults. Continued reform and change will be needed to meet the needs of this growing population, especially around issues of cost control, management, and efficiency and around the benefits currently excluded, such as some preventive services, and long-term-care coverage.

MEDICAID

The federal government became involved with health care for individuals with low income through the 1965 congressional enactment of Title 19 of the Social Security Act. Medicaid provides health insurance for low-income families with children and people with disabilities, long-term care for older adults and people with disabilities, and supplemental coverage for low-income Medicare beneficiaries for services not covered by Medicare, such as outpatient prescription drugs, Medicare premiums, deductibles, and cost sharing. Each state sets its own guidelines as to who qualifies for assistance and determines funding levels for its Medicaid recipients. The Medicaid program functions as a safety net for older adults but in order to qualify, older adults must meet a "means test" demonstrating that their income is under a certain level as determined by federal and state governments.[54]

Coverage for Nursing Home and Custodial Care

Medicaid covers more than two thirds of nursing home residents who require long-term care for chronic medical conditions. Because Medicare does not cover nursing home care for chronic conditions, many middle-income adults who enter a nursing home enter it as a private pay patient and then "spend down" almost all of their assets to eventually qualify for Medicaid.[55] Although this long-term care is important, Medicaid coverage for this care is limited to services provided within an institutional setting. Medicaid provides limited home services that would enable older adults to live at home with help. Some states are testing new models of care that have increased Medicaid funding for community- and home-based services to minimize nursing homes costs.[55,56] These models of more efficient use of funds and payment reforms are steps toward improving care provided to lower-income older adults.

Dual Coverage

"Dual eligibles" are low-income older adults with disabilities who qualify for Medicare Part A and need both Medicare and Medicaid programs to help pay for their care. Dual eligibles typically have extensive health care needs, and rely on both programs to help pay for care. Medicare provides primary health benefits such as physician and hospital care under Medicare Part A and Medicaid pays for the Medicare B premium, cost-sharing, and critical benefits that Medicare does not cover, such as long-term-care services. Because Medicaid is a state-administered program with varying levels of state and federal financing depending on the state, states take on an additional financial burden for low-income older adults.[57]

Medicaid's Value-Based Purchasing: Controlling Costs and Improving Quality

Value-based purchasing initiatives are also an integral part of the Medicaid program.[58,59] The Center for Medicaid and State Operations (CMSO) has infused incentives throughout the state-managed programs, including the State Children's Health Insurance Program (SCHIP).[60] The value-based purchasing programs are critical to identify appropriate utilization of limited program dollars.

The CMSO, in its role as an organization that transfers information from the federal government to the states, recognizes that each state may approach its value-based purchasing decisions differently. Managed care Medicaid model health plans have also been included in the program's design for promotion of value-based purchasing. Despite state differences, the basic elements of the plan include attention to (1) evidence-based care and quality measurement, (2) pay-for-performance, (3) health information technology, (4) partnerships, (5) information and technical assistance, and (6) health care disparities.[58]

In 2007, the CMS announced its intent to develop a National Medicaid Quality Framework.[61] The CMS has supported the ongoing "Medicaid and SCHIP Promising Practices" initiatives taking place in a number of states.[62] For example, in Louisiana, a phone-based disease management program for asthma has effectively decreased unnecessary, expensive emergency room visits. Washington State has developed strict criteria for bariatric surgery after recognizing that the surgeries were costly and mortality rates were high. Other states have designed programs dealing with dental issues, health literacy, obesity, disease management, and care coordination.

As Medicaid programs increasingly look at costs and outcomes over an episode of care, it will be important for rehabilitation professionals to advocate for recognition that the services they provide are valuable in managing high-cost chronic conditions such as cardiovascular diseases, pulmonary disease, and diabetes. Participation by rehabilitation professionals in programs that are designed to address value-based purchasing initiatives will be critical. Ultimately, payment for services may depend on participation in the effective management of certain conditions by a team of skilled professionals.

Reimbursement in Other Settings

At Home: Family and Community Services

Older adults who live at home may find activities of daily living such as personal care or preparing meals difficult to accomplish alone. Medicare, Medicaid, and private insurance cover some of these needs through home health aides but typically only in the context of the person's medical home care needs as it relates to a medical problem. As a result, many older adults who need such long-term-care services pay for it themselves and/or receive it from friends and family.[63] It is estimated that 28 million people provide informal care to older adults and in 1996, estimated to total 21.5 billion hours of help per year, which approaches a value of $200 billion.[64] Average costs in the United States in 2008 for some home services were $29 per hour for a home health aide, $18 per hour for a homemaker service, and $59 per day for care in an adult day health care center.[65] Only the very wealthy can afford to pay out of pocket for such services, and these costs support the need for health care reform in long-term-care services.

Nursing Home and Chronic Custodial Care

Long-term care, although sometimes provided in a nursing home, includes the services and supports needed when the ability to care for oneself has been reduced by chronic illness, disability, or aging. Long-term care is provided in a number of different settings, including at home by family and friends, in the community through services such as home health and adult day care, or in institutional settings, such as nursing homes. Often, long-term-care users will need a combination of these types of care over the course of their lifetimes.

Custodial or maintenance care is not a covered service in nursing homes under Medicare or most private insurances. However, low-income older adult who need ongoing 24-hour maintenance care can qualify for coverage under Medicaid. Higher-income older adults must first "spend down" their savings by paying privately in a nursing home before qualifying for Medicaid as a person with low income. Medicaid is the safety net for coverage for nursing home custodial care and on an aggregate level covers some 49% of long-term care in nursing homes.[5]

The yearly cost estimate of a nursing home in 2009 was $219 per day for a semiprivate room or almost $80,000 annually.[66] Lack of long-term-care coverage, that is, nursing home care when older adults need 24-hour custodial care, is a serious omission in health care coverage. As an attempt to fill this void, private insurers for many years have been promoting private policies to ensure for the need for long-term care. Only a small percentage of older adults have purchased this costly insurance, with only 9% of long-term-care costs covered by such insurance.[5]

THE FUTURE: IMPROVING THE HEALTH OF OLDER ADULTS

First, improving the health of older adults requires integration of financing across all settings and a whole-system approach to improve access, quality, and cost.[67] Medicare is conducting innovative demonstration projects to measure the effect of potential program changes. For example, one project is using nurse practitioners to partner with primary care physicians to provide care for homebound frail older adults to prevent unnecessary hospitalizations. Second, more data are needed to better quantify and understand services that best improve the function of people who have limitations and require rehabilitation services. Post–acute care providers (IRFs, SNFs, long-term-care hospitals, and home health agencies) all have relatively new prospective payment systems and each have different classes of providers as well as separate payment systems and outcome measurement tools. Comparing outcome data from one setting to the next is difficult and, although payment incentives exist, they are not necessarily based on research of what services most change patient function.[68] Further research is needed to collect functional outcome data to provide the evidence needed to advocate for financing rehabilitation services.

Third, increasing preventive services would improve older adult's health. Research is indicating the secondary preventive efforts in this population that focus on lifestyle changes are worthwhile, and predictions are that better prevention and investments in public health would be more effective than investment in technologies.[69] For example, the projected 10-year impact on national spending (for all ages) by reducing obesity through taxes invested in prevention programs is estimated to be $283 billion. Instituting positive incentives for health behavior through federally funded wellness programs are estimated to have the potential to save $19 billion.[70] Health is shown to be affected by genetics, social circumstances, environmental exposures, behavioral patterns, and health care; behavioral patterns are estimated to contribute 40% toward premature death.[71] Focusing on preventive behavior changes could have a significant impact on risk reduction resulting in improved population health, and if these efforts also targeted children and young adults, the impact on spending could be significantly greater.

A number of Web-based resources are available to help the reader stay updated on current federal health insurance regulations, research, and health reform for older adults. Box 30-9 details these resources.

BOX 30-9	Useful Websites to Stay Updated on Current Federal Health Insurance Regulations for Older Adults

Centers for Medicare & Medicaid Services
  www.cms.hhs.gov

Medicare Consumer Handbook
  www.medicare.gov/Publications/Pubs/pdf/10050.pdf

Centers for Medicare & Medicaid Services: Medicare benefit policy manual. www.cms.hhs.gov/Manuals/IOM/itemdetail.asp?itemID=CMS012673

American Physical Therapy Association. Federal regulatory affairs
  www.apta.org

Kaiser Family Foundation www.kff.org

National Institute on Aging http://www.nia.nih.gov/

SUMMARY

Opportunities exist for health professionals to advocate changing the health care system for older adults. Understanding health insurance programs provided to older adults as well as methods used for reimbursing providers and for controlling health care costs, is foundational for advocating for change. Legislators, insurers, health care providers, and consumers all need to have a voice in the discussion of how best to improve the health care system in the United States. Chapter 31 that follows will discuss advocacy and health policy and provide the reader with tools and resources to effectively advocate as a health care professional.

REFERENCES

To enhance this text and add value for the reader, all references are included on the companion Evolve site that accompanies this text book. The reader can view the reference source and access it online whenever possible. There are a total of 71 cited references and other general references for this chapter.

CHAPTER 31

Health Policy and Advocacy in the United States:
A Perspective for Geriatric Physical Therapy

Justin Moore, PT, DPT

INTRODUCTION

The desired outcome of policy and the advocacy process is to influence decisions aimed to improve the health of the individuals physical therapists serve. Health policy and advocacy are interwoven together with the policy decisions that determine how health care professionals practice linked with the advocacy processes that influence these decisions. Physical therapists who provide services to older adults are subject to a number of policies that range from determining the scope of practice through state licensure laws to the payment for services delivered through entitlement programs, such as Medicare and Medicaid. Many health care professionals actively engage in the advocacy process to improve current policies or to enact new policies to enable physical therapists to better serve this growing population of Americans.

For the purposes of this chapter, it is important to understand the concepts of policy and advocacy. Policy refers to the decisions issued by government bodies with which health care professionals have to comply. The process to arrive at these decisions is informed and influenced by the advocacy process. Another way to think of it is that policy is an outcome and describes a current status; advocacy is the plan or desire to change this policy or status.

PUBLIC POLICY, HEALTH POLICY, AND ADVOCACY

Public policy is whatever the government chooses to do or not to do and covers action, inaction, decision, and nondecisions as it implies a very deliberate choice between alternatives.[1] Public policy are the laws promulgated by government entities that authorize specific rules and regulations with which individuals must comply or appropriate funds to implement specific actions. This definition is an amalgamation of several contemporary definitions and provides a pragmatic approach to a broad and diverse discipline that is without a consensus definition. *Health policy*, as it is used in this chapter, is consistent with this public policy definition but also can be understood in a multidimensional way, with its impacts extending beyond the formal system of laws promulgated by government entities. Health policies can be as basic as handwashing procedures for a restaurant, which is a voluntary health policy based on scientific evidence and backed by public interest, or as complex as payment based on the adherence to clinical guidelines.

Health policy is the decisions, usually developed by government policy makers, for determining present and future objectives pertaining to the health care system.[2] Health policy comprises the decisions policy makers make to establish laws and regulations with which health care professionals must comply or outline the use of finite resources within the health care delivery system. Advocacy is the process to change or influence these decisions. Advocacy supplies the process and framework to enact, change, or advance health policy and therefore is dependent on the sociopolitical construction of the community, state, or country in which one is trying to shape public policy. In many venues, the advocacy process is itself governed by public policies that define how you can influence or impact policies. Regardless of the venue, whether it is local, state, or federal, the right to petition government and to exercise freedom of speech is well protected and is the foundation of advocacy in the United States. This chapter will describe the multidimensional aspects of health policy and the advocacy process by which individuals attempt to shape health policy. Interwoven throughout the text will be examples specific to physical therapists and the health policies that guide physical therapist practice, education, and research.

COMPONENTS OF HEALTH POLICY

The National Library of Medicine describes the components of health policy as legislation, regulation, professional guidelines/standards/protocols, public health policy, and health advocacy. For the purposes of this chapter, we will consider these components of health policy, but discuss health advocacy as part of the advocacy process at the conclusion of the chapter[3] (Figure 31-1).

The components of health policy provide a multidimensional construct of health policy that applies across all venues. Each venue involves a recognized authority that is empowered to make these decisions by adjudicating among the varied opinions and priorities of the multiple stakeholders who will be affected by these decisions. Although not covered in detail in this chapter, it is important to note that health policy can be promulgated or implemented by an organization, a place of work, a local school district or community, or by the more traditionally understood jurisdictions, such as cities, states, or countries. For example, a school district might author a policy that all children will participate in 30 minutes of organized and supervised physical education, which incorporates elements of both health policy and public health advocacy. This chapter will focus on the formal recognized jurisdictions that can promulgate policies that determine how health care professionals can practice. These formal jurisdictions are primarily state and federal legislatures and the executive branch agencies that enforce the laws, regulations, and rules that the legislative body authors.

The components of health policy of legislation and regulation occur in a defined process and public forum. When the legislative process yields a determination on a particular health policy, this determination becomes law with statutory authority. Regulation is an administrative process defined by the regulatory agency with the authority to issue policies within the parameters of the law.

When the regulatory process issues a policy that is not consistent with an individual or group's objectives, they can petition the agency for policy change or seek legislative change to alter the parameters within which this regulation was authored.

Health policies issued by formally established governmental entities seek to impact the health of individuals and communities. These policy bodies have to make decisions across varied populations and with finite resources. Setting priorities and choosing among numerous policy proposals are key functions of these policy bodies with recognized jurisdictional authority. Among the concerns that health policies seek to address, remediate, or impact across the broadest population possible are public safety, disparities and inequities, and allocation of resources.

Health policy development also draws from several fields of study, including law, economics, sociology, and ethics, as well as health and medical research findings. Data and insights from these disciplines assist the determination of resource allocation, a perennial pressure point on health policy. Health policy formulation also involves making a case for the economics of a course of action, establishing the legality and ethics of the proposed action if implemented, and identifying the most likely outcome on the health status of the individuals affected by the action. All three of these considerations are crucial to many decisions in health-related public policy (Figure 31-2).

The individuals who serve in formal policy-making roles in health care include elected officials, appointed government officials, and bureaucrats within government entities. Because these policy makers (such as members of Congress) are educated, influenced, and informed by citizen advocates, community activists, lobbyists, public policy analysts, academics, and business leaders, the development and implementation of health policy is interconnected to the advocacy process.

Examining each of these three critical considerations in depth during the formulation of specific health policy adds greatly to our understanding of public policy development in general. In the United States, health policy also must make the case for adoption within a closed economic market, where scarce or limited resources must be allocated across a diverse population. The

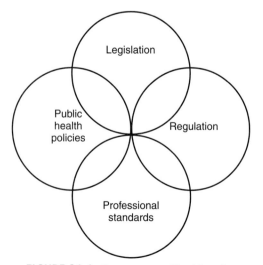

FIGURE 31-1   Components of health policy.

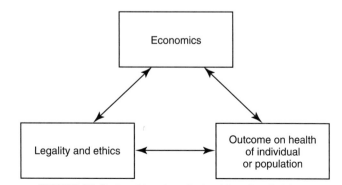

FIGURE 31-2   Considerations for health policy decisions.

economics of health policy must speak to issues of cost-effectiveness and resource allocations while detailing the specific features of the payment policies that will support the health policy. The intended outcome of policies to improve the health status of a population should be responsive to issues of health disparities, accessibility and availability of services, and provide incentives to encourage the adoption of specific practices that are linked to improving health care. Health policies can also be used to build and continuously improve the infrastructure and capacity of the health care system by promoting structural elements, such as the adoption of health information technology or the recruitment of individuals to study in the health professions.

DOMAINS OF HEALTH POLICY

Access, quality, and cost are the three major domains that are commonly used to evaluate health services in our country[4] (Figure 31-3). The first domain of access encompasses health policies that ensure individuals have accessibility and availability of health care services to meet their own needs and the needs of the broader community in which they live. We define this domain first as it is the entry point into the health care delivery system in the United States. The implementation of health policy decisions begins with accessibility and availability policies. Individuals' abilities to access health care from an available and qualified health care professional is essential to the overarching goal of most health policies, that is, to improve the health status of the population the policy seeks to serve.

The second domain of health policy is quality and outcomes. Once an individual can access services from available and qualified health care professionals, policies are needed to ensure that the services meet basic standards for care and do not jeopardize the individual's

health, safety, and welfare. The classic Hippocratic Oath "I will do no harm or injustice to them" is the ethical foundation of the charge to health policies to advance quality.[5] The domain of quality is on a continuum that begins with doing no harm and transitions to advancing the health status of a population through evidence and clinical judgment. If we can regard health policy as making determinations and decisions to improve health, then those decisions that have a defined impact are critical to health policy determinations. Quality measurement and outcomes are currently still in their infancy but represent a growing area in health policy development, the evaluation of health care professionals and facilities, and resource allocation.

The third domain covers the cost and financing of health policies, or the economics of the decision. This domain is the arena in which the priorities or values upon which the policy is based are highly debated. In the United States, the cost and financing of health care has been a long-standing, and often contentious, public debate. Distributing a finite set of resources in a way that is acceptable to the public, health care providers, payers, and policy makers is the primary challenge in health policy today. Financing or cost in health policy can broadly be divided into its inputs, that is, how we finance health care, and its outputs, that is, how we distribute the resources that are available to the system. The inputs into health care in the United States come primarily from taxes that are paid to support federal programs and the funding of private insurance by employers and employees. The outputs or health care expenditures are primarily to hospitals, physicians and health care professionals, and prescription drugs. Balancing the supply of the inputs with the demand of the outputs is critical to our economy and public health.

Further investigation of the three domains of health policy uncovers many examples in the current environment of policies that affect physical therapists and health care providers in each domain. Each domain has specific policy ramifications for the physical therapist whose practice is oriented toward an older adult population. The three domains of health policy are also interrelated; for example, policies that affect accessibility and availability of services have an impact on the quality and cost. Successful health policy systematically balances the three domains to achieve the best possible outcome for the desired population.

Accessibility and Availability

The public's ability to access health care services from the individual of their choice has long been a health policy issue. If health policy's goal is to improve the health status of the population it seeks to serve, then accessibility to services and the availability of health care professionals to serve this objective are critical issues for policy makers to address in their efforts to author and

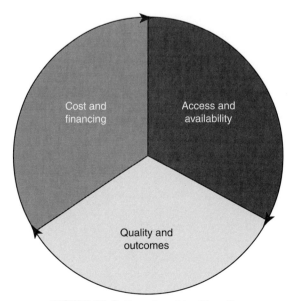

FIGURE 31-3 Domains of health policy.

implement health policy. Access can be looked at in three ways: denial of care, delays in service provision, and disparities in health care. All three elements have been identified as problems in the United States health delivery system.

Access to comprehensive health care services is currently limited and denied to a significant portion of Americans. In 2007, the U.S. Census Bureau estimated that 45.7 million Americans, or one in seven individuals, lacked health care insurance for the calendar year.[6] Other studies, including one by Families USA, estimated that this number grows to 86.7 million individuals when one considers those persons who lacked health insurance for some period of time over a 2-year calendar period in 2006 and 2007.[7] Although debate exists on the exact number of individuals who lack health insurance, it is unquestionable that the ability of these individuals to access available health care services has been substantially curtailed, if not completely blocked. Access to health care insurance is a major determinant of individuals' ability to obtain health care services.

Health policies in the United States previously attempted to address this problem of limited access by implementing a safety net through the authorization of the Emergency Medical Treatment and Labor Act (EMTALA). On a very basic level, all Americans have access to health care services through EMTALA. Congress enacted EMTALA in 1986 to ensure public access to emergency services regardless of ability to pay. Section 1867 of the Social Security Act imposes specific obligations on Medicare-participating hospitals with emergency services to provide a medical screening examination (MSE) when a request is made for examination or treatment for an emergency medical condition (EMC), including active labor, regardless of an individual's ability to pay. Hospitals are then required to provide stabilizing treatment for patients with EMCs. An appropriate transfer should be implemented if a hospital is unable within its capability to stabilize a patient, or if the patient requests a transfer.[8] Although this EMTALA requirement provides access to health care through emergency services, it does not address the continuum of health services or ensure the accessibility of services. Many times these services are limited solely to emergency cases, bounded by geographical considerations, and do not meet the health care needs of individuals. In addition, this access has substantial ramifications for the costs of health care services and jeopardizes the precarious balance of access, quality, and cost.

On March 23, 2010, President Barack Obama signed into law health care reform legislation, the Patient Protection and Affordable Care Act, now Public Law 111-148. This law has been estimated to increase coverage to 32 million more Americans, representing 95% of the population.[9] This will provide near universal coverage to health care services beyond those provided in the emergency room. This coverage is achieved through an expansion of Medicaid, access to health care insurance exchanges to purchase coverage, and an individual and employer mandate to enforce coverage. These proposals would also attempt to reform current insurance through health policies to eliminate practices such as denial or rescission of coverage based on health status or a preexisting condition or placement of limitations on benefits such as annual or lifetime caps, to enhance access to services.

Health policy to eliminate arbitrary limits on benefits is of particular interest to rehabilitation health care professionals that serve a geriatric population. Since 1997, a per beneficiary per year financial limitation on therapy services has been placed on seniors and individuals with disabilities under the Medicare program. This "therapy cap" in 2010 limits a patient to $1860 of physical therapy and speech–language pathology services and $1860 of occupational therapy services per calendar year. Although Congress has interceded several times since 1997 to place a moratorium on therapy caps or to provide a clinically based exceptions process, efforts to fully repeal the cap have been unsuccessful. This particular health policy has ramifications for Medicare beneficiaries and their abilities to access clinically appropriate rehabilitation services provided by physical therapists and other rehabilitation health care professionals.

During the health care reform debate of 2009 and 2010, health policies under consideration sought to address the expansion of services that should be available to our populations by enacting policies to ensure the availability of qualified health care professionals to provide these services. To ensure the United States has a qualified workforce available to meet the need created through increased access, the health care reform law (Public Law 111-148) authored a framework to develop a comprehensive plan of workforce initiatives to match these health policies.

Expanding health care to include prevention and chronic care management programs would have a significant impact on the health policy goal of improving the health status of Americans at a lower per capita or system cost. Policies to prevent falls are another example of increasing the accessibility of prevention services that geriatric physical therapists might provide. The Centers for Disease Control and Prevention (CDC) report that more than one third of adults age 65 years and older fall each year in the United States and also that falls are the leading cause of injury-related deaths among older adults.[10] To reduce cost and improve health quality, programs and initiatives to reduce falls in older Americans are critical prevention initiatives and health policies for physical therapists who serve this at-risk population. On April 23, 2008, President George W. Bush signed legislation, the Safe Seniors Act (now Public Law 110-202), that amends the Public Service Act and authorized the Department of Health and Human Services to implement a comprehensive plan to reduce falls in older

Americans. To implement this plan, the Department of Health and Human Services must conduct research, implement a national awareness campaign, and improve the diagnosis, treatment, and rehabilitation of individuals at risk for falls or repeat falls.

Access to health care services is further complicated by disparities across racial and ethnic groups and by geographical and socioeconomic factors. Currently in the United States, one in three Americans identies themselves as being African American, American Indian/Alaska Native, Asian, Native Hawaiian/Pacific Islander, Hispanic/Latino, or multiracial. This number is expected to increase by 2050 to one in two.[11] In its report, Unequal Treatment, the Institute of Medicine outlined the extent of racial and ethnic disparities that exist in health care, including access to services. Although there has been substantial progress in public policies to advance civil rights, health care has continued to demonstrate gaps in access to quality health care services for underrepresented racial or ethnic minorities.[12]

Achieving universal coverage in the United States does not guarantee that services will be accessible if a sufficient number of health care providers are not available to provide the services that are now accessible. Compounding the gaps in access for minorities is the corresponding gap in representation of these minorities as health care professionals. In physical therapy, despite a sustained effort through minority initiatives by the professional society and leaders in the field, racial and ethnic minorities only represent 7% of the populations surveyed for the American Physical Therapy Association membership profile. Of this 7%, more than half identify their ethnic group representation as Asian.[13] Physical therapy is similar to other health professions in that whites continue to represent the vast majority of practicing professions. This disparity can be a contributing factor to the unavailability of services for underrepresented population subgroups. Health policy should consider directing resources toward the recruitment and retention of underrepresented populations to meet the growing problems of accessibility and availability of health care for racial and ethnic groups as part of a commitment to social justice within the professions.

Where one lives also has a significant effect on one's ability to access health care services. Currently, one in four Americans lives in a rural area. Rural areas have been demonstrated to have higher rates of poverty, a larger percentage of older Americans, and a diminished health status. Not only is access to health services limited in rural areas, these communities have fewer physicians, health care professionals, hospitals, and health resources than urban and suburban areas of the United States.[14] Limited access and scarce available resources and professionals to meet the increasing health care needs in rural areas are a major public health issue for the United States. Health care policy to address this issue should continue to improve accessibility to

services. Increasing the availability of health care resources and providers to rural populations is a critical health policy issue because of the poor health status and limited resources available to this population.

Recruiting and retaining qualified health care professionals, such as physical therapists, in rural areas is a policy challenge. Various proposals are examples of health policy whose objective is to ensure accessibility and availability of health care in underserved areas. If pending legislation, the Physical Therapist Student Loan Repayment Eligibility Act is adopted, physical therapists will be eligible for the National Health Services Corps, a federal program that places qualified health care professionals and physicians in underserved areas. The incentive to recruit and retain health care professionals to this program and to service in underserved areas is student loan repayment. In 2010, a health care professional who is selected and completes the required service in the National Health Service Corp is eligible for up to $50,000 in student loan repayments.

Critical to the accessibility of individuals and programs is their availability. Health policy can authorize decisions and reach determinations to make health services more accessible, but there could be a limitation on the resources to make these services available. Currently, workforce shortages in health professions highlight the differing concepts of accessibility and availability. As formalized medicine developed in the United States, health policies were grounded in the authorization of services by medical doctors. This requirement limited access to health services through a finite number of individuals who were authorized to direct this care and created disparities, delays, and denials of access of health services. Furthermore, the growth of specialization in medicine and health care reduced the number of primary care providers available in the health care system, creating another limitation on access to services.

Health policies over the past several decades have made care from health care professionals more readily accessible. These policies have capitalized on the increasing educational and clinical training qualifications of some health professionals. Health policies have recognized osteopathic physicians, some doctorally educated practitioners, and advanced clinical practice nurses qualified to serve as entry points to the health care system. These policies have increased access but also increased demand for services with corresponding strains on the availability of qualified practitioners.

Balancing the public's safety with individual autonomy and self-determination has been critical to the decisions that policy makers have had to make in meeting the objectives of health policy. A prime example of this responsibility is seen in the licensure of health care professionals to serve the health needs of the population. Licensure has been seen as the purview of the police powers of individual states. The core of licensure is found in the limitations on practice that are promulgated to protect the public's health, safety, and welfare. Licensure signifies to the public that one is qualified to practice a certain profession and has met the qualification standards. Traditionally, licensure provides the public protection through title and term protection and through scope of practice of the individual authorized to use the title and term to the public. Physical therapy has achieved licensure laws in all 50 states, the District of Columbia, Puerto Rico, and the U.S. Virgin Islands. This legislative achievement provides term and practice protection, although overlap in term and practice protection with complementary and competing professions exists.

In recent decades, emerging professions have used licensure as a form of professional recognition over and above its purpose of public protection. In many instances, professional recognition is a prerequisite for payment in return for providing health care services, and therefore licensure is a priority of emerging professions. Licensure laws, considered as a type of health policy, seek to appropriately limit a profession and its practitioners to their education and training in the best interests of the public. However, using a policy whose objective is public protection through appropriate limitations on practice for the purposes of gaining recognition or opening access to payment pulls this form of health policy into conflict and public debate.

Licensure is also an important consideration from the perspective of availability. Licensure limits the pool of individuals who are recognized as able to meet the health care needs of the population. This limitation is important as it ensures a level of patient safety and public confidence in the health care delivery system. However, licensure, and its corresponding scope of practice restrictions, limits access to the public and the availability of individuals to meet the health care needs of the population.

Health policy must seek decisions and determinations to improve access to health care with an equal commitment to improving the availability of qualified health care professionals. Access to health care for older Americans is a subset of issues in health policy debate. Currently, all Americans over the age of 65 have access to health care coverage through Medicare, Medicaid, or both. Access to services is reported to be good for a vast majority of older Americans, but the availability of health care professionals to serve their health needs will continue to be a pressure point for policy makers to address.

Access to and the availability of health care services is basic to health policy. Policies to achieve improved access or to increase availability must be balanced to ensure patient safety, enhance quality, and to utilize scarce resources in an efficient and effective manner.

Quality and Outcomes

"Quality is the degree to which health services for individuals and populations increase the likelihood of desired health outcomes and are consistent with current professional knowledge."[15] The United States health care delivery system has been plagued by issues of quality and its impact on the health status of Americans or outcomes. In 2001, the Institute of Medicine issued a landmark study, *Crossing the Quality Chasm,* and stated "The U.S. health care delivery system does not provide consistent, high quality medical care to all people."[16] This report, along with other health policy studies, indicated a high degree of variance in health care delivery in the United States. In 1998, a Rand report found that U.S. adults receive about half of recommended health care services.[17] Other studies have found that women, older adults, members of racial and ethnic minorities, poorer, less educated, or uninsured are less likely to receive needed care, largely as a result of lack of access to care in addition to variance in quality.

The Institute of Medicine in another report, *To Err Is Human,* found that almost 100,000 deaths occur each year in the United States health care system as a result of medical errors.[18] The data are clear that we need health policies to reduce the errors and improve the poor quality of health care services in our delivery system. Improving the quality of health care is a multidimensional issue and challenge for health care policy makers. With one of the most expensive health care systems in the world, getting an adequate return on this investment and changing the health status of our population are the key elements of quality in health policy.

The six dimensions of quality or quality improvement in health care as defined by the Institute of Medicine are safety, effectiveness, patient-centeredness, timeliness, efficiency, and equity (Figure 31-4).[16]

Safety is the practice that ensures patients are not harmed by the health care they receive or where they

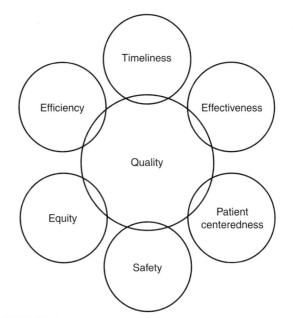

FIGURE 31-4 Institute of Medicine's multidimensional nature of quality in health care.

receive it. Effectiveness is the use of evidence and practice standards to match the care delivered with the best available scientific data with resource allocation and utilization. Patient-centeredness is respect for individuals and their wishes in the health care experience. Timeliness is ensuring that health status is not detrimentally affected by waiting times and delays in access. Efficiency is the reduction of fraud, waste, and abuse in the health care system. Equity is ensuring that disparities in the health care system are reduced.[16]

One dimension especially worth exploration because of its relevance to physical therapy is the dimension of effectiveness. Effectiveness can be divided into the elements of overuse and underuse. The use of interventions in physical therapy that are not proven to provide therapeutic value is a classic overutilization issue. Many physical agents are consistently utilized without the evidence to support their use leading to overutilization. The lack of use of those interventions for which there is better support leads to underutilization. Manual therapy and manipulation for individuals with some presentations of low back pain could be considered as examples of underutilization.

Looking at quality across the six dimensions is critical in health policy as it illustrates the complexity of measuring "quality." These six dimensions also have varying impacts on the other domains of access and cost and must be balanced with these domains. The highest quality might be the most costly and hardest to access. Clinicians must always keep these six dimensions in focus as they strive to deliver high-quality care.

Measuring quality can proceed along several lines, such as structure, process, and outcome. Structure looks at the system in which the health care experience occurs and those features that enhance quality of care. An example of a structural measure of quality is the use of health information technology. Process measures investigate the method of delivery and assure that critical steps are taken. An example of a process measure of quality can be found in ensuring that a critical question is posed as part of the patient history, such as has the patient fallen in the past month. Outcome measures, the patient-critical level of quality measurement, document the impact of the intervention on the patient's health status. In physical therapy, the functional improvement of the patient is the primary focus of many outcome measures. An example of a treatment outcome measure for population subgroups would be the reduction of falls in patients who have undergone a standardized balance program. The challenge of interpreting outcome measures in order to compare patients with different risk profiles can often complicate interpretation of findings across groups. Assessment tools and outcome measures in physical therapy have existed in many forms, for example, the Outpatient Physical Therapy Improvement in Movement Assessment Log, the Uniform Data System of Medical Rehabilitation and its outcome measurement tool, the

Functional Independence Measure, and the Medical Outcomes Study–Short Form (SF-36). These instruments provide ways for clinicians to measure improvement in patient outcomes following intervention.[4]

Currently, outpatient physical therapists can participate in quality reporting under the Medicare program called the Physician Quality Reporting Initiative. Although this program is currently limited to physical therapists in private practice, it provides a glimpse of efforts to improve our health care delivery system by measuring outcomes and rewarding quality. The Physician Quality Reporting Initiative measures at this stage are limited primarily to process measures but allow the federal government to begin to improve quality of health care by moving incentives toward measures of treatment quality and patient outcomes. Physical therapists currently have access to eight different quality reporting measures, and the battery of appropriate measures will most certain expand in the coming years.

Ensuring quality in health policy decisions is a difficult exercise in balancing the multiple dimensions of quality and then reconciling quality with its impact on the domains of access and cost. Health care is at its very core personal and individualized. The uniformity that ensures quality in many other areas of our economy is not always applicable to health care. Assembly lines in manufacturing created advancement in many of the dimensions of quality from efficiency, timeliness, uniformity and safety, but many of these approaches in health care would not likely have the same result.

Cost and Financing of Health Care

The third domain of health policy is the cost and financing of health care. The cost of health care continues to be a significant health and public policy issue for the United States. The National Health Expenditures data showed that health care spending grew 6.1% in 2007, costs the average person in our country $7421, and accounts for 16.2% of our economy as measured by the gross domestic product (GDP). Health costs are also projected to grow significantly without significant changes through health policy. Health care spending is expected to grow by appropriately 6% annually over the next decade, reaching 20.3% of the economy as measured by GDP in 2018.[19] The recently passed health care reform legislation (Public Law 111-148) seeks to "bend this cost curve" down from its current projection, and its ability to do so will be closely monitored in the years to come.

The increasing cost of health care is consistent across many sectors of the industry, although to varying degrees. In 2007, Medicare spending grew 7.2%, Medicaid spending increased by 6.4%, and personal health care spending grew by 5.8%. Besides the variance in spending growing between federal programs and personal health care spending, geographical differences in health care costs also show a level of inconsistency. In 2010, the highest state in the country, Massachusetts, spends more than double in personal health care costs ($6683) than the lowest state in the country, Utah ($3972). In Medicare spending, this variance continues with the highest state, Louisiana, spending double compared to the lowest state, South Dakota.[19] This disparity in the cost of health care across the United States is one of today's health policy priorities.

Increasing utilization and costs have been seen in physical therapy as well. Data from a 2002 Advanced Med/Computer Sciences Corporation (CSC) study reported that 3.75 million individuals utilized therapy services (physical therapy, occupational therapy, and speech–language pathology services) under the Medicare program. Of these individuals, 88% received physical therapy services. From 2000 to 2002, therapy services experienced 4.4% growth in users compared to only 1.9% growth in the total number of beneficiaries. Total expenditures for therapy services were $3.4 billion at an average patient cost of $896, an increase from $581 in 2000. The increasing number of individuals accessing therapy services and amount paid per patient present health policy challenges for rehabilitation therapy professionals in the area of cost and financing.[20]

Health policies center primarily on how to contain the outputs or expenditures. The government and private insurance companies issue policies to regulate practice and to set mechanisms of payment aimed to control the cost or limit the demand for health care services. These policies can have detrimental impacts on the quality of care or access to services. The major pressure point in health care today are the policies of cost containment and their impact across all domains of health policy. Physical therapists experience cost-containment strategies in two forms, regulations and mechanisms of payment. Regulations that set criteria for what is payable by the government or private insurance help to control costs. These regulations can set criteria for the use of support personnel, set minimum time requirements for certain interventions, and limit what interventions can be utilized for certain diagnoses. Mechanisms of payment are designed to help control costs and manage resource allocation in physical therapy. Mechanisms of payment range from fee for service, where a fee is charged for each intervention utilized, to case-rate payments, where a single preset fee is paid for a certain clinical condition to cover all services provided, whether the actual cost of care falls within the case rate or not.

As defined at the beginning of the chapter, health policy comprises the decisions, usually developed by government policy makers, for determining present and future objectives pertaining to the health care system. Balancing access, quality, and cost are extremely difficult in health care. The consumer wants the highest quality at the lowest cost immediately available. The complexity of this balancing act is only compounded by the varied

stakeholders who bring different perspectives and interests to this challenge. If health policy is intended to balance quality, access, availability, and cost, then the process to achieve this balance in a manner consistent with professional perspectives and beliefs is advocacy.

ADVOCACY

Advocacy is the pursuit of influencing outcomes—including public-policy and resource allocation decisions within political, economic, and social systems and institutions—that directly affect people's current lives.[21] In the United States the advocacy process is clearly articulated in the United States Constitution and its First Amendment. The First Amendment, ratified on December 15, 1791, outlines the freedoms of religion, press, and expression and states:

> Congress shall make no law respecting an establishment of religion, or prohibiting the free exercise thereof; or abridging the freedom of speech, or of the press; or the right of the people peaceably to assemble, and to petition the Government for a redress of grievances.[22]

This right of individuals to bring issues before government entities sets the framework for a majority of health policy initiatives and decisions. Through the process of advocacy, individuals or groups approach recognized individuals, organizations, or governments that are authorized to issue such policies and empowered to promulgate specific guidelines, rules, regulations, or laws. Advocacy exists at the level of the individual and the group. Self-advocacy is an important personal attribute that is a recognized characteristic of a competent adult. In addition to self-advocacy in which one acts on behalf of oneself, it is also an essential characteristic of health care professionals to advocate as individuals in the best interest of the patient or client. Self-advocacy and patient-focused advocacy are core principles in health care and in physical therapy. APTA's Code of Ethics, Principle 3, states, "A physical therapist shall comply with laws and regulations governing physical therapy and shall strive to effect changes that benefit patients/clients." This principle clearly establishes that compliance with public policies governing health care and health professions is required for ethical practice, but also indicates that there is an ethical obligation to advocate for changes in laws and regulations that benefit patients.[23]

Margaret Mead once remarked, "Never doubt that a small group of thoughtful, committed citizens can change the world; indeed, it's the only thing that ever does."[24] This statement is the core of advocacy at the systems or community level. Health care professionals have long banded together to advance their profession and hopefully change the world through the policies they seek to advance. One of health policy's first focal points began as advocacy to license health care professionals in order to provide assurance to the public that health care was being delivered by qualified individuals who met basic standards for practice.

An Advocacy Framework

Legal, legislative, and regulatory advocacy is the process of educating, implementing, influencing, and enacting policy changes to effect the desired outcome, whether that is to improve the health through health policy initiatives or to enable professional advancement. As a health care professional, advocacy is a critical role for physical therapists to provide and essential for the enactment of policies that enable physical therapists to practice to the full extent of education, experience, and expertise. Advocacy in public or health policy includes the process of setting a plan to influence an authorized body to issue a decision.

Advocacy is the process to get to a policy decision. The advocacy process is cyclical and continuous as it depends on the particular policy decision sought and its congruity with shifting priorities for both the advocate and the decision maker. To effectively advocate for changes that match a desired outcome, a systematic plan of action is required. Although there are many different textbooks and articles to assist with formulating an advocacy plan, one approach is outlined in the 6-step advocacy framework (Figure 31-5).

The first step is problem identification or development of the idea. This step is critical as it defines the deficit that advocacy efforts will seek to correct through policy change. This step is not limited solely to the process of problem identification and then outlining a path to the solution. New ideas can also be developed within the advocacy process. The formulation of these new ideas also represents the initial step in this process of problem identification. The clear articulation of the problem

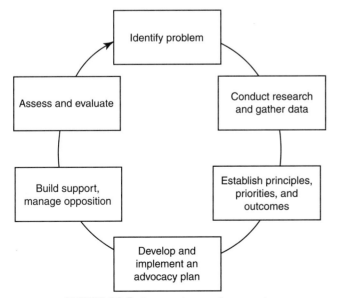

FIGURE 31-5 6-step advocacy framework.

becomes the case statement and represents step 1 in the 6-step advocacy framework.

The second step is to compile the necessary research, data, and background on the issue. Problem identification only pinpoints the issue an individual or group seeks to change. It is then necessary to collect data and conduct the research to begin to build the case for change. Public health data, consumer opinions, surveys, and other data are needed to build the foundation for the reasons for seeking the change. Defining the issue and supporting it with strong and sound evidence increases the potential for success. This step requires considerable understanding of the legal and policy background of the issue. One of the essential elements of this second step is identification of the policy that will need to be changed to achieve the desired outcome and also the venue in which the change can occur. The legislative body is often the venue of last resort. Many times, policies can be changed at the regulatory level and this is an important assessment of step 2 in the advocacy framework. The regulatory process, although as complex and as difficult to navigate as the legislative process, can make many policy determinations and provide some flexibility in approaches and outcomes. This step can involve consultants and attorneys who are experienced in identifying the options and policy bodies involved in making the decision to effect the outcome of a change in health policy.

Following the data-gathering step, principles, priorities, and outcomes are outlined in the third step. This step can be used to establish short, intermediate, and long-range goals. In the mid-1990s, the biomedical research establishment determined from their data that funding at the National Institutes of Health was insufficient. This community developed the policy principle that federal funding to the National Institutes of Health should be doubled over a 10-year period. This principle described the desired outcome, but also set incremental goals that needed to be achieved over several years of annual appropriations to meet the ultimate goal. The steps taken over legislative victories across several years resulted in success. The third step is critical for identifying key advocacy champions and constituencies.

The fourth step in the advocacy process is the establishment and implementation of an action plan. This step articulates what needs to be done in order to present the case for change to the body that has the authority to make a determination consistent with the desired outcome. This process can involve an in-depth strategic plan or be an informal process. The action plan should consider the individuals or parties involved in making the decision, how the case should be presented to them, a timeline for the desired determination, and the process that the policy will be subject to before it can be issued. The plan should be built upon the research and data gathered in step 2 and consistent with the priorities outlined in step 3. Part of this step could also identify that additional research is needed and further study is incorporated into the action plan. This step sets the course for implementing advocacy efforts. A growing field of grassroots advocacy consultation is developing in the United States to assist organizations in outlining their action plans and identifying key steps to be successful in making changes to policies.

Although the fifth step could be a significant part of step 4, it is singled out because of its importance. Broadening the community of advocates behind the action plan is essential. In today's electronic communications world, advocacy plans can be put into action in quick order. Rising above the rank-and-file advocacy initiatives takes a concerted effort to build a community of support and diminish opposition. Coalitions, alliances, and partnerships are as much the fabric of policy development and advocacy world as lobbyists, elected officials, and think tanks. The successful implementation of coalition efforts can build momentum, establish consistency in the plan, and show broad public support. Campaigns have long used opposition research to inform their strategy and approach. The best way to counter any opposition to an advocacy plan is first to understand the source of the opposition. Once the opposition is understood, negotiations to seek a policy alternative that meets both groups' needs can be initiated or the opposition can be engaged in a public debate on the policy. Coalitions, alliances, and partners are the force multiplier in advocacy plans with and without opposition and are a key element to a successful advocacy plan.

The final step is the assessment and evaluation process and it is essential in a process that is cyclical. The advocacy process never ends at a destination. Although there should be evaluative measures in each step of the advocacy process, there is the need to take the necessary time to assess what worked and what could have been done more effectively or efficiently. This assessment and evaluation will feed into the data collection efforts described in step 2 to inform the next round of advocacy efforts or possibly identify new venues in which to make the case for change.

A good example of the steps in action can be found by reviewing the process used by the National Council on Aging (NCOA) with the Home Safety Council on falls prevention. The recognition that falls prevention programs could improve health outcomes for older adults and other populations served as a catalyst for the development of an advocacy plan. The NCOA and Home Safety Council built their policy case and priorities around government data on the impact of falls on cost and quality in health care with a desire to improve access to programs to prevent these adverse events in health care. The NCOA and Home Safety Council convened stakeholders to develop a National Action Plan and a corresponding blueprint for health policies to reduce falls and increase falls prevention within the health care system and in the community. These stakeholders developed the plan and built a coalition to implement its

objectives, the Falls Free Coalition. This coalition and its advisory committee continue to explore strategies and assess its progress. The coalition has also developed resources to expand their advocacy reach with manuals and guides for state action on falls prevention. The advocacy framework from problem identification to setting a plan of action to assessing the progress by the National Council on Aging and its partners provide an effective model for advocacy success.[25]

Advocacy: Seeking to Influence a Desired Audience

Essential to an advocacy plan is identification of the arena that is most appropriate to address the policy concern and the corresponding determination of the audiences to be influenced. Understanding whether the issue is best addressed at the local, state, or national level is critical. It also must be determined if the policy change is best addressed by administrative procedurals, regulations, or by legislation. As outlined in this chapter, the legislative process is the most formal approach as it requires the passage of a bill to become a law. Regulatory agencies can rule on policies within the existing parameters of the law and are often an appropriate venue to advocate for policy changes. At other times, the policy change might only take a decision by the administrative body that has been given the authority to make rulings on policies. It is important to note that policy always has another option of the judiciary branch of government. Although not utilized often, when legislative and regulatory bodies have not been able to meet the objectives of your action plan, legal options can be pursued. The Supreme Court of the United States is the pinnacle of policy issues that have exhausted all other policy venues for addressing the issue under debate.

Once the appropriate arena and venue have been identified, the next step is to identify the audience to which the case must be made. An audience might be the body that has the power to promulgate policy. The primary audience in an advocacy plan is typically the policy maker, who should have been correctly identified in the action plan as the appropriate policy body with the authority to issue policy to meet the principles and outcomes also articulated in the action plan. There are laws, rules, and regulations that govern how you interact with these authorities and the implementation of the plan. The research stage of the advocacy process should consider compliance with the regulations that affect how this audience may be addressed. Alternatively, the "best" audience might be the group that welds power to influence the decision makers. A secondary audience that can be used to influence promotion of the desired outcome is the media. Building public support for your policy issue is essential to the advocacy process. These audiences usually are identified in step 4 using the advocacy framework. If the desired policy encompasses a broad issue that appeals to multiple constituents, the likelihood for success is enhanced. Engaging the press and other media in the issue is vital for success of the advocacy plan.

To achieve policy change, one needs to set forth a well-conceived plan. This plan should identify the issue that the policy body should solve; establish a clear path that identifies the arena, audience, and authority for policy change; and establish evidence and support for the issue and proposed policy solution. This advocacy process will help inform and engage policy makers, both elected and appointed. This advocacy process can help physical therapists become a participant in the nation's representative democracy at all levels. Health policy and changes to health policy are only as effective as the individuals who participate in the advocacy process are at making their case for their principles and priorities.

CONCLUSION

Policy and advocacy go hand in hand. To enact or change policy takes a concerted effort to influence the bodies that possess the power to make these changes. Health policy is a complex balancing act of decisions that policy makers must make to improve access, enhance quality, and reduce cost. Understanding health policy will assist understanding the limitations and possibilities of the health care delivery system. Health policies should also outline the need for policy changes to enable all health care professionals to serve to their fullest capabilities and for patients to be assured safety and access. Balancing these policy objectives in health care continues to challenge our policy makers and advocacy organizations.

It is essential regardless of setting of practice, political perspective, or policy expertise that physical therapists engage in the health policy and advocacy process. As health care professionals, physical therapists are obligated to comply with existing laws, regulations, and policies. Advocacy is part of your professional responsibility. Competency in health policy and advocacy will only further the profession's ability to serve patients and help them reach their full potential.

REFERENCES

To enhance this text and add value for the reader, all references are included on the companion Evolve site that accompanies this text book. The reader can view the reference source and access it online whenever possible. There are a total of 25 cited references and other general references for this chapter.

Page numbers followed by f, t or b indicate figures, tables, or boxes, respectively.

594